LANCHESTER LIBRARY
3 8001 00554 9716
D1761433
LANCHESTER LIBRARY, Co
Gosford Street, Coventry CV1 5DD

Movement, Stability & Lumbopelvic Pain

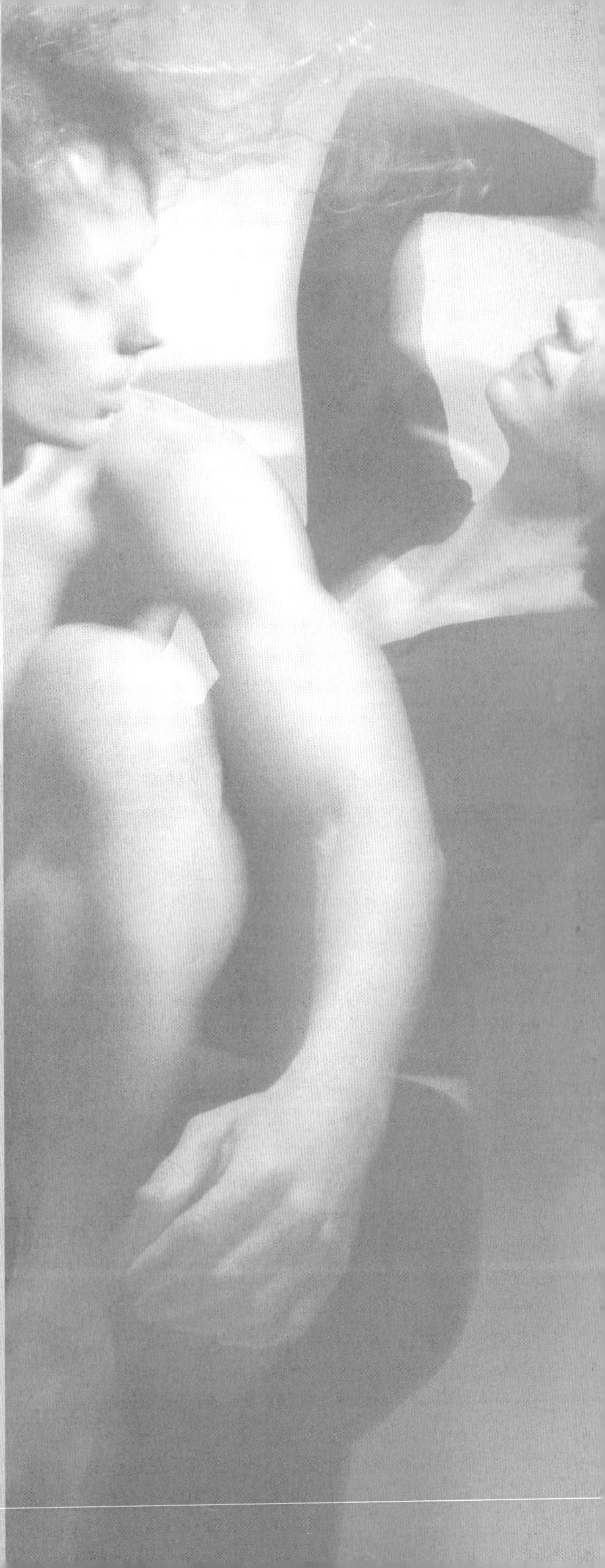

For Churchill Livingstone:

Senior Commissioning Editor: **Sarena Wolfaard**
Associate Editor: **Claire Wilson; Claire Bonnett**
Project Manager: **David Fleming; Jane Dingwall**
Design: **Stewart Larking**
Illustration Manager: **Bruce Hogarth**

2nd Edition

Movement, Stability & Lumbopelvic Pain

Integration of Research and Therapy

Edited by

Andry Vleeming PhD
Clinical Anatomist and Founder
Spine and Joint Center, Rotterdam, The Netherlands

Vert Mooney MD
Measurement Driven Rehabilitation Systems, San Diego, CA, USA

Rob Stoeckart PhD
Department of Neuroscience, Erasmus MC, Rotterdam,
The Netherlands

Illustrations by
Philip Wilson
Chartwell

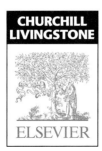

CHURCHILL LIVINGSTONE

ELSEVIER

Edinburgh London New York Oxford Philadelphia St Louis Sydney Toronto 2007

CHURCHILL
LIVINGSTONE
ELSEVIER

CHURCHILL LIVINGSTONE
An imprint of Elsevier Limited

© Pearson Professional Limited 1997
© Harcourt Publishers Limited 1999
© 2007, Elsevier Limited. All rights reserved.
Ch 26 © SV Paris 2007
Ch 35 © SM McGill 2007

The right of Andry Vleeming, Vert Mooney and Rob Stoeckart to be identified as editors of this work has been asserted by them in accordance with the Copyright, Designs and Patents Act 1988

No part of this publication may be reproduced, stored in a retrieval system, or transmitted in any form or by any means, electronic, mechanical, photocopying, recording or otherwise, without either the prior permission of the publishers or a licence permitting restricted copying in the United Kingdom issued by the Copyright Licensing Agency, 90 Tottenham Court Road, London W1T 4LP. Permissions may be sought directly from Elsevier's Health Sciences Rights Department in Philadelphia, USA: phone: (+1) 215 238 7869, fax: (+1) 215 238 2239, e-mail: healthpermissions@elsevier.com. You may also complete your request on-line via the Elsevier Science homepage (http://www.elsevier.com), by selecting 'Customer Support' and then 'Obtaining Permissions'.

First edition 1997
Reprinted 1999
Second edition 2007

ISBN 978 0 443 10178 6

British Library Cataloguing in Publication Data
A catalogue record for this book is available from the British Library

Library of Congress Cataloging in Publication Data
A catalog record for this book is available from the Library of Congress

ELSEVIER your source for books, journals and multimedia in the health sciences
www.elsevierhealth.com

Working together to grow libraries in developing countries
www.elsevier.com | www.bookaid.org | www.sabre.org
ELSEVIER BOOK AID International Sabre Foundation

The publisher's policy is to use **paper manufactured from sustainable forests**

Printed in China

Coventry University Library

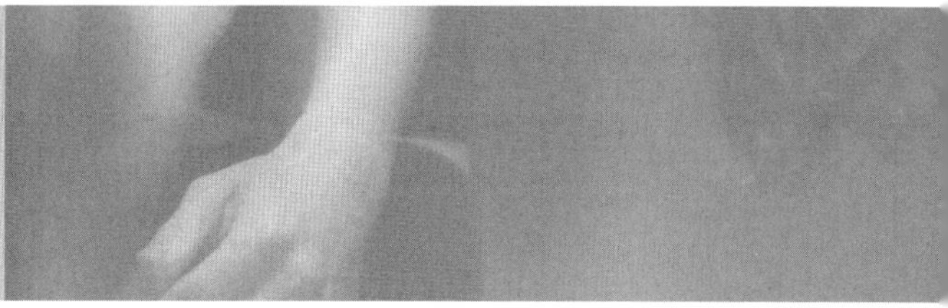

Contents

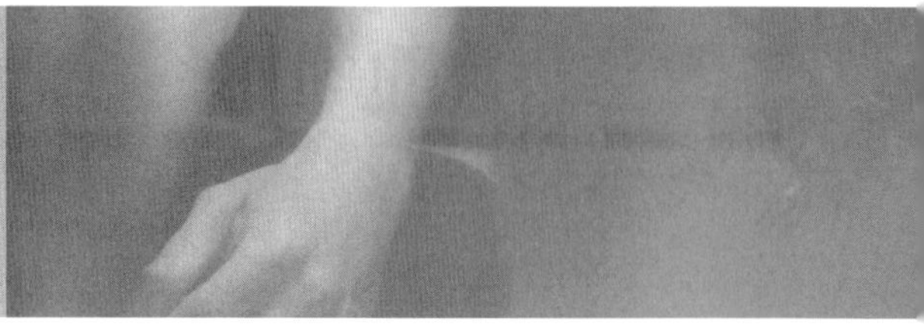

Contributors

MA Adams BSc PhD
Senior Research Fellow, Department of Anatomy, University of Bristol, Bristol, UK

PJ Barker BAppSc(Physio) PhD
Senior Tutor, Department of Anatomy and Cell Biology, The University of Melbourne, Victoria, Australia

M Benjamin PhD
Professor of Musculoskeletal Biology and Sports Medicine Research, School of Biosciences, Cardiff University, Cardiff, UK

CA Briggs BSc Dip Ed MSc PhD
Associate Professor and Deputy Head, Department of Anatomy and Cell Biology, The University of Melbourne, Victoria, Australia

L Chaitow ND DO
Honorary Fellow, School of Integrated Health, University of Westminster, London, UK; Editor-in-Chief, Journal of Bodywork & Movement Therapies

J Cholewicki
Associate Professor, Department of Orthopaedics & Rehabilitation, Yale University School of Medicine, New Haven, CT, USA

HJ Dananberg DPM
Podiatrist, private practice, Catholic Medical Centre, Bedford, New Hampshire, USA; Contributing Editor, Journal of the American Podiatric Medical Association

L Danneels PT PhD
Professor of Rehabilitation Sciences and Physiotherapy, Faculty of Medicine and Health Sciences, Ghent, Belgium

C DeRosa PT PhD
Professor of Physical Therapy, Northern Arizona University, Flagstaff, Arizona, USA

PF Dijkstra MD DIC PhD
Former Radiologist, Academic Medical Centre, Amsterdam, The Netherlands; Former Head of Department of Radiology, Jan van Breemen Institute for Skeletal Disease, Amsterdam, The Netherlands

P Dolan PhD
Reader in Biomechanics, Department of Anatomy, University of Bristol, Bristol, UK

RL DonTigny PT
Physical Therapist, Havre, Montana, USA

S Gibbons BSc (Hons) PT MSc MCPA
Stability Physiotherapy, Mt. Pearl, Newfoundland, Canada

W Gilleard PhD
Senior Lecturer in Biomechanics, School of Exercise & Sports Management, Southern Cross University, Lismore, Australia

S Gracovetsky PhD
Retired, Concordia University, Montreal, QC, Canada

PW Hodges BPhty (Hons) PhD MedDr
Professor and NHMRC Principal Research Fellow, Division of Physiotherapy, The University of Queensland, Brisbane, Australia

S Holm
Professor, Department of Orthopaedics, Sahlgrenska University Hospital, Goteborg, Sweden

B Hungerford PhD
Consultant Musculoskeletal Physiotherapist, Sydney Spine & Pelvis Centre, Drummoyne, NSW, Australia

A Huson MD PhD
Professor Emeritus, Maastricht University, The Netherlands

A Indahl MD PhD
Consultant, Specialist in physical medicine and rehabilitation, Department of Physical Medicine and Rehabilitation, Hospital for Rehabilitation, Stavern, Norway

RE Irvin DO
Clinical Associate Professor, Dept of Osteopathic Manipulative Medicine, College of Osteopathic Medicine, Oklahoma State University Health Science Center, Tulsa, Oklahoma, USA

E Jurriaans BSc MBChB DTM&H FRCR(UK) FRCP(C)
Associate Professor, McMaster University, Faculty of Health Sciences, Hamilton, Ontario, Canada; Staff Radiologist, St. Joseph's Healthcare, Hamilton, Ontario, Canada

B Koes PhD
Professor of General Practice, Head of Research Department, Department of General Practice, Erasmus MC, University Medical Centre, Rotterdam, The Netherlands

M Laslett PhD NZRP Dip MT Dip MDT
Senior Clinician, PhysioSouth @ Moorhouse Medical Clinic, Christchurch, New Zealand

D Lee BSR FCAMT
Clinical and Education Consultant, Diane Lee & Associates, Canada

SM Levin MD FACS
Director, Ezekiel Biomechanics Group, McLean, VA, USA

CO Lovejoy MA PhD
University Professor of Anthropology, Department of Anthropology and Division of Biomedical Sciences, Kent State University and Northeast Ohio Universities College of Medicine, Ohio, USA

AT Masi MD DRPH
Professor of Medicine, University of Illinois College of Medicine at Peoria (UICOMP), Illinois, USA

SM McGill
Professor, Faculty of Applied Health Sciences, Dept of Kinesiology, University of Waterloo, Ontario, Canada

V Mooney MD
Clinical Professor of Orthopaedics, USSD, Private Practitioner, San Diego, California, USA

G Lorimer Moseley PhD BAppSc(Phty)(Hons)
Nuffield Medical Research Fellow, Centre for fMRI of the Brain and Dept of Human Anatomy & Genetics, University of Oxford, UK

G Müller
Orthopaedic Surgeon, Sports Medicine, Manual Therapy, Chairman of Rueckenzentrum Am Michel, Hamburg, Germany

JMD O'Neill MB BAO BCh MRCPI MSc FRCR(UK)
Assistant Professor, McMaster University, Faculty of Health Sciences, Hamilton, Ontario, Canada; Staff Radiologist & Director – Musculoskeletal Imaging, St. Joseph's Healthcare, Hamilton, Ontario, Canada

HC Östgaard MD PhD
Associate Professor, Chief of Dept of Orthopaedics, Sahlgren University Hospital, Molndal, Sweden

SV Paris PT PhD FAPTA
President, University of St. Augustine for Health Sciences, St. Augustine, Florida, USA

JA Porterfield PT MA ATC
Owner, Rehabilitation and Health Center, Inc., Akron, Ohio; CEO, Venture Practice Services Ltd., Akron, Ohio, USA

T Ravin MD
Physician; President of the American Association of Musculoskeletal Medicine, Denver, Colorado, USA

R Stoeckart PhD
Department of Neuroscience, Erasmus MC, Rotterdam, The Netherlands

B Stuge PT PhD
Senior Researcher, Institute of Nursing & Health Sciences, University of Oslo, Norway

B Sturesson MD PhD
Head of Spine Unit, Department of Orthopaedics, Angelholm Hospital, Angelholm, Sweden

M van Tulder PhD
Professor, Institute for Research in Extramural Medicine (EMGO) and Institute for Health Sciences (HIS), VU University Medical Centre, Amsterdam, The Netherlands

DM Urquhart BPhysio(Hons) PhD
Dept of Epidemiology & Preventive Medicine, Monash University, Victoria, Australia

LMG Vancleef MSc
Dept Medical, Clinical and Experimental Psychology, Maastricht University, The Netherlands

J Viti
Assistant Professor, University of St. Augustine for Health Sciences, St. Augustine, Florida, USA

JWS Vlaeyen PhD
Dept Medical, Clinical and Experimental Psychology, Maastricht University, The Netherlands

A Vleeming PhD
Clinical Anatomist and Founder, Spine and Joint Center, Rotterdam, The Netherlands

NK Vøllestad PhD
Professor, Head of Institute of Nursing & Health Sciences, University of Oslo, Norway

FH Willard PhD
Professor, College of Osteopathic Medicine, Family Medicine, University of New England, Biddeford, Maine, USA

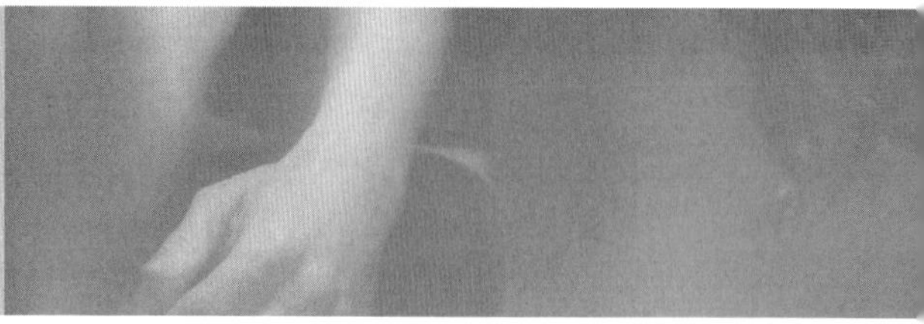

Preface

There are a large number of books dealing with the lumbar spine and pelvis, so why this book on *Movement, Stability and Lumbopelvic Pain*? This question is pertinent as there are several excellent books available which cover these topics. Our reasons are diverse.

Firstly, several distinguished scientists, physicians and other specialists have lately provided evidence-based, relevant new data on the lumbopelvic area. This forces us to look afresh at the adequacy of current diagnostic and therapeutic methods. Secondly, most books deal either with the low back or with the pelvic girdle; our aim is to collect all relevant material in one book. Thirdly, most books on the subject are written by one expert or by a small team of experts. This makes it difficult to get a grip on the vast wealth of information available. Finally, and probably most importantly, notwithstanding all efforts to treat patients adequately, large numbers of patients still suffer chronically from low back pain and/or pelvic girdle pain. It is our hope and ambition to provide, together with all contributors, an integrated book that can be of help to people involved in the diagnosis or treatment of patients with lumbopelvic pain.

The contributors to this book include scientists of internationally renowned clinical groups and departments dealing with basic sciences. Their contributions are from different disciplines embracing anthropology, orthopedic surgery, biomechanical engineering, chiropractic practice, anatomy, osteopathy, physical therapy, podiatry, gynecology, rehabilitation medicine, epidemiology and several others. In the book they are grouped into the following parts:

1. Biomechanical, clinical–anatomical and evolutionary aspects of lumbopelvic pain and dysfunction
2. Insights in function and dysfunction of the lumbopelvic region
3. Diagnostic methods
4. Guidelines
5. Effective training and treatment
6. Integrating different views and opinions when dealing with a complex system.

The studies reviewed in this book reflect the specialties of the contributors, their backgrounds, styles, approaches and specific ideas about how lumbopelvic structures function and dysfunction. Several chapters were written by authors with a unique concept about the origin of pain and dysfunction of lumbopelvic structures and about the therapy requested. In a way this is hazardous since certain authors were invited, not because of their evidence-based approach, but since in the opinion of the editors their audacious and sometimes controversial ideas merit attention. Their concepts should invite sound research that can confirm, refute, or adapt the ideas presented. We are convinced that the wealth of information presented by the contributors will help to create rational and effective treatment programs for the management of lumbopelvic pain and dysfunction.

Andry Vleeming, Vert Mooney and
Rob Stoeckart

PART ONE

Section One

Biomechanical, clinical–anatomical and evolutionary aspects of lumbopelvic pain and dysfunction: Clinical–anatomical aspects

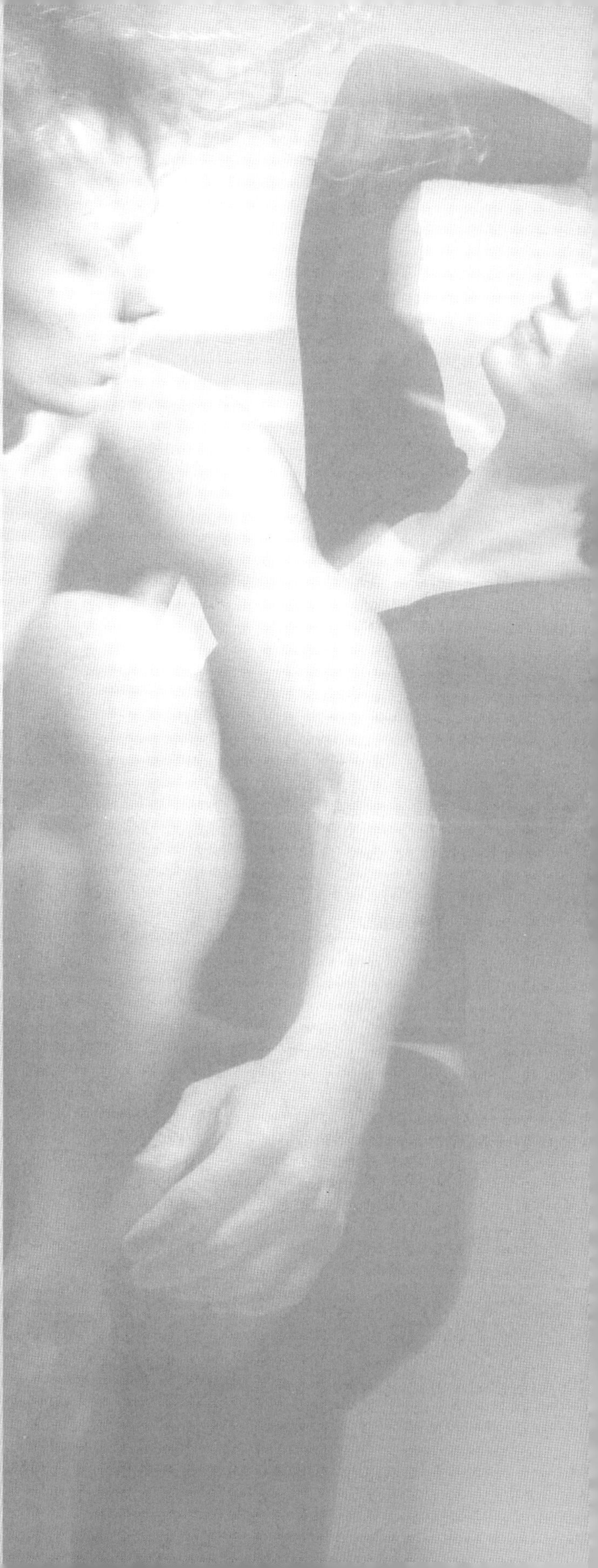

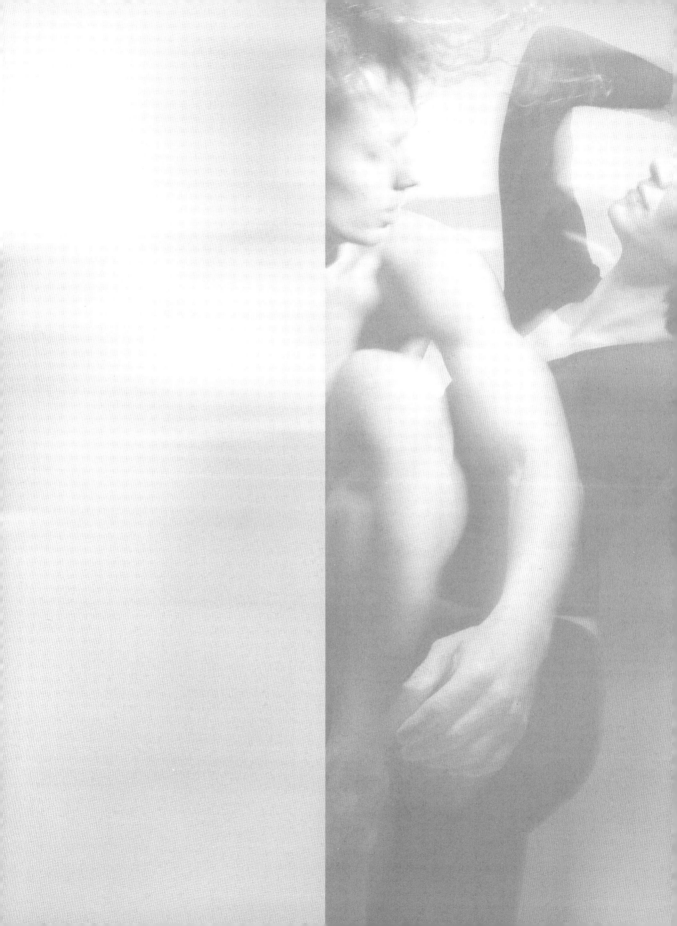

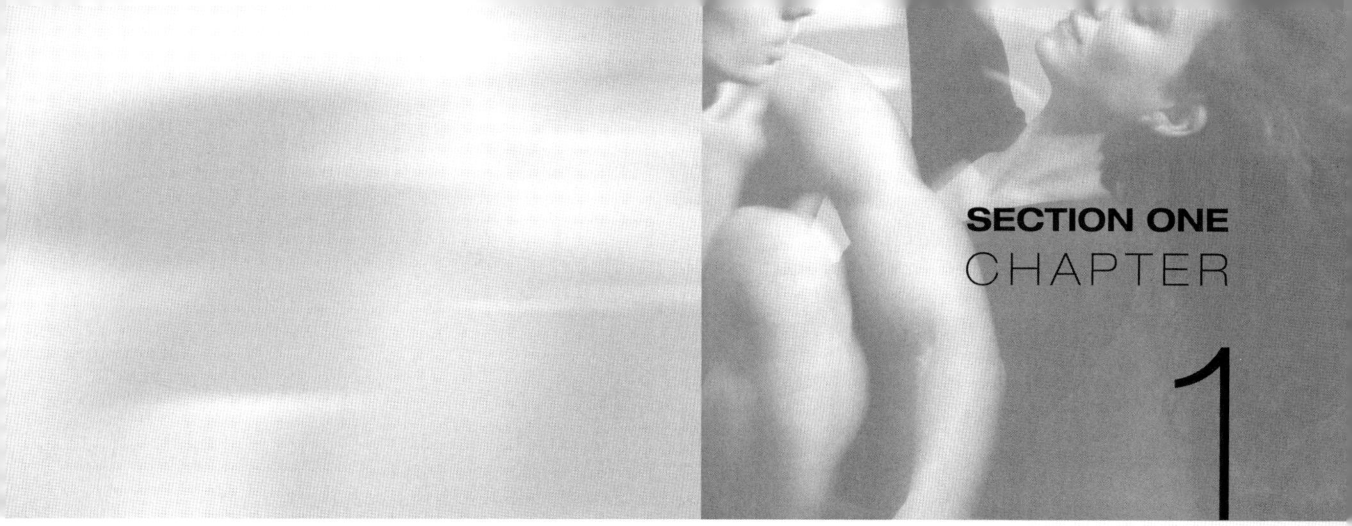

SECTION ONE

CHAPTER 1

The muscular, ligamentous, and neural structure of the lumbosacrum and its relationship to low back pain

FH Willard

INTRODUCTION

The lumbosacral spinal column performs a key role in the transfer of weight from the torso and upper body into the lower extremities, both in static positions and during mobility. The primary bony structures involved in this force transduction are: five lumbar vertebrae, a sacrum, two innominate bones, and the two femoral heads. Critical to the stability of these bony components is a complex arrangement of dense connective tissue. Although typically described as separate entities in most textbooks of anatomy, these fibrous, soft-tissue structures actually form a continuous ligamentous stocking in which the lumbar vertebrae and sacrum are positioned. The major muscles representing the prime movers in this region – such as the multifidus, gluteus maximus, and biceps femoris – have various attachments to this elongated, ligamentous stocking. The muscular and ligamentous relationships composing the lumbosacral connection are of extreme importance in stabilizing the lumbar vertebrae and sacrum during the transfer of energy from the upper body to the lower extremities. This arrangement has been termed a 'self-bracing mechanism' (Vleeming et al 1995c) and, as such, its dysfunction is critical to the failure of the lower back.

A critical relationship also exists between the neural components of the lumbosacral region and the surrounding ligamentous structures. Traumatic, inflammatory, and degenerative disease processes affect the structure of the lumbosacral region and impact on the surrounding nerves. Current research, using immunohistochemical techniques to identify specific types of axons, suggests that all of these connective tissue structures receive a supply of small-caliber, primary afferent fibers (Aδ and C-fibers), typical of those involved in nociception. Irritation of these primary afferent nociceptive axons initiates the release of neuropeptides that interact with fibroblasts, mast cells, and immune cells present in the surrounding connective tissue (Levine et al 1993). The resultant cascade of events, referred to as a neurogenic inflammatory response, is thought to play a major role in degenerative diseases and the development of low back pain (Garrett et al 1992, Kidd et al 1990, Schaible et al 2005, Weidenbaum & Farcy 1990, Weinstein 1992). Sensitization of these small-caliber, primary afferent fibers, along with sensitization of their central connections in the dorsal horn of the spinal cord, appears to play a crucial role in the evolution of chronic painful conditions (Coderre et al 1993, Ji et al 2003, Woolf & Chong 1993). This chapter examines recent advances in our knowledge of the lumbosacral region structural architecture, pathology, and innervation.

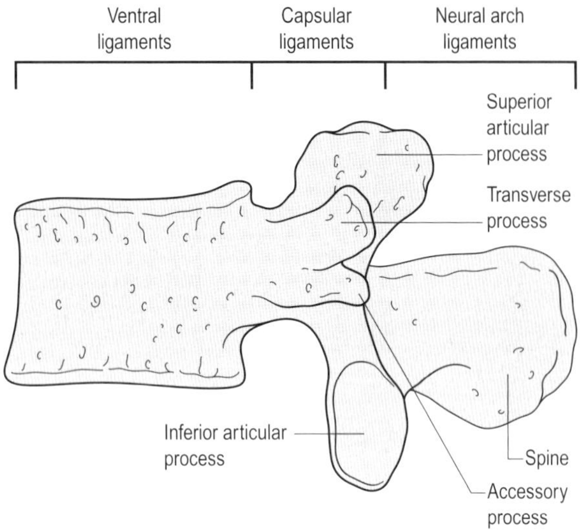

Fig. 1.1 A lateral view of a lumbar vertebra illustrating the position of the neural arch ligaments, capsular ligaments, and ventral ligaments.

Ligamentous structure of the lumbar region

The various ligaments of the lumbar vertebral column form a continuous, dense, connective-tissue stocking surrounding the vertebrae and extending into the sacral area. For ease of description, the vertebral connective tissue sheath can be divided into three parts: (1) the neural arch structures; (2) the capsular structures; and (3) the ventral or vertebral body structures (Fig. 1.1). However, it should be noted that the partitions between each of these three divisions are for convenience only, as the connective tissue of the dorsal and ventral components is essentially continuous across the pedicles of the vertebrae.

Neural arch ligaments

The neural arch of each lumbar vertebra is composed of the pedicles, laminae, transverse processes, and spine (Figs 1.1 and 1.2). Two major ligaments participate in surrounding the neural arch: the ligamentum flavum and the interspinous ligament; two additional small ligaments are also described: the supraspinous ligament posteriorly and the intertransverse ligament laterally. To view the ligaments of the neural arch, the multifidus muscle must be completely removed from the lumbosacral region (Figs 1.2 and 1.3). Although most of these ligaments have a distinct biochemical make-up when analyzed in isolation (Ballard & Weinstein 1992, Fujii & Hamada 1993, Fujii et al 1993, Yahia et al 1990a, 1990b) *in vivo* they grade together at their boundaries to unite and function as a single unit. To demonstrate this concept, the osseous components of the neural arch were removed with minimal disturbance to the associated ligamentous structures (Figs 1.4 and 1.5). The unitary nature of the supraspinous and intraspinous ligaments and of the ligamentum flavum is obvious because these soft tissue structures maintain their continuity despite the lack of supporting osseous material.

Ligamentum flavum

The ligamentum flavum, located between individual laminae, represents a medialward continuation of the articular capsule of the facet joint (Fig. 1.4). This elastic ligament forms a significant portion of the roof of the spinal canal. Superiorly, it attaches to the anterior surface of the lamina above and inferiorly it establishes a cup-like grasp on the superior margin of the lamina below (Olszewski et al 1996). The medial fibers of the ligament bridge the gap between the laminae of adjacent vertebra, fusing with the interspinous ligament, whereas the lateral fibers attach to the facet joint capsule (Figs 1.4B and 1.5; see also Behrsin & Briggs 1988, Bogduk & Twomey 1991, Ramsey 1966). This distensible ligament is composed of elastic fibers (80%) and collagenous fibers (20%), the elastic fibers imparting the ligament its yellow color and flexible nature (Bogduk & Twomey 1991). A significant function for the ligamentum flavum is

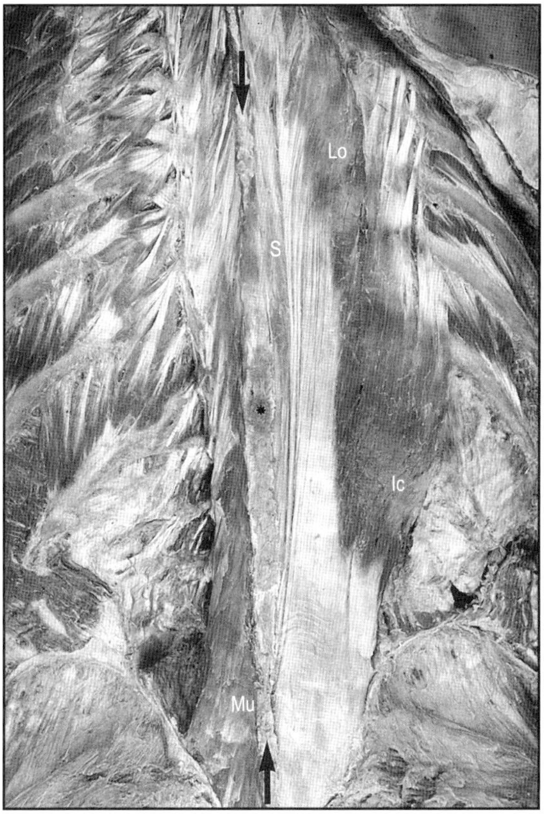

Fig. 1.2 The three lumbar paravertebral muscles in a male. On the individual's right side is the iliocostalis muscle (Ic) laterally and the longissimus muscle (Lo) medially. Note that the spinalis muscle (S) does not extend into the lumbar region beyond L2 or L3. On the individual's left side, the iliocostalis and longissimus have been removed to reveal the medially positioned multifidus muscle (Mu). Arrows top and bottom are aligned along the spinous processes of the thoracic and lumbar vertebrae (midline). The thick lumbar multifidus muscle is seen differentiating into the thin, flattened semispinalis muscle at the superior end of the lumbar vertebral column (asterisk).

to provide a roof for the vertebral canal that will not buckle during extension–flexion movements of the vertebral column (Bogduk & Twomey 1991). At rest (in a neutral position), the ligaments have a pretension, ideally keeping the ligaments from buckling (Nachemson & Evans 1968).

Despite the elasticity of the ligamentum flavum, it is known to be a significant source of root compression in the lumbar region (Okuda et al 2005). A component of this neural compression appears to be related to buckling of the ligament inferiorly secondary to age-related intervertebral disc collapse or other degenerative processes. A second component can be related to an age-related loss of elastic fibers and elasticity of the ligamentum flavum, contributing to their progressive loss of tension in the elderly (Nachemson & Evans 1968, Ramsey 1966). Specifically, there is a decrease in elastic fibers and a concomitant increase in the density of collagen fibers, along with a shift to high-molecular-weight proteoglycans (Kashiwagi 1993, Okada et al 1993). These events favor the deposition of calcium (Kashiwagi 1993), thus nearly all flaval ligaments in a sampling of patients with lumbar spinal stenosis had histological signs of ossification (Schrader et al 1999). Calcification of the ligament leads to its hypertrophy and to subsequent lumbar spinal stenosis (Yoshida et al 1992). These age-related changes in the ligamentum flavum have been related to specific neurologic sequelae such as the cauda equina syndrome and lumbar radiculopathy (Baba et al 1995, Ryan 1993). Whereas ossification of the ligament is associated with increasing age and the presence of cauda equina syndrome, chondrogenesis in the ligament appears more associated with the presence of spondylolisthesis (Okuda et al 2004). Finally, failure of the elastic properties of this ligament has also been related to the development of adolescent idiopathic scoliosis (Hadley-Miller et al 1994). Unfortunately, there is little or no regenerative capacity in the elastic tissue of the ligamentum flavum; thus a damaged ligament is replaced by a dense connective tissue cicatrix (Ramsey 1966).

Interspinous ligament

The interspinous ligament extends between borders of the spines of adjacent vertebrae (Figs 1.5 and 1.6). Its anterior border is a continuation of the ligamentum flavum. The posterior border of the ligament thickens to form the supraspinous ligament, which is, in turn, anchored to the thoracolumbar fascia. The orientation of fibers in the interspinous ligament has been given multiple, conflicting descriptions. In humans, the ligament can best be described as a fan (Fig. 1.6; see also Fig. 1.11 below). The narrow or proximal end of the fan blends with the ligamentum flavum and contains elastic fibers (Yahia et al 1990b), whereas the broad end of the fan extends in a posterior direction towards the tips of the spines and is composed primarily of collagen fibers. In the center of the ligament, the collagen fibers are oriented parallel to the vertebral spines; distally, the peripheral collagen fibers flare posterocranially and posterocaudally (Aspden et al 1987, Hukins et al 1990). This fan-like arrangement

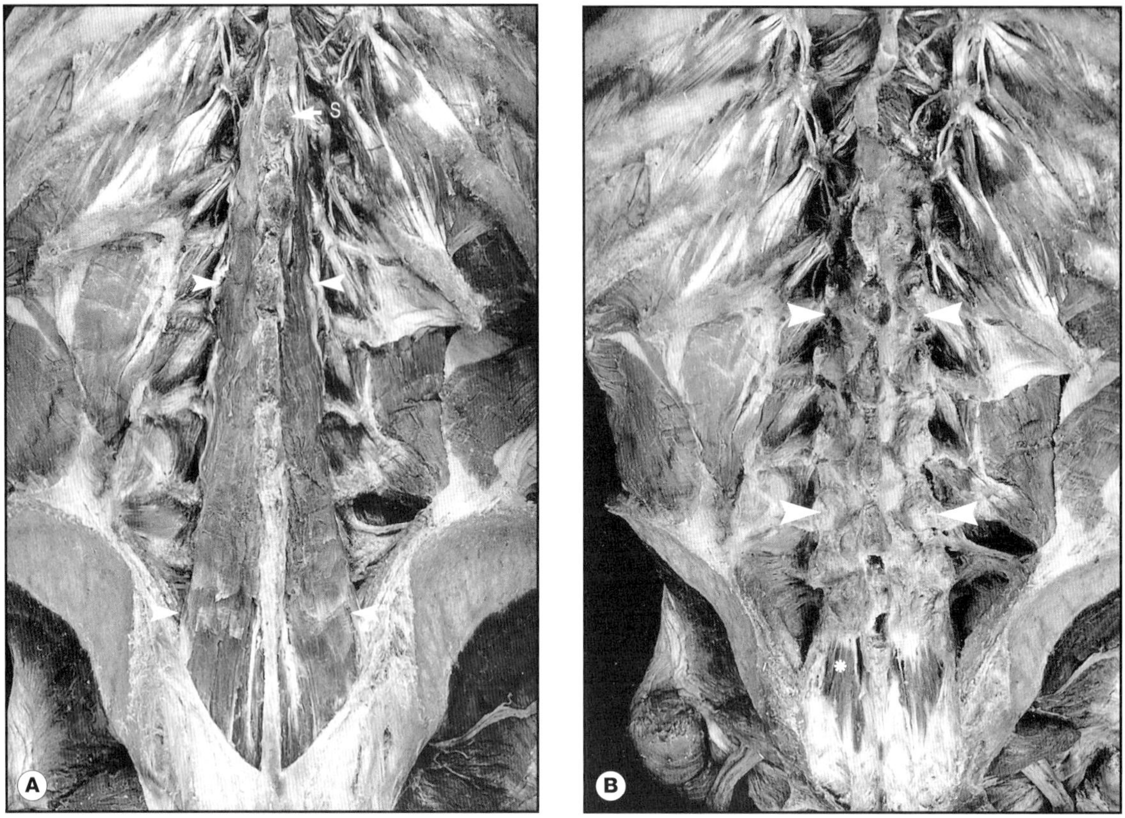

Fig. 1.3 The multifidus muscle and its bed. (A) The pyramidal-shaped multifidus muscle is demonstrated between the four arrowheads (S, lumbar spinous processes). (B) The multifidus muscle has been removed to reveal a continuous ligamentous stocking surrounding the neural arch components of the lumbar vertebrae (between arrowheads). On the sacrum, only the deepest laminae of the multifidus remain (asterisk).

allows the ligament to expand without rupture as the vertebral spines separate during flexion. The fibers of this ligament are described as resisting the separation of the vertebral spines during flexion (Bogduk & Twomey 1991); however, the most likely function of these ligaments, given their anteroposterior fiber orientation, is to act as an anchor, transmitting the anteroposterior pull of the thoracolumbar fascia, into which it is attached via the supraspinous ligament (Hukins et al 1990), into an increased tension in the ligamentum flavum (Fig. 1.7). This increased tension would assist in preventing the latter ligament from buckling onto the spinal cord and would also serve to assist in alignment of the lumbar vertebrae. Chondrocytes are present along the osseous borders of the interspinous ligaments and age-related chondrification of the interspinous ligament occurs after the third decade of life (Yahia et al 1990b). Degenerative processes in the motion segment of the vertebrae appear to coincide with the chondrification of the ligament and evidence for degenerative events in the interspinous ligament has recently been demonstrated with CT and MRI imaging (Jinkins 2004). All of these pathologic events occurring to the interspinous ligament should diminish the ability of the thoracolumbar fascia to influence the alignment of the lumbar vertebrae, and thereby increase their risk of destructive injury.

Supraspinous ligament

The supraspinous ligament lies along the posterior border of the interspinous ligament (Fig. 1.8). Throughout its lumbar course, it is tightly adherent to the posterior border of the lumbar spines and to the interspinous ligament. This creates an interspinous–supraspinous thoracolumbar (IST) ligamentous complex that anchors the major fascial planes of the back to the lumbar spines. Traction placed on the thoracolumbar fascia will destroy the thoracolumbar sheath before it will separate

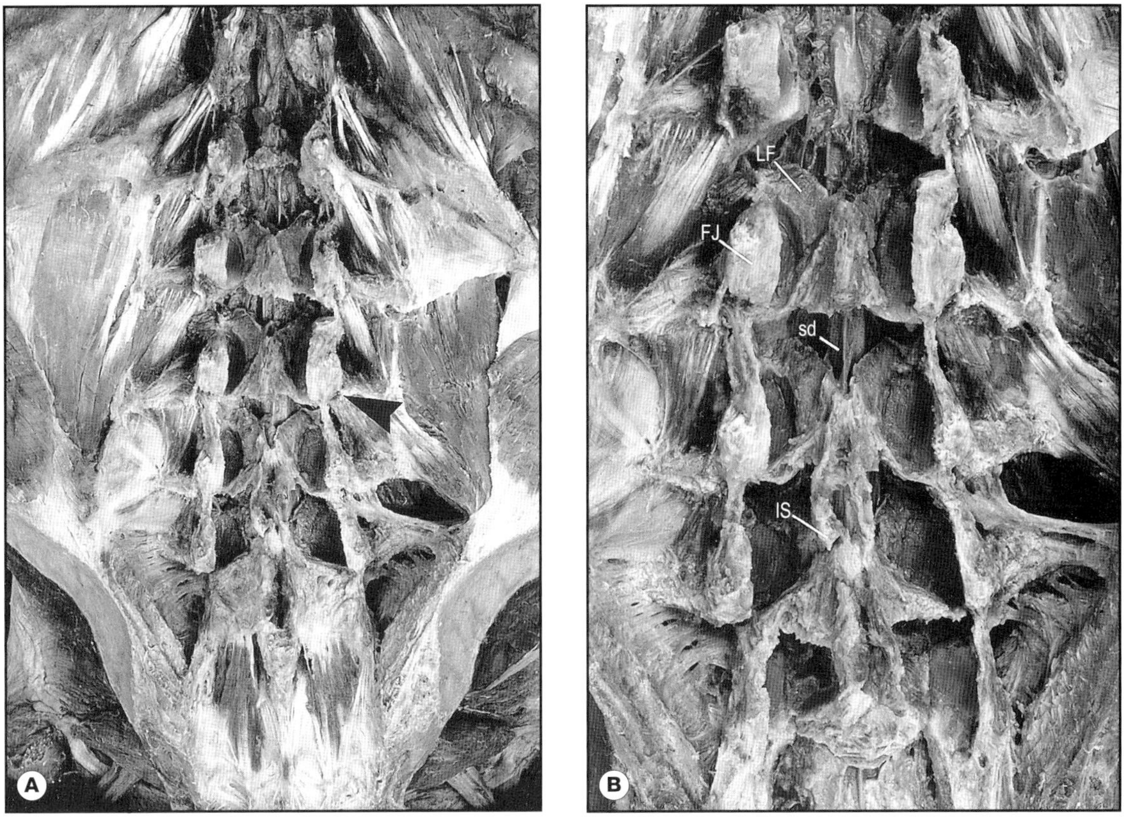

Fig. 1.4 The ligamentous stocking of the lumbar vertebrae. (A) This orientation photograph is a posterior view of the lumbar spinal column, similar to that in Fig. 1.3. The spinous processes, laminae, and inferior articular processes of the facet joint have been removed. (B) Detailed view of the ligamentous stocking illustrating the ligamentum flavum (LF) extending between the interspinous ligament (IS) medially and the facet joint capsule (FJ) laterally. The arrowhead indicates the same facet joint capsule in both photographs. The epidural space and spinal dural (sd) can be seen between the flaval ligaments.

the IST complex (Fig. 1.8). Thus it is possible for the interspinous and supraspinous ligaments to act as force transducers, translating the tension of the thoracolumbar fascia, developed in the extremities and torso, into the lumbar vertebral column. At lower lumbar levels, the supraspinous ligament becomes progressively less organized as it grades into the distal attachments of the thoracolumbar fascia, and in some individuals it might not be recognizable caudal to L4 (Bogduk & Twomey 1991). This ligament often presents with fatty involution late in life (Heylings 1978) and can also ossify (Mine & Kawai 1995).

Articular capsular ligament

The articular processes of the lumbar vertebrae form the facet or zygapophyseal joints. Each joint consists of two opposed and vertically oriented plates surrounded by a dense connective-tissue fibrous capsule (Lewin et al 1962). The plates are curved such that the inferior articular process (from the above vertebrae) presents a convex process to the concave superior articular process (of the vertebrae below) (Fig. 1.9). These joints contain a true synovial space, a connective tissue rim and a complicated array of surrounding adipose tissue pads and fibroadipose menisci (Engel & Bogduk 1982). The articular surface of the facet joints is covered with a hyaline cartilage. The joint capsule represents a connective-tissue bridge between the neural arch ligaments and those of the vertebral body. As such, the capsule is encased in a thin sheet of dense, irregular investing fascia, which is continuous dorsally with that surrounding the ligamentum flavum and ventrally with the investing fascia of the vertebral body. The capsule itself has two components: an outer layer of dense connective

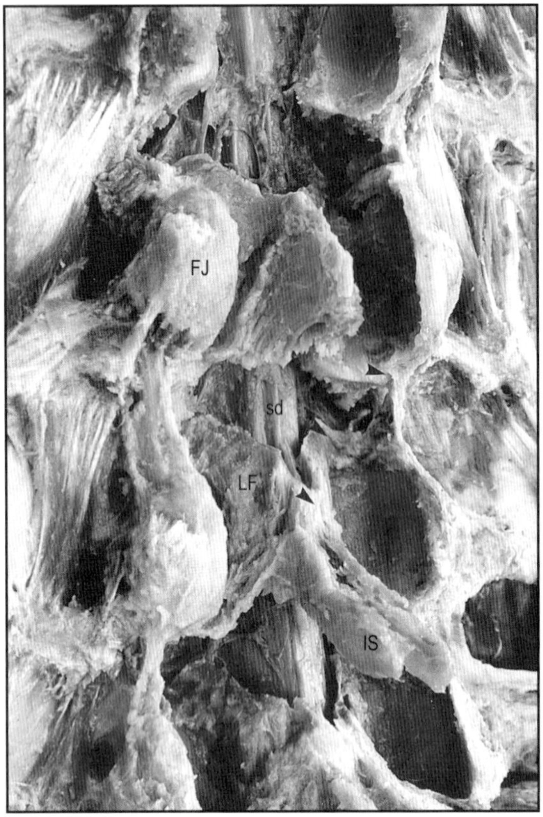

Fig. 1.5 Lateral view of the lumbar ligamentous stocking. The facet joint (FJ) is the same as the marked FJ in Fig. 1.4B. The continuity of the flaval ligament (LF) with the facet joint capsule and interspinous ligament (IS) is indicated by the arrowheads. The spinal dura (sd) can be seen in the epidural space.

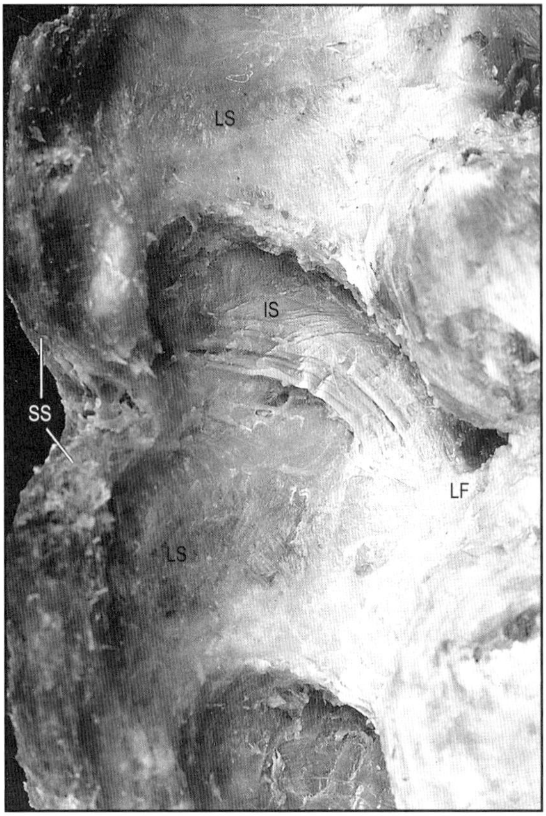

Fig. 1.6 A magnified view of the interspinous ligament. The lumbar spinous processes (LS) are seen superior and inferior to the ligament. Note the fan-like orientation of the collagenous fibers in the ligament. The proximal end of the ligament is continuous with the ligamentum flavum (LF) and the distal end of the ligaments is embedded in the supraspinous ligament (SS). This latter structure is attached to the thoracolumbar fascia. This arrangement would serve to transform any increased tension in the thoracolumbar fascia into increased tension on the ligamentum flavum, resulting in an alignment of the lumbar vertebrae (see Fig. 1.7).

tissue and an inner layer composed of elastic fibers similar to the ligamentum flavum (Yamashita et al 1996). The outer layer is composed of dense, regularly arranged connective tissue in which the predominant orientation of the collagenous fibers is orthogonal to the joint line, the plane on which the two facet plates oppose each other (Fig. 1.10). The capsule is bound tightly to the articular processes with the exception of its inferior and superior recesses, each of which consists of a loosened fold in the capsule wall (Figs 1.9C and 1.11). This arrangement of the capsule allows for a gliding movement in the sagittal plane but restricts its range of motion in the horizontal plane. Each recess has a small defect that is capable of transmitting fat from the capsular space outward (Bogduk & Twomey 1991). The capsule is reinforced dorsally by the multifidus muscle and ventrally by the ligamentum flavum. It is weakest around the superior recess, which can burst from effusion during arthrography (Dory 1981). The inferior border of the capsule is continuous with the ligamentum flavum, the medial border with the periosteum of the lamina, and the lateral border with the periosteum of the pedicle and body.

The intervertebral disc and its two associated facet joints make up a triad representing the load-bearing joint surfaces at each lumbar vertebral level (Lewin et al 1962). Logic suggests that anatomical abnormalities or degenerative changes of one component would lead to changes in other

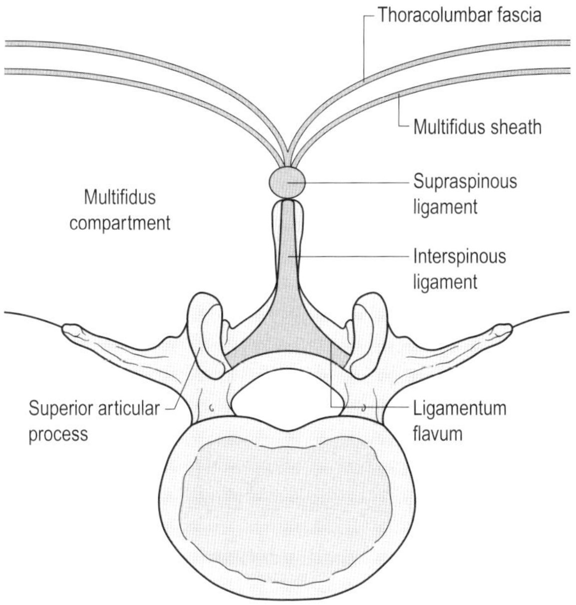

Fig. 1.7 A horizontal view of a lumbar vertebra illustrating the interspinous–supraspinous–thoracolumbar (IST) ligamentous complex. By anchoring the thoracolumbar fascia and multifidus sheath to the facet joint capsules, the IST complex becomes the central support system for the lumbar spine.

components of the unit; however these relationships have been difficult to prove. Anatomical changes, such as trophisms (asymmetry of the planar joint surfaces) of the facet joints, have not demonstrated a strong relationship to disc degeneration or herniation (except the L4–L5 disc); however, facet orientation – particularly in the sagittal plane – has been associated with herniation and degenerative spondylolisthesis (Boden et al 1996, Fujiwara et al 2001, Vanharanta et al 1993). Facet trophism does not even appear to be strongly associated with degeneration of facet cartilage or subcortical bone either (Grogan et al 1997).

Age-related degenerative processes of the intervertebral disc have also proved difficult to relate to the condition of the facet joint. The facet joint is subject to an age-related process of degeneration that might begin early in life (Gries et al 2000); however, unlike the intervertebral discs, facet joints maintain the proteoglycans of their articular cartilage surface, which actually thickens through a process of increased hydration with age (Tobias et al 1992). These changes are accompanied by an increase in coarse fibrillation of the facet joint surface, more pronounced on the superior than the inferior process (Tobias et al 1992, Ziv et al 1993), osteophyte formation, and sclerosis of the subchondral bone (Vernon-Roberts 1992). The degenerative changes of the facet joint

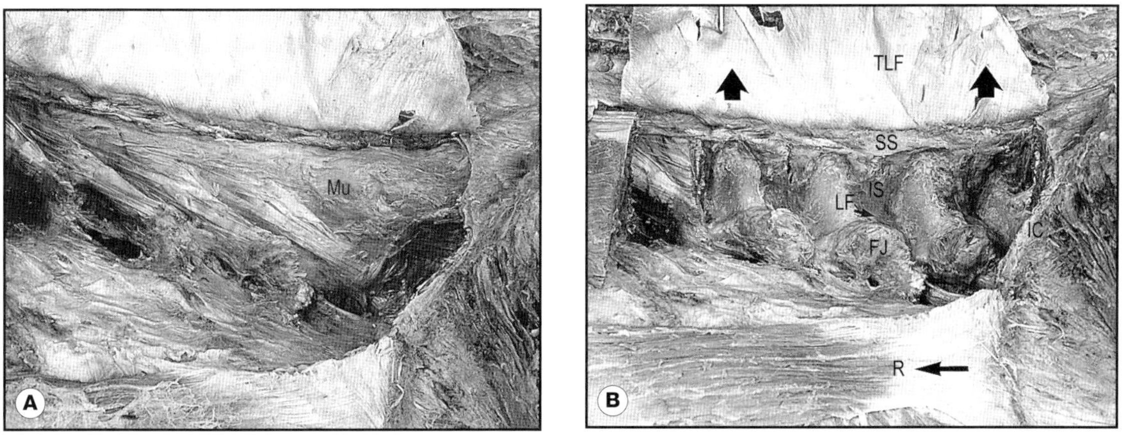

Fig. 1.8 The attachment of the multifidus sheath to the supraspinous ligament. The thoracolumbar fascia (TLF) and multifidus sheath have been sectioned longitudinally to reveal the multifidus muscle (Mu). (A) The iliocostalis and longissimus muscles have been removed. (B) The multifidus muscle has also been removed to illustrate the continuity between the thoracolumbar fascia (and multifidus sheath), supraspinous ligament (SS), ligamentum flavum (LF), and facet joint capsule (FJ). Traction in the posterior direction on the TLF (see hemostat tips) shreds the fascial sheath long before it ever separates this fascial complex. The arrow in the lower right points rostral (R) and the iliac crest (IC) is seen on the right side.

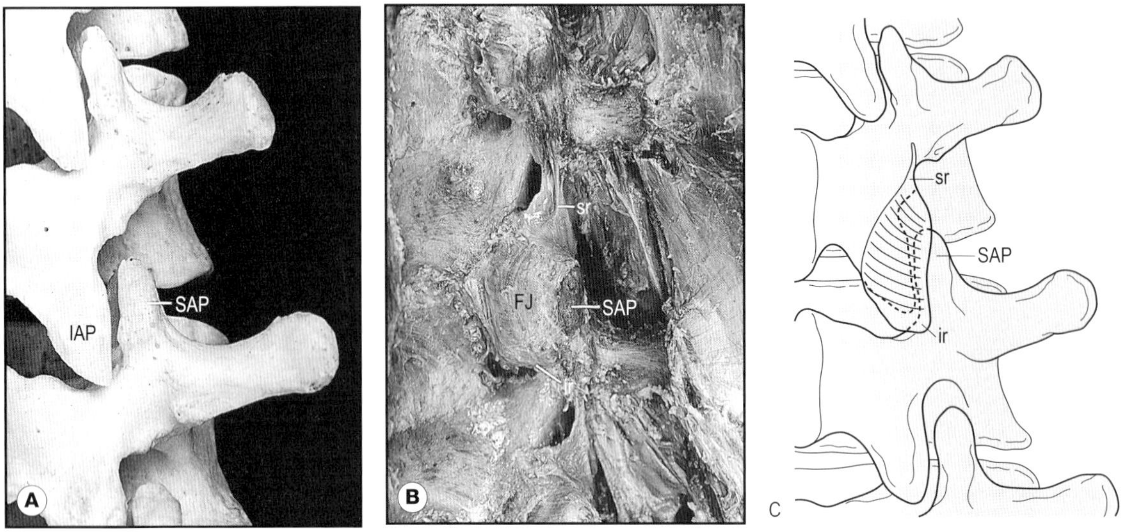

Fig. 1.9 The lumbar facet joint capsule recesses. (A) Orientation view of an articulated lumbar column illustrating the superior articular process (SAP) and inferior articular process (IAP) of the lumbar facet joint (rostral is towards the top of the figure). (B) Same orientation as (A). The facet joint (FJ) capsule is seen with the superior (sr) and inferior (ir) recesses. (C) A schematic illustrating the facet joint capsule (shading) with the superior (sr) and inferior (ir) recesses.

are regional (Gries et al 2000, Swanepoel et al 1995, Taylor & Twomey 1986), being greatest for the articular surface of the superior (concaved) process peripherally, superiorly, and inferiorly; but in the inferior process it is peripheral and posterior (Swanepoel et al 1995).

Recent identification of inflammatory cytokines in the facet joint suggests a possible mechanism of inflammation in the degenerative process (Igarashi et al 2004a). Interleukin-1β, interleukin-6 (IL-6) and tumor necrosis factor-α have been demonstrated in the lumbar facet joints of individuals with degenerative lumbar spinal disorders; IL-6 was present in the highest concentrations. This finding correlates with the previously documented presence of phospholipase A2 and prostaglandins – stimulants of the proinflammatory cytokines – in these joints as well (Willburger & Wittenbeg 1994).

Ligaments ventral to the facet joints

Anterior longitudinal ligament

The vertebral bodies are surrounded by a well-developed periosteum. This sheath can be envisioned as a dense connective tissue stocking that houses the vertebrae and the annular ligaments of the intervertebral discs. Dorsally, the periosteum of the body is continuous with that of the pedicles, facet joint capsule, and laminae. Embedded in the periosteal sheath of the vertebrae are two longitudinal thickenings: the anterior longitudinal ligament and the posterior longitudinal ligament.

The anterior longitudinal ligament, the stronger of the two vertebral body ligaments in the lumbar region (Panjabi & White 1990), consists of a thickened band of vertically oriented collagenous fibers that extends from the basiocciput to the sacrum, where it is continuous with the anteromedial aspect of the sacroiliac joint (SIJ) capsule. The deepest bands of collagenous fibers are the shortest and extend from one vertebral body to the next, forming only loose attachments to the annular ligament of the intervertebral disc. The more superficial bands of the ligament span longer distances (Bogduk & Twomey 1991). A superficial annular ligament of vertically oriented collagenous fibers fuses the anterior longitudinal ligament to the annulus fibrosus of the L5–S1 disc (Hanson et al 2000). In the lumbar region, the fibrous organization of the anterior longitudinal ligament is disrupted where it serves as an attachment for the two crura of the diaphragm (Fig. 1.12). Although the main attachments of the crura are in the region of the upper three lumbar vertebrae, some of the crural fibers extend as low as L3 or below. The lateral borders of the anterior longitudinal ligament are attachment sites for the psoas muscle (Fig. 1.12) and the lumbar sympathetic trunk courses along the border of the psoas attachment.

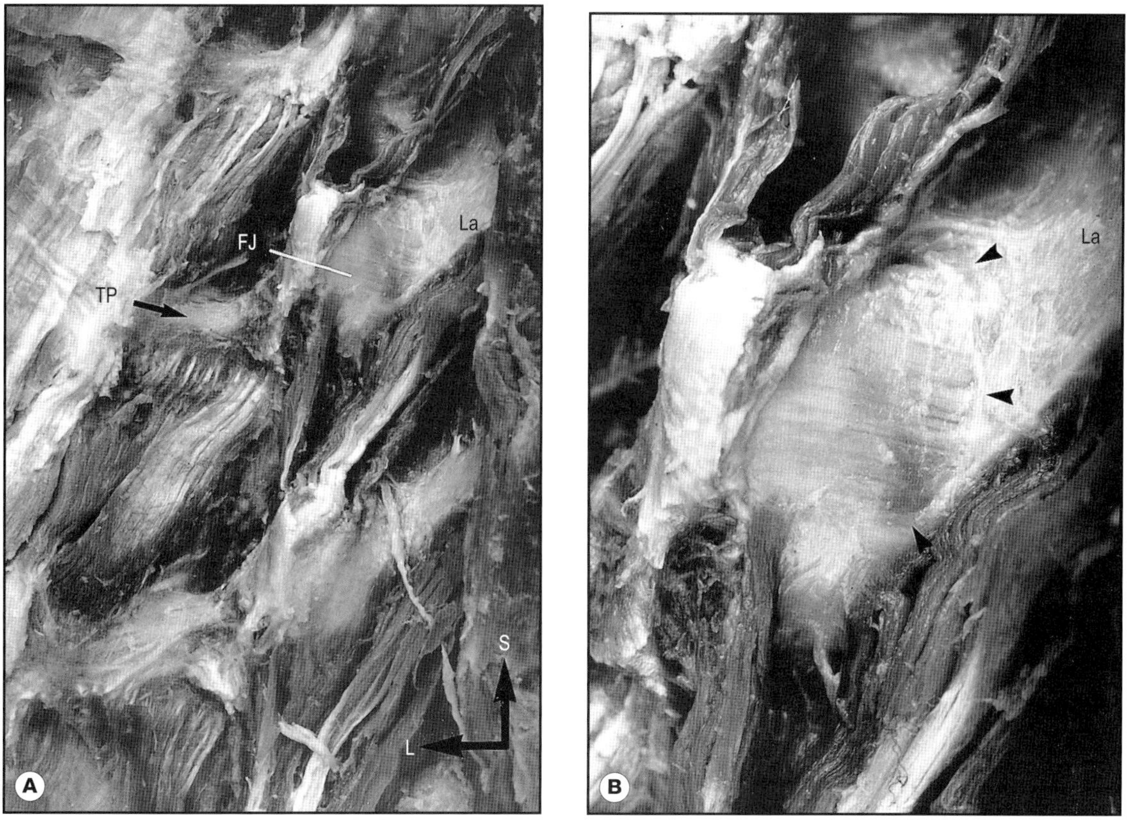

Fig. 1.10 The lumbar facet joint capsule. (A) Dorsal view of the lumbar spinal column with all but the deepest laminae of the multifidus muscle removed to reveal the facet joint capsule (FJ), vertebral laminae (La), and transverse processes (TP) of a lumbar vertebra. The right side is aligned along the midline of the body. The orientation figure (lower right) indicates superior (S) and lateral (L) directions. (B) An enlarged view of the lumbar facet joint capsule marked FJ in (A). Arrowheads mark the medial border of the capsule as it attaches to the vertebral laminae (La). Note the horizontal orientation to the collagenous fibers in the capsule. This orientation is orthogonal to the long axis of the joint. The capsule is strongest on its posterior (current view) and anterior sides, and weakest superiorly and inferiorly. The deepest laminae of the multifidus muscle can be seen attaching to the inferior and superior recesses of the capsule.

The anterior longitudinal ligament undergoes age-related changes. Its energy-absorbing and elastic properties decrease with age, as does the strength of the bone into which it is attached (Neumann et al 1994, Panjabi & White 1990). As the mineral content of the surrounding bone decreases with age, the strength of the ligament also decreases (Neumann et al 1994). Occasionally, the anterior longitudinal ligament calcifies, with extreme cases resulting in compression of the spinal cord and peripheral nerve entrapment (McCafferty et al 1995).

Posterior longitudinal ligament

The posterior longitudinal ligament is also embedded in the periosteum of the vertebrae and extends from the basiocciput (as the membrana tectoria) cervically to the sacrum caudally. As this ligament descends along the anterior wall of the vertebral canal, it narrows to pass around the bases of the pedicles and expands over the annular ligament of the intervertebral discs. This undulating margin imparts a serrated appearance to the longitudinal profile of the ligament (Fig. 1.13). In contradiction to its anterior counterpart, the attachments of the posterior longitudinal ligament are strongest to the outer layer of the annulus fibrosus of the intervertebral disc and weakest to the vertebral body, where the ligament arches over the opening of the foramen for the central vein (basivertebral vein) of the body (Hogan 1991). The lumbar posterior longitudinal ligament is much

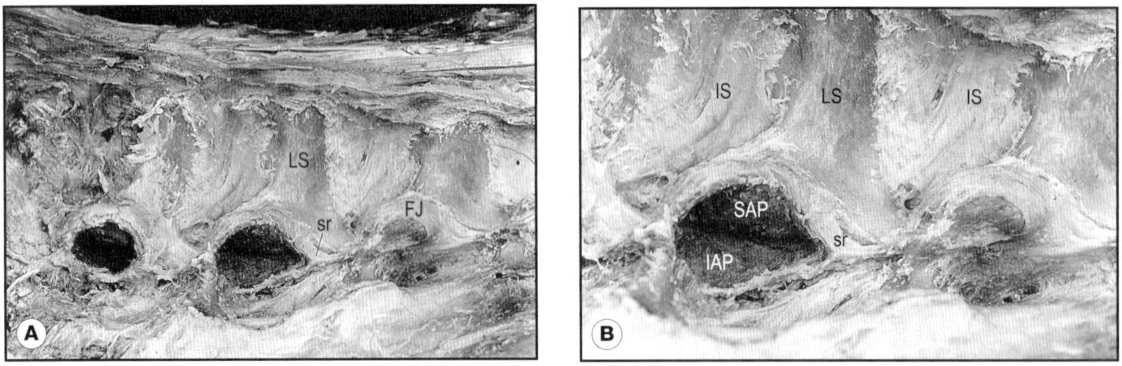

Fig. 1.11 The lumbar facet joint cavity. (A) Lateral view of the middle lumbar vertebra after removing the multifidus muscle. The spines (LS) of the lumbar vertebrae are oriented vertically, the cadaver is prone, with rostral positioned to the right. The lower two facet joints (FJ) have had the superior articular process drilled away to expose the joint cavity and its superior recesses (sr). (B) Magnified view of the middle facet joint in (A). The superior articular process (SAP) can be seen forming the posteromedial wall of the joint and the remains of the inferior articular process (IAP) can be seen in an anterolateral position. The superior recess (SR) extends upward toward the facet joint above. A lumbar spine (LS) and two interspinous ligaments are visible. Note the orientation of the fibers in the interspinous ligament, parallel to the long axis of the lumbar spine.

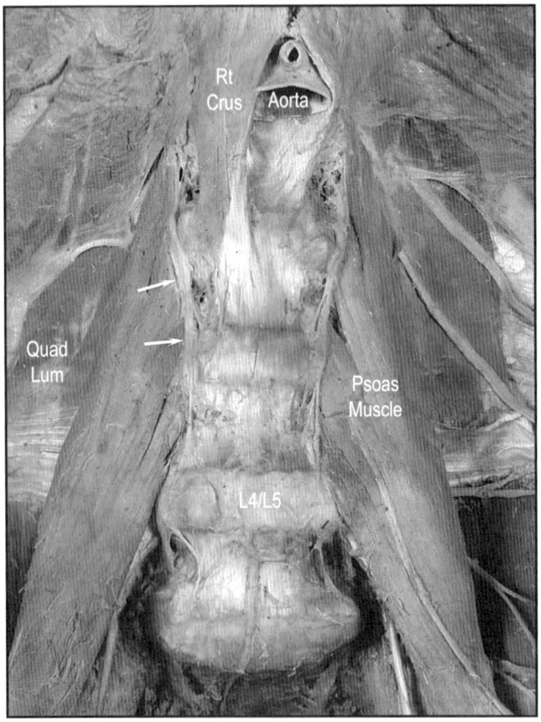

Fig. 1.12 An anterior view of the lumbar anterior longitudinal ligament. The crura of the diaphragm can be seen disrupting the fibrous structure of the anterior longitudinal ligament in the upper lumbar segments. The psoas muscle can be seen attaching the anterior longitudinal ligament laterally in close relationship to the sympathetic trunk.

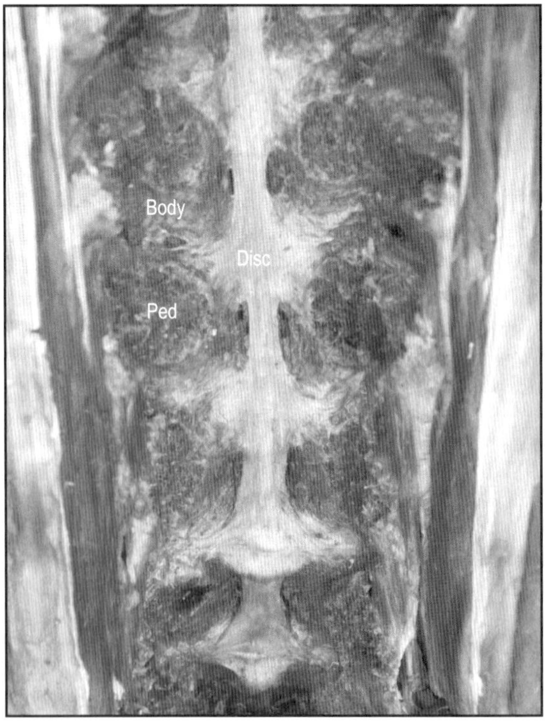

Fig. 1.13 A posterior view of the lumbar posterior longitudinal ligament. The undulating margin of the ligament is clearly seen on this figure. The widest portion of the ligament attaches to the posterior aspect of the intervertebral disc. The narrow portion of the ligament arches over the body of the vertebra allowing the central vein of the body to drain into the epidural plexus of veins.

thinner, both in width and thickness, than its anterior counterpart; therefore, the main opposition to flexion of the lumbar spine comes from the ligamentum flavum (Panjabi & White 1990). Throughout its lumbosacral distribution, the posterior longitudinal ligament acts as an attachment site for the spinal dural sac (Dupuis 1992, Parke & Watanabe 1990, Spencer et al 1983). These attachments are accomplished in part through a series of ventral adhesions referred to as Hoffmann ligaments, as well as through more generalized fascial adhesions. Medial and lateral dural attachment ligaments are recognized (Firooznia et al 1993). Wadhwani et al (2004) re-evaluated the extent and distribution of the Hoffman ligaments. The ligaments are seen from C7 to L5; some were segmental, others were multi-segmental, and the density of the ligaments is more than previously thought. The Hoffman ligaments appear shortly before birth (Hamid et al 2002) and are suspected in playing a role in the stabilization of the spinal cord and dural sac in the spinal canal; in the adult they firmly fuse the anterior surface of the dura to the posterior longitudinal ligament in the lumbar region of the spinal canal (Hogan 1991).

The two longitudinal ligaments and the ligamentum flavum function to stabilize the lumbar vertebral column in flexion (posterior longitudinal ligament and ligamentum flavum) and extension (anterior longitudinal ligament). The ligaments, especially the anterior longitudinal ligament, are most vulnerable to injury when in rotation (Roaf 1960). Of particular interest is the observation that data on load-deformation values for the anterior longitudinal ligament are similar to those data obtained from the ligamentum flavum, suggesting that the two major stabilizing ligaments are balanced in their design (Panjabi & White 1990). The anterior longitudinal ligament comes under its greatest strain in extension (Panjabi et al 1982) and its injury is associated with instability of the spinal column in extension (Oxland et al 1991).

Ligaments of the sacral region

Iliolumbar ligament (lumbo-ilio-sacral ligament)

A large fan-shaped, complex ligament extends laterally from the transverse processes of the lower two lumbar vertebrae and reaches the iliac crest and the SIJ capsule (Figs 1.14, 1.15 and 1.16). Traditionally, this structure is termed the iliolumbar ligament, but components of this structure have been renamed as the lumbosacral ligament and recently the entire structure was referred to as the lumbo-ilio-sacral ligament (Hanson & Sorensen 2000). The structure has received numerous and varied descriptions. *Gray's anatomy* (Standing 2005) describes upper and lower bands in the ligament and, although the text does not use the term 'lumbosacral ligament' for the inferior band, it is labeled as such in a figure (see Standing 2005, Fig. 111.11). Kapandji (1974) describes superior and inferior bands with an occasional sacral band below the inferior band. O'Rahilly (1986) describes anterior, superior, and inferior bands, whereas Bogduk and Twomey (1991) describe anterior, posterior, superior, inferior, and vertical iliolumbar divisions. A study based on 100 specimens reported only two parts to the ligament: anterior and posterior (Hanson & Sonesson 1994). A recent study has described a dorsal band, ventral band, sacroiliac part, and a lumbosacral band (Pool-Goudzwaard et al 2001). My experience with the iliolumbar ligament is that the individual bands of fascia are highly variable in their number and their form, but that they consistently blend superiorly with the intertransverse ligaments of the lumbar vertebrae and inferiorly with both the posterior (Figure 1.15) and anterior (Fig. 1.16) aspects of the SIJ capsule as well as attach laterally to the iliac crest (Fig. 1.14).

The iliolumbar ligament arises from the transverse processes of L4 and L5 in some individuals (Figs 1.14 and 1.15; see also Pool-Goudzwaard et al 2001, Standing 2005); this is contrary to the observations of Hanson and Sonesson (1994) that it attaches only to L5. The iliolumbar ligament has previously been described as developing out of the inferior border of the quadratus lumborum muscle in the second decade of life (Luk et al 1986). However, this was refuted with the observation that the ligament is present in the fetus as early as 11–15 weeks gestational age (Uhthoff 1993), a finding that has been verified by Hanson & Sonesson (1994). The taut bands of the iliolumbar ligament form hoods over the L4 and L5 nerve roots. These hoods are capable of compressing the associated nerve roots (Briggs & Chandraraj 1995). The iliolumbar ligament is subject to fatty degeneration after the first decade of life and has been reported to ossify on occasion (Lapadula et al 1991).

The major function of the iliolumbar ligament is to restrict motion at the lumbosacral junction, particularly that of side bending (Chow et al 1989, Leong et al 1987, Yamamoto et al 1990). After bilateral transection of the iliolumbar ligament,

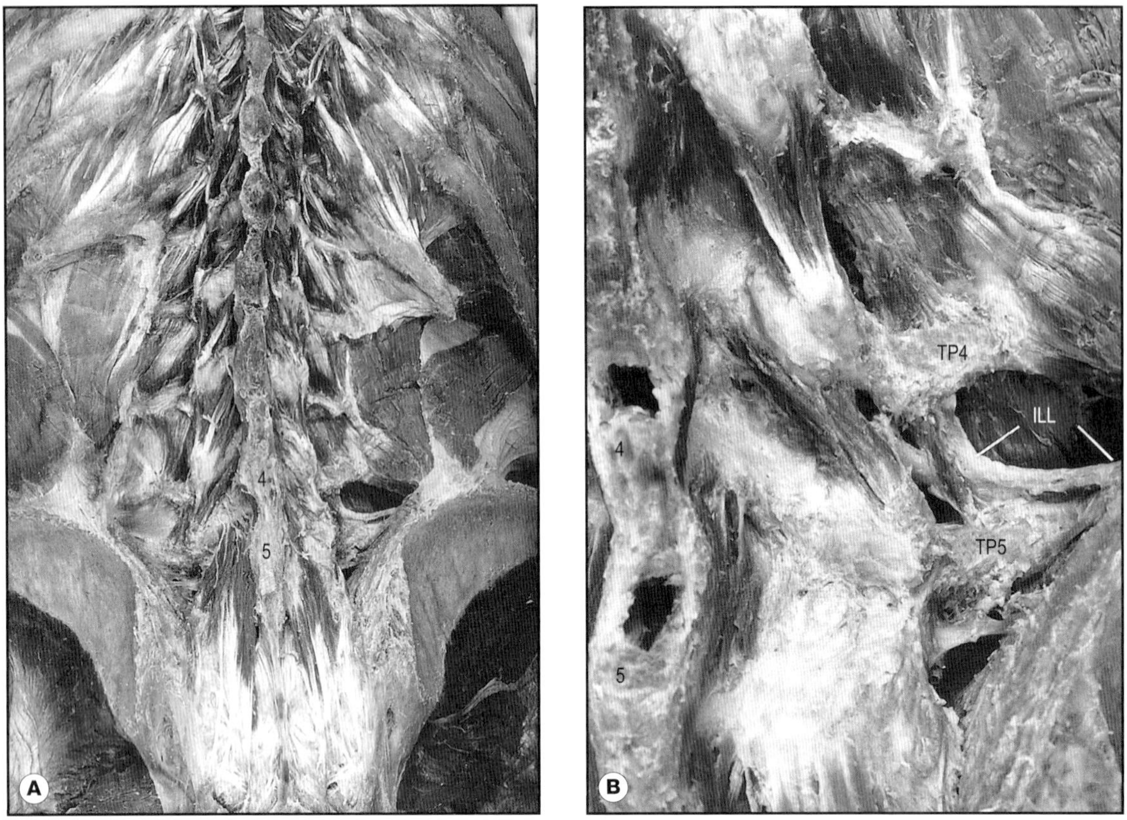

Fig. 1.14 Dorsal view of the sacrum and iliolumbar ligament. (A) In this orientation view, note that the multifidus muscle, except for its deepest laminae, has been removed. The spinous processes of L4 and L5 are indicated. (B) Enlarged view of the iliolumbar ligament (ILL) in (A). The ligament (ILL) can be seen attaching to the transverse processes of L4 and L5 (TP4 and TP5). The spinous processes of L4 and L5 are indicated.

rotation about the vertebral axis is increased by 18%, extension by 20%, flexion by 23%, and lateral bending by 29% (Yamamoto et al 1989). Thus the iliolumbar ligament represents a critical structure for stabilizing the lumbar vertebrae on the sacral base.

Articular capsule of the sacroiliac joint

At the caudal end of the lumbar spine, the ligamentous stocking surrounding the spine expands to form the capsular structure of the SIJ. This joint is partially synovial in nature, having a C-shaped articular surface, with the longer limb of the joint oriented posteriorly and the shorter limb superiorly (Fig. 1.17). The lower portion of the superior limb and the inferior limb are synovial in construction; the upper portion of the superior limb is not (as described in the review by Cole et al 1996). As such, the joint has a limited range of motion (Brunner et al 1991, Vleeming et al 1992). There is a renewed interest in understanding the structure (Bernard & Cassidy 1991) and biomechanics (Jacob & Kissling 1995, Kissling 1995, Kissling & Jacob 1996) of this joint because it is now realized that its dysfunction represents a major source of low back pain (Cole et al 1996, Daum 1995, Fortin et al 1994a, 1994b, Schwarzer et al 1995, Vleeming et al 1995c). The joint surface is derived, in part, from the first three sacral vertebrae; its sacral surface is lined with a thickened hyaline cartilage and its ileal surface with a thinner fibrocartilage (see Fig. 1.17; McLauchlan & Gardner 2002).

The SIJ is surrounded by a tough capsule presenting several remarkably different surfaces (see Figs 1.15–1.17). The superior aspect of the joint capsule is a caudalward extension of the iliolumbar ligament, specifically the lumbosacral band of the ligament. The anterior aspect of this capsule (also termed the anterior sacroiliac ligament) is composed

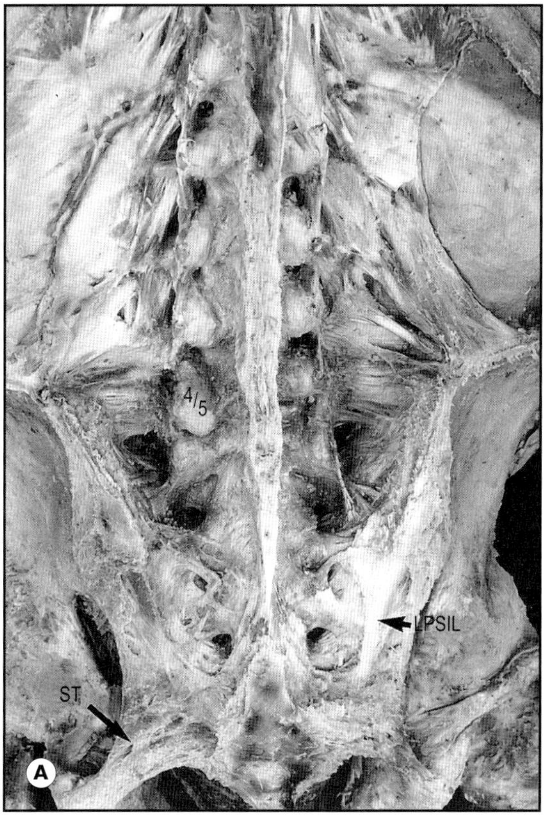

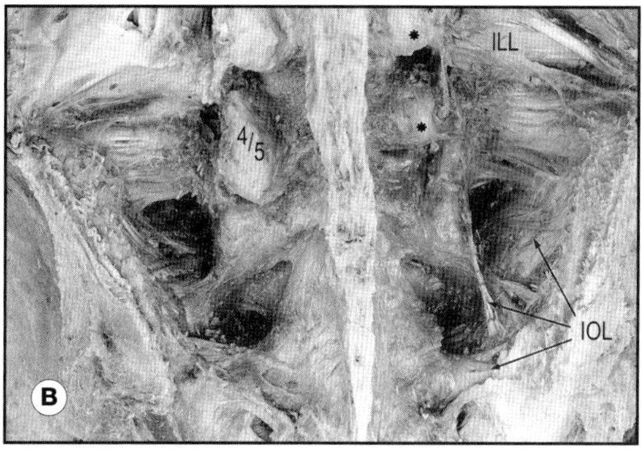

Fig 1.15 Dorsal view of the female sacroiliac joint (SIJ). (A) In this orientation view the multifidus muscle has been entirely removed to reveal the interosseous ligaments of the SIJ. The long dorsal (posterior) SI ligament (LPSIL), the facet joint between the 4th and 5th lumbar vertebrae (4/5), and the sacrotuberous ligament (ST) are indicated as landmarks. (B) In this enlarged view of the SIJ, the interosseous ligaments (IOL), the facet joint between the 4th and 5th lumbar vertebrae (4/5), and the iliolumbar ligaments (ILL) are indicated. The iliolumbar ligament is seen attaching to the transverse processes of L4 and L5. Each process is located opposite the facet joint capsule marked with an asterisk.

of a smooth sheet of dense connective tissue stretched between the ventral surface of the sacral alar and that of the ilium (see Fig. 1.17). The caudal border of the anterior SI capsule blends with the rostral edge of the sacrospinous ligament. The posterior aspect of the joint capsule is much more complex than its anterior counterpart (see Fig. 1.15) and is composed of two groups of ligaments. Around the margins of the joint are numerous, discontinuous interwoven bands of dense connective tissue; these comprise the first group. These short interosseous sacroiliac ligaments arise on the intermediate and lateral sacral crest and attach to the rough sacropelvic surface of the ilium. Conversely, the second group, the dorsal (posterior) sacroiliac ligaments, extends from the median and lateral sacral crests, diagonally in a superior direction across the sacral gutter, and attach to the posterior superior spine of the ilium. Particularly prominent is the long dorsal sacroiliac ligament, which is a thickened band extending from the posterior superior iliac spine to the lower transverse tubercle on the lateral sacral crest (Fig. 1.18). Several structures anchor into these tough ligaments of the SIJ. A portion of the sacrotuberous ligament attaches laterally to the sacrum where its fibers blend with the long dorsal sacroiliac ligaments of the joint capsule (Figs 1.19 and 1.20), and the thoracolumbar fascia anchors to these same interosseous ligaments from its medial side. This anchoring portion of the thoracolumbar fascia also forms a prominent raphe separating the multifidus and gluteus maximus muscle (see Fig. 1.22 below).

The articular surfaces of the SIJ are smooth and flattened at birth, and the long axis of the joint is oriented parallel to that of the lumbar spine (Bernard & Cassidy 1991). Remodeling of the joint into the adult, C-shaped orientation with roughened surface occurs after puberty (Schunke 1938 as cited in Cole et al 1996). The ileal surface develops a crescent-shaped ridge along its long axis (see Fig. 1.17A) and the sacral surface forms a concavity complementary to the convexity of the ileal surface in the second decade of life (see Fig. 1.17B). These changes in the surface of the joint contribute to its stability and limited range of motion (Simonian et al 1994). The interlocking surfaces of the joint form the centerpiece in the self-bracing model of

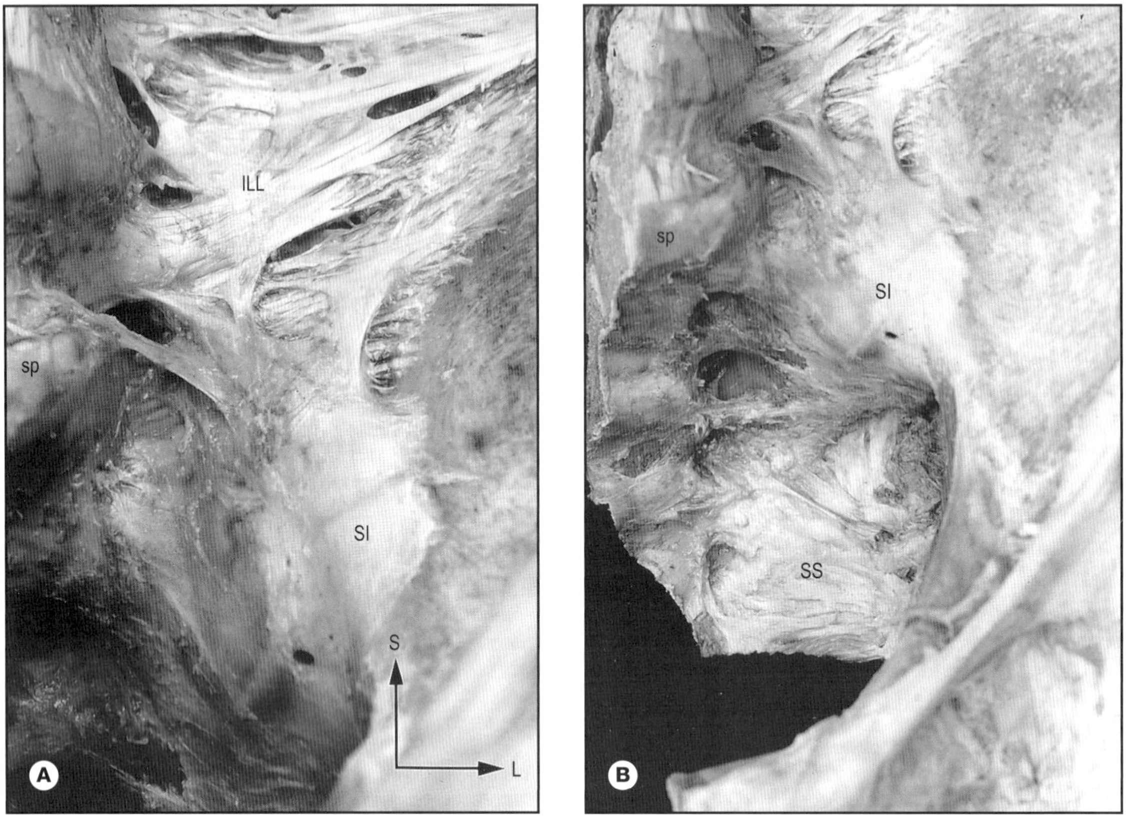

Fig. 1.16 Anterior views of the sacroiliac joint (SIJ) taken into a bisected female pelvic basin after removing all the pelvic contents and endopelvic fascia. (A) The superior portion of the SIJ (SI), demonstrating its smooth surface and its continuity with the iliolumbar ligament (ILL). (B) The inferior portion of the SIJ (SI), demonstrating its continuity with the sacrospinous ligament (SS). In both (A) and (B), the sacral promontory (sp) is marked for reference. The orientation figure in the lower right of (A) indicates superior (S) and lateral (L) directions.

SIJ function (Snijders et al 1993, Vleeming et al 1995c).

The SIJ capsule frequently has defects that allow fluid substances in the joint space to leak out onto surrounding structures. In 61% of 76 joints examined by injection and imaging, leakage of injected contrast was reported (Fortin et al 1999b). Notably, contrast leaked into the dorsal sacral foramina, where it could be in contact with the dorsal sacral plexus, and into the ventral region in close juxtaposition with the lumbosacral plexus. These represent intriguing pathways whereby the proinflammatory contents of an inflamed joint could leak into the surrounding neural structures of the pelvis (Fortin et al 1999b).

A series of age-related degenerative changes occur to the joint, especially after the fifth decade of life. In this age range, the cartilaginous surfaces of the joints begin to degenerate and ossification occurs between the two articular surfaces, especially in males (Bernard & Cassidy 1991). These changes eventually lead to further restricted motion of the joint. Finally, asymmetric laxity in the SIJ in women with pregnancy-related pelvic pain can be a risk factor for the persistence of moderate pain in the postpartum period (Damen et al 2001, 2002). Modern imaging has cast doubt on the degree of ankylosis that is reported to occur in the joint after 50 years of age (see citations in Cole et al 1996 and Chapter 20).

Sacrotuberous ligament

The sacrotuberous ligament is a specialization derived from the posteroinferior aspect of the SIJ capsule. It is a triangular-shaped structure extending between the posterior iliac spines, the SIJ

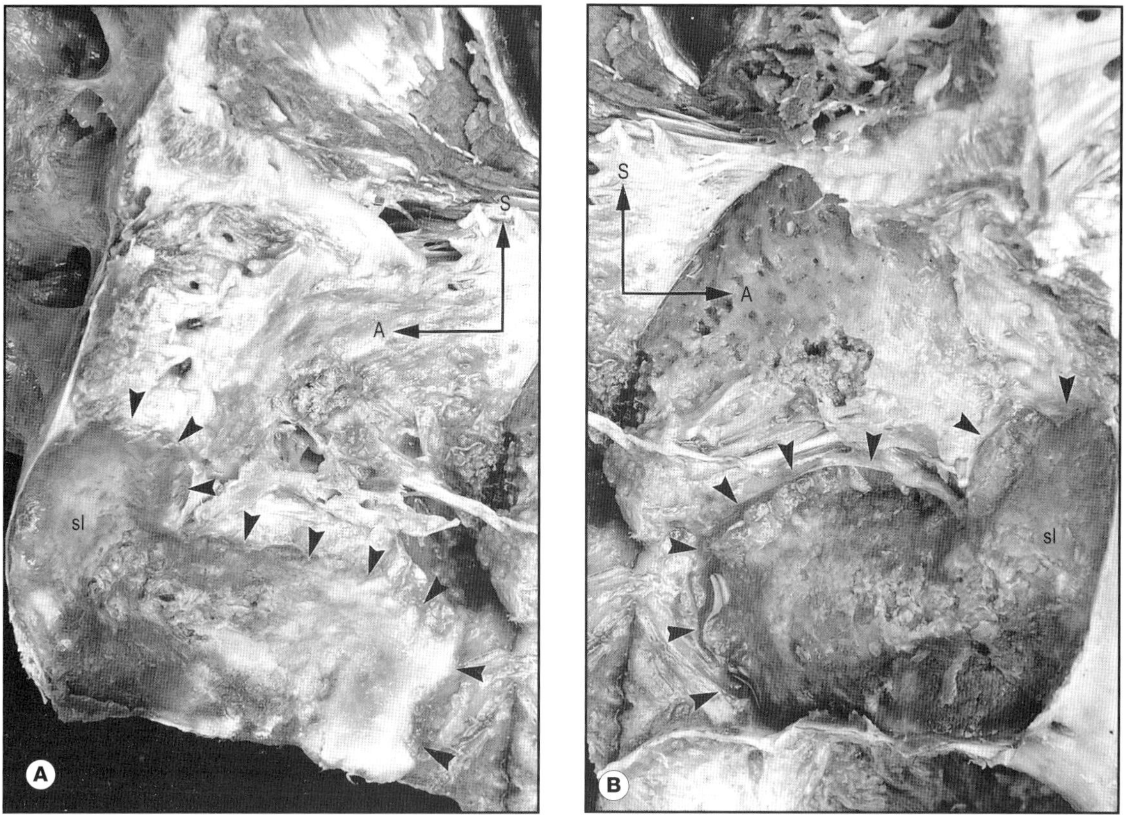

Fig. 1.17 The internal features of the sacroiliac joint (SIJ). The female SIJ in Fig. 1.16 was opened to display (A) its medial (or sacral) and (B) its lateral (or iliac) surfaces. The boundaries of the joint are marked with arrowheads in (A) and (B). The anterior boundary is formed by a precise capsule, the posterior boundary being formed by the interweaving of the interosseous ligaments. The joint has a superior limb (sl) and inferior limb. The orientation arrows in both (A) and (B) indicate the superior (S) and anterior (A) directions. The medial surface is concave and covered with hyaline cartilage with associated fatty deposits; the lateral surface is convex and covered with fibrocartilage.

capsule, the coccygeal vertebrae, and the ischial tuberosity (see Fig. 1.19). The tendon of the biceps femoris often reaches over the tuberosity to attach to the sacrotuberous ligament (Vleeming et al 1989a), and an occasional aberrant extension derived from the biceps femoris establishes the attachment of its entire superior head to this ligament (Akita et al 1992). The tendons of the deepest laminae of the multifidus often extend under the long dorsal sacroiliac ligament to embed in the sacrotuberous ligament from its superior surface (see Fig. 1.19). The sacrotuberous ligament can be divided into several large fibrous bands (Fig. 1.20). Its prominent lateral band reaches from the posterior inferior iliac spine to the ischial tuberosity and its medial band connects the coccygeal vertebrae with the ischial tuberosity. The superior band is the thinnest and forms a plate stretching between the posterior iliac spines and the coccygeal vertebrae. Several central bands arise from the lateral band and attach to the lower transverse tubercle of the lateral sacral crest. They share this attachment with the inferior border of the long dorsal SI ligament. Along its medial and superior borders, the sacrotuberous ligament merges with the interosseous ligaments of the SIJ capsule. The body of the sacrotuberous ligament is made up from the fusion of its multiple bands and is occasionally penetrated by branches from the inferior gluteal neurovascular bundle.

The sacrotuberous ligament is positioned to resist nutation of the sacrum and is opposed by the long dorsal SI ligament that is portioned to resist counternutation (Vleeming et al 1995a). Several studies have examined the stability of the pelvis after sectioning the sacrotuberous ligament (Borrelli et al 1996, Dujardin et al 2002, Le Blanche

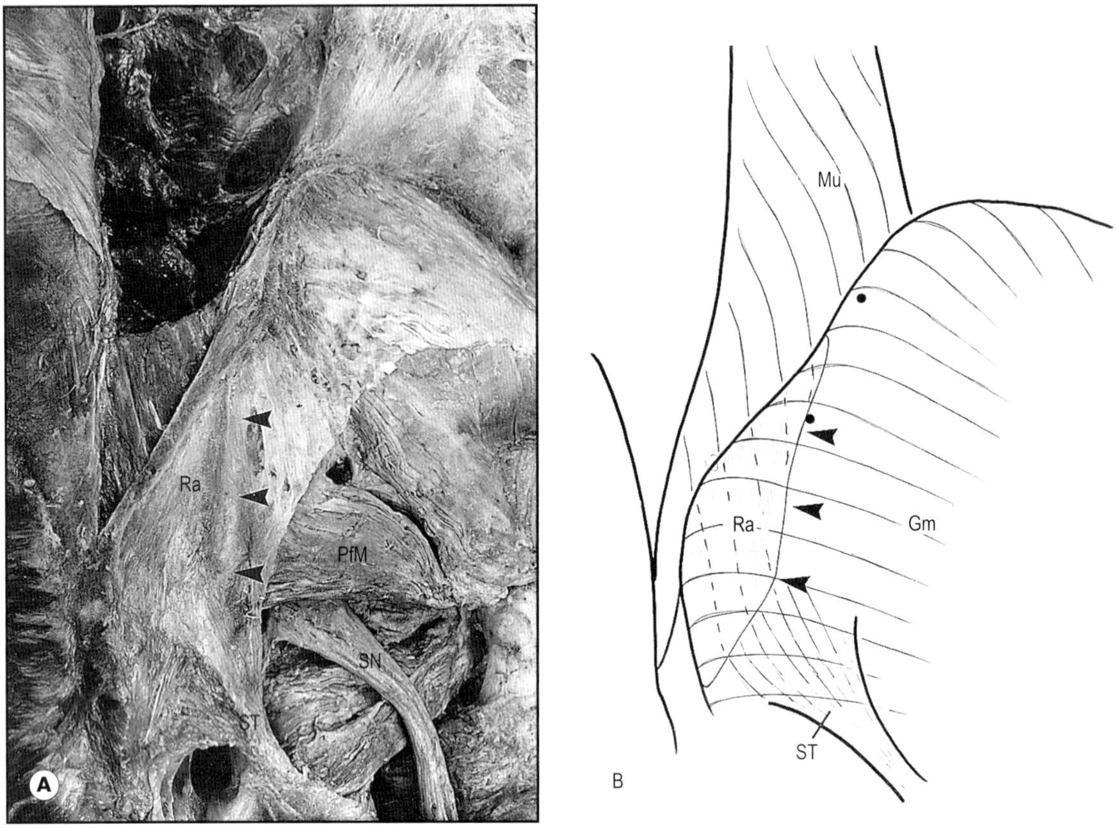

Fig. 1.18 Posterior attachments of the sacroiliac joint (SIJ). (A) Posterior view of the sacral region with the multifidus sheath open. Most of the multifidus muscle has been removed, as has the entire gluteus maximus muscle. The raphe (Ra) overlaying the inferior end of the multifidus muscle is present. The posterior surface of the raphe is the attachment of the gluteus maximus muscle. A ridge in the raphe (arrowheads) indicates its attachment to the long posterior interosseous ligament of the SIJ. The interior border of the raphe blends into the sacrotuberous ligament (ST). The piriformis muscle (PfM) and sciatic nerve (SN) are seen emerging from the greater sciatic foramen under the raphe. (B) The raphe (Ra) as it separates the multifidus (Mu) and gluteus maximus (Gm) muscles. The deep border of the raphe lies along the long posterior interosseous ligament (arrowheads). The posterior superior iliac spine and posterior inferior iliac spine are indicated by black dots.

et al 1996, Vrahas et al 1995). The consensus of these studies is that the sacrotuberous ligament helps to stabilize the pelvis in the vertical axis. Occasional ossification of the sacrotuberous ligament has been reported outside the more obvious cases of general ossification, such as occurs in diffuse idiopathic skeletal hyperostosis (Prescher & Bohndorf 1993).

Sacrospinous ligament

The sacrospinous ligament is a specialization of the anteroinferior aspect of the SIJ capsule. It is a triangular-shaped structure (see Fig. 1.14B) arising from the lateral margin of the lower sacral and coccygeal vertebrae and the inferior aspect of the SIJ capsule. Its distal attachment is to the spine of the ischium. Proximally, its superior fibers blend with those of the SIJ capsule and the sacrotuberous ligament (Standing 2005). The ligament is thought to be a degenerate portion of the coccygeus muscle (Standing 2005). Although initially involved in movements of the tail in quadrupeds, this ligament has evolved into a support mechanism for the pelvic floor in humans (Abitbol 1988). As such, the ligament forms the posterolateral border of the pelvic outlet and has been used as an anchor into which the pelvic floor is secured in situations involving eversion of the vagina (Dofferhof & Vink 1985, Morley & DeLancey 1988, Nichols 1985, Porges & Smilen 1994).

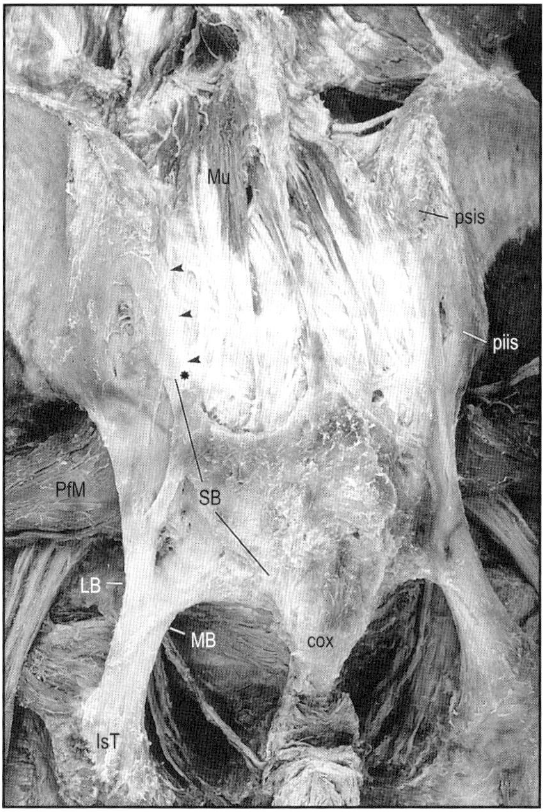

Fig. 1.19 Dorsal view of the male sacroiliac joint (SIJ) and sacrotuberous ligament. All but the deepest laminae of the multifidus muscle (Mu) have been removed. The sacrotuberous ligaments seen stretching from the ischial tuberosity (IsT) to the coccyx (cox) medially and the posterior iliac spines superolaterally. The posterior superior iliac spine (psis) and the posterior inferior iliac spine (piis) are marked on the contralateral side. The asterisk marks the transverse tuberosity of the lateral sacral crest and the arrowheads mark the course of the long posterior interosseous ligament under the lateral band of the sacrotuberous ligament. Three major bands of the ligament are seen: lateral (LB), medial (MB), and superior (SB). The lateral band spans the piriformis muscle (PfM) to reach the ilium inferior to the (piis). As the lateral band climbs toward the (psis), it blends with the raphe (see Fig. 1.18). The medial band attaches to the coccyx, and the superior band courses superficial to the long dorsal SI ligament to connect the coccyx with the posterior ileal spines. Tendons of the multifidus pass between the superior band and the long dorsal SI ligament to insert into the body of the sacrotuberous ligament.

Summary of the ligamentous structures

The ligamentous structures of the lumbosacral connection form a continuous, dense connective tissue stocking that houses the lumbar vertebrae and sacrum and provides attachment sites for the associated muscles. This complicated ligamentous structure plays a key role in the self-bracing mechanism of the pelvis, a mechanism that functions to maintain the integrity of the low back and pelvis during the transfer of energy from the spine to the lower extremities (Vleeming et al 1989a, 1989b). Tension in the sacrotuberous and long dorsal SI ligaments varies with rocking movements of the sacrum in its joint capsule (Vleeming et al 1995a), and unilateral lesions of the SIJ capsule increase the range of motion (decrease the stability) of the joint under compressive loads (Simonian et al 1994). The ligamentous support mechanism of the lumbosacral region is influenced by several major muscle groups in the low back and pelvis; each of these groups will be discussed below.

Major muscle groups associated with the lumbosacral ligamentous structures

Multifidus muscle

The paravertebral muscles in the lumbar region are represented by three large muscles (see Fig. 1.2), each in its own fascial compartment and arranged from lateral to medial: the iliocostalis, longissimus, and multifidus (Bogduk 1980a). The lateral two muscles, iliocostalis and longissimus, arise from the iliac crest and thoracolumbar fascia, but, with the exception of a few medial slips from the longissimus, do not attach to the lumbar vertebrae. The multifidus is divided into five bands (Fig. 1.21), each band arising from the spine of a lumbar vertebrae and associated tissues (Macintosh et al 1986). Its distal attachments are the sacrum, interosseous SI ligaments, thoracolumbar fascia, and extreme medial edge of the iliac crest. The attachment of the muscles to the thoracolumbar fascia represents a raphe separating the multifidus from the gluteus maximus muscle (Figs 1.18 and 1.22). The anterior border of the raphe is anchored in the SIJ capsule, and the posterior border of the raphe becomes part of the thoracolumbar fascia. Finally, tendinous slips of the multifidus muscle pass under the long dorsal SI ligament to join with the sacrotuberous ligament (see Fig. 1.19). These connections integrate the multifidus into the ligamentous support system of the SIJ.

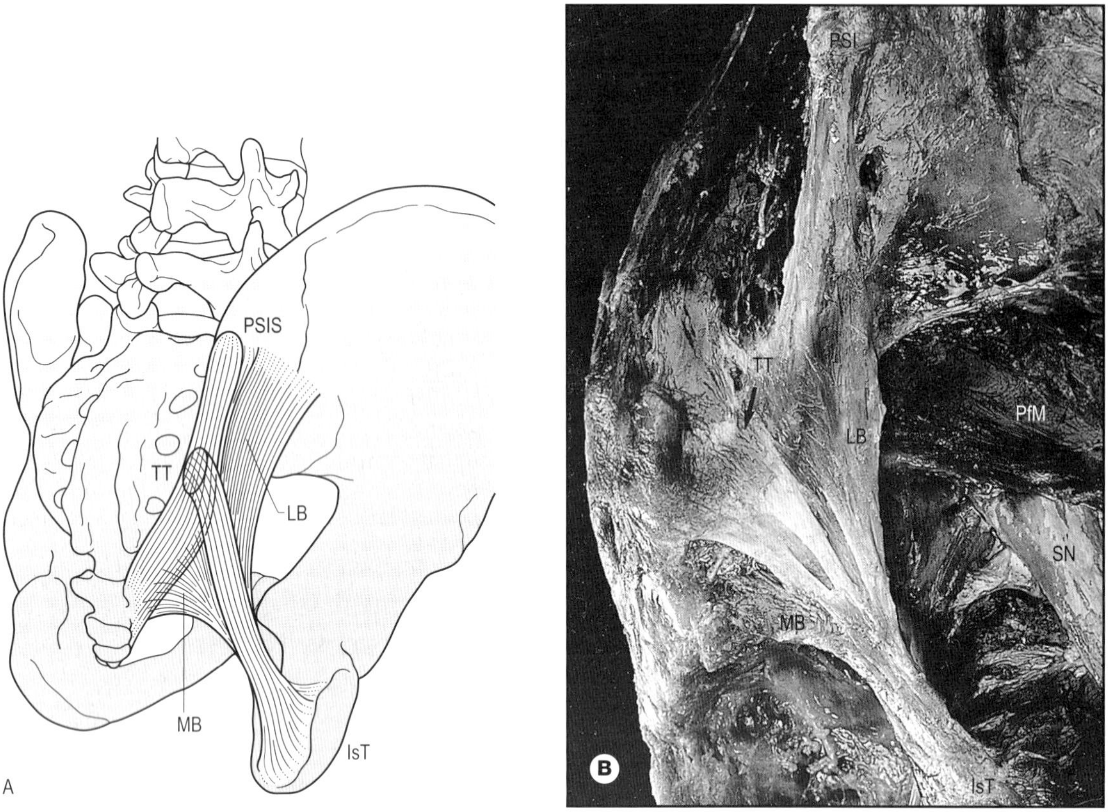

Fig. 1.20 Relationships between the sacrotuberous ligament and the sacroiliac joint (SIJ). (A) Schematic illustrating the three groups of bands forming the sacrotuberous ligament. The lateral band (LB) overlays the long posterior interosseous ligament (arrowheads) and reaches upward toward the posterior superior iliac spine. The firmest attachment of the lateral band is to the transverse tubercle (TT) of the lateral sacral crest. The medial band (MB) bends toward the coccygeal vertebra. Both of these bands arise on the ischial tuberosity (IsT). A superior band courses upward from the coccygeal attachments to blend with the lateral band over the long posterior interosseous ligament. (B) Photograph of the sacrotuberous ligament similar to that depicted in (A). The piriformis muscle (PfM) and sciatic nerve (SN) are marked for reference.

The fibers of the multifidus are aligned in the vertical plane with only very slight horizontal deviations. This arrangement is specific for movement in the sagittal plane, making the multifidus a significant lumbar spine extensor muscle, along with the erector spinae muscles (Bogduk et al 1992, Macintosh & Bogduk 1986). However, owing to its geometry, only slight movements in the horizontal plane can be accomplished by this muscle. The long fibers in the body of the muscle span multiple segments, thus giving this portion of the multifidus muscle an additional role as a stabilizer of the lumbar spine (Crisco & Panjabi 1991, Macintosh & Bogduk 1986). Finally, by increasing tension on the thoracolumbar fascia, SI ligaments and sacrotuberous ligaments, activation of the multifidus also contributes to the self-bracing mechanism (Snijders et al 1995) of the pelvis and to the transfer of energy from the upper body to the lower extremities.

The multifidus muscle plays an important role in standing or seated posture (Bogduk et al 1992, Moseley et al 2003, O'Sullivan et al 2002), gait (Dofferhof & Vink 1985, Moseley et al 2002), trunk movement (Andersson et al 2002, Macintosh et al 1993a, 1993b, Ng et al 1997) and when lifting or carrying a load (Cholewicki et al 1997, Danneels et al 2001) as based on electromyographic studies. Given the importance of this muscle it is easy to understand how its dysfunction could lead to injury of the low back and to low back pain. Alteration in the structure of the multifidus muscle occurs

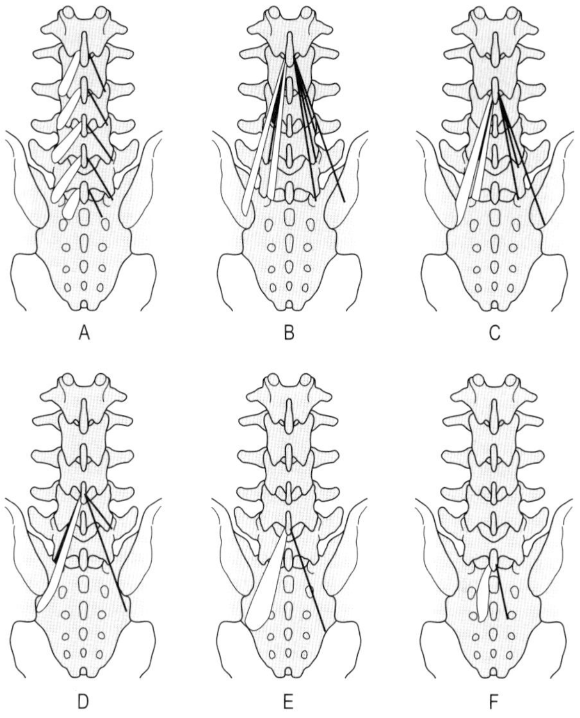

Fig. 1.21 The laminae of the multifidus muscle. (A) The shortest laminae of the multifidus muscle. (B–F) The five laminae of the multifidus muscle (B, L1; C, L2; D, L3; E, L4; F, L5). Each lamina arises from a lumbar spine and attachment is to the sacrum. (Adapted from Macintosh et al 1986.)

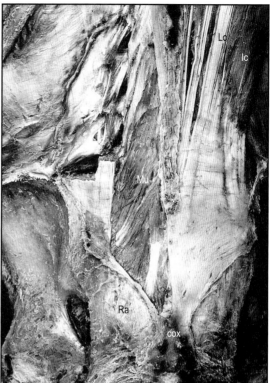

Fig. 1.22 Dorsal view of the sacroiliac (SI) region with the gluteus maximus muscle removed. The thoracolumbar fascia and the tendinous insertion of the iliocostalis (Ic) and longissimus (Lo) muscles have been opened to expose the multifidus muscle (Mu). The raphe (Ra) separating the multifidus and gluteus muscles is seen stretching from the coccyx (cox) to the posterior superior ilial spine (asterisk). Its anterior border is blended with the SI joint capsule and its posterior border with the thoracolumbar fascia. The rough surface visible on this raphe represents the attachment site for the gluteal muscle.

either with aging or in association with pathologic processes. Size changes have been reported for the multifidus muscle in idiopathic scoliosis, the side of the lumbar spinal convexity being reduced in cross-sectional area on imaging (Kennelly & Stokes 1993). In addition, structural changes in the muscle histochemistry, the muscle fiber type, and the myotendinous junction have been reported for the multifidus on the concave side of the lumbar scoliotic curve (Khosla et al 1980). Lumbar disc herniation is also associated with histochemical changes in the multifidus muscle consistent with atrophy and fibrosis (Bajek et al 2000, Lehto et al 1989, Mattila et al 1986, Rantanen et al 1993, Yoshihara et al 2001, 2003, Zhao et al 2000). Low back pain has been associated with reduction in size of the multifidus muscle (Hides et al 1994, Kader et al 2000, Lee et al 1999, Parkkola et al 1993, Sihvonen et al 1997). Finally, there is with aging a pronounced fatty metaplasia in the muscle, this event being exacerbated in neuromuscular diseases involving the multifidus (Hadar et al 1983). Reduced size of the muscle and increased fatty deposits typified a population of low back pain patients when compared with a population of healthy volunteers (Parkkola et al 1993).

Latissimus dorsi muscle

The upper extremity is anchored to the body through an anterior muscular hood, the pectoralis muscles, and a posterior muscular hood, the latissimus dorsi. This latter muscle has its axial attachment to the thoracolumbar fascia (Fig. 1.23), the iliac crest, and to the caudal three or four ribs. Its appendicular attachment is to the intertubercular

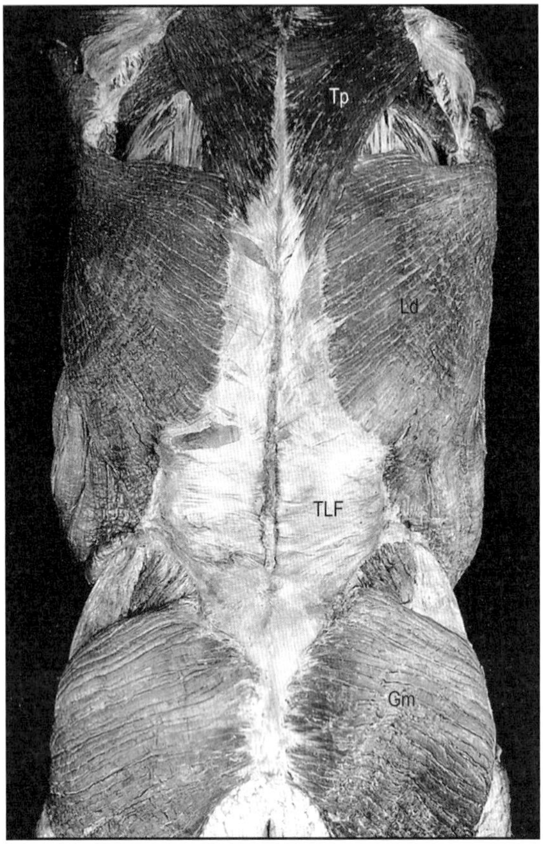

Fig. 1.23 Posterior view of the thoracolumbar fascia in a male cadaver. The superficial fat and fascia have been removed to demonstrate the diamond shape of the thoracolumbar fascia (TLF). A small window is present in the fascial sheath on the left, revealing the paravertebral muscles underneath. Large muscles of the upper extremity (trapezius, Tp; latissimus dorsi, Ld) and lower extremity (gluteus maximus, Gm) attach along the borders of the thoracolumbar fascia. The iliac crest and gluteus medius muscle can be seen emerging from under the superolateral border of the gluteus maximus.

groove of the humerus. This broad, fan-shaped muscle can be divided into four parts based on its attachments (Bogduk et al 1998): the thoracic portion attaches to the lower six thoracic spines, a transitional portion that attaches to the upper two lumbar spines, a raphe portion that attaches to the lateral raphe of the thoracolumbar fascia and an iliac portion that attaches to the iliac crest. Considerable debate exists concerning the role of the latissimus dorsi in assisting the lumbar spine through its connections to the thoracolumbar fascia (Barker et al 2004, Bogduk et al 1998, Danneels et al 2001, Granata & Marras 1995, McGill & Norman 1988, Vakos et al 1994, van Wingerden et al 2004, Vleeming et al 1996). Agreement seems to be centered around the concept that the muscle is primarily involved in movement of the arm and its influence on movement of the lumbar spine, although slight (Bogduk et al 1998), might provide some stabilizing activity (Barker et al 2004, van Wingerden et al 2004).

Gluteus maximus muscle

The gluteus maximus is the largest skeletal muscle of the body. It is attached to the posterior surface of the iliac blade and crest, the thoracolumbar fascia (see Fig. 1.23) and its associated raphe (which also functions as an attachment for the multifidus), the sacrotuberous ligament, and the lateral crest of the sacrum and coccygeal vertebrae. Its appendicular attachment involves the iliotibial band and the gluteal tuberosity of the femur. This muscle, through its attachment to the raphe of the thoracolumbar fascia, is coupled to the ipsilateral multifidus muscle and to the contralateral latissimus dorsi muscle (Vleeming et al 1995b). Electromyographic data and results from color Doppler studies support the role of the gluteus maximus, multifidus, and biceps femoris in trunk extension (Clark et al 2002, van Wingerden et al 2004). Thus, through its attachments to the ligaments and fascia of the SIJ, the gluteus maximus muscle can become a contributing force to the self-bracing mechanism of the pelvis (Snijders et al 1993).

Biceps femoris muscle (long head)

In many individuals, the long head of the biceps femoris muscle reaches over the posterior surface of the ischial tuberosity to attach to the sacrotuberous ligament (Vleeming et al 1989a). Its inferior attachment is to the lateral aspect of the fibular head, to the lateral condyle of the tibia, and to a sheet of fascia covering the lateral aspect of the leg. This muscle represents a continuum from the SI ligaments to the fibula and investing fascia of the leg. During gait, electromyographic activity of the biceps femoris is most prominent at heel strike (Ericson et al 1986). Contraction of the biceps femoris, along with extending the thigh, will pull the sacrum against the ilium, compressing and stabilizing the SIJ. Thus, at heel strike, this self-bracing mechanism in the pelvis can best assist in stabilizing the SIJ during the force transfer from spine to lower extremity (Vleeming et al 1989a).

Piriformis muscle

Inside the pelvic basin, another extremity muscle, the piriformis, influences the integrity of the SIJ. Proximally, the piriformis muscle attaches to the sacrum, the sacrotuberous ligament, the margin of the greater sciatic foramen, and the medial edge of the SIJ capsule. Distally, the muscle reaches through the greater sciatic foramen to attach to the greater trochanter of the femur. Contraction of the piriformis, besides laterally rotating the thigh and stabilizing the head of the femur in the acetabulum, also places tension on the SIJ capsule, pulling the sacrum against the ilium and thereby contributing to the self-bracing mechanism (Vleeming et al 1989a).

Summary of the muscular and ligamentous structures

The ligamentous stocking of the lumbar spine and the SIJ capsule fuse to the anterior surface of the thoracolumbar fascia. This large sheet of fascia and these lumbosacral ligaments serve as attachment sites for the major prime movers and stabilizing muscles of the spine. Activation of these muscles helps to tighten the connective tissue support structures, stabilizing the lumbosacral spine, and thereby contributing to a mechanism that has been referred to as self-bracing (Snijders et al 1993). The multifidus, gluteus maximus, and biceps femoris muscles play major roles, whereas minor contributions most likely arise in the latissimus dorsi and piriformis muscles. This arrangement of muscles and fascia facilitates the transfer of energy, generated by movement of the upper extremities, through the spine and into the lower extremities. The close coupling of these extremity and back muscles through the thoracolumbar fascia and its attachments to the ligamentous stocking of the spine, allow the motion in the upper limbs to assist in rotation of the trunk and movement of the lower extremities in gait, creating an integrated system (Vleeming et al 1995a).

Innervation of the lumbosacral region

The ligaments of the lumbosacral region are innervated predominantly with small-caliber primary afferent fibers and sympathetic fibers, carried by branches of the dorsal rami of lumbar and sacral spinal nerve roots and the lower portion of the sympathetic trunk. The primary afferent fibers are typical of those involved with the detection of nociception and the initiation of inflammatory processes; they have been termed 'primary afferent nociceptors' (reviewed in Levine et al 1993). The nerve supply to the lumbosacral ligaments plays a key role in the integrity of this region. There are three separate sources of innervation to the tissue of the lumbosacral region: the dorsal rami of the spinal nerves, the sinu vertebral nerve or recurrent meningeal nerve (a branch of the spinal nerve), and the somatosympathetic nerves derived from the sympathetic trunk and its communicating rami (Bogduk 1983, Groen et al 1990, Imai et al 1995, Jinkins et al 1989, Stilwell 1956). Each nerve supply covers a different area of tissue and, based on its distribution, creates a different pattern of pain perception when irritated.

Spinal nerve roots and spinal nerves

The lumbosacral spinal cord gives rise to numerous nerve rootlets from its dorsolateral and ventrolateral sulci. In the subarachnoid space of the vertebral canal, between five and seven dorsal rootlets from each lumbar segment bundle together to form a dorsal spinal nerve root, which joins with a similarly derived ventral spinal nerve root (de Peretti et al 1989). These nerve roots descend in the vertebral canal, exiting at each intervertebral foramen. At the level of the foramen, a complex relationship occurs. The nerve roots enter a funnel-shaped lateral recess of the spinal canal that narrows to form the lumbar nerve root canal (Firooznia et al 1993). The distal end of the root canal is the intervertebral foramen. The walls of the nerve root canal are composed of the pedicle and pars interarticularis of the vertebra, the ligamentum flavum, and the lateral aspect of the intervertebral disc (Bose & Balasubramanian 1984). From L1 to S1, the obliquity of the canals and their length increase (Bose & Balasubramanian 1984). As the nerve root enters this canal, it is enveloped by a sheath of spinal dura termed the 'epineurium.' In the canal, the nerve root is deflected laterally around the pedicle and over the surface of the intervertebral disc. The dorsal root ganglion is located at the point where the root passes around the pedicle and can leave an impression in the bony structure of the pedicle (de Peretti et al 1989). The dorsal root ganglion contains the primary afferent cell bodies; distal to this structure, the dorsal and ventral roots fuse to form the spinal nerve and the dural layer seals to the spinal nerve. In the lumbar region, as the spinal nerves leave their canals, they are attached to the foramen by several fibrous expansions of the canal wall (de Peretti et al 1989). As the nerve root traverses the canal and foramen, it is at risk from several structures: the pedicles and intervertebral discs (Hasegawa et al 1995, Hasue et al 1983), the ligamentum flavum (Yoshida et al 1992), the capsule of the facet joint (Kirkaldy-Willis 1984), and the foramenal ligaments (Golub & Silverman 1969, Nowicki & Haughton 1992).

In addition, the intervertebral canal transmits branches of the spinal artery into the spinal canal along with veins draining the epidural plexus and associated lymphatic vessels (Garfin et al 1995, Nohara et al 1991, Olmarker et al 1989, Rydevik 1992, Rydevik et al 1984, Sato et al 1994). Venous congestion, arteriovenous malformation, and epidural hematoma have all been demonstrated to mimic disc herniation or lumbar spinal stenosis (Hanley et al 1994, LaBan et al 2001, Parke 1991). Whether by mechanical compression or fluid congestion, the traumatized lumbosacral nerve roots experience edema and ischemia, which lead to inflammatory and fibrotic alterations in the neural tissue with concomitant loss of motor function, paresthesia, and hypesthesia (Garfin et al 1995, Olmarker et al 1989, Rydevik 1992, Rydevik et al 1984, Sato et al 1994). Finally, an additional nonmechanical method for irritating neural tissue in the foraminal area appears to involve the release of nuclear fluids containing such proinflammatory compounds as the proteoglycans and tumor necrosis factor-α from a leaky disc (Cuellar et al 2004, Olmarker & Larsson 1998, Olmarker & Myers 1998, Olmarker et al 1993, 1995).

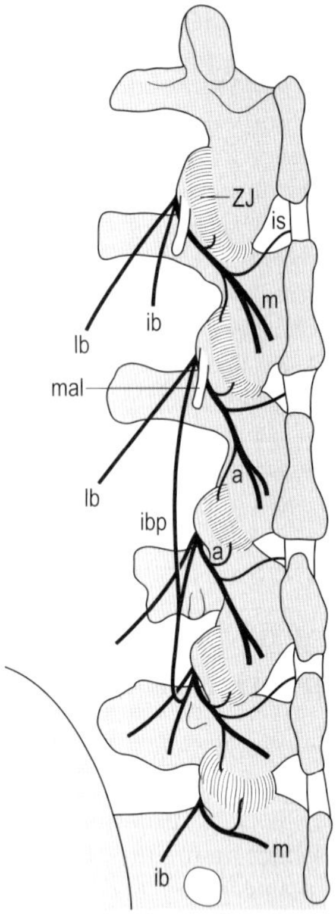

Fig. 1.24 Dorsal view of the lumbar spine showing the three major branches of the dorsal ramus. a, articular twigs from medial branch; ib, intermediate branch; ibp, intermediate branch plexus; is, interspinous twig from medial branch; lb, lateral branch; m, medial branch; mal, mamillio-accessory ligament; ZJ, zygoapophyseal joint. (Reproduced from Bogduk 1983.)

Lumbosacral dorsal rami

The dorsal ramus leaves the spinal nerve as the nerve exits the lumbar intervertebral canals. As this ramus wraps around the facet joint directly below, it divides into several main branches: the lateral branch, which innervates the lateral fascial compartment containing the iliocostalis muscle; the intermediate branch, which innervates the intermediate fascial compartment containing the longissimus muscle; and several medial branches, which innervate the medial fascial compartment containing the multifidus muscle, as well as the ligaments and intrinsic muscles of the lumbar and sacral vertebrae (Fig. 1.24) (Bogduk 1983). Specifically, the medial compartment contains the multifidus, interspinalis, and intertransversarii medialis muscles; it also contains skeletal elements such as the interspinous ligament, the facet joints, and the ligament flavum. Inferiorly, the dorsal and possibly ventral rami of L5 and of the sacral roots provide innervation of the SIJ capsule (Ikeda 1991). Recent studies have confirmed the innervation of the joint from dorsal rami, but not from branches of the ventral rami (Fortin et al 1999a, Grob et al 1995, Willard et al 1998). Irritation of the small-caliber, primary afferent fibers of the dorsal ramus innervating these tissue results in the perception of pain. This perception is usually a sharp, burning pain that is similar to spinal root pain and can refer to the area supplied by the corresponding ventral ramus, thus mimicking sciatica. As the dorsal ramus also innervates muscle groups in the back, compression or damage to this nerve can present with signs of denervation weakness, as well as with pain. Several descriptions of the dorsal ramus syndrome exist (Bogduk 1980b, Gonzalez-Darder 1989, Helbig & Lee 1988, Shao et al 1996, Sihvonen & Partanen 1990).

Sinu vertebral or recurrent meningeal nerves

Distal to the dorsal root ganglion, but prior to the division into dorsal and ventral rami, the spinal nerve gives off a small branch that recurs into the intervertebral foramen to reach the vertebral canal (Pedersen et al 1956b; Fig. 1.25). This small branch is termed the 'sinu vertebral' or 'recurrent meningeal' nerve. The terminal branches of this nerve supply the posterior longitudinal ligament, the periosteum on the posterior aspect of the vertebral body, the outer layers of the intervertebral discs, and the anterior surface of the spinal dura (Bogduk 1983, Groen et al 1990, Pedersen et al 1956a, Stilwell 1956, for a review see Jinkins et al 1989 or Jinkins 1993). In an elegant study of the sinu vertebral nerve Groen et al (1990) demonstrated that this nerve can travel up and/or down the vertebral canal at least two or three segments from the point of entry (Fig. 1.25, parts 1–5). In addition, it can cross the midline to innervate tissue on the contralateral side (Fig. 1.25, parts 6a–c). Notably, some sinu vertebral fibers cross the vertebral canal and subsequently pass outward through the contralateral intervertebral foramina (Fig. 1.25, part 6c). Microscopic dissection of the dorsal root ganglion region in the lumbar spine has demonstrated that the L1 and L2 roots have a complex array consisting of multiple branches of the sinu vertebral nerve re-entering the intervertebral foramen, whereas the lower lumbar vertebrae had only a few branches of the nerve at each level (Raoul et al 2003).

Small-caliber, primary afferent nociceptors – as well as sympathetic fibers – appear to be contained within the sinu vertebral nerve. Sympathetic fibers have been suggested by staining techniques (Groen et al 1990, Raoul et al 2003) whereas primary afferent nociceptors have been detected by electrophysiology (Sekine et al 2001). Based on this pattern of innervation, irritation of the small-caliber, primary afferent fibers in the sinu vertebral nerve can refer pain several segments up or down the spinal cord, as well as referring pain to the contralateral side of the body. In addition, very slight movements of any obstacle in the vertebral canal or intervertebral foramina could irritate sinu vertebral fibers from either or both of the left or right sides of the body. This arrangement also offers a possible explanation for the apparent shifting of pain presentation patterns from side to side in a given patient. Finally, the sinu vertebral nerve does not supply any skeletal muscle or skin, so compression or other damage to

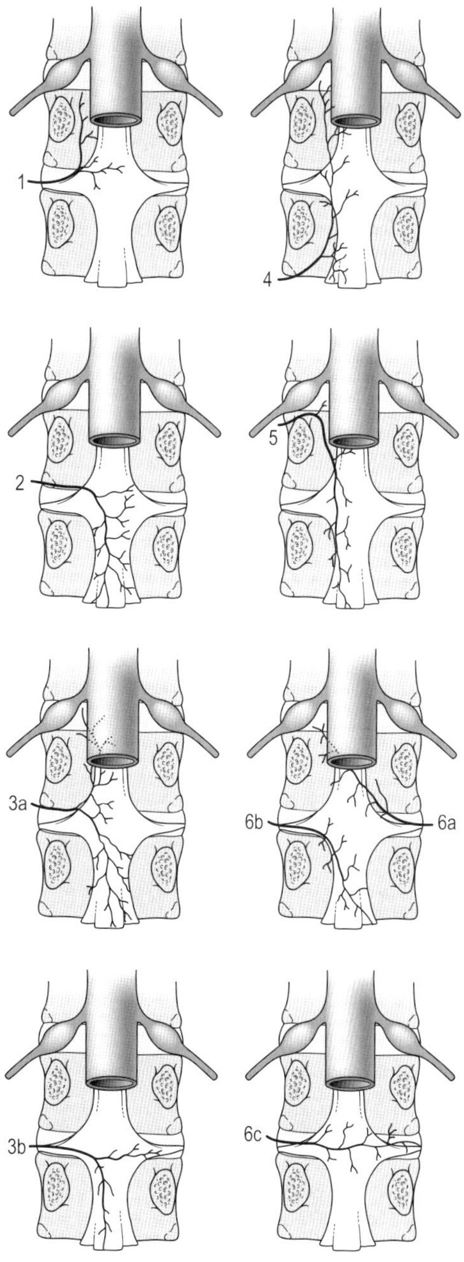

Fig. 1.25 The sinu vertebral nerve. The eight diagrams represent variations in the distribution of the sinu vertebral nerve. (Reproduced from Groen et al 1990.)

this nerve alone does not present with the signs of denervation weakness or cutaneous analgesia.

Somatosympathetic nerves

No somatic nerves (direct branches of the dorsal or ventral rami or spinal nerves) reach the anterior aspect of the vertebral bodies. However, this area is richly supplied by sensory fibers traveling in branches of the sympathetic trunk (Bogduk 1983, Groen et al 1990, Jinkins et al 1989, Stilwell 1956). These small-caliber, primary afferent nociceptors wrap around the anterior longitudinal ligament and the periosteum on the anterior aspect of the vertebral body and penetrate into the outer layers of the intervertebral discs (Fig. 1.26). To return to the spinal cord these sensory fibers follow the sympathetic trunk and appear to use white rami when gaining access to the spinal nerve and dorsal root ganglia. Therefore sensory fibers entering the trunk below L2 pass must superiorly in the trunk to reach the L1–L2 white rami located at the thoracolumbar junction (Jinkins et al 1989). Thus, noxious stimuli in the lower lumbar and sacral levels will ascend in the sympathetic trunk, presenting to the spinal cord at the thoracolumbar junction (the region of the lowest white rami). This circuitous route results in referral of pain and subsequent facilitation of spinal segments in the lower thoracic and upper lumbar region from dysfunction of lumbosacral and pelvic structures.

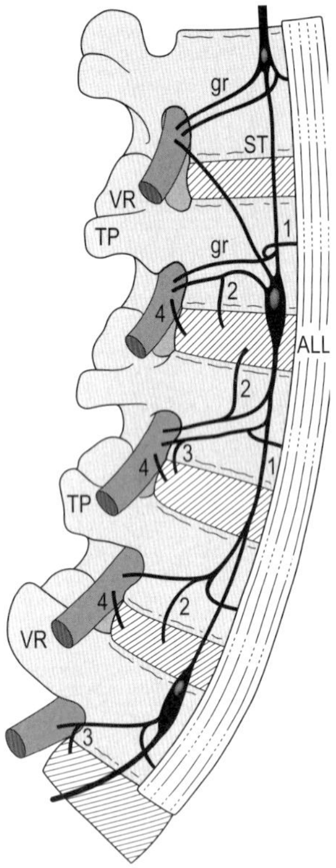

Fig. 1.26 Side view of the lumbar spine illustrating the somatosympathetic nerve. The sympathetic trunk communicates with the ventral ramus (VR) through gray rami (gr). Small branches (1) from the sympathetic trunk provide sympathetic efferent and primary afferent fibers to the anterior longitudinal ligament (ALL). Small branches (2 and 3) from the gray rami and ventral ramus (4) reach the intervertebral disc. TP, transverse process. (Reproduced from Bogduk 1983.)

Noxious stimuli activating somatosympathetic fibers result in what has been described as a diffuse, dense, boring pain that refers to the zones of Head in the thoracolumbar region (Jinkins et al 1989). In a population chosen because the individuals were experiencing pain, individuals with vertebral lesions involving the anterior territory (anterior longitudinal ligament) generally described the pain as deep, dense, and hard to localize. The referral zones involved upper lumbar segments along the flank of the body extending downward onto the thigh. This pattern was present even in individuals with anterior disc lesions as low as L5. The somatosympathetic pattern of pain was in contrast to that in patients suffering pain and having posterior lesions that irritated axons in the sinu vertebral nerve or dorsal ramus. The pain pattern in these latter patients of Jinkins was better related to the segment of injury and was of a sharp or burning quality. As with the sinu vertebral nerve, the somatosympathetic axons do not supply any skeletal muscle or skin, so damage to these nerves alone will not present with signs of denervation weakness or cutaneous analgesia.

Innervation of specific lumbosacral structures

The general innervation patterns described in the previous section demonstrate that most structures in the lumbosacral region receive a generous nerve supply. However, a critical question involves the exact types of axons and terminals found in specific connective tissues. The types of nerve fiber present will influence the function of the tissue as well as its susceptibility to neurogenic inflammatory processes (Basbaum & Levine 1991, Levine et al 1993, Schaible & Grubb 1993). There are three general innervation patterns for tissue other than skeletal muscle: (1) large, myelinated sensory axons with encapsulated endings involved with discriminative touch and proprioception; (2) small, lightly myelinated or unmyelinated sensory axons with naked nerve endings involved in nociception; and (3) small, lightly myelinated efferent axons involved in the autonomic nervous system. Of the latter two types of axon, the small primary afferent axons (nociceptors) often contain neuropeptides such as substance P, calcitonin gene-related polypeptide, or somatostatin. Axons associated with the autonomic nervous system often contain norepinephrine (which can be indicated by the presence of tyrosine hydroxylase) and neuropeptide Y. Both small, primary afferent fibers and sympathetic fibers play critical roles in the induction and maintenance of neurogenic inflammatory processes (Basbaum & Levine 1991, Levine et al 1993).

Neural arch ligaments

The use of immunohistochemical procedures to label and identify axons found in connective tissue has allowed the characterization of the innervation of neural arch ligaments. These ligaments are serviced by the medial branch of the dorsal ramus. Small-caliber axons from this nerve have been detected in the supraspinous ligament and interspinous ligament (Jiang et al 1995, Rhalmi et al 1993) and ligamentum flavum (Rhalmi et al 1993), these fibers being identified with an antibody for neurofilament protein, which is a nonspecific marker for the neural process. Electrical stimulation of the lumbar supraspinous ligament in the cat initiated spinal reflexes that involved electromyographically recorded activity bilaterally in the surrounding paraspinal muscle. This activity was seen most intensely in the segment below the stimulation, but was also present at as far away as two levels above or below the stimulation (Stubbs et al 1998). It is suggested by the authors that these are protective reflexes and, if dysfunctional, that they might contribute to low back pain.

The innervation of the ligamentum flavum and its potential role in the genesis of low back pain is of special note. Nerve fibers have been detected in sections of the flaval ligament stained with protein S100, a calcium-binding protein that is not entirely specific for neural tissue (Viejo-Fuertes et al 1998). Small-caliber sensory nerve fibers immunoreactive for protein gene product 9.5 (a pan-neuronal marker) were detected in a sample of flaval ligaments taken from patients with low back pain at surgery (Bucknill et al 2002). A subset of these fibers also stained immunopositive for the voltage-gated sodium channel SNS/PN3, a tetrodotoxin-resistant channel found particularly in primary afferent nociceptors (Sangameswaran et al 1996). Several previous studies have failed to demonstrate any detectable innervation of the ligamentum flavum by small primary afferent nociceptors and the study by Bucknill et al used tissue from patients suffering from low back pain. Thus, it is possible that the normal ligament has a paucity of sensory fibers that could increase in distribution in pathological conditions.

Small, primary afferent fibers have also been found in the thoracolumbar fascia (Rhalmi et al 1993, Yahia et al 1992). Frequently, the small axons were seen to leave the areas of the blood vessels and course through the matrix of the surrounding connective tissue. Small-caliber fibers containing substance P, suggesting a role in nociception, have been demonstrated in the supraspinous ligament (El-Bohy et al 1988). Larger-caliber fibers in the supraspinous and interspinous ligaments, reactive for neurofilament protein, were seen associated with Pacinian and Ruffini endings (Jiang et al 1995), suggesting a role in proprioception. In addition, fibers positive for tyrosine hydroxylase and neuropeptide Y, suggesting that they are sympathetic axons, have been described in the interspinous ligaments (Ahmed et al 1993). Electrophysiologic recordings from neural processes in the supraspinous and interspinous ligaments and in the ligamentum flavum have been described (Yamashita et al 1990) and, based on their activation thresholds and conduction velocities, both proprioceptive and nociceptive axons were present. These results collectively demonstrate the presence of both primary afferent proprioceptors and nociceptors and efferent sympathetic axons in the neural arch ligaments of the lumbar spine.

Articular capsule ligaments

Lumbar facet joints have long been thought to represent a source of low back pain (Helbig & Lee 1988, Mooney & Robertson 1976); recent facet injection studies have strongly supported this contention (Dreyfuss et al 1997, Kaplan et al 1998, Manchikanti et al 2004, Schwarzer et al 1994). The facet joint is innervated by branches from the medial divisions of the dorsal rami above and below the joint (Bogduk & Long 1979). This observation suggests that inflammatory or degenerative diseases of any facet joint will activate multiple segments in the spinal cord. Recent studies demonstrate an even broader range of facet innervation (Ohtori et al 2003). Fluorogold (a retrogradely transported neuronal marker) was injected into the L5–L6 facet of a rat, labeled neurons were present in the dorsal root ganglia from T13–L6; a wider range of innervation than would be expected from conventional models of joint innervation.

Neurophysiologic studies of the lumbar facet joints of rabbits have demonstrated the presence of both high-threshold, slow-conducting fibers and low-threshold, fast-conducting fibers (Avramov et al 1992, Cavanaugh et al 1997, McLain 1994, Yamashita et al 1990). The former represent potential nociceptive axons and are more prevalent in the joint capsule, whereas the latter are probably proprioceptive axons and are found in larger numbers in the surrounding muscle (Cavanaugh et al 1997; for reviews of joint innervation and nociception, see Cavanaugh et al 1996, Wyke 1967, 1976). Electrophysiologic recordings of primary afferent fibers from joints under varying loads also demonstrate the presence of proprioceptive and nociceptive components (Avramov et al 1992). Encapsulated nerve endings, suggestive of proprioceptors, have been observed histologically in facet joint capsules (Jackson et al 1966, McLain 1994). The presence of small-caliber, primary afferent fibers containing sensory neuropeptides, such as substance P and calcitonin gene-related polypeptide, in the joint capsule and synovial plica have also been confirmed in several anatomical studies (Ahmed et al 1993, Beaman et al 1993, El-Bohy et al 1988, Suseki et al 1996). Many of these primary afferent fibers are present in the connective tissue of the joint capsule, separate from the vasculature (Ahmed et al 1993). In addition, fibers containing tyrosine hydroxylase and neuropeptide-Y – markers for sympathetic axons – have been reported in the joint capsule; however, these axons remain close to the vasculature (Ahmed et al 1993). The presence of afferent neurons in the dorsal root ganglia that innervate the lumbar facet joints demonstrates the presence of brain-derived neurotrophic factor and vanilloid receptor subtype 1 immunoreactivity, strongly suggesting that these neurons are primary afferent nociceptors (Ohtori et al 2003). Finally, the presence of small-caliber, primary afferent nociceptors in the ligamentum flavum, facet joint capsule, intervertebral disc, and spinal roots has been strongly suggested by the demonstration that many of these fibers express the SNS/PN3 and NAN/SNS2 sodium channel transcripts (Bucknill et al 2002); these channel forms are fairly specific to small dorsal root ganglion cells of the nociceptive type (Waxman 1999).

Facet joints contain proinflammatory cells such as monocytes and reactive fibroblasts – cells positive for CD11 antigens (Konttinen et al 1990b). When an inflammatory substance, such as carrageenan, is injected into these joints, it produces sensitized primary afferent fibers (increased firing rates) and recruits 'silent nociceptors,' the smallest of the primary afferent fibers and those typically associated with pain (Ozaktay et al 1994). The presence of small-caliber, primary afferent fibers in the capsule of the facet joints, responding to inflammatory challenge, supports the contention that dysfunction of these joints is a source of low back pain (Bernard & Kirkaldy-Willis 1987, Carette et al 1991, Mooney & Robertson 1976). This is consistent with the relief of pain experienced by some patients following anesthetization of the lumbar facet joints (Schwarzer et al 1994).

Plasticity of phenotype can be a significant feature in the development of a facet pain syndrome. The bone and articular cartilage of normal human facet joints contains small-caliber fibers, positive for the neuropeptide substance P (Beaman et al 1993) and calcitonin gene-related polypeptide (CGRP; Ashton et al 1992), but these have been shown to be present only in very low numbers. However, neuropeptide-containing axons were present in increased quantity in specimens that were undergoing degenerative diseases involving the facet joints. These fibers were found in erosion channels accompanying the vasculature deep into the bone underlying the articular surface. Such observations suggest that normal facet joints can be relatively refractive to pain as the result of a limited supply of small-caliber fibers under pressure-bearing surfaces, and that degenerative joints become painful because of an increase in nociceptive fibers associated with pressure-bearing surfaces. The possible plasticity of the facet joint innervation in noxious situations was further supported by studies looking at the phenotypic stability of joint afferent fibers (Ohtori et al 2001). Exposure of rat facet joints to Freund's adjuvant – a proinflammatory substance – resulted in the expression of CGRP in large primary afferent axons that normally would not contain this marker for nociceptive fibers. A similar study demonstrated that joint inflammation can induce the expression of brain-derived neurotrophic factor, another marker for primary afferent nociceptors, in large afferent fibers (Ohtori et al 2002).

The projection of afferent fibers from the lumbar facets to the spinal cord has been investigated in a series of very intriguing studies (Sameda et al 2001, Suseki et al 1996, 1997). Using the retrograde transport of fluorescent dyes, it was found that the L5–L6 facet joint in the rat (*note*: rats have six lumbar vertebrae) receives primary afferent fibers from neurons located in the L1–L6 dorsal root ganglion, demonstrating the potentially very wide ranging influence the facet joint has on the spinal cord (up to six segments or more). Some, but not all, of these axons travel in the sympathetic trunk and communicating rami to reach the joint, thus supporting the contention that the trunk contains sensory fibers and can be a source of pain. Finally, quite remarkably, up to 3–4% of these dorsal root ganglion neurons have a bifurcated axon, one portion going to the facet joint and the second portion of the axon coursing down the lower extremity in the sciatic nerve, thus suggesting a possible source of referred pain from the facet joint to the lower extremity.

Vertebral body ligaments and intervertebral discs

An extensive nerve plexus is present in the posterior and anterior longitudinal ligaments of the lumbar region (Bogduk 1983, Cavanaugh et al 1995, Groen et al 1988, 1990, Imai et al 1995, Jackson et al 1966, Kojima et al 1990a, 1990b, Korkala et al 1985, Pedersen et al 1956b, Pionchon et al 1986, Stilwell 1956, von During et al 1995). Despite the density of small-caliber fibers present along these ligaments, very few large fibers with encapsulate endings have been demonstrated to date (Cavanaugh et al 1995, Jackson et al 1966). Small primary afferent axons, containing neuropeptides, have been identified in the posterior longitudinal ligament and the peripheral portion of the annulus fibrosus (Imai et al 1995, Konttinen et al 1990a, Korkala et al 1985) and substance P has been detected in the small fibers of anterior longitudinal ligament samples from degenerate lumbar discs (Coppes et al 1997). Similar distribution of neuropeptide-containing axons has been documented in the rabbit (Kallakuri et al 1998). Electrophysiological recordings have been taken from fibers arising in the posterior longitudinal ligament in the cat (Sekine et al 2001). Such fibers responded to mechanical stimuli and their conduction velocity was in the group III (Aδ-fiber) and group IV (C-fiber) range. As many of these axons travel in the sinu vertebral nerve, these observations support the theory that this nerve is capable of nociception (Korkala et al 1985). Axons positive for tyrosine hydroxylase and neuropeptide Y – suggesting that they are sympathetic axons – have also been detected in the posterior longitudinal ligament (Imai et al 1995), the ventral dura, the periosteum of the vertebral body, the intervertebral disc, and the vertebral body, where they reach into the marrow cavities (Ahmed et al 1993).

Imai and colleagues (1995) have described a dual plexus of fibers in the rat posterior longitudinal ligament. The superficial plexus ascends and descends along the margins of the ligament whereas the deep plexus is present only over the intervertebral segments of the ligament and reaches inward to serve the outer layers of the annulus fibrosus. Axons containing CGRP, suggesting nociceptive sensory functions, are present in both plexuses, whereas axons containing tyrosine hydroxylase, suggesting sympathetic activity, are present only in the superficial plexus.

Based on the density of small-caliber fiber (nociceptive) innervation for the longitudinal ligaments, one would expect that the commonly observed large disc and osteophyte distortions present in these ligaments would be painful. This is, however, not often the case, as these large protrusions are frequently 'clinically silent' when detected in imaging studies. An explanation of this conundrum might lie in the observation that the degree of pain perceived from injury of the spinal ligaments is related to the speed of the injury and not to its extent; thus a slow-growing distortion could give the neural plexus ample time to accommodate and not trigger afferent barrages on nociceptive afferent fibers. Support for this concept comes from the observation that the degree of nerve injury in experimental compression neuropathies is proportional to the speed of onset of the compressive force (Olmarker et al 1990).

The intervertebral discs are innervated by fibers from an elaborate plexus supplied by the sinu vertebral nerve on the posterior longitudinal ligament and the somatosympathetic nerve on the anterior longitudinal ligament (Antonacci et al 1998, Bogduk 1983, Bogduk et al 1981, Groen et al 1990, Jinkins 1993, Jinkins et al 1989, Stilwell 1956). In a normal, healthy disc, branches from this plexus penetrate through the outer one-third to reach to the middle third of the annulus fibrosus (Freemont et al 1997). These branches are primarily composed of small-caliber fibers having unencapsulated endings (Jackson et al 1966). Many of these fibers contain neuropeptides such as substance P and CGRP, as demonstrated through immunohistochemical staining of disc tissue from rats (Ahmed et al 1993, von During et al 1995), rabbits (Cavanaugh et al 1995), and humans (Konttinen et al 1990a). Cell bodies of these fibers in the dorsal root ganglia have been demonstrated to express brain-derived neurotrophic factor and the vanilloid receptor VR1, both markers of small nociceptive neurons (Ohtori et al 2003). There is no evidence of any of these nociceptive fibers innervating the nucleus pulposus in the central portion of the disc. The recent findings demonstrating neuropeptides in the outer one-third of the annulus support a sensory role for the sinu vertebral–somatosympathetic plexus present in the periosteum and ligaments surrounding the vertebral column.

The widespread and anastomotic nature of the plexus surrounding the lumbar vertebral column is best illustrated by its projection back to the spinal cord through the dorsal root ganglia. As previously noted, studies using a retrogradely transported neuronal marker, injected in the most lateral aspect of the L5–L6 disc in a rat was found to be present in neurons bilaterally in the dorsal root ganglia from T12 to L6 (Aoki et al 2004c; *note*: rats have 13 thoracic vertebrae and 6 lumbars). This widespread representation has also been seen in the contributions of the sinu vertebral and somatosympathetic system to the spinal cord. The sinu vertebral nerve contributions appeared to be more restricted in distribution and segmentally arranged; conversely the afferent fibers of the somatosympathetic system (paravertebral sympathetic trunk) broadly spread over seven spinal segments when entering the spinal cord (Ohtori et al 1999). This widespread distribution of lumbar disc input to the spinal cord, and its bilateral nature, can explain the difficulties encountered in localizing the exact source of vertebral pain in a patient. Pain-generating lesions can easily be several segments above or below, as well as on the contralateral side to the patient's perception of the pain.

Further confusion in interpreting pain patterns can arise as a result of the plastic changes in the small-fiber system that occur consequent to injury. In degenerate disc material, taken at surgery, the small-caliber fibers have expanded their territory into the inner third of the annulus fibrosus (Freemont et al 1997) and increased their presence in the associated dorsal root ganglia (Aoki et al 2004a, 2004b). The expansion in axonal territory is related to the growth of collateral axonal branches associated with the invasion of vascular buds. Interestingly, the growing vascular trees secreted nerve growth factor and the expanding collaterals expressed the receptors for nerve growth factor (Freemont et al 2002). The increase in nociceptor presence involved an increase in the number of neurons that produced CGRP in the dorsal root ganglia, as well as an increase in the expression of Schwann cell markers in the disrupted disc material (Johnson et al 2001). As these neurons are not known to divide, the increase in number most likely developed from a process termed 'phenotypic modulation.' The convergence of Aβ-fibers to peptide-producing sensory neurons similar to C-fibers in their ability to excite the spinal cord has been described in other inflammatory pain situations (Neumann et al 1996) as well as in rat models of inflammatory lumbar facet joints (Ohtori et al 2001, 2002).

The vertebral plexus of nerves raises the problem of why discography is generally a nonpainful procedure in normal individuals, but a painful one in patients with degenerative discs. It is possible that this is due to the distance separating the nuclear material in the normal individual from the nerve endings in the outer portion of the disc. However, an additional consideration could be that most of the disc fibers are 'silent nociceptors,' that is, they are normally unexcitable even by some noxious stimuli. If provoked by prolonged exposure to proinflammatory chemical insult, they can become active and have a threshold of activation well within the range of non-noxious stimuli. This concept is supported by the observation that autologous material from the nucleus pulposus is proinflammatory and an irritant to nerve endings (Aoki et al 2002, McCarron et al 1987, Olmarker et al 1993, 1995, Saal 1995, Saal et al 1990). Thus discographic materials delivered to the center of a normal disc for a temporary period of time would not be expected to activate the normally quite silent nociceptors. The same material delivered to a degenerative disc might be reaching and activating previously sensitized primary afferent nociceptors.

Sacral region ligaments

Although the SIJ has long been thought to be involved in low back pain (Beal 1982, Bernard & Kirkaldy-Willis 1987, Bogduk 1995, Borenstein 1996, Daum 1995, Fortin et al 1994a, 1994b, 1999a, Kirkaldy-Willis 1992, Schwarzer et al 1995, Wyke 1976), very few studies have examined its innervation. Ikeda reports that the anterior superior aspect of the joint receives twigs from spinal nerve L5, and the inferior anterior aspect of the joint is supplied by sacral spinal nerve S2 and other sacral nerves (Ikeda 1991). The posterior superior aspect of the joint is supplied by lateral branches from the fifth lumbar dorsal ramus and the inferior posterior aspect from a plexus of lateral branches from the sacral dorsal rami. In similar studies, Grob et al (1995) and Willard et al (1998) identified fine branches from the dorsal rami S1–S4 reaching the joint, but were unable to confirm any innervation from the ventral rami.

The posterior innervation of the SIJ is the only one consistently seen by investigators. These fibers arise from the lateral arcades of the dorsal sacral plexus located on the floor of the sacral gutter and coursing in between the sacroiliac ligaments (Fig. 1.27). A recent study using gross dissection and fluoroscopic imaging of small metal wires placed on the lateral branches of the dorsal sacral plexus has demonstrated small twigs entering the SIJ along its medial and inferior boundaries (Fig. 1.28; Yin et al 2003).

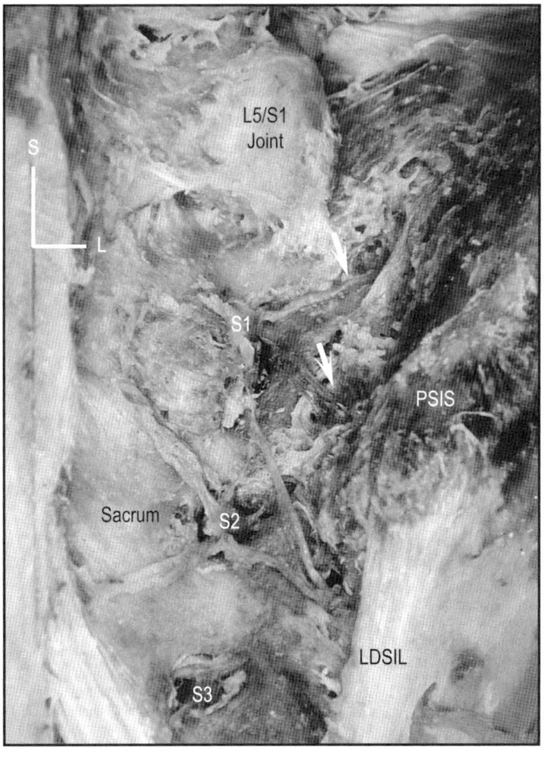

Fig. 1.27 A dorsal view of the dorsal sacral rami coursing on the fused lamina of the sacrum. As the rami exit the sacral foramina, they divide, giving off medially and laterally directed fibers. The medial fibers innervate the multifidus muscle whereas the lateral branches form an arcade. From the arcade, laterally directed branches pass under or through the long dorsal sacroiliac ligament (LDSIL), enter the sacrotuberous ligament and eventually become cutaneous on the buttock. Small, laterally oriented twigs form the arcade (arrows) and weave through the short sacroiliac ligaments to reach the sacroiliac joint directly deep to the posterior superior iliac spine (PSIS).

The articular nerves reach the joint capsule and invade the surrounding ligaments. Thick myelinated fibers, thin lightly myelinated fibers, and unmyelinated fibers are all present in the SI branches (Grob et al 1995). Many axons in the nerves to the SIJ were approximately 0.2–2.5 μm in diameter, placing them well within the range of the group IV (C-fibers) and possibly within the smaller end of the group III (A-delta) fiber range (Ikeda 1991). Electrophysiological recordings for SIJ axons in the cat reveal that most fibers are high-threshold, group III in nature (Sakamoto et al 2001). Axons of this size and with these physiologic properties are associated with nociception and most likely are involved in the perception of pain from the SIJ. However, these caliber axons are not likely to play a role in proprioception. Thus the role of the SIJ in the generation of low back pain seems well supported by these findings.

Neurogenic inflammation

The recent studies of the lumbosacral ligamentous structure using immunohistochemical techniques have provided evidence that much of the structure, if not the entire connective tissue stocking, receives a small-caliber, primary afferent fiber innervation. Not only are these sensory neurons organized to supply the spinal cord with nociceptive stimuli but they are also typical of the small afferent neural system (Prechtl & Powley 1990), that is, many of them are capable of secreting proinflammatory neuropeptides from their distal processes (Levine et al 1993). Irritation of these primary afferent nociceptor fibers and the subsequent release of such peptides as substance P and CGRP can result in the degranulation of mast cells and the release of histamine (Fig. 1.29). This biogenic amine promotes vasodilation, leukocyte recruitment, and proliferation, and can further irritate primary afferent fibers, initiating the release of more substance P (Basbaum & Levine 1991, Julius & Basbaum 2001). In addition, substance P stimulates macrophages and monocytes to increase phagocytosis, to release proinflammatory compounds such as thromboxane and hydrogen peroxide, and to increase the production of cytokines such as interleukin-1 (Payan 1989, 1992). Thus a vicious cycle of events is begun, the

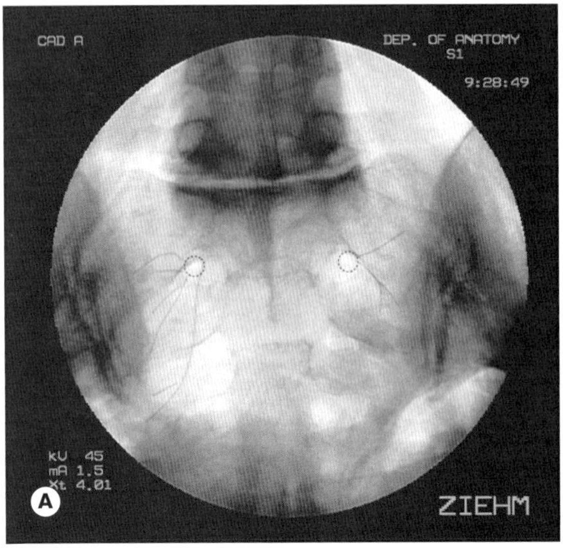

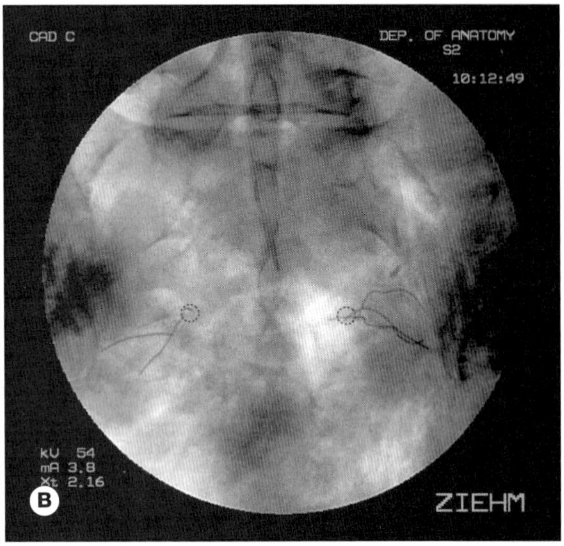

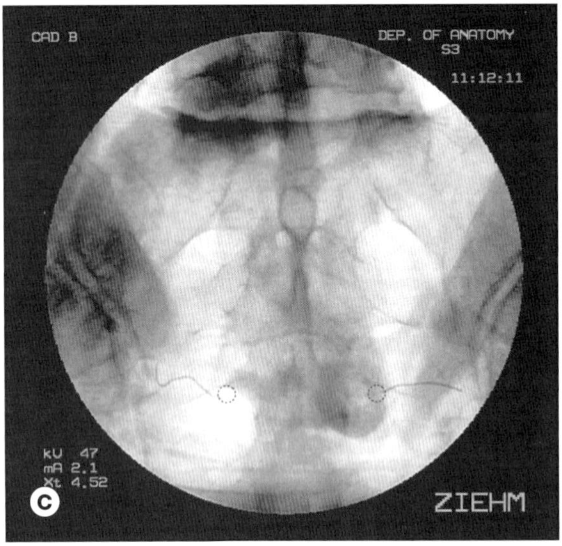

Fig. 1.28 Representative sacral lateral branch (LB) topographic fluoroscopic anatomy. Common reference in articular process (AP) imaging with superior endplate of S1 'square.' Dotted lines have been drawn, marking the bony boundary of the dorsal sacral foramina. Wires have been placed over LB nerves arising from the dorsal sacral foramina and seen entering the sacroiliac joint capsule. Each image demonstrates LB topography from a single representative cadaver. Note the variation in number and course of LB nerves. (A) S1 lateral branches. (B) S2 lateral branches. (C) S3 lateral branches. (Taken from Yin et al 2003.)

final product of this sequence being tissue inflammation and edema (Willard 2003). This cascade of events, involving neural–immune interactions, typifies the neurogenic inflammatory process and produces a condition of peripheral sensitization in the primary afferent nociceptors (Schaible et al 2005, Woolf 2004). Peripheral sensitization underlies the development of hyperalgesia around inflamed tissue.

Inflammation plays a large role in the destruction of tissue in the musculoskeletal system. Inflammatory cells are present in the synovial plica of lumbar facet joints (Igarashi et al 2004b, Konttinen et al 1990b) and in the nucleus pulposus of herniated disc material (Gronblad et al 1994, Iwabuchi et al 2001). In addition, the proteoglycans-rich fluid in the nucleus pulposus is inflammatory to nondisc tissue (Olmarker et al 1995, 2002). It has been shown that material from degenerate facet joints or intervertebral discs can initiate changes in the neurochemicals in the dorsal root ganglion of the lumbar nerves (Larsson et al 2005, Onda et al 2005). Thus the elements are present in the lumbosacral musculoskeletal system to facilitate chronic inflammatory processes (Weinstein 1991), leading to tissue degeneration and chronic pain syndromes.

Several observations also suggest that the population of sensory neurons innervating connective tissue is dynamic and can respond to changing states of the tissue. The thoracolumbar fascia in

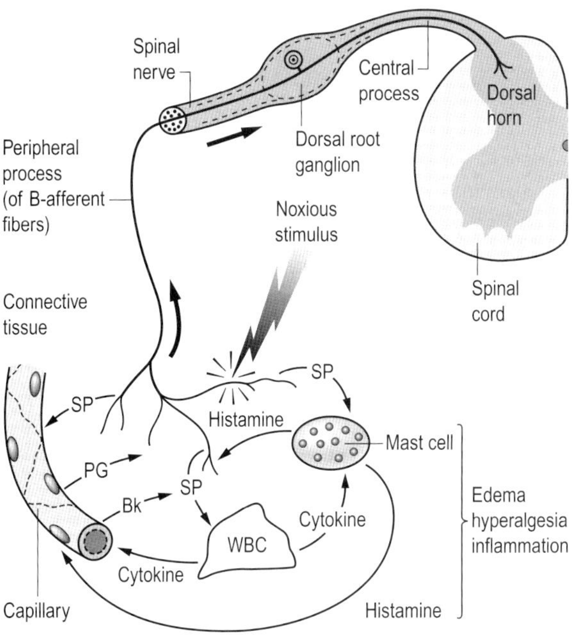

Fig. 1.29 The cascade effect of neurogenic inflammation. A primary afferent nociceptor, its central termination in the dorsal horn and its peripheral termination near a blood vessel in the local tissue, is shown. A noxious stimulus has irritated the terminal end of the primary afferent, causing it to depolarize. Action potentials are being sent to the central nervous system and neuropeptides (e.g. substance P, SP) are being released into the tissue surrounding the terminal. In response to the neuropeptides, mast cells degranulate, releasing histamine, and in response to this neuropeptide–histamine cocktail, blood vessels dilate, extravasating fluid and initiating edema and swelling. Prostaglandins (PG) and bradykinin (Bk) are released into the tissue. This chemical cocktail is chemoattractant for white blood cells (WBC), which then release cytokines [e.g. interleukin-1 (IL-1) and IL-6], furthering the inflammatory process. The chemical soup so created irritates the primary afferent nociceptor, thereby propagating the neurogenic inflammation. (Adapted from Willard 1995).

patients without back pain has both fibers with small, naked nerve endings and larger fibers with encapsulated endings (Pedersen et al 1956a, Yahia et al 1992), whereas patients who required surgery for treatment of low back pain were missing the myelinated fibers and encapsulated endings in the thoracolumbar fascia (Bednar et al 1995). Small, unmyelinated fibers with naked endings remained detectable in the fascia of the surgical cohort. From this study, it is impossible to say which happened first, the initiation of low back pain or the shift in sensory fiber population. However, studies of normal tissue that has been deafferented suggest that the loss of sensory innervation destabilizes the tissue, predisposing it to other damage such as degenerative disease processes (O'Connor et al 1985).

In addition to the primary afferent fibers, sympathetic axons have been detected in much of the connective tissue of the lumbosacral spine. A balanced interaction between these two neural systems is thought to be important for the maintenance of normal tissue texture and the normal trafficking of cells through the extracellular matrix of the tissue (Holzer 1988, Kidd et al 1992, Levine et al 1990). Abnormal activity in either or both of these systems, increasing the output of neuropeptides and catecholamines, has been associated with increased susceptibility to degenerative connective tissue diseases (Basbaum & Levine 1991, Garrett et al 1992, Kidd et al 1989, 1990, 1992, Lam & Ferrell 1991, Levine et al 1985a, 1985b, 1993). Thus the activity of the primary afferent nociceptors and sympathetic fiber systems represents an important consideration in maintenance of the integrity of the lumbosacral ligamentous structures.

Finally, evidence has accumulated suggesting that sympathetic fibers can activate, either directly or indirectly, sensitized primary afferent fibers (Kinnman et al 1997, Liu et al 1996, Roberts & Kramis 1990, Wang et al 2004). These findings raise the possibility that the sympathetic fiber is involved in either the genesis and/or the maintenance of chronic pain states in connective tissue of the lumbosacral spine.

Summary

1. This chapter has examined the anatomy and innervation of the ligamentous stocking that forms the lumbosacral connection. Although there are numerous regional ligaments in this stocking, their continuity with each other has been emphasized, thereby giving the structure a unitary function.
2. The ligamentous stocking supports the osseous elements of the lumbosacral spine. In turn, this stocking is anchored to the thoracolumbar fascia of the back. This large sheet of aponeurotic fascia serves as an attachment site for the major muscle groups of the spine, the abdomen, and the upper and lower extremities. Through these connections, the thoracolumbar fascia can

assist in the transfer of energy from the upper to the lower body, minimizing stress on the lumbosacral spine. It can also facilitate the upper body's ability to assist in lower body motion, forming the integrated system described by Vleeming et al (1995b).

3. Not surprisingly, the thoracolumbar fascia has been demonstrated to contain both a small-caliber fiber system, typical of nociceptors and sympathetic axons, and a large-caliber fiber system with encapsulated endings typical of mechanoreception and proprioception. Thus the force transformation occurring through the thoracolumbar fascia might be under proprioceptive control by neural elements in this tissue.
4. It has also been demonstrated that most of the component tissues in the ligamentous stocking of the lumbosacral spine receive a primary afferent nociceptor and sympathetic axon supply.
5. There are at least three separate sources of the small-caliber, primary afferent fibers in the lumbosacral region. Each fiber source has a differential distribution within the tissues of the back. Thus several different pain presentation patterns in the low back are established.
6. A possible interactive role of these neural elements in the normal trophic activity of the tissue has also been proposed. Besides their role in the maintenance of normal tissue, it is clear that these neural systems are also instrumental in orchestrating neurogenic inflammatory processes when they become irritated and sensitized.
7. Thus the tissues of the lumbosacral connection receive a nerve supply that is capable of sustaining a prolonged inflammatory response, contributing to the progressive breakdown of function in the back and the initiation of chronic pain conditions.

Acknowledgement

I would like to thank Jane Carreiro, DO, for critical discussion both in the preparation of the dissected material and the manuscript.

References

Abitbol MM 1988 Evolution of the ischial spine and of the pelvic floor in the Hominoidea. American Journal of Physical Anthropology 75:53–67

Ahmed M, Bjurholm A, Kreicbergs A, Schultzberg M 1993 Neuropeptide Y, tyrosine hydroxylase and vasoactive intestinal polypeptide–immunoreactive nerve fibers in the vertebral bodies, disc, dura mater, and spinal ligaments of the rat lumbar spine. Spine 18:268–273

Akita K, Sakamoto H, Sato T 1992 Innervation of an aberrent digastric muscle in the posterior thigh: stratified relationships between branches of the inferior gluteal nerve. Journal of Anatomy 181:503–506

Andersson EA, Grundstrom H, Thorstensson A 2002 Diverging intramuscular activity patterns in back and abdominal muscles during trunk rotation. Spine 27: E152–E160

Antonacci MD, Mody DR, Heggeness MH 1998 Innervation of the human vertebral body: a histologic study. Journal of Spinal Disorders 11:526–531

Aoki Y, Rydevik B, Kikuchi S, Olmarker K 2002 Local application of disc-related cytokines on spinal nerve roots. Spine 27:1614–1617

Aoki Y, Ohtori S, Takahashi K et al H 2004a Innervation of the lumbar intervertebral disc by nerve growth factor-dependent neurons related to inflammatory pain. Spine 29:1077–1081

Aoki Y, Takahashi Y, Ohtori S et al 2004b Distribution and immunocytochemical characterization of dorsal root ganglion neurons innervating the lumbar intervertebral disc in rats: a review. Life Sciences 74: 2627–2642

Aoki Y, Takahashi Y, Takahashi K et al 2004c Sensory innervation of the lateral portion of the lumbar intervertebral disc in rats. Spine Journal 4:275–280

Ashton IK, Ashton BA, Gibson SJ et al 1992 Morphological basis for back pain: the demonstration of nerve fibers and neuropeptides in the lumbar facet joint capsule but not in ligamentum flavum. Journal of Orthopaedic Research 10:72–78

Aspden RM, Bornstein NH, Hukins DWL 1987 Collagen organisation in the interspinous ligament and its relationship to tissue function. Journal of Anatomy 155:141–151

Avramov AI, Cavanaugh JM, Ozaktay CA et al 1992 The effects of controlled mechanical loading on group-II, III, and IV afferent units from the lumbar facet joint and surrounding tissue. An in vitro study. Journal of Bone and Joint Surgery (Am) 74:1464–1471

Baba H, Maezawa Y, Furusawa N et al 1995 The role of calcium deposition in the ligamentum flavum causing a cauda equina syndrome and lumbar radiculopathy. Paraplegia 33:219–223

Bajek S, Bobinac D, Bajek G et al 2000 Muscle fiber type distribution in multifidus muscle in cases of lumbar disc herniation. Acta Medica Okayama 54:235–241

Ballard WT, Weinstein JN 1992 Biochemistry of the intervertebral disc. In: Kirkaldy-Willis WH, Burton CV

(eds) Managing low back pain. Churchill Livingstone, New York, p39–48
Barker PJ, Briggs CA, Bogeski G 2004 Tensile transmission across the lumbar fasciae in unembalmed cadavers: effects of tension to various muscular attachments. Spine 29:129–138
Basbaum AI, Levine JD 1991 The contributions of the nervous system to inflammation and inflammatory disease. Canadian Journal of Physiology and Pharmacology 69:647–651
Beal MC 1982 The sacroiliac problem: review of anatomy, mechanics, and diagnosis. Journal of the American Osteopathic Association 81:667–679
Beaman DN, Graziano GP, Glover RA, Wojtys EM, Vhang V 1993 Substance P innervation of lumbar spine facet joints. Spine 18:1044–1049
Bednar DA, Orr FW, Simon GT 1995 Observations on the pathomorphology of the thoracolumbar fascia in chronic mechanical back pain: a microscopic study. Spine 20:1161–1164
Behrsin JF, Briggs CA 1988 Ligaments of the lumbar spine: a review [Review]. Surgical and Radiologic Anatomy 10:211–219
Bernard TN, Cassidy JD 1991 The sacroiliac joint syndrome: pathophysiology, diagnosis, and management. In: Frymoyer JW (ed) The adult spine: principles and practices. Raven Press, New York, p2107–2130
Bernard TN, Kirkaldy-Willis WH 1987 Recognizing specific characteristics of nonspecific low back pain. Clinical Orthopaedics and Related Research 217:266–280
Boden SD, Riew KD, Yamaguchi K, Branch TP, Schellinger D, Wiesel SW 1996 Orientation of the lumbar facet joints: association with degenerative disc disease. Journal of Bone and Joint Surgery (Am) 78:403–411
Bogduk N 1980a A reappraisal of the anatomy of the human lumbar erector spinae. Journal of Anatomy 131:525–540
Bogduk N 1980b Lumbar dorsal ramus syndrome. Medical Journal of Australia 2:537–541
Bogduk N 1983 The innervation of the lumbar spine. Spine 8:286–293
Bogduk N 1995 The anatomical basis for spinal pain syndromes [Review] [27 refs]. Journal of Manipulative & Physiological Therapeutics 18:603–605
Bogduk N, Long DM 1979 The anatomy of the so-called 'articular nerves' and their relationship to facet denervation in the treatment of low-back pain. Journal of Neurosurgery 51:172–177
Bogduk N, Twomey LT 1991 Clinical anatomy of the lumbar spine. Melbourne: Churchill Livingstone
Bogduk N, Tynan W, Wilson AS 1981 The nerve supply to the human lumbar intervertebral discs. Journal of Anatomy 132:39–56
Bogduk N, Macintosh JE, Pearcy MJ 1992 A universal model of the lumbar back muscles in the upright position. Spine 17:897–913
Bogduk N, Johnson G, Spalding D 1998 The morphology and biomechanics of latissimus dorsi. Clinical Biomechanics 13:377–385
Borenstein D 1996 Epidemiology, etiology, diagnostic evaluation, and treatment of low back pain [Review] [27 refs]. Current Opinion in Rheumatology 8:124–129
Borrelli JJ, Koval KJ, Helfet DL 1996 Operative stabilization of fracture dislocations of the sacroiliac joint. Clinical Orthopaedics and Related Research 329:141–146
Bose K, Balasubramanian P 1984 Nerve root canals of the lumbar spine. Spine 9:16–18
Briggs CA, Chandraraj S 1995 Variations in the lumbosacral ligament and associated changes in the lumbosacral region resulting in compression of the fifth dorsal root ganglion and spinal nerve. Clinical Anatomy 8:339–346
Brunner C, Kissling RO, Jacob HAC 1991 The effects of morphology and histopathologic findings on the mobility of the sacroiliac joint. Spine 16:1111–1117
Bucknill AT, Coward K, Plumpton C, Tate S, Bountra C, Birch R, Sandison A, Hughes SP, Anand P 2002 Nerve fibers in lumbar spine structures and injured spinal roots express the sensory neuron-specific sodium channels SNS/PN3 and NaN/SNS2. Spine 27:135–140
Carette S, Marcoux S, Truchon R, Grondin C, Gagnon J, Allard Y, Latulippe M 1991 A controlled trial of corticosteroid injections into facet joints for chronic low back pain. New England Journal of Medicine 325: 1002–1007
Cavanaugh JM, Kallakuri S, Özaktay AC 1995 Innervation of the rabbit lumbar intervertebral disc and posterior longitudinal ligament. Spine 20:2080–2085
Cavanaugh JM, Özaktay AC, Yamashita HT, King AI 1996 Lumbar facet pain: Biomechanics, neuroanatomy and neurophysiology. Journal of Biomechanics 29:1117–1129
Cavanaugh JM, Özaktay AC, Yamashita T, Avramov A, Getchell TV, King AI 1997 Mechanisms of low back pain: a neurophysiologic and neuroanatomic study. Clinical Orthopaedics and Related Research 335:166–180
Cholewicki J, Panjabi MM, Khachatryan A 1997 Stabilizing function of trunk flexor–extensor muscles around a neutral spine posture. Spine 22:2207–2212
Chow DH, Luk KDK, Leong JC, Woo CW 1989 Torsional stability of the lumbosacral junction. Significance of the iliolumbar ligament. Spine 14:611–615
Clark BC, Manini TM, Mayer JM et al 2002 Electromyographic activity of the lumbar and hip extensors during dynamic trunk extension exercise. Archives of Physical Medicine and Rehabilitation 83:1547–1552
Coderre TJ, Katz J, Vaccarina AL, Melzack R 1993 Contribution of central neuroplasticity to pathological pain: review of clinical and experimental evidence. Pain 52:259–285
Cole AJ, Dreyfuss P, Statton SA 1996 The sacroiliac joint: a functional approach. Critical Reviews in Physical and Rehabilitation Medicine 8:125–152
Coppes MH, Marani E, Thomeer RT, Groen GJ 1997 Innervation of 'painful' lumbar discs. Spine 22:2342–2349
Crisco JJ, Panjabi MM 1991 The intersegmental and multisegmental muscles of the lumbar spine: a biomechanical model comparing lateral stabilizing potential. Spine 16:793–799
Cuellar JM, Montesano PX, Carstens E 2004 Role of

TNF-alpha in sensitization of nociceptive dorsal horn neurons induced by application of nucleus pulposus to L5 dorsal root ganglion in rats. Pain 110:578–587

Damen L, Buyruk HM, Guler-Uysal F et al 2001 Pelvic pain during pregnancy is associated with asymmetric laxity of the sacroiliac joints. Acta Obstetrica Gynecologica Scandinavica 80:1019–1024

Damen L, Buyruk HM, Guler-Uysal F et al 2002 The prognostic value of asymmetric laxity of the sacroiliac joints in pregnancy-related pelvic pain. Spine 27: 2820–2824

Danneels LA, Vanderstraeten GG, Cambier DC et al 2001 A functional subdivision of hip, abdominal, and back muscles during asymmetric lifting. Spine 26:E114–E121

Daum WJ 1995 The sacroiliac joint: an underappreciated pain generator. American Journal of Orthopedics 24:475–478

de Peretti F, Micalef JP, Bourgeon A et al 1989 Biomechanics of the lumbar spinal nerve roots and the first sacral root within the intervertebral foramina. Surgical Radiologic Anatomy 11:221–225

Dofferhof AS, Vink P 1985 The stabilising function of the mm. iliocostales and the mm. multifidi during walking. Journal of Anatomy 140:329–336

Dory MA 1981 Arthrography of the lumbar facet joints. Radiology 140:23–27

Dreyfuss P, Schwarzer AC, Lau P, Bogduk N 1997 Specificity of lumbar medial branch and L5 dorsal ramus blocks. A computed tomography study. Spine 22:895–902

Dujardin FH, Roussignol X, Hossenbaccus M, Thomine JM 2002 Experimental study of the sacroiliac joint micromotion in pelvic disruption. Journal of Orthopedics and Trauma 16:99–103

Dupuis P 1992 The anatomy of the lumbosacral spine. In: Kirkaldy-Willis WH, Burton CV (eds) Managing low back pain. Churchill Livingstone, New York, p7–25

El-Bohy AA, Cavanaugh JM, Getchell ML et al 1988 Localization of substance P and neurofilament immuno-reactive fibers in the lumbar facet joint capsule and supraspinous ligament of the rabbit. Brain Research 460:379–382

Engel R, Bogduk N 1982 The menisci of the lumbar zygo-apophysial joints. Journal of Anatomy 135:795–809

Ericson MO, Nisell R, Ekholm J 1986 Quantified electro-myography of lower-limb muscles during level walking. Scandinavian Journal of Rehabilitation Medicine 18:159–163

Firooznia H, Rauschning W, Rafii M, Golimbu C 1993 Normal correlative anatomy of the lumbosacral spine and its contents. Neuroimagimaging Clinics of North America 3:411–423

Fortin JD, Aprill CN, Ponthieux B, Pier J 1994a Sacroiliac joint: pain referral maps upon applying a new injection/arthrography technique: Part II: clinical evaluation. Spine 19:1483–1489

Fortin JD, Dwyer AP, West S, Pier J 1994b Sacroiliac joint: pain referral maps upon applying a new injection/arthrography technique. Part I: asymptomatic volunteers. Spine 19:1475–1482

Fortin JD, Kissling RO, O'Connor BL, Vilensky JA 1999a Sacroiliac joint innervation and pain. American Journal of Orthopedics 28:687–690

Fortin JD, Washington WJ, Falco FJ 1999b Three pathways between the sacroiliac joint and neural structures. American Journal of Neuroradiology 20:1429–1434

Freemont AJ, Peacock TE, Goupille P et al 1997 Nerve ingrowth into diseased intervertebral disc in chronic back pain. Lancet 350:178–181

Freemont AJ, Watkins A, Le Maitre C et al 2002 Nerve growth factor expression and innervation of the painful intervertebral disc. Journal of Pathology 197:286–292

Fujii H, Hamada H 1993 A CNS-specific POU transcription factor, Brn-2, is required for establishing mammalian neural cell lineages. Neuron 11:1197–1206

Fujii Y, Yoshida H, Sakou T 1993 Immunohistochemical studies on tenascin in human yellow ligament. In Vivo 7:143–146

Fujiwara A, Tamai K, An HS et al 2001 Orientation and osteoarthritis of the lumbar facet joint. Clinical Orthopaedics and Related Research 385:88–94

Garfin SR, Rydevik BL, Lind B, Massie J 1995 Spinal nerve root compression. Spine 20:1810–1820

Garrett NE, Mapp PI, Cruwys SC et al 1992 Role of substance P in inflammatory arthritis. Annals of the Rheumatic Diseases 51:1014–1018

Golub BS, Silverman B 1969 Transfrominal ligaments of the lumbar spine. Journal of Bone and Joint Surgery 51:947–956

Gonzalez-Darder JM 1989 Thoracic dorsal ramus entrap-ment. Case report. Journal of Neurosurgery 70:124–125

Granata KP, Marras WS 1995 The influence of trunk muscle coactivity on dynamic spinal loads. Spine 20:913–919

Gries NC, Berlemann U, Moore RJ, Vernon-Roberts B 2000 Early histologic changes in lower lumbar discs and facet joints and their correlation. European Spine Journal 9:23–29

Grob KR, Neuhuber WL, Kissling RO 1995 Innervation of the sacroiliac joint of the human. Zeitschrift für Rheumatologie 54:117–122

Groen GJ, Baljet B, Drukker J 1988 The innervation of the spinal dura mater: anatomy and clinical implications. Acta Neurochirurgica 92:39–46

Groen GJ, Baljet B, Drukker J 1990 Nerves and nerve plexuses of the human vertebral column. American Journal of Anatomy 188:282–296

Grogan J, Nowicki BH, Schmidt TA, Haughton VM 1997 Lumbar facet joint tropism does not accelerate degeneration of the facet joints. American Journal of Neuroradiology 18:1325–1329

Gronblad M, Virri J, Tolonen J et al 1994 A controlled immunohistochemical study of inflammatory cells in disc herniation tissue. Spine 19:2744–2751

Hadar H, Gadoth N, Heifetz M 1983 Fatty replacement of lower paraspinal muscles: normal and neuromuscular disorders. American Journal of Roentgenology 5: 895–898

Hadley-Miller N, Mims B, Milewicz DM 1994 The potential role of the elastic fiber system in adolescent idiopathic scoliosis. Journal of Bone and Joint Surgery (Am) 76:1193–1206

Hamid M, Fallet-Bianco C, Delmas V, Plaisant O 2002 The human lumbar anterior epidural space: morphological comparison in adult and fetal specimens. Surgical and Radiologic Anatomy 24:194–200

Hanley EN, Howard BH, Brigham CD et al 1994 Lumbar epidural varix as a cause of radiculopathy. Spine 19:2122–2126

Hanson P, Sonesson B 1994 The anatomy of the iliolumbar ligament. Archives of Physical Medicine and Rehabilitation 75:1245–1246

Hanson P, Sorensen H 2000 The lumbosacral ligament. An autopsy study of young black and white people. Cells Tissues Organs 166:373–377

Hanson P, Qvortrup K, Magnusson SP 2000 The superficial anulus fibrosus ligament. An incipient description of a separate ligament between the lumbar anterior longitudinal ligament and the intervertebral disc. Cells Tissues Organs 167:259–265

Hasegawa T, An HS, Haughton VM, Nowicki BH 1995 Lumbar foraminal stenosis: Critical heights of the intervertebral discs and foramina. A cryomicrotome study in cadavera. Journal of Bone and Joint Surgery (Am) 77A:32–38

Hasue M, Kikuchi S, Sakuyama Y, Ito T 1983 Anatomic study of the interrelation between lumbosacral nerve roots and their surrounding tissues. Spine 8:50–58

Helbig T, Lee CK 1988 The lumbar facet syndrome. Spine 13:61–64

Heylings DJA 1978 Supraspinous and interspinous ligaments of the human lumbar spine. Journal of Anatomy 125:127–131

Hides JA, Stokes MJ, Saide M et al 1994 Evidence of lumbar multifidus muscle wasting ipsilateral to symptoms in patients with acute/subacute low back pain. Spine 19:165–172

Hogan QH 1991 Lumbar epidural anatomy. A new look by cryomicrotome section. Anesthesiology 75: 767–775

Holzer P 1988 Local effector functions of capsaicin-sensitive sensory nerve endings: involvement of tachykinins, calcitonin gene-related polypeptide and other neuropeptides. Neuroscience 24:739–768

Hukins DWL, Kirby MC, Sikoryn TA et al 1990 Comparison of structure, mechanical properties, and function of lumbar spinal ligaments. Spine 15:787–795

Igarashi A, Kikuchi S, Konno S, Olmarker K 2004a Inflammatory cytokines released from the facet joint tissue in degenerative lumbar spinal disorders. Spine 29:2091–2095

Igarashi A, Kikuchi S, Konno S, Olmarker K 2004b Inflammatory cytokines released from the facet joint tissue in degenerative lumbar spinal disorders. Spine 29:2091–2095

Ikeda R 1991 Innervation of the sacroiliac joint. Macrosopical and histological studies. Nippon Ika Daigaku Zasshi 58:587–596

Imai S, Hukuda S, Maeda T 1995 Dually innervating nociceptive networks in the rat lumbar posterior longitudinal ligaments. Spine 20:2086–2092

Iwabuchi M, Rydevik B, Kikuchi S, Olmarker K 2001 Effects of anulus fibrosus and experimentally degenerated nucleus pulposus on nerve root conduction velocity: relevance of previous experimental investigations using normal nucleus pulposus. Spine 26:1651–1655

Jackson HC, Winkelmann RK, Bickel WH 1966 Nerve endings in the human lumbar spinal column and related structures. Journal of Bone and Joint Surgery (Am) 48:1272–1281

Jacob HAC, Kissling RO 1995 The mobility of the sacroiliac joints in healthy volunteers between 20 and 50 years of age. Clinical Biomechanics 10:352–361

Ji RR, Kohno T, Moore KA, Woolf CJ 2003 Central sensitization and LTP: do pain and memory share similar mechanisms? Trends in Neuroscience 26:696–705

Jiang HX, Russell G, Raso VJ et al 1995 The nature and distribution of the innervation of human supraspinal and interspinal ligaments. Spine 20:869–876

Jinkins JR 1993 The pathoanatomic basis of somatic and autonomic syndromes originating in the lumbosacral spine. Neuroimaging Clinics of North America 3: 443–463

Jinkins JR 2004 Acquired degenerative changes of the intervertebral segments at and suprajacent to the lumbosacral junction. A radioanatomic analysis of the nondiscal structures of the spinal column and perispinal soft tissues. European Journal of Radiology 50:134–158

Jinkins JR, Whittermore AR, Bradley WG 1989 The anatomic basis of vertebrogenic pain and the autonomic syndrome associated with lumbar disk extrusion. Americal Journal of Radiology 152:1277–1289

Johnson WE, Evans H, Menage J et al 2001 Immunohistochemical detection of Schwann cells in innervated and vascularized human intervertebral discs. Spine 26:2550–2557

Julius D, Basbaum AI 2001 Molecular mechanisms of nociception. Nature 413:203–210

Kader DF, Wardlaw D, Smith FW 2000 Correlation between the MRI changes in the lumbar multifidus muscles and leg pain. Clinical Radiology 55:145–149

Kallakuri S, Cavanaugh JM, Blagoev DC 1998 An immunohistochemical study of innervation of lumbar spinal dura and longitudinal ligaments. Spine 23:403–411

Kapandji IA 1974 The physiology of the joints. Volume 3: The trunk and the vertebral column. Edinburgh: Churchill Livingstone

Kaplan M, Dreyfuss P, Halbrook B, Bogduk N 1998 The ability of lumbar medial branch blocks to anesthetize the zygapophysial joint. A physiologic challenge. Spine 23:1847–1852

Kashiwagi K 1993 Histological changes of the lumbar ligamentum flavum with age. Nippon Seikeigeka Gakkai Zasshi 67:221–229

Kennelly KP, Stokes MJ 1993 Pattern of asymmetry of paraspinal muscle size in adolescent idiopathic scoliosis examined by real-time ultrasound imaging. A preliminary study. Spine 18:913–917

Khosla S, Tredwell SJ, Day B et al 1980 An ultrastructural study of multifidus muscle in progressive idiopathic scoliosis. Changes resulting from a sarcolemmal defect at the myotendinous junction. Journal of Neurological Science 46:13–31

Kidd BL, Mapp PI, Gibson SJ et al 1989 A neurogenic mechanism for symmetrical arthritis. Lancet 2(8672): 1128–1130

Kidd BL, Mapp PI, Blake DR et al 1990 Neurogenic influences in arthritis. Annals of the Rheumatic Diseases 49:649–652

Kidd BL, Cruwys S, Mapp PI, Blake DR 1992 Role of the sympathetic nervous system in chronic joint pain and inflammation. Annals of the Rheumatic Diseases 51:1188–1191

Kinnman E, Nygårds EB, Hansson P 1997 Peripheral α-adrenoreceptors are involved in the development of capsaicin induced ongoing and stimulus evoked pain in humans. Pain 69:79–85

Kirkaldy-Willis WH 1984 The relationship of structural pathology to the nerve root. Spine 9:49–52

Kirkaldy-Willis WH 1992 Pathology and pathogenesis of low back pain. In: Kirkaldy-Willis WH, Burton CV (eds) Managing low back pain. Churchill Livingstone, New York, p49–79

Kissling RO 1995 The mobility of the sacro-iliac joint in healthy subjects. In: Vleeming A et al (eds) Second Interdisciplinary World Congress on Low Back Pain. San Diego, CA. ECO, Rotterdam, p411–422

Kissling RO, Jacob HA 1996 The mobility of the sacroiliac joint in healthy subjects. Bulletin – Hospital for Joint Diseases 54:158–164

Kojima Y, Maeda T, Arai R, Shichikawa K 1990a Nerve supply to the posterior longitudinal ligament and the intervertebral disc of the rat vertebral column as studied by acetylcholinesterase histochemistry. I. Distribution in the lumbar region. Journal of Anatomy 169:237–246

Kojima Y, Maeda T, Arai R, Shichikawa K 1990b Nerve supply to the posterior longitudinal ligament and the intervertebral disc of the rat vertebral column as studied by acetylcholinesterase histochemistry. II. Regional differences in the distribution of the nerve fibres and their origins. Journal of Anatomy 169:247–255

Konttinen YT, Gronblad M, Antti-Poika I et al 1990a Neuroimmunohistochemical analysis of peridiscal nociceptive neural elements. Spine 15:383–386

Konttinen YT, Gronblad M, Korkala O et al 1990b Immunohistochemical demonstration of subclasses of inflammatory cells and active, collagen-producing fibroblasts in the synovial plicae of lumbar facet joints. Spine 15:387–390

Korkala O, Gronblad M, Liesi P, Karaharju E 1985 Immunohistochemical demonstration of nociceptors in the ligamentous structures of the lumbar spine. Spine 10:156–157

LaBan MM, Wilkins JC, Wesolowski DP et al 2001 Paravertebral venous plexus distention (Batson's): An inciting etiologic agent in lumbar radiculopathy as observed by venous angiography. American Journal of Physical Medicine and Rehabilitation 80:129–133

Lam FY, Ferrell WR 1991 Neurogenic component of different models of acute inflammation in the knee joint. Annals of the Rheumatic Diseases 50:747–751

Lapadula G, Covelli M, Numo R, Pipitone V 1991 Iliolumbar ligament ossification as a radiologic feature of reactive arthritis. Journal of Rheumatology 18:1760–1762

Larsson K, Rydevik B, Olmarker K 2005 Disc related cytokines inhibit axonal outgrowth from dorsal root ganglion cells in vitro. Spine 30:621–624

Le Blanche AF, Mabi C, Bigot JM et al 1996 The sacroiliac joint: anatomical study in the coronal plane and MR correlation. Surgical and Radiologic Anatomy 18: 215–220

Lee JH, Hoshino Y, Nakamura K et al 1999 Trunk muscle weakness as a risk factor for low back pain. A 5-year prospective study. Spine 24:54–57

Lehto M, Hurme M, Alaranta H et al 1989 Connective tissue changes of the multifidus muscle in patients with lumbar disc herniation. An immunohistologic study of collagen types I and III and fibronectin. Spine 14: 302–309

Leong JC, Luk KD, Chow DH, Woo CW 1987 The biomechanical functions of the iliolumbar ligament in maintaining stability of the lumbosacral junction. Spine 12:669–674

Levine JD, Collier DH, Basbaum AI et al 1985a Hypothesis: the nervous system may contribute to the pathophysiology of rheumatoid arthritis. Journal of Rheumatology 12:406–411

Levine JD, Moskowitz MA, Basbaum AI 1985b The contribution of neurogenic inflammation in experimental arthritis. Journal of Immunology 135:843s–847s

Levine JD, Coderre TJ, Covinsky K, Basbaum AI 1990 Neural influences on synovial mast cell density in rat. Journal of Neuroscience Research 26:301–307

Levine JD, Fields HL, Basbaum AI 1993 Peptides and the primary afferent nociceptor. Journal of Neuroscience 13:2273–2286

Lewin T, Moffett B, Viidik A 1962 The morphology of the lumbar synovial intervertebral joints. Acta Morphologica Neerl Scandinavia 4:299–319

Liu MW, Max MB, Parada S et al 1996 The sympathetic nervous system contributes to capsaicin-evoked mechanical allodynia but not pinprick hyperalgesia in humans. Journal of Neuroscience 16:7331–7335

Luk KDK, Ho HC, Leong JCY 1986 The iliolumbar ligament: a study of its anatomy, development and clinical significance. Journal of Bone and Joint Surgery (UK) 68:197–200

Macintosh JE, Bogduk N 1986 The biomechanics of the lumbar multifidus. Clinical Biomechanics 1:205–213

Macintosh JE, Valencia FP, Bogduk N, Munro RR 1986 The morphology of the human lumbar multifidus. Clinical Biomechanics 1:196–204

Macintosh JE, Bogduk N, Pearcy MJ 1993a The effects of flexion on the geometry and actions of the lumbar erector spinae. Spine 18:884–893

Macintosh JE, Pearcy MJ, Bogduk N 1993b The axial torque of the lumbar back muscles: torsion strength of the back muscles. Australia and New Zealand Journal of Surgery 63:205–212

Manchikanti L, Boswell MV, Singh V et al 2004 Prevalence of facet joint pain in chronic spinal pain of cervical, thoracic, and lumbar regions. Musculoskeletal Disorders 5:15

Mattila M, Hurme M, Alaranta H et al 1986 The multifidus muscle in patients with lumbar disc herniation. A histochemical and morphometric analysis of intra-operative biopsies. Spine 11:732–738

McCafferty RR, Harrison MJ, Tamas LB, Larkins MV 1995 Ossification of the anterior longitudinal ligament and Forestier's disease: an analysis of seven cases. Journal of Neurosurgery 83:13–17

McCarron RF, Wimpee MW, Hudkins PG, Laros GS 1987 The inflammatory effects of nucleus pulposus: a possible element in the pathogenesis of low back pain. Spine 12:760–764

McGill SM, Norman RW 1988 Potential of the lumbodorsal fascia forces to generate back extension movements during squat lifts. Journal of Biomedical Engineering 10:312–318

McLain RF 1994 Mechanoreceptor endings in human cervical facet joints. Spine 19:495–501

McLauchlan GJ, Gardner DL 2002 Sacral and iliac articular cartilage thickness and cellularity: relationship to subchondral bone end-plate thickness and cancellous bone density. Rheumatology (Oxford) 41:375–380

Mine T, Kawai S 1995 Ultrastructural observations on the ossification of the supraspinous ligament. Spine 20:297–302

Mooney V, Robertson J 1976 The facet syndrome. Clinical Orthopaedics and Related Research 115:149–156

Morley GW, DeLancey JOL 1988 Sacrospinous ligament fixation for eversion of the vagina. American Journal of Obstetrics and Gynecology 158:872–881

Moseley GL, Hodges PW, Gandevia SC 2002 Deep and superficial fibers of the lumbar multifidus muscle are differentially active during voluntary arm movements. Spine 27:E29–E36

Moseley GL, Hodges PW, Gandevia SC 2003 External perturbation of the trunk in standing humans differentially activates components of the medial back muscles. Journal of Physiology 547:581–587

Nachemson A, Evans J 1968 Some mechanical properties of the third lumbar intervertebral ligament (ligamentum flavum). Journal of Biomechanics 1:211

Neumann P, Ekstrom LA, Keller TS et al 1994 Aging, vertebral density, and disc degeneration alter the tensile stress–strain characteristics of the human anterior longitudinal ligament. Journal of Orthopaedic Research 12:103–112

Neumann S, Doubell TP, Leslie T, Woolf CJ 1996 Inflammatory pain hypersensitivity mediated by phenotypic switch in myelinated primary sensory neurons. Nature 384:360–364

Ng JK, Richardson CA, Jull GA 1997 Electromyographic amplitude and frequency changes in the iliocostalis lumborum and multifidus muscles during a trunk holding test. Physical Therapy 77:954–961

Nichols DH 1985 Vaginal prolapse affecting bladder function. Urologic Clinics of North America 12:329–338

Nohara Y, Brown MD, Eurell JA 1991 Lymphatic drainage of epidural space in rabbits. Orthopedics Clinics of North America 22:189–194

Nowicki BH, Haughton VM 1992 Neural foraminal ligaments of the lumbar spine: appearance at CT and MR imaging. Radiology 183:257–264

O'Connor BL, Palmoski MJ, Brandt KD 1985 Neurogenic acceleration of degenerative joint lesions. Journal of Bone and Joint Surgery (Am) 67A:562–572

O'Rahilly R 1986 Anatomy: a regional study of human structure. Philadelphia, PA: WB Saunders

O'Sullivan PB, Grahamslaw KM, Kendell M et al 2002 The effect of different standing and sitting postures on trunk muscle activity in a pain-free population. Spine 27:1238–1244

Ohtori S, Takahashi Y, Takahashi K et al 1999 Sensory innervation of the dorsal portion of the lumbar intervertebral disc in rats. Spine 24:2295–2299

Ohtori S, Takahashi K, Chiba T et al 2001 Phenotypic inflammation switch in rats shown by calcitonin gene-related peptide immunoreactive dorsal root ganglion neurons innervating the lumbar facet joints. Spine 26:1009–1013

Ohtori S, Takahashi K, Moriya H 2002 Inflammatory pain mediated by a phenotypic switch in brain-derived neurotrophic factor-immunoreactive dorsal root ganglion neurons innervating the lumbar facet joints in rats. Neuroscience Letters 323:129–132

Ohtori S, Takahashi K, Moriya H 2003 Existence of brain-derived neurotrophic factor and vanilloid receptor subtype 1 immunoreactive sensory DRG neurons innervating L5/6 intervertebral discs in rats. Journal of Orthopedic Science 8:84–87

Okada A, Harata S, Takeda Y et al 1993 Age-related changes in proteoglycans of human ligamentum flavum. Spine 18:2261–2266

Okuda T, Baba I, Fujimoto Y et al 2004 The pathology of ligamentum flavum in degenerative lumbar disease. Spine 29:1689–1697

Okuda T, Fujimoto Y, Tanaka N et al 2005 Morphological changes of the ligamentum flavum as a cause of nerve root compression. European Spine Journal 14:277–286

Olmarker K, Larsson K 1998 Tumor necrosis factor alpha and nucleus-pulposus-induced nerve root injury. Spine 23:2538–2544

Olmarker K, Myers RR 1998 Pathogenesis of sciatic pain: role of herniated nucleus pulposus and deformation of spinal nerve root and dorsal root ganglion. Pain 78:99–105

Olmarker K, Rydevik BL, Holm S 1989 Edema formation in spinal nerve roots induced by experimental, graded compression: an experimental study on the pig cauda equina with special reference to the differences in effects between rapid and slow onset of compression. Spine 14:569–573

Olmarker K, Holm S, Rydevik BL 1990 Importance of compression onset rate for the degree of impairment of impulse propergation in experimental compression of the porcine cauda equina. Spine 15:416–419

Olmarker K, Rydevik BL, Nordborg C 1993 Autologous nucleus pulposus induces neurophysiologic and histologic changes in porcine cauda equina nerve roots. Spine 18:1425–1432

Olmarker K, Blomquist J, Strömberg J et al 1995 Inflammatogenic properties of nucleus pulposus. Spine 20:665–669

Olmarker K, Storkson R, Berge OG 2002 Pathogenesis of sciatic pain: a study of spontaneous behavior in rats exposed to experimental disc herniation. Spine 27: 1312–1317

Olszewski AD, Yaszemski MJ, White AA, III 1996 The anatomy of the human lumbar ligamentum flavum – new observations and their surgical importance. Spine 21:2307–2312

Onda A, Murata Y, Rydevik B et al 2005 Nerve growth factor content in dorsal root ganglion as related to changes in pain behavior in a rat model of experimental lumbar disc herniation. Spine 30:188–193

Oxland TR, Panjabi MM, Southern EP, Duranceau JS 1991 An anatomic basis for spinal instability: a porcine trauma model. Journal of Orthopaedic Research 9: 452–462

Ozaktay AC, Cavanaugh JM, Blagoev DC et al 1994 Effects of a carrageenan-induced inflammation in rabbit lumbar facet joint capsule and adjacent tissues. Neuroscience Research 20:355–364

Panjabi MM, White AA 1990 Physical properties and functional biomechanics of the spine. In: White AA, Panjabi MM (eds) Clinical biomechanics of the spine. JB Lippincott, Philadelphia, PA, p1–84

Panjabi MM, Goel VK, Takata K 1982 Physiologic strains in the lumbar spinal ligaments. An in vitro biomechanical study. Spine 7:192–203

Parke WW 1991 The significance of venous return impairment in ischemic radiculopathy and myelopathy. Orthopedic Clinics of North America 22:213–221

Parke WW, Watanabe R 1990 Adhesions of the ventral lumbar dura: an adjunct source of discogenic pain? Spine 15:300–303

Parkkola R, Rytokoski U, Kormano M 1993 Magnetic resonance imaging of the discs and trunk muscles in patients with chronic low back pain and healthy control subjects. Spine 18:830–836

Payan DG 1989 Substance P: a neuroendocrine-immune modulator. Hospital Practics (Office Edition) 24(2): 67–80

Payan DG 1992 The role of neuropeptides in inflammation. In: Gallin JI, Goldstein IM, Snyderman R (eds) Inflammation: basic principles and clinical correlations. Raven Press, New York, p177–192

Pedersen HE, Blunck CJF, Gardner E 1956a Innervation of the lumbar spine. Journal of Bone and Joint Surgery (Am) 38:377–391

Pedersen HE, Blunck FJ, Gardner E 1956b The anatomy of lumbosacral posterior rami and meningeal branches of spinal nerves (sinu-vertebral nerves). Journal of Bone and Joint Surgery (Am) 38:377–391

Pionchon H, Tommasi M, Pialat J et al 1986 Study of the innervation of the spinal ligaments at the lumbar level [in French]. Bulletin de l'Association des Anatomistes 70:63–67

Pool-Goudzwaard AL, Kleinrensink GJ, Snijders CJ et al 2001 The sacroiliac part of the iliolumbar ligament. Journal of Anatomy 199:457–463

Porges R, Smilen SW 1994 Long-term analysis of the surgical management of pelvic support defects. America Journal of Obstetrics and Gynecology 171: 1518–1528

Prechtl JC, Powley TL 1990 B-afferents: a fundamental division of the nervous system mediating homeostasis? Behavioural and Brain Science 13:289–331

Prescher A, Bohndorf K 1993 Anatomical and radiological observations concerning ossification of the sacrotuberous ligament: is there a relation to spinal diffuse idiopathic skeletal hyperostosis (DISH)? Skeletal Radiology 22:581–585

Ramsey RH 1966 The anatomy of the ligamenta flava. Clinical Orthopaedics and Related Research 44:129–140

Rantanen J, Hurme M, Falck B et al 1993 The lumbar multifidus muscle five years after surgery for a lumbar intervertebral disc herniation. Spine 18:568–574

Raoul S, Faure A, Robert R et al 2003 Role of the sinu-vertebral nerve in low back pain and anatomical basis of therapeutic implications. Surgical and Radiologic Anatomy 24:366–371

Rhalmi S, Yahia LH, Newman N, Isler M 1993 Immunohistochemical study of nerves in lumbar spinae ligaments. Spine 18:264–267

Roaf R 1960 A study of the mechanics of spinal injuries. Journal of Bone and Joint Surgery (UK) 42B:810

Roberts WJ, Kramis RC 1990 Sympathetic nervous system influence on acute and chronic pain. In: Fields HL (ed) Pain syndromes in neurology. Butterworth Heineman, Oxford, UK, p85–106

Ryan LM 1993 Calcium pyrophosphate dihydrate crystal deposition and other crystal deposition diseases. Current Opinion in Rheumatology 5:517–521

Rydevik BL 1992 The effects of compression on the physiology of nerve roots. Journal of Manipulative and Physiological Therapeutics 15:62–66

Rydevik BL, Brown MD, Lundborg G 1984 Pathoanatomy and pathophysiology of nerve root compression. Spine 9:7–15

Saal JS 1995 The role of inflammation in lumbar pain. Spine 20:1821–1827

Saal JS, Franson RC, Dobrow R et al 1990 High levels of inflammatory phospholipase A2 activity in lumbar disc herniation. Spine 15:674–678

Sakamoto N, Yamashita T, Takebayashi et al 2001 An electrophysiologic study of mechanoreceptors in the sacroiliac joint and adjacent tissues. Spine 26:E468–E471

Sameda H, Takahashi Y, Takahashi K et al 2001 Primary sensory neurons with dichotomizing axons projecting to the facet joint and the sciatic nerve in rats. Spine 26:1105–1109

Sangameswaran L, Delgado SG, Fish LM et al 1996 Structure and function of a novel voltage-gated, tetrodotoxin-resistant sodium channel specific to sensory neurons. Journal of Biological Chemistry 271:5953–5956

Sato K, Olmarker K, Cornefjord M et al 1994 Effects of chronic nerve root compression on intraradicular blood flow: an experimental study in pigs. Neuro-Orthopedics 16:1–7

Schaible HG, Grubb BD 1993 Afferent and spinal mechanisms of joint pain. Pain 55:5–54

Schaible HG, Del Rosso A, Matucci-Cerinic M 2005 Neurogenic aspects of inflammation. Rheumatological Diseases Clinics of North America 31:77–101

Schrader PK, Grob D, Rahn BA et al 1999 Histology of the ligamentum flavum in patients with degenerative lumbar spinal stenosis. European Spine Journal 8:323–328

Schwarzer AC, Aprill CN, Derby R et al 1994 Clinical features of patients with pain stemming from the lumbar zygapophysial joints. Is the lumbar facet syndrome a clinical entity? Spine 19:1132–1137

Schwarzer AC, Aprill CN, Bogduk N 1995 The sacroiliac joint in chronic low back pain. Spine 20:31–37

Sekine M, Yamashita T, Takebayashi T et al 2001 Mechanosensitive afferent units in the lumbar posterior longitudinal ligament. Spine 26:1516–1521

Shao Z, Chen Z, Zhou L et al 1996 Spinal dorsal ramus syndrome. Chinese Medical Journal 109:317–321

Sihvonen T, Partanen J 1990 Segmental hypermobility in lumbar spine and entrapment of dorsal rami. Electromyography & Clinical Neurophysiology 30:175–180

Sihvonen T, Lindgren KA, Airaksinen O, Manninen H 1997 Movement disturbances of the lumbar spine and abnormal back muscle electromyographic findings in recurrent low back pain. Spine 22:289–295

Simonian PT, Routt MLC, Harrington RM et al 1994 Biomechanical simulation of the anteroposterior compression injury of the pelvis. Clinical Orthopaedics and Related Research 309:245–256

Snijders CJ, Vleeming A, Stoeckart R 1993 Transfer of lumbosacral load to iliac bones and legs. Part I: Biomechanics of self-bracing of the sacroiliac joints and its significance for treatment and exercise. Clinical Biomechanics 8:285–294

Snijders CJ, Vleeming A, Stoeckart R et al 1995 Biomechanics of sacroiliac joint stability: validation experiments on the concept of self-locking. In: Vleeming A et al (eds) The integrated function of the lumbar spine and sacroiliac joints. ECO, Rotterdam, p77–91

Spencer DL, Irwin GS, Miller JAA 1983 Anatomy and significance of fixation of the lumbosacral nerve roots in sciatica. Spine 8:672–679

Standing S 2005 Gray's anatomy, the anatomical basis of clinical practice. Edinburgh: Churchill Livingstone

Stilwell DL 1956 The nerve supply of the vertebral column and its associated structures in the monkey. Anatomical Record 125:139–169

Stubbs M, Harris M, Solomonow M et al 1998 Ligamento-muscular protective reflex in the lumbar spine of the feline. Journal of Electromyography and Kinesiology 8:197–204

Suseki K, Takahashi Y, Takahashi K et al 1996 CGRP-immunoreactive nerve fibers projecting to lumbar facet joints through the paravertebral sympathetic trunk in rats. Neuroscience Letters 221:41–44

Suseki K, Takahashi Y, Takahashi K et al 1997 Innervation of the lumbar facet joints. Origins and functions. Spine 22:477–485

Swanepoel MW, Adams LM, Smeathers JE 1995 Human lumbar apophyseal joint damage and intervertebral disc degeneration. Annals of the Rheumatic Diseases 54:182–188

Taylor JR, Twomey LT 1986 Age changes in lumbar zygapophyseal joints. Observations on structure and function. Spine 11:739–745

Tobias D, Ziv I, Maroudas A 1992 Human facet cartilage: swelling and some physico-chemical characteristics as a function of age Part 1: Swelling of human facet joint cartilage. Spine 17:694–700

Uhthoff HK 1993 Prenatal development of the iliolumbar ligament. Journal of Bone and Joint Surgery (UK) 75: 93–95

Vakos JP, Nitz AJ, Threlkeld AJ, Shapiro R, Horn T 1994 Electromyographic activity of selected trunk and hip muscles during a squat lift. Effect of varying the lumbar posture. Spine 19:687–695

van Wingerden JP, Vleeming A, Buyruk HM, Raissadat K 2004 Stabilization of the sacroiliac joint in vivo: verification of muscular contribution to force closure of the pelvis. European Spine Journal 13:199–205

Vanharanta H, Floyd T, Ohnmeiss DD, Hochschuler SH, Guyer RD 1993 The relationship of facet tropism to degenerative disc disease. Spine 18:1000–1005

Vernon-Roberts B 1992 Age-related and degenerative pathology of intervertebral discs and apophyseal joints. In: Jayson MIV (ed) The lumbar spine and back pain. Churchhill Livingstone, Edinburgh, p17–41

Viejo-Fuertes D, Liguoro D, Rivel J et al 1998 Morphologic and histologic study of the ligamentum flavum in the thoraco-lumbar region. Surgical and Radiologic Anatomy 20:171–176

Vleeming A, Stoeckart R, Snijders CJ 1989a The sacrotuberous ligament: a conceptual approach to its dynamic role in stabilizing the sacroiliac joint. Clinical Biomechanics 4:201–203

Vleeming A, van Wingerden J-P, Snijders CJ et al 1989b Load application to the sacrotuberous ligament; influences on sacroiliac joint mechanics. Clinical Biomechanics 4:204–209

Vleeming A, Stoeckart R, Snijders CJ 1992 General introduction (to the sacroiliac joint). In: Vleeming A et al (eds) The sacroiliac joint: First Interdisciplinary World Congress on Low Back Pain. San Diego, CA. ECO, Rotterdam, p3–63

Vleeming A, Pool-Goudzwaard AL, Hammudoghlu D et al 1995a The function of the long dorsal sacroiliac ligament: its implication for understanding low back pain. In: Vleeming A et al (eds) The integrated function of the lumbar spine and sacroiliac joints. ECO, Rotterdam, p125–137

Vleeming A, Pool-Goudzwaard AL, Stoeckart R et al 1995b The posterior layer of the thoracolumbar fascia: its function in load transfer from spine to legs. Spine 20:753–758

Vleeming A, Snijders CJ, Stoeckart R, Mens JMA 1995c A new light on low back pain: The selflocking mechanism of the sacroiliac joints and its implication for sitting, standing and walking. In: Vleeming A et al (eds) Second Interdisciplinary World Congress on Low Back Pain. San Diego, CA. ECO, Rotterdam, p149–168

Vleeming A, Pool-Goudzwaard AL, Hammudoghlu D et al 1996 The function of the long dorsal sacroiliac ligament - Its implication for understanding low back pain. Spine 21:556–562

von During M, Fricke B, Dahlmann A 1995 Topography and distribution of nerve fibers in the posterior longitudinal ligament of the rat: an immunocytochemical and electron-microscopical study. Cell and Tissue Research 281:325–338

Vrahas M, Hern TC, Diangelo D et al 1995 Ligamentous contributions to pelvic stability. Orthopedics 18: 271–274

Wadhwani S, Loughenbury P, Soames R 2004 The anterior dural (Hofmann) ligaments. Spine 29:623–627

Wang J, Ren Y, Zou X et al 2004 Sympathetic influence on capsaicin-evoked enhancement of dorsal root reflexes in rats. Journal of Neurophysiology 92:2017–2026

Waxman SG 1999 The molecular pathophysiology of pain: abnormal expression of sodium channel genes and its contributions to hyperexcitability of primary sensory neurons. Pain (suppl 6):S133–S140

Weidenbaum M, Farcy J-P 1990 Pain syndromes of the lumbar spine. In: Floman Y (ed) Disorders of the lumbar spine. Aspen Publishing, Rockville, MD, p85–115

Weinstein JN 1991 Neurogenic and nonneurogenic pain and inflammatory mediators. Orthopedic Clinics of North America 22:235–246

Weinstein JN 1992 The role of neurogenic and non-neurogenic mediators as they relate to pain and the development of osteoarthritis. Spine 105:S356–S361

Willard FH 1995 Neuroendocrine–immune network, nociceptive stress, and the general adaptive response. In: Everett T, Dennis M, Ricketts E (eds) Physiotherapy in mental health: a practical approach. Butterworth Heinemann, Oxford, UK, p102–126

Willard FH 2003 Nociception, the neuroendocrine immune system and osteopathic medicine. In: Ward RC (ed) Foundations for osteopathic medicine. Lippincott, Williams & Wilkins, Philadelphia, PA, p137–156

Willard FH, Carreiro JE, Manko W 1998 The long posterior interosseous ligament and the sacrococcygeal plexus. Proceedings of the Third Interdisciplinary World Congress on Low Back & Pelvic Pain, p207–209

Willburger RE, Wittenbeg RH 1994 Prostaglandin release from lumbar disc and facet joint tissue. Spine 19: 2068–2070

Woolf CJ 2004 Pain: moving from symptom control toward mechanism-specific pharmacologic management. Annals of Internal Medicine 140:441–451

Woolf CJ, Chong M-S 1993 Preemptive analgesia— treating postoperative pain by preventing the establishment of central sensitization. Anesthesia and Analgesia 77: 362–379

Wyke BD 1967 The neurology of joints. Annals of the Royal College of Surgeons 41:25–50

Wyke BD 1976 Neurological aspects of low back pain. In: Jayson MIV (ed) The lumbar spine and back pain. Sector Publishing Limited, London, p189–256

Yahia LH, Drouin G, Newman N 1990a Structure–function relationship of human spinal ligaments. Zeitschrift für mikroskopisch-anatomische Forschung 104:33–45

Yahia LH, Garzon S, Strykowski H, Rivard C-H 1990b Ultrastructure of the human interspinous ligament and ligamentum flavum. a preliminary study. Spine 15: 262–268

Yahia LH, Rhalmi S, Newman N, Isler M 1992 Sensory innervation of the human thoracolumbar fascia. Acta Orthopedica Scandinavia 63:195–197

Yamamoto I, Panjabi MM, Oxland TR, Crisco JJ 1990 The role of the iliolumbar ligament in the lumbosacral junction. Spine 15:1138–1141

Yamamoto N, Kurotani T, Toyama K 1989 Neural connections between the lateral geniculate nucleus and visual cortex in vitro. Sci 245:192–194

Yamashita T, Cavanaugh JM, El-Bohy AA et al 1990 Mechanosensitive afferent units in the lumbar facet joint. Journal of Bone and Joint Surgery (Am) 72-A: 865–870

Yamashita T, Minaki Y, Ozaktay AC et al 1996 A morphological study of the fibrous capsule of the human lumbar facet joint. Spine 21:538–543

Yin W, Willard F, Carreiro J, Dreyfuss P 2003 Sensory stimulation-guided sacroiliac joint radiofrequency neurotomy: technique based on neuroanatomy of the dorsal sacral plexus. Spine 28:2419–2425

Yoshida M, Shima K, Taniguchi Y et al 1992 Hypertrophied ligamentum flavum in lumbar spinal canal stenosis. Pathogenesis and morphologic and immunohistochemical observation. Spine 17:1353–1360

Yoshihara K, Shirai Y, Nakayama Y, Uesaka S 2001 Histochemical changes in the multifidus muscle in patients with lumbar intervertebral disc herniation. Spine 26:622–626

Yoshihara K, Nakayama Y, Fujii N et al 2003 Atrophy of the multifidus muscle in patients with lumbar disk herniation: histochemical and electromyographic study. Orthopedics 26:493–495

Zhao WP, Kawaguchi Y, Matsui H et al 2000 Histochemistry and morphology of the multifidus muscle in lumbar disc herniation: comparative study between diseased and normal sides. Spine 25:2191–2199

Ziv I, Maroudas C, Robin G, Maroudas A 1993 Human facet cartilage: swelling and some physico-chemical characteristics as a function of age Part 2: Age changes in some biophysical parameters of human facet joint cartilage. Spine 18:136–146

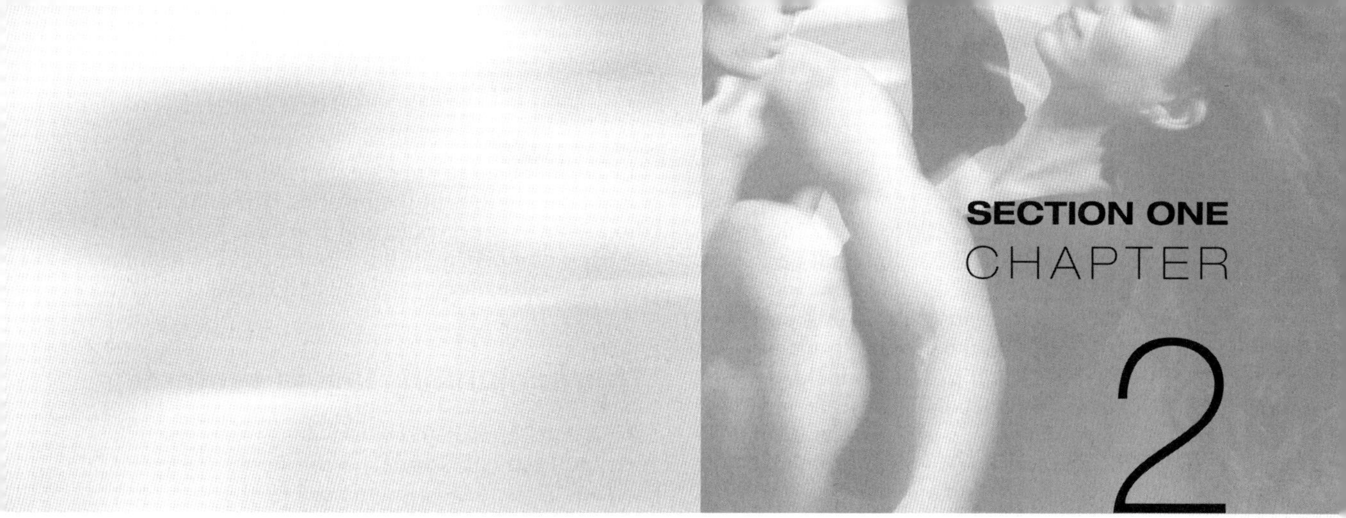

SECTION ONE

CHAPTER 2

Anatomical linkages and muscle slings of the lumbopelvic region

Carl DeRosa and James A Porterfield

Introduction

Nonspecific low back pain continues to be a complex medical and societal problem. It is complicated by the fact that, in most low back conditions, a precise anatomical tissue cannot be identified as the source of the pain. Due to the synergistic relationships of spinal structures and tissues, the likelihood that one tissue alone is the pain generator in most nonspecific low-back-pain conditions is probably not that high, but instead the pain response is due to the loss of load-attenuating capacity of multiple tissues that work in concert with one another. The physiological loading capacity of tissues is lowered by the aging and degenerative processes, as well as by injury. When the physiological limits of tissue loading are exceeded, nonspecific low back pain can result. Consequently, larger-scale, functional anatomical models of the spine must be considered to gain a better appreciation as to how function is disrupted in the presence of low back pain and – conversely – how disruption of the uniquely linked functional anatomical units ultimately contributes to the onset and propagation of low back pain.

The focus of this chapter is on the linkages between different muscles of the trunk, pelvic girdle, and shoulder girdle and the muscular slings they form over the lumbopelvic region. The spine devoid of muscle and relying primarily on its osteoligamentous framework is an inherently unstable structure and buckles very quickly under compressive loading (Bergmark 1989). The muscles, in particular the neuromotoric drive that contributes to the varying contractile states of muscle, act to stiffen the spine and thus influence its stability. The musculature, both in conditions of low back pain and in its absence, therefore assumes significant clinical importance. It is not just a loss of strength, power, and endurance of muscle that affects spinal function. The slings and linkages of the shoulder girdle to the trunk, and of the hip to the trunk, are also an integral part of the sophisticated array of reflexes that allow for precise motion while simultaneously providing for spinal stability. Deficiencies in timely muscle activation in response to sudden loading of the trunk (Magnusson et al 1996) and in association with upper and lower limb movement (Hodges & Richardson 1998, 1999) in patients with low back pain further illustrate the importance of the musculature associated with the spine. The implication is that the highly sophisticated, coordinated, and instantaneously changing activation patterns of the muscles associated with the spine profoundly influence spinal stability.

Earlier work postulated that muscles of the spine can be grouped into: (1) 'local muscles,' which span and consequently act over only a few segments; and (2) 'global muscles,' which extend over much greater regions of the spine and act regionally over a much greater area of the spine (Crisco & Panjabi 1991, Panjabi et al 1989, Wilke et al 1995). However, recent studies have suggested that it is not a single local or global muscle that is responsible for spine stability, but rather muscle activity over the spine changes instantaneously in response to the loads applied and the tasks required (Cholewicki & McGill 1996, Cholewicki & VanVlier 2002, Kavcic et al 2004). The diverse roles of the trunk musculature suggest that rather than focus a rehabilitation program on one or two isolated muscles, training efforts should be designed to target multiple muscles that can influence spinal loading conditions and the various motor programs that multiple muscle groups are responsible for. Thus the importance of understanding the muscular slings and anatomical linkages that are associated with the lumbopelvic region.

This chapter examines how muscles are linked to each other through fascial and ligamentous connections, and how the force of muscle contraction is potentially passed via specialized connective tissues to the skeletal structures and lumbopelvic articulations. Rather than looking at isolated muscle action over the lumbar spine, the focus will be on the neuromuscular apparatus of the trunk, hips, and shoulder girdle, as the optimal prescription for low back pain might in fact simply be the conditioning of the muscular linkages of the trunk, pelvic girdle, and shoulder girdle. This chapter examines these anatomical linkages with the intent of providing the anatomical basis for the design of exercise programs, specifically, resistance exercise programs that are intended to improve strength, stiffness, and functional abilities of the muscles. The anatomical discussion will occur around the three key fascial systems influencing the lumbopelvic region: thoracolumbar, fascia lata, and abdominal.

Thoracolumbar fascia system

The thoracolumbar fascia is a dense network that extends from the sacrum to the upper back and neck. It is especially prominent in the low back region and is generally described as consisting of three layers of connective tissue, which enclose the erector spinae, multifidus, and quadratus lumborum muscles. The three layers merge laterally to serve as points of attachment for several different muscles, most notably the external oblique, internal oblique, and transversus abdominis (Fig. 2.1).

The posterior layer of the thoracolumbar fascia, attached to the spinous processes, is a bilaminar layer consisting of superficial and deep portions. It is the thickest and strongest of the three layers. It lies posterior to the erector spinae and multifidus muscles, and is the only layer of the thoracolumbar fascia to extend into the thoracic region. The middle layer, which is attached to the lumbar transverse processes, separates the deeper, lumbar portion of the erector spinae muscle from the quadratus lumborum muscle. The thinner anterior layer covers the anterior surface of the quadratus lumborum muscle. This results in the anterior layer of the thoracolumbar fascia lying directly posterior to the psoas major muscle. The anterior layer of the fascia becomes thicker as it is followed cranialward, whereby it contributes to the formation of the lateral lumbocostal arch, which gives rise to the attachment of the diaphragm. The diaphragm, working in conjunction with the transversus abdominis and pelvic floor, plays an important role in increasing stiffness of the lumbar spine by increasing intra-abdominal pressure (Hodges et al 2003).

The posterior layer of the thoracolumbar fascia is designed to transmit forces between the shoulder girdle, lumbar spine, pelvic girdle, and lower extremity (Barker & Briggs 1999, Hodges & Richardson 1996, Vleeming et al 1995). Contraction of muscles that are attached to the fascial network, e.g. the latissimus dorsi, gluteus maximus, and abdominal muscles, results in increased fascial tension (Barker et al 2004, Gracovetsky et al 1985, Hodges & Richardson 1997, Tesh et al 1987). Muscles within the fascial envelope also increase fascial tension by virtue of the broadening effect

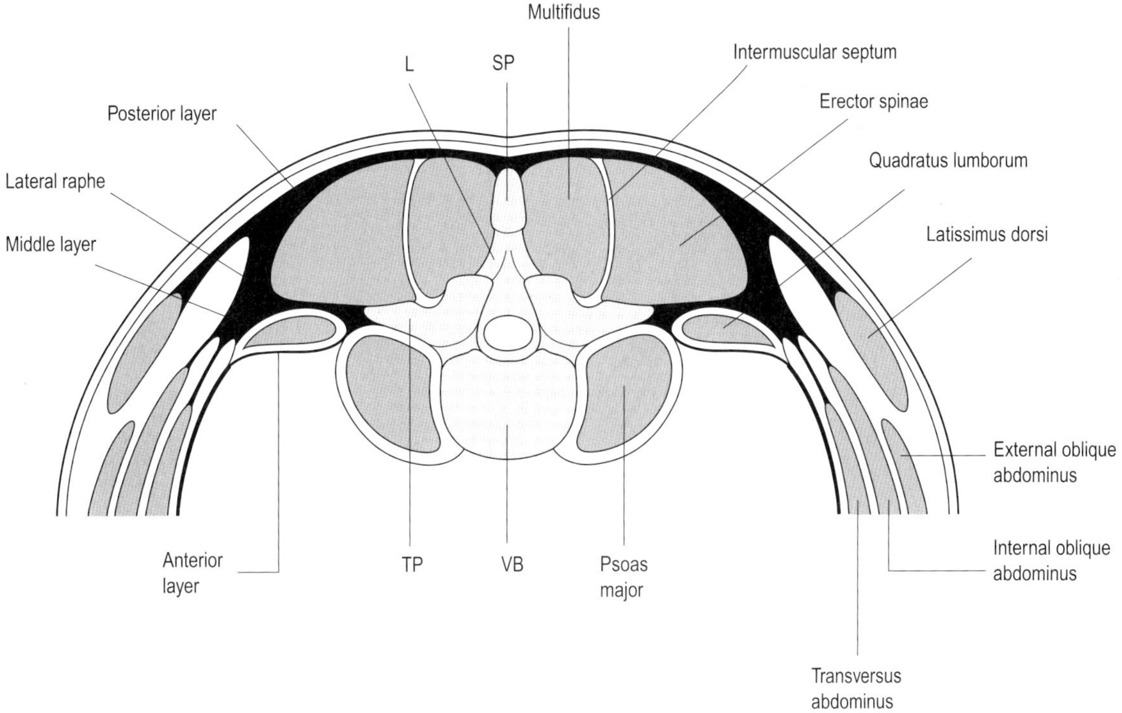

Fig. 2.1 Cross-section of the lumbar spine illustrating the anatomical relationships of the thoracolumbar fascia. The lateral extent where the anterior, middle, and posterior layers converge is the lateral raphe. L, lamina; SP, spinous process; TP, transverse process; VB, vertebral body. (From Porterfield & DeRosa 1998, p 64.)

of the muscle's contraction. This is described as a 'pushing' effect of the muscles within the fascial cylinder which further increases fascial tension and results in stiffening of the spinal column (Fig. 2.2) (Gracovetsky et al 1977, Hukins et al 1990). Several linkages between the thoracolumbar fascia and selected muscles are especially noteworthy in considering the mechanisms by which spinal stability might be augmented and are discussed in the following sections.

Latissimus dorsi–gluteus maximus linkage

The latissimus dorsi and gluteus maximus muscles are linked to the superolateral and inferolateral aspects of the posterior layer of the thoracolumbar fascia, respectively (Fig. 2.3). Individually, each muscle has the potential to increase tension to the thoracolumbar fascia contralaterally as well as ipsilaterally (Vleeming et al 1995). As the thoracolumbar fascia is attached to each lumbar vertebra and spans the upper aspect of the sacroiliac articulation, 'cinching' the fascia through contraction of these two muscles stiffens the lumbar spine over multiple spinal segments, potentially minimizing aberrational translatory motion between the lumbar vertebrae. Because the fascial complex crosses the upper aspect of the sacroiliac joint, compression is increased between the sacrum and ilium, enhancing the ability of this joint to attenuate shear loads (Porterfield & DeRosa 1998, Vleeming et al 1990). Adaptive changes in the connective tissue matrix of the posterior layer might occur as a result of strengthening of the latissimus dorsi and gluteus maximus. More likely, however, strengthening programs not only improve muscle strength but result in changes in motor programs due to enhanced neural drive. Such training increases stiffness of the muscle with a resultant increased resting muscle tension, which, in the case of the latissimus dorsi and gluteus maximus, increases tension to the posterior layer of the thoracolumbar fascia.

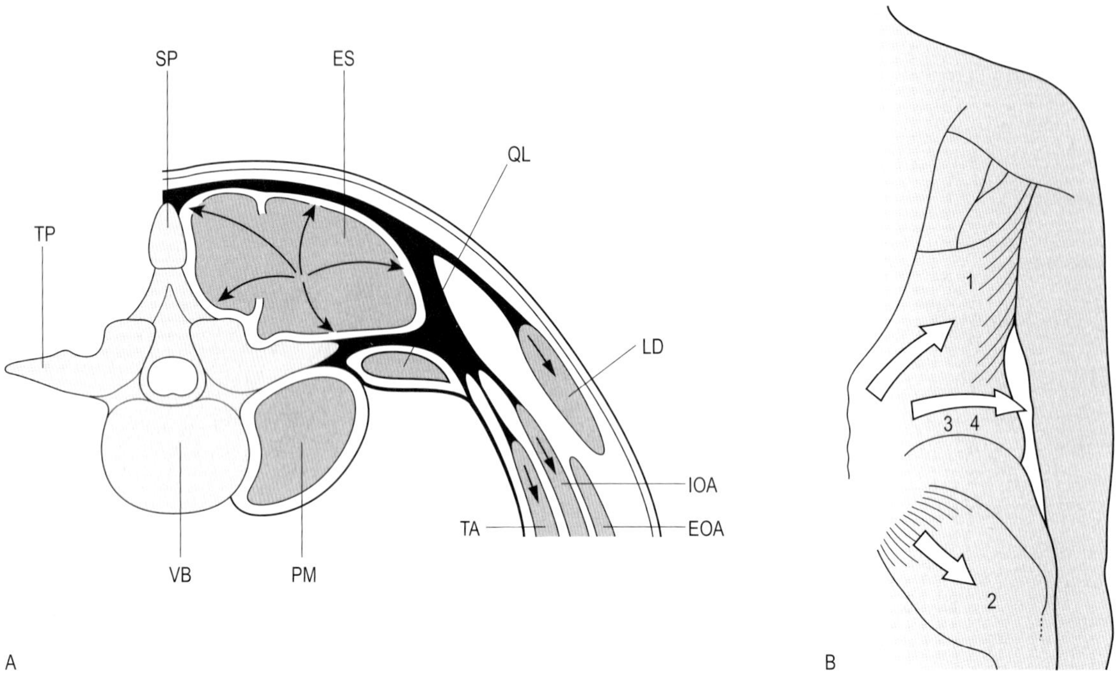

Fig. 2.2 (A) Muscle contraction resulting in increased tension to thoracolumbar fascia. EOA, external oblique; ES, erector spinae; IOA, internal oblique; LD, latissimus dorsi; PM, psoas major; QL, quadratus lumborum; SP, spinous process; TA, transversus abdominis; VB, vertebral body; TP, transverse process. (B) Posterior view of the musculature that attaches to the thoracolumbar fascia. Note the forces that are generated to the fascia from the latissimus dorsi muscle (1) from above, the gluteus maximus muscle (2) from below, and the internal oblique abdominis muscle (3) and transversus abdominis muscle (4) from the front. (From Porterfield & DeRosa 1998, p 67.)

Obliques and transversus abdominis muscles

Posteriorly, the external abdominal oblique, internal abdominal oblique, and transversus abdominis muscles attach at the lateral raphe, which is the junction of the posterior and middle layers of the thoracolumbar fascia. The transversus abdominis attachment is quite extensive and results in the muscle influencing all lumbar levels, whereas the internal oblique has primary influence over the lower lumbar levels and the external oblique over the upper lumbar levels (Barker et al 2004). The attachments of the transversus abdominis to the fascia at the lower lumbar levels is of clinical importance because contraction of the transversus abdominis stabilizes the spine to provide a stable axial platform from which the upper and lower extremities can act. Intramuscular electromyography (EMG) analysis suggests that the transversus abdominis exhibits contraction prior to perturbations of the trunk and before rapid limb movements are initiated (Hodges & Richardson 1997, 1998). The especially strong attachment of the internal oblique and the transversus abdominis to the middle layer of the thoracolumbar fascia provides a nearly direct pull to the lumbar transverse processes, which – in particular – provides effective stabilization of the spinal segments of the lumbar spine in the transverse and frontal planes. The linkage of the abdominal mechanism with the shoulder girdle, and the linkage of the obliques and transversus abdominis to the rectus abdominis, are discussed later.

The erector spinae and multifidus muscles

Anatomically, the erector spinae muscles – both the superficial and deep portions – consist of an iliocostalis portion and a more medially placed longissimus portion. The erector spinae and the multifidus are discussed in the context of the thoracolumbar fascia to fully appreciate the multiple roles they serve in mobility and stability of the lumbopelvic region. For the purposes of this chapter,

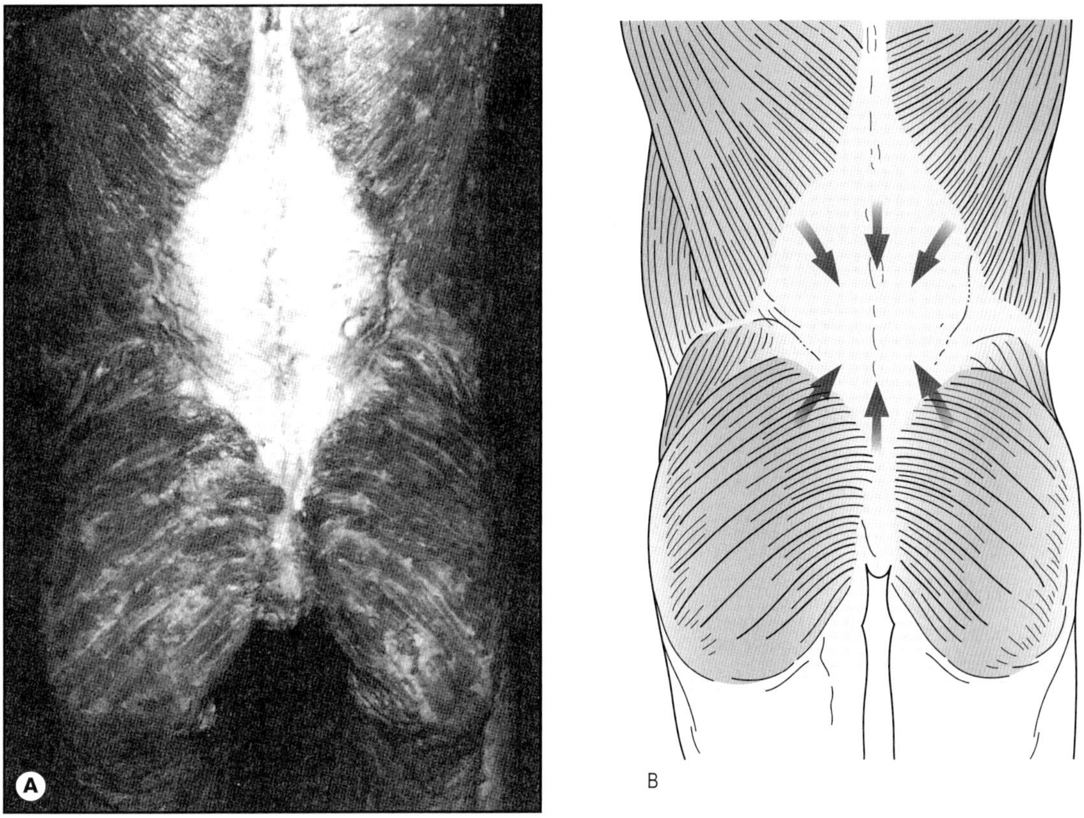

Fig. 2.3 Dissection and drawing of the latissimus dorsi and gluteus maximus attachments to thoracolumbar fascia. (From Porterfield & DeRosa 1998, p 66.)

the superficial erector spinae is the component that attaches to the thoracic spine and ribs (the thoracic erector spinae), whereas the deep erector spinae is that part attached to the transverse processes of the lumbar vertebrae (lumbar erector spinae). The caudal fascicles of the thoracic part form a strong, broad tendinous attachment to the ilium and the sacrum referred to as the erector spinae aponeurosis (Fig. 2.4). As a result of its attachments, the thoracic erector spinae muscle acts over the lumbar spine, but not via direct attachments to it. Contraction of the muscle moves the thorax posteriorly over the lumbar spine, resulting in an extension moment to the lumbar region and a compressive load to the lumbar segments. The superficial thoracic erector spinae muscle and the anteroinferior portion of the internal oblique muscle have been shown to be preferentially activated in erect standing and sitting postures and less active in passive trunk postures (O'Sullivan et al 2002).

The broad erector spinae aponeurosis has a direct attachment to the kyphotically oriented sacrum, and exerts a flexion or nutation moment on the sacrum. Sacral nutation serves to increase the tension of the key ligamentous structures of the sacroiliac joint, most notably the sacrotuberous, sacrospinous, and interosseous ligaments, thus enhancing sacroiliac joint stability via the pull of the thoracic erector spinae on the sacrum through the erector spinae aponeurosis (Fig. 2.5).

The lumbar portion of the erector spinae has been dissected and described but with slightly conflicting results (Bustami 1986). Most recently, the attachments of the lumbar portion of the erector spinae have been described as originating from the ventral surface of the erector spinae aponeurosis and the ilium along the area of the posterior superior iliac spine from which they course cranially toward the accessory and transverse processes of the lumbar vertebrae (Daggfeldt et al 2000). The anteriorly placed attachment to the transverse processes serves as a dynamic check for anterior shear of the lumbar vertebrae (Porterfield & DeRosa 1998). Note the posterior–anterior 'guy wire' effect that the orientation of the deep erector spinae and the psoas major has in contributing to the stability

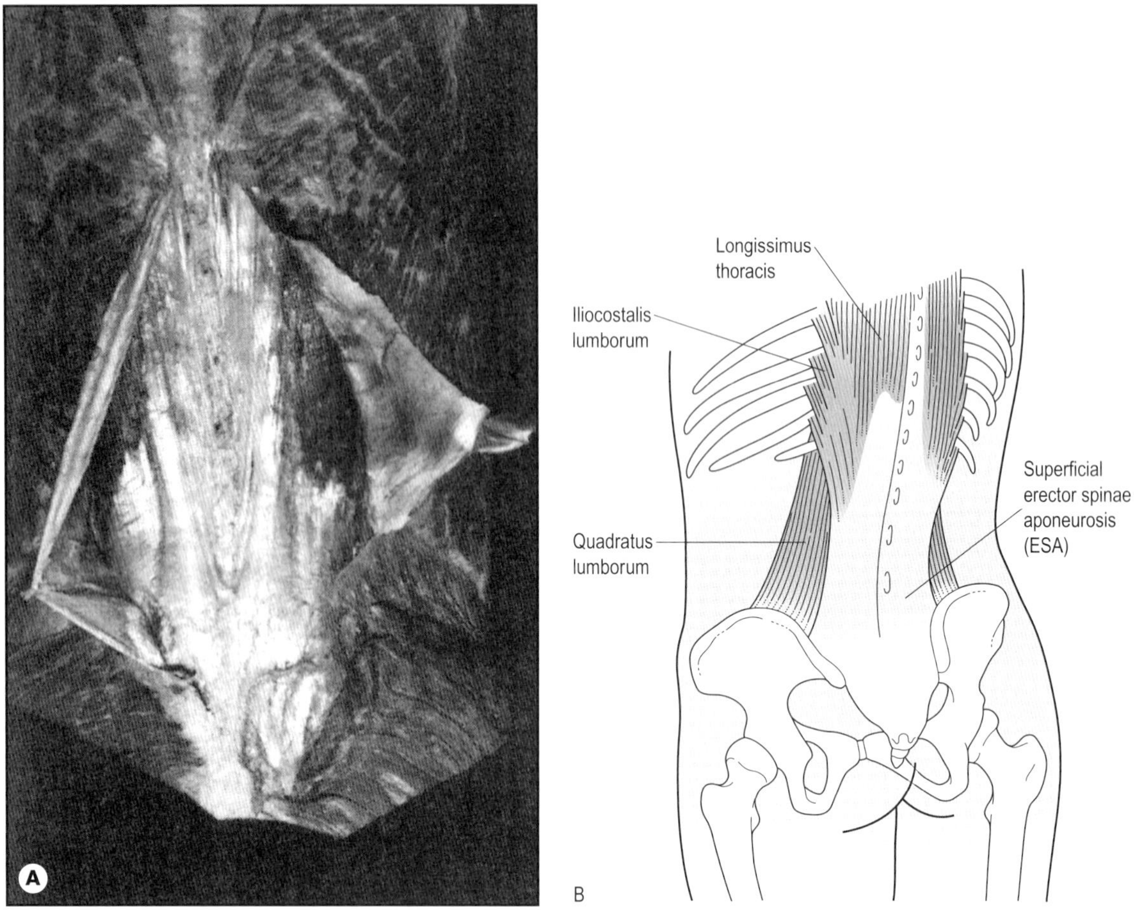

Fig. 2.4 Erector spinae aponeurosis. (From Porterfield & DeRosa 1998, p 71.)

of the lumbar spine (Fig. 2.6). These two muscles form a muscle sling that simultaneously contributes to compression of the lumbar spinal segments and provides a dynamic restraint to anterior–posterior shear stresses in the lumbar spine. The lumbar erector spinae muscles have been described as being more active than the thoracic erector spinae in patients with low back pain, presumably because of their more direct effect in contributing to lumbar stability (van Dieen et al 2003).

The multifidus muscle is recognized as an important stabilizer of the lumbar spine, which has been seen to undergo various morphologic changes in conditions of low back pain (Hides et al 1996, Moseley et al 2002, Yoshihara et al 2001). The superficial aspect of the multifidus serves as an extensor of the lumbar spine due to its spinous process attachments. This spinous process attachment, lying well posterior to the axis motion in the lumbar spine, gives the muscle an excellent lever arm for lumbar extension. The deeper part of the multifidus acts over individual lumbar spinal segments in compression rather than torque as its attachments to the inferior border of the lamina, mamillary processes, and facet joint capsules of the lumbar vertebrae are nearer the axis of motion of the lumbar spine. Relative to the thoracolumbar fascia, contraction of the multifidus and the erector spinae results in increased tension to the thoracolumbar fascia by virtue of the broadening effect of muscle as it contracts (see Fig. 2.2A). Atrophy of the multifidus is seen in patients with chronic back pain, and with such a deficit, one might assume loss of the stabilization role of the multifidus as well as loss of fascial tension generating ability within the thoracolumbar fascial envelope (Cooper et al 1992, Kader et al 2000, Rantanen et al 1993). The most effective training method that influences the cross sectional area (hypertrophy) of the multifidus muscle in patients

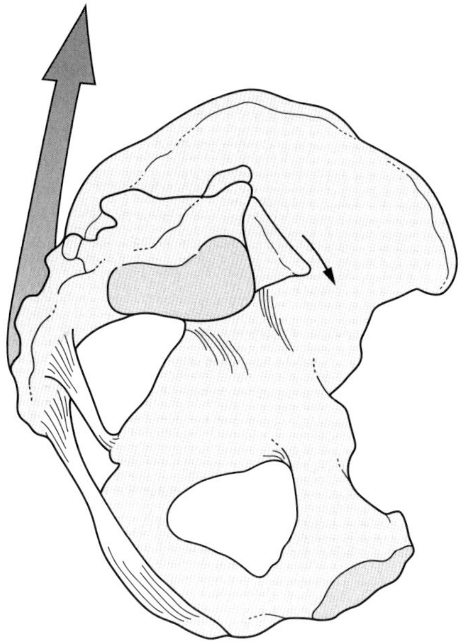

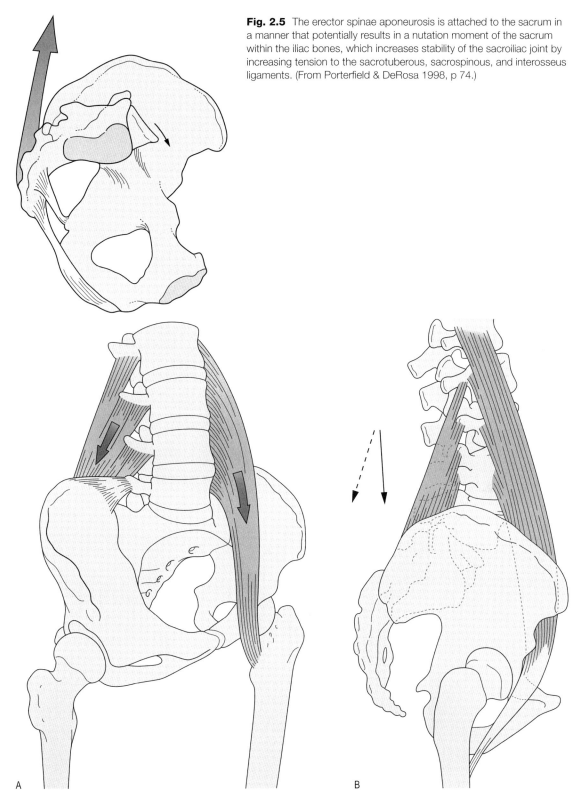

Fig. 2.5 The erector spinae aponeurosis is attached to the sacrum in a manner that potentially results in a nutation moment of the sacrum within the iliac bones, which increases stability of the sacroiliac joint by increasing tension to the sacrotuberous, sacrospinous, and interosseus ligaments. (From Porterfield & DeRosa 1998, p 74.)

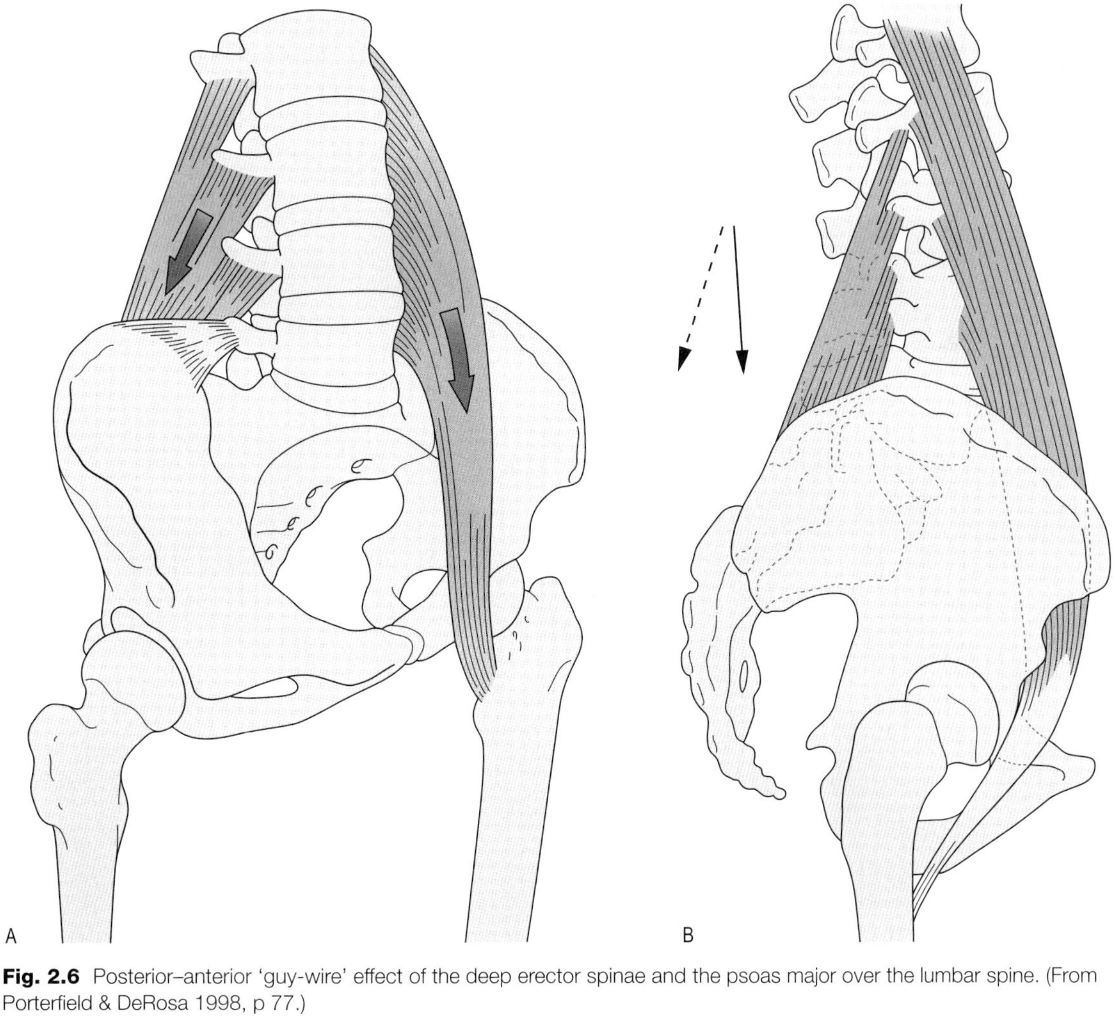

Fig. 2.6 Posterior–anterior 'guy-wire' effect of the deep erector spinae and the psoas major over the lumbar spine. (From Porterfield & DeRosa 1998, p 77.)

with low back pain is dynamic motion of the spine against resistance combined with a static hold between the concentric and eccentric phases of the exercise (Danneels et al 2001).

Fascia lata system

The muscles, fascial networks, and ligaments of the hips and pelvis form several important slings and anatomical linkages that contribute to the stability of the lumbar spine and sacroiliac joint. Exercise therapy, specifically through strengthening of the gluteus maximus, hamstrings, and quadriceps is an integral component of a comprehensive rehabilitation program for mechanical low back pain due to these linkages. The fascia lata serves as the point from which the discussion of the linkage between the lower extremity and the spine can take place.

The fascia lata is a strong network of connective tissue that surrounds the thigh musculature. It is thickest in its lateral aspect and this aspect is often referred to as the iliotibial tract. Muscles attach to the fascia lata – most notably the gluteus maximus and the tensor fascia lata – and several large muscles are encased within the fascia. These include the quadriceps, the hamstrings, and the adductor group.

Gluteus maximus linkage

The linkage between the gluteus maximus and the latissimus dorsi through the thoracolumbar fascia was described in the preceding sections. This section focuses on the distal attachment of the gluteus maximus. The primary distal attachment of the gluteus maximus as it courses from the pelvis to the lower extremity is into the fascia lata. Only the deeper third of this large muscle is attached to the femur; the larger part of the muscle blends in with the lateral aspect of the fascia lata. Thus the gluteus maximus serves as a muscular linkage between the two major fascial systems of the lumbopelvic region – the thoracolumbar fascia and the fascia lata (Fig. 2.7). This creates one of the most important muscle slings over the lumbopelvic region. Both fascial networks envelope large muscle masses, the thoracolumbar fascia encasing the erector spinae and multifidus (as described above), and the fascia lata encasing the quadriceps, hamstrings, and adductors (described below).

Therefore the gluteus maximus links more than a one-dimensional fascial sheet that crosses several areas of the spine. Instead, it links two fascial complexes that are essentially three-dimensional compartments containing the key muscles of the

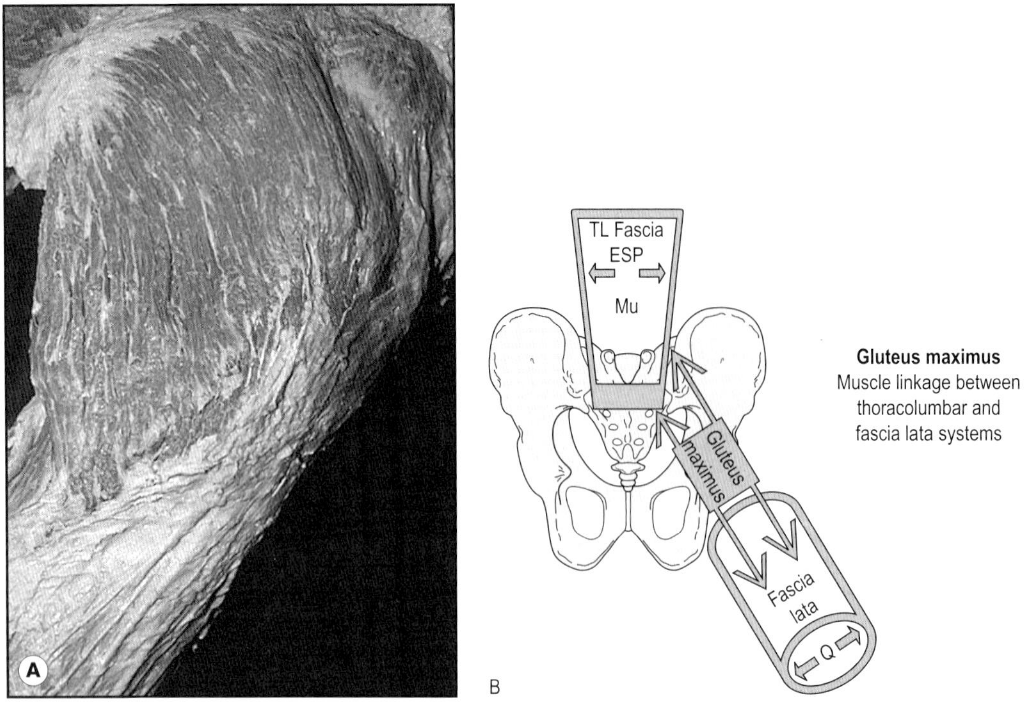

Fig. 2.7 The gluteus maximus muscle serves as the muscular linkage between the thoracolumbar fascial system and the fascia lata system. ESp, erector spinae; Mu, multifidus; Q, quadratus lumborum; TL, thoracolumbar.

spine and of the thigh. Contraction of the gluteus maximus, or an increase in its stiffness, results in enhanced tension of these two important fascial networks that span the lumbar spine, sacroiliac joint, and hips.

Thigh musculature within the fascia lata and the relationship to the muscle slings of the gluteus maximus

Several large muscle groups are encased within the fascia lata envelope. As the quadriceps take origin from the posterior aspect of the femur (linea aspera) and subsequently converge to the anterior aspect of the femur, they are a significant muscle mass within the fascia lata cylinder. Like the multifidus and erector spinae within the thoracolumbar fascial network, the contraction of the quadriceps within the fascia lata results in increased tension to the fascia by virtue of the broadening effect of the muscle contraction (Fig. 2.8). Note that tension in the fascia lata is augmented through two different powerful mechanisms: (1) the pull from the externally placed gluteus maximus; and (2) the push from the internally placed quadriceps.

This increased stiffness of the fascia lata serves an important role in lumbopelvic mechanics because the gluteus maximus exerts a powerful influence over the pelvis through its attachments to the sacrotuberous ligament, the pelvis, and the lumbar spine through the lumbopelvic fascial connections to the lumbar spine. This is especially relevant when one is in the standing position. Lumbopelvic extension to an upright position from a forward, flexed position initially occurs primarily through the actions of the musculature at the hip (McClure et al 1997). The efficient control of dynamic motion of the pelvis and lumbar spine in the standing position is in part dependent on the action of the gluteus maximus, which extends the pelvis over the femur as a result of the stable fascial platform provided from the stiffness generated within the fascia lata as a result of the action of the quadriceps.

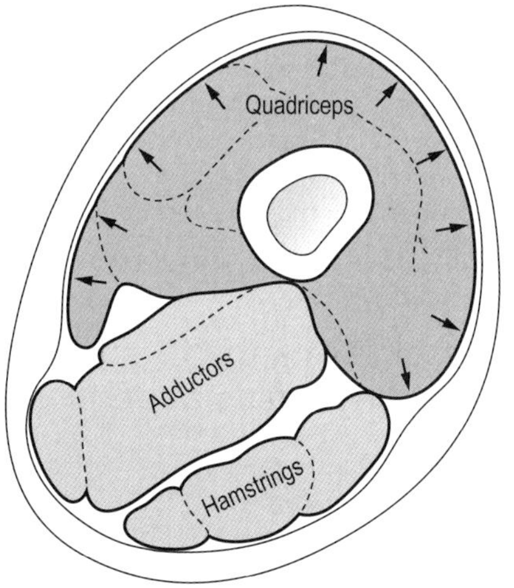

Fig. 2.8 Contraction of the quadriceps within the fascia lata system results in a 'pushing' effect within the fascia lata complex, increasing the tension to the fascia. (From Porterfield & DeRosa 1998, p 113.)

The hamstrings

The hamstrings lie within the fascia lata envelope, and the girth of the muscle and resting state of muscle tension also contribute to the tension of the fascia lata. The hamstrings act directly over the pelvis through their attachments to the ischial tuberosity, and contribute to the stability of the sacroiliac joint through their linkage with the sacrotuberous ligament (Fig. 2.9). Increased tension to the sacrotuberous ligament enhances stability of the sacroiliac joint because the sacrotuberous ligament minimizes nutation of the sacrum and posterior torsion of the ilium. Increased tension in the sacrotuberous ligament during nutation can be due to nutation itself, but with the available motion of the sacroiliac joint being so small, increased ligamentous tension occurs by way of contraction of the biceps femoris and/or the gluteus maximus muscle (Vleeming et al 1996). These mechanisms ultimately assist in helping to control the torque and shear of the sacrum within the ilium.

Abdominal fascial system

Like the thoracolumbar and fascia lata systems, the abdominal fascial system features muscles encased within the fascial network, the paired abdominis muscles, and muscles that are attached to the fascial network, the transversus abdominis, internal abdominal, and the external abdominal (Fig. 2.10). Contraction of these latter muscles increases tension to the abdominal fascia in the same way that the latissimus dorsi and gluteus maximus increase tension to the thoracolumbar fascia. In addition to the abdominal muscles, the pectoralis major muscle is linked to the abdominal fascia and the serratus anterior is linked to the external

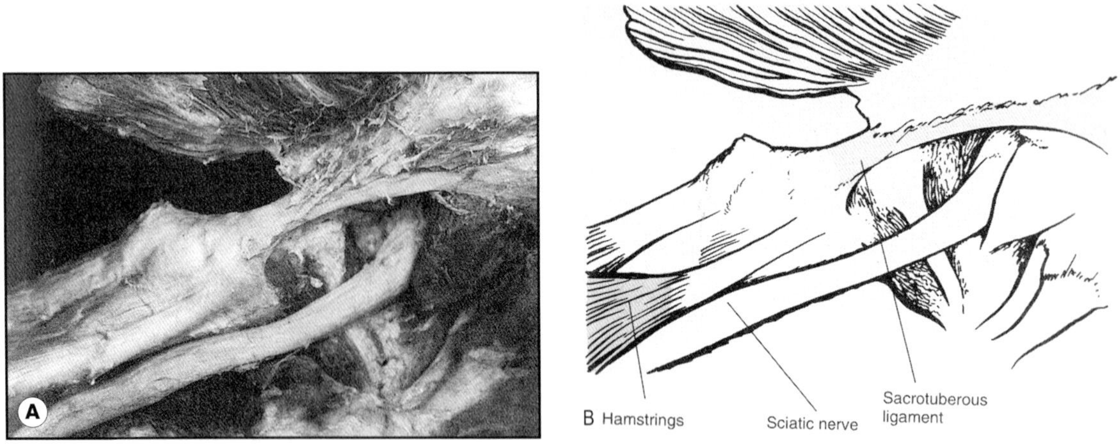

Fig. 2.9 The hamstrings – primarily the biceps femoris – are seen to be continuous with the sacrotuberous ligament. Contraction of the hamstrings increases tension to this extrinsic sacroiliac ligament, checking nutation of the sacrum and posterior torsion of the ilium. (From Porterfield & DeRosa 1998, p 107.)

abdominal oblique muscle. This in effect forms a muscle sling from the shoulder girdle through the abdominal mechanism and pelvis (this is described further below).

The abdominal fascia is directly related to the abdominal muscles, and presents as the aponeuroses of the external and internal abdominal oblique and transverse abdominis muscles, and the rectus sheath, which is related to the rectus abdominis muscle (Porterfield & DeRosa 1998). As the aponeuroses of the obliques and transversus abdominis muscles course anteriorly, they enclose the rectus abdominis to form the rectus sheath. However, the formation of the rectus sheath by the different layers of aponeuroses is different in the region above the umbilicus, and also below the umbilicus. The anteriorly placed lattice-work arrangement of the abdominal fascia is similar to the lattice-work of the thoracolumbar fascia posteriorly.

The rectus abdominis muscle is surrounded by its own fascial layer (the rectus sheath), formed by the individual aponeurotic contributions of the transversus abdominis, external oblique, and internal oblique muscles as they converge toward the linea alba. Cranial/superior to the umbilicus the external oblique muscle sends its aponeurosis anterior to the rectus abdominis. The aponeurosis of the internal abdominal oblique muscle splits at the lateral border of the rectus abdominis, and the aponeurosis passes anterior and posterior to it. The aponeurosis of the transversus abdominis muscle travels on the posterior side of the rectus abdominis muscle.

Below the umbilicus, all three lateral abdominal muscles pass aponeurotic expansions anterior to the rectus abdominis muscle. Such an arrangement offers additional connective tissue support to counter the anterior shear stress of the lumbar spine and abdominal visceral in this region. The extra fascial support can be viewed as a response to the forces generated from the lordotic angle at the corresponding level in the lumbar spine (i.e. the L4–L5 and L5–S1 region). In this region of the lumbar spine, the rate of curvature is greater than the rate of curvature of the upper lumbar spine. Accompanying this lordotic curve is the increased caudally and anteriorly directed force of the abdominal contents, which helps to create the need for the additional connective tissue support (Porterfield & DeRosa 1998).

Rectus abdominis linkage to obliques and transversus abdominis

The rectus abdominis muscle extends vertically from the pubic tubercles to attach to the lower rib cage on either side of the sternum and features intermuscular connective tissue bands. The oblique muscles attach to the rectus sheath at the level of these tendinous intersections, thereby exerting a laterally directed force to the rectus sheath and anchoring these tendinous intersections

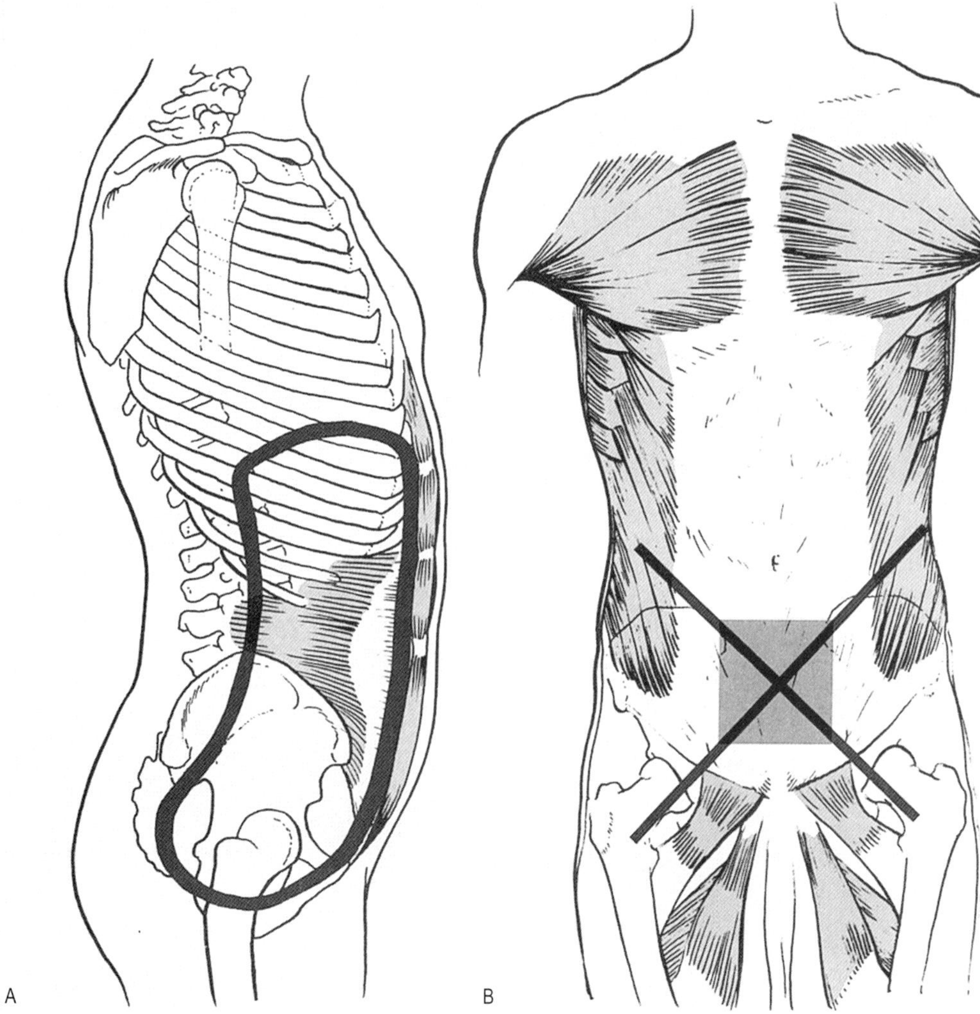

Fig. 2.10 The abdominal fascia formed from the aponeuroses of the abdominal muscles. Note the linkage of the pectoralis major muscle to the fascia. (From Porterfield & DeRosa 2004, p 86.)

(Fig. 2.11). Note how such a muscular sling affords a mechanical link between the pull of the obliques and the pull of the rectus abdominis. A lateral pull at the intermuscular septa stabilizes the rectus attachments and in essence results in the rectus abdominis functioning segmentally rather than simply as one long strap muscle.

External abdominal oblique, pectoralis major, and serratus anterior muscles

The abdominal muscles are extremely important muscles with regard to stability of the lumbar spine and pelvis and there is good evidence that the recruitment of the abdominal muscles is altered in the presence of low back pain (Ferreira et al 2004, Hungerford et al 2003). Fig. 2.12 illustrates the anterior and lateral extent of the abdominal fascia. The most superficial muscles contributing to the anterior and anterolateral abdominal wall include the external oblique, the pectoralis major, and the serratus anterior. The latter two shoulder girdle muscles provide an important muscular sling that links the shoulder girdle to the abdominal mechanism and will be detailed below following a description of all of the abdominal muscles. Note that the line of pull on the abdominal fascia of the external oblique muscle would be cranial-

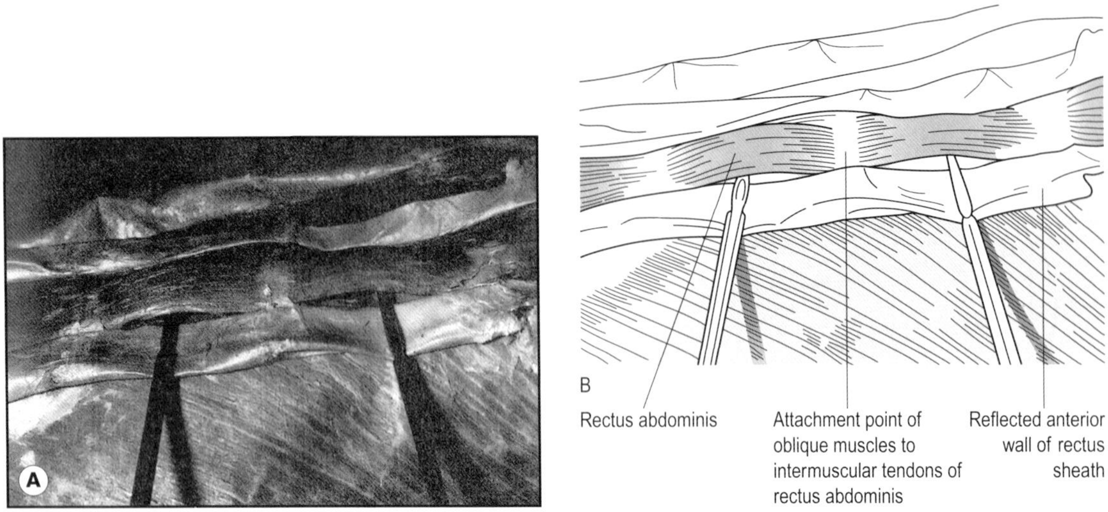

Fig. 2.11 Anchoring of the intermuscular septa of the rectus abdominis is via the oblique muscles and the transversus abdominis muscles. This linkage enhances the efficiency of the rectus abdominis muscles by creating fixed tendinous points from which it can then act. (From Porterfield & DeRosa 1998, p 97.)

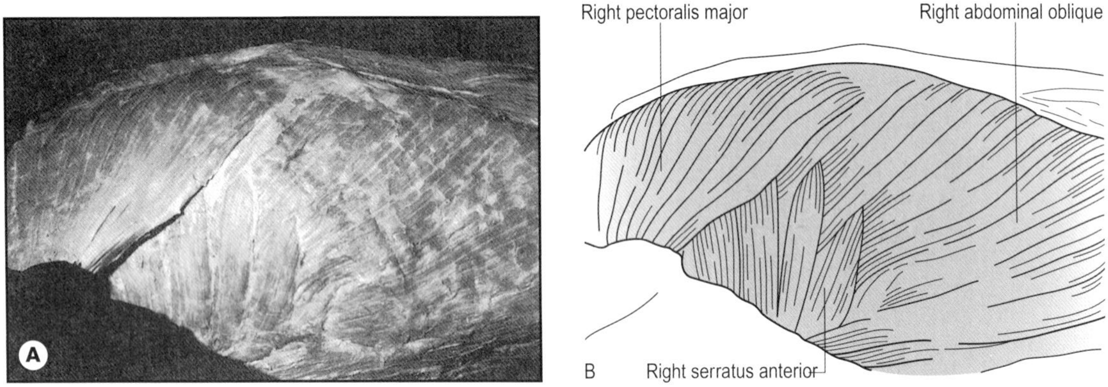

Fig. 2.12 The serratus anterior muscle interdigitates with the external abdominal oblique muscle. There is a strong linkage with the pectoralis major, serratus anterior, and abdominal muscles. (From Porterfield & DeRosa 1998, p 92.)

ward and posterior. In addition, close inspection of the pectoralis major muscle reveals that its lower attachment is also to the abdominal fascia and that contraction of the pectoralis major muscle also increases the tension to the upper aspect of the abdominal fascia. Whereas a small component of the external oblique attaches to the upper aspect of the thoracolumbar fascia, the primary attachment of this muscle is to the ribs, where the serrated edges of the external oblique interdigitate with the serratus anterior muscle.

Internal abdominal oblique muscle

The internal oblique is a substantial muscle, often thicker than the transversus abdominis or the external oblique. It has a large attachment to the iliac crest and the thoracolumbar fascia. Its attachment to the thoracolumbar fascia is primarily at the key lower lumbar segments. The more inferiorly placed portion of the muscle exerts a pull on the pelvis, a motion that is medially directed, effectively increasing compression of the pubic

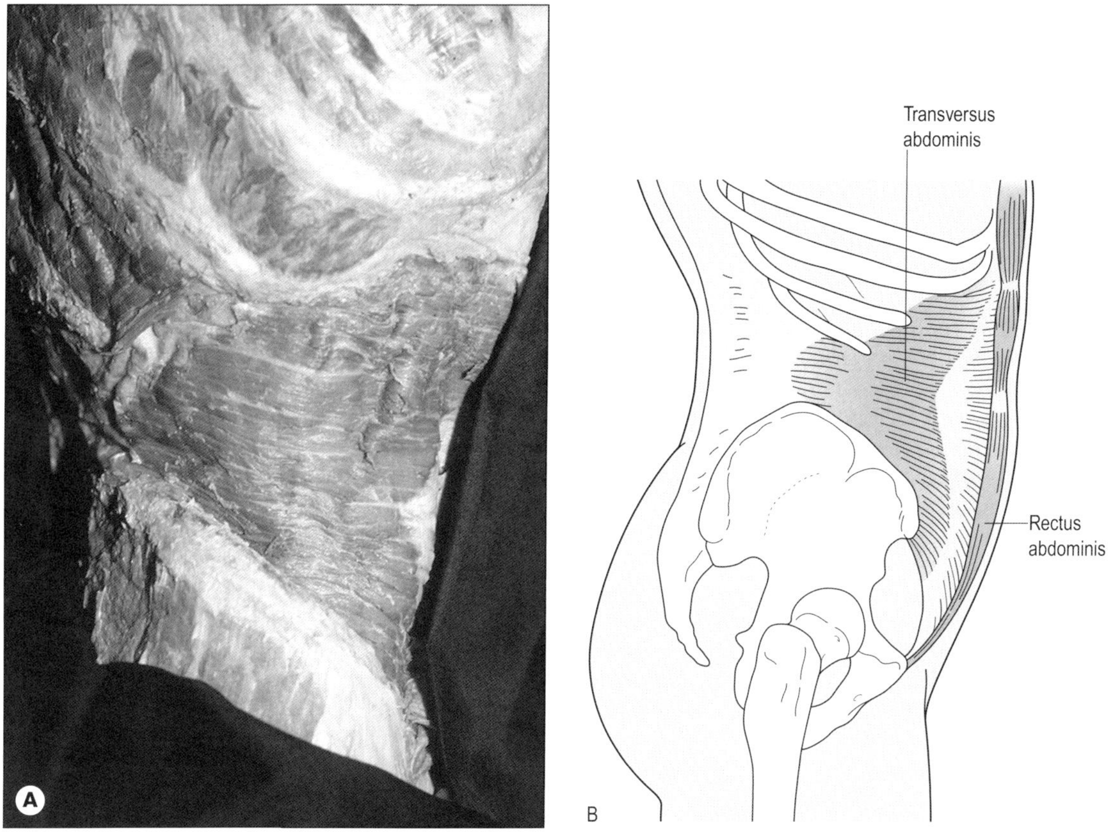

Fig. 2.13 The transversus abdominis is attached posteriorly to the thoracolumbar fascia and anteriorly to the abdominal fascia. Note that it has an optimal muscle fiber orientation to pull posteriorly on the abdominal fascia, complimenting the more angled forces on the fascia exerted by the external and internal abdominal oblique muscles. (From Porterfield & DeRosa 1998, p92.)

symphysis. This muscular sling is complimented by the muscle pull of the hip adductors, which also act to increase compression at the region of the pubic symphysis via a muscle pull that is caudal and medialward (Hungerford et al 2003). Note, however, that the internal abdominal oblique component of this sling requires the transference of the force of muscle contraction through the abdominal fascia. The superior and middle extent of this muscle can exert a powerful forward and elevation movement of the pelvis – a motion that is essential in sprinting, for example. This aspect of the internal abdominal oblique can also exert a caudal and posterior-directed force to the abdominal fascia. Thus its line of force over the abdominal fascia is approximately at right angles to the pull of the external abdominal oblique.

Transversus abdominis muscle

The transversus abdominis is a key stabilizer of the lumbar spine and evidence suggests that a rehabilitation focus on its role in stabilization of the spine helps to decrease low back pain and enhance function (O'Sullivan et al 1997, Richardson et al 2002, Shaughnessy & Caulfield 2004). The transversus abdominis is optimally aligned for a posterior pull on the abdominal fascial complex (see Fig. 2.13). This posteriorly directed pull, especially around the slightly pressurized abdominal cylinder, compliments the more angled pulls of the external and internal abdominal oblique muscles. Thus the pull of the abdominal muscles 'cinches' the abdomen with a corset-like effect and brings the abdominal contents posterior against the lumbar spine, which serves as another check to anterior shear of the lumbar vertebrae. In addition, this posterior pull, combined with the contraction of the diaphragm and the pelvic floor, increases intra-abdominal pressure, further assisting in stabilization of the lumbar spine.

Linkage of the shoulder girdle and abdominal mechanism

Like the linkage of the lower extremity to the trunk muscles, the shoulder girdle is also intimately linked to the abdominal mechanism. On the posterior aspect of the spine, the rhomboid major and minor muscles angle inferiorly and laterally from their thoracic spinous processes origin to reach the medial border of the scapula. This area of the scapula is the precise region where the serratus anterior is attached and the two muscles can be seen to be anatomically linked to each other (Fig. 2.14). When the serratus anterior is followed laterally around the trunk from this scapular attachment, it can be seen to interdigitate and often fuse with the external abdominal oblique (see Fig. 2.12). If the line of direction of the muscle fibers in the external abdominal oblique is followed across the midline of the body, it can be seen to lie parallel to the muscle fiber direction of the contralateral internal abdominal oblique, thus forming a continuous muscle sling from the shoulder girdle to the abdominal wall (Fig. 2.15).

Summary

As muscles are largely responsible for our ability to assume and maintain postures, and they control the acceleration and deceleration of movement, an optimal balance between stabilizing and moving the spinal segments must occur instantaneously as well as continuously. In the clinical setting, the spectrum of exercise is often a continuum of care that starts with pain-modulating activities and progresses to patient instruction on postural positioning and 'how to' contract individual muscles. Ultimately, training of the neuromuscular system through carefully prescribed overload serves to influence strength, power, coordination, endurance, and stiffness of the muscles, and thus enhances the physical condition and overall health of the patient. Often, exercise programs begin with isolated training of specific muscles. However, although a good starting point in the rehabilitation process,

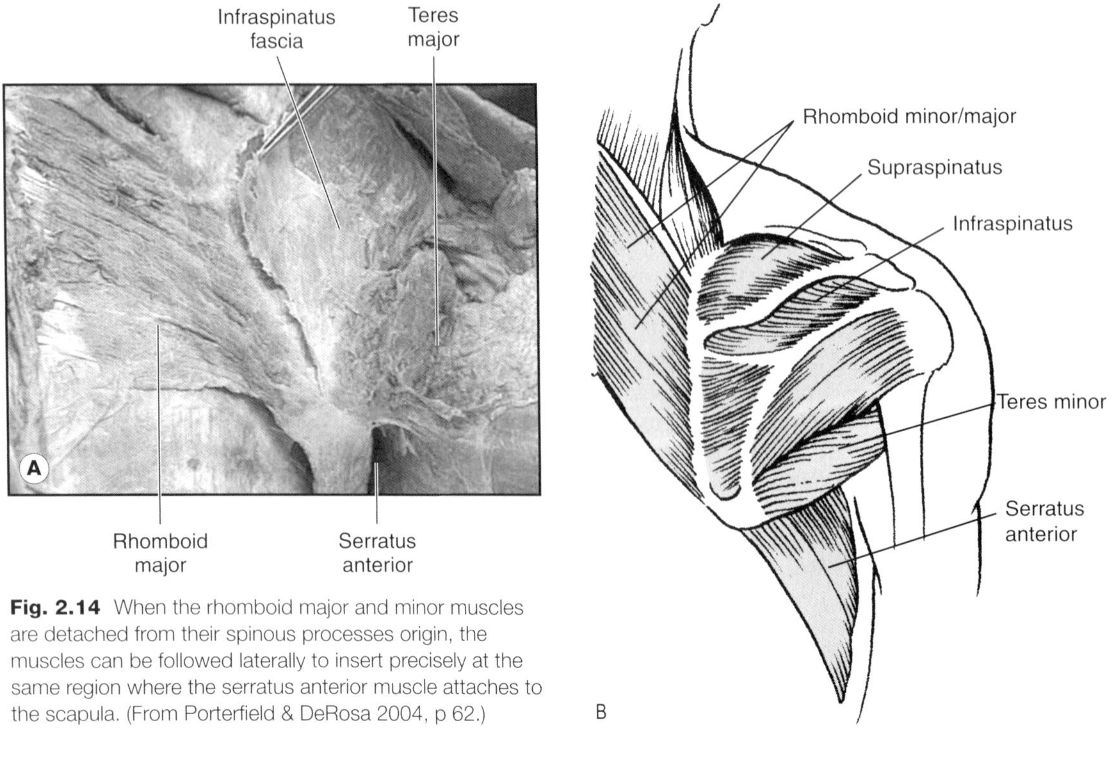

Fig. 2.14 When the rhomboid major and minor muscles are detached from their spinous processes origin, the muscles can be followed laterally to insert precisely at the same region where the serratus anterior muscle attaches to the scapula. (From Porterfield & DeRosa 2004, p 62.)

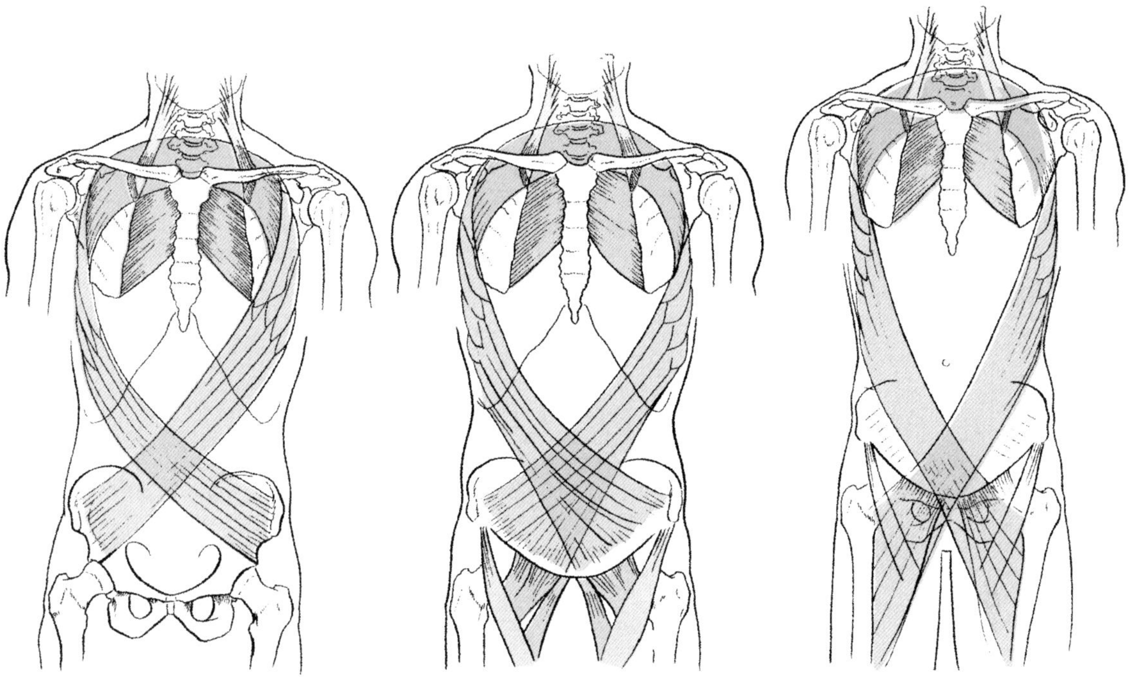

Fig. 2.15 Muscle sling of the shoulder girdle and abdominal mechanism. The muscle fiber line of the rhomboids is continuous with the line of pull of the serratus anterior. The serratus anterior interdigitates and is often fused with the external abdominal oblique, which has a muscle fiber line of force in parallel with the internal abdominal oblique on the opposite side of the body. (From Porterfield & DeRosa 2004, p 63.)

ultimately training multiple muscle groups and motor patterns through the muscle slings and anatomical linkages that tie the muscles of the pelvic girdle and shoulder girdle to the spine should be the rehabilitation focus.

References

Barker P, Briggs C 1999 Attachments of the posterior layer of lumbar fascia. Spine 24:1757–1764

Barker PJ, Briggs CA, Bogeski G 2004 Tensile transmission across the lumbar fasciae in unembalmed cadavers. Spine 29:129–138

Bergmark A 1989 Mechanical stability of the human lumbar spine: a study in mechanical engineering. Acta Orthopaedica Scandinavica 60:1–54

Bustami FM 1986 A new description of the lumbar erector spinae in man. Journal of Anatomy 144:81–91

Cholewicki J, McGill S 1996 Mechanical stability of the in vivo lumbar spine: implications for injury and chronic low back pain. Clinical Biomechanics 11:1–15

Cholewicki J, VanVlier J 2002 Relative contributions of trunk muscles to the stability of the lumbar spine during isometric exertions. Clinical Biomechanics 17:99–105

Cooper RG, St Clair Forbes W, Jayson MIV 1992 Radiographic demonstration of paraspinal muscle wasting in patients with chronic low back pain. British Journal of Rheumatology 31:389–394

Crisco JJ, Panjabi M 1991 The intersegmental and multisegmental muscles of the lumbar spine: a biomechanical model comparing lateral stabilizing potential. Spine 16:793–799

Daggfeldt K, Huang QM, Thorstensson A 2000 The visible human anatomy of the lumbar erector spinae. Spine 25:2719–2725

Danneels LA, Vanderstraeten GG, Cambier DC et al 2001 Effects of three different training modalities on the cross sectional area of the lumbar multifidus muscle in patients with chronic low back pain. British Journal of Sports Medicine 35:186–191

Ferreira P, Ferreira ML, Hodges PW 2004 Changes in recruitment of the abdominal muscles in people with low back pain: ultrasound measurement of muscle activity. Spine 29:2560–2566

Gracovetsky S, Farfan H, Lamy C 1977 A mathematical model of the lumbar spine using an optimized system to control muscles and ligaments. Orthopaedic Clinics of North America 8:135–153

Gracovetsky S, Farfan H, Helleur C 1985 The abdominal mechanism. Spine 10:317–324

Hides JA, Richardson CA, Jull G 1996 Multifidus muscle recovery is not automatic after resolution of acute first-episode low back pain. Spine 21:2763–2769

Hodges PW, Richardson CA 1996 Inefficient stabilization of the lumbar spine associated with low back pain: a motor control evaluation of transverses abdominis. Spine 21:2640–2650

Hodges PW, Richardson CA 1997 Feedforward contraction of transverses abdominis is not influenced by direction of arm movement. Experimental Brain Research 114:362–370

Hodges PW, Richardson CA 1998 Delayed postural contraction of transverses abdominis in low back pain associated with movement of the lower limb. Journal of Spinal Disorders 11:46–56

Hodges PW, Richardson CA 1999 Altered trunk recruitment in people with low back pain with upper limb movement at different speeds. Archives of Physical Medicine and Rehabilitation 80:1005–1012

Hodges P, Holm AK, Holm S et al 2003 Intervertebral stiffness of the spine is increased by evoked contraction of transversus abdominis and the diaphragm: In vivo porcine studies. Spine 28:2594–2601

Hukins DWL Aspden RM, Hickey DS 1990 Thoracolumbar fascia can increase the efficiency of the erector spinae muscles. Clinical Biomechanics 5:30–34

Hungerford B, Gilleard W, Hodges P 2003 Evidence of altered lumbopelvic muscle recruitment in the presence of sacroiliac pain. Spine 28:1593–1600

Kader DF, Wardlaw D, Smith FW 2000 Correlation between the MRI changes in the lumbar multifudus muscles and leg pain. Clinical Radiology 55(2):145–149

Kavcic N, Grenier S, McGill S 2004 Determining the stabilizing role of individual torso muscles during rehabilitation exercises. Spine 29:1254–1265

Magnusson ML, Aleksiev A, Wilder DG et al 1996 Unexpected load and asymmetric posture as etiologic factors in low back pain. European Spine Journal 5: 23–35

McClure P W, Esola M, Schreier R, Siegler S 1997 Kinematic analysis of lumbar and hip motion while rising from a forward, flexed position in patients with and without a history of low back pain. Spine 22:552–558

McIntosh JE, Bogduk N 1991 The morphology of the lumbar erector spinae. Spine 16:783–792

Moseley GL, Hodges PW, Gandevia SC 2002 Deep and superficial fibers of the lumbar multifidus muscle are differentially active during voluntary arm movements. Spine 27:E29–E36

O'Sullivan PB, Twomey LT, Allison GT 1997 Evaluation of specific stabilizing exercise in the treatment of chronic low back pain with radiologic diagnosis of spondylolysis or spondylolisthesis. Spine 22:2959–2967

O'Sullivan PB, Grahamslaw KM, Kendell MM et al 2002 The effect of different standing and sitting postures on trunk muscle activity in a pain-free population. Spine 27:1238–1244

Panjabi M, Abumi K, Duranceau J et al 1989 Spine stability and intersegmental muscle forces: a biomechanical model. Spine 14:194–200

Porterfield JA, DeRosa C 1998 Mechanical low back pain. Perspectives in functional anatomy. Philadelphia, PA: WB Saunders

Porterfield JA, DeRosa C 2004 Mechanical low back pain. Philadelphia, PA: WB Saunders

Rantanen J, Hurme M, Falck B et al 1993 The lumbar multifidus five years after surgery for a lumbar intervertebral disc herniation. Spine 18:568–574

Richardson CA, Snijders CJ, Hides JA et al 2002 The relation between transversus abdominis muscles, sacroiliac joint mechanics, and low back pain. Spine 27:399–405

Shaughnessy M, Caulfield B 2004 A pilot study to investigate the effect of lumbar stabilization exercise training on functional ability and quality of life in patients with chronic low back pain. International Journal of Rehabilitation Research 27:297–301

Tesh KM, Dunn JS, Evans JH 1987 The abdominal muscles and vertebral stability. Spine 12:501–508

van Dieen J, Cholewicki J, Radebold A 2003 Trunk muscle recruitment patterns in patients with low back pain enhance the stability of the lumbar spine. Spine 28: 834–841

Vleeming A, Stoeckart R, Volkers ACW, Snijders CJ 1990 Relation between form and function in the sacroiliac joint. Spine 15:130–132

Vleeming A, Pool-Goudzwaard AL, Stoeckart R et al 1995 The posterior layer of the thoracolumbar fascia: its function in load transfer from spine to legs. Spine 20:753–758

Vleeming A, Pool-Goudzwaard A, Hammudoghlu D et al 1996 The function of the long dorsal sacroiliac ligament: Its implication for understanding low back pain. Spine 21:556–562

Wilke HJ, Wolf S, Claes LE et al 1995 Stability increase of the lumbar spine with different muscle groups: a biomechanical in vitro study. Spine 20:192–198

Yoshihara K, Shirai Y, Nakayama Y, et al 2001 Histochemical changes in the multifidus muscle in patients with lumbar intervertebral disc herniation. Spine 26:622–626

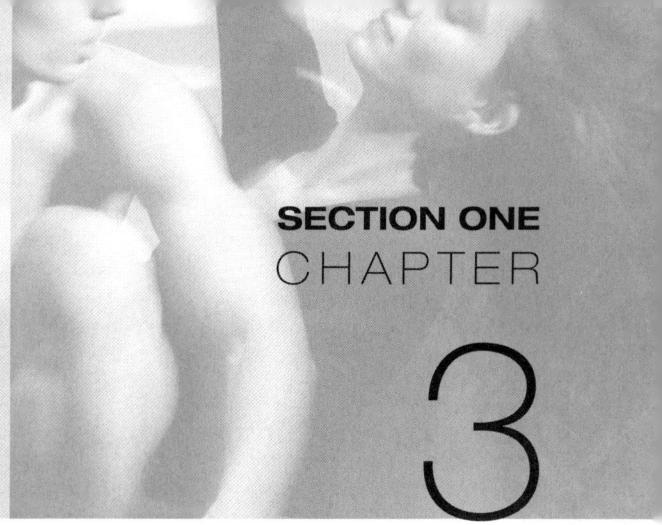

SECTION ONE
CHAPTER 3

Anatomy and biomechanics of the lumbar fasciae: implications for lumbopelvic control and clinical practice

Priscilla J Barker and Christopher A Briggs

Introduction

This chapter describes the anatomy and biomechanics of the lumbar fasciae in detail, reviewing evidence for their potential roles in lumbopelvic support and incorporating current clinical knowledge on management of lumbopelvic pain.

Our interest was initially drawn to the posterior layer of lumbar fascia (PLF, or thoracolumbar fascia) when preparing cavaderic dissections. We observed that its superficial lamina had an attachment of variable thickness to the lower border of rhomboid major (Barker & Briggs 1999), a point not noted in current anatomy textbooks, yet documented in very early anatomical texts (Eisler 1912, Poirier 1901). This greater extent of the PLF had implications for manual tests.

Concurrent studies indicated that changes occurred in the cross-sectional area and electromyographic (EMG) behavior of related muscles in patients with low back pain (LBP) (Hides et al 1996, Hodges & Richardson 1996, 1998). Dysfunction was noted in several trunk muscles attached to or enclosed by the lumbar fasciae, particularly 'local' muscles with segmental attachments. Local muscles are proposed to control segmental movement and forces (Bergmark 1989) and tension generated in the lumbar fasciae by the local muscle transversus abdominis (TrA) was hypothesized to influence segmental motion (Hodges & Richardson 1997). This drew our focus to the lumbar region, to clarify the anatomy and tensile capacity of myofascial tissues and to determine whether fascial tensile transmission could influence segmental stiffness.

The clinical application of this research is in determining the biomechanical basis of specific exercises used to retrain motor control in local trunk muscles (Jull & Richardson 2000, Richardson & Jull 1995). By integrating anatomical and biomechanical knowledge with evidence-based treatment, researchers and clinicians are provided with a common framework to understand myofascial influences on the spine, which might further improve management of lumbopelvic pain.

Anatomy and biomechanics

Of the three layers of lumbar fasciae, the anterior layer (ALF) is thin and membranous whereas the middle and posterior layers (MLF, PLF) are fibrous, forming aponeurotic attachments for attached muscles. The MLF and PLF attach to lumbar transverse and spinous processes respectively, enclosing the paraspinal muscles. All three layers meet and fuse at the lateral raphe, between the twelfth rib and iliac crest (Farfan 1995). Muscular attachments at this raphe include fascicles from TrA, internal oblique (IO) and external oblique (EO) as well as latissimus dorsi (LD) (Bogduk et al 1998, Bogduk & Macintosh 1984, Tesh 1986) (Fig. 3.1). Only the PLF extends above T12.

Anterior layer of lumbar fascia

The ALF covers quadratus lumborum (QL), joins the MLF at the lateral raphe and inserts medially on the anterior surface of each lumbar transverse process. It is thin (~0.1 mm) and membranous (Barker 2005) with minimal capacity for tensile transmission.

Middle layer of lumbar fascia

The MLF has attachments inferiorly to the iliac crest and iliolumbar ligament, superiorly to the twelfth rib and lumbocostal ligament, and medially to the lumbar transverse processes and intertransverse ligaments (Bogduk & Macintosh 1984, Tesh et al 1987, Williams et al 1995). The average thickness of the MLF is 0.55 mm; being considerably thicker at its transverse process attachments (0.62 mm) than between them (0.4 mm; Barker 2005). Via these attachments, the moment arm of the MLF on the segmental axis of rotation is approximately 7 cm (Tesh 1986). The MLF extends only 2–3 cm laterally from the processes before its posterior surface fuses with the PLF to form the lateral raphe, yet this junction is indistinguishable anteriorly, where the MLF appears directly continuous with the aponeurosis of TrA, which extends another 5–6 cm laterally (Barker 2005). Most fibers of the MLF are oriented inferolaterally (10–25° below horizontal), continuous with the middle fascicles of TrA (Barker 2005, Urquhart et al 2005; Fig. 3.2).

A fiber orientation closer to horizontal indicates the MLF's directional stiffness (Hukins 1985,

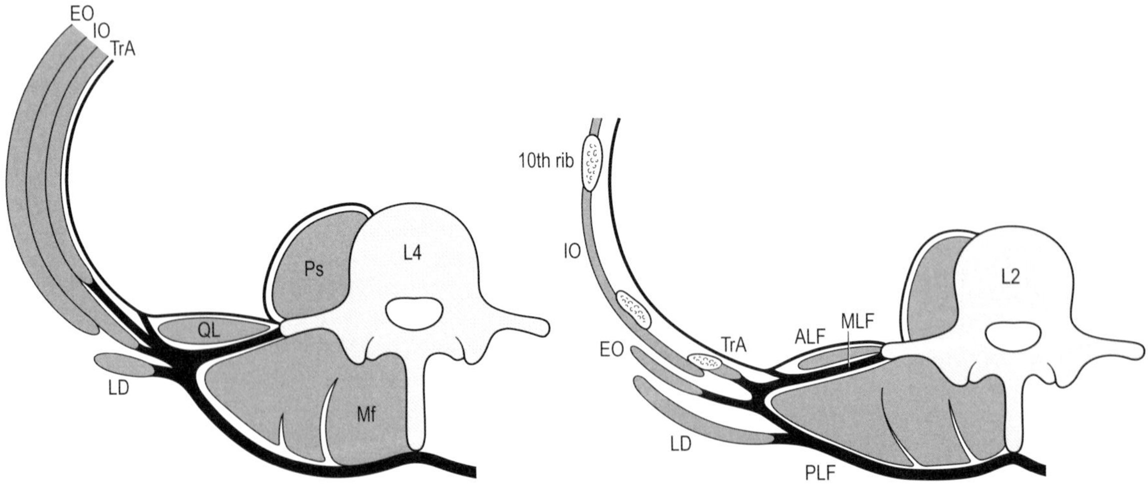

Fig. 3.1 The lumbar fasciae in cross section at L4 and L2 levels. The left figure shows the more typically depicted level (L4) with internal oblique (IO) attaching to the lateral raphe but external oblique (EO) ending freely. The right figure shows that above L3, IO ends freely and EO is attached to the lateral raphe. ALF, anterior layer of lumbar fasciae; LD, latissimus dorsi; Mf, multifidus; MLF, middle layer of lumbar fasciae; PLF, posterior layer of lumbar fasciae; Ps, psoas; QL, quadratus lumborum; TrA, transversus abdominis. (Reproduced from Barker et al 2004, with permission from Lippincott, Williams & Wilkins.).

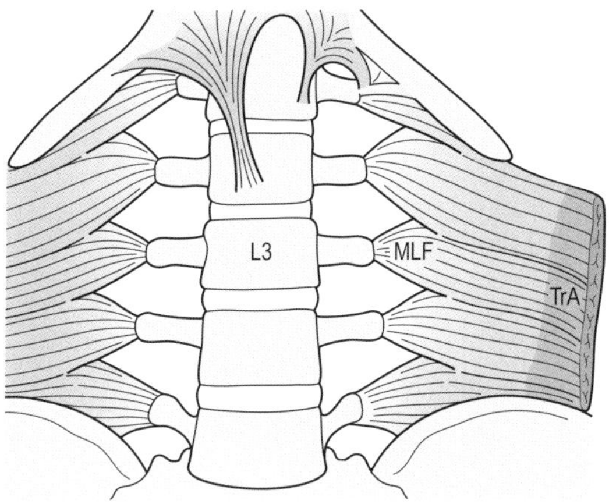

Fig. 3.2 Middle layer of lumbar fascia (MLF). Note the MLF is continuous with the transversus abdominis (TrA) via inferolateral fibers and has thick attachments to the transverse processes. MLF, middle layer of lumbar fasciae; TrA, transversus abdominis. (Reproduced from Barker et al 2006, with permission.)

Minns et al 1973). Rapid transverse traction on the MLF can avulse the tips of the lumbar transverse processes, with either fascia or bone failing at a mean tension of 82 N in embalmed cadavers (Barker 2005). This tensile capacity would be predicted to be higher in young, healthy individuals *in vivo*. The finding is consistent with mathematical predictions that a transverse (hoop) tension of at least 50 N per segment would be generated in this layer during maximal intra-abdominal pressure (IAP; Barker et al 2004). Despite its fiber orientation, the MLF can also generate considerable longitudinal tension. Tesh et al (1987) applied lateral flexion torques to cadavers and then varied pressure in an intra-abdominal balloon confined to the lumbar region. Increasing pressure tended to right the trunk against the applied force, requiring restraining forces of up to 14.5 N/m, or approximately 40% of the moment produced by body weight when standing in lateral flexion. This force was attributed to longitudinal tension in the MLF (Tesh et al 1987).

The main muscular attachments of the MLF include fascicles of TrA, LD (Bogduk & Macintosh 1984), EO and IO (Barker et al 2004, Bogduk & Macintosh 1984, Vleeming et al 1995a). EO attaches to it above the level of the transverse process of L3, IO below this level and TrA to the full length of the lateral raphe (Barker et al 2004). The attachment of TrA is extensive and aponeurotic laterally, its fascicles being directly continuous with fibers of the MLF. By contrast, the attachments of LD, IO, and EO are relatively small and muscular, with fascicles of IO and LD oriented almost perpendicular to fibers of the MLF. Studies indicate that all of these attachments can transmit tension to the lumbar fasciae (Barker et al 2004, Vleeming et al 1995a).

Passive tension applied to the attachment of TrA is noted to displace greater areas of fasciae than tension on the oblique muscles and to resist higher applied tension before failure (Barker et al 2004). Strain gauge readings at fascial vertebral attachments (L3) indicate that applied tension to TrA is transmitted almost twice as effectively to the MLF as the PLF (Fig. 3.3) and directly to vertebrae rather than across the midline (Barker et al 2004). Intra-abdominal pressure is similarly indicated to generate more tensile force in the MLF than PLF, since simulated IAP using a balloon was noted to be sustained even when the PLF was incised (Tesh 1986).

The MLF is also noted to effectively transmit small tensile loads to vertebrae, conveying the majority (95%) of applied passive tension to the TrA aponeurosis. Application of 20 N tension (simulating a 50% contraction of TrA) is capable of influencing segmental motion and stiffness in the sagittal plane at all lumbar levels (Barker et al 2006). Tension on the aponeurosis significantly increases resistance to flexion and decreases resistance to extension, particularly at the onset of loading, so that initial stiffness is increased or decreased (Fig. 3.4), yet the final stiffness minimally altered (Barker et al 2006). The actual difference in stiffness (obtained by comparing point gradients of curves on Fig. 3.4) is much greater (3–5 times) for flexion than extension (6 N/mm or 44% at 25 N for flexion, compared with 2 N/mm or 8% at 25 N for extension). These findings indicate that even moderate fascial tension can influence segmental motion.

Whereas the above study merely simulated contraction of TrA, in-vivo evidence indicates that contraction of TrA produces fascial tension capable of influencing segmental stiffness. Imaging studies in humans note that during voluntary contraction of TrA, its fascicles shorten bilaterally and symmetrically, drawing the MLF and PLF anterolaterally (Richardson & Hides 2004, Tesh 1986), whereas porcine studies report that electrical stimulation of TrA (producing MLF tension) increases resistance to simulated flexion at L3/4 (Hodges et al 2003).

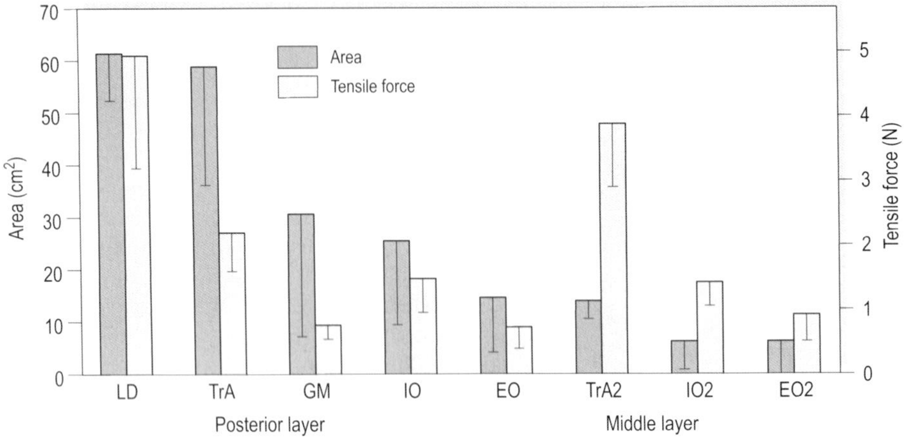

Fig. 3.3 Total areas of fascia displaced and tensile forces produced in fascia with 10 N applied tension. 'Tensile force' indicates the transverse component of tensile force at L3. EO, external oblique; GM, gluteus maximus; IO, internal oblique; LD, latissimus dorsi; TrA, transversus abdominis. (Reproduced from Barker et al 2004, with permission from Lippincott, Williams & Wilkins.)

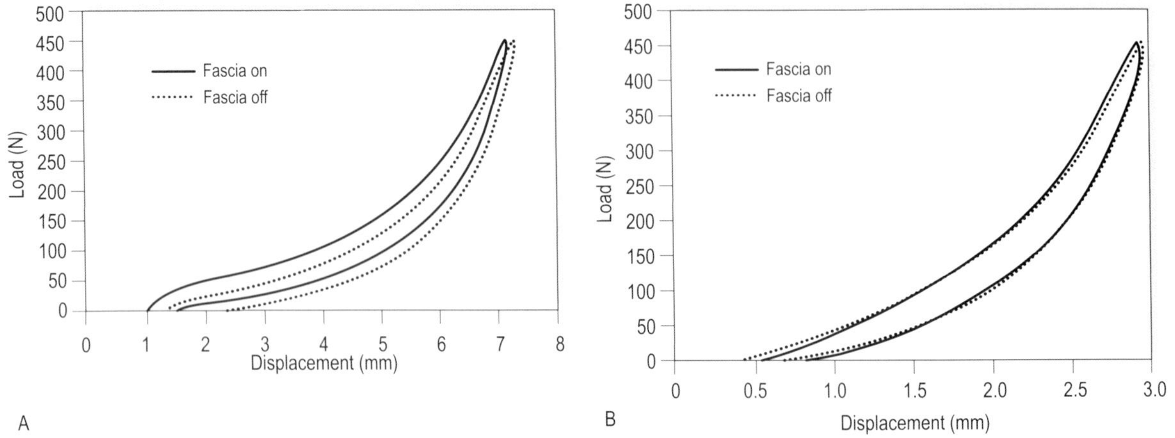

Fig. 3.4 Typical load–displacement curve at L4–L5 during flexion (A) and L2–L3 during extension (B). Applied tension of 20 N to the transversus abdominis (TrA) aponeurosis acts mainly via the middle layer of lumbar fasciae (MLF) to decrease initial displacement and, to lesser extent, final displacement at 450 N (by ~29%:2%, respectively) during flexion. During extension (B) fascial tension increases initial displacement and slightly decreases final displacement at 450 N (by ~23% and 1%, respectively). The initial segment of the loading curve (< 25 N) should be ignored due to end effects. (Reproduced from Barker et al 2006, with permission from Lippincott, Williams & Wilkins.)

The MLF is well structured to transmit tension from TrA to all lumbar vertebrae. It possesses thickenings via which it can transmit high loads (> 190 N) capable of avulsion fracture of the lumbar transverse processes. Lower (~20 N) loads are also effectively transmitted through the MLF and can influence segmental motion and stiffness in the sagittal plane.

Posterior layer of lumbar fascia

The PLF surrounds the paraspinal muscles and consists of two laminae that are increasingly fused below T12 (Barker & Briggs 1999, Bogduk & Macintosh 1984). Both have distinct fiber directions and muscle attachments (Fig. 3.5).

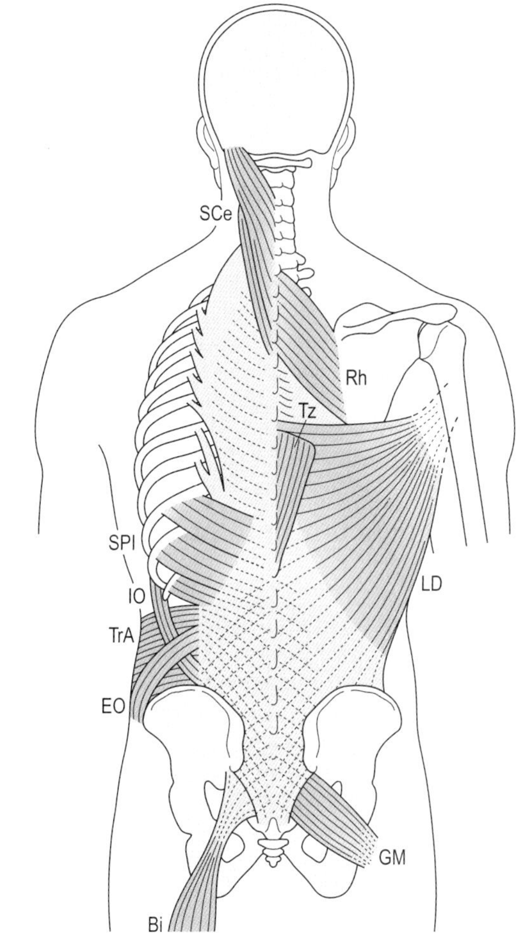

Fig. 3.5 Attachments to the superficial (right) and deep (left) laminae of the PLF. Note the attachments of the external oblique (EO) and internal oblique (IO) above and below L3 (respectively) and of the transversus abdominis (TrA) to the entire lateral raphe. Bi, biceps femoris; GM, gluteus maximus; LD, latissimus dorsi; Rh, rhomboids; SCe, splenius cervicis; SPI, serratus posterior inferior; TrA, transversus abdominis; Tz, trapezius. (Reproduced from Barker et al 2004, with permission from Lippincott, Williams & Wilkins.)

The PLF attaches in the midline to thoracic and lumbar spinous processes and their intervening ligaments, although less evidently below L3 (Bogduk & Macintosh 1984, Vleeming et al 1995a). It also attaches to the posterior ilium and, via fibers crossing the midline, to the opposite ilium (Bogduk & Macintosh 1984, Tesh et al 1987). The deep lamina attaches superolaterally at each rib angle (Barker & Briggs 1999) and inferiorly both laminae may be continuous with the long dorsal sacroiliac and sacrotuberous ligaments (Vleeming et al 1995a).

Fiber angles of the PLF vary across the regions of the spine (up to 40 degrees from horizontal) (Fig. 3.5), lying most obliquely in the lower lumbar region. They are, however, consistently oriented closer to horizontal than vertical (Barker & Briggs 1999). Fibers of the superficial lamina that cross the midline give it a cross-hatched appearance below T12 (Tesh et al 1987). This has been attributed to fibers in its superficial lamina aligning superolaterally with LD and inferolaterally with the contralateral gluteus maximus (GM) (Vleeming et al 1995a). Other muscles with fascicles closely oriented to fibers of the PLF and that might contribute to fascial fiber direction are serratus posterior inferior (SPI) and TrA (see Fig. 3.5). Fibers in the deep lamina are consistently directed superolaterally (~20 degrees above horizontal; Barker & Briggs 1999).

The PLF is a similar thickness to the MLF in the lumbar region (mean 0.52–0.55 mm; Barker & Briggs 1999, Barker 2005). It is thickened at its vertebral attachments, but only slightly (6%) compared with the MLF (55%). Both laminae of the PLF are thinner in the thoracic region, the superficial being of variable thickness and fibrosity towards its attachment to rhomboid major whereas the deep has a largely membranous attachment to splenius cervicis (Barker & Briggs 1999). The deep lamina thus forms an enclosed compartment surrounding the paraspinal and splenius muscles and running the length of the spine, verifiable using dye injection (Peck et al 1986).

The PLF is approximately 7 cm wide on each side (Barker et al 2004) and lies ~7 cm behind the instantaneous axis of rotation, possessing an excellent moment arm to resist flexion (Tesh et al 1987). Mechanical testing indicates samples of PLF increase in stiffness with deformation (Tesh 1986, Yahia et al 1993) and are up to four times stiffer transversely than longitudinally (Tesh 1986) with a maximum (transverse) stiffness of 113 MPa. This is relatively unimpressive compared with other fasciae (Tesh 1986), yet testing of isolated samples is likely to significantly underestimate their true tensile capacity (Adams & Green 1993). The PLF can withstand at least 50 N transverse tension (Barker et al 2004) but its maximal capacity is uncertain and should not be mathematically estimated using IAP, as the MLF appears to be the primary restraint for this (Tesh 1986).

Relatively small (10 N) tensile loads applied to attached muscles are easily transmitted to the PLF and its vertebral attachments (Barker et al 2004). Tension in the TrA aponeurosis is likely partly transmitted to vertebrae via the PLF, because cutting this layer during segmental testing slightly (~5%) reduces it (Barker et al 2005), yet the remainder passes via the MLF. Similarly, during balloon simulations of raised IAP, cutting the PLF caused its cut edges to spring apart, yet pressure was retained by the MLF (Tesh 1986). Although these observations suggest a diminished role for the PLF in segmental control, 20 N lateral tension applied directly to the PLF is reported to increase resistance to axial distraction of the spinous processes (simulating flexion), particularly at the onset of loading (Tesh 1986). This is similar to the effect noted from tensioning the TrA aponeurosis (and mainly the MLF) in flexion (Barker et al 2006). *In vivo*, more than 5% of TrA tension might, however, be transmitted via the PLF, as the erector spinae are noted to contract prior to flexion perturbations of the upper limb (Hodges et al 1999) and contraction of the paraspinal muscles is noted *in vivo* (using CT studies) to tension the PLF (Tesh 1986).

The PLF receives the same attachments as the MLF, via the lateral raphe, from TrA, EO, and IO (see Fig. 3.1). It also receives attachments from many extrinsic back muscles, as illustrated in Fig. 3.5. In the thoracic region, the superficial lamina is attached to the lowest fascicles of trapezius and at the origin of the rhomboids. It receives a broad, oblique attachment from LD in the lumbar region and has thick attachments to both ipsilateral and contralateral fascicles of GM inferiorly. Fibers of the deep lamina are continuous with fascicles of SPI in the upper lumbar region and have an attachment of variable thickness to the lumbar erector spinae aponeurosis below L5 (Hutchinson & Dall 1994). The deep lamina can also be indirectly attached to biceps femoris via the sacrotuberous ligament (Vleeming et al 1989).

Applied tension to attached muscles can reveal the extent of their influence on the lumbar fasciae and the vertebral segments. Vleeming et al (1995) applied 50 N tension to the PLF attachments in embalmed cadavers, reporting that both LD and GM transmitted tension to the PLF contralaterally, up to 4 cm past the midline, whereas traction to SPI and EO, biceps femoris and trapezius and gluteus medius produced variable, limited or no fascial displacement, respectively. A similar study used a lower (10 N) applied tension in unembalmed cadavers and found greatly increased tensile transmission, with every muscle tested (LD, GM, TrA, IO, EO) producing fascial movement and tensile force (Barker et al 2004; and see Fig. 3.3). Tension on LD and TrA displaced the PLF bilaterally between T12 and S1, whereas tension on GM and IO caused fascial displacement below L3 and tension on EO above it. Tension on the obliques often produced only unilateral displacement. Tensile force passing transversely in the PLF (measured using a strain gauge adjacent to L3) was also found to be greatest when tension was applied to LD and TrA, with up to 50% of applied force being transmitted to the midline (Barker et al 2004; and see Fig. 3.3).

The PLF has a long axial extent with broad muscle attachments to LD and TrA and a thick attachment to GM. Its numeric stiffness is uncertain but is likely to be greatest transversely. All muscle attachments appear capable of generating tension in the PLF and, via it, can contribute to spinal stability. Transverse tension in the PLF increases stiffness to segmental flexion in early range.

Comparative features of MLF and PLF

Both MLF and PLF are capable of transmitting tension from TrA to all lumbar vertebrae, with fibers of the MLF being directly continuous with fascicles of TrA laterally and thickened at their medial attachments to the transverse processes. From the lateral raphe, the MLF provides a relatively short, direct route to vertebrae that is likely to transmit the majority of tension from an isolated contraction of TrA (see Fig. 3.1). The MLF is well structured to transmit a wide range of tensile loads from TrA and even relatively small amounts of tension in this layer are capable of influencing segmental stiffness.

By contrast, the PLF's multiple fiber orientations indicate its suitability for tensile transmission from several attached muscles. The PLF is stiffest in the transverse direction, yet it forms a less direct route (than the MLF) between TrA and vertebrae that transmits less tensile force. While segmental studies indicate that the PLF resists flexion and that it has a greater moment arm to do so than the MLF, its midline attachments are relatively unthickened and mobile, so its efficiency in influencing segmental motion may be dependent on activation of the paraspinal muscles.

Biomechanical roles of the lumbar fasciae

Lumbar segmental control

Attachments to the vertebral processes maximize the leverage of both MLF and PLF on segmental movement. Along with obliquely oriented fibers, they permit the MLF and PLF to contribute to stability in all three movement planes. Anatomical and biomechanical findings suggest that the effects of fasciae on segmental motion will be greatest in the transverse plane.

Contraction of TrA can limit segmental movement by generating tension in the MLF and PLF (Hodges & Richardson 1997) and is documented to produce a small extension moment in cadaver segments (Barker et al 2005, Tesh 1986) and *in vivo* porcine models (Hodges et al 2003). Fascial tension can prevent injury by restricting vertebral displacement (Hodges & Richardson 1997; and see Fig. 3.6) as indicated by load displacement curves in flexion, where fascial tension increases initial stiffness and reduces the segment's neutral zone (see Fig. 3.4A). Fascial tension is also noted to reduce the proportion of shear to rotation (instability factor; Weiler et al 1990) in flexion and extension (KT Guggenheimer et al, unpublished work, 2005). Transversus abdominis and the lumbar fasciae therefore influence features of segmental motion used to define biomechanical instability.

Segmental testing studies (Barker et al 2006) simulate a relatively isolated, bilateral, symmetrical and submaximal contraction of TrA, as is indicated to precede trunk perturbations *in vivo* (Cresswell et al 1992, Hodges et al 1999, Hodges & Richardson 1997).

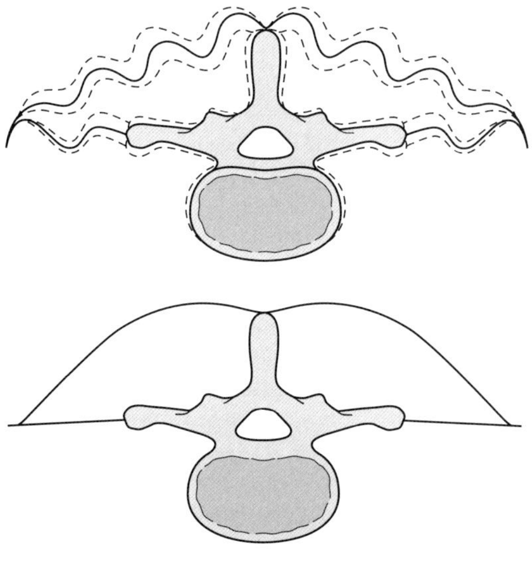

Fig. 3.6 Control of segmental motion via tension in the lumbar fasciae. Motion of the vertebrae is associated with changes in the length of the fasciae (top image) and can be limited by tensioning the fasciae (bottom image). (Adapted from Hodges 2004.)

Imaging studies confirm that fascial lengthening occurs during similar (voluntary, submaximal) contractions of TrA (Richardson & Hides 2004). Documentation of this myofascial contribution to segmental stability may help explain the effectiveness of retraining motor control of TrA in the management of lumbopelvic pain (Hides et al 2001, O'Sullivan et al 1997, Stuge et al 2004b).

Proprioception

The lumbar fasciae might play a proprioceptive role in lumbar stability (Willard 1997, Yahia et al 1992). Attached to ligaments and muscles as well as containing mechanoreceptors (Yahia et al 1992), they are closely related with each of Panjabi's (1992) passive, active and neural subsystems. The fasciae can form functional interfaces between these subsystems and are ideally placed to contribute to sensorimotor control at a segmental level. Feedback from mechanoreceptors on the status of tension in related muscles and ligaments might be incorporated by the neural subsystem and tension in muscles modified to help prevent excess segmental movement (Panjabi 1992). Investigation of patients during spinal surgery demonstrates that such interactions do occur. Stimulation of the supraspinous ligament, which is continuous with the PLF, was reported to elicit reflex activity in the underlying multifidus (Solomonow et al 1998), whereas studies in decerebrate cats indicate that mechanical stimulation of the PLF produces reflex activity in the dorsal spinal muscles (Pederson et al 1956).

Disruption of this sensorimotor mechanism might alter proprioceptive feedback and segmental control. Studies indicate that proprioceptive awareness (Leinonen et al 2002, O'Sullivan et al 2003, Parkhurst & Burnett 1994) and postural control (Mok et al 2004) are reduced in patients with LBP. This could be partly due to deficient innervation of the lumbar fasciae, as suggested by microscopic and immunohistochemical findings from the PLF of patients with chronic LBP (Bednar et al 1995). Further investigation in control subjects is required to confirm these results. Fascial denervation might contribute to the increased difficulty observed in motor control retraining of local muscles in patients with lumbopelvic pain (Richardson 2004a).

Longitudinal tension generation

The PLF was initially thought to possess longitudinal fibers (Fairbank & O'Brien 1980) that might help to oppose flexion moments (Gracovetsky et al 1981). Its fibers are, however, oriented closer to horizontal than vertical and it is mainly thick and fibrous in the lumbar region, so not optimally structured to generate axial tension.

Nonetheless, the PLF does have a limited capacity for longitudinal tension generation via its crossing oblique fibers. Lateral tension generated by TrA, IO, and EO was proposed to increase longitudinal tension in the PLF (Bogduk & Macintosh 1984) and simulation of this in cadavers produced a small amount of lumbar extension (Fairbank & O'Brien 1980). During lateral flexion, the MLF might similarly contribute to longitudinal tension generation in the coronal plane, as indicated by cavaderic studies using intra-abdominal balloons (Tesh 1986). Longitudinal tension in the MLF can resist considerable (14.5 N/m) lateral flexion torques, although as with the PLF, its fiber orientation suggests it is better oriented to generate transverse tension.

The 'hydraulic amplifier' effect

By enclosing the paraspinal muscles and restricting their radial expansion, the MLF and PLF might enhance their contraction and the extension moment generated by them. This is known as the 'hydraulic amplifier' effect (Aspden 1992, Farfan 1973, Gracovetsky et al 1977). Mathematical analysis predicts that this effect might increase the efficiency of paraspinal muscle contraction by up to 30% (Hukins et al 1990).

It is difficult to test the hydraulic amplifier effect in humans without invasive in-vivo testing and fasciectomy. Nonetheless, intramuscular pressure recordings from the erector spinae (Carr et al 1985, Konno et al 1994, Styf & Lysell 1987) support that the lumbar fasciae restrict and enhance activity of the paraspinal muscles. Studies on dog and rat limb muscles indicate that fasciotomy can reduce muscle force-generating capacity by 10–16% (Garfin et al 1981, Huijing & Baan 2001) and recommend that muscle function always be assessed with overlying fascia intact.

Load transfer across the midline

It is proposed that the PLF assists in load transfer between the limbs and trunk and across the midline with contraction of LD and GM, particularly during activities involving contralateral limb extension or trunk rotation, such as walking (Snijders et al 1993). This is supported by tensile transmission from LD and GM across the midline (Vleeming et al 1995a) and EMG evidence that these muscles are coactivated contralaterally during gait, trunk rotation (Mooney et al 2001), running (Montgomery et al 1994), and lifting (Noe et al 1992). They form an 'oblique dorsal sling' (Vleeming et al 1995b) that can be recruited to brace the sacroiliac joint (SIJ) and help dissipate forces across the midline with activities at high loads. Because the erector spinae are often concurrently contracted (Oddsson & Thorstensson 1987, Tan et al 1993, Vogt et al 2003), the hydraulic amplifier effect would also be increased (Hukins et al 1990, Noe et al 1992).

Sacroiliac stability

Contraction of attached muscles can help counter shear forces at the SIJ by generating tension in the PLF to actively compress the joint, also known as 'force closure' (Vleeming et al 1995a). Biomechanical analysis indicates that LD produces a limited effect via the PLF at the SIJ (Bogduk et al 1998), with tensile testing reporting effects on fascia only as low as S1 (Barker et al 2004). The GM is, however, estimated to have greater capacity for force closure via the PLF (Barker 2005) and is noted to transmit tension directly behind the SIJ, as low as S3 (Barker et al 2004).

In vivo studies support GM making a greater contribution than LD to force closure. GM displays greater (surface EMG) signal amplitude than LD during gait and trunk rotation (Mooney et al 2001) and its contraction is noted to correspond with an increase in SIJ stiffness two to three times that noted with contraction of LD (Wingerden et al 2004). GM's onset of contraction is also altered with sacroiliac dysfunction (Hungerford et al 2003).

Whereas regular general exercise (e.g. walking, running, swimming) often incorporates contraction of the contralateral GM and LD and is indicated to be beneficial for LBP, management regimes for sacroiliac dysfunction based on specifically training these muscles have produced inconsistent outcomes and in some cases might worsen symptoms (Mens et al 2000, Mooney et al 2001). This might be due to global muscles normally being required only for activities involving greater loading through the SIJ, yet being excessively recruited with lumbopelvic pain. Prioritizing restoration of function in local muscles (Richardson 2004b) might lead to better outcomes, as supported by clinical trials in women with postpartum pelvic girdle pain (Stuge et al 2004a).

The PLF might primarily contribute to force closure of the SIJ during high-load activities involving contraction of attached and enclosed global muscles (LD, GM, and erector spinae) by transmitting transverse tension behind the joint.

Summary

The MLF and PLF have suitable morphology for generating transverse tension and are capable of transmitting tensile loads from attached muscles to all lumbar vertebrae. Whereas the MLF provides a more direct route and is indicated to transmit the majority of tension from TrA, tension in both layers can influence features of segmental control in the sagittal plane and would be predicted to have greater effects in the transverse plane. The PLF might provide a greater contribution in the presence of paraspinal muscle contraction. In healthy subjects, an early onset of contraction of TrA prior to trunk perturbations is likely to act via the MLF and PLF to limit excess intersegmental movement occurring in all planes. The influence of the lumbar fasciae and their attached muscles should be incorporated into current biomechanical models of lumbopelvic control.

Conversely, disruption of an early onset of contraction of TrA, as observed with LBP, would eliminate fascial influences on segmental neural zone motion and shear and could increase predisposition to injury. The MLF and PLF also provide a mechanism for continuous proprioceptive feedback from each lumbar segment, with disruption of innervation possibly contributing to reduced segmental control in patients with chronic LBP. Together with clinical findings, an understanding of musculofascial anatomy, histology, function, and biomechanics can help form the basis of effective management and/or preventative strategies for these clinical conditions.

In addition to the segmental roles of fasciae, the PLF can have effects across multiple segments during activities that recruit its attached or enclosed global muscles. These may contribute to compression across the SIJ and lumbar spine as well as increase the effectiveness of paraspinal muscle contraction. Such global roles are effected on an underlying requirement for restriction of segmental movement, influenced by local muscle activity and transverse fascial tension from TrA. Further research clarifying the effects of TrA via the MLF and PLF on segmental movement in other planes, and the consequences of fascial disruption, will provide greater insight into the roles of these tissues in segmental control and in lumbopelvic pain.

References

Adams MA, Green TP 1993 Tensile properties of the annulus fibrosus. Part I: The contribution of fibre–matrix interactions to tensile stiffness and strength. European Spine Journal 2:203–208

Aspden RM 1992 Review of the functional anatomy of the spinal ligaments and the lumbar erector spinae muscles. Clinical Anatomy 5:372–387

Barker PJ 2005 Applied anatomy and biomechanics of the lumbar fasciae: implications for segmental control. PhD thesis, University of Melbourne, Australia, 1–227

Barker PJ, Briggs CA 1999 Attachments of the posterior layer of lumbar fascia. Spine 24(17):1757–1764

Barker PJ, Briggs CA, Bogeski G 2004 Tensile transmission across the lumbar fasciae in unembalmed cadavers: effects of tension to various muscular attachments. Spine 29(2):129–138

Barker PJ, Guggenheimer KT, Grkovic I et al 2006 Effects of tensioning the lumbar fasciae on segmental stiffness during flexion and extension. Spine 31(4):397–405

Bednar DA, Orr FW, Simon GT 1995 Observations on the pathomorphology of the thoracolumbar fascia in chronic mechanical back pain. A microscopic study. Spine 20(10):1161–1164

Bergmark A 1989 Stability of the lumbar spine. A study in mechanical engineering. Acta Obstetricia et Gynecologica Scandinavica Supplement 230:1–54

Bogduk N, Macintosh JE 1984 The applied anatomy of the thoracolumbar fascia. Spine 9(2):164–170

Bogduk N, Johnson G, Spalding D 1998 The morphology and biomechanics of latissimus dorsi. Clinical Biomechanics 13(6):377–385

Carr D, Gilbertson L, Frymoyer J et al 1985 Lumbar paraspinal compartment syndrome. A case report with physiologic and anatomic studies. Spine 10(9): 816–820

Cresswell AG, Grundstrom H, Thorstensson A 1992 Observations on intra-abdominal pressure and patterns of abdominal intra-muscular activity in man. Acta Physiologica Scandinavica 144(4):409–418

Eisler P 1912 Die Muskeln des Stammes. Handbuch der Anatomie des Menschen 2(2):1. K von Bardeleben, Gustav Fisher, Jena, p352

Fairbank JC, O'Brien JP 1980 The abdominal cavity and thoraco-lumbar fascia as stabilisers of the lumbar spine in patients with low back pain. Engineering aspects of the spine. Mechanical Engineering Publications, London, p83–88

Farfan HF 1973 Mechanical disorders of the low back. Lea & Febiger, Philadelphia, PA, p1–39, p171–197

Farfan HF 1995 Form and function of the musculoskeletal system as revealed by mathematical analysis of the lumbar spine. An essay. Spine 20(13):1462–1474

Garfin SR, Tipton CM, Mubarak SJ et al 1981 Role of fascia in maintenance of muscle tension and pressure. Journal of Applied Physiology 51(2):317–320

Gracovetsky S, Farfan HF, Lamy C 1977 A mathematical model of the lumbar spine using an optimized system

to control muscles and ligaments. Orthopedic Clinics of North America 8(1):135–153
Gracovetsky S, Farfan HF, Lamy C 1981 The mechanism of the lumbar spine. Spine 6(3):249–262
Hides JA, Richardson CA, Jull GA 1996 Multifidus muscle recovery is not automatic after resolution of acute, first-episode low back pain. Spine 21(23):2763–2769
Hides JA, Jull GA, Richardson CA 2001 Long-term effects of specific stabilizing exercises for first-episode low back pain. Spine 26(11):E243–E248
Hodges PW 2004 Abdominal mechanism and support of the lumbar spine and pelvis. In: Richardson CA, Hodges PW, Hides JA (eds) Therapeutic exercise for lumbopelvic stabilization. Churchill Livingstone, Edinburgh, p31–57
Hodges PW, Cresswell A, Thorstensson A 1999 Preparatory trunk motion accompanies rapid upper limb movement. Experimental Brain Research 124(1):69–79
Hodges PW, Richardson CA 1996 Inefficient muscular stabilization of the lumbar spine associated with low back pain. A motor control evaluation of transversus abdominis. Spine 21(22):2640–2650
Hodges PW, Richardson CA 1997 Feedforward contraction of transversus abdominis is not influenced by the direction of arm movement. Experimental Brain Research 114(2):362–370
Hodges PW, Richardson CA 1998 Delayed postural contraction of transversus abdominis in low back pain associated with movement of the lower limb. Journal of Spinal Disorders 11(1):46–56
Hodges PW, Kaigle Holm A, Holm S et al 2003 Intervertebral stiffness of the spine is increased by evoked contraction of transversus abdominis and the diaphragm: in vivo porcine studies. Spine 28(23):2594–2601
Huijing PA, Baan GC 2001 Myofascial force transmission causes interaction between adjacent muscles and connective tissue: effects of blunt dissection and compartmental fasciotomy on length force characteristics of rat extensor digitorum longus muscle. Archives of Physiology and Biochemistry 109(2):97–109
Hukins DWL 1985 Composition and properties of connective tissues. Trends in Biochemical Sciences 10:260–264
Hukins DWL, Aspden RM, Hickey DS 1990 Thoracolumbar fascia can increase the efficiency of the erector spinae muscles. Clinical Biomechanics 5:30–34
Hungerford B, Gilleard W, Hodges PW 2003 Evidence of altered lumbopelvic muscle recruitment in the presence of sacroiliac joint pain. Spine 28(14):1593–1600
Hutchinson MR, Dall BE 1994 Midline fascial splitting approach to the iliac crest for bone graft. A new approach. Spine 19(1):62–66
Jull GA, Richardson CA 2000 Motor control problems in patients with spinal pain: a new direction for therapeutic exercise. Journal of Manipulative and Physiological Therapeutics 23(2):115–117
Konno S, Kikuchi S, Nagaosa Y 1994 The relationship between intramuscular pressure of the paraspinal muscles and low back pain. Spine 19(19):2186–2189
Leinonen V, Maatta S, Taimela S et al 2002 Impaired lumbar movement perception in association with postural stability and motor- and somatosensory-evoked potentials in lumbar spinal stenosis. Spine 27(9):975–983
Mens JM, Snijders CJ, Stam HJ 2000 Diagonal trunk muscle exercises in peripartum pelvic pain: a randomized clinical trial. Physical Therapy 80(12):1164–1173
Minns RJ, Soden PD, Jackson DS 1973 The role of the fibrous components and ground substance in the mechanical properties of biological tissues: a preliminary investigation. Journal of Biomechanics 6(2):153–165
Mok NW, Brauer SG, Hodges PW 2004 Hip strategy for balance control in quiet standing is reduced in people with low back pain. Spine 29(6):E107–E112
Montgomery WH 3rd, Pink M, Perry J 1994 Electromyographic analysis of hip and knee musculature during running. American Journal of Sports Medicine 22(2):272–278
Mooney V, Pozos R, Vleeming A et al 2001 Exercise treatment for sacroiliac pain. Orthopedics 24(1):29–32
Noe DA, Mostardi RA, Jackson ME et al 1992 Myoelectric activity and sequencing of selected trunk muscles during isokinetic lifting. Spine 17(2):225–229
O'Sullivan PB, Twomey LT, Allison GT 1997 Evaluation of specific stabilizing exercise in the treatment of chronic low back pain with radiologic diagnosis of spondylolysis or spondylolisthesis. Spine 22(24):2959–2967
O'Sullivan PB, Burnett A, Floyd AN et al 2003 Lumbar repositioning deficit in a specific low back pain population. Spine 28(10):1074–1079
Oddsson L, Thorstensson A 1987 Fast voluntary trunk flexion movements in standing: motor patterns. Acta Physiologica Scandinavica 129(1):93–106
Panjabi MM 1992 The stabilizing system of the spine. Part I. Function, dysfunction, adaptation, and enhancement. Journal of Spinal Disorders 5(4):383–389
Parkhurst TM, Burnett CN 1994 Injury and proprioception in the lower back. Journal of Orthopaedic and Sports Physical Therapy 19(5):282–295
Peck D, Nicholls PJ, Beard C et al 1986 Are there compartment syndromes in some patients with idiopathic back pain? Spine 11(5):468–475
Pederson HE, Blunck CJF, Gardner E 1956 Innervation of the lumbar spine. Journal of Bone and Joint Surgery 38A:377–391
Poirier P 1901 Myologie. Traite d'Anatomie Humaine 2(1). P Poirer and A Charpy Masson et Compagnie, Paris, p189–190, p497
Richardson CA 2004a Impairments in muscles controlling pelvic orientation and weightbearing. In: Richardson CA, Hodges PW, Hides JA (eds) Therapeutic exercise for lumbopelvic stabilization. Churchill Livingstone, Edinburgh, p163–171
Richardson CA 2004b The time to move forward. In: Richardson CA, Hodges PW, Hides JA (eds) Therapeutic exercise for lumbopelvic stabilization. Churchill Livingstone, Edinburgh, p3–7
Richardson CA, Hides JA 2004 Stiffness of the lumbopelvic region for load transfer. In: Richardson CA, Hodges PW,

Hides JA (eds) Therapeutic exercise for lumbopelvic stabilization. Churchill Livingstone, Edinburgh, p77–92

Richardson CA, Jull GA 1995 Muscle control–pain control. What exercises would you prescribe? Manual Therapy 1(1):2–10

Snijders CJ, Vleeming A, Stoeckart R 1993 Transfer of lumbosacral load to iliac bones and legs. Part 1: Biomechanics of self-bracing of the sacroiliac joints and its significance for treatment and exercise. Clinical Biomechanics 8:285–294

Solomonow M, Zhou BH, Harris M et al 1998 The ligamento-muscular stabilizing system of the spine. Spine 23(23):2552–2562

Stuge B, Laerum E, Kirkesola G et al 2004a The efficacy of a treatment program focusing on specific stabilizing exercises for pelvic girdle pain after pregnancy: a randomized controlled trial. Spine 29(4):351–359

Stuge B, Veierod MB, Laerum E et al 2004b The efficacy of a treatment program focusing on specific stabilizing exercises for pelvic girdle pain after pregnancy: a two-year follow-up of a randomized clinical trial. Spine 29(10):E197–E203

Styf J, Lysell E 1987 Chronic compartment syndrome in the erector spinae muscle. Spine 12(7):680–682

Tan JC, Parnianpour M, Nordin M et al 1993 Isometric maximal and submaximal trunk extension at different flexed positions in standing. Triaxial torque output and EMG. Spine 18(16):2480–2490

Tesh KM 1986 The abdominal muscles and vertebral stability. PhD thesis. University of Strathclyde, Glasgow, p166–349

Tesh KM, Dunn JS, Evans JH 1987 The abdominal muscles and vertebral stability. Spine 12(5):501–508

Urquhart DM, Barker PJ, Hodges PW et al 2005 Regional morphology of the transversus abdominis and obliquus internus and externus abdominis muscles. Clinical Biomechanics 20(3):233–241

Vleeming A, Stoeckart R, Snijders CJ 1989 The sacrotuberous ligament: a conceptual approach to its dynamic role in stabilizing the sacroiliac joint. Clinical Biomechanics 4(4):201–203

Vleeming A, Pool-Goudzwaard AL, Stoeckart R et al 1995a The posterior layer of the thoracolumbar fascia. Its function in load transfer from spine to legs. Spine 20(7):753–758

Vleeming A, Snijders CJ, Stoeckart R et al 1995b A new light on low back pain: the selflocking mechanism of the sacroiliac joints and its implications for sitting, standing and walking. 2nd Interdisciplinary World Congress on Low Back Pain and its relation to the sacroiliac joint. San Diego, European Conference Organizers, p149–169

Vogt L, Pfeifer K, Banzer W 2003 Neuromuscular control of walking with chronic low-back pain. Manual Therapy 8(1):21–28

Weiler PJ, King GJ, Gertzbein SD 1990 Analysis of sagittal plane instability of the lumbar spine in vivo. Spine 15(12):1300–1306

Willard FH 1997 The muscular, ligamentous and neural structure of the low back and its relation to low back pain. In: Vleeming A et al (eds) Movement, stability and low back pain: The essential role of the pelvis. Churchill Livingstone, New York, p3–35

Williams PL, Bannister LH, Berry MM et al (eds) 1995 Gray's anatomy (38th edn). Churchill Livingstone, New York, p809–829

Wingerden JP, Vleeming A, Buyruk HM et al 2004 Stabilization of the sacroiliac joint in vivo: verification of muscular contribution to force closure of the pelvis. European Spine Journal 13(3):199–205

Yahia L, Rhalmi S, Newman N et al 1992 Sensory innervation of human thoracolumbar fascia. An immunohistochemical study. Acta Orthopaedica Scandinavica 63(2):195–197

Yahia LH, Pigeon P, DesRosiers EA 1993 Viscoelastic properties of the human lumbodorsal fascia. Journal of Biomedical Engineering 15(5):425–429

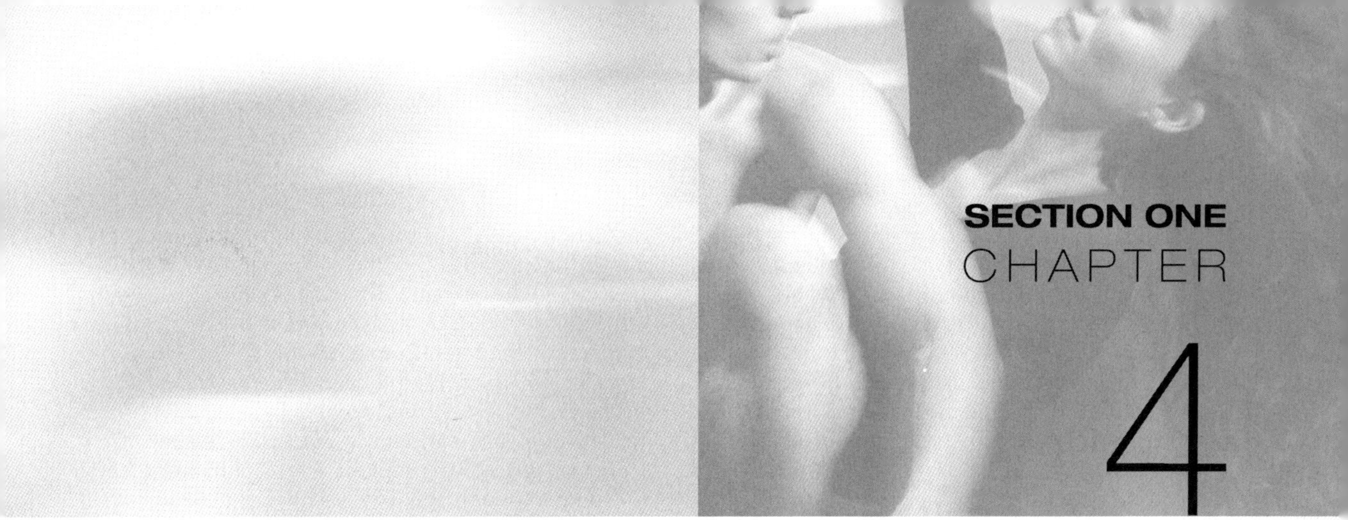

SECTION ONE
CHAPTER
4

Clinical anatomy of the anterolateral abdominal muscles

Donna M Urquhart and Paul W Hodges

Introduction

There is increasing evidence to indicate the importance of the abdominal muscles in the management of lumbopelvic pain. Electromyographic (EMG) and biomechanical studies have shown that these muscles have a fundamental role in movement and control of the lumbar spine and pelvis (Cholewicki et al 1999, Cresswell et al 1992, Hodges & Gandevia 2000). Deficits in the motor control of the superficial and deep abdominal muscles have also been reported in patients with low back pain (LBP) (Hodges & Richardson 1996, Radebold et al 2000) and a new approach, which involves specific retraining of the deep spinal muscles (Richardson et al 1999), has been shown to be effective in the management of LBP (Hides et al 1996, O'Sullivan et al 1997, 1998). However, a number of key aspects related to abdominal muscle function remain unclear. For instance, the mechanisms by which the deep and superficial abdominal muscles stabilize the spine and pelvis are not completely understood and the contribution of the abdominal muscles to the development and resolution of LBP has not been clearly defined. A detailed knowledge of the clinical anatomy of the abdominal muscles is fundamental to further understanding these mechanisms, and ultimately, to improving therapeutic exercise approaches for lumbopelvic pain.

The anatomy of the anterolateral abdominal muscles is complex. Each muscle arises from a number of different structures, which include the costal cartilages, thoracolumbar fascia (TLF), iliac crest, and inguinal ligament, and contributes to an interconnecting, bilaminar aponeurosis anteriorly. Our knowledge of abdominal muscle anatomy has traditionally been based on textbook descriptions. However, quantitative data from well-designed studies have more recently been reported and novel findings are apparent. Of note, differences in the morphology between regions of transversus abdominis (TrA), obliquus internus abdominis (OI), and obliquus externus abdominis (OE) have been reported (Askar 1977, McGill et al 1991, Sakamoto et al 1996, Urquhart et al 2005a), and these suggest the existence of functionally distinct muscles and regions. This chapter examines traditional and current descriptions of abdominal muscle anatomy and discusses the significance of new morphological findings.

Anterolateral abdominal wall

The anterolateral abdominal wall consists of three distinct muscles: the most superficial muscle, OE, overlays the intermediate and deep muscles, OI and TrA respectively (Eisler 1912, Poirier & Charpy 1901, Williams et al 1999). A layer of connective tissue, the transversalis fascia, lies between the undersurface of TrA and the peritoneum. The aponeurotic fibers of OE, OI, and TrA fuse anteriorly to form a sheath, which invests the most ventral abdominal muscle, rectus abdominis.

Fibro-osseous attachments

The anterolateral abdominal muscles have extensive attachments to the rib cage, spine, and pelvis (Poirier & Charpy 1901, Schafer et al 1923, Williams et al 1999). Most attachments of the abdominal muscles are well documented and consistently described in anatomical texts (Poirier & Charpy 1901, Schafer et al 1923, Williams et al 1999). However, some features remain controversial, even though they have been reported in detail.

Obliquus externus abdominis

The fascicles of OE are consistently reported to arise from the lower eight ribs and fuse with the linea alba and the anterior half of the iliac crest (Williams et al 1999). However, there are conflicting reports regarding the attachments of OE to TLF (Barker 2005, Knox 2002, Williams et al 1999). Several anatomical variations of OE have been identified, including an absence of the highest and lowest costal digitations (Schafer et al 1923) and a doubling and detachment of slips to the ribs (Eisler 1912); tendinous intersections between OE fascicles have been documented (Schafer et al 1923).

Anatomical texts describe OE to have a free posterior border (Williams et al 1999) and a recent dissection study indicates that only the muscle's sheath blends with the dorsal aponeurosis of TrA (just below the eleventh rib) (Knox 2002). However, other cadaveric data indicate that OE consistently attaches to the lateral raphe of the TLF above the level of the third lumbar vertebra (Barker 2005). Whereas the two earlier reports indicate that OE cannot influence stiffness of the spine, the results from Barker (2005) suggest that contraction of OE might tension the TLF and control motion of the upper lumbar spine. Further investigation is required to resolve this controversy.

Obliquus internus abdominis

The fascicles of OI originate from the anterior two thirds of the iliac crest and insert into the lower three or four costal cartilages, the linea alba, the lateral third of the inguinal ligament, and the pubic crest (Williams et al 1999). As detailed for OE, the connection of OI with the TLF has been documented differently by authors (Bogduk & Macintosh 1984, Knox 2002). Anatomical variations in the attachments of lower OI include absence of the lower fascicles of OI that attach to the inguinal ligament [below the anterior superior iliac spine (ASIS)] (Macalister 1875, Schafer et al 1923) and fusion of the fascicles of OI with those of TrA in the inguinal region (Macalister 1875, McVay 1971, Schafer et al 1923).

Barker (2005) examined the attachments of the abdominal muscles to the TLF and reported OI to consistently attach to the lateral raphe below the level of the third lumbar vertebra. These results are consistent with reports that indicate approximately half of the posterior fascicles of OI fuse with the lower section of the lateral raphe (Knox 2002). However, Bogduk & Macintosh (1984) reported that in one of eight specimens all the fascicles of OI fused with the lateral raphe, whereas in two cadavers no connection was evident. Thus, discrepancy remains regarding the capacity of OI to influence spinal motion.

Transversus abdominis

The fascicles of TrA originate from the inner surface of the lower six costal cartilages (interdigitating with the diaphragm), the lumbar spine via the TLF, the anterior two thirds of the inner lip of the iliac crest, and the lateral third of the inguinal ligament.

They insert into the linea alba (with the exception of the lower fascicles that attach to the pelvis) (Williams et al 1999). Anatomical variations associated with the attachments of TrA have also been documented. These indicate that TrA may occasionally be fused with OI (Macalister 1875, McVay 1971, Schafer et al 1923, Urquhart et al 2005a), be completely or partially detached from the iliac crest (Urquhart et al 2005a), have no attachment of the muscle to the lateral raphe (Jemmett et al 2004), terminate above the ASIS (Macalister 1875, Schafer et al 1923, Urquhart et al 2005a), be absent in the upper and lower regions of the abdominal wall (Jemmett et al 2004) or be completely absent (Macalister 1875, Schafer et al 1923). However, these variations have been described to be rare and present in a small number of specimens.

Innervation

The abdominal muscles are segmentally innervated by the anterior rami of the thoracic and lumbar spinal nerves (Bardeen 1902, Eisler 1912, Sakamoto et al 1996, Schafer et al 1923, Williams et al 1999). Early descriptions indicate that OE, OI, and TrA are innervated by the fifth to the twelfth (T5–T12) (Bardeen 1902), tenth to the twelfth (T10–T12), and sixth to the twelfth (T6–T12) intercostal trunks, respectively, as well as the first lumbar spinal nerve (L1) (Eisler 1912, Schafer et al 1923). Eisler (1912) also reported OI to be innervated by the genitofemoral nerve (second lumbar spinal nerve; L2). However, current anatomical texts describe OE, OI, and TrA to be segmentally innervated by the anterior primary rami of the lower six thoracic spinal nerves and the first lumbar spinal nerve (T7–L1) (Moore & Dalley 1999, Snell 2000). By contrast, a cadaveric study that involved minute dissection of the anterior rami of the thoracic and lumbar nerves indicated that OE is innervated by the lower eight thoracic spinal nerves and the first two lumbar nerves (T5–L2), OI by the lower three thoracic spinal nerves and the first lumbar nerve (T10–L1), and TrA by the lower seven thoracic spinal nerves and the first lumbar spinal nerve (T6–L1) (Sakamoto et al 1996). Although Sakamoto and coworkers (1996) reported cadaveric data for only one specimen, this comprehensive investigation provides empirical evidence of the innervation of the abdominal muscles. The differing descriptions of abdominal muscle innervation might be a result of normal variability between individuals, anatomical features of the spine and/or developmental factors (Bardeen 1902, 1903). It is clear that further investigation is warranted to determine the extent of variability associated with abdominal muscle innervation.

Fascicle orientation

Anatomical texts generally describe the fascicles of OE, OI, and TrA to be consistently inferomedial, superomedial, and horizontal in orientation respectively (with the exception of the lower fascicles of TrA and OI, which are inferomedial) (Moore & Dalley 1999, Snell 2000, Williams et al 1999). By contrast, descriptions from two large cadaveric studies indicate that the fascicles of these muscles vary in their orientation between regions of the abdominal wall (Askar 1977, Urquhart et al 2005a). Regional variation in the anatomy of the abdominal muscles has been evaluated in terms of three distinct anatomical areas: the upper region from the sixth costal cartilage to the inferior border of the rib cage, the middle region from the inferior border of the rib cage to a line connecting the superior borders of the iliac crest, and the lower region from this line to the pubic symphysis (Urquhart et al 2005a) (Fig. 4.1).

A recent dissection study indicated that the fascicles of TrA are horizontal in the upper region, and become increasingly inferomedial in the middle and lower regions (Urquhart et al 2005a) (Fig. 4.2). By contrast, the upper and middle fascicles of OI are oriented superomedially, whereas the lower fascicles were directed inferomedially below the ASIS (Urquhart et al 2005a). Consistent with

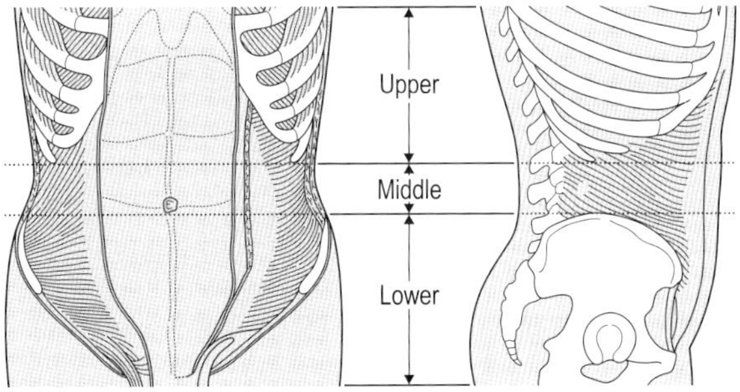

Fig. 4.1 Anterior and lateral view of the upper, middle and lower regions of the abdominal wall and transversus abdominis (TrA). Horizontal lines indicate the borders of the regions. Note the different fibro-osseous attachments for each region of TrA; the costal cartilages in the upper region, the thoracolumbar fascia (TLF) in the middle region, and the pelvis in the lower region. (Reprinted from Urquhart et al 2005a, with permission from Elsevier.)

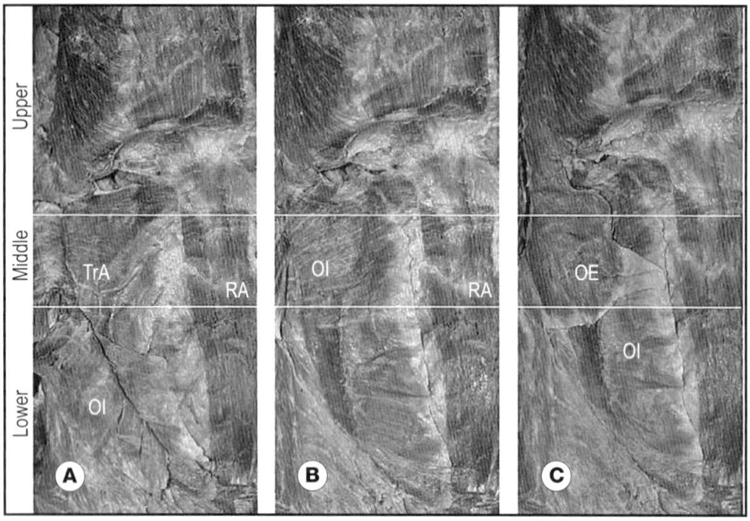

Fig. 4.2 Fascicle orientation of the abdominal muscles. Serial dissections of the right abdominal wall showing right (A) transversus abdominis (TrA), (B) internal oblique (OI), and (C) external oblique (OE) for a single specimen. Horizontal lines divide the upper, middle, and lower abdominal regions in each panel. Differences in fascicle orientation can be observed between muscles (compared between panels) and between regions (compared within each panel). In the middle region, fascicles of TrA are the most horizontal. The fascicles of OI radiate superomedially and inferomedially from the iliac crest. Fascicles of OE are inferomedial in all regions. RA, rectus abdominus. (Reprinted from Urquhart et al 2005a, with permission from Elsevier.)

previous reports by Ng and colleagues (1998), the lower fascicles of OI were found to be horizontal at the level of the ASIS (Urquhart et al 2005a). Although all fascicles of OE were reported to be inferomedial in orientation, the middle fascicles had a greater angulation than the upper fascicles (Urquhart et al 2005a). Consistent with the data from that study, other authors have reported differences in fascicle orientation between regions of TrA and OI, with the upper fascicles superomedially angulated, the middle fascicles almost transverse, and the lower fascicles inferomedially directed (Askar 1977). Variation in results between these studies might be due to the lack of empirical data and reference to bony landmarks in the latter study and/or variation in fascicle orientation between specimens (Ng et al 1998, Urquhart et al 2005a). The fascicle orientation of upper and middle OI and OE is consistent with their role in flexion and rotation of the trunk (Carman et al 1972, Cresswell et al 1992, Goldman et al 1987) and the horizontal fascicle orientation of TrA and OI in the middle and lower regions, respectively, supports their role in provision of stability to the lumbopelvic region (Richardson et al 2002, Snijders et al 1995) with minimal contribution to torque generation (Hodges & Richardson 1996).

Muscle thickness

The thickness of a muscle can provide an indication of its force-generating capacity (Bergmark 1989, Williams et al 1999). Differences in thickness between the abdominal muscles have been reported in both real-time ultrasound and dissection studies (Table 4.1). Four studies have reported the middle region of OI to be thicker than OE, and OE thicker than TrA (Cresswell et al 1992, De Troyer et al 1990, McGill et al 1996, Urquhart et al 2005a). By contrast, one study reported OE to be thinner than both OI and TrA at functional residual capacity (Misuri et al 1997). These differences in results can be explained by variation in subject positioning and suggest that the effect of body posture needs to be considered when comparing the structure, and potentially the function, of the abdominal muscles.

Regional differentiation in abdominal muscle thickness has also been reported (Table 4.1). The upper region of TrA was found to be thicker than the lower and middle regions (Urquhart et al 2005a), while the lower regions did not differ in their thickness (McGill et al 1996, Urquhart et al 2005a). Similarly, the upper OI was thicker than the lower region when a single layer of lower OI was measured

Table 4.1 Thickness of the abdominal muscles. Comparison of thickness measures of OE, OI and TrA in the middle region of the abdominal wall (between the iliac crest and the costal margin)

Studies	Mean (SD) muscle thickness (mm)		
	OE	OI	TrA
Cresswell et al 1992[a,u]	6–9	11–15	4–7
De Troyer et al 1990[u]	7.2 (0.9)	11.5 (2.7)	4.6 (1.0)
McGill et al 1996[u]	7.4 (1.9)	12.7 (2.5)	4.9 (1.2)
Misuri et al 1997[u]	5.5 (1.7)	11.1 (3.8)	5.8 (1.3)
Urquhart et al 2005a[d]	1.7 (0.8)	1.8 (0.9)	0.7 (0.2)

[a] indicates a range of thickness measures are presented for each muscle; [d] dissection study; OE, obliquus externus abdominis; OI, obliquus internus abdominis; SD, standard deviation; TrA, transversus abdominis; [u] real-time ultrasound imaging study.

(refer to 'Subdivisions of OI' below) (Carman et al 1972, Urquhart et al 2005a). In contrast, the middle region of OE was thicker than the upper region of this muscle (Urquhart et al 2005a). Although the absolute thickness values for the dissection studies are considerably smaller than that of the real-time ultrasound studies, these data provide a relative indication of the capacity of different muscles and regions to generate force (Williams et al 1999).

Fascicle length

The fascicle length of a muscle provides an indication of its functional role. Long fascicles undergo greater absolute changes in length than shorter fascicles (Gans & de Vree 1987, Williams et al 1999). Thus, long fascicles tend to be more effective in the production of torque for movement, while short fascicles tend to sustain isometric tension for joint stability (Bergmark 1989). Fascicle length differs between the abdominal muscles and between muscle regions. A recent dissection study reported the lower fascicles of TrA and OI to be the shortest, and OE fascicles the longest (Urquhart et al 2005a). Similar data comparing regions were provided by McGill (1991). However, the lengths of the muscle aponeuroses were included in these measures. Although an anatomical text has also described the length of TrA in different abdominal regions, no empirical data were provided (Williams et al 1999). These results indicate that the fascicles of OE might have a greater role in trunk movement, whereas the lower fascicles of TrA and OI might contribute to the control of joint motion (Hodges et al 1999, Snijders et al 1995).

Distal fibers of the abdominal muscles

Knowledge of the inferior extent of the abdominal muscles is important for understanding their contributions to sacroiliac joint (SIJ) control and support of the lower abdominal contents. The terminations of the fascicles of TrA and OI are reported to be highly variable (Anson et al 1960, Condon 1996, Chandler & Schadewald 1944, Zimmerman et al 1944). Two extensive dissection studies (n >200 specimens) also describe considerable variation between specimens (Anson et al 1960, Chandler & Schadewald 1944). These findings indicate that structures contributing to the functions of the lower abdominal region, such as the support of the abdominal contents, might differ between individuals. A recent dissection study examined the fascicles of OI and TrA at the level of the iliac crest and midpoint of the inguinal ligament (Urquhart et al 2005a). The fascicles of OI and TrA were reported to extend below the iliac crest in 100% and 96% of specimens, respectively. Given that biomechanical models suggest that muscles arising from the iliac crest have the capacity to generate compressive forces to control the SIJ (Snijders et al 1995), these findings provide anatomical evidence for the contribution of these muscles to SIJ stability (Richardson et al 2002, Snijders et al 1995).

Intramuscular septa

Septa or divisions between the muscle fascicles of TrA and OI have been reported (Fig. 4.3). Although

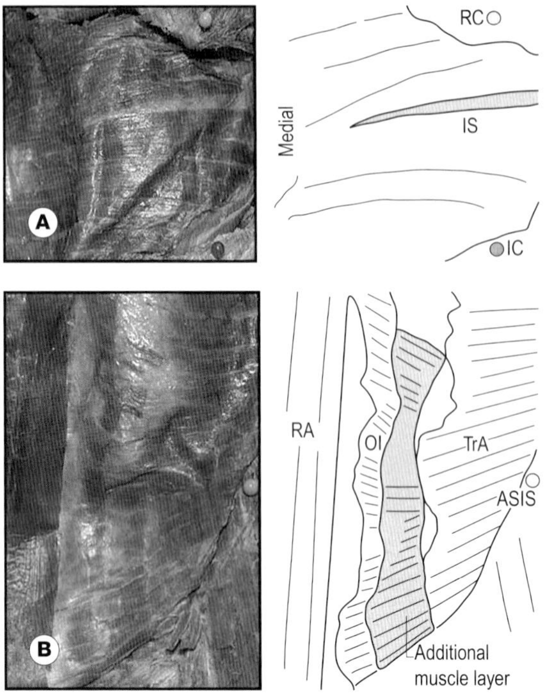

Fig. 4.3 Features of the deep abdominal muscles. (A) Intramuscular septa separating the fascicles of transversus abdominis (TrA) in the middle and upper regions. The right panel shows a line drawing highlighting the extent of the septa, from the lateral raphe around the lateral abdominal wall to three-quarters along the length of the TrA fascicles. IC, iliac crest; IS, intramuscular septa; RC, rib cage. (B) Anterior fascial attachment of TrA and the two distinct muscle layers of internal oblique (OI) in the lower and middle abdominal region. From left to right: RA (rectus abdominis), attachment of superficial fascicles of OI, deeper fascicles of OI (additional muscle layer), and TrA medial to the ASIS (anterior superior iliac spine). The additional muscle layer is shaded in the right panel. Note the tiered arrangement of the muscle layers as they become aponeurotic, with the fascicles of TrA being the shortest and deepest. (Reprinted from Urquhart et al 2005a, with permission from Elsevier.)

these septa have not been mentioned in recent anatomical texts, they have been described in early French and German texts (Eisler 1912, Poirier & Charpy 1901) and more recent dissection studies (Geller & Machado Da Costa 1970, Urquhart et al 2005a, Zimmerman et al 1944). The septa have been reported between the fascicles of TrA just below the ribcage (Urquhart et al 2005a) and at the level of the iliac crest (Eisler 1912, Urquhart et al 2005a). It has been proposed that these septa might: (1) prevent the lateral transmission of force at the interface between adjacent muscle regions, allowing independent function; (2) be the result of incomplete fusion of myotomes that are separated by connective tissue septa during development (Keith 1921, Schafer et al 1923); or (3) be a sign of atrophy or pathology (Eisler 1912). Additional studies are required to determine their etiology and function.

Subdivisions of internal oblique

The OI has been reported to divide into two separate muscle layers in the middle and lower regions of the abdominal wall (Anson & McVay 1938, Chouke 1935, Urquhart et al 2005a) (see Fig. 4.3). However, there is controversy regarding the characteristics and frequency with which this division of the muscle is present. Chouke (1935) observed the muscle layer to be present bilaterally in 63% of 136 specimens and unilaterally in 35%, whereas Anson & McVay (1938) reported its presence in 40% of 125 cadavers. More recently, Urquhart and colleagues (2005a) reported the division of OI into two layers in 100% of 24 cadavers bilaterally. Chouke (1935) reported the additional muscle layer to be 5–8 cm wide, to fuse with TrA before inserting into the linea alba, and to extend inferiorly as far as the linea semicircularis (Chouke 1935). However, the muscle has also been observed to vary in width, extend from the umbilicus to at least the midpoint of the inguinal ligament, and to insert medial to TrA and lateral to OI (Urquhart et al 2005a). Whereas similarities in fascicle orientation with the lower region of OI might suggest a synergistic function, the muscle layer has been reported to be distinct from the more superficial portion of OI with a different site of insertion (Urquhart et al 2005a). It is likely that contraction of this additional layer, in conjunction with lower TrA and OI, might prevent the abdominal contents being displaced by hydrostatic pressure and/or the stability of the SIJ being compromised by shear forces.

Regional variation in abdominal muscle morphology

There are distinct differences in morphology between regions of each of the abdominal muscles. Current data indicate variation in attachments, fascicle orientation and length, and muscle thickness between regions of OE, OI, and TrA, along with segmental innervation and the presence of septa dividing the fascicles of TrA and OI. For example, the upper fascicles of TrA arising from the costal cartilages have been reported to be thicker, have a horizontal orientation and be separated by septa from the middle and lower fascicles, which are attached to the TLF and iliac crest and are increasingly directed inferomedially (Urquhart et al 2005a) (Table 4.2). These findings are fundamental to understanding the functions of the abdominal muscles and evaluating the mechanical effect of each muscle and region on the lumbar spine and pelvis.

Regional differentiation in anatomy of the abdominal muscles suggests variation in function between muscle regions. Given that the abdominal muscles have different fibro-osseous attachments, it has been proposed that fascicles with varying attachments may differ in their recruitment (Urquhart et al 2005a). For example, all regions of TrA might contribute to increasing intra-abdominal pressure, but the upper region might stabilize the rib cage (DeTroyer et al 1990, Urquhart et al 2005a), the middle region tension the TLF (Bogduk & Macintosh 1984, Tesh et al 1987, Urquhart et al 2005a), and the lower region compress the SIJ

Table 4.2 Summary of similarities and differences in morphology between regions of transversus abdominis (TrA)

Anatomical features	Regional differences	Regions of TrA			Type and source of evidence
		Upper	Middle	Lower	
Origin	Yes – all differ	Lower 6 costal cartilages	Lumbar spine via TLF	Iliac crest/ inguinal ligament	Textbook[1] * Dissection studies[2,3,4]
Insertion	Yes – upper/ middle ≠ lower	Linea alba	Linea alba	Pelvis	Textbook[1] Dissection studies[5,6]
Innervation	Yes – different spinal nerves to different regions	Segmental	Segmental	Segmental	Textbooks[1,7,8] Dissection studies[9,10]
Vertical dimensions	Yes – lower > upper > middle	Intermediate	Smallest	Largest	Dissection study[11]
Fascicle orientation	Yes – all differ	Horizontal Superomedial Horizontal	Inferomedial + Horizontal Horizontal	Inferomedial ++ Inferomedial Inferomedial	Dissection: quantitative[11] Dissection: qualitative[5] Textbook[1]
Muscle thickness	Yes – upper > lower = middle	Thickest	Thinner	Thinner	Dissection studies[11,12]
Fascicle length	Yes – middle > upper > lower	Intermediate	Longest	Shortest	Dissection study[11]
	Middle > lower > upper	Shortest	Longest	Intermediate	Textbook[1]
Additional features	Yes Intramuscular septa	Divides this region from the middle region	Divides this region from the upper and/or lower regions	Divides this region from the middle region	Textbooks[1,7,13] Dissection studies[11,14]

TLF, thoracolumbar fascia.
** Refers to attachment in the middle region.*
1, Williams et al 1999; 2, Barker 2005; 3, Knox 2002; 4, Bogduk & Macintosh 1984; 5, Askar 1977; 6, Rizk 1980; 7, Eisler 1912; 8, Schafer et al 1923; 9, Sakamoto et al 1996; 10, Bardeen 1902; 11, Urquhart et al 2005a; 12, McGill et al 1996; 13, Poirier & Charpy 1901; 14, Zimmerman et al 1944.

(Snijders et al 1995, Urquhart et al 2005a). This is consistent with a number of other human muscles, such as trapezius (Rasch & Burke 1977) and gluteus medius (Soderberg & Dostal 1978), which have anatomically distinct regions that differ in their recruitment.

Growing evidence from EMG studies confirms this hypothesis. Regional differences in TrA and OI have been reported during trunk rotation, postural challenges involving upper limb movements, and therapeutic exercises used in clinical practice. During trunk rotation, the upper region of TrA has been reported to be active with contralateral rotation, in contrast to activity of the lower and middle regions during ipsilateral rotation (Urquhart and Hodges 2005). Similarly, the lower and middle regions of TrA were recruited prior to the upper region during rapid shoulder movement (Urquhart et al 2005b) and greater tonic activity of lower TrA has been reported during repetitions of arm movement (Hodges et al 1999). The activation of lower and middle TrA has also been shown to be independent to that of upper TrA during inward movement of the lower abdominal wall in supine (an exercise currently used in clinical practice) (Urquhart et al 2005c) and greater activity of lower OI relative to middle OI has been observed during unilateral straight leg raise and pelvic tilt in standing (Carman et al 1972).

These results have several important implications. First, they indicate that the abdominal muscles are not single structural and functional entities, but they are muscles with anatomically distinct regions that differ in their functional roles. Second, the results emphasize the importance of using multivector methods in biomechanical models to ensure that the mechanical effect of the entire muscle on the lumbopelvic region is examined. Third, as alignment of the electrode parallel with the fascicle orientation of the muscle has been recommended, these normative data are important for obtaining accurate surface recordings of regions of the abdominal muscles (Loeb & Gans 1986, Masuda & Sadoyama 1987). Finally, the findings highlight the need to further consider the functions of regions of OE, OI, and TrA, as well as the effect of pain on different muscle regions and their role in therapeutic exercise approaches.

Summary

1. Although there is growing evidence to indicate the importance of the abdominal muscles in lumbopelvic movement and control, the functions of these muscles are not clearly defined. A precise understanding of the morphology of OE, OI, and TrA is essential in furthering our understanding of spinal control mechanisms.
2. Our knowledge of abdominal muscle anatomy has largely been based on descriptions from anatomical textbooks; empirical data on the fibro-osseous attachments, innervation, fascicle orientation and length, and muscle thickness of the abdominal muscles have only been reported more recently. Specific issues remain controversial and require further investigation.
3. Differences in the morphology between regions of TrA, OI, and OE have been reported. In conjunction with evidence from EMG studies, these data indicate that the regions of the abdominal muscles cannot be considered as having a single common function but consist of anatomically distinct regions with varying functions.
4. Current morphological findings have implications for muscle classification and future biomechanical and EMG studies of the lumbopelvic region. They also suggest that future work might consider the role of different regions of TrA and OI in therapeutic exercise for lumbopelvic pain.

Acknowledgements

We would like to thank Dr Priscilla Barker and Associate Professor Chris Briggs from The University of Melbourne Department of Anatomy and Cell Biology for their contribution to this work. The authors of this chapter were funded by National Health and Medical Research Council.

References

Anson BJ, McVay CB 1938 Inguinal hernia I. The anatomy of the region. Surgery, Gynecology and Obstetrics 66:186–191

Anson BJ, Morgan EH, McVay CB 1960 Surgical anatomy of the inguinal region based upon a study of 500 body-halves. Surgery, Gynecology and Obstetrics 111: 707–725

Askar OM 1977 Surgical anatomy of the aponeurotic expansions of the anterior abdominal wall. Annals of Royal College of Surgeons of England 59:313–321

Bardeen CR 1902 A statistical study of the abdominal and border-nerves in man. American Journal of Anatomy 1:203–228

Bardeen CR 1903 Variations in the internal architecture of the m. obliquus abdominis externus in certain mammals. Anatomischer Anzeiger 10(2):241–249

Barker PJ 2005 Applied anatomy and biomechanics of the lumbar fasciae: implications for segmental control. PhD thesis. University of Melbourne, Australia, p1–227

Bergmark A 1989 Stability of the lumbar spine. A study in mechanical engineering. Acta Orthopaedica Scandinavica Supplementum 230(60):1–54

Bogduk N, Macintosh JE 1984 The applied anatomy of the thoracolumbar fascia. Spine 9:164–170

Carman DJ, Blanton PL, Biggs NL 1972 Electromyographic study of the anterolateral abdominal musculature utilizing indwelling electrodes. American Journal of Physical Medicine 51:113–129

Chandler SB, Schadewald M 1944 Studies on the inguinal region. I. The conjoined aponeurosis versus the conjoined tendon. Anatomical Record 89:339–343

Cholewicki J, Juluru K, McGill SM 1999 Intra-abdominal pressure mechanism for stabilizing the lumbar spine. Journal of Biomechanics 32:13–17

Chouke KS 1935 The constitution of the sheath of the rectus abdominis muscle. Anatomical Record 61:341–349

Condon RE 1996 Reassessment of groin anatomy during evolution of preperitoneal hernia repair. American Journal of Surgery 172(1):5–8

Cresswell AG, Grundstrom H, Thorstensson A 1992 Observations on intra-abdominal pressure and patterns of abdominal intra-muscular activity in man. Acta Physiologica Scandinavica 144:409–418

De Troyer A, Estenne M, Ninane et al 1990 Transversus abdominis muscle function in humans. Journal of Applied Physiology 68:1010–1016

Eisler P 1912 Die muskeln des stammes. Verlag von Gustav Fischer, Jena

Gans C, de Vree F 1987 Functional bases of fiber length and angulation in muscle. Journal of Morphology 192:63–85

Geller M, Machado Da Costa R 1970 Anatomic considerations of a variable tendinous intersection in the obliquus abdominis internus muscle. Hospital 77: 1005–1016

Goldman JM, Lehr RP, Millar AB et al 1987 An electromyographic study of the abdominal muscles during postural and respiratory manoeuvres. Journal of Neurology, Neurosurgery and Psychiatry 50:866–869

Hides JA, Richardson CA, Jull GA 1996 Multifidus muscle recovery is not automatic after resolution of acute, first-episode low back pain. Spine 21(23):2763–2769

Hodges PW, Richardson CA 1996 Inefficient muscular stabilization of the lumbar spine associated with low back pain. A motor control evaluation of transversus abdominis. Spine 21:2640–2650

Hodges PW, Gandevia SC 2000 Changes in intra-abdominal pressure during postural and respiratory activation of the human diaphragm. Journal of Applied Physiology 89:967–976

Hodges P, Cresswell A, Thorstensson A 1999 Preparatory trunk motion accompanies rapid upper limb movement. Experimental Brain Research 124:69–79

Jemmett RS, Macdonald DA, Agur AM 2004 Anatomical relationships between selected segmental muscles of the lumbar spine in the context of multi-planar segmental motion: a preliminary investigation. Manual Therapy 9(4):203–210

Keith A 1921 Human embryology and morphology. Edward Arnold, London, p66–73

Knox JJ 2002 The functional anatomy of the thoracolumbar fascia and associated muscles and ligaments. Masters Thesis. University of Otago, Dunedin, New Zealand

Loeb GE, Gans C 1986 Electromyography for experimentalists. The University of Chicago Press, Chicago, IL

Macalister A 1875 Observations on muscular anomalies in the human anatomy. Third series with a catalogue of the principal muscular variations hitherto published. The Transactions of the Royal Irish Academy of Science 25:1–130

Masuda T, Sadoyama T 1987 Skeletal muscles from which the propagation of motor unit action potentials is detectable with a surface electrode array. Electroencephalography and Clinical Neurophysiology 67(5): 421–427

McGill SM 1991 Kinetic potential of the lumbar trunk musculature about three orthogonal orthopaedic axes in extreme postures. Spine 16:809–815

McGill SM, Jaker D, Axler C 1996 Correcting trunk muscle geometry obtained from MRI and CT scans of supine postures for use in standing postures. Journal of Biomechanics 29:643–646

McVay CB 1971 The normal and pathologic anatomy of the transversus abdominis muscle in inguinal and femoral hernia. Surgical Clinics of North America 51(6):1251–1261

Misuri G, Colagrande S, Gorini M et al 1997 In vivo ultrasound assessment of respiratory function of abdominal muscles in normal subjects. The European Respiratory Journal 10:2861–2867

Moore KL, Dalley AF 1999 Clinically oriented anatomy. Lippincott, Williams and Wilkins, Philadelphia, PA

Ng JK-F, Kippers V, Richardson CA 1998 Muscle fibre orientation of abdominal muscles and suggested surface EMG electrode positions. Electromyography and Clinical Neurophysiology 38:51–58

O'Sullivan PB, Twomey LT, Allison GT 1997 Evaluation of specific stabilizing exercise in the treatment of chronic low back pain with radiologic diagnosis of spondylolysis or spondylolisthesis. Spine 22(24):2959–2967

O'Sullivan PB, Twomey LT, Allison GT et al 1998 Specific stabilizing exercise in the treatment of chronic low back pain with a clinical and radiological diagnosis of lumbar segmental 'instability'. In: Proceedings of Third Interdisciplinary World Congress on Low Back and Pelvic Pain, Vienna, Austria, 366–367

Poirier P, Charpy A 1901 Traité d'anatomie humaine. Masson et Cie, Paris

Radebold A, Cholewicki J, Panjabi MM et al 2000 Muscle

response pattern to sudden trunk loading in healthy individuals and in patients with chronic low back pain. Spine 25(8):947–954

Rasch PJ, Burke RK 1977 Kinesiology and applied anatomy, 7th edn. Lea and Febiger, Philadelphia, PA

Richardson CA, Jull GA, Hodges PW et al 1999 Therapeutic exercise for spinal segmental stabilization in low back pain: Scientific basis and clinical approach. Churchill Livingstone, London

Richardson CA, Snijders CJ, Hides JA et al 2002 The relation between the transversus abdominis muscles, sacroiliac joint mechanics, and low back pain. Spine 27:399–405

Rizk NN 1980 A new description of the anterior abdominal wall in man and mammals. Journal of Anatomy 131(3):373–385

Sakamoto H, Akita K, Sato T 1996 An anatomical analysis of the relationships between the intercostal nerves and the thoracic and abdominal muscles in man. II. Detailed analysis of innervation of the three lateral abdominal muscles. Acta Anatomica 156(2):143–150

Schafer ES, Symington J, Bryce TH (eds) 1923 Quain's elements of anatomy. Longmans Green and Co, London

Snell RS 2000 Clinical anatomy for medical students. Lippincott, Williams and Wilkins, Baltimore, MD

Snijders CJ, Vleeming A, Stoeckart R et al 1995 In: Dorman TA (ed) State of the art reviews. Hanley and Belfus, Philadelphia, PA, p419–432

Soderberg GL, Dostal WF 1978 An electromyographic study of three parts of the gluteus medius during activities of daily living. Journal of the American Physical Therapy Association 58:691–696

Tesh KM, Shaw Dunn SJ, Evans JH 1987 The abdominal muscles and vertebral stability. Spine 12:501–508

Urquhart DM, Hodges PW 2005 Differential activity of regions of transversus abdominis during trunk rotation. European Spine Journal 14(4):393–400

Urquhart DM, Barker PJ, Hodges PW et al 2005a Regional morphology of transversus abdominis, and obliquus internus and externus abdominis. Clinical Biomechanics 20(3):233–241

Urquhart DM, Hodges PW, Story IH 2005b Postural activity of the abdominal muscles varies between regions of these muscles and between body positions. Gait and Posture 22(4):295–301

Urquhart DM, Hodges PW, Allen TJ et al 2005c Abdominal muscle recruitment during a range of voluntary exercises. Manual Therapy 10(2):144–153

Williams PL, Bannister LH, Berry MM et al (eds) 1999 Gray's anatomy. The anatomical basis of medicine and surgery. Churchill Livingstone, London

Zimmerman LM, Anson BJ, Morgan EH et al 1944 Ventral hernia due to normal banding of the abdominal muscles. Surgery, Gynecology and Obstetrics 78: 535–540

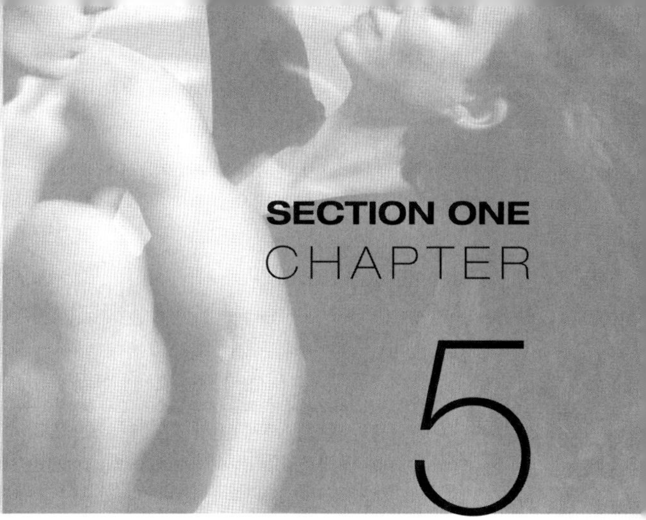

SECTION ONE CHAPTER 5

Clinical anatomy of the lumbar multifidus

L Danneels

Introduction

For thorough clinical examination and adequate treatment of chronic low back pain (LBP) physiotherapists and manual therapists need knowledge of the clinical anatomy of the lumbar multifidus muscle. The purpose of this chapter is to give a better insight into its functional anatomy.

The lumbar back muscles

Morphological and functional subdivision

As described by Bogduk (1997), the lumbar back muscles are those muscles that lie behind the plane of the transverse processes and which exert an action on the lumbar spine. They include muscles that attach to the lumbar vertebrae and thereby act directly on the lumbar spine, and certain other muscles that, although not attaching to the lumbar vertebrae, nevertheless exert an action on the lumbar spine. For descriptive purposes Bogduk made an anatomical classification of the back muscles into three groups:

- The short intersegmental muscles: the mm. interspinales and the mm. intertransversarii mediales.
- The polysegmental muscles that attach to the lumbar vertebrae: the m. multifidus and the lumbar components of m. longissimus and m. iliocostalis.
- The long polysegmental muscles, represented by the thoracic components of m. longissimus and m. iliocostalis lumborum,

which in general do not attach to the lumbar vertebrae, but cross the lumbar region from the thoracic levels to find attachments to the ilium and the sacrum.

The provision of functional spinal stability involves a complex interaction between many muscles of the trunk and limb girdles. Whereas some muscles perform and control the primary action, other muscles must work in synergy to balance any asymmetrical forces, control unwanted movements, and offer support to articular structures (Twomey & Taylor 1994).

Bergmark (1989) proposed the concept of different trunk muscles playing different roles in the provision of dynamic stability to the lumbar spine and introduced the concept of two muscular systems: the global and the local systems. The global muscle system consists of large, torque-producing muscles that act on the trunk and spine without being directly attached to it. In addition to allowing movement of the spine, the global muscles provide general trunk stabilization, but they do not have a direct influence on the spinal segments. The local muscular system consists of muscles that directly attach to the lumbar vertebrae and are responsible for providing segmental stability, directly controlling the lumbar segments.

Many researchers agree with this idea and state that the muscles of the local system have the greatest potential to prevent segmental buckling and control the motion segment (O'Sullivan et al 1997a). However, extrapolation of this anatomical subdivision to a functional one has to be treated with caution. From a biomechanical point of view, the more superficial muscles are suited architecturally not only to the control of spine orientation, they have a large potential to create compression. The distance of these muscles to the center of rotation means that they have an effective moment arm to produce both torque movement and compression. When the torque movement is countered by antagonistic muscle work, activity of the large superficial muscle results in global trunk stabilization and compression forces contribute to segmental stability. In this manner, it appears that the local and global muscles of the trunk combine to exert compressive loading of the spine, thereby enhancing its stiffness and functional stability.

Macintosh & Bogduk (1987) were the first to describe that the polysegmental back muscles are not one muscle mass that connects the sacrum and ilium with lumbar and thoracic vertebrae and ribs. In contrast with the descriptions given in several standard books, they made a clear distinction between the m. multifidus and the different parts of the mm. erector spinae.

The lumbar paravertebral muscles: the multifidus and erector spinae

The lumbar multifidus

The lumbar multifidus is the most medial of the lumbar muscles, and consists of repeating series (five separate bands) of fascicles that stem from the laminae and spinous processes of the lumbar vertebrae and exhibit a constant pattern of attachments caudally (Fig. 5.1). This arrangement of predominantly vertebra-to-vertebra attachments within the lumbar spine and between the lumbar and sacral vertebrae (Macintosh et al 1986), gives this muscle the unique morphological capacity to provide lumbopelvic stability.

The erector spinae

The lumbar erector spinae lies lateral to the multifidus and forms the prominent dorsolateral contour of the back muscles in the lumbar region. It consists of two muscles: the m. longissimus thoracis and the m. iliocostalis lumborum. Furthermore, each of these muscles has two components: a lumbar part, consisting of fascicles arising from the lumbar vertebrae, and a thoracic part, consisting of fascicles arising from thoracic vertebrae or ribs (Bogduk 1997, Macintosh & Bogduk 1987). These four parts can be referred to, respectively, as: longissimus thoracis pars lumborum, iliocostalis lumborum pars lumborum, longissimus thoracis pars thoracis, and iliocostalis lumborum pars thoracis.

Although the thoracic erector spinae has no essential attachments to the lumbar spine, it has an optimal lever arm for lumbar extension. By pulling the thorax posteriorly, it creates an extension moment at the lumbar spine. The thoracic erector spinae functions eccentrically – to control the descent of the trunk during forward bending – and isometrically – to control the position of the lower thorax with respect to the pelvis during functional movements (Danneels et al 2001). As mentioned above, when counterbalanced by antagonistic muscle activity, these muscles have a major capacity to create compression.

The lumbar erector spinae has a poor lever arm for spine extension but is aligned to provide a dynamic counterforce to the anterior shear force imparted to the lumbar spine from gravitational force.

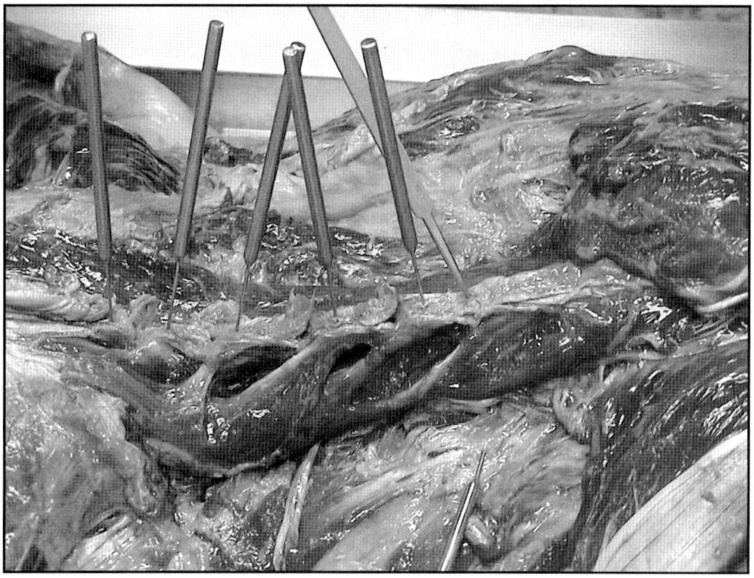

Fig. 5.1 A posterolateral view of the repeating series (five separate bands) of fascicles which stem from the top and the lateral side of the spinous processes of the lumbar vertebrae and exhibit a constant pattern of attachments caudally.

Due to their morphology, the thoracic parts of the erector spinae are traditionally considered as global muscles; the lumbar parts are classified as local muscles. The discussion above illustrates that this subdivision has to be interpreted with caution. All different paravertebral muscles work together in function of segmental stiffness, global trunk stability, and movement during static and dynamic loading.

Clinical anatomy of the lumbar multifidus

Morphology of the lumbar multifidus

(Bogduk 1997, Jemmett et al 2004, Kay 2000, Macintosh et al 1986, Twomey & Taylor 1994)

The lumbar multifidus muscle is the largest and most medial of the lumbar back muscles. The deepest fibers of the multifidus muscle in the lumbar spine (the laminar fibers) arise from the posteroinferior aspect of each vertebral lamina and articular capsule of the zygapophyseal joint and insert into the mamillary process two levels below (Fig. 5.2). The L5 laminar fibers have no mamillary process into which they can insert; instead they insert into an area on the sacrum just above the first dorsal sacral foramen.

The greater muscle mass is from the other five fascicles radiating from the lumbar spinous processes and a common tendon. At each segmental level, a fascicle arises from the base and caudolateral edge of the spinous process, and several fascicles arise, by way of a common tendon, from the caudal tip of the spinous process. Jemmet et al (2004) agree that the more superficial fibers of each fascicle attach to the caudolateral tip of the spinous process, but they described that the deeper fibers from the same central tendon attach to the caudolateral base of the spinous process of the lower level. However, preliminary findings from our research group confirm the description of Bogduk et al (see Fig. 5.2). As neither Jemmet et al ($n = 1$) nor Bogduk ($n = 3$) studied a large number of cadavers, further work in this regard is warranted.

These much larger fascicles are arranged in five overlapping groups such that each lumbar vertebra gives rise to one of these groups. These superficial fascicles diverged caudally to the mamillary processes, the iliac crest, and sacrum.

The fascicle arising from the base of the L1 spinous process attaches to the L4 mamillary process, whereas those from the common tendon insert into the mamillary processes of L5–S1 as well as to the medial aspect of the iliac crest (PSIS) (Fig. 5.3).

The fascicle from the base of the spinous process of L2 attaches caudally to the mamillary process

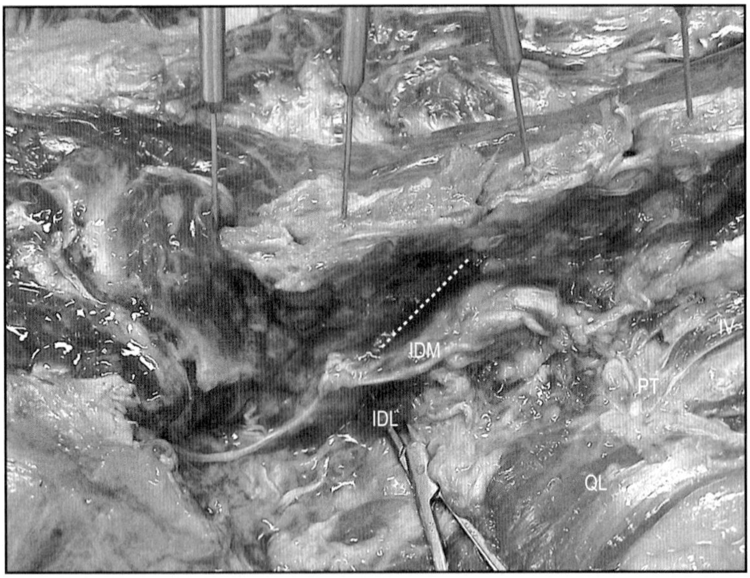

Fig. 5.2 A posterolateral view of the laminar fibers (dotted line) of the right multifidus muscle in the lumbar spine arising from the posteroinferior aspect of the vertebral lamina and articular capsule of the zygapophyseal joint and inserting into the mamillary process of two levels below. The mamillary process lies at the same height of the processus spinosus of the level above. (IDM: intertransversarius dorsalis medialis – IDL: intertransversarius dorsalis lateralis – IV: intertransversarius ventralis – PT: processus transversus – QL: quadratus lumborum.)

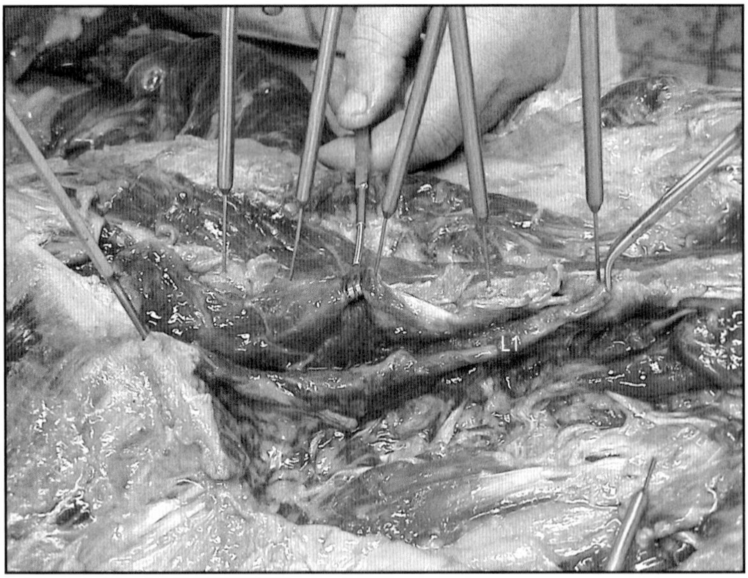

Fig. 5.3 A posterolateral view of the fascicle arising from the base of the L1 spinous process attaches to the L4 mamillary process, while those from the common tendon insert into the mamillary processes of L5–S1 as well as into the medial aspect of the iliac crest (the posterior superior iliac spine).

of L5, whereas those of the common tendon insert into the mamillary process of S1 vertebrae and the PSIS of the innominate, and an area on the iliac crest just caudoventral to the PSIS (Fig. 5.4).

The fascicle from the base of the L3 spinous process inserts into the mamillary process of the sacrum, whereas those fascicles of the common tendon insert into the superolateral aspect (costal element) of the S1 and S2 segments and the iliac crest. The multifidus from the L4 spinous process attaches more medially to the L3 insertion area, but still lateral to the dorsal sacral foramina. The multifidus from the L5 level inserts into the intermediate sacral crest inferiorly to S3, onto an area medial to the dorsal sacral foramina.

Functional anatomy of the lumbar multifidus (Bogduk 1997, Jemmett et al 2004, Kay 2000, Macintosh et al 1986, Moseley et al 2002, Twomey & Taylor 1994)

Typical for the morphology of the multifidus is that the different fascicles are arranged segmentally. The muscle is arranged for individual control of vertebrae. Because of their morphology, the laminar fibers can be considered to stabilize the two overlying functional segments. These deep fibers are near the centers of lumbar vertebra rotation, and thus have a limited ability to extend the spine. Furthermore, because the moment arm of this muscle is small, it might exert its effect throughout the range of motion without compromise from its length–tension relation. The deep fibers are ideally placed to control intervertebral shear and torsion via intervertebral compression. The proximity of the deep multifidus to the center of rotation also means that it produces compression with minimal movement torque, which would need to be overcome by antagonistic muscle activity. The attachment of these deep fibers to the facet capsule allows the multifidus to aid in keeping the capsule from being pinched during movements caused by the multifidus.

In a posterior view the oblique, caudolateral line of action of the five fascicles radiating from the lumbar spinous processes can be resolved into a large vertical and a smaller horizontal vector.

The primary vector is to provide spinal extension, as the insertion comes into the spinous process from caudal at a right angle to the long axis of the spinous process. During forward-bending motions, this muscle contributes to controlling the rate and magnitude of flexion and anterior shear. The small horizontal vector suggests that the multifidus could pull the spinous processes sideways, and therefore produce horizontal rotation. However, horizontal rotation of lumbar vertebrae is impeded

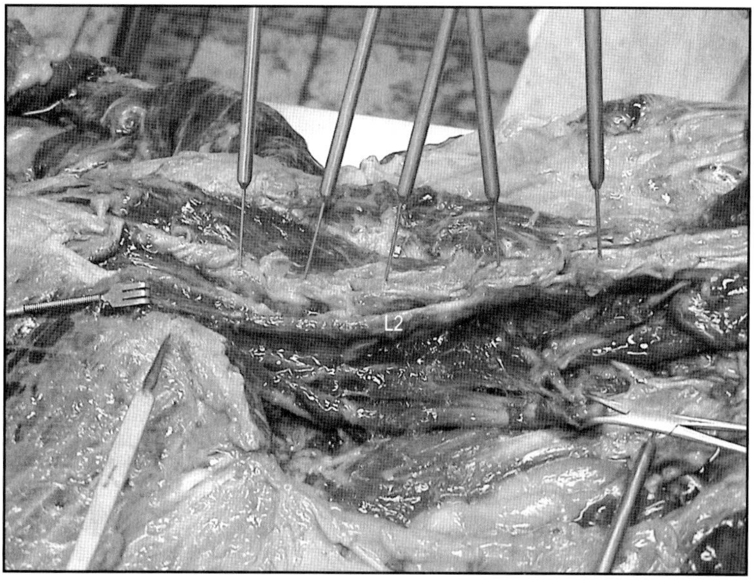

Fig. 5.4 A posterolateral view of the fascicle from the base of the spinous process of L2 attaches caudally to the mamillary process of L5, while those of the common tendon insert into the mamillary process of S1 and the PSIS, and an area on the iliac crest just caudoventral to the posterior superior iliac spine.

by the impaction of the contralateral facet joints. Horizontal rotation occurs after impaction of the joints only if an appropriate shear force is applied to the intervertebral discs. The horizontal vector of the multifidus, however, is so small that it is unlikely that the multifidus would be capable of exerting such a shear force on the disc by acting on the spinous process. The primary rotators of the trunk are the oblique abdominals that, by virtue of their vertical vector, cause a flexion moment as well as rotation, which is stabilized by the lumbar multifidus.

Surface electromyographic (EMG) studies reveal that the multifidus is active in both ipsilateral and contralateral rotation, suggesting a stabilizing role during rotation (Donisch & Basmajian 1972). An EMG study by our group showed symmetric activation of the multifidus during the performance of low-load asymmetric lifting tasks, which confirms its stabilizing role during these torsional maneuvers (Danneels et al 2001).

These findings support the idea that bilateral patterns of cocontraction of the deep abdominal muscles and the multifidus exert a stiffening effect on the lumbar spine during asymmetric lifting tasks. However, differences in the symmetry of multifidus activation were detected between the lifting and lowering tasks. The pattern of activity was almost perfectly symmetric during the downward phase, whereas an asymmetric activity tended to occur during the upward phase in the one-handed lifting condition. Many studies have emphasized the stabilizing role of the multifidus (Goel et al 1993, Kaigle et al 1995, Panjabi 1992, Wilke et al 1995). Wilke examined the effect of the simulated force of the multifidus on the motion segment stiffness. When compared with the erector spinae and the psoas major, the multifidus accounted for two thirds of the increased motion segment stiffness produced by the simulated contraction of the muscles. In the study by our group, the almost perfectly symmetric activity during weight lowering was consistent with the findings of Saudek & Palmer (1987), who suggested that the eccentric function of the multifidus serves to stabilize the spine during flexion and rotation movements. Conversely, the multifidus appears to act as a prime mover during the upward phase of the one-handed lifting task, with a trend towards greater activity of the contralateral multifidus when compared to the ipsilateral multifidus. This could indicate that in the concentric phase of lifting, the multifidus participates in the torque production.

EMG data obtained from intramuscular electrodes placed superficially in the multifidus have also shown direction-specific activity during standing trunk movements, and limb movements in prone subjects (Morris et al 1962).

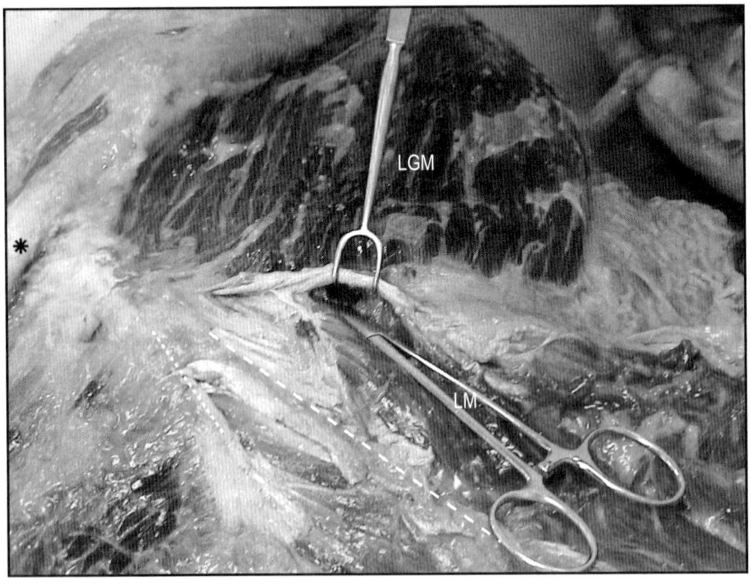

Fig. 5.5 A craniocaudal view (from the right to the left side) of the raphe separating the multifidus and the gluteus maximus. The raphe on the right site is marked with a dotted line, the midline with a striped line (LM: left multifidus – LGM: left gluteus maximus – *: os coccyx).

In contrast to all the findings of the superficial fibers, the EMG activity of the deep fibers of the multifidus is independent of reactive force direction and has a nondirection-specific pattern of activity (Moseley et al 2002).

In conclusion, it can be stated that the primary role of the laminar fibers is to control intersegmental rotational and shear forces through the exertion of compressive force between segments. The superficial fibers have a combined function: exerting compressive loading of the spine to enhance its stiffness, and producing an effective moment arm for extension of the lumbar spine and control of the lumbar lordosis. The results of many studies support both functions.

In addition to these functions, the multifidus also attaches to the deep laminae of the posterior thoracolumbar fascia. This occurs through a raphe separating the multifidus and the gluteus maximus (Willard 1997; Fig. 5.5). The anterior border of the raphe is anchored to the sacroiliac joint (SIJ) capsule and the posterior border of the raphe becomes part of the thoracolumbar fascia. Tendinous slips of the multifidus pass between the superior band of the sacrotuberous ligament and the long dorsal sacroiliac ligament to join with the sacrotuberous ligament (Fig. 5.6); these connections are thought to integrate the multifidus into the ligamentous support system of the SIJ (Willard 1997).

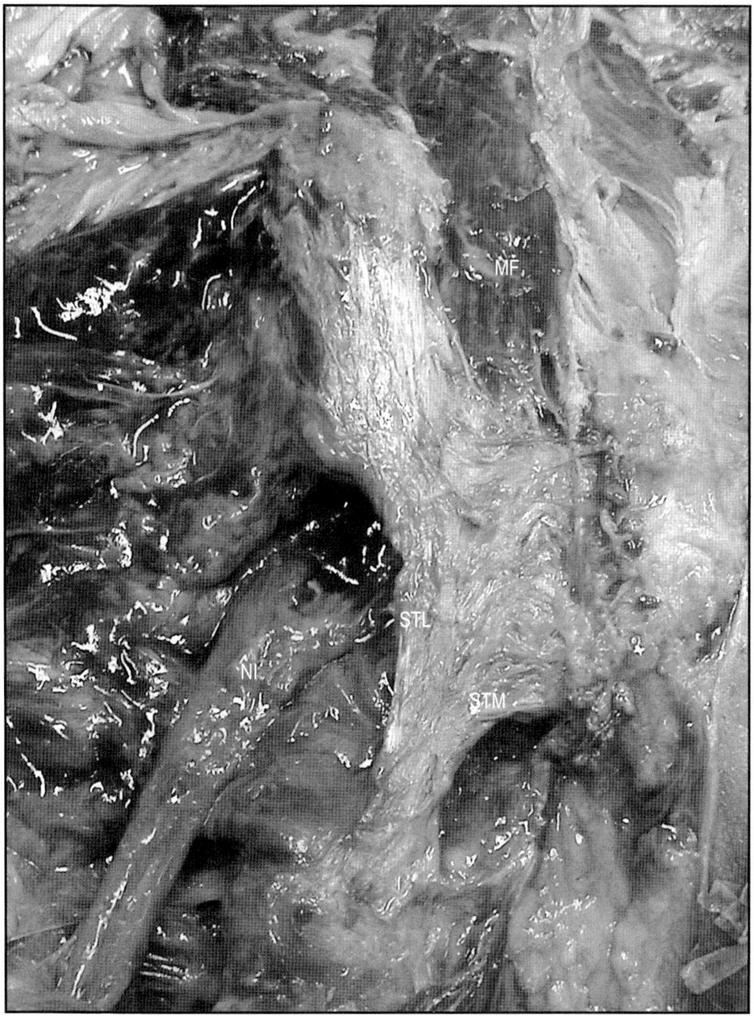

Fig. 5.6 A posterior view of the tendinous slips of the left multifidus (MF) pass under the long dorsal SI ligament to join with the lateral part of the sacrotuberous ligament (STL). (NI: nervus ischiadicus – STM: medial part of the sacrotuberous ligament.)

In the pelvis, this muscle is contained between the dorsal aspect of the sacrum and the deep layers of the thoracodorsal fascia (Vleeming et al 1995).

Neural control of the lumbar multifidus

Not only is the multifidus arranged segmentally from a morphological point of view, but also on the basis of the innervation. The fascicles are innervated by the medial branch of the dorsal ramus such that all fascicles arising from the same spinous process are innervated by the same nerve regardless of the inferior extent of their insertion (Bogduk 1997). Thus, the muscles that directly act on a particular vertebral segment are innervated by the nerve of that segment.

More recent research demonstrated that in addition to this segmental innervation differences in neural control mechanism exist between the more superficial fascicles and the deep fibers. Moseley et al (2002) have shown that the deep fibers of the multifidus muscle are anticipatory for stabilization of the lumbar region and are feedforward recruited prior to the initiation of any movement of the upper extremity when the timing of the load is predictable. By contrast, the superficial fibers of the multifidus muscle were shown to be direction dependent. On the basis of these results, they concluded that the superficial multifidus contributes to the control of the spine orientation, while the deep fibers are active in a nondirection-specific manner to modulate spine compression for the control of intervertebral shear and rotation forces.

Dysfunction of the lumbar multifidus

Trunk muscle dysfunction is being implicated as a contributory factor in the development or recurrence of subacute and chronic mechanical back complaints. Although most studies provide data on gross muscle function, more specific information is required concerning the pattern and degree to which individual muscles contribute to the dysfunction. It has been shown that the muscular response to back pain might not be uniform among all muscles of the back: it is mainly the action of the deep muscle system, which is disturbed and inhibited in the presence of LBP (Barker et al 2004, Danneels et al 2000, Hides et al 1994, 1996, Hodges & Richardson 1998).

Several investigators have studied the response of the multifidus in LBP and found that the fatigue rate of the multifidus muscle was greater in patients with chronic low back pain (CLBP) than in control subjects without back pain, whereas no such difference was evident for the thoracic part of the iliocostalis lumborum (Biedermann et al 1991). Others noted that the multifidus becomes inhibited and reduces in size in LBP (Barker et al 2004, Danneels et al 2000, 2002, Hides et al 1994, 1996, Hodges & Richardson 1998, O'Sullivan et al 1997a, 1997b).

Within this context, our research group demonstrated an atrophy of the multifidus and not of the lumbar erector spinae and hip flexor muscles in normal active CLBP patients. As disuse and immobilization related to back pain leads to atrophy of both flexors and extensors (Danneels et al 2000), the question arose as to whether reflex inhibition, pain, and/or inflammation arising in the lumbar spine could hamper activation of the multifidus and could thus have caused the observed selective atrophy of this muscle. Using real-time ultrasound imaging, Hides et al (1994) detected unilateral wasting of the multifidus in acute and subacute LBP patients. The fact that reduced cross-sectional area was unilateral and isolated to one level suggested that the mechanism of wasting was not generalized disuse atrophy or spinal reflex inhibition. Inhibition due to perceived pain, via a long loop reflex, which targeted the vertebral level of pathology to protect the damaged tissues, was the likely mechanism of wasting in the acute stage. In a following study, Hides et al (1996) showed that multifidus recovery did not occur spontaneously on remission of painful symptoms.

Therefore, based on the available literature, we suggested that after the pain onset and possible pain inhibition of the multifidus, in the subacute and chronic stage a combination of reflex inhibition and changes in coordination of the trunk muscles work together (Danneels et al 2000). The reflex inhibition hampers alpha motor neuron activity in the anterior horn of the spinal cord and inhibits accurate activity of the multifidus. Moreover, already in the early stage, different recruitment patterns install, other muscles become active and try to substitute for the stabilizing muscles, particularly the multifidus (O'Sullivan et al 1997c). This mechanism becomes chronic and results in selective atrophy of the multifidus. Diminished ability to recruit the multifidus, as found in another study on a chronic LBP population, supports these results (Danneels et al 2002).

Another explanation could be that the atrophy of the multifidus is not secondary to LBP but that there is an etiological relationship. Further prospective studies are required to resolve this question (Danneels et al 2000).

Summary

Recent research suggests that besides the typical segmental structure of the multifidus, which is supported by its innervation, differences between deep and superficial fibers exist. Functionally, the deep laminar fibers control intersegmental rotational and shear forces through the exertion of compressive force between segments, while the superficial fibers have a combined function. They exert compressive loading of the spine to enhance its stiffness and produce an effective moment arm for extension of the lumbar spine and control the lumbar lordosis.

LBP is a complex disorder in which muscle dysfunction seems to play an important role. Currently, multifidus dysfunction is being increasingly implicated as a contributory factor in the development or recurrence of subacute and chronic mechanical back complaints.

Insight into the anatomical structure of the multifidus and its response to LBP are crucial components for the development of accurate preventive and intervention strategies for LBP patients. To restore the integrity of the stability of the lumbopelvic region, evaluation and rehabilitation of the condition and activation patterns of the multifidus have to be a point of attention.

Acknowledgement

The author thanks Dr Erik Barbaix for his advice and the dissections.

References

Barker KL, Shamley DR, Jackson D 2004 Changes in cross-sectional area of multifidus and psoas in patients with unilateral back pain. The relation to pain and disability. Spine 29:E515–E519

Bergmark A 1989 Stability of the lumbar spine. A study in mechanical engineering. Acta Orthop Scand 60:20–24

Biedermann H, Shanks G, Forrest W, Inglis J 1991 Power spectrum analyses of electromyographic activity. Discriminators in the differential assessment of patients with chronic low back pain. Spine 16:1179–1184

Bogduk N 1997 Clinical anatomy of the lumbar spine and sacrum. Edinburgh, Churchill Livingstone

Danneels LA, Vanderstraeten GG, Cambier DC et al 2000: CT imaging of trunk muscles in chronic low back pain patients and healthy control subjects. Eur Spine J 9:266–272

Danneels LA, Vanderstraeten GG, Cambier DC et al 2001 A functional subdivision of hip, abdominal, and back muscles during asymmetric lifting. Spine 26: E114–E121

Danneels LA, Coorevits PL, Cools AM et al 2002 Differences in multifidus and iliocostalis lumborum activity between healthy subjects and patients with subacute and chronic low back pain. Eur Spine J 11:13–19

Donisch EW, Basmajian JV 1972 Electromyography of deep back muscles in man. Am J Anat 133:15–36

Goel V, Kong W, Han J et al 1993 A combined finite element and optimization investigation of lumbar spine mechanics with and without muscles. Spine 18: 1531–1541

Hides J, Stokes M, Saide M et al 1994 Evidence of lumbar multifidus muscle wasting ipsilateral to symptoms in patients with acute/subacute low back pain. Spine 19:165–172

Hides J, Richardson C, Jull G 1996 Multifidus recovery is not automatic following resolution of acute first episode of low back pain. Spine 21:2763–2769

Hodges PW, Richardson C 1996 Inefficient muscular stabilization of the lumbar spine associated with low back pain: A motor control evaluation of transversus abdominis. Spine 21:2640–2650

Hodges PW, Richardson C 1998 Delayed postural contraction of the transversus abdominis in low back pain associated with movement of the lower limb. J Spinal Disord 11:46–56

Jemmett RS, MacDonald DA, Agur AMR 2004 Anatomical relationships between selected segmental muscles of the lumbar spine in the context of multi-planar segmental motion: a preliminary investigation. Man Ther 9: 203–210

Kaigle A, Holm S, Hansson T 1995 Experimental instability in the lumbar spine. Spine 20:421–430

Kay AG 2000 An extensive literature review of the lumbar multifidus: anatomy. Journal of Manual and Manipulative Therapy 8:102–114

Macintosh J, Bogduk N 1987 Volvo award in basic science: the morphology of the lumbar erector spinae. Spine 12:658–668

Macintosh J, Valencia F, Bogduk N, Munro R 1986 The morphology of the human lumbar multifidus. Clin Biomech 1:196–204

Morris J, Brenner F, Lucas D 1962 An electromyographic study of the intrinsic muscles of the back in man. J Anat 96:509–520

Moseley GL, Hodges PW, Gandavia SC 2002 Deep and superficial fibers of the lumbar multifidus muscle are differentially active during voluntary arm movements. Spine 27:E29–E36

O'Sullivan P, Twomey L, Allison G 1997a Dynamic

stabilization of the lumbar spine. Crit Rev Phys Rehab Med 9:315–330

O'Sullivan P, Twomey L, Allison G 1997b Dysfunction of the neuro-muscular system in the presence of low back pain – Implications for physical therapy management. J Man Manip Ther 5:20–26

O'Sullivan P, Phyty G, Twomey L, Allison G 1997c Evaluation of specific stabilizing exercise in the treatment of chronic low back pain with radiologic diagnosis of spondylolysis or spondylolisthesis. Spine 22:2959–2967

Panjabi M 1992 The stabilising system of the spine: Part I, Function, dysfunction, adaptation and enhancement. Part II, Neutral zone and instability hypothesis. J Spinal Disord 5:383–397

Saudek CE, Palmer KA 1987 Back pain revision. JOSPT 12:556–566

Twomey L, Taylor J (eds) 1994 Physical therapy of the low back, 2nd edn. Churchill Livingstone, New York

Vleeming A, Pool-Goudzwaard A, Stoeckart R et al 1995 Posterior layer of the thoracolumbar fascia: its function in load transfer from spine to legs. Spine 20:753–759

Wilke H, Wolf S, Claes L et al 1995 Stability increase of the lumbar spine with different muscle groups. A biomechanical in vitro study. Spine 20:192–198

Willard FH 1997 The muscular, ligamentous and neural structure of the low back and its relation to back pain. In: Vleeming A et al (eds) Movement, stability and low back pain. Churchill Livingstone, Edinburgh

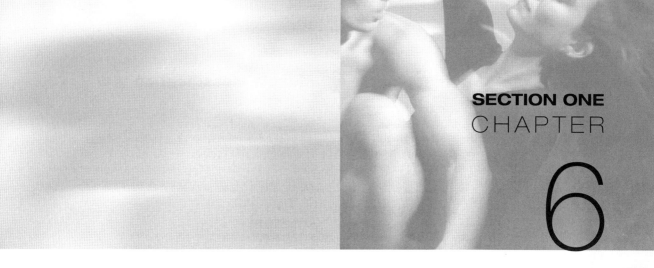

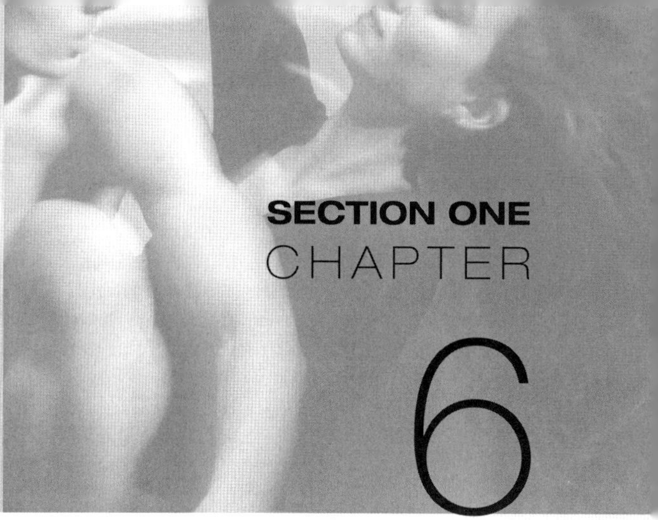

SECTION ONE
CHAPTER
6

Clinical anatomy and function of psoas major and deep sacral gluteus maximus

S Gibbons

Introduction

Research since the 1990s has brought a new understanding of muscle function, and the role of muscles in providing stability is now well recognized. The concept of stability in itself is somewhat controversial and there are different schools of thought (Comerford & Mottram 2001a, McGill 2002, Richardson et al 2004, Sahrmann 2002). Some conflict has arisen because muscles can have a primary role in providing stability or can have multiple roles in movement and stability. This is further complicated by what demands are required under normal low load daily activities versus higher loads required for manual handling, and contact sports (low load versus high load stability) (Gibbons & Comerford 2001). Our understanding has been enhanced by a better awareness in anatomy, physiology, biomechanics, imaging techniques, and how to interpret the results of research studies.

Psoas major (PM) is a unique muscle. It originates on the lumbar spine with segmental attachments, attaches to the sacroiliac joint as it crosses it, and inserts into the hip. This anatomical position places PM in an ideal position to function as an important stability muscle for the lumbar spine (Gracovetsky et al 1981, Nachemson 1968). Despite this, it is not fully understood and there is still considerable debate regarding its functional role (Aspinal 1993, Bachrach et al 1991, McGill 2002, Richardson et al 2004). A mechanism to simultaneously flex the hip and stabilize the lumbopelvic region is needed. It does not seem logical that a muscle such as PM would have a detrimental effect to the lumbopelvic region.

Conversely, there is little debate regarding the importance of gluteus maximus (GM). It is considered an important stability muscle of the lumbopelvic region (Lee 2004), as well as of the hip (Sahrmann 2002). This is supported by motor control studies (Bullock-Saxton et al 1994, Hungerford et al 2003) and biomechanical analysis (Pool-Goudzwaard et al 1998). One issue of confusion involves overactivity and shortness of GM (Lee 2004, Sahrmann 2002). This can have an effect on such things as postural alignment, recruitment strategies, and compensatory movement patterns. A mechanism to understand how a very important stability muscle can become potentially harmful has not been described.

The purpose of this chapter is to present evidence of a stability role for PM and introduce a new role for GM in sacroiliac joint (SIJ) stability. A better understanding of the implications of the function of PM and GM on the stability of the lumbopelvic region might improve clinical management of related dysfunction. This could also highlight new areas of research in the field.

Muscle function

Muscle function is more complex than considering 'origin to insertion,' or assessing activity profiles with electromyography (EMG). Information regarding muscle function can be obtained from four key sources (Gibbons 2005b). These are listed in Table 6.1.

Table 6.1 Sources of information for understanding muscle function in order to functionally classify muscles (reproduced with permission from Kinetic Control)

Function	Dysfunction
• Anatomical location & structure • Biomechanical potential • Neurophysiology	• Consistent & characteristic changes in the presence of pain or pathology

Muscle classification

A new classification system of muscle function has been presented (Comerford & Mottram 2001b). This divides muscles into local stabilizers, global stabilizers, and global mobilizers. Of particular interest to this chapter are the local stability muscles. Their characteristics are presented in Table 6.2.

Anatomy

Psoas major

PM has anterior and posterior fibrous attachments to the spine (Fig. 6.1). The anterior attachment is to the anteromedial aspect of all the lumbar discs and adjoining bodies with the exception of the L5–S1 disc. The posterior attachment is on the anteromedial aspect of all the lumbar transverse processes (Bogduk et al 1992, Gibbons 2004). The fasciculii of PM are about the same length within specimens and have a unipennate fiber orientation. This ranges from 75° in the superior aspect of the fasciculii to 45° in the inferior aspect of the fasciculii. The fiber length ranges from 3 to 8 cm and 3 to 5 cm in the anterior and posterior fasciculii, respectively (Gibbons 2004). The fasciculii run inferolaterally to reach a central tendon, where they descend over the pelvic brim and share a common insertion with iliacus to the lesser trochanter (Bogduk et al 1992, Gibbons 2004, Santaguida & McGill 1995).

PM also has significant fascial relations. The medial arcuate ligament is a continuation of the superior PM fascia that continues superiorly to the diaphragm. The right and left crus comprise the spinal attachment of the diaphragm. They attach to the anterolateral component of the upper three vertebrae and bodies. The crus and their fascia overlap PM and appear continuous with the muscle until they come more anterior and blend with the

Table 6.2 Characteristics of local stability muscles in normal function and after the presence of pain (dysfunction) (Review: Comerford & Mottram, 2001)

Function	Dysfunction
• ↑Muscle stiffness to control segmental translation • No or minimal length change in functional movements • Anticipatory recruitment prior to functional loading provides protective stiffness (as required) • Activity may be continuous and independent of the direction of movement	• Uncontrolled segmental translation • Segmental change within cross-sectional area • Altered pattern of low-threshold recruitment • Motor recruitment timing deficit

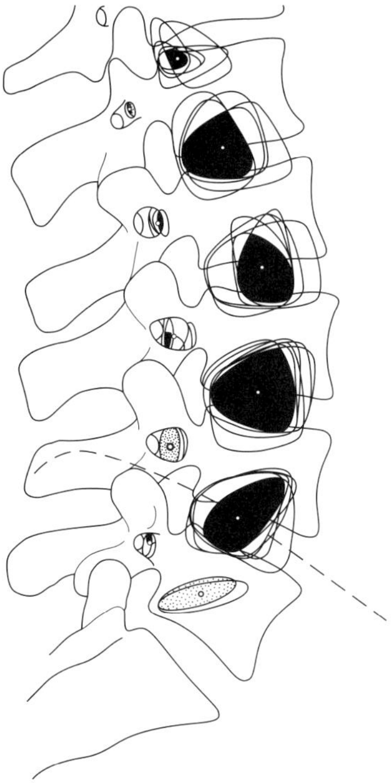

Fig. 6.1 The spinal attachments of psoas major. The attachment on the disc and adjoining body and transverse process have been termed 'anterior' and 'posterior', respectively. (Reproduced with permission from PSPR Ltd.)

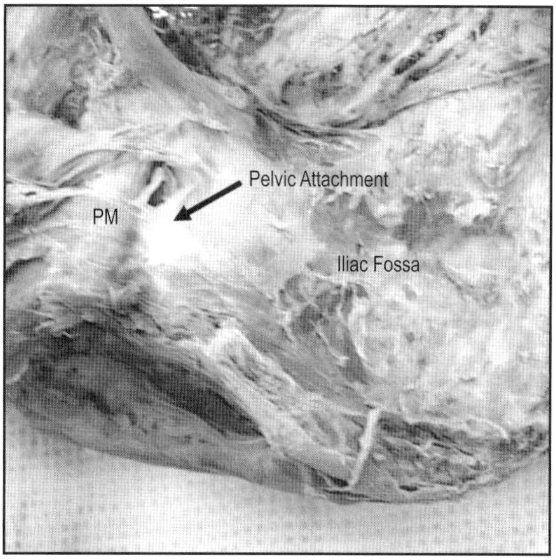

Fig. 6.2 Psoas major and iliacus descend over the iliopectineal eminence and have a strong attachment to the pelvic brim (identified by the arrow). This attachment may constitute an innominate ligament. (Reproduced with permission from PSPR Ltd.)

anterior longitudinal ligament. As PM descends, its inferomedial fascia becomes thick at its lower portion and is continuous with the pelvic floor fascia. This also forms a strong link with transversus abdominus (TrA) and the internal oblique (OI). PM attaches firmly to the pelvic brim as it passes over it (Gibbons 2004). This attachment may constitute an 'innominate ligament' (Fig. 6.2) (Gibbons 2005a).

The nerve supply to PM is not reported consistently because most anatomical texts list two or three different variations. These are listed under PM (at the hip and lumbar spine), the lumbar plexus, and the femoral nerve (Moore 1992, Romanes 1987, Williams et al 1989). In a dissection study of 24 cadavers, all specimens had a separate nerve supply for the anterior and posterior fasciculii. The anterior fasciculii were supplied by branches of the femoral nerve from L2, L3, and L4, whereas the posterior fasciculii were supplied by branches of the ventral rami. In 13 specimens the nerve supply was segmental from T12, L1, L2, L3, and L4 (Gibbons 2005a). In light of this, PM should be considered as two distinct parts: anterior and posterior. Also, the term 'iliopsoas' should be reconsidered. This pattern of separate functional roles within PM may be similar to the superficial and deep lumbar multifidus, which have been shown to have different EMG to spinal perturbations (Moseley et al 2002).

Deep sacral gluteus maximus

GM has been previously subdivided into superficial and deep (Kapandji 1987) and cranial and caudal (Jaegers et al 1992, Moore & Dalley 1999). Recently, it was found that GM has three subdivisions: superficial sacral fibers, deep sacral fibers, and deep ilium fibers. The superficial sacral fibers run to the iliotibial band in 7–10 fascicular arrangements; some of these fibers also attach to the gluteal tuberosity. The deep ilium fibers run predominately to the gluteal tuberosity. Superiorly, the deep sacral fibers cross the SIJ and attach to the posterior pelvic brim just lateral to the posterior superior iliac spine. These are present in approximately two thirds of specimens. Inferiorly, they are short and are orientated inferolaterally. These deep sacral fibers cross from the lateral sacrum to the posterior ischial spine, the ischial tuberosity, and the sacrotuberous ligament. The deep fibers are present in all muscles. No separate nerve supply could be located for individual groups of fibers (Gibbons & Mottram 2004).

Biomechanics

Psoas major

The studies that have investigated the biomechanics of PM are limited by using incorrect or incomplete anatomy and unsubstantiated assumptions. Of the studies with merit, a consistent finding is that the primary force of PM on the lumbar spine is axial compression and that the compression force is always greater than shear (Bogduk et al 1992, Gibbons 2004, Rab et al 1977, Santaguida & McGill 1995). Compression from PM can create segmental stiffness (Janevic et al 1991) and can resist shear forces (McGill 2002). Due to the size, most of the force will come from the anterior fasciculii (Bogduk et al 1992, Gibbons 2004). The line of action of PM is too close to the axis of rotation to contribute to significant spinal movement (Fig. 6.3) (Bogduk et al 1992, Gibbons 2004, Santaguida & McGill 1995). There is a small amount of extension at L1, L2, and L3, whereas there is a small amount of flexion from L4 and L5 (Bogduk et al 1992, Gibbons 2004). This closely resembles a neutral lumbar lordosis.

PM crosses the pelvis and therefore must exert a force on the SIJ. It has been generally thought that PM produced a force to anteriorly rotate the innominate (Bachrach et al 1991, Snijders et al 1995); however, this has recently been called into question. The PM muscle was modeled as a pulley over the pelvic brim in the erect posture (Gibbons et al 2001).

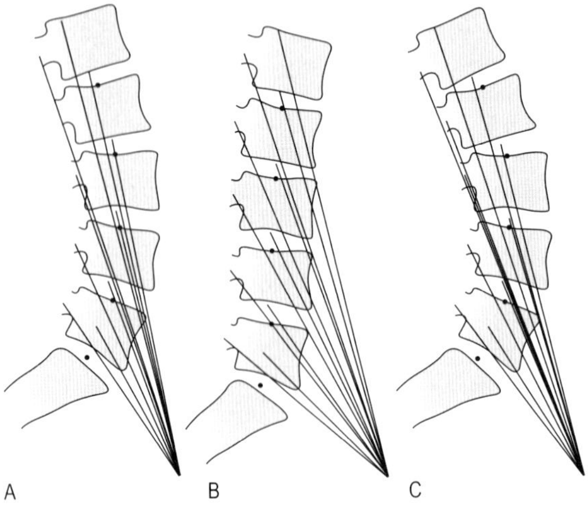

Fig. 6.3 The psoas major lines of action from the individual fascicle attachments to the lumbar spine and a straight line to the iliopubic eminence. (Reproduced with permission from PSPR Ltd.)

Several scenarios were considered to include the PM attachment to the innominate described above. In all scenarios, the resultant force was posterior rotation of the innominate.

PM is unipennate muscle, not a fusiform muscle, and the fiber length and ability of the muscle to shorten is less than believed. This calls into question its efficiency as a hip flexor. Yoshio et al (2002) conducted a detailed morphological and biomechanical study of PM at the hip. They concluded that the primary role of PM was for lumbar stability and that PM contributed very little to hip flexion. The primary role for PM at the hip was for stability. This was achieved through maintaining the femoral head in the acetabulum. Their findings are summarized in Table 6.3.

Neurophysiology

Psoas major

Although EMG has been used in more than 20 studies to assess the function of PM, very little information has been obtained. This is because PM cannot be assessed with superficial EMG and the EMG from iliacus cannot be considered the same as EMG from PM. Further, normalization concerns exist, and the methodologies used have been unable to provide useful information regarding the complex function of PM.

After assessing the articles that have used EMG, there is evidence to suggest that PM plays a role in hip flexion but is not the dominant hip flexor; iliacus appears to be more active than PM during hip flexion. Andersson et al (1995) found that, during hip flexion, PM EMG ranged from 49%, 69%, and 86% as active as iliacus during hip flexion to 30°, 60°, and 90° respectively. It is not known if the EMG activity of PM is active to stabilize the lumbar spine, pelvis, or hip; to produce hip flexion; or all of these. Similar comments could also be made regarding the activity of iliacus during hip flexion. It should be noted that other hip flexors, such as rectus femoris, tensor fascia latae and sartorius, also contribute to hip flexion (Andersson et al 1997). All these are more efficient hip flexors than PM and iliacus (Dostal et al 1986). Both Andersson et al (1995) and Juker et al (1998) found that PM is minimally involved in producing spinal movement, but it might contribute to maintaining or producing the lumbar lordosis (Andersson et al 1995). It might lower the spine eccentrically during side flexion (Andersson et al 1995) and control side flexion during

Table 6.3 Summary of the functions of psoas major as a function of hip flexion angle. Hip stability is created due to psoas major maintaining the femoral head in the acetabulum. Psoas major is an effective hip flexor between 45°–65°. Lumbar stability is created because psoas major maintains the lumbar curve (Yoshio et al 2002)

Hip flexion angle	Function of psoas major
0°–15°	• Hip stability • Lumbar stability
15°–45°	• Hip stability • Lumbar stability
45°–60°	• Hip flexion • Hip stability • Lumbar stability
60° +	• No action on femoral head • Lumbar stability

gait (Andersson et al 1997). It should be noted that the recordings appear to have been taken from the anterior fasciculii, hence the functions mentioned above should be considered from anterior PM and not posterior PM.

Deep sacral gluteus maximus

During an initial pilot study, it was hypothesized that the deep sacral gluteus maximus (DSG) would be active in positions of counternutation when the sacrotuberous ligament was not tensioned. Fine-wire EMG was placed in the cranial and caudal aspects of gluteus maximus (Jaegers et al 1992) and the DSG just posterior to the sacrotuberous ligament. This was confirmed with real-time ultrasound imaging. Slouched sitting was used because this has been shown to produce a position of counternutation of the sacrum (Snijders et al 2004). When a vertical force was placed through the shoulders of subjects, the activity of DSG suggested it may have a separate role in vertical loading from the cranial and caudal GM fibers.

During gait, it has been suggested that the sacrum torsions (or rotates) to face the innominate that is posteriorly rotated. In the existing biomechanical theory of the gait cycle, when the femur is extended and internally rotated, the innominate is relatively anteriorly rotated on that side. Conversely, when the femur is flexed and externally rotated, the innominate is relatively posteriorly rotated on that side (Lee 2004). During a trunk twist to the left in normal standing, the right femur will be relatively extended and internally rotated, whereas the right innominate is in relative anterior rotation. Here the sacrum will torsion, or rotate to the left. During trunk twisting (to create pelvic torsion), increased activity was observed in the DSG that was different from the cranial or caudal GM fibers. These observations suggest that the DSG might be involved in controlling aspects of vertical loading and pelvic torsion. It should be cautioned that these are preliminary observations and further investigation is needed before conclusions can be drawn (unpublished pilot study, Gibbons et al 2004).

Consistent changes in the presence of pain and pathology

Local stability muscles show consistent and characteristic changes following a significant episode of pain (Comerford & Mottram 2001b); these are listed in Table 6.2. The characteristics that are revelant for PM include segmental atrophy and altered patterns of low threshold recruitment.

Segmental atrophy

Psoas major

Dangaria & Naesh (1998) assessed the cross-sectional area (CSA) of PM in unilateral sciatica caused by disc herniation. There was significant reduction in the CSA of PM at the level and ipsilateral to the site of disc herniation. Barker et al (2004) assessed the CSA of PM and lumbar multifidus in subjects with unilateral LBP. There was a significant reduction of the CSA on the side of symptoms. The decrease in CSA was largest at the level of symptoms, with smaller changes one level above and below for both muscles. A similar pattern of atrophy is seen in lumbar multifidus in acute LBP (Hides et al 1994).

It has been proposed that the posterior aspect of PM plays a more specific role in spinal stability (Gibbons 2004, Gibbons et al 2001, 2002a). A protocol was developed to observe and measure the width of the posterior fascicles of the PM muscle utilizing a helical scan and a coronal oblique view with computed tomography (CT) imaging (Gibbons & Whalen 2003). A pilot study found reliability to be high, and the validity of this technique was demonstrated in cadavers (Gibbons et al 2002b). The preliminary results of a current investigation show a trend towards more specific atrophy in the posterior fasciculii in PM in subjects with first-time acute unilateral LBP.

Altered pattern of low-threshold recruitment

Psoas major

Indirect methods of measurement of muscle function have been used in research when direct methods have been invasive or difficult due to the deep location of certain muscles (Jull 2000, O'Sullivan et al 1997). A specific low-threshold exercise was developed for PM (Gibbons et al 2002a). Briefly, this is a hip-shortening exercise where there is vertical shortening of the femoral head into the acetabulum. Superficial EMG was recorded during the exercise from multi-joint hip muscles that could potentially contribute to the movement. Subjects either had a history of LBP and were pain free at the time or did not have a history of LBP. PM was observed via ultrasound imaging at the pelvic brim and the neutral spine position was monitored with a pressure biofeedback. The subjects with a history of LBP exhibited significantly higher amounts of EMG activity during the exercise and tended to loose the neutral spine position. It was hypothesized that one of the reasons this may have occurred was due to poor function in PM in the LBP subjects (Gibbons et al 2005).

Deep sacral gluteus maximus

A specific low-threshold exercise was developed for the DSG. This involved a medial swelling contraction of GM without a lateral swelling contraction. A pilot study was conducted similar to the above study (with regard to subject criteria). Superficial EMG was recorded during the exercise from the medial GM region over the sacrotuberous ligament, the lateral GM region between the ischial tuberosity and the greater trochanter, biceps femoris, rectus femoris and tensor fascia latae. GM was observed via ultrasound imaging over the sacrotuberous ligament and subjects had to achieve a 1-cm swelling contraction. The subjects with a history of LBP exhibited higher amounts of EMG activity during the exercise, particularly in rectus femoris and the hamstrings (unpublished pilot study, Gibbons et al 2003).

Purpose of this research

Movement dysfunction and specific motor control stability exercise has been growing in its research base since the 1990s. Existing paradigms of muscle function and advances in technology have facilitated new ideas for research. A pattern has emerged in which some muscles, or specific fibers of muscles, have a separate role in providing stability. Two such muscles are PM and GM. We should aim to investigate these further and explore other muscles for their roles in stability. It is hoped that our group can collaborate with other researchers to share ideas and gain a better understanding of the mechanisms of specific muscle function in spinal stability. From this, we might be able to provide enough evidence to facilitate a change, improve clinical interventions and the management of related musculoskeletal disorders.

Summary

There appears to be evidence of a stability role for PM. The anatomy of PM suggests that it: (1) does not significantly change length; (2) can provide compression to the sacroiliac joint; and (3) has two separate components, which might have individual roles. The biomechanics of PM show that it: (1) does not contribute significantly to spinal motion except to produce a lumbar lordosis; and (2) produces axial compression in the lumbar spine. At the hip, it produces vertical shortening into the acetabulum and does not contribute significantly to hip flexion. At the SIJ, it has the potential to produce posterior rotation of the innominate. The neurophysiology suggests a separate role for iliacus and PM. It appears that PM is not the dominant hip flexor. With dysfunction, it has a segmental change in cross-sectional area and it exhibits an altered pattern of low-threshold recruitment during a specific exercise.

The DSG is a recent finding, therefore little is known about its function. The anatomy of the DSG suggests it does not contribute to physiological movement. The neurophysiology suggests a specific role that is separate from the cranial and caudal fibers. In dysfunction, it might have an altered pattern of low-threshold recruitment during a specific exercise. However, as noted, these were pilot studies and any interpretation from these results should be made with caution.

A new description of PM is that the anterior and posterior fasciculii have separate functions and that the posterior fasciculii might have a separate function in controlling lumbar segmental translation. No direct evidence comes from neurophysiology, although there are some unique findings. First, the separate nerve supplies for the anterior and posterior fasciculii suggest a different function. Second, the posterior fasciculii have segmental attachments and are located in an ideal position to control intersegmental motion. Third, they are much smaller and cannot generate much force or contribute significantly to range of motion. Further, the vast fascial connections of PM to the diaphragm, TrA, and the pelvic floor place it in an ideal position for cocontraction mechanisms to enhance stability.

It is proposed that GM consists of three separate functional subdivisions. It is likely that the superficial sacral fibers of GM are the ones involved in dysfunction of overactivity (Lee 2004) and prone to shortness, which can lead to compensatory movements (Sahrmann 2002). This is because these fibers continue into the iliotibial band and thus constitute a multi-joint muscle and might be prone to overactivity (Comerford & Mottram 2001b).

Further research is warranted to investigate the role of PM and DSG in lumbopelvic stability. This might help dispel some common myths and misconceptions regarding PM and provide new avenues for research in the field.

References

Andersson E, Oddsson L, Grundstrom H et al 1995 The role of the psoas and iliacus muscles for stability and movement of the lumbar spine, pelvis and hip. Scandinavian Journal of Medicine, Science and Sports 5:10–16

Andersson EA, Nilsson J, Thorstensson A 1997 Intramuscular EMG from the hip flexor muscles during human locomotion. Acta Physiologica Scandinavica 161:361–370

Aspinall W 1993 Clinical implications of iliopsoas dysfunction. The Journal of Manual and Manipulative Therapy; 1(2):41–46

Bachrack RM, Nicelorra J, Winuk C 1991 The relationship of low back pain to psoas insufficiency. Journal of Orthopedic Medicine 13(2):34–40

Barker KL, Shamley DR, Jackson D 2004 Changes in the cross sectional area of multifidus and psoas in patients with unilateral back pain. Spine 29(22):E515–E519

Bogduk N, Pearcy M, Hadfield G 1992 Anatomy and biomechanics of psoas major. Clinical Biomechanics 7:109–119

Bullock-Saxton JE, Janda V, Bullock M 1994 The influence of ankle injury on muscle activation during hip extension. International Journal of Sports Medicine 15:330–334

Comerford MJ, Mottram SL 2001a Functional stability retraining: Principles and strategies for managing mechanical dysfunction. Manual Therapy 6(1):3–14

Comerford MJ, Mottram SL 2001b Movement and stability dysfunction – contemporary developments. Manual Therapy 6(1):15–26

Dangaria T, Naesh O 1998 Changes in cross-sectional area of psoas major muscle in unilateral sciatica caused by disc herniation. Spine 23(8):928–931

Dostal WF, Soderberg GL, Andrews JG 1986 Actions of hip muscles. Physical Therapy 66(3):351–361

Gibbons SGT 2004 A hypothetical link between psychosocial factors, pain and sensory motor function using a biomechanical model of psoas major. MSc Thesis in Health Ergonomics, University of Surrey, UK

Gibbons SGT 2005a Anatomy and functional relations of psoas major. Submitted

Gibbons SGT 2005b Muscle function – a critical evaluation. Proceedings of the Second International Conference on Movement Dysfunction. 'Pain and Performance: Evidence & Effect.' 23–25 September, Edinburgh, UK

Gibbons SGT, Comerford MJ 2001 Strength versus stability. Part I: Concepts and terms. Orthopaedic Division Review. March/April, 21–27

Gibbons SGT, Mottram SL 2004 Functional anatomy of gluteus maximus: deep sacral gluteus maximus – a new muscle? Proceedings of: The 5th Interdisciplinary World Congress on Low Back Pain. November 7–11, Melbourne, Australia

Gibbons SGT, Whalen B 2003 Computed tomography imaging of posterior psoas major. Proceedings of the 52nd Annual Conference of the Newfoundland and Labrador Association of Medical Radiation Technologists. St John's, Newfoundland

Gibbons SGT, Pelley B, Molgaard J 2001 Biomechanics and stability mechanisms of psoas major. Proceedings of the Fourth Interdisciplinary World Congress on Low Back Pain. 9–11 November, Montreal, Canada

Gibbons SGT, Comerford MJ, Emerson P 2002a Rehabilitation of the stability function of psoas major. Orthopaedic Division Review Jan/Feb: 7–16

Gibbons SGT, Comerford MJ, Whalen B 2002b Inter and intra tester reliability of posterior psoas major. Proceedings of the Thirteenth Annual Orthopaedic Symposium. Canadian Physiotherapy Association Orthopaedic Division. 21–22 September, Saskatoon, Canada

Gibbons SGT, Holmes MWR, Grandy C et al 2005 Altered hip and trunk muscle recruitment in subjects with chronic low back pain during a specific exercise for the psoas major muscle. Submitted

Gracovetsky S, Farfan HF, Lamy C 1981 The mechanism of the lumbar spine. Spine 6(3):249–262

Hides JA, Stokes MJ, Saide M et al 1994 Evidence of lumbar multifidus muscle wasting ipsilateral to symptoms in patients with acute/subacute low back pain. Spine 19(2):165–172

Hungerford B, Gilleard W, Hodges PW 2003 Evidence of altered lumbopelvic muscle recruitment in the presence of sacroiliac joint pain. Spine 28(14):1593–1600

Jaegers S, Dantuma R, de Jongh HJ 1992 Three-dimensional reconstruction of the hip muscles on the basis of magnetic resonance images. Surgical and Radiologic Anatomy 14(3):241–249

Janevic J, Ashton-Miller JA, Schultz AB 1991 Large compressive pre-loads decrease lumbar motion segment flexibility. Journal of Orthopedic Research 19:228–236

Juker D, McGill S, Kropf P et al 1998 Quantitative intramuscular myoelectric activity of lumbar portions of psoas and the abdominal wall during a wide variety of tasks. Medicine & Science in Sports and Exercise 30(2):301–310

Jull G 2000 Deep cervical flexor muscle dysfunction in whiplash. Journal of Musculoskeletal Pain 8(1/2): 143–154

Kapandji IA 1987 The physiology of the joints. Volume two: lower limb, 5th edn. Churchill Livingstone, Edinburgh

Lee D 2004 The pelvic girdle, 3rd edn. Churchill Livingstone, Edinburgh

McGill S 2002 Low back disorders. Evidence-based prevention and rehabilitation. Human Kinetics, Champaign, IL

Moore KL 1992 Clinically oriented anatomy, 3rd edn. Williams & Wilkins, Baltimore, MD

Moore KL, Dalley AF 1999 Clinically oriented anatomy, 4th edn. Williams & Wilkins, Philadelphia, PA

Nachemson A 1968 The possible importance of the psoas muscle for stabilisation of the lumbar spine. Acta Orthopaedica Scandinavica 39:47–57

O'Sullivan PB, Twomey L, Allison G et al 1997 Altered patterns of abdominal muscle activation in patients with chronic low back pain. Australian Journal of Physiotherapy 43(2):91–98

Pool-Goudzwaard AL, Vleeming A, Stoeckart R et al 1998 Insufficient lumbopelvic stability: a clinical, anatomical and biomechanical approach to 'a-specific' low back pain. Manual Therapy 3(1):12–20

Rab GT, Chao EYS, Stauffer RN 1977 Muscle force analysis of the lumbar spine. Orthopedic Clinics of North America 8(1):193–199

Richardson C, Jull G, Hodges PW et al 1999 Therapeutic exercise for spinal segmental stabilization in low back pain: scientific basis and clinical approach. Churchill Livingstone, Edinburgh

Richardson C, Hodges PW Hides 2004 Therapeutic exercise for lumbopelvic stabilization, 2nd edn. Churchill Livingstone, Edinburgh

Romanes GJ 1987 Cunningham's manual of practical anatomy, 15th edn. Vol II: Thorax and abdomen. Oxford University Press, Oxford, UK

Sahrmann S A 2002 Diagnosis and treatment of movement impairment syndrome. CV Mosby, St Louis, MO

Santaguida PL, McGill SM 1995 The psoas major: a three dimentional geometric study. Journal of Biomechanics 28:339–345

Snijders CJ, Vleeming A, Stoeckart R et al 1995 Biomechanical modeling of sacroiliac joint stability in different postures. Spine: State of the Art Reviews 9(2):419–432

Snijders CJ, Hermans PFG, Niesing R et al 2004 The influence of slouching and lumbar support on iliolumbar ligaments, intervertebral discs and sacroiliac joints. Clinical Biomechanics 19(4):323–329

Williams PL, Warwick R, Dyson M et al 1989 Gray's anatomy, 37th edn. Churchill Livingstone, Edinburgh

Yoshio M, Murakami G, Sato T et al 2002 The function of the psoas major muscle: passive kinetics and morphological studies using donated cadavers. Journal of Orthopaedic Science 7:199–207

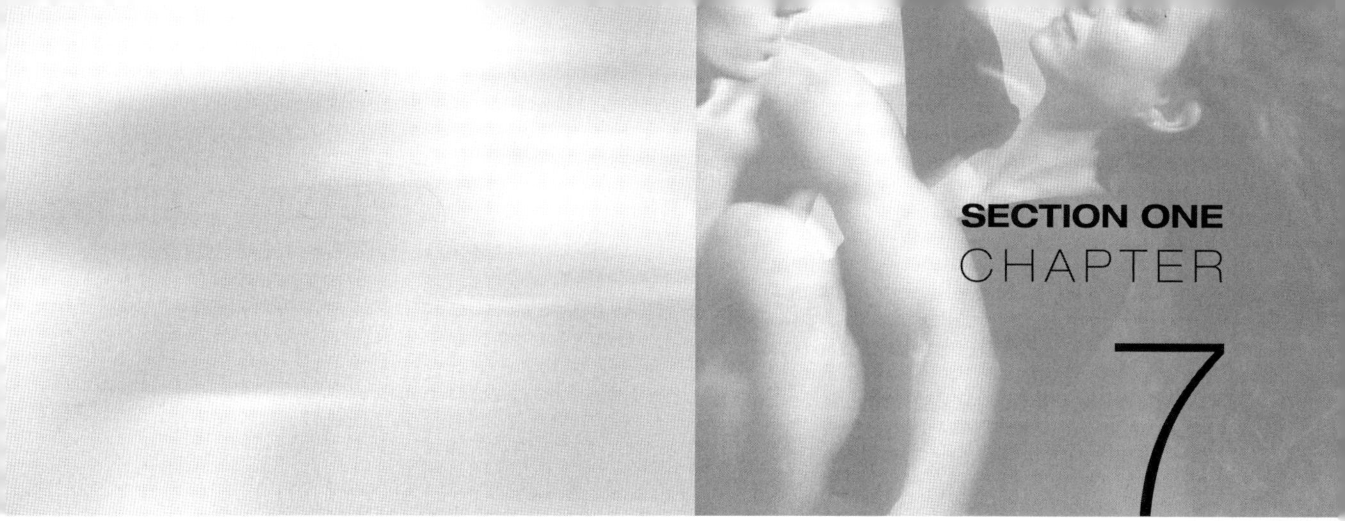

SECTION ONE
CHAPTER 7

The sacroiliac joint: sensory–motor control and pain

Aage Indahl and Sten Holm

Introduction

At the turn of the twentieth century, the sacroiliac joint (SIJ) was thought of as the main pain generator of the back and sacroiliac dysfunction was described (Albee 1909). In the search for causes of low back pain (LBP), the SIJ has gained renewed interest as a possible pain generator (Daum 1995, Schwarzer et al 1995). There is a special awareness of the SIJ as a source of pain in pregnant and postpartum women, and although the mechanism is not understood, relaxation of the SIJ before childbirth is believed to play a role (MacLennan et al 1986). As mechanisms behind sacroiliac dysfunction, instability and/or subluxation have most often been suggested (Calvillo et al 2000, DonTigny 1985, Mooney 1993). Despite any proven clinical finding or clearly defined function of the joint, 'sacroiliac dysfunction' has been established as a clinical entity (Bernard & Cassidy 1991, DonTigny 1979, Dreyfuss et al 1996, Mooney 1993).

'Stability' and 'instability' have been important parts of most theories and hypotheses regarding painful low back and pelvic conditions. On the one hand, these terms seem to indicate that something is proper and confined to its normal range of motion or, on the other hand, that pathological motion exists. Despite the popularity of these terms, they have been difficult to define and, in our opinion, there are no fully accepted definitions. Without a proper definition, and thereby the possibility of measuring the nature of the pathology, the terms are useless in scientific work. However, there is little doubt that pain in the low back and pelvic area has something to do with disturbances in or around the SIJ. Despite many trials, we feel that the function of the SIJ in locomotion is not well established.

The joint is relatively small, considering the forces transmitted across it, and looking at it from a purely mechanical point of view has not led to significant better treatments for patients, as results from trials are conflicting (Nilsson-Wikmar et al 2005, Stuge 2004). Perhaps we can look at the SIJ from another perspective than the purely mechanical? Could there be other explanations for pelvic pain than some kind of pathological motion in the SIJ? Could it be that the hypothesis of 'instability' is basically wrong? What, then, could be the cause of pain and what else could produce the clinical picture described as 'instability'? This chapter deals with different factors involved in sensory–motor control to see if it can offer an alternative hypothesis for painful conditions of the SIJ and its adjacent structures.

For a joint so centrally located and considering the amount of forces transmitted through it, it is feasible to believe that the SIJ must have a role in sensory motor control during locomotion. Normal locomotion requires the involvement of multiple levels of neural control to support the body against gravity, maintain posture, and propel it forward. During all this, balance must be maintained and the locomotion must be adapted to the environment and purpose. This task is accomplished by coordination of muscle contractions at many joints. The basis for this coordination is sensory information. The proper moment-to-moment functioning of the motor system depends on a continuous inflow of sensory information.

Sensory input, especially proprioceptive information, is integral to both feedback and feedforward mechanisms, which provide flexibility in the control of motor output.

Anatomical aspects

The SIJ is a true synovial joint with an auricular shape and a very limited amount of motion (Fig. 7.1). The movement of the SIJ seems to be very limited and has so far not been able to be detected by objective methods apart from invasive techniques. No proven clinical tests have been shown to be reliable in detecting increased or decreased motion of the joint. Roentgen stereophotogrammetric analysis has shown the amount of SIJ motion to range from 0.5 to 1.6 mm for translation and up to 4 degrees for rotation (Sturesson et al 1989, 2000).

The SIJ does, however, have an extensive network of strong ligaments that maintain its integrity. Its limited motion gives flexibility to the pelvic ring and the large twisting forces applied during locomotion can be buffered by the joint (Bogduk 1997). The shape and position of the joint are probably ideal only for weight-bearing and the proposed interlocking mechanism made by the ridges and grooves in the joint would possibly make the joint less efficient as a stress reliever. However, the position and shape of the SIJ, together with the extensive ligamentous structures, provide an ideal system for efficient walking by relieving stress and storing energy; the torsional forces might be stored in ligamentous structures as elastic energy and in a spring-like action make walking more efficient energy-wise (see Chapter 8).

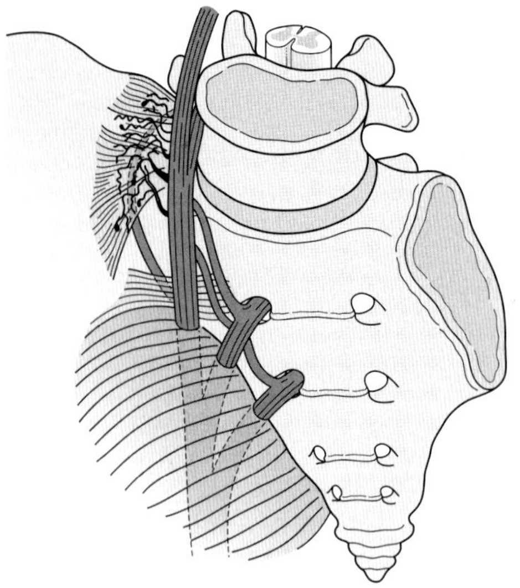

Fig. 7.1 Schematic representation of the lumbar–sacral area indicating the SIJ position on the right hand side. (Reproduced from Indahl 1999, with permission.)

Ligaments

The different ligaments and the capsule of the SIJ are responsible for the integrity of the joint and have been described in detail elsewhere. All ligaments seem to be innervated, even the ligamentum flavum (Bucknill et al 2002), but the exact innervation is still being studied (see also Chapter 1).

Musculature

There are no muscles that cross only the SIJ; the muscles that cross the joint exert their forces on the spine and/or the hip joint. The lumbar musculature is formed by a network of smaller

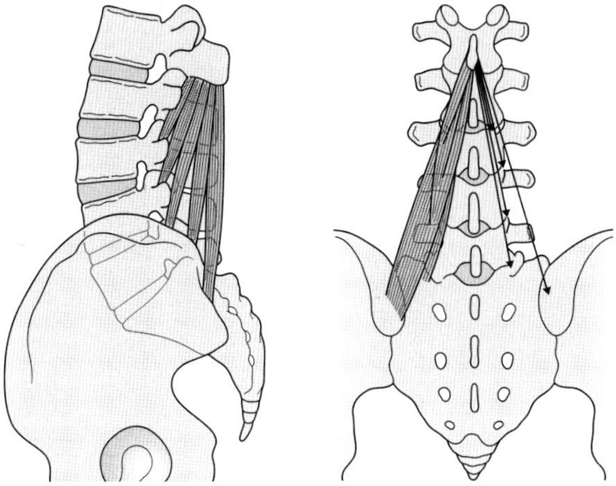

Fig. 7.2 The intersegmental musculature forms a network capable of fine-tuning load transfer in the lumbar spine and SIJ. (Reproduced from Indahl 1999, with permission.)

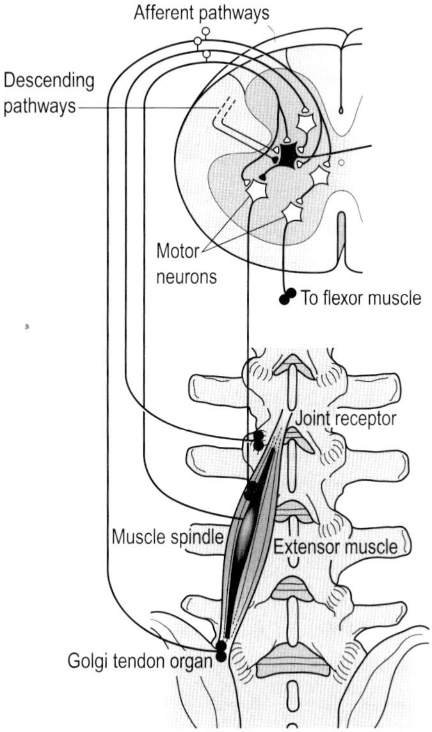

Fig. 7.3 Neuromuscular feedback system depicting the afferent sensory information from joint receptors, muscle spindles, and Golgi tendon organs for regulating muscle tension. (Reproduced from Indahl 1999, with permission.)

and larger muscles that exert various forces on the spinal motion segments. The function of these muscles is to support the spine and transfer loading while providing mobility. The functions of the larger muscle groups, such as the erector spinae and multifidus muscles, have been determined experimentally but, for some of the smaller muscles, the functions have only been inferred from their architectural arrangement. Due to the relatively small size and lever arm, these muscles are not considered to be large generators of force. Their function is perhaps better considered as adjusters, where they are capable of fine-adjusting loads on the spinal structures (Fig. 7.2). Along with the multifidus, this network of muscles is capable of adjusting not only the loading on a single segment, but also polysegmentally.

The hip muscles not only move the hip but are also important in keeping balance of the moving body. In muscle and tendon, the motor and sensory functions of the neural structures for controlling posture and movements are well established. The load-sensitive nerve endings, or mechanoreceptors, found in muscle (muscle spindles) and tendon (Golgi tendon organs), provide proprioceptive information regarding tension levels, position and motion, essential for controlling muscle tone (Fig.7.3).

Neural structures

The SIJ appears to be richly innervated, although there seems to be some uncertainty as to the exact innervation patterns. Solonen (1957) found the SIJ to be predominantly innervated by the L4–S1 nerve roots, with some contribution from the superior gluteal nerve, but with a lesser contribution from S2, and rarely from L3 nerve roots. Grob et al (1995), in a study on adult human cadavers, found the SIJ to be innervated by fine nerve branches derived exclusively from dorsal rami of the S1–S4 spinal nerves. Ikeda (1991) reported that the upper ventral portion of the SIJ was mainly supplied by the ventral ramus of the fifth lumbar nerve, whereas the lower ventral portion was mainly supplied by the ramus of the S2 nerve. Thick, thin, and unmyelinated nerve fibers have been reported, and are compatible with a broad repertoire of sensory receptors, including encapsulated mechanoreceptors (Grob et al 1995, Ikeda 1991). Various studies (Atlihan et al 2000, Fortin et al 1999b) have also demonstrated the close physical relationships between the SIJ capsule and adjacent neural structures, including the lumbosacral nerves and sympathetic nerves. Given the wide range of innervations of the SIJ and its adjacent neural structures, SIJ capsular stimulation might refer various pain patterns to the buttock, groin, thigh, calf, or foot (Dreyfuss et al 1996, Fortin et al 1994, 1999a, Schwarzer et al 1995).

Experimental studies

Several experiments, using a porcine model, have studied a possible interaction between the lumbar intervertebral disc, zygapophyseal joints, SIJ, and paraspinal and gluteal muscles.

In the first two experiments, stimulation of the outer disc annulus or facet joint capsule produced paraspinal muscular responses on various levels, thereby demonstrating the existence of neural pathways between these structures. Introduction of saline or local anesthetics into the zygapophyseal joint interfered in the stimulation pathway from the disc to the musculature. This effect was most likely an inhibitory stretch reflex from the capsule that stimulated inhibitory interneurons, thus inhibiting motorneurons (Indahl et al 1995, 1997).

A porcine model was then used to determine if stimulation of nerves in the SIJ and the sacroiliac capsule could elicit contractions in the porcine gluteal or lumbar muscles.

When stimulating within the ventral area of the SIJ 5–10 mm deep, responses were found to occur in the gluteus medius, maximus and quadratus lumborum muscles, whereas only minor effects were observed in the remaining muscles (Fig. 7.4). However, when simulating on the dorsal site of the SIJ capsule, the greatest muscular responses were detected in the multifidus, with the predominant response in the fascicles lateral to L5, which was closest to the SIJ; minor responses were observed in the remaining muscles (Fig. 7.5).

In conclusion, stimulation of nerves and mechanoreceptors in the SIJ and SIJ capsule elicited muscular responses in various muscle groups. These findings suggest that the SIJ might be involved in activating muscles responsible for overall posture control, as well as control on the segmental level in the lumbar spine (Indahl et al 1999b).

In a recent experiment, the same model was used to determine if muscle activity in the paraspinal muscles caused by disc stimulation could be altered by either mechanical compression or distraction of the SIJ (Holm et al 2005). The aim of that investigation was to measure the SIJ involvement in activation of muscles in the lumbar spine. Adolescent domestic pigs were used. Two pairs of fixating screws were inserted into the ilium. A mechanical exciter was attached to the screws and a load was applied. Stimulating electrodes were placed in the L4–L5 disc. EMG needles were in the lumbar muscles from L3–L6. The application of a load on the SIJ resulted in inhibition of muscle activity in the monitored muscles. This inhibition varied in magnitude in different areas of the muscles (Fig. 7.6). Significant

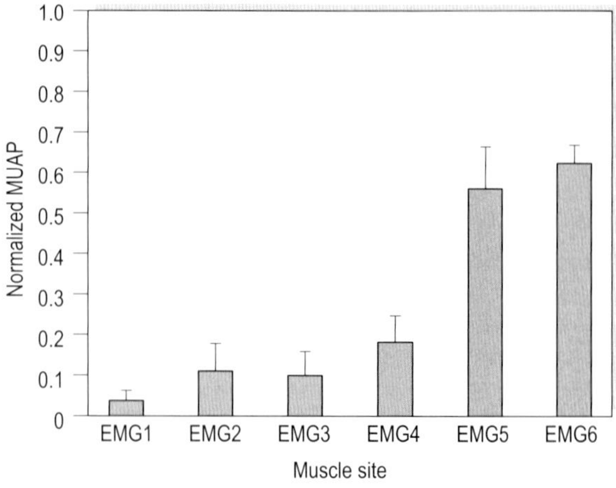

Fig. 7.4 The mean and standard error of the normalized muscle responses at each muscle site found when stimulating on the dorsal site of the sacroiliac joint capsule. Muscle sites: EMG1, multifidus (L3 level); EMG2, multifidus (L4 level); EMG3, multifidus (L5 level); EMG4, gluteus medius; EMG5, gluteus maximus; EMG6, quadratus lumborum. (Reproduced from Indahl et al 1999, with permission.)

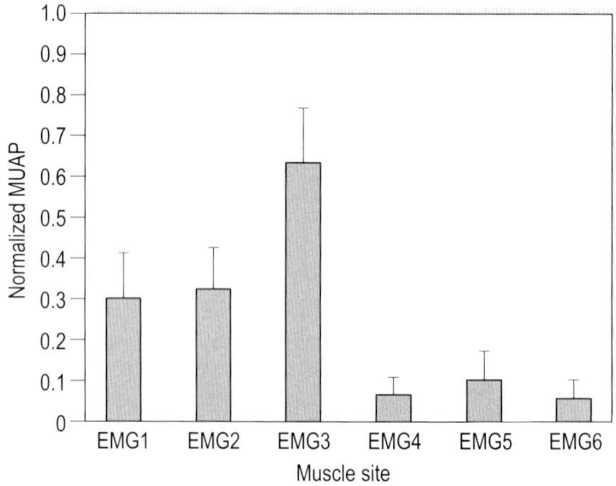

Fig. 7.5 The mean and standard error of the normalized muscle responses at each muscle site found when stimulating within the SIJ 5 to 10 mm deep. Muscle sites: EMG1, multifidus (L3 level); EMG2, multifidus (L4 level); EMG3, multifidus (L5 level); EMG4, gluteus medius; EMG5, gluteus maximus; EMG6, quadratus lumborum. (Reproduced from Indahl et al 1999, with permission.)

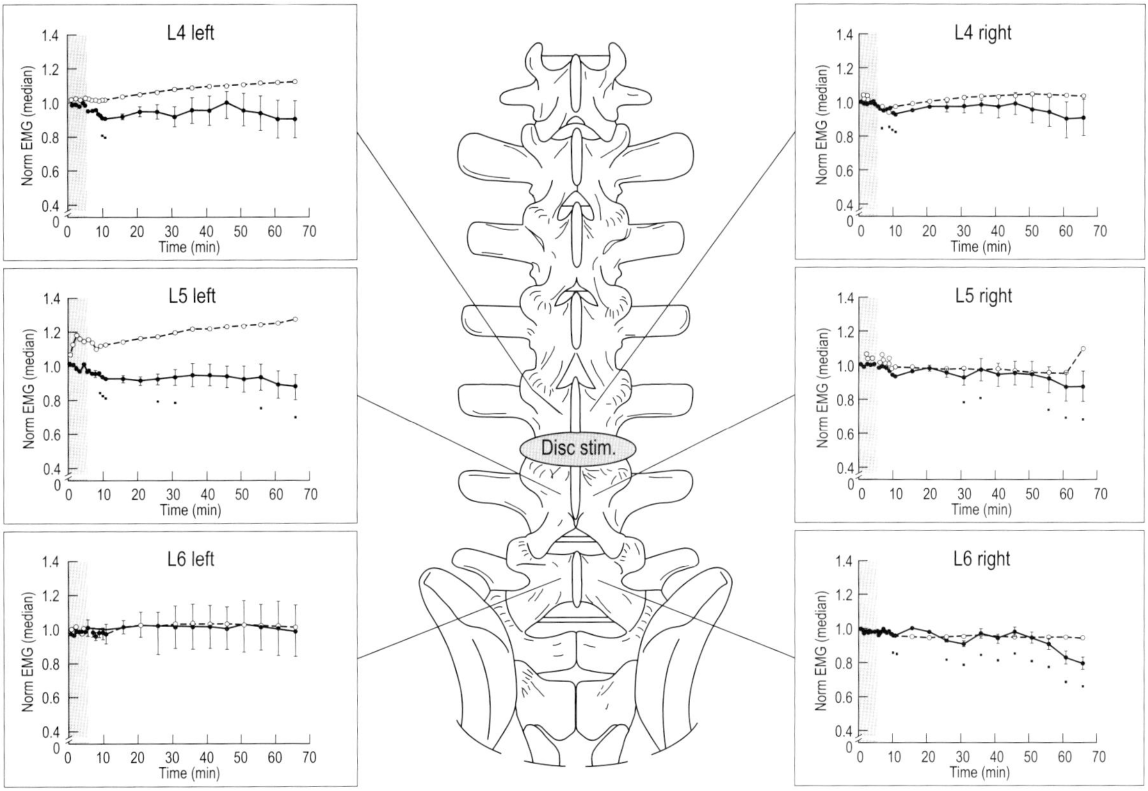

Fig. 7.6 The muscular responses with disc stimulation in controls and with loading of the sacroiliac joint. (Reproduced from Holm et al 2005, with permission.)

inhibition was also recorded at the contralateral side (L4 and L6) of the stimulated disc. Changes in muscle activation on the same side as the stimulation were found one to two levels caudally. After finishing the stimulation periods, the muscle activity gradually returned to initial levels. Thus changes in loading on the SIJ might result in altered activation of the controlling lumbar muscles and thus play an important regulatory function in spinal stabilization, load transfer, balance and movement of the upper body during postural changes.

Sensory–motor control

Normal gait seems so easy and effortless, yet it is a complicated and very much automatic behavior. For this to happen, sensory information is essential for adequate motor response and the functioning of the motor system is therefore intimately related to that of the sensory system. During activity, the proper moment-to-moment functioning of the motor system depends on a continuous inflow of a large variety of sensory information (Gordon 1991). This continuous flow of sensory information influences motor output in many ways and at all levels of the motor system. The system responsible for muscle coordination around a joint is called the 'myotactic unit.' Muscle spindle afferents make direct connection to motor neurons responsible for activation of synergist muscles and to interneurons inhibiting motorneurons of antagonist muscles. By these divergent connections to the different muscles around a joint, a strong neural network is established so that muscles do not act independently of each other. It is such arrangements that are responsible for joint stiffness.

Mechanoreceptors are thought to play an important role in the function of monitoring position and movements of joints by regulating and modifying muscle tension. The descending signals that initiate muscle action are modified by the sensory input from the proprioceptive nerve endings. Recruitment of the paraspinal and hip muscles can thus be coordinated in such a manner that the forces applied to the various structures are properly distributed and in such a pattern that the loading on the motion segment is optimal regardless of position. In such a system, the action of these muscles can provide the different structures with the support that is needed in order to counteract detrimental forces and prevent injury. Overload on specific parts can, by high threshold nerve endings, be detected and in due process, inhibit muscle actions responsible for the increased loading, and thereby prevent injury. This might be the reason why heavy physical loading does not seem to have the impact on degeneration of the spine as earlier assumed (Battie et al 1995, Lundberg et al 1994, Nachemson 1992).

The range of motion and innervation of the SIJ seem well suited for detecting various loading patterns during locomotion. In man, the slanted position of the L5–S1 motion segment and the relative position of the SIJ might have physiological importance for load detection, balance, and mobility. Not only can this system detect the load transferred and the stresses applied, but also calculate the vectors of the forces. The afferent input from SIJ receptors, as well as mechanoreceptors in the intervertebral discs and zygapophyseal joints, might contribute by feedback mechanisms to the modification of different muscle activations. The multi-segmental innervation indicates that sensory information from these structures is essential on many levels of the spinal cord. Feedback from the various structures enables us to develop efficient feedforward mechanisms that activate different muscles at different times thus making the movement (motion) elegant and at the same time distribute the loading on structures capable of handling the load. Spinal reflexes, where the 'myotactic units' are the building blocks, provide the nervous system with a set of elementary patterns of coordination that can be activated, either by sensory stimuli or by descending signals from the brain stem and cerebral cortex (Fig. 7.7).

For the activation and optimalization of the motor responses, particularly when it comes to postural adjustments, the body relies on both feedforward and feedback mechanisms. The feedforward or anticipatory mechanisms make us activate groups of muscles so that we can meet the challenges ahead. With anticipatory responses we can manage to stand on the deck of a rocking boat; and the more we do it, the more efficient our feedforward responses become. Before we become experienced standing on the deck, we refine our response by feedback or compensatory responses. Some of the feedback responses are rapid spinal reflexes, like the stretch reflex that helps us keep our balance in challenging situations. Other feedback

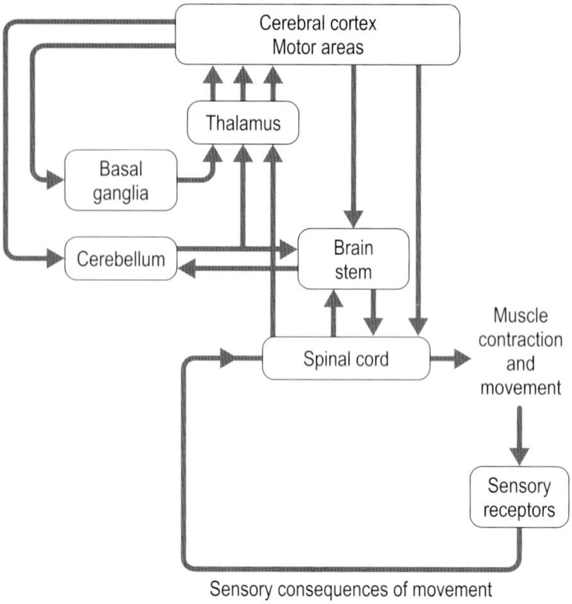

Fig. 7.7 Flowchart showing control of movement and the interaction between the different levels of the sensory–motor system. (Reproduced with permission from Ghez 1991 in Kandel et al, Principles of Neural Science, 3rd edn, © The McGraw-Hill Companies, Inc.)

mechanisms are slower and involve higher central nervous centers like the brain stem, cerebellum, and the cortex. Sensory input, especially proprioceptive information, is integral to both feedback and feedforward mechanisms, which provide flexibility in the control of motor output (Fig. 7.8). For instance, both feedforward control and rapid feedback compensatory corrections maintain postural balance during standing and walking. For most of the time we use a combination of these mechanisms during activity, like when we practice to improve our putting skills in golfing. If the feedforward response is not precise and adequate enough, there is sensory feedback that modifies our next response and in that way our putting improves. The feedforward or anticipatory response is a central process that engages different areas of the brain. The location of the 'feedforward controller' is probably in the premotor cortex area. The function has to do with planning and executing activity and behavior. This process relies on incoming sensory signals from all joints, muscles, and the balance system. It uses our experiences related to earlier similar activity and it anticipates what is going to happen during the planned activity. If a certain activity is about to be carried out that we have experienced to have caused pain, not only will our experience have an

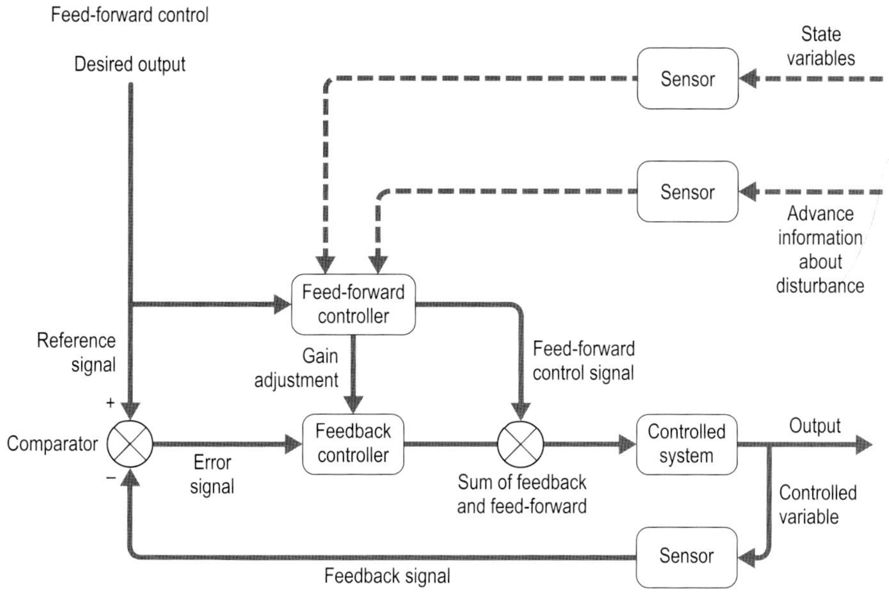

Fig. 7.8 Flowchart showing the functioning of the motor system involving feedforward control in relation to feedback compensatory corrections. (Reproduced with permission from Ghez 1991 in Kandel et al, Principles of Neural Science, 3rd edn, © The McGraw-Hill Companies, Inc.)

influence on the planning of the movement, but we will most likely anticipate that pain will be provoked again and the activity might therefore have the character of an avoidance behavior. Most of this function of the feedforward controller is subconscious and we do not have to think how we walk or ride a bike after we have learned it. We do not control specific muscles, we decide over activity. Once we have decided on a particular activity, the automatic system takes over, e.g. when we ride a bike; if you start thinking about how you are able to keep your balance on the bike you are likely to roll over and fall. This indicates that the automatic systems are necessary for most of our activity and enable us to carry out a complicated activity, but the activity can be taken under central control at any moment, which will result in less efficient and less refined performance.

Therefore the position of the SIJ, its pattern of movement and its nerve supply give us reason to believe that the joint plays an important role in the coordination of the back and pelvic musculature so that we can move normally. The joint's position and nerve supply are ideal for measuring the vectors of the various forces that act through the joint in walking and other strain. In a way, the joint might act as the body's 'bathroom scale', which measures loading and thereby controls the switching-on of musculature that in turn controls and moves the pelvis and torso during activity.

Pain and the SIJ: possible mechanisms

The multisegmental sensory innervation of the SIJ, discs, and zygapophyseal joints has several implications for the clinical evaluation of patients with low back and pelvic pain. It certainly does not make our job of finding where the pain comes from any easier. Also, the response of pain provocation of different structures might be difficult to evaluate. Responses could just as well be an effect of changes in the complex sensory motor control system as it also could be a local response; the difference will be difficult to differentiate.

Pain from the SIJ can come from a local structure that is injured or altered in such a manner that pain signals are generated. Pain can also be a result of a change in the complex sensory motor control system. Disturbances affecting the sensory nerve endings around the joint might lead to alteration of the control system. This can be caused by trauma, such as a fall, or it could be physiological changes as experienced during pregnancy or spontaneous derangements of unknown origin. Such a lesion must occur in an innervated region of the annulus fibrosus. Depending on the size of the lesion, the density of the neural structures and damage done to them, and the degree of irritation on the surrounding nerve endings, the firing pattern from these nerve endings might be altered in such a manner so as to cause increased activation of the paraspinal and hip muscles. For a minor transient change that more or less repairs itself, the sensory motor control system might also return to its normal activity. Changes of a more permanent character or long-lasting might require adaptation of the sensory motor control system to the new environment. How effective this adaptation is might not only have an impact on function, but also on pain. An adaptation resulting in increased muscle activation and coactivation might lead to increased pain. This muscle activation might occur in a 'bracing pattern' and subject the muscles to static work, which is thought to be responsible for muscle pain (Edwards 1988). Although it is not known which the responsible processes for muscle pain are, it is a common human experience that muscles can be painful (Ursin et al 1988).

During pregnancy the changes in the pelvic structures necessary for a safe delivery might certainly lead to altered environment for the sensory nerve endings in the area. In some women, these changes are well adjusted for and accommodated and no pain or problem arises. In others, the changes might be of greater magnitude or happen during a shorter time and thus an increased challenge for the adaptation is needed. There is normally no awareness of any movement of the pelvic girdle itself during activity. Alterations that affect the sensory nerve endings might lead to pain, but also to an awareness of the motion taking place. The changes of the range of motion might be minute, but as mechanoreceptors are capable of detecting changes down to a few thousandths of a millimeter, it might be experienced as substantial. If the normal translation in a SIJ is 1 mm and this is altered over a short period of time to 2 mm, it represents a change in the range of motion for the mechanoreceptors of 100%. This alteration might be too small to detect for any clinical testing or even for most advanced imaging techniques but would still have a huge impact on the sensory–motor control system and make the adaptation to this new environment challenging.

An awareness of increased motion might result in increased central control of the back and hip muscles. The focus of muscle activation might be altered from locomotion, balance, and weight transfer to that of keeping the pelvis 'in place.' This could lead to more coactivation and a static load on the muscles involved gaining control and resulting in a maladaptive behavior with increased pain as a result. These same mechanisms may be responsible for maladaptive processes regardless of what caused the changes around the sensory nerve endings to take place.

The mechanisms by which psychosocial factors have an impact on low back and pelvic pain and the transition from acute to chronic pain is not clear, although it can be explained on the basis of spinal reflexes. These factors probably have their major influence on the feedforward mechanisms or anticipatory responses. The muscular response is triggered by what we anticipate. If we anticipate that a certain movement will result in pain or injury our feedforward response will try to prevent this. If we have a feeling that the pelvis is 'unstable,' this will affect our muscle activation pattern. Most likely it will result in a 'bracing' pattern of the lumbar paraspinal and hip muscles. What we *think* is taking place in the SIJ might be of greater impact on the feedforward responses than what *actually* takes place. The picture we have in our head of what is taking place in the pelvis will determine our behavior; the more threatening the picture is, the greater the impact on behavior will be.

This suggests that movement and movement-related pain should be considered as complex behaviors; not solely as a biomechanical, psychiatric, or a neurological problem, but rather as a problem related to the integration of nervous and biomechanical mechanisms. This involves the control of movements, with feedback from muscles, discs, and joints, all in a complex interaction with psychological mechanisms.

Summary

In conclusion, the position of the SIJ, its pattern of movement and its nerve supply give us reason to believe that the joint plays an important role in the coordination of the back and pelvic musculature so that we can move normally. The joint's position and nerve supply are ideal for measuring the vectors of the various forces that act through the joint in walking and other strains. In a way, the joint acts as the body's 'bathroom scale', measuring loading and thereby controlling the switching-on of musculature that in turn controls and moves the pelvis and torso during activity. An alteration of the environment around the sensory nerve endings might lead to a need for readjustments in the sensory–motor control system. How effective an adaptation to changes takes place will depend on the nature and magnitude of the change and the time involved, as well as the conception of what is wrong. Misconceptions of what really takes place in the pelvis might, for the individual trying to re-establish adequate feedforward responses, result in a maladaptive behavior and increased pain. Movement and movement pathophysiology might therefore be understood as a complex result of a network involving the peripheral and central nervous systems, psychological processes, as well as the traditional peripheral pain mechanisms.

References

Albee FH 1909 A study of the anatomy and the clinical importance of the SIJ. JAMA 53:1273–1276

Atlihan D, Tekdemir I, Ates Y, et al 2000 Anatomy of the anterior SIJ with reference to lumbosacral nerves. Clin Orthop 376:236–241

Battie MC, Videman T, Gibbons LE et al 1995 Determinants of lumbar disc degeneration: a study relating lifetime exposures and magnetic resonance imaging findings in identical twins. Spine 20:2601–2612

Bernard PN, Cassidy JD 1991 SIJ syndrome: Pathophysiology, diagnosis and management. In: Frymoyer JW (ed) The adult spine: principles and practice. Raven Press, New York, p2107–2131

Bogduk N 1997 Clinical anatomy of the lumbar spine and sacrum. Churchill Livingstone, New York

Bucknill AT, Covard K, Plumton C et al 2002 Nerve fibers in lumbar spine structures, and injured spinal roots express the sensory neuron specific sodium channels SNS/PN3 and NaN/SNS2. Spine 27:135–140

Calvillo O, Skaribas I, Turnipseed J 2000 Anatomy and pathophysiology of the SIJ. Curr Rev Pain 4(5):356–361

Daum WJ 1995 The sacroiliac joint: an underappreciated pain generator. Am J Orthop 24:475–478

DonTigny RL 1979 Dysfunction of the SIJ and its treatment. J Ortho Sports Phys Ther 1:23–35

DonTigny RL 1985 Function and pathomechanics of the SIJ. A review. Phys Ther 65:35–44

Dreyfuss P, Michalsen M, Pauza K et al 1996 The value of medical history and physical examination in diagnosing SIJ pain. Spine 21:2594–2602

Edwards RHT 1988 Hypotheses of peripheral and central mechanisms underlying occupational muscle pain and injury. Eur J Appl Physiol 57:275–281

Fortin JD, Dwyer AP, West S et al 1994 SIJ: pain referral maps upon applying a new injection/arthrography technique: part 1, asymptomatic volunteers. Spine 19(13):1475–1482

Fortin JD, Kissling RO, O'Connor BL et al 1999a SIJ innervation and pain. Am J Orthop 28(12):687–690

Fortin JD, Washington WJ, Falco FJ 1999b Three pathways between the SIJ and neural structures. AJNR Am J Neuroradiol 20(8):1429–1434

Ghez C 1991 Control of movement. In: Kandel ER, Schwartz JH, Jessel TM (eds) Principles of neural science, 3rd edn. Appleton and Lange, Norwalk, CT, p535

Gordon G 1991 Spinal mechanisms of motor coordination. In: Kandel ER, Schwartz JH, Jessel TM (eds) Principles of neural science, 3rd edn. Appleton and Lange, Norwalk, CT, p581–595

Grob KR, Neuberger WL, Kisslig RO 1995 Die innervation des sacroiliacgelenkes beim menschen. Zeitschrift für Rheumatologie 54:117–122

Holm S, Indahl A, Kaigle Holm A et al 2005 The influence of sacroiliac joint loading on lumbar muscle response induced by intradiscal stimulation. ISSLS Meeting, New York

Ikeda R 1991 Innervation of the sacroiliac joint. Macroscopical and histological studies [in Japanese]. J Nippon Medical School 58:587–596

Indahl A 1999 Low back pain – a functional disturbance. Physiology and treatment. Thesis. Centre for Orthopaedics, National Hospital University of Oslo, Norway

Indahl A, Kaigle A, Reikerås O, Holm S 1995 Electromyographic response of the porcine multifidus musculature after nerve stimulation. Spine 20:2652–2658

Indahl A, Kaigle A, Reikerås O, Holm S 1997 Interaction between the porcine lumbar intervertebral disc, zygapophysial joints, and paraspinal muscles. Spine 22:2834–2840

Indahl A, Kaigle A, Reikerås O, Holm S 1999 Sacroiliac joint involvement in activation of the porcine spinal and gluteal musculature. J Spin Disord 12:325–330

Lundberg U, Mardberg B, Frankenhauser M 1994 The total work load of male and female white collar workers as related to age, occupational level, and number of children. Scand J Psychol 35:315–337

MacLennan AH, Green RC, Nicolson R, Bath M 1986 Serum relaxin and pelvic pain of pregnancy. Lancet 2:243–245

Mooney V 1993 Understanding, examining for, and treating sacroiliac pain. J Musculoskel Med 37–49

Nachemson AL 1992 Newest knowledge of low back pain. Clin Orthop 279:8–20

Nilsson-Wikmar L, Holm K, Oijerstedt R, Harms-Ringdahl K 2005 Effect of three different physical therapy treatments on pain and activity in pregnant women with pelvic girdle pain: a randomized clinical trial with 3, 6, and 12 months follow-up postpartum. Spine 30(8):850–856

Schwarzer AC, Aprill CN, Bogduk N 1995 The sacroiliac joint in chronic low back pain. Spine 20:31–37

Solonen KA 1957 The sacroiliac joint in light of anatomical, roentgenological and clinical studies. Act Orthop Scand 27(suppl):1–27

Stuge B, Laerum E, Kirkesola G, Vollestad N 2004 The efficacy of a treatment program focusing on specific stabilizing exercises for pelvic girdle pain after pregnancy: a randomized controlled trial. Spine 29(4):351–359

Sturesson B, Selvik G, Uden A 1989 Movements of the sacroiliac joints: a roentgen stereophotogrammetric analysis. Spine 14:162–165

Sturesson B, Uden A, Vleeming A 2000 A radiostereometric analysis of the movements of the sacroiliac joints in the reciprocal straddle position. Spine 25(2):214–217

Ursin H, Endresen I, Ursin G 1988 Psychological factors and self-reports of muscle pain. Eur J Appl Physiol 57:282–290

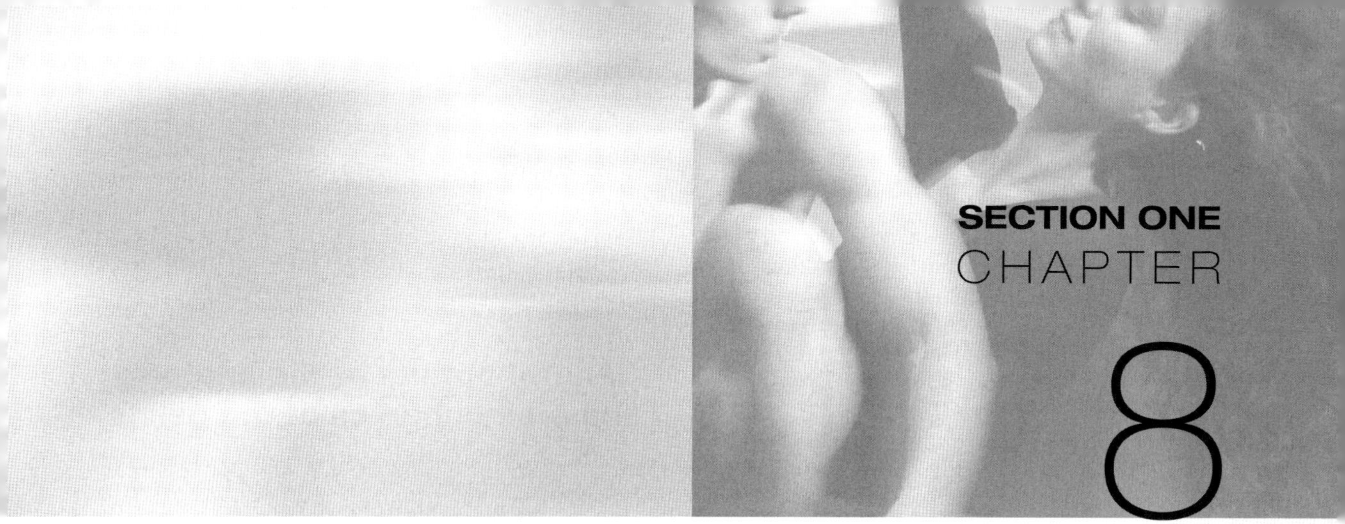

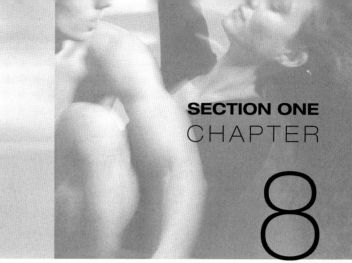

SECTION ONE
CHAPTER

8

The role of the pelvic girdle in coupling the spine and the legs: a clinical–anatomical perspective on pelvic stability

Andry Vleeming and Rob Stoeckart

Introduction

Musculoskeletal disorders, and particularly low back pain (LBP), are very expensive in today's modern society. The causes of LBP are not well understood and therapy frequently fails. Appropriate models to explain nonspecific LBP are not sufficiently available, probably due to the nature of these models.

For the past few decades, research on LBP has focused on the anatomical structures that could generate and explain pain, and so a search for pain generators and less focus on functional kinematical relations. However, such a functional approach could help to understand the real causes of lumbopelvic pain. In other words, we have to deepen our knowledge of complex kinematical chains, particularly the role of motor control in optimizing body function.

When we started clinical lumbopelvic studies in our research group, we were hampered by our knowledge; it was primarily based on topographic anatomy. This branch of anatomy has been developed to map the body, to answer the question of what structures our body consists of, and to categorize them. The use of topographic anatomy is not satisfactory for answering complex questions such as 'Why are there so many LBP patients?' and 'How do the spine, pelvis, and legs function as an integrated system?'; in fact, categories such as 'spine' and 'pelvis' are already confusing. 'Spine' muscles are strongly connected to the pelvis and to the ligaments around the sacroiliac joint (SIJ). Officially, in the *terminologia anatomica*, the pelvic joints and ligaments are classified as belonging to the legs. However, although classifications such as 'legs', 'pelvis', and 'spine' might serve a didactic purpose, they impede our understanding of the functional mechanisms operating in this region.

In scrutinizing the literature on spine and pelvis, our attention was triggered by the studies of the American therapist DonTigny (see Chapter 18). DonTigny (1979) consistently reported that the SIJ is essential for understanding spinal function, whereas Bowen & Cassidy (1981) described a peculiar cartilage pattern of the human SIJ. However, the literature did not give sufficient clues to enable understanding of the mechanisms that might lead to 'nonspecific' LBP.

Our research started on the function of the SIJs as the essential joints transferring load between spine and legs. The pelvis is regarded as the main bony platform, connected to three levers (spine and legs) that have to be stabilized under altering conditions. New studies showed that the SIJ adapts to new loading situations with altered levels of stiffness (Fig. 8.1). This was a contradictory view because the accepted characteristic of a joint is its capacity to function smoothly. There is now ample evidence for the view that the SIJ, like other joints, can change its stiffness characteristics under altering load conditions. This concept helped us to think differently about the stabilizing mechanisms of the human body at rest and during movement, and about the question of how stability of the pelvis is warranted by a coupled action of spine, pelvis, legs, and even arms.

This chapter considers in more detail the anatomy and biomechanics (see also Chapters 13, 14, 39 and 40) of the pelvic girdle and the implications for diverse situations such as stability of the pelvic girdle in standing, sitting, walking, and forceful trunk rotation. It also deals with the implications for pelvic girdle pain (PGP) itself. PGP has recently been shown to be a subcategory of LBP and can be regarded as a specific form of LBP (see Chapter 31).

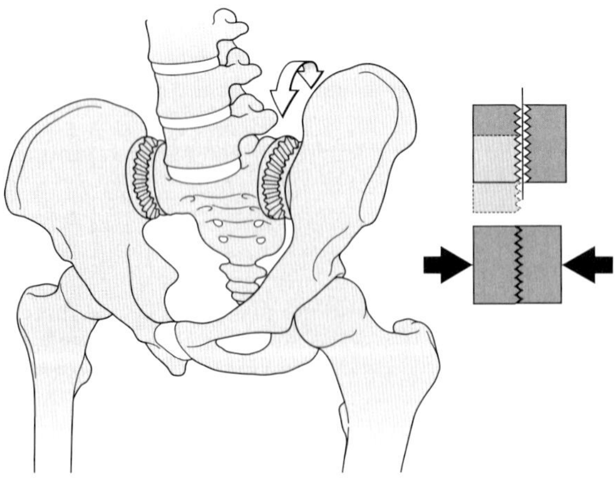

Fig. 8.1 Whimsical depiction of sacroiliac joints with friction device.

General outline of the anatomy and biomechanics of the pelvis

In all quadrupeds and bipeds, the pelvic girdle forms a firm connection between the spine and the lower extremities. In bipeds, the pelvis has to serve as a basic platform with three large levers acting on it (the spine and the legs). To allow bipedal gait in humans, evolutionary adaptations of the pelvis have been necessary, i.e. changing the shape of the ilia, flaring out into the sagittal plane, providing a more optimal lateral attachment site for the gluteus medius as an important muscle for hip pelvic stability. In particular, a dramatically increased attachment site for the gluteus maximus muscle has changed this muscle – a relatively minor muscle in the chimpanzee – into one of the largest muscles of the human body (Lovejoy 1988). Thus the human pelvis evolved quite differently to that of the chimpanzee (see Chapter 12).

Additional evolutionary changes in humans are the muscular and ligamentous connections between the sacrum and ilia: (1) muscles, like the lower lumbar multifidi, that insert into the sacrum and also into the medial cranial aspects of the ilium; (2) changes in the position of the coccygeus and the piriform muscles, and of the gluteus maximus muscle originating from the sacrum and sacrotuberous ligaments; (3) extensive fibrous connections adapted to the typical anatomy of the SIJ, like the interosseous ligaments, surrounding an iliac protrusion fitting in a dorsal sacral cavity, called the axial joint just behind the auricular surfaces of the SIJ (Bakland & Hansen 1984); (4) ventral and dorsal SIJ ligaments, sacrotuberous and sacrospinous ligaments between sacrum and lumbar spine (anterior longitudinal ligaments). In addition, direct fibrous connections exist between the iliac bone and L4 and L5, the iliolumbar ligaments. A recent study has described the influence of the iliolumbar ligaments on SIJ stability (Pool-Goudzwaard et al 2003). Due to the above-mentioned muscular and ligamentous connections, movement of the sacrum with respect to the iliac bones, or vice versa, affects the joints between L5–S1 and between the higher lumbar levels. Anatomical and functional disturbances of the pelvis or lumbar region influence each other. Due to the tightness of the fibrous connections and the specific architecture of the SIJ, mobility in the SIJ is normally very limited, but movement does occur and has not been scientifically challenged (Egund et al 1978, Lavignolle et al 1983, Miller et al 1987, Solonen 1957, Sturesson et al 1989, 2000a, 2000b, Vleeming et al 1990a, 1990b, 1996, Weisl 1955).

The main movements in the SIJ are forward rotation of the sacrum relative to the iliac bones (nutation) and backward rotation of the sacrum relative to the ilia (counternutation) (Fig. 8.2). It was shown that even at advanced age (> 72 years) the combined movement of nutation and counternutation can amount to 4°; normally movements are less than 2° (Vleeming et al 1992a). In the latter study, the SIJ with the lowest mobility showed radiologically marked arthrosis. Ankylosis of the SIJ was found to be an exception, even at advanced age. This finding is in agreement with studies of Stewart (1984) and Miller et al (1987).

Nutation is increased in load-bearing situations, e.g. standing and sitting. In lying prone, nutation is also increased compared to supine positions (Egund et al 1978, Sturesson et al 1989, 2000a, 2000b, Weisl 1955). Counternutation normally occurs in unloaded situations like lying down (supine). Counternutation in supine positions can be altered to nutation by maximal flexion in the hips, using the legs as levers to posteriorly rotate the iliac bones relative to the sacrum, as in a labour position, creating space for the head of the baby during delivery.

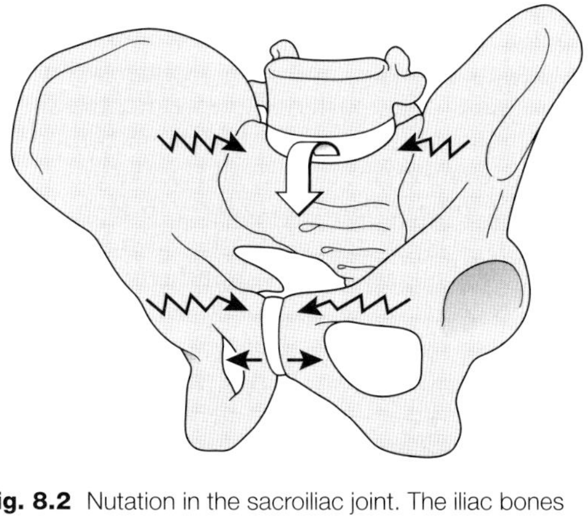

Fig. 8.2 Nutation in the sacroiliac joint. The iliac bones are pulled to each other due to ligament tension (among others) and compress the sacroiliac joints (upper black arrows). It can be expected that especially the upper (anterior) part of the pubic symphysis is compressed.

The anatomy of the sacroiliac joint

The SIJs are relatively flat, unlike ball and socket joints such as the hip. Generally speaking, flat articular surfaces are less resistant to shear forces and therefore the presence of flat surfaces in the pelvis seems surprising. This anatomical configuration gives rise to three questions: (1) 'Why did nature create a seemingly flat SIJ?'; (2) 'What specific adaptations are available to prevent shear in the SIJs?'; and (3) 'Why is the SIJ not perpendicularly orientated to the forces of gravitation?'

Why did nature create a seemingly flat SIJ?

A large transfer of forces is required in the human SIJ, and indeed flat joints are theoretically well suited to transfer large forces (Snijders et al 1993a, 1993b). An alternative for effective load transfer by these flat joints would be a fixed connection between sacrum and iliac bones, for instance by ankylosis of the SIJ. The SIJs in humans serve a purpose: to economize gait, to allow shock and shear absorption, and to alleviate birth of (in the evolutionary sense) abnormally large babies. The principal function of the SIJs is to act as stress relievers, ensuring that the pelvic girdle is not a solid ring of bone that could easily crack under the stresses to which it is subjected (Adams et al 2002).

What specific adaptations are available to prevent shear in the SIJs?

The SIJs are abnormal compared to other joints because of cartilage changes that are present already before birth. These occur especially at the iliac side of the joint and were misinterpreted as degenerative arthrosis (Bowen & Cassidy 1981, Sashin 1930). These cartilage changes are more prominent in men than in women and, according to Salsabili et al (1995), the sacral cartilage is relatively thick in females. This gender difference might be related to childbearing and possibly to a different localization of the center of gravity in relation to the SIJ (Dijkstra et al 1989, Vleeming et al 1990a, 1990b). Vleeming et al (1990a, 1990b) considered these changes to reflect a functional adaptation. The features seem to be promoted by the increase in body weight during the pubertal growth spurt and concern a coarse cartilage texture and a wedge and propeller-like form of the joint surfaces.

Studies of frontal slides of intact joints of embalmed specimens show the presence of cartilage-covered bone extensions protruding into the joint.

These protrusions seemed irregular but are in fact complementary ridges and grooves. Joint samples taken from normal SIJ with both coarse texture and complementary ridges and grooves were characterized by high-friction coefficients (Vleeming et al 1990b). All these features are expected to reflect adaptation to human bipedality, contributing to a high coefficient of friction and enhancing the stability of the joint against shear (Vleeming et al 1990a). As a consequence, less muscle and ligament force is required to bear the upper part of the body (Fig. 8.3).

The 'keystone-like' bony architecture of the sacrum further contributes to its stability within the pelvic ring. The bone is wider cranially than caudally, and wider anteriorly than posteriorly. Such a configuration permits the sacrum to become 'wedged' cranially and dorsally into the ilia within the pelvic ring (Vleeming et al 1990a, 1990b). The SIJ has evolved from a relatively flat joint into a much more stable construction (Fig. 8.4).

To illustrate the importance of friction in the SIJ, the principles of form and force closure were introduced (Vleeming et al 1990a, 1990b). Form closure refers to a theoretical stable situation with closely fitting joint surfaces, where no extra forces are needed to maintain the state of the system, given the actual load situation. If the sacrum would fit in the pelvis with perfect form closure, no lateral forces would be needed. However, such a construction would make mobility practically impossible. With force closure (leading to joint compression) both a lateral force and friction are needed to withstand vertical load. Shear in the SIJ is prevented by the combination of the specific anatomical features (form closure; see Fig. 8.5) and the compression generated by muscles and ligaments that can be accommodated to the specific loading situation (force closure). Force closure is the effect of changing joint reaction forces generated by tension in ligaments, fasciae, and muscles and ground reaction forces (Fig. 8.5).

Why is the SIJ not perpendicularly orientated to the forces of gravitation?

Force closure ideally generates a perpendicular reaction force to the SIJ to overcome the forces of gravity (Vleeming et al 1990b). This shear prevention system was named the self-bracing mechanism and such a mechanism is present elsewhere in the body, e.g. in the knee, foot, and shoulder. When a larger lever is applied and/or coordination time becomes less, the general effect in the locomotor system will be closure or reduction of the degrees of freedom of the kinematic chain, leading to a reduction of the chain's mobility or a gain of stability by increasing force closure (Huson 1997; see Chapter 10).

In self-bracing of the pelvis, nutation of the sacrum is crucial. This movement can be seen as an anticipation for joint loading. Hodges et al (2003) use the terminology 'preparatory motion' for a comparable phenomenon in the lumbar spine. So, nutation is seen as a movement to prepare the pelvis for increased loading by tightening most of the SIJ ligaments, among which are the vast interosseous and short dorsal sacroiliac ligaments. As a consequence the posterior parts of the iliac bones are pressed together, enlarging compression of the SIJ.

Ligaments and their role in self-bracing the pelvis

In self-bracing the pelvis, nutation in the SIJ is crucial (see above); this involves several ligaments. To further explain self-bracing of the pelvis we will discuss two sets of ligaments (Fig. 8.6): the sacrotuberous ligaments (Vleeming et al 1989a, 1989b, van Wingerden et al 1993) and the long dorsal SI ligaments (Vleeming et al 1996, 2002). In the literature, specific data on the functional and clinical relevance of the long ligaments are not available. In several anatomical atlases and textbooks, the long ligament and the sacrotuberous ligament are portrayed as fully continuous ligaments. The drawings generally convey the impression that the ligaments have identical functions. As shown by the contrasting effects of nutation and contranutation on these ligaments (see below), this is not the case. Essentially, the long ligament connects the sacrum and posterior superior iliac spine (PSIS), whereas the main part of the sacrotuberous ligament connects the sacrum and ischial tuberosity. However, some of the fibers derived from the ischial tuberosity pass to the iliac bone. Generally, they are denoted as part of the sacrotuberous ligament, although 'tuberoiliac ligament' would be more appropriate. In the *terminologia anatomica* such a ligament does not exist. In fact, this also holds for the long (dorsal SI) ligament, reflecting one of the problems of topographical anatomy.

Sacrotuberous ligaments

In embalmed human specimens, we could demonstrate a direct relation between nutation and

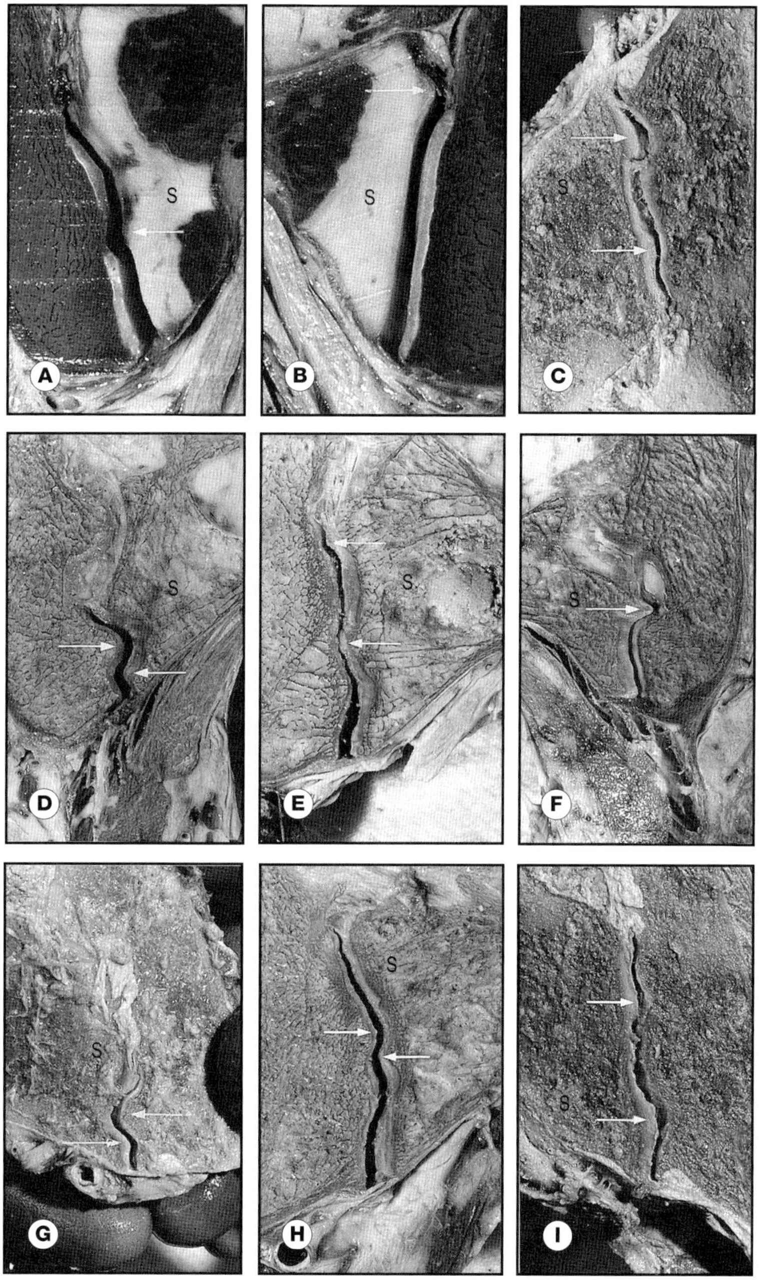

Fig. 8.3 Frontal sections of the sacroiliac joint (SIJ) of embalmed male specimen. S indicates the sacral side of the SIJ. (A) and (B) concern a 12-year-old boy; (C) to (I) concern specimen older than 60 years. Arrows are directed at complementary ridges and depressions. They are covered by intact cartilage, as was confirmed by opening the joints afterwards.

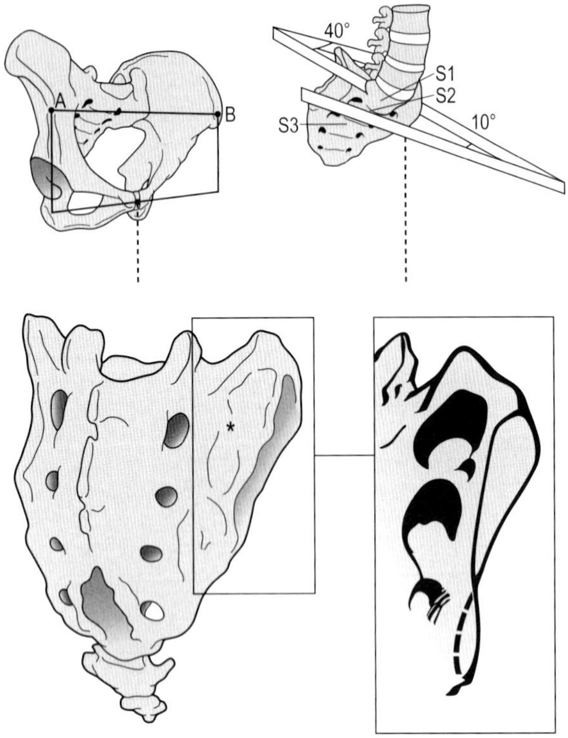

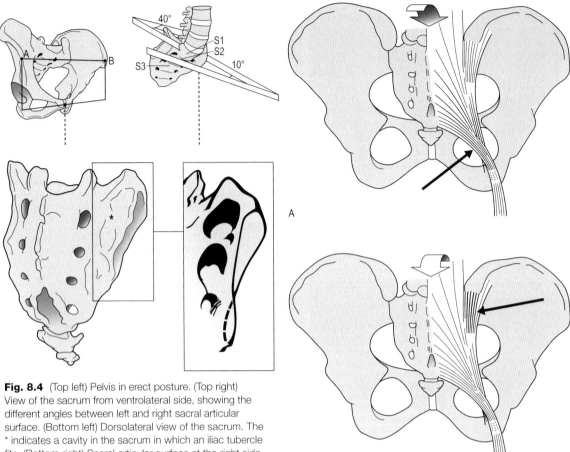

Fig. 8.4 (Top left) Pelvis in erect posture. (Top right) View of the sacrum from ventrolateral side, showing the different angles between left and right sacral articular surface. (Bottom left) Dorsolateral view of the sacrum. The * indicates a cavity in the sacrum in which an iliac tubercle fits. (Bottom right) Sacral articular surface at the right side. The different angles reflect the propeller-like shape of an adult sacroiliac joint.

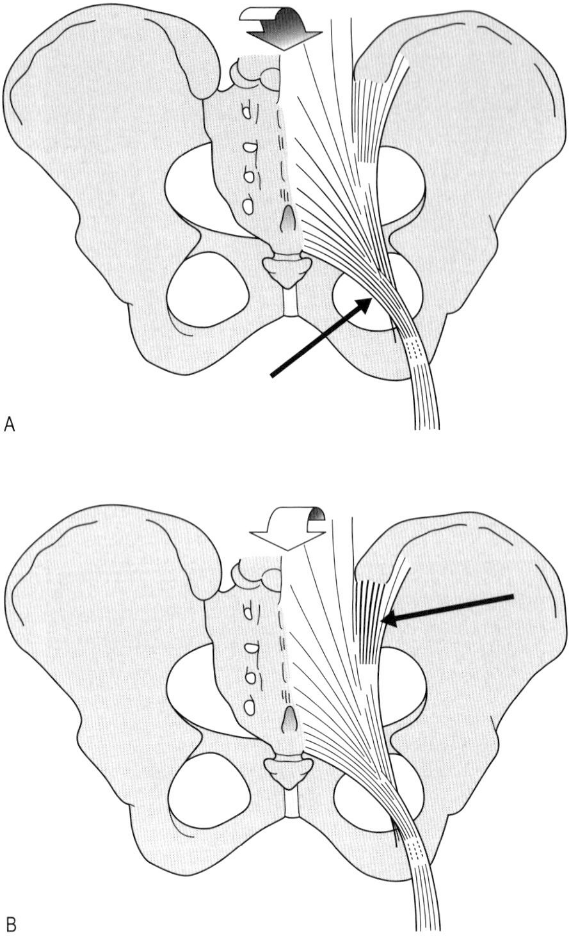

Fig. 8.6 (A) Nutation winds up the sacrotuberous ligament. (B) Counternutation winds up the long dorsal sacroiliac ligament.

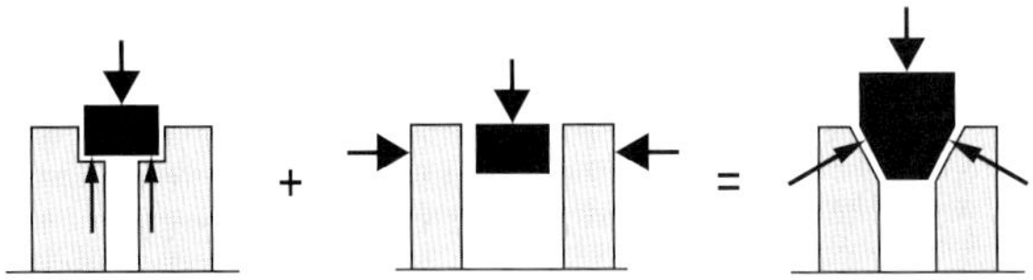

Fig. 8.5 Model of the self-locking mechanism. The combination of form closure and force closure establishes stability in the sacroiliac joint.

tension of the sacrotuberous ligament (Fig. 8.6A). By straining this ligament, we found a decrease of nutation (Vleeming et al 1989a, 1989b), indicating that these ligaments are well suited to restrict nutation. It can be expected that the opposite (diminished ligament tension) will increase nutation.

Long dorsal sacroiliac ligaments

In view of the capability of the sacrotuberous ligaments to restrict nutation, we wondered which ligament(s) could restrict counternutation. Because of its connection to the PSIS and to the lateral part of the sacrum (Fig. 8.6B), we expected that the long dorsal SI ligament could fulfill this function. The ligament can be easily palpated in the area directly caudal to the PSIS and is of special interest since women complaining of lumbopelvic back pain during pregnancy frequently experience pain within the boundaries of this ligament (Mens et al 1992, Njoo 1996, Vleeming et al 1996). Pain in this area is also not uncommon in men. The ligament is the most superficially located SIJ ligament and therefore well suited to mirror asymmetric stress in the SIJ. As this ligament is not well known in medical practice, we will summarize data from an anatomical and biomechanical study (Vleeming et al 1996) that assessed the function of the ligament by measuring its tension during incremental loading of biomechanically relevant structures.

For that purpose, the tension of the long ligament ($n = 12$) was tested under loading. Tension was measured with a buckle transducer. Several structures, including the erector spinae muscle and the sacrum itself, were incrementally loaded (with forces of 0–50 N). The sacrum was loaded in two directions (nutation and counternutation).

Anatomical aspects

At the cranial side, the long ligament is attached to the PSIS and the adjacent part of the iliac bone, at the caudal side to the lateral crest of the third and fourth sacral segments. In some specimens, fibers also pass to the fifth sacral segment. From the sites of attachment on the sacrum, fibers pass to the coccyx. These are not considered to be part of the long ligament.

The lateral expansion of the long ligament directly caudal to the PSIS varies between 15 and 30 mm. The length, measured between the PSIS and the third and fourth sacral segments, varies between 42 and 75 mm. The lateral part of the long ligament is continuous with fibers of the sacrotuberous ligament, passing between the ischial tuberosity and the iliac bone. The variation is wide. Fibers of the long ligament are connected to the deep lamina of the posterior layer of the thoracolumbar fascia, to the aponeurosis of the erector spinae muscle and to the multifidus muscle.

Biomechanical aspects

Forced incremental nutation in the SIJ diminished the tension in the long ligament, whereas forced counternutation increased the tension. Tension increased also during loading of the ipsilateral sacrotuberous ligament and erector spinae muscle. Tension decreased during traction on the gluteus maximus muscle. Tension also decreased during traction on the ipsilateral and contralateral posterior layer of the thoracolumbar fascia in a direction simulating contraction of the latissimus dorsi muscle.

Obviously, the long dorsal SI ligament has close anatomical relations with the erector spinae/multifidus muscle, the posterior layer of the thoracolumbar fascia, and a specific part of the sacrotuberous ligament (tuberoiliac ligament). Functionally, it is an important link between legs, spine, and arms. The ligament is tensed when the SIJs are counternutated and slackened when nutated. Slackening of the long dorsal SI ligament can be counterbalanced by both the sacrotuberous ligament and the erector spinae muscle.

Pain localized within the boundaries of the long ligament could indicate, among others, a spinal condition with sustained counternutation of the SIJ. In diagnosing patients with a specific LBP or PGP, the long dorsal SI ligament should not be neglected. Even in cases of arthrodesis of the SIJ, tension in the long ligament can still be altered by different structures.

This observation implies that the tension of the long ligament can be altered by displacement in the SIJ as well as by action of various muscles. Obviously, nutation in the SIJ induces relaxation of the long ligament, whereas counternutation increases tension. This is in contrast to the effect on the sacrotuberous ligament (see Fig. 8.6). Increased tension in the sacrotuberous ligament during nutation can be due to SIJ movement itself as well as to increased tension of the biceps femoris and/or gluteus maximus muscle. This mechanism can help to control *nutation*. As counternutation increases tension in the long ligament, this ligament can assist in controlling *counternutation* (see Fig. 8.6).

Ligaments with opposite functions, such as the long and sacrotuberous ligaments, apparently do not interact in a simple way. After all, loading of the sacrotuberous ligament also leads to a small increased tension of the long ligament. This effect will be due to the connections between long ligament and tuberoiliac (part of the sacrotuberous ligament) ligament, and possibly also to a counternutating moment generated by the loading of the sacrotuberous ligament.

A comparable complex relation might hold for the long ligament and the erector spinae, or more specifically the multifidus muscle. As the multifidus is connected to the sacrum (MacIntosh & Bogduk 1986, 1991; see Chapter 1), its action induces nutation. As a result, the long ligament will slacken. However, the present study shows an increase of tension in the long ligament after traction to the erector spinae muscle. This counterbalancing effect is due to the connections between the erector spinae muscle and the long ligament, and opposes the slackening. *In vivo*, this effect might be smaller because the moment of force acting on the sacrum is raised by the pull of the erector spinae muscle and the resulting compression force on the spine (Snijders et al 1993b). This spinal compression was not applied in this study. Both antagonistic mechanisms – between long and sacrotuberous ligaments and between the long ligament and the erector spinae muscle – might serve to preclude extensive slackening of the long ligament. Such mechanisms could be essential for a relatively flat joint such as the SIJ, which is susceptible to shear forces (Snijders et al 1993a, 1993b). It can be safely assumed that impairment of a part of this interconnected ligament system will have serious implications for the joint as load transfer from spine to hips and vice versa is primarily transferred via the SIJ (Snijders et al 1993a, 1993b).

As shown earlier (Vleeming et al 1996), traction to the biceps femoris tendon hardly influences tension of the long ligament.This is in contrast to the effect of the biceps on the sacrotuberous ligament (Vleeming et al 1989a, 1989b, van Wingerden et al 1993). The observations might well be related to the spiraling of the sacrotuberous ligament. Most medial fibers of the ligament tend to attach to the cranial part of the sacrum, whereas most fibers arising from a lateral part of the ischial tuberosity tend to the caudal part of the sacrum (see Fig. 8.6A). The fibers of the biceps tendon, which approach a relatively lateral part of the ischial tuberosity, pass mainly to the caudal part of the sacrum. As a consequence, the effect of traction to the biceps femoris on the tension of the long ligament can only be limited.

The effect on the long ligament of loading the posterior layer of the thoracolumbar fascia depends on the direction of the forces applied. Artificial traction to the fascia mimicking the action of the transverse abdominal muscle has no effect. Traction in a craniolateral direction, mimicking the action of the latissimus dorsi muscle, results in a significant decrease in tension in the ipsilateral and contralateral long ligaments. As shown in another study (Vleeming et al 1995), traction to the latissimus dorsi influences the tension in the posterior layer of the thoracolumbar fascia, ipsilaterally as well as contralaterally, especially below the level of L4. Thus slackening of the long ligament could be the result of increased tension in the posterior layer by the latissimus dorsi. This might itself lead to a slight nutation, leading to more compression and force closure of the SIJ. As shown in this study, slackening of the long ligament can also occur due to action of the gluteus maximus muscle, which is ideally suited to compress the SIJ.

It is inviting to draw conclusions when palpation, directly caudal to the PSIS, is painful. However, pain in this area might be due to pain referred from the SIJ itself (Fortin et al 1994a, 1994b), but also due to counternutation in the SIJ. Counternutation is part of a pattern of flattening the lumbar spine (Egund et al 1978, Lavignolle et al 1983, Sturesson et al 1989) that occurs in particular late in pregnancy when women counterbalance the weight of the fetus (Snijders et al 1976). However, such a posture combined with counternutation could also result from a pain-withdrawal reaction to impairment elsewhere in the system. Hence, only specific pain within the boundaries of the long ligament can be used as a diagnostic criterion (Vleeming et al 2002). An example of a pain-withdrawal reaction could be the following: pain of the pubic symphysis following delivery (Mens et al 1992) could preclude normal lumbar lordosis and hence nutation owing to pain of an irritated symphysis. After all, lumbar lordosis leads to nutation in the SIJ (Egund et al 1978, Lavignolle et al 1983, Sturesson et al 1989, Weisl 1955). Nutation implies that the left and right PSISs approach each other slightly while the pubic symphysis is caudally extended and cranially compressed (Lavignolle et al 1983, Walheim & Selvik 1984). In this example the patient will avoid nutation and flattens the lower spine, leading to sustained tension and pain in the long ligament. In a study by Mens et al (1999), it was shown that a positive active straight leg raise test coincides with a counternutated position of the SIJ in many patients.

In conclusion: functionally, the long dorsal SI ligament is an important link between legs, spine, and arms. In women with lumbopelvic back pain frequently pain is experienced within the boundaries of this ligament, which is tensed with counternutation and slackened with nutation. The erector muscle and the sacrotuberous ligament can counterbalance this slackening. The connections between ligaments and muscles with opposing functions could serve as a mechanism to preclude excessive slackening of ligaments.

Before focusing on the role of the muscles, we will draw attention to the thoracolumbar fascia.

The role of the thoracolumbar fascia in stabilizing the lumbopelvic area

To deepen our knowledge of the role of the thoracolumbar fascia the posterior layer of the thoracolumbar fascia was loaded by simulating the action of various muscles (Vleeming et al 1995).

Anatomical aspects

The posterior layer of the thoracolumbar fascia covers the back muscles from the sacral region, through the thoracic region as far as the fascia nuchae. At the level of L4–L5 and the sacrum, strong connections exist between the superficial and deep lamina. The transverse abdominal and internal oblique muscles are indirectly attached to the thoracolumbar fascia through a dense raphe formed by fusion of the middle layer (Bogduk & MacIntosh 1984) of the thoracolumbar fascia and both laminae of the posterior layer. This 'lateral raphe' (Bogduk & MacIntosh 1984, Bogduk & Twomey 1987) is localized laterally to the erector spinae and cranial to the iliac crest.

Superficial lamina (Fig. 8.7)

The superficial lamina of the posterior layer of the thoracolumbar fascia is continuous with the latissimus dorsi, gluteus maximus, and part of the external oblique muscle of the abdomen and the trapezius muscle. Cranial to the iliac crest, the lateral border of the superficial lamina is marked by its junction with the latissimus dorsi muscle. The fibers of the superficial lamina are orientated from craniolateral to caudomedial. Only a few fibers of the superficial lamina are continuous with the aponeurosis of the external oblique and the trapezius. Most of the fibers of the superficial lamina derive from the aponeurosis of the latissimus dorsi and attach to the supraspinal ligaments and spinous processes cranial to L4. Caudal to L4–L5, the superficial lamina is generally loosely (or not at all) attached to midline structures, such as supraspinal ligaments, spinous processes and median sacral crest. In fact, they cross to the contralateral side, where they attach to sacrum, PSIS, and iliac crest. The level at which this phenomenon occurs varies; it is generally caudal to L4 but in some preparations already occurs at L2–L3.

Barker & Briggs (1999) (see also Chapters 3 and 4) showed that the superficial lamina is also continuous superiorly with the rhomboids. They could not confirm the findings of Bogduk et al (1998) in relation to thickening of the fascia and the presence of posterior accessory ligaments. This is in agreement with the findings of Vleeming et al (1995).

At sacral levels, the superficial lamina is continuous with the fascia of the gluteus maximus. These fibers are orientated from craniomedial to caudolateral. Most of these fibers attach to the median sacral crest. However, at the level of L4–L5, and in some specimens even as caudally as S1–S2, fibers *partly or completely* cross the midline, attaching to the contralateral PSIS and iliac crest. Some of these fibers fuse with the lateral raphe and with fibers derived from the fascia of the latissimus dorsi. Owing to the different fiber directions of the latissimus dorsi and the gluteus maximus, the superficial lamina has a cross-hatched appearance at the level of L4–L5, and in some preparations also at L5–S2. The lamina becomes thicker and stronger especially over the lower lumbar spine and SIJ.

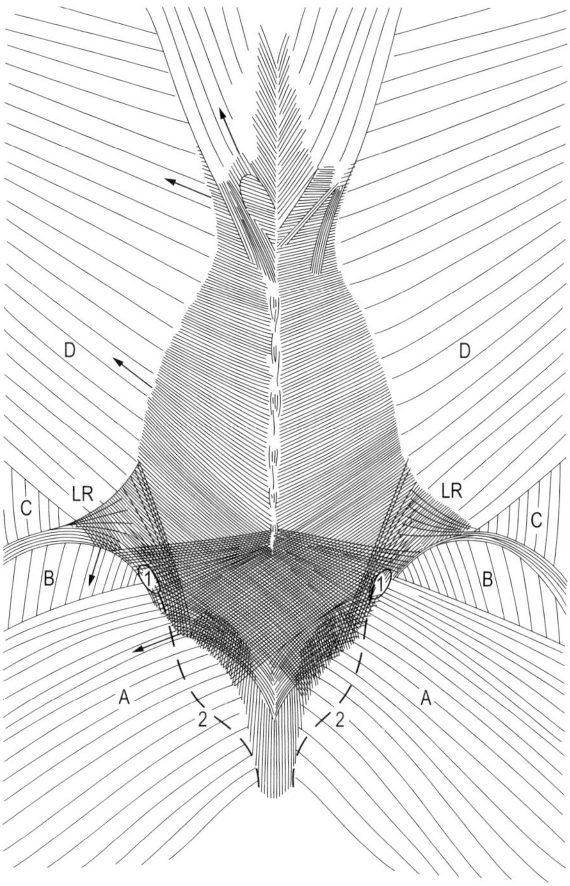

Fig. 8.7 The superficial lamina. A, fascia of the gluteus maximus; B, fascia of the gluteus medius; C, fascia of external oblique; D, fascia of latissimus dorsi; 1, posterior superior iliac spine (PSIS); 2, sacral crest; LR, part of lateral raphe. Arrows (at left) indicate, from cranial to caudal, the site and direction of the traction (50 N) given to trapezius, cranial and caudal part of the latissimus dorsi, gluteus medius and gluteus maximus muscles, respectively. (Reproduced from Vleeming et al 1995, with permission from *Spine*.)

Deep lamina (Fig. 8.8) (see also Chapters 3 and 4)

Barker & Briggs (1999) showed that the deep lamina is continuous cranially with the tendons of

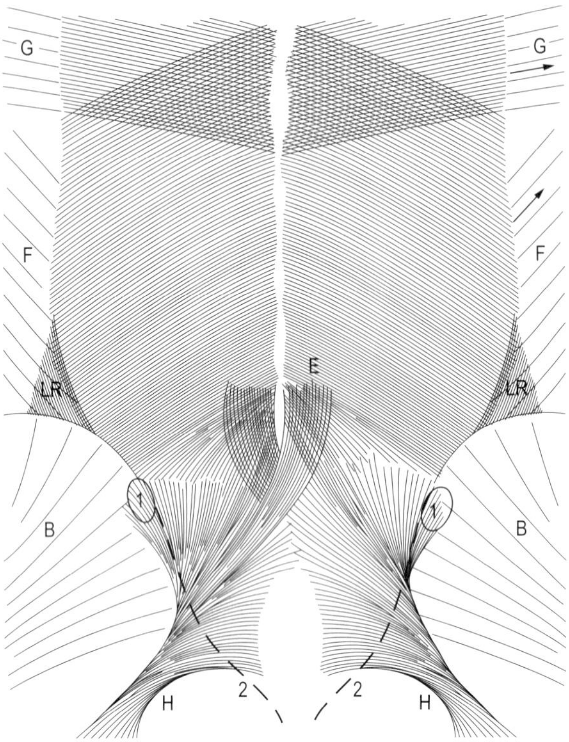

Fig. 8.8 The deep lamina. B, Fascia of the gluteus medius; E, connections between the deep lamina and the fascia of the erector spinae; F, fascia of the internal oblique; G, fascia of the serratus posterior inferior; H, sacrotuberous ligament; 1, the posterior superior iliac spine (PSIS); 2, sacral crest; LR, part of lateral raphe. Arrows (right) indicate, from cranial to caudal, traction to serratus posterior inferior and internal oblique muscles, respectively. (Reproduced from Vleeming et al 1995, with permission from *Spine*.)

the splenius cervicis and capitis muscles. At lower lumbar and sacral levels, the fibers of the deep lamina are oriented from craniomedial to caudolateral. At sacral levels, these fibers are fused with those of the superficial lamina. As, in this region, fibers of the deep lamina are continuous with the sacrotuberous ligament, an indirect link exists between this ligament and the superficial lamina. There is also a direct connection with some fibers of the deep lamina. In the pelvic region, the deep lamina is connected to the PSIS, iliac crests, and long dorsal SI ligament. This ligament originates from the sacrum and attaches to the PSIS. In the lumbar region, fibers of the deep lamina derive from the interspinous ligaments. They attach to the iliac crest and more cranially to the lateral raphe, to which the internal oblique is attached. In some specimens, fibers of the deep lamina cross to the contralateral side between L5 and S1. In the depression between the median sacral crest and the posterior superior and inferior iliac spines, fibers of the deep lamina fuse with the fascia of the erector. More cranially, in the lumbar region, the deep lamina becomes thinner and freely mobile over the back muscles. In the lower thoracic region, fibers of the serratus posterior inferior muscle and its fascia fuse with fibers of the deep lamina.

Biomechanical aspects

Traction to the superficial lamina

Depending on the site of the traction, quite different results were obtained (Vleeming et al 1995). Traction to the cranial fascia and muscle fibers of the latissimus dorsi muscle showed limited displacement of the superficial lamina (homolaterally up to 2–4 cm). Traction to the caudal part of the latissimus dorsi caused displacement up to the midline. This midline area is 8–10 cm removed from the site of traction. Between L4–L5 and S1–S2, displacement of the superficial lamina occurred even contralaterally. Traction to the gluteus maximus also caused displacement up to the contralateral side. The distance between the site of traction and visible displacement varied from 4 to 7 cm. The effect of traction to the external oblique muscle varied markedly between the different preparations. In all preparations, traction to the trapezius muscle resulted in a relatively small effect (up to 2 cm).

Traction to the deep lamina

Traction to the biceps femoris tendon, applied in a lateral direction, resulted in displacement of the deep lamina up to the level L5–S1. Obviously, this load transfer is conducted by the sacrotuberous ligament. In two specimens, displacement occurred at the contralateral side, 1–2 cm away from the midline. Traction to the biceps tendon directed medially showed homolateral displacement in the deep lamina, up to the median sacral crest.

As shown by the traction tests, the tension of the posterior layer of the thoracolumbar fascia can be influenced by contraction or stretch of a variety of muscles. It is noteworthy that especially muscles such as the latissimus dorsi and gluteus maximus are capable of exerting a contralateral effect especially to the lower lumbar spine and pelvis. This implies that the ipsilateral gluteus maximus muscle and contralateral latissimus dorsi muscle both can tension the posterior layer.

Hence, parts of these muscles provide a pathway for mechanical transmission between pelvis and trunk. One could argue that the lack of connection between the *superficial* lamina of the posterior layer and the supraspinous ligaments in the lumbar region is a disadvantage for stability. However, it would be disadvantageous only in case strength, coordination, and effective coupling of the gluteus maximus muscle and the caudal part of the contralateral latissimus dorsi muscle are diminished. It can be expected that increased strength of these mentioned muscles accomplished by torsional training could influence the quality of the posterior layer. Following this line of thinking, the posterior layer of the thoracolumbar fascia could play an integrating role in rotation of the trunk and in load transfer, and hence instability of the lower lumbar spine and pelvis.

Barker & Briggs (1999) make the interesting comment that the posterior layer is ideally positioned to receive feedback from multiple structures involved in lumbar movements and may regulate ligamentous tension via its extensive muscular attachments to both deep stabilizing and more superficial muscles. They also report that the fascia displays viscoelastic properties and thus is capable of altering its structure to adapt to the stresses placed on it. The posterior layer has been reported to stiffen with successive loading and adaptive fascial thickening is possible.

Barker & Briggs (1999) also comment that when adaptive strengthening of the posterior layer takes place, one might expect to facilitate this by using exercises that strengthen its attaching muscles, both deep and superficial. Adaptive strengthening therefore would be expected to occur with exercises using contralateral limbs such as swimming and walking and torsional training. It also might occur with recovery of muscle bulk and function (erector spinae/multifidus) during lumbopelvic stabilization exercises.

Bogduk et al (1998) do not agree with the concept that the latissimus dorsi has a role in rotating the spine and comment that the muscle is designed to move the upper limb and its possible contribution to bracing the SIJ via the thoracolumbal fascia is trivial. In contrast to this, Kumar et al (1996) show that axial rotation of the trunk involves agonistic activity of the contralateral external obliques, and ipsilateral erector spinae and latissimus dorsi as agonistic muscles to rotate the trunk.

Mooney et al (2001) used the anatomical relation of the latissimus dorsi and the contralateral gluteus maximus muscles to study their coupled effect during axial rotation exercises and walking. They concluded that in normal individuals, walking a treadmill, the functional relationship between the mentioned muscles could be confirmed. It was apparent that the right gluteus maximus muscle had on average a lower signal amplitude compared to the left ($n = 15$; 12 right-handed). This reciprocal relationship of muscles correlates with normal reverse rotation of shoulders versus the pelvis in normal gait. They showed that during right rotation of the trunk the right latissimus dorsi muscle is significantly more active than the left, but the left gluteus maximus muscle is more active than the right. In patients with SIJ problems a strikingly different pattern was noticed. On the symptomatic side the gluteus maximus was far more active compared with the healthy subjects. The reciprocal relation between latissimus and gluteus maximus muscles, however, was still present. After an intense rotational strengthening training program, the patients showed a marked increase of latissimus dorsi muscle strength and diminished activity of the gluteus muscle on the symptomatic side.

The importance of these findings could be that rotational trunk muscle training is important particularly for stabilizing the SIJ and lower spine. These findings contradict the conclusion of Bogduk et al (1998) that the latissimus dorsi muscle has no function besides upper limb movement.

Pelvic girdle pain (see Chapter 24) can be partially relieved by application of a pelvic belt, a device that 'self-braces' the SIJ (Vleeming et al 1992b). By exerting compression on the lower lumbar spine and pelvis, the posterior layer of the thoracolumbar fascia and its attached muscles can accomplish self-bracing physiologically. It is noteworthy that, as shown in this study, the coupled function of the gluteus maximus and the contralateral latissimus dorsi muscles creates a force perpendicular to the SIJ.

Attention is drawn to a possible role of the erector muscle and multifidus in load transfer. Between the lateral raphe and the interspinous ligaments, the deep lamina encloses the erector muscle and multifidus. It can be expected that contraction of the erector/multifidus will longitudinally increase the tension in the deep lamina. In addition, the whole posterior layer of the thoracolumbar fascia will be 'inflated' by contraction of the erector spinae/multifidus (Vleeming et al 1995), comparable to pumping up a ball. Consequently, it can be assumed that the training of muscles such as the gluteus maximus, latissimus dorsi and erector spinae, and the multifidus can assist in increasing force closure also by strengthening the posterior layer of the thoracolumbar fascia. However, for a proper sequence of training methods please see the therapeutic chapters in Parts 5 and 6 of this book and Chapter 3.

In conclusion: the posterior layer of the thoracolumbar fascia could play an important role in transferring forces between spine, pelvis, and legs, especially in rotation of the trunk and stabilization of lower lumbar spine and SIJ. The gluteus maximus and the latissimus dorsi merit special attention because they can conduct forces contralaterally via the posterior layer. Because of the coupling between the gluteus maximus and the contralateral latissimus dorsi via the posterior layer of the thoracolumbar fascia, one must be very cautious when categorizing certain muscles as arm, spine, or leg muscles. Rotation of the trunk is mainly a function of the oblique abdominals. However, a counter muscle sling in the back helps to preclude deformation of the spine. Rotation against increased resistance will activate the posterior oblique sling of latissimus and gluteus maximus.

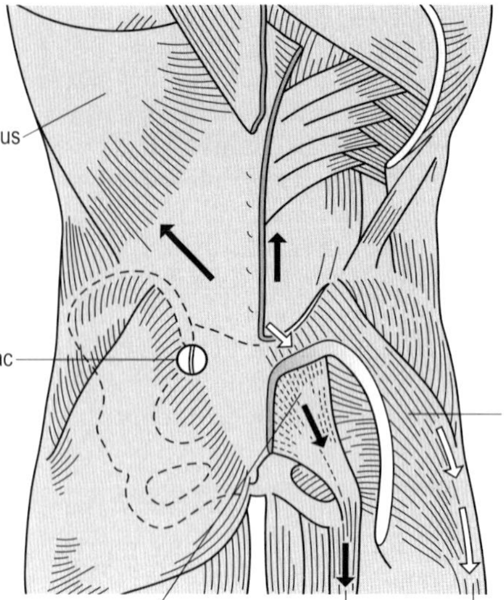

Fig. 8.9 Schematic dorsal view of the low back. The right side shows a part of the longitudinal muscle–tendon–fascia sling. Below this is the continuation between biceps femoris tendon and sacrotuberous ligament, above this is the continuation of the erector spinae. To show the right erector spinae, a part of the thoracolumbar fascia has been removed. The left side shows the sacroiliac joint and the cranial part of the oblique dorsal muscle–fascia–tendon sling, latissimus dorsi muscle and thoracolumbar fascia. In this drawing the left part of the thoracolumbar fascia is tensed by the left latissimus dorsi and the right gluteus maximus muscle.

Muscles and self-bracing

Various muscles are involved in force closure of the SIJ. With respect to SIJ function, we focus here on four muscles: the erector spinae/multifidus, gluteus maximus, latissimus dorsi, and biceps femoris (Fig. 8.9). Core lumbopelvic stability in relation to other muscles is discussed elsewhere (see Chapters 4, 6, 13, 33, 34 and 36).

The erector spinae/multifidus is the pivotal muscle that loads and extends spine and pelvis. The sacral connections of the erector/multifidus induce nutation in the SIJ, tensing ligaments such as the interosseous, sacrotuberous, and sacrospinal. Nutation is anticipatory for preloading the SIJ (preparatory movement; Hodges et al 2003 and see above). These muscles have a double function because their iliac connections pull the posterior sides of the iliac bones towards each other, constraining nutation. This implies that during nutation, due to action of the erector spinae/multifidus, the cranial side of the SIJ tends to be compressed whereas the caudal side has a tendency to widen. The latter is restricted by the sacrotuberous ligament, tensed by nutation, which has direct fascial connections with the erector spinae. A comparable process will occur in the pubic symphysis where the largest symphyseal ligament passes caudally to the joint (see Fig. 8.2).

Owing to its perpendicular orientation to the SIJ, the gluteus maximus can compress the joints directly and also indirectly by its vast muscular connections with the sacrotuberous ligament. Gibbons (2004; see also Chapter 6) speculates that the caudal part of the gluteus maximus, originating from the sacrotuberous ligament, can function in conjunction with the pelvic floor. Vleeming et al (1995) noted in a study on the SIJ that compression, among others, also can be established by coupling of the gluteus maximus with the contralateral latissimus dorsi muscle via the thoracolumbar fascia (Fig. 8.9).

Tension in the sacrotuberous ligament is increased by caudal traction to the long head of the biceps femoris. This is possible because not all fibers of the long head of the biceps attach to the ischial tuberosity; partly, and occasionally completely, its proximal tendon is continuous with the sacrotuberous ligament (Fig. 8.9). This tension mechanism of the biceps femoris depends on body position (van Wingerden et al 1993). In most specimens, a higher percentage of force was transferred from the biceps to the sacrotuberous ligament in a flexed, stooped position than in an erect stance. This could be expected because the flexion torque on the lumbar spine increases when changing from an erect to a flexed stance. Consequently, in stooped positions, larger compression forces are needed to prevent the sacrum from tilting forward. This force can be derived in part from the biceps femoris but also from other muscles attached to the sacrotuberous ligament (the sacral part of the aponeurosis of the erector spinae and gluteus maximus). Barker (2005) showed that besides the biceps muscle also part of the semimembranosus muscle regularly is connected to the sacrotuberous ligament. In her studies, Barker confirmed the biceps connection with the sacrotuberous ligament.

Comparable to the erector muscle, a double function of the hamstrings (including the biceps femoris muscle) can be described. Particularly in stooped positions and in sitting with straight legs, sitting upright, the hamstrings are well positioned to rotate the iliac bones posteriorly relative to the sacrum. This nutating effect (Sturesson et al 1989) can be constrained by the biceps femoris with its connections to the sacrotuberous ligament. Nutation in stooped positions can help to avoid excessive loading of the posterior part of the lumbar discs.

This polyarticular coupling effect of muscles can also be seen in the arm where the long tendon of the biceps brachii, forming an integrated part of the glenohumeral joint, is one of the key structures for shoulder stabilization.

Self-bracing during forward bending

When stooped, the sacrum assumes a more or less horizontal position. When lifting objects in this posture, the vertical force from the upper part of the body and the object acts almost perpendicularly to the longitudinal axis of the sacrum. In this situation, the joint also becomes loaded in the transverse plane and stability will depend on effective compression of the SIJ in a transverse plane. The transverse diameter is small in comparison with the longitudinal diameter, so additional forces are needed to protect the SIJ. An EMG study found that, during lifting, the activity of the gluteus maximus muscle paralleled that of latissimus dorsi and erector spinae muscles (Noe et al 1992). These observations indicate that, in this position, self-bracing of the pelvis can be established by contraction of the mentioned muscles and core muscles like the transversus, multifidus, the pelvic floor, and the diaphragm (Hodges et al 2003).

Self-bracing in unconstrained positions

The question of how the SIJ can be stabilized in unconstrained sitting and standing led to the following experiment: we expected that during unconstrained sitting, especially the oblique abdominals would be active to self-brace the pelvis, to deliver the necessary compression force. Using electromyography (EMG) the abdominal muscle activity was recorded in different positions (supine, unconstrained standing, and sitting with and without crossed legs on an office chair with the use of a backrest and armrests). For both the external and internal obliques, the activity was significantly higher in standing than in sitting. The activity of particularly the internal obliques turned out to be significantly higher in sitting than in a supine position (Fig. 8.10). Surprisingly, the activity of the oblique abdominals was lowered by crossing the legs (Snijders et al 1995; cross-legged or ankle on knee as preferred by the individual; Fig. 8.10). By contrast, the activity of the rectus abdominis was not altered by leg-crossing. We concluded that to stabilize the pelvis: (1) unconstrained sitting and standing initiates an oblique ventral muscle–tendon sling; and (2) leg-crossing is a functional habit. Crossing the legs causes rotation in the pelvis and possibly tenses the thoracolumbar fascia. Due to creep of tissues (elongation), leg-crossing is only temporarily functional; as a consequence the legs are crossed to the other side (Snijders et al 1995).

Failed self-bracing

The different mechanisms that warrant stability of the SIJ can become less effective as a result of a decline in muscle performance and/or increased laxity of ligaments. This could occur in people withdrawing from sports or undertaking sedentary work. A characteristic case could be a young girl performing top-level gymnastics. Through excessive training, the mobility of spine and pelvis is markedly enhanced and the girl will develop extremely strong muscles. Thus the mobile pelvis can be adequately constrained with force closure. If such an athlete abruptly terminates high-level training, the muscles rapidly decline. The muscles are not up to their task and form closure will be limited because of enlarged mobility and laxity.

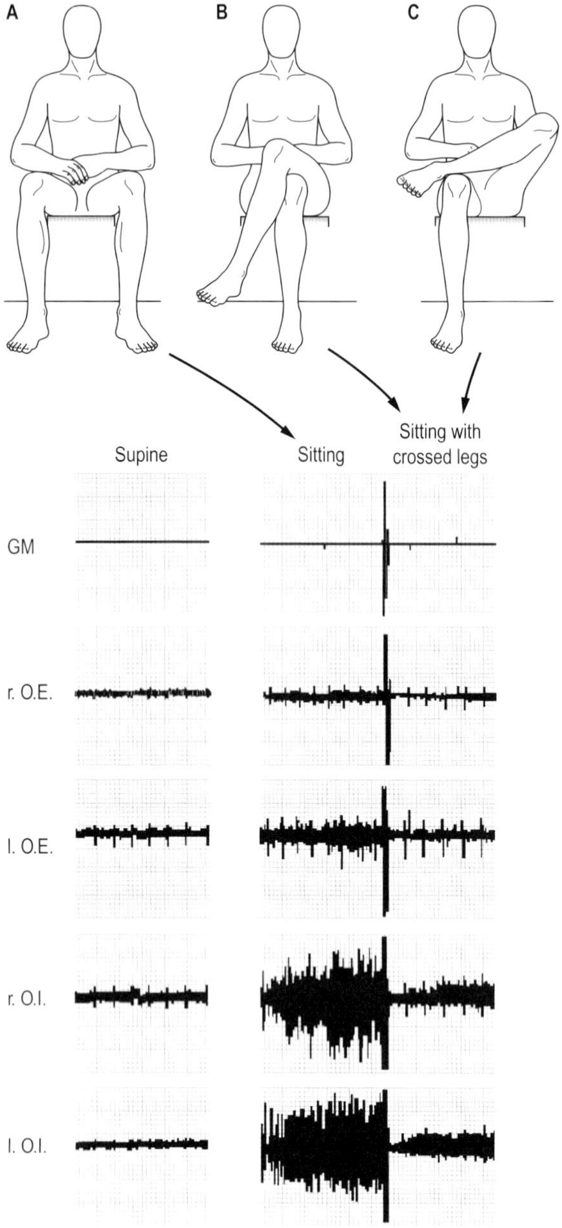

Fig. 8.10 Normal sitting (A) and sitting with crossed legs (B and C). The electromyographic data show a remarkable increase of the internal obliques during sitting with uncrossed legs (A). The activity diminishes when the legs are crossed (B and C). GM, gluteus maximus; lOE, left external oblique; lOI, left internal oblique; rOE, right external oblique; rOI, right internal oblique.

Laxity of pelvic ligaments especially occurs during pregnancy, due to relaxin. In addition, patients with a painful pubic symphysis will avoid nutation because this strains the symphysis. Consequently, these women will 'choose' a counternutated position.

One method to facilitate pelvic stability and reduce pain is the use of a pelvic belt (Mens et al 1996). In a loading experiment on embalmed human preparations, nutation of the sacrum decreased by about 20% when applying a belt force of only 50 N. Based on the biomechanical model presented here, such a belt must be applied with a small force, like the laces of a shoe. This will be sufficient to generate a self-bracing effect in the SIJ under heavy load (Snijders et al 1993a, 1993b, Vleeming et al 1992a, 1992b). The model indicates that the belt must be positioned just cranial to the greater trochanters; it crosses the SIJ caudally, and can assist in preventing gapping of the caudal part of the SIJ. However, this is not what we propose to our patients. Only in very severe cases do patients wear belts for a short period in the beginning and during training. See also the comments on training of the core muscles like the deep abdominal obliques, the transversus and multifidus (see Chapters 33, 36 and 40).

We like to emphasize that, according to the model presented here, weakening of the erector spinae/multifidus (insufficient nutation) and the gluteus maximus muscles (insufficient ligament pull and SIJ compression) will lead to diminished straining of the sacrotuberous ligament. Weakness of these muscles has in addition implications for the strength of the thoracolumbar fascia, especially if combined with a weak latissimus dorsi muscle. Weakening or inadequate use of the tranversus abdominis muscle precludes, among others, sufficient tension of the thoracolumbar fascia (see Chapters 3 and 4). This leads to diminished self-bracing of the SIJ. With insufficient bracing, the body can be expected to use other strategies, e.g. tensing the sacrotuberous ligament through activation of the biceps femoris or exaggerated contraction of parts of the gluteus maximus. Although definite experimental data are lacking, we presume that tension of the biceps and other hamstring muscles can be increased over an extended period. Hungerford et al (2003) showed altered firing patterns of these muscles in SIJ patients. Higher tension of the hamstrings will force the pelvis to rotate backwards, leading to flattening of the lumbar spine. The biceps femoris muscle, in particular, will strain the sacrotuberous ligament, diminishing nutation. Both processes will be harmful if hamstring tension is continuously increased because, in this relatively counternutated position, load will be unnaturally distributed to the lower lumbar discs. In our opinion, it is important to realize that counternutation of the SIJ seems to be a pain-withdrawal reaction that disengages the normal self-bracing of the pelvis. The patient seeks to compress the SIJ in a new joint position, with less adequate and strong ligaments to be tensed. Hence, the lower spine can become unstable and prone to infringement, leading to LBP.

We tried to define a simple exercise that could assist in preventing LBP and counteract the detrimental effects of modern life. The exercise shown in Fig. 8.11 facilitates nutation of the SIJ and couples the action of biceps femoris, erector spinae, and gluteus maximus. We suppose this to be an effective and natural way to stretch the hamstring. To evaluate its effectiveness, the exercise needs further practical study. This is an exercise that has to be demonstrated carefully to patients with the main movement occurring in the hip joints with a relaxed spine. In case of lumbar impairments, of course, care has to be taken with this exercise (see also Chapter 18).

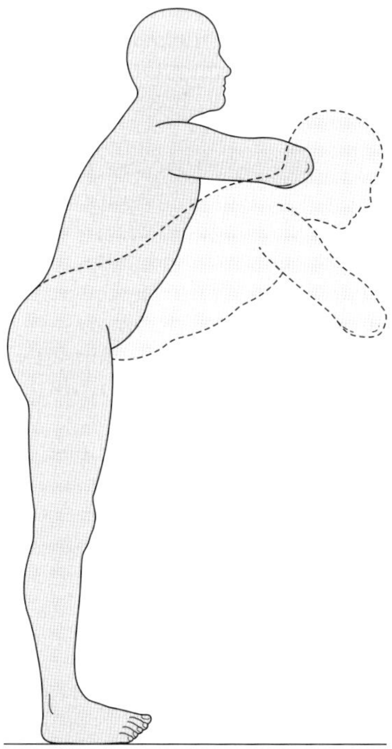

Fig. 8.11 A suggested exercise with lordosis of the lumbar spine and nutation of the sacroiliac joint. The biceps femoris, gluteus maximus and erector muscle are simultaneously activated.

Optimal and non-optimal pelvic girdle stability

Since the mid-1990s, several clinicians and researchers have studied PGP and its causes (see Chapter 31). In the past, PGP research focused on the functional and clinical analysis, mainly in women; this was a consequence of former publications emphasizing relaxation of the pelvic girdle as a primary cause for instability of the pelvic ring. By the 1870s, Snelling was of the impression that relaxation of the pelvic articulations becomes apparent either suddenly after parturition or gradually during pregnancy, permitting mobility which hinders locomotion and gives rise to distressing and alarming sensations (in Svensson et al 1990).

Abramson et al (1934) described pelvic pain and instability and made the distinction between symptoms related to the pubic joint, to the SIJ, or to a combination. They also described pain in the symphyseal region with radiation to the thighs. The SIJ symptoms are presented as low (lowest) backache and localized pain in the SIJ. Furthermore, they noted a waddling gait and a positive Trendelenburg sign (during walking the patient shows inability to hold the pelvis in the horizontal plane). The authors used, among others, screening techniques like X-rays of the pubic symphysis, even in women who were 8 months pregnant (Abramson et al 1934). So before the hazards of X-rays were realized, increased mobility and widening of the symphysis in relation to PGP were well documented. Post-mortem studies in former days, when mortality during pregnancy and labor was not exceptional, showed increased mobility of the SIJ and an increased amount of synovial SIJ and symphyseal fluid in pregnant women (Brooke 1924).

After these studies on pelvic instability in the nineteenth and twentieth centuries, analysis of pelvic pain shifted towards a more functional approach. By contrast, the study of lumbar pain after Mixter and Barr's (1934) study (which explained that radiating pain in the leg is the consequence of a rupture of the intervertebral disc) has been particularly addressed to the study of pain generators that could generate the symptoms. Since the 1980s there have been increasing efforts to study the lumbar and pelvic area as an integrated part of a complex kinematic system.

More recent functional pelvic studies have stated that pelvic girdle pain can be related to nonoptimal stability, which is underpinned by the fact that a pelvic belt reduces pain symptoms and influences the laxity of the pelvic ring. Vleeming et al (1992b) conclude that pelvic belts enhance pelvic stability because they reduce SIJ laxity. Mens et al (1999) suggest that, after initial provocative pelvic tests, these tests should be repeated with application of a pelvic belt to assess possible differences. In these studies, only a small tension (50 N) is applied to the belt, just above the greater trochanter. Larger forces did not yield better results, as predicted in a biomechanical study (Vleeming et al 1990a, 1990b). The efficacy of the pelvic belt was primarily determined by the location of the belt and the effects were explained by increased compression of the SIJ.

Buyruk et al (1995a, 1995b, 1999) applied unilateral oscillations to the anterior superior iliac spine to assess laxity of the pelvic joints. With sonoelasticity, using Doppler imaging of vibrations (DIV), they measured the stiffness/laxity ratio of artificially unstabilized SIJ in comparison with stabilized pelvices. The new method was objective and repeatable. *In vivo* studies have used the same technology in healthy subjects (Damen et al 2002a, 2002b). It was shown that pelvic belts are effective to alter the laxity of the SIJ with an applied force of the pelvic belt of maximally 50 N. Subsequently, they showed that the laxity values of the SIJ decreased after application of a pelvic belt in patients with pelvic pain (Damen et al 2002a). In another study (Damen et al 2002b), patients with asymmetric SIJ laxity reported significantly more pain during pregnancy when compared with patients with symmetric laxity. According to the authors, increased general laxity is not associated with pelvic pain. Pregnant women with moderate or severe pelvic pain have the same laxity of the SIJ as pregnant women with no or mild pain. According to these studies, the *asymmetry* of laxity correlates with the symptomatic individual. In keeping with these data, perhaps manual motion testing should focus more on the (a)symmetry of SIJ motion. However, up to now, there has been no evidence that manual motion tests have a sufficient level of intra- and intertester reliability.

In 1999, Mens et al developed a new diagnostic test. They studied the relation between impaired active straight leg raising (ASLR) and the mobility of pelvic joints with and without the application of a pelvic belt (testing the hypothesis that the pelvis is the basic bony platform that has to be stabilized before levers, like the legs and spine, can be used effectively). They conclude that impairment of the ASLR test correlates highly with the level of laxity of the pelvis, because application of a pelvic belt generally reduces the impairment of the ASLR test. The sensitivity and specificity of the test is high for PGP (pelvic girdle pain) and the test is suitable to discriminate between PGP patients and healthy individuals (Mens et al 2002).

The same authors (Mens et al 1999) showed – by means of X-rays taken after pregnancy – that the pubic bone on the symptomatic side shifts caudally relative to the other side when the symptomatic leg is freely hanging down in a standing position. This procedure differs from the classical Chamberlain X-ray method, which screens the symptomatic loaded side. The authors conclude that this symphyseal shift is the result of an anterior rotation of the iliac bone relative to the sacrum on the symptomatic side (counternutation in the SIJ).

Hungerford et al (2001) came to the same conclusion. Using an external motion analysis system, they studied (three dimensionally) the angular and translational displacements in patients with SIJ problems and in healthy persons. They concluded that posterior rotation of the iliac bones relative to the sacrum (nutation) occurs in normals on the weightbearing side. By contrast, the iliac bones rotated anteriorly relative to the sacrum (counternutation; see Fig. 8.6B) in the patient group. They found the same in the standing flexion test. Only on the loaded (standing) symptomatic side did an anterior rotation of the iliac bone occur (see Chapter 25).

The conclusion of these recent studies is that a relation exists between pelvic asymmetric laxity and the severity of complaints (Buyruk et al 1999, Damen et al 2002b). Damen et al state that subjects with asymmetric laxity of the SIJ during pregnancy have a threefold higher risk of moderate to severe pelvic pain persisting into the postpartum period, compared to subjects with symmetric laxity during pregnancy. They also conclude that pelvic belt application can diminish the laxity and stiffen the pelvis and influence an impaired ASLR test with application of the DIV method. Based on the studies mentioned here a dysfunctional SIJ is normally not related to a subluxated position of the joint, but to an altered position within the normal range of motion due to asymmetric forces acting on the joint.

Stability

The following model could help to explain the relation between optimal stability and laxity. Living on earth requires a constant response to gravity and bipedality requires that the gravitational forces are transferred through the pelvis and hip joints to the legs, and that the resultant forces are dealt with effectively. How well this load is transferred over a lifetime, dictates the efficiency of function (Lee & Vleeming 1998).

Static and dynamic stability throughout the body is achieved when the passive, active, and control systems work together to transfer load (Panjabi 1992, Snijders et al 1993a, 1993b). Adequate approximation of the joint surfaces must be the result of forces acting across the joint, if stability is to be ensured (Vleeming et al 1990a, 1990b). 'Adequate' means ideally tailored to the existing situation, using the least amount of compression to guarantee stability. Consequently, the ability to effectively transfer load through joints is a dynamic process and depends on many factors. These factors include: (1) optimal function of the bones, joints, and ligaments (form closure or joint congruency; Vleeming et al 1990a, 1990b); (2) optimal function of the muscles and fascia (force closure; O'Sullivan et al 2002, Richardson et al 2002, Vleeming 1990, Vleeming et al 1990a, 1990b, 1995); and (3) appropriate neural function (motor control, emotional state and body awareness; Gandavia et al 2002, Hodges 1997, Hodges & Richardson 1997, Holstege et al 1996).

Stability is not merely about how much a joint is moving (quantity of motion) or how resistant structures are; it is also about motion control allowing load to be transferred and movement to be smooth and effortless. This brings us to a definition of joint stability (Vleeming et al 2004a). Effective joint control is the property that the joint returns to its initial position after perturbation. In particular, the translational stability is important. Translations are normally small and rotations generally large and mainly limited near the end of the range of motion. Increased muscle cocontractions, proprioceptive muscle reflexes, increased ligament tension, gravity and the shape of the articular surfaces and the actual joint position, will modify the joint reaction and determine the level of force closure/stiffness of the joint.

Given a translationally stable joint, joint admittance is the property that describes how much the joint will dislocate after force perturbation. A lax joint will permit large translations (high admittance), a stiff joint small (low admittance; van der Helm, 2004, personal correspondence). To help understanding laxity of the lumbopelvic area, the theoretical concepts of neutral zone and elastic zone are helpful. The *neutral zone*, according to Panjabi (1992), is a small range of movement near the joint's neutral position where minimal resistance is given by the osteoligamentous structures. The *elastic zone* is that part of the motion from the end of the neutral zone up to the physiological limit. Panjabi notes that a joint has nonlinear load–displacement curves. The nonlinearity results in relative laxity in the neutral zone and increased stiffness toward the end of the range of motion. Laxity in the neutral zone can lead to repositioning of the joint to a position in the elastic zone to seek higher compression forces to stiffen the joint. Panjabi describes that the size of the neutral zone alters with injury, articular degeneration, and/or weakness of the stabilizing musculature and that this is a more sensitive indicator (laxity/versus stiffness) than angular range of motion for detecting instability. Panjabi's model, however, does not include that the neutral zone can be influenced by compression.

It was hypothesized (Lee & Vleeming 1998) that the neutral and elastic zone properties are affected qualitatively by altering the force closure (compression forces) across the joint. Also, neutral zone *movement* can be influenced by altered compression. This implies that joint force closure/compression can be too much, too little, or optimal.

If the articular surfaces of the sacrum and the iliac bones fitted together with perfect form closure, displacement in the joint would be impossible. However, form closure of the SIJ is not perfect

Box 8.1

A functional description of joint stability

The effective accommodation to each specific load demand, through an adequate tailored joint compression, as a function of gravity, coordinated muscle and ligament forces, to produce effective joint reaction forces under altering conditions to maintain stability.

Optimal stability is achieved when the balance between performance (the level of optimal stability) and effort is optimized to economize the use of energy.

Sub/nonoptimal joint stability implicates altered laxity/stiffness values leading to increased joint translations resulting in a new joint position or/and exaggerated joint compression, with a disturbed performance/effort ratio (Vleeming et al 2004a).

and displacement is possible, albeit small, and therefore stabilization during loading the pelvic joints is required. This is achieved by increasing compression across the joint surface at the moment of loading. The anatomical structures responsible for this are the ligaments and muscles, together with their fascia.

Ligaments are tensed when bones move in directions that lengthen them and when muscles that attach to them contract. When the joint is compressed, friction increases (Vleeming et al 1990b) and consequently augments, what is coined self-bracing of the joint (Snijders et al 1993a, 1993b, Vleeming et al 1990a, 1990b). This is seen as a prerequisite in all joints and the effective application of compression is the decisive factor, besides the anatomical factors, for joint stabilization. Compression reduces the size of the joint's neutral zone and increases the stiffness value of the joint. Shear forces are thereby controlled, facilitating stabilization of the joint.

In all joints, it is the combination of regional and local ligaments, muscles, fascial systems, and gravity that contribute to force closure (Snijders et al 1993a, 1993b, Vleeming et al 1990a, 1990b), and not only the deep stabilizing muscles. Muscles with a bigger lever arm to the joint also add to joint reaction forces. When this mechanism works efficiently in the pelvis, the shear forces between the iliac bones and sacrum are adequately controlled and loads can be transferred between the trunk, pelvis, and legs (Snijders et al 1993a, 1993b).

Van Wingerden et al (2004) studied several muscles that could contribute to force closure of the pelvis and influence the stiffness characteristics of the joint. In six healthy women, SIJ stiffness was measured using DIV. SIJ stiffness was measured both in a relaxed situation and during EMG-recorded isometric voluntary contractions. The biceps femoris, gluteus maximus, erector spinae, and contralateral latissimus dorsi muscles were included in this study, whereas deeper muscles such as the internal obliques, the transversus abdominis, and the multifidus muscle were omitted. Pelvic stiffness significantly increased when the individual muscles were activated. This held especially for activation of the erector spinae, the biceps femoris, and the gluteus maximus. During some tests, significant cocontraction of other muscles occurred. The study concludes that SIJ stiffness increased even with slight muscle activity, supporting the notion that effective load transfer from spine to legs is possible when muscle forces actively compress the SIJ, preventing shear. This is in agreement with the work of Cholewicki et al (2000), showing that sufficient stability of the spine is achieved in most people with modest levels of coactivation of the paraspinal and abdominal wall muscles. Furthermore, Hodges et al (2003) demonstrated in porcine experiments that contractions of both the transversus abdominis muscle and the diaphragm increase the stiffness of the spine.

Van Wingerden et al (2004) also mention that during manual test procedures, the influence of muscle activation patterns must be considered, because both inter- and intratester reliability can be directly altered by muscle activity.

Richardson et al (2002) further elaborated on the force closure model by showing that contractions of the transversus abdominis and multifidus muscles significantly decrease SIJ laxity. However, in their study influences of other muscles were not measured or controlled.

O'Sullivan et al (2002) showed elegantly how the pelvic floor and diaphragm directly can influence the active straight leg raise by a different strategy of motor control of the pelvis and diaphragm, influencing force closure and stabilizing the pelvis.

A study by Indahl et al (1999), using pigs, revealed that stimulation with bipolar wire electrodes in the ventral SIJ capsule, initiated a muscular response of the gluteus maximus and the quadratus lumborum muscles. Stimulation directly dorsal of the SIJ capsule provoked a response in the deep medial multifidus fascicles lateral to the L5 spinous process (see Chapter 7). The latter study could help to broaden our knowledge of muscular control of SIJ.

Damen et al (2002b) concludes her studies with the notion that the term 'pelvic instability' should not be used because increased symmetric laxity (based on the DIV methodology) is not properly related to pelvic pain, although asymmetric laxity is. However, Damen et al, although using a proper method for inclusion of pelvic patients, did not specify for left or right leg differences of a positive ASLR test and did not specifically study the relation between positive ASLR test and laxity.

It is important to realize that the DIV method enables us to study joint play *in vivo*: the study of neutral zone movement. Many clinicians use a joint play test to fathom joint play. By contrast, the elastic zone movement is not specifically measured by DIV; DIV measures stiffness only in the neutral zone. Therefore it would be a mistake to use DIV studies as the single method for analyzing pelvic girdle mobility.

A problem of the DIV method is that laxity is strongly influenced by altered muscle tension, as shown by the study of Richardson et al (2002) and van Wingerden et al (2004). This implies that altered motor patterns influence the dynamics of stiffness. For that reason asymmetric stiffness/laxity can shift to the other side when another muscular (defense) strategy is used. As a consequence, the findings of anatomists and gynecologists in older studies, describing the relation between pelvic pain and increased mobility of the SIJ, cannot be refuted by the outcome of DIV laxity studies. Simply stated, they studied another quality of pelvic girdle motion.

In this respect, the studies of Sturesson et al (1989, 1999, 2000a, 2000b) applying Roentgen stereo photogrammetric analysis (RSA) of the SIJ, deal with the overall movement characteristics (elastic zone movements) of the SIJ. This technique was developed by Selvik (1990) to study kinematics of the skeletal system. Sturesson et al (1989, 1999, 2000a, 2000b) found, in practically all their studies, that an anterior rotation of the sacrum (nutation) was observed when patients loaded their spine by means of rising from a supine towards a sitting or standing position. Sturesson et al (2000a) acknowledge that nutation is a prerequisite for the described self-bracing mechanism. Although Sturesson et al conclude that movements measured in the SIJ do not differ between the symptomatic and asymptomatic side, it was shown that movements of the SIJ are reduced by increased loads. Sturesson et al (1999) note that SIJ movement in most patients can be reduced by applying an external Hoffman Slatis frame and that this will in all probability reduce the pain. This is in line with studies on pelvic belts; use of a pelvic belt normalizes the ASLR test (Mens et al 1999) and influences the amount of laxity in the joint (Damen et al 2002a).

Conclusion of stability research

To be able to comprehend the movement characteristics of the SIJ, both elastic zone research (RSA, quantitative study of movement, and the outcome of former studies) and neutral zone research (DVI, quality of movement) are needed. The RSA and DIV approaches deal with different characteristics of joint movement. However, both methods show that increased stiffness correlates with increased performance (pelvic belt, ASLR test and application of the external frame). Furthermore, the studies by Richardson et al (2002) and van Wingerden et al (2004) illustrate that muscle force directly influences and diminishes the laxity of the SIJ (increasing SIJ stiffness).

Static and dynamic stability is achieved when the passive, active and control systems work together to transfer load (Panjabi 1992, Snijders et al 1993a, 1993b). *Adequate* approximation of the joint surfaces must be the result of all forces acting across the joint if stability is to be ensured (Vleeming et al 1990a, 1990b). Here, 'adequate' implies ideally tailored to the existing situation and using the least amount of compression to guarantee stability: the ability to effectively transfer load through joints is a dynamic process and depends on many factors.

The reversal of nonoptimal stability depends on normalizing displacement in the SIJ (which implies nutation of the sacrum during loading), on proper functioning ligaments, and on the controlled use of muscles to effectively compress the SIJ. Studies by both Mens et al (1999) and Hungerford et al (2003), which used different methods to study the kinematics of the pelvic girdle, noticed, in patients with pelvic girdle pain, a pattern with anteriorly rotated iliac bones relative to the sacrum, implying a counternutated position. Mens et al (1999) note significant differences between symptomatic and reference side, with the symptomatic side showing a caudal shift of the pubic bone with respect to the reference side. Hungerford et al (2003) note the same mechanism on the supporting leg, during a standing hip flexion task, comparing normals with patients with SIJ complaints. These findings need further investigation and might have implications for the studies of Sturesson & Udén (1999) and Sturesson et al (2000a, 2000b), who studied patients exclusively. If counternutation is a regular finding in patients with PGP, Sturesson et al's measurements could be an underestimation of the displacement values for normals because of the counternutated SIJ in the loaded postures of the patients.

Treatment of sub/nonoptimal stability has to focus on restoring key stability of the pelvic girdle. This implicates that the patient has to be trained initially without the use of large levers, like spine and legs, and has to start with core exercises of the trunk. Only when basic stability is achieved through adequate muscle control, is the use of larger lever exercises advised.

Gait

Directly after birth, the general orientation of the human SIJ is comparable to that in quadrupeds. The articular surfaces are orientated in the sagittal plane as the synovial joints of the vertebral arches of most lumbar vertebrae. Changes in the joint appear when the child starts to walk. The sacrum enlarges laterally and the orientation of the articular surfaces transforms into the adult curvatures (see Fig. 8.4, bottom right). These changes are brought about by mechanical factors such as body weight, load on the femur, and strain on the pubic symphysis (Schunke 1938, Solonen 1957). We wonder which stabilizing mechanisms operate during gait, when muscle function has to be adjusted to the various stages of walking.

Swing phase

During the swing of the right leg forwards, the cranial part of the right iliac bone tends to rotate dorsally with respect to the sacrum as suggested by Greenman (1992; Fig. 8.12B). Stated otherwise, at the right side, the top of the sacrum inclines forward relative to the iliac bones. Nutation increases ligament tension and SIJ compression, whereas at the left the opposite occurs. These movements are normally very small. Increased nutation at the end of the swing phase will prepare the joint for the impact of heel strike. At this moment, the leg and the ipsilateral SIJ become weight bearing. Gait analysis shows that the hamstrings become active just before heel strike (Weil & Weil 1966). As a consequence, knee extension is limited at the right side, and tension of the sacrotuberous ligament increases due to biceps femoris activation and nutation.

What would be the effect of activation of the biceps femoris on its distal connection? The biceps is connected to the head of the fibula (Fig. 8.12B) and also partially to the strong fascia of the peroneus muscles. To answer the question, we loaded the biceps femoris in embalmed specimens and measured tension in the peroneus fascia (van Wingerden et al 1996, unpublished data). About 18% of the applied load was transferred to the fascia. We questioned what would happen to the fibula during the impact. Fortunately, this had already been described by Weinert et al (1973). In contrast to what is commonly believed, they showed a downward movement of the fibula during heel strike. This fits in nicely with the concept of a spine–pelvis–leg mechanism. The downward movement of the fibula will further 'load' the already tensed biceps femoris muscle and sacrotuberous ligament.

Is this mechanism confined to the lateral part of the leg? An important muscle attached to the medial part of the foot is the tibialis anterior. To keep the point of the foot raised during the swing phase (inversion/dorsiflexion of the foot), this muscle contracts prior to heel strike. What a smart trick of nature that this muscle is attached to the plantar

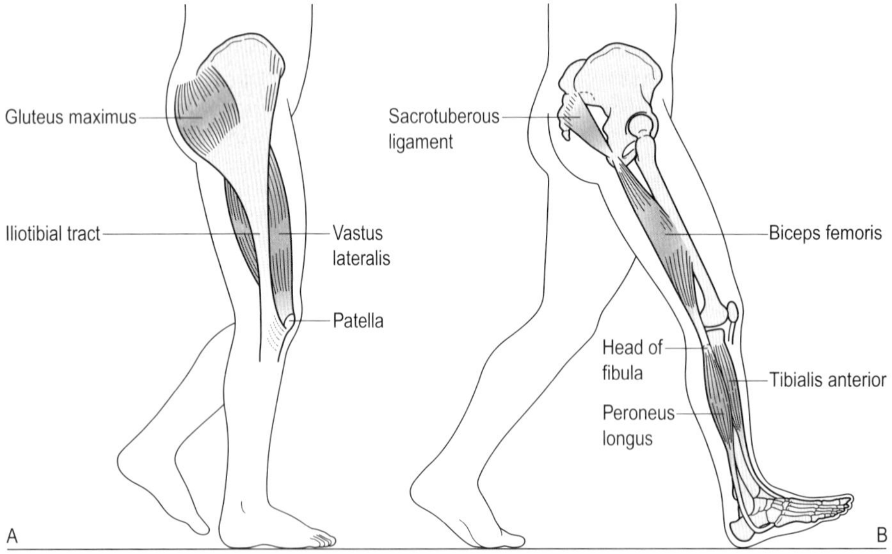

Fig. 8.12 (A) Lower part of the oblique dorsal muscle–fascia–tendon sling. Relationship between gluteus maximus muscle, iliotibial tract, vastus lateralis muscle, and knee in the single support phase. The iliotibial tract can be tensed by action of the dorsally located gluteus maximus and ventrolaterally located tensor fascia latae muscle. The tract can also be tensed by contraction of the vastus lateralis muscle. (B) The longitudinal muscle–tendon–fascia sling. Relations at the end of the swing phase.

side of the large first metatarsal bone, where it blends with the peroneus longus muscle that crosses the foot underneath. Together they form a long longitudinal muscle–tendon–fascia sling (Fig. 8.12B). The action of tibialis anterior and biceps femoris are smartly coupled to load the longitudinal sling, which could serve to store energy.

Single support phase

Heel strike is followed by the single support phase. The action of the biceps femoris muscle diminishes. The ipsilateral iliac bone gradually starts to rotate forward (minimal displacement in the direction of counternutation) and subsequently the loading of the vast majority of the ligaments diminishes. The gluteus maximus muscle gradually replaces biceps femoris activity. The gluteus maximus muscle is better positioned to compress the SIJ than the biceps because it compresses the SIJ both directly and indirectly (by straining the sacrotuberous ligament).

As in quadrupeds, the arms and legs of bipeds move rhythmically. Before right-sided heel strike, the trunk already shows counter-rotation (left arm forwards). This is distinct in energetic movements such as jumping. As mentioned above, the gluteus maximus and contralateral latissimus dorsi muscles are coupled via the thoracolumbar fascia. The counter-rotation of the trunk and anteflexion of the arm assist in tensing the latissimus dorsi and consequently the thoracolumbar fascia. In combination with the action of the gluteus maximus muscle, an oblique dorsal muscle–fascia–tendon sling is active, which crosses the spine.

The tension of the gluteus maximus muscle is partly transferred downwards in the vast iliotibial tract (see Fig. 8.12A). Like the thoracolumbar fascia, this is a strong and large sheath of connective tissue, tensed by the gluteus maximus and tensor fasciae latae muscle. In addition, the iliotibial tract can be tensed by expansion of the huge vastus lateralis muscle during its contraction. The vastus, an important part of the extensor muscle of the knee (the quadriceps), is active during the single support phase to counteract flexion in the knee. As a result, the iliotibial tract is pushed aside (to lateral) and further stretched. Counter to what is described in many textbooks, the distal end of the tract participates in the outer lateral capsule of the knee (see Fig. 8.12A). The direction of the collagenous fibers is perpendicular to the patella tendon, the distal part of the quadriceps muscle that is attached to the tibial bone. In the single support phase, when the knee is fully loaded by body weight, forward shear of the femur (Gracovetsky, personal communication) in the knee joint can be precluded by the tension through the thoracolumbar fascia, gluteus maximus muscle, and iliotibial tract.

This system, involving left and right parts of the body, could also function as a smart spring. It is based on trunk torsion, action of the latissimus dorsi and gluteus maximus, and expansion of the vastus lateralis muscle. Because of its length it is suited to store ample energy and can assist among others in unwinding the trunk.

Energy storage as a concept was raised by Margaria (1968) and needs explanation. According to Margaria, energy is accumulated during gait. He describes that the work done by muscles in active tension is partly stored as elastic energy. This energy can be utilized if the muscle is allowed to shorten immediately afterwards. Dorman compares this mechanism with maximally extending a finger and releasing it (Dorman 1992). Alexander (1984) raised the question of where energy is stored during gait. He supposed that the elastic strain is stored in tendons, and that the extensor muscles of knee and ankle, particularly, could serve as springs. Dorman expected that the fasciae are the main structures to store energy. However, it is open to question whether the topographic division between muscle, tendon, and fascia is functional. By functional coupling of these seemingly separate structures, the longitudinal sling might be an effective energy storage system. The energy stored can be used to minimize muscle action.

All slings, the longitudinal and both obliques, overcome the shortcoming of relatively small individual tendons and muscle fibers; they can conserve only limited amounts of energy. The slings are coupled to the function of the SIJ and the lower lumbar spine. We assume that these slings reflect our capacity to use our legs and trunk for energizing the body. According to Dorman (1992), defects in this system might lead to a higher oxygen demand. We also assume that, without defects, activities such as sluggish strolling inadequately energize the slings. This could explain why shopping is such a hardship for many people.

The single support phase is followed by the double support phase. In this, the SIJs are less loaded because both legs carry the weight. The gluteus maximus muscle becomes less active. At the start of the new swing phase, nutation in the SIJ is diminished, the joint is unloaded and the leg can freely swing forward.

Summary

We emphasize that functional anatomical models are required to attack a complex puzzle as nonspecific LBP. Such an approach can help to understand that seemingly different structures are functionally related. In this respect, we like to quote Radin (1990), who perceptively remarked, 'Functional analysis, be it biological, mechanical or both, of a single tissue will fail to give a realistic functional analysis as, in all complex constructs, the interaction between the various components is a critical part of their behavior.'

The focus in this chapter has been to clarify the anatomy and biomechanics of the pelvic girdle and SIJ. However, spinal function and pelvic function are fully coupled. Any SIJ movement has consequences for the lumbar spine and vice versa. Nutation of the SIJ is coupled to extension of the lumbar spine. The spine and pelvis cannot be studied in isolation.

Nutation of the sacrum generally is the result of load bearing and a functional adaptation to stabilize the pelvic girdle.

The intervertebral discs are loaded by compression, bending, and torsion. As a result of body weight and force moments, the largest force acts perpendicularly to the discs. By contrast, this force is almost parallel to the surfaces of the practically flat SIJ. As a result, there is considerable shear loading in the SIJ and a risk of damaging the ligaments. In general, the ligamentous structures surrounding the SIJ are assumed to be sufficient to prevent shear and stabilize the joints. We do not agree with this view. We put forward evidence that the ligaments alone are not capable of transferring lumbosacral load effectively to the iliac bones. This holds especially for heavy loading situations and for conditions with sustained load resulting in creep, such as standing and sitting.

According to the self-bracing mechanism, resistance against shear results from the specific properties of the articular surfaces of the SIJ (form closure) and from the compression produced by body weight, muscle action, and ligament force (force closure). Different aspects of this mechanism are operating in standing, sitting, and walking and during actions such as forceful rotation and lifting in a stooped posture. The study reveals a functional relation between the biceps femoris, gluteus maximus, latissimus dorsi, and erector spinae/multifidus muscles. Also, a relation exists with core muscles like the transversus abdominis and internal obliquus abdominis muscles, pelvic floor, and diaphragm. In understanding their coupled function, the SIJ plays a central role.

We state that knowledge of the coupling mechanisms between spine, pelvis, legs, and arms is essential to understand dysfunction of the human locomotor system, particularly the lower back. It has led us to describe three muscle slings (one longitudinal and two oblique) that can be energized.

We have provided evidence that nonoptimal pelvic connections can be a main cause of complaints in patients with LBP. Diminished and/or unbalanced muscle function can lead to sustained counternutation in the SIJ. According to the model, the SIJ becomes especially prone to shear forces if loaded in a counternutation position. Counternutation, which is coupled to a supine position and to flattening of the spine in standing and sitting, could lead to abnormal loading of the lumbar discs and, in the end, herniation. Based on the data presented, disc herniation is not necessarily a separate syndrome but could be the result of failed stabilization of the pelvis and lower spine.

As a consequence, 'nonspecific LBP' can be prevented and treated by modifying posture and by specific training methods. On the basis of the model presented above, advice is to treat and prevent LBP by appropriately strengthening and coordinating trunk and leg muscles to reach core stability. Initially, big levers like the legs and spine in the case of sub/nonoptimal stability should not be used and only trained when core stability is sufficiently established.

Acknowledgement

We would like to extend our gratitude to Frans van der Helm, Cees de Vries, Annemarie van Randen, Jan-Paul van Wingerden, Annelies Pool, Ria van Kruining, Eddy Dalm, Jan Velkers, and Cees Entius.

References

Abramson D, Roberts SM, Wilson PD 1934 Relaxation of the pelvic joints in pregnancy. Surgical Gynecology and Obstetrics 58:595–613

Adams MA, Dolan P, Burton K, Bodguk N 2002 The biomechanics of back pain. Churchill Livingstone, Edinburgh

Alexander RMCN 1984 Walking and running. American Scientist 72:348–354

Bakland O, Hansen JH 1984 The axial sacroiliac joint. Anatomica Clinica 6:29–36

Barker J 2005 The thoralumbar fascia. Thesis. University of Melbourne, Australia

Barker J, Briggs CA 1999 Attachments of the posterior layer of the lumbar fascia. Spine 24(17):1757–1764
Bogduk N, Twomey LT 1987 Clinical anatomy of the lumbar spine. Churchill Livingstone, Melbourne
Bogduk N, Johnson G, Spalding D 1998 The morphology and biomechanics of the latissimus dorsi. Clinical Biomechanics 13:377–385
Bogduk N, MacIntosh JE 1984 The applied anatomy of the thoracolumbar fascia. Spine 9(2):164–170
Bowen V, Cassidy JD 1981 Macroscopic and microscopic anatomy of the sacroiliac joints from embryonic life until the eighth decade. Spine 6:620
Brooke R 1924. The sacroiliac joint. Journal of Anatomy 58:299–305
Buyruk HM, Stam HJ, Snijders CJ et al 1995a The use of colour Doppler imaging for the assessment of sacroiliac joint stiffness: a study on embalmed human pelvises. European Journal of Radiology 21:112–116
Buyruk HM, Snijders CJ, Vleeming A et al 1995b The measurements of sacroiliac joint stiffness with colour Doppler imaging: a study on healthy subjects. European Journal of Radiology 21:117–121
Buyruk HM, Stam HJ, Snijders CJ et al 1999 Measurement of sacroiliac joint stiffness in peripartum pelvic pain patients with Doppler imaging of vibrations (DIV). European Journal of Obstetrics, Gynecology and Reproductive Biology 83(2):159–163
Cholewicki J, Simons APD, Radebold A 2000 Effects of external trunk loads on lumbar spine stability. Journal of Biomechanics 33(11):1377–1385
Damen L, Spoor CW, Snijders CJ, Stam HJ 2002a Does a pelvic belt influence sacroiliac laxity? Clinical Biomechanics 17(7):495–498
Damen L, Buyruk HM, Guler Uysal F et al 2002b The prognostic value of asymmetric laxity of the sacroiliac joint in pregnancy related pelvic pain. Spine 27(24): 2820–2824
Dijkstra PF, Vleeming A, Stoeckart R 1989 Complex motion tomography of the sacroiliac joint: an anatomical and roentgenological study. Fortschritte auf dem Gebiete der Rontgenstrahlen und der Nuklearmedizin 150: 635–642
DonTigny RL 1979 Dysfunction of the sacroiliac joint and its treatment. Journal of Orthopedics and Sports Physical Therapy 1:23–35
Dorman TA 1992 Storage and release of elastic energy in the pelvis: dysfunction, diagnosis and treatment. In: Vleeming A et al (eds) First interdisciplinary world congress on LBP and its relation to the sacroiliac joint. San Diego, CA, 5–6 November, p585–600
Egund N, Ollson TH, Schmid H, Selvik G 1978 Movements in the sacroiliac joints demonstrated with roentgen stereophotogrammetry. Acta Radiologica, Diagnosis 19:833
Fortin JD, Dwyer AP, West S, Pier J 1994a Sacroiliac joint: pain referral maps upon applying a new injection/ arthrography technique. 1: Asymptomatic volunteers. Spine 19:1475–1482
Fortin JD, Aprill CN, Ponthieux B, Pier J 1994b Sacroiliac joint: pain referral maps upon applying a new injection/ arthrography technique. 2: Clinical evaluation. Spine 19:1483–1489
Gandavia SC, Butler JE, Hodges PW, Taylor JL 2002 Balance acts: respiratory sensations, motor control and human posture. Clinical and Experimental Pharmocology and Physiology 29 (1–2):118–121
Gibbons S 2004 The caudomedial part of the gluteus maximus and its relation to the sacrotuberous ligament. Fifth Interdisciplinary World Congress on Low Back Pain. Melbourne, Australia
Greenman PE 1992 Clinical aspects of sacroiliac function in human walking. In: Vleeming A et al (eds) First Interdisciplinary World Congress on Low Back Pain and its relation to the sacroiliac joint. San Diego, CA, 5–6 November, p353–359
Hodges PW 1997 Feedforward contraction of transversus abdominis is not influenced by the direction of arm movement. Experimental Brain Research 114:362–370
Hodges PW, Richardson CA 1997 Contraction of the abdominal muscles associated with movement of the lower limb. Physical Therapy 77:132–144
Hodges PW, Kaigle A, Holm S et al 2003 Intervertebral stiffness of the spine is increased by evoked contraction of transversus abdominus and the diaphragm; in vivo porcine studies. Spine 28(23):2594–2601
Holstege G, Bandler R, Saper C B 1996 The emotional motor system. Elsevier Science, Amsterdam
Hungerford B, Gilleard W, Lee D 2001 Alteration of sacroiliac joint motion patterns in subjects with pelvic motion asymmetry. In: Proceedings from the Fourth World Interdisciplinary Congress on Low Back and Pelvic Pain. Montreal, Canada
Hungerford B, Gilleard W, Hodges PW 2003 Evidence of altered lumbo–pelvic muscle recruitment in the presence of sacroiliac joint pain. Spine 28(14):1593–1600
Huson A 1997 Kinematic models and the human pelvis. In: Vleeming A et al (eds) Movement stability and low back pain. Churchill Livingstone, Edinburgh p123–131
Indahl A, Kaigle A, Reikeras O, Holm S 1999 Sacroiliac joint involvement in activation of the porcine spinal and gluteal musculature. Journal of Spinal Disorders 12(4):325–330
Kumar S, Narayan BS, Zedka M 1996 An electromyographic study of unresisted trunk rotation with normal velocity among healthy subjects. Spine 21(13):1500–1512
Lavignolle B, Vital J M, Senegas J et al 1983 An approach to the functional anatomy of the sacroiliac joints in vivo. Anatomica Clinica 5:169
Lee D, Vleeming A 1998 Impaired load transfer through the pelvic girdle. A new model of altered neutral zone function. In: Proceedings of the Third Interdisciplinary World Congress on Low Back and Pelvic Pain. Vienna, Austria
Lovejoy CO 1988 Evolution of human walking. Scientific American 259:118–125
MacIntosh JE, Bogduk N 1986 The biomechanics of the lumbar multifidus. Clinical Biomechanics 1:205–213

MacIntosh JE, Bogduk N 1991 The attachments of the lumbar erector. Spine 16:783–792
Margaria R 1968 Positive and negative work performances and their efficiencies in human locomotion. Internationale Zeitschrift für angewandte Physiologie einschliesslich Arbeitsphysiologie 25:339–351
Mens JMA, Stam HJ, Stoeckart R et al 1992 Peripartum pelvic pain: a report of the analysis of an inquiry among patients of a Dutch patient society. In: Vleeming A et al (eds) First Interdisciplinary World Congress on Low Back Pain and its Relation to the Sacroiliac Joint. San Diego, CA, 5–6 November, p521–533
Mens JMA, Vleeming A, Stoeckart R et al 1996 Understanding peripartum pelvic pain: implications of a patient survey. Spine 21(11):1303–1369
Mens JMA, Vleeming A, Snijders CJ et al 1999 The active straight leg raising test and mobility of the pelvic joints. European Spine 8:468–473
Miller JA, Schultz AB, Andersson GB 1987 Load displacement behavior of sacroiliac joint. Journal of Orthopaedic Research 5:92
Mixter WJ, Barr JS 1934 Rupture of the intervertebral disc with involvement of the spinal canal. New England Journal of Medicine 211:210–215
Mooney V, Pozos R, Vleeming A et al 2001 Exercise treatment for sacroiliac joint pain. Orthopedics 24(1):29–32
Njoo KH 1996 Nonspecific LBP in general practice: a delicate point. Thesis, Erasmus University, Rotterdam
Noe DA, Mostardi RA, Jackson ME et al 1992 Myoelectric activity and sequencing of selected trunk muscles during isokinetic lifting. Spine 17(2):225
O'Sullivan PB, Beales DJ, Beetham JA et al 2002 Altered motor control strategies in subjects with sacroiliac pain during the active straight leg raise test. Spine 27(1): E1–E8
Panjabi MM 1992 The stabilizing system of the spine. Part I: function, dysfunction, adaptation, and enhancement. Journal of Spinal Disorders 5(4):383–389
Pool-Goudzwaard A, Hoek van Dijke G, Mulder P et al 2003 The iliolumbar ligament: its influence on stability of the sacroiliac joint. Clinical Biomechanics 18(2): 99–105
Radin EL 1990 The joint as an organ: physiology and biomechanics. Abstracts of the first world congress on biomechanics, La Jolla, CA, September, 2:1
Richardson CA, Snijders CJ, Hides JA et al 2002 The relationship between the transversus abdominus muscle, sacroiliac joint mechanics and LBP. Spine 27(4):399–405
Salsabili N, Valojerdy MR, Hogg DA 1995 Variations in thickness of articular cartilage in the human sacroiliac joint. Clinical Anatomy 8:388–390
Sashin D 1930 A critical analysis of the anatomy and the pathological changes of the sacroiliac joints. Journal of Bone and Joint Surgery 12:891
Selvik G 1990 Roentgen stereophotogrammetric analysis. Acta Radiologica 31(2):113–126
Snijders CJ, Seroo JM, Snijder JGN, Hoedt HT 1976 Change in form of the spine as a consequence of pregnancy. Digest of the Eleventh International Conference on Medical and Biological Engineering, May 1976, Ottawa, Canada, p670–671
Snijders CJ, Vleeming A, Stoeckart R 1993a Transfer of lumbosacral load to iliac bones and legs. 1: Biomechanics of self-bracing of the sacroiliac joints and its significance for treatment and exercise. Clinical Biomechanics 8: 285–294
Snijders CJ, Vleeming A, Stoeckart R 1993b Transfer of lumbosacral load to iliac bones and legs. 2: Loading of the sacroiliac joints when lifting in a stooped posture. Clinical Biomechanics 8:295–301
Snijders CJ, Slagter AHE, Strik R van et al 1995 Why leg-crossing? The influence of common postures on abdominal muscle activity. Spine 20(18):1989–1993
Solonen KA 1957 The sacroiliac joint in the light of anatomical, roentgenological and clinical studies. Acta Orthopaedica Scandinavica 27:1–127
Stewart TD 1984 Pathologic changes in aging sacroiliac joints. Clinical Orthopaedics and Related Research 183:188
Sturesson B, Udén A 1999 Can an external frame fixation reduce the movements in the sacroiliac joints? A radiostereometric analysis of 10 patients. Acta Orthopedica Scandinavica 70(1):42–46
Sturesson B, Selvik G, Udén A 1989 Movements of the sacroiliac joints. A roentgen stereophotogrammetric analysis. Spine 14:162–165
Sturesson B, Udén A, Vleeming A 2000a A radiostereometric analysis of movements of the sacroiliac joints during the standing hip flexion test. Spine 25(3):364–368
Sturesson B, Udén A, Vleeming A 2000b A radiostereometric analysis of the movements of the sacroiliac joints in the reciprocal straddle position. Spine 25(2): 214–217
Svensson HO, Andersson GBJ, Hagstad A, Jansson PO 1990 The relationship of low-back pain to pregnancy and gynaecologic factors. Spine 15:371–375
Vleeming A 1990 The sacroiliac joint. A clinical–anatomical, biomechanical and radiological study. Thesis, Erasmus University, Rotterdam
Vleeming A, Stoeckart R, Snijders CJ 1989a The sacrotuberous ligament: a conceptual approach to its dynamic role in stabilizing the sacroiliac joint. Clinical Biomechanics 4:201–203
Vleeming A, Wingerden JP van, Snijders CJ et al 1989b Load application to the sacrotuberous ligament: influences on sacroiliac joint mechanics. Clinical Biomechanics 4:204–209
Vleeming A, Stoeckart R, Volkers ACW, Snijders CJ 1990a Relation between form and function in the sacroiliac joint. 1: Clinical anatomical aspects. Spine 15:130–132
Vleeming A, Volkers ACW, Snijders CJ, Stoeckart R 1990b Relation between form and function in the sacroiliac joint. 2: Biomechanical aspects. Spine 15(2):133–136
Vleeming A, Wingerden JP van, Dijkstra PF et al 1992a Mobility in the SI-joints in old people: a kinematic and radiologic study. Clinical Biomechanics 7:170–176
Vleeming A, Buyruk HM, Stoeckart R et al 1992b An

integrated therapy for peripartum pelvic instability. American Journal of Obstetrics and Gynecology 166(4):1243–1247

Vleeming A, Pool-Goudzwaard AL, Stoeckart R et al 1995 The posterior layer of the thoracolumbar fascia: its function in load transfer from spine to legs. Spine 20:753–758

Vleeming A, Pool-Goudzwaard A, Hammudoghlu D et al 1996 The function of the long dorsal sacroiliac ligament: its implication for understanding LBP. Spine 21(5): 556–562

Vleeming A, de Vries HJ, Mens JMA, van Wingerden JP 2002 Possible role of the long dorsal sacroiliac ligament in women with peripartum pelvic pain. Acta Obstetrica et Gynecologica Scandinavica 81:430–436

Vleeming A, Albert H, Lee D et al 2004a A definition of joint stability. In: European COST guideline report, working group 4 (submitted)

Vleeming A, Albert H, Östgaard HC et al 2004b A definition of pelvic girdle pain. In: European COST guideline report, working group 4 (submitted)

Walheim GG, Selvik G 1984 Mobility of the pubic symphysis. In vivo measurements with an electromechanic method and a roentgen stereophotogrammetric method. Clinical Orthopaedics and Related Research 191:129–135

Weil S, Weil UH 1966 Mechanik des Gehens. Georg Thieme Verlag, Stuttgart

Weinert CR, MacMaster JH, Ferguson RJ 1973 Dynamic function of the human fibula. American Journal of Anatomy 138:145–150

Weisl H 1955 The movements of the sacroiliac joints. Acta Anatomica 23:80

Wingerden JP van, Vleeming A, Snijders CJ, Stoeckart R 1993 A functional–anatomical approach to the spine–pelvis mechanism: interaction between the biceps femoris muscle and the sacrotuberous ligament. European Spine Journal 2:140–144

Wingerden JP van, Vleeming A, Buyruk HM, Raissadat K 2004 Stabilization of the SIJ in vivo: verification of muscular contribution to force closure of the pelvis. European Spine Journal 13(3):199–205

PART ONE

Section Two

Biomechanical, clinical–anatomical and evolutionary aspects of lumbopelvic pain and dysfunction: Evolution, biomechanics and kinematics

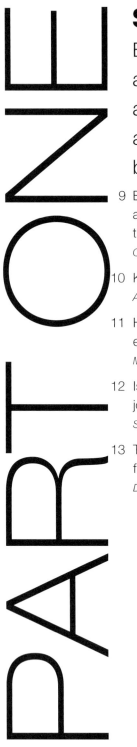

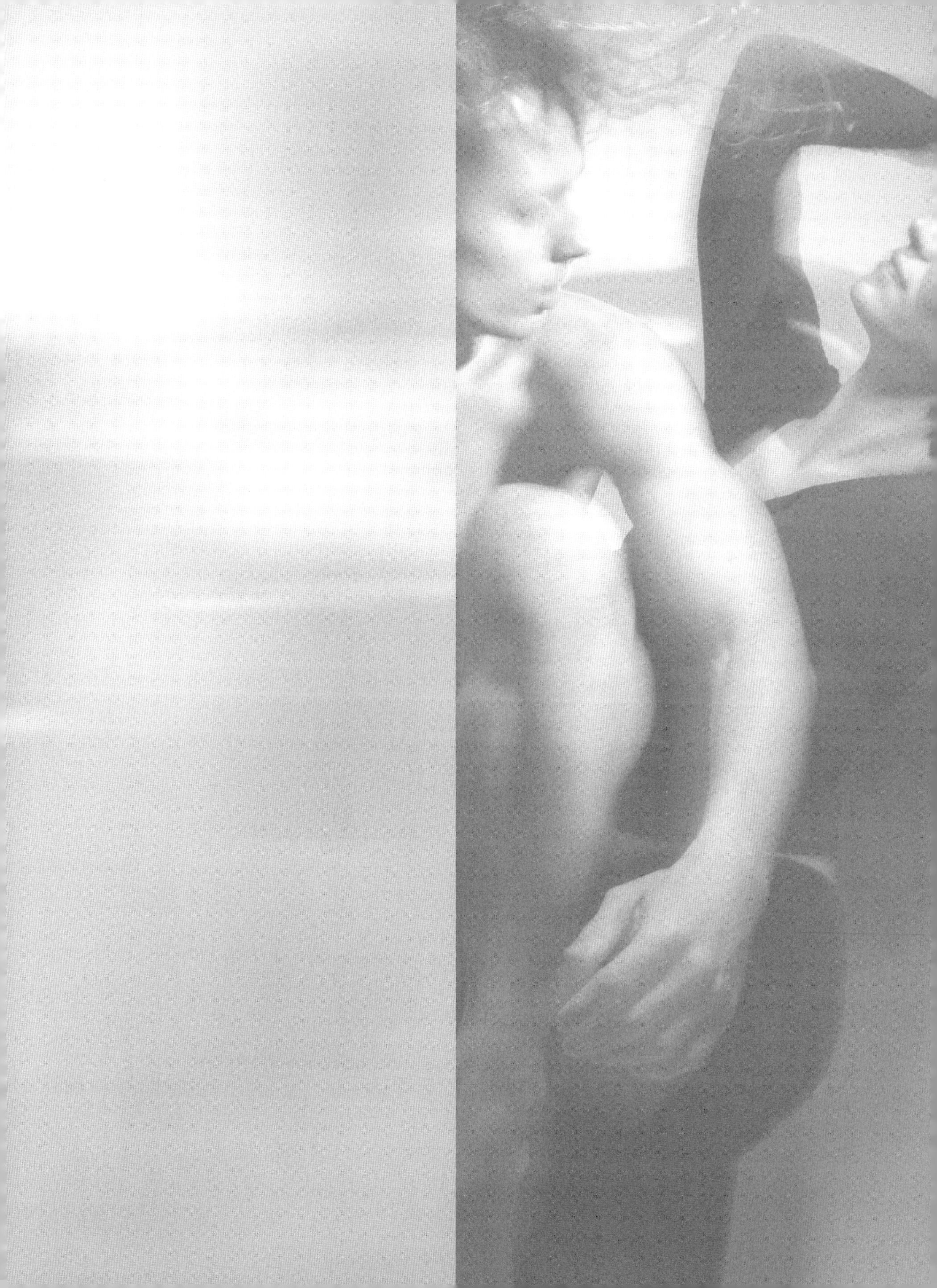

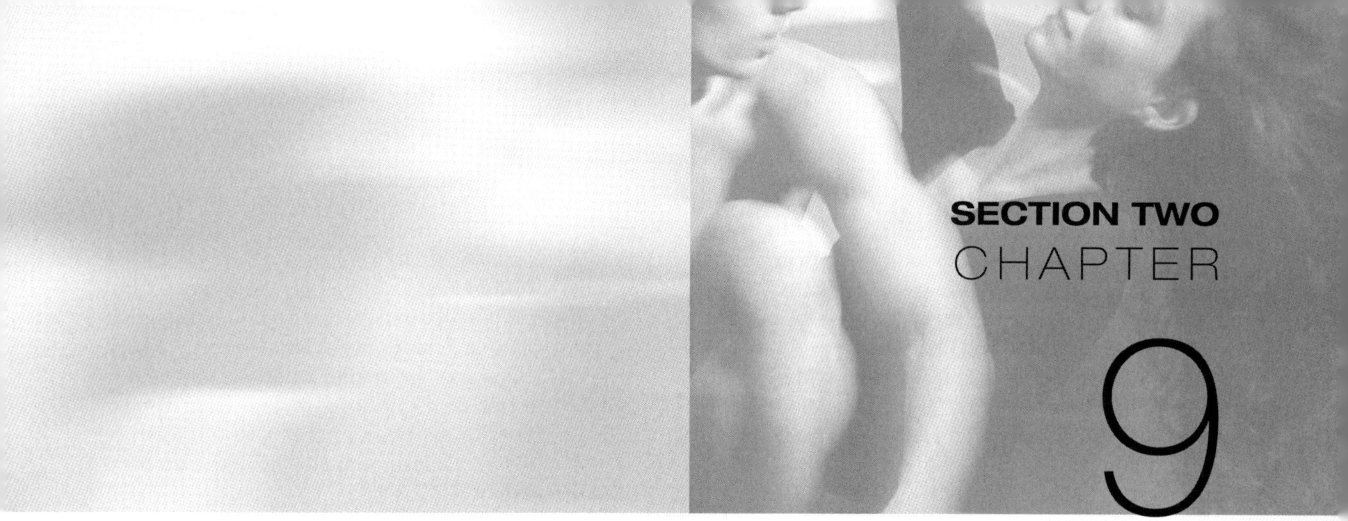

SECTION TWO
CHAPTER
9

Evolution of the human lumbopelvic region and its relationship to some clinical deficits of the spine and pelvis

C Owen Lovejoy

Introduction

Tracing the evolutionary origin of structures can often broaden our understanding of their function and thereby provide a clearer picture of why they will, in some cases, suffer a clinical deficit. The human lower back and pelvis are unique among mammals and knowledge of their evolutionary origin might therefore improve our understanding of the etiologies of some of the disorders that affect them.

All anatomical structures are derived by the interaction between variations in their underlying morphogenesis and their musculoskeletal expression and function. The biomechanical effectiveness of any structure is ultimately 'judged' by natural selection. In the past, however, functional interpretations of typical morphological variants have often been excessive, and have led to 'adaptationism,' which is the assignment of too great an impact on differential reproductive success to only minor musculoskeletal variants. The latter are often merely simple 'byproducts' of the underlying developmental genomic basis of a 'target' adaptation (Gould & Lewontin 1979, Lovejoy et al 2003, Reno et al 2000). The role of the evolutionary biologist is therefore to provide a *broad* evolutionary background for anatomical complexes that best explains their origin, variation, and morphogenesis without excessive attribution of significance to inconsequential variations (Lovejoy et al 2003).

The lower back, pelvis, and hip have played a primary and unique role in human evolution. In fact, adaptations to upright walking are the oldest phyletic indicator of the human evolutionary lineage, preceding all other human specializations (such as tool making and encephalization). The human fossil record today includes an abundance of fossils that can be used to trace the origin and development of these anatomical structures (and occasionally even their morphogenesis) and their role in human bipedality, which is not only unique to primates but to mammals in general (Lovejoy 2005a, 2005b).

Upright walking is now known to be quite ancient and our adaptations to it are far more 'advanced' than has been claimed in the past by some observers (see, for example, Wood 1996). Indeed, the earliest evidence of habitual upright progression in hominids now dates to as early as 6 million years ago (MYA) (Brunet et al 2002, Galik et al 2004, Ohman et al 2005, Pickford 2001). Here, we will briefly outline the origins of some of the specialized human adaptations to upright walking in the spine and pelvis, and note their chronology so as to provide a more accurate assessment of their true antiquity.

Evolutionary framework

The hominid fossil record is one of the best known and most complete of any mammal. This has been the product of intensive search for appropriate fossils, by the highly favorable taphonomic conditions of East and South Africa, and by the fact that early hominids were unusually demographically successful. Although a variety of taxonomic issues remain the subject of intense current debate, a broad picture of early hominid evolution has emerged and is summarized in Fig. 9.1. A combination of current paleogeographic and DNA hybridization data suggest that humans last shared a common ancestor (LCA) with the African apes (*Pan troglodytes, Pan paniscus, Gorilla gorilla*) in the range of 6–9 MYA (Sibley & Ahlquist 1987). There is little question that this LCA was geographically African. Although a smattering of fossils have begun to appear from time depths within this range (or at least its most recent boundary), fossil samples sufficient to permit designation of actual taxa are still more limited, but have been burgeoning in recent years, especially as a consequence of activities of teams working in Chad, Ethiopia, and Kenya.

Only a few years ago, fossils of such great age and primitive structure were recovered from Ethiopia that they justified a new early hominid genus designated *Ardipithecus ramidus* (White et al 1994, 1995). An additional chronospecies is now known (*Ardipithecus kadabba*) (Haile-Selassie et al 2004) and the genus now ranges in age from about 5 to 4.4 MYA. A more derived species recovered from Kenya is *Australopithecus anamensis* (Ward et al 2001). This now serves as the horizon species of the genus first defined in 1925 by Dart with the recovery of fossils from South African caves and named *Australopithecus africanus* (Dart 1925). A number of other fossils have been recovered from similar caves but all can now reasonably be assigned to two distinct clades (phyletic lines), which probably diverged from one another between 3 and 2 MYA (see Fig. 9.1). Both phyletic lines appear to have shared a common ancestor in the form of *Australopithecus afarensis*, which is now known from the time span of 3.5–2.8 MYA.

Although there are still major gaps in our understanding of the emergence of the modern human locomotor system, systematically combining all of the evidence from each of these fossil taxa provides an unusually clear picture of many aspects of early human bipedality. Fossils assigned to *A. ramidus* have received only cursory description and thus cannot yet contribute to that picture. Moreover, the remains of *Au. anamensis* are still rare, and with respect to the locomotor skeleton comprise only fragments of the radius, tibia, and isolated bones of the foot (Ward et al 2001).

By contrast, the remains of *Au. afarensis* are extensive and unusually complete and include the partial skeleton AL-288-1 ('Lucy'; Johanson et al 1982). In addition, the clear existence of two subsequent clades (see Fig. 9.1), which probably diverged from this parent species, gives us special insight into any locomotor characters that were shared because of common ancestry. Certainly, a fuller understanding of the two species – *A. ramidus* and *Au. anamensis* – holds great promise for enhancing our understanding of the earlier phases of the emergence of human locomotion. Even so, however, the record made available by *Au. afarensis*, although more recent, still allows many insights into the earliest emergence of the modern human frame.

It is a common practice among some current authors to argue that *Au. afarensis* was in some fashion 'poorly adapted' to upright walking and running, that running was difficult or impossible for members of the species, or that its bipedality was in some fashion 'facultative' (Bramble & Lieberman 2004, Wood 1996). However, such a view is wholly incorrect and the species demonstrates a number of advanced specializations to upright locomotion not seen in other primates (except descendant hominids) and which are obvious, substantial adaptations to both walking *and* running. A partial list of these is presented in Box 9.1. Although only some of these adaptations concern either the lower

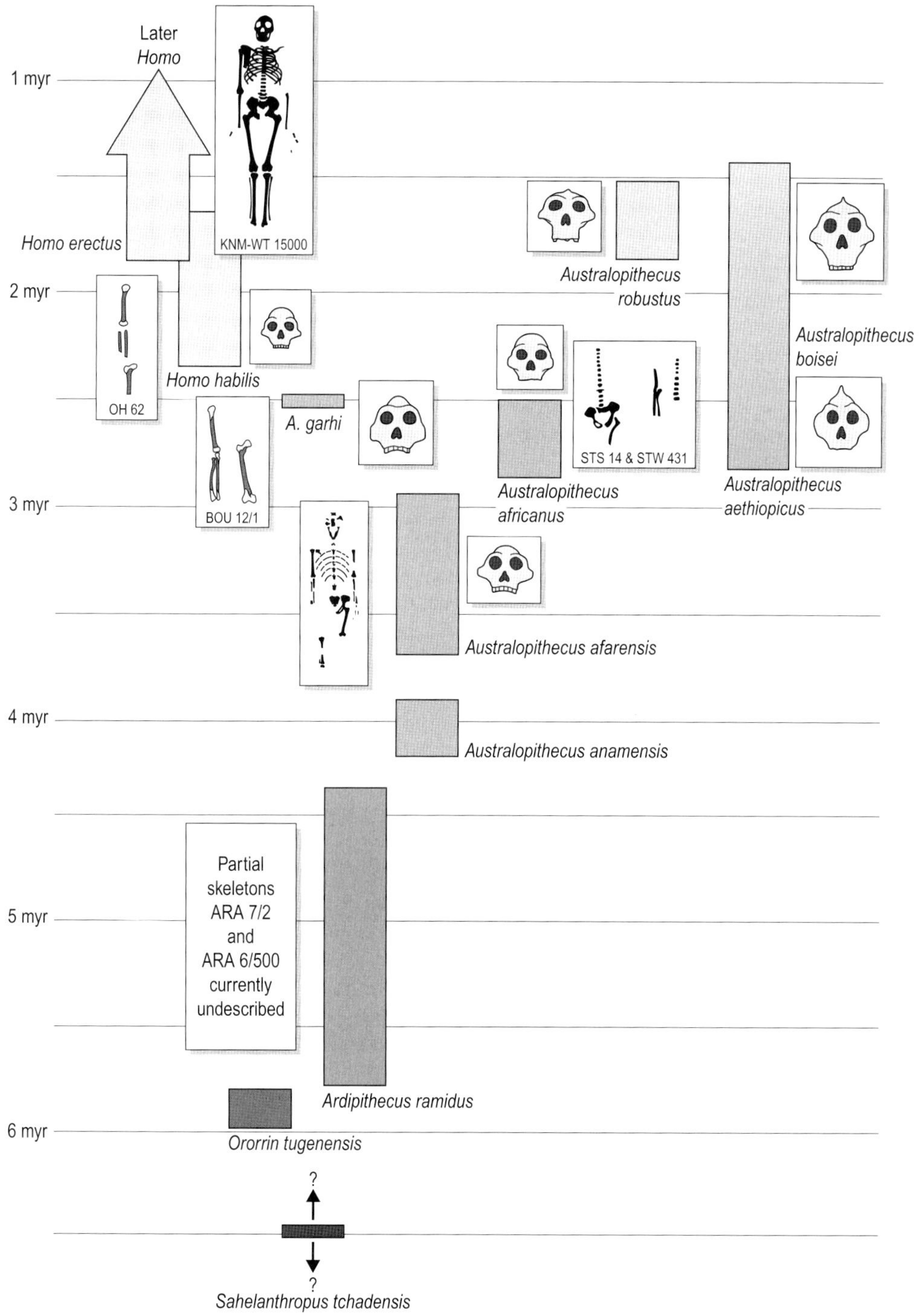

Fig. 9.1 Broad phylogenetic relationships between current 'major' early hominid taxa (i.e. those recognized almost universally). The pictograms next to each specimen show approximate completeness of important postcrania (only specimens with associated postcrania are illustrated here). There is a strong probability that only two major phyletic lines emerged between 6 and 2 MYA. One of these led to several extinct species of *Australopithecus* whereas the other led to *Homo habilis* and its eventual successors: *H. erectus* and *H. sapiens*. (Reproduced with permission from Lovejoy 2005a. © LB Spurlock/MA McCollum.)

Box 9.1

Partial list of distinct lower limb morphological characters that reflect advanced bipedality in early hominids (including all species of *Australopithecus*)

1. Reduction of iliac height, preventing 'capture' of L6 and facilitation of lumbar lordosis
2. Broadest sacrum of any primate for combining effective abduction with adequate pelvic volume
3. Laterally flared ilia for effective abduction, with novel sigmoid curvature to iliac crest (only in hominids)
4. Ischial length reduced for effective action of hamstrings at the end of the stance phase
5. Long femoral neck for advantageous position of abductors during single support phase
6. Anterior inferior iliac spine from separate center of ossification: growth pattern typical only of hominids
7. Expanded retroauricular area of ilium for enlargement of sacroiliac joint (SIJ) capsule
8. Distinct greater and lesser sciatic notches
9. Anterior iliac pillar position consistent with degree of lateral iliac flare
10. Elongated pubis for effective pelvic volume with reduced iliac height (platypelloidy)
11. Shortened pubic corpus and symphysis consistent with overall superoinferior pelvic shortening
12. Greatly reduced distance from auricular surface to acetabulum: shortens moment arm of thorax in single support and heel strike
13. Angular differentiation of ischial tuberosity reflecting transformation of hamstring function during gait
14. Six lumbars for substantial lumbar lordosis including distinct imbrication facets
15. Distinct superoinferior gradient of facet joint spacing in lumbar column for maximum flexibility and lordosis
16. Distinct trabecular pattern within proximal femur typical of modern humans and inconsistent with Trendelenberg gait
17. Lowered and prominent greater trochanter for effective abductor lever arm (compresses femoral neck)
18. Distinct third trochanter and hypotrochanteric fossa in femur showing modern disposition of gluteus maximus
19. Distinct obturator externus groove
20. True linea aspera reflecting transformation of quadriceps to modern proportions
21. Elongated femur compared to those of other hominoids
22. Elliptical profile of both condyles of distal femur reflecting increasing cartilage contact during extension
23. High anterolateral lip of lateral femoral condyle providing patellar retention with fully extended knee
24. Moderate to high bicondylar angle reflecting normal knee valgus with full extension
25. Expanded trabecular architecture in proximal tibia
26. Eccentric meniscal axis in knee
27. Tibial (versus patellar) dominance of cartilage modeling in knee
28. Transverse distal tibial plafond
29. Wedged talar dome
30. Longitudinal and transverse pedal arches
31. Permanently adducted first ray
32. Vertical groove for tibialis anterior
33. Distinct dorsiflexion profile in metatarsophalangeal joints for all five rays
34. Markedly expanded calcaneal tuber for energy dissipation at heel strike

back or hip; others that are listed in the box are equally demonstrative of the fact that adaptation to bipedality was profound as early as 3.5 MYA.

The modern human skeleton *does* differ from that of australopithecines, and some of these differences do represent further adaptations to bipedality. However, the marked degree of adaptation seen in australopithecines confirms that if we were able somehow to see them locomote today, their fundamental gait pattern in both walking and running would not differ significantly from our own – the changes that have occurred in the human skeleton over the past 3.5 million years have been largely restricted to mechanical modifications that improve our capacity to walk and run without skeletal degradation or injury. They have been largely '*protective*' rather than '*enabling*' for bipedality.

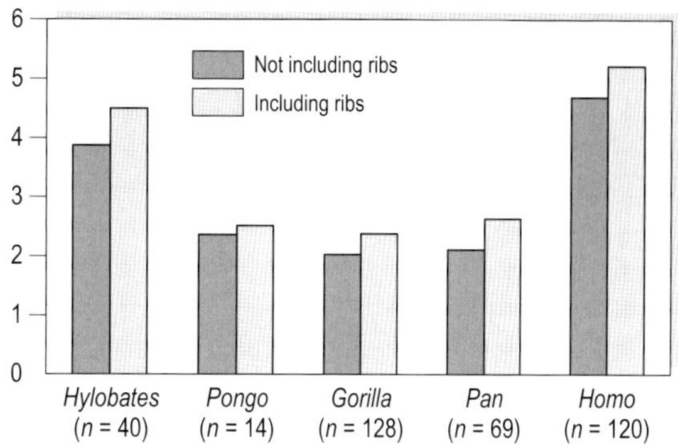

Fig. 9.2 Results of recent survey of functional status of lumbar vertebrae in living hominoids. The *y* axis shows the average number of vertebrae considered anatomically mobile, i.e. each vertebra must have met three requirements: (1) exhibit transverse processes rather than ribs (both sides); (2) exhibit both left and right zygapophyses in lumbar rather than thoracic orientation; (3) be free from entrapment by either or both ilia. Relaxation of the rib requirement increased mobility totals only slightly. Sample sizes are provided for each taxon.

Evolutionary background of the human spine

The lumbar spine has been a primary focus of change and adaptation in human evolution, so much so that despite the proviso made immediately above (that bipedality and our adaptations to it are both very old), there are many aspects of their evolution that clearly underlie modern pathologies and which also allow functional identification of major 'problem areas' of spinal function. Understanding this aspect of our evolution requires that we first revisit some structural aspects of the Miocene LCA of apes and humans.

One of the most striking differences between evolved hominid bipeds and their contemporary hominoid relatives is the lengths and mobility of their lumbar spines (Sanders 1998, Ward et al 1997). All living hominoids (chimpanzee, bonobo, gorilla, orangutan) share a demonstrably similar vertebral structure that distinguishes them from gibbons ('lesser apes') and Old World monkeys (OWMs), our next closest 'relatives,' and which are *generally* representative of the primitive Miocene apes from which all living hominoids evolved (i.e. the LCA of all hominoids) (Ward et al 1993). Many of these changes are currently thought to have appeared in the middle Miocene, although there is also evidence for an even earlier appearance in some Miocene species (MacLatchy et al 2000, Young & MacLatchy 2004).

In stark contrast to humans, each of the contemporary great apes exhibits an especially stiff, virtually immobile, lumbar spine. Indeed, a recent survey of potential functional mobility in the hominoid lumbar spine has revealed that, on average, apes have only about two potentially mobile lumbar vertebrae (Fig. 9.2) (Stevens & Lovejoy 2004).

This reduction of the lumbar spine is believed to be a specialized adaptation to a novel form of locomotion that progressively appeared in the Miocene hominoid ancestors of humans and apes (Lovejoy 2005a). OWMs, which are generally anatomically representative of the basal Miocene apes (although it is clear that the latter were already tail-less) (Nakatsukasa et al 2004), have between six and seven lumbar vertebrae, almost all of which have substantial mobility (Hartman & Straus 1933). Spinal flexion and extension are an important part of locomotion in OWMs, because they are, for the most part, small bodied 'above-branch quadrupeds' and therefore share many locomotor features with other typical terrestrial cursors. Why did the apes so dramatically change basic lumbar morphology?

The most likely reasons for this change were a substantial increase in body mass and modifications of longevity that herald major shifts in demographics, feeding strategy, and social structure. Miocene apes are often (but not always) significantly larger than most contemporary, arboreal OWMs (Kelley 1997, Lovejoy 1981). They probably became too large to remain above-branch quadrupeds, one reason being that they were also becoming increasingly 'K adapted', i.e. they were evolving elongated life phases (especially the periods of infant dependency and 'childhood'), so as to increase the time period over which learning could occur – a common adaptation in many derived mammals and one that is most extremely expressed in living humans (Pianka 1988).

In response to these selection pressures, later Miocene apes developed a form of locomotion called 'bridging', in which all four limbs became specialized for grasping (as opposed to the typical digitigrade 'fulcrumation' of most terrestrial quadrupeds and OWMs; Cartmill & Milton 1978). Some descendants of Miocene forms further enhanced such bridging and became primarily suspensory (e.g. orangutans and small-bodied gibbons).

By the late middle Miocene, hominoids had developed a high range of pronation and supination in their forelimbs by 'withdrawing' the ulna from direct participation in the ulnocarpal joint (the ulna in livings apes and humans is now separated from their carpals by a meniscus, and their ulnar styloid is extremely short; Lewis 1974, Moya-Sola et al 2004). This permitted much greater ulnar deviation of the hand and greatly expanded its range of 'grasping.' Other changes included enhanced grasping capacity of the foot, especially increased robusticity in the first ray, and several other changes that further improved the range of motion and suspensory capacity of the forelimb. The latter included a reduction of the olecranon process of the ulna, which allowed complete extension of the elbow, and a posterior translation of the scapula on the thoracic wall, which relocated the forelimb to a more posterior position such that it faces more laterally in apes than it does in OWMs in which if tends to face anteriorly (Fig. 9.3).

Changes in the spine and pelvis of Miocene apes played the central role in these dramatic reorganizations. Instead of acting in its original propulsive role in locomotion, the lumbar spine became fixed so as to serve as a stable, rigid, axis from which the more mobile fore and hind limbs could extend (Lovejoy & Latimer 1997). This involved several major modifications critical to understanding modern human structure.

First, the lumbar spine was shortened by reducing the actual number of lumbar vertebrae (from 6–7 in OWMs to 3–4 in living apes; see earlier; Schultz 1930a). Via genetic changes that quite obviously involve shifts in *Hox* gene expression boundaries, some lower lumbars were converted to sacrals (the sacrum of apes is generally 6–7 segments in length) and often one upper lumbar was converted

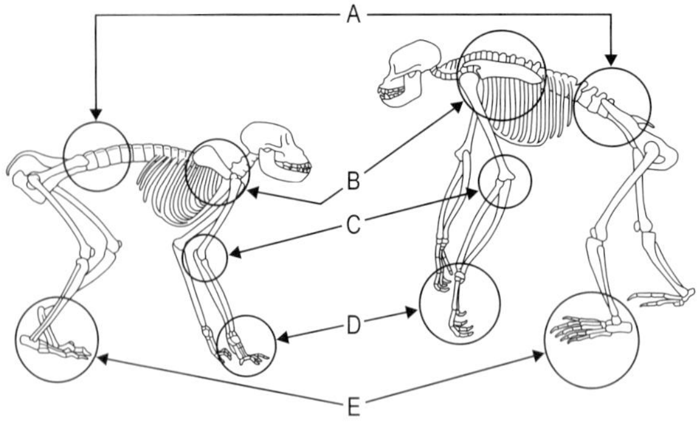

Fig. 9.3 Stylized skeletons of an Old World Monkey (OWM; left) and chimpanzee (right) in typical standing postures for illustration of major locomotor changes adopted in the last shared common ancestor (LCA) of modern apes and humans. The OWM, while still retaining a tail (shown abbreviated here), which was lost in early apes, illustrates many of the generalized features sacrificed by later Miocene apes to evolve 'bridging.' The primary anatomic regions most affected have been circled in each specimen. All substantially reduce the capacity to dissipate ground reaction in the ape compared to the OWM. (A) The long, flexible lumbosacral region of the OWM has been replaced by a short, invaginated, immobilized spine in the ape. (B) The anteriorly oriented scapular blade and glenoid in the OWM (which allow the serratus anterior to contract eccentrically at ground contact without danger of shoulder subluxation) have been more laterally oriented in the ape (this is also a byproduct of vertebral column invagination). (C) The long olecranon in the OWM (which allows the triceps surae to eccentrically resist flexion induced by ground reaction) has been greatly shortened in the ape to permit full extension at the elbow. (D) The stable wrist joint of the digitigrade OWM, which enjoys a long, distally projecting ulnar styloid (which functions similarly to the malleoli of the ankle mortise) has been replaced in the ape by a new form of digitigrade in which energy dissipation is accomplished by means of eccentric contraction of the long digital and wrist flexors when its metacarpus is forcefully dorsiflexed during ground contact. (E) The OWM's digitigrade posterior pedal metacarpus has been replaced by a plantagrade posture in the ape, in which grasping has been enhanced by greater opposition and robusticity in the foot. Each of these energy dissipating mechanisms available to OWMs was lost in the LCA of humans and apes, and necessitated radical new energy mechanisms when their descendants became terrestrial, i.e. knuckle walking in the African apes, and a variety of hindlimb specializations in bipedal hominids. Virtually all of these hominid mechanisms were already present in australopithecines. For discussion see text.

to a thoracic (Pilbeam 2004, Rosenman et al 2002). In addition, the superoinferior height of the ilium appears to have also been increased, permitting the frequent 'capture' of two lumbars by the iliac blades

– their close proximity and dense ligamentous attachment preventing virtually any movement of the 'entrapped' vertebrae. As just noted, these changes almost entirely eliminated any motion within the lumbar spine – indeed it is so short in modern apes that the distance between the iliac crest and the most caudal rib is normally a single intercostal space (Fig. 9.4; Schultz 1930a).

A second modification is especially important in understanding the natural history of the human spine. Spinal mobility was also eliminated in hominoids by a ventral invagination of the entire column into the thorax (Fig. 9.5; Schultz 1930b, 1961, Schultz & Straus 1945). In OWMs, the transverse processes of the lumbar vertebrae originate from the approximate anteroposterior midpoint of each vertebral centrum, whereas in apes and humans they take origin from the pedicles. There has thus been a dramatic shift in the position of the anatomical location and physical structure of the spine. The (new) more ventral position of the spine (both lumbar and thoracic) has structurally 'rigidified' it (Benton 1967). At the same time, however, such passive rigidity has also resulted in a remarkable loss in the size of the erector spinae musculature (Fig. 9.6; Benton 1967). In OWMs these muscles are involved in primary locomotion (e.g. leaping), whereas in apes, they have become much smaller and are only used to secondarily aid spinal stabilization.

Whether these changes were the product of selection for a stiffer frame with which Miocene apes could 'bridge' gaps in the arboreal canopy, or whether they simply prevented injury to the lower spine during forelimb suspension because of a 'whiplash effect' from the greater mass of their lower limbs is largely irrelevant here. What *is* relevant, however, is how crucial lower back mobility is to upright walking – to walk bipedally, early hominids had to *reverse* some of these changes.

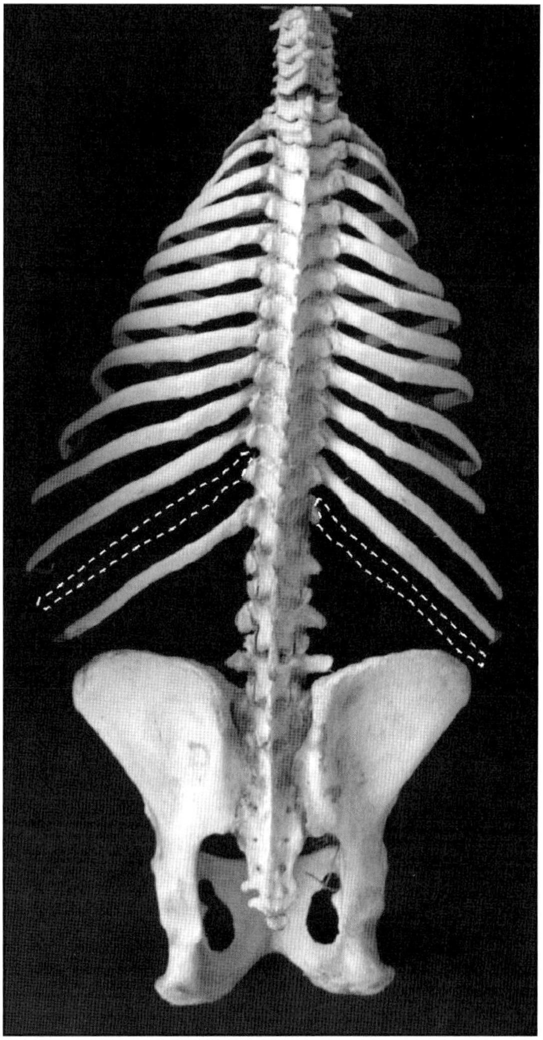

Fig. 9.4 Ligamentous specimen of *Pan troglodytes (schweinfurthii)* (Royal Museum for Central Africa, Tervuren, Belgium) showing typical thoracic and pelvic relationships. Two ribs were lost postmortem whose locations are indicated by dotted lines. Note the presence of 13 thoracics and four lumbars, as well as the proximity of the thirteenth rib to the iliac crest laterally, being separated only by about one intercostal space. This specimen is unusual because only one lumbar is 'entrapped by its ilia' (for discussion, see text and data in Fig. 9.2), although the proximity of the right transverse process of its third lumbar would have likely ensured that its mobility was greatly restricted. However, this specimen would receive a 'score' of three in the survey presented in Fig. 9.2.

The unique structure of the human spine

In the final analysis, all of the changes described above, which substantially reduced the fundamental quadrupedal adaptations typical of other primates, would have a substantial effect on their descendants when they once again became partially terrestrial (apes) or completely so (humans). As the changes in the forelimbs described earlier substantially compromised both their energy-absorbing capacity [i.e. eccentric contractions of triceps surae at the elbow and of serratus magnus (or s. anterior in humans) in the shoulder] and joint stability (elimination of ulnar styloid from the wrist joint), unique forms of locomotion

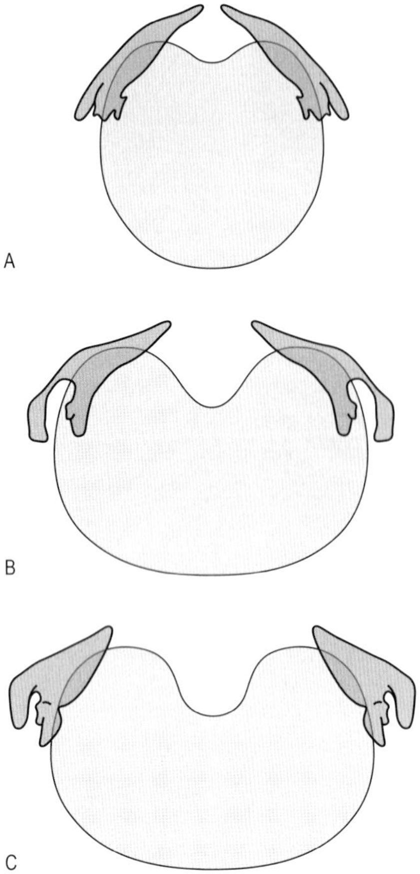

Fig. 9.5 Invagination of the vertebral column into the thorax and its effects on the structural integrity of the spine. (A) Old World Monkey (macaque); (B) chimpanzee; (C) human. In the two hominoids (B and C), column invagination has 'rigidified' the thorax and made it elliptical in cross section. This has also caused the scapular blade to become more mediolaterally oriented. Invagination is most dramatic in humans because of lumbar lordosis. (Reprinted from Gaitand Posture, V21(1):95-112, Lovejoy CO: 'The natural history of human gait and posture': Part 2 Hip and Thigh © Elsevier BV.)

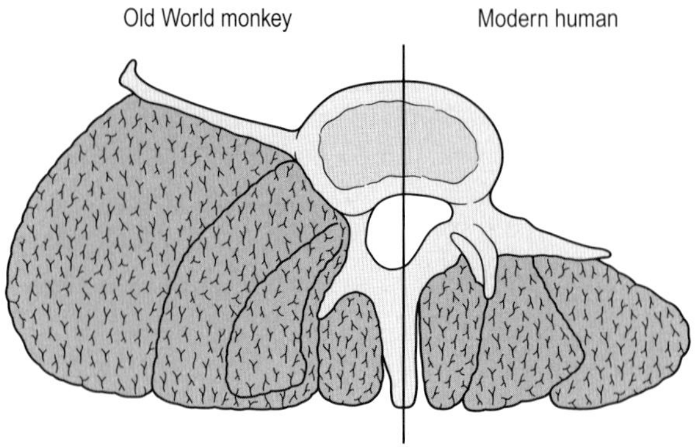

Fig. 9.6 'Hybrid' erector spinae of an OWM (*Cercopithecus*) (right) and human (left). The two vertebrae have been scaled to the same anteroposterior overall dimension of their centra. The massive erector spinae of the monkey extends its transverse process well anterior onto the vertebral body while that of the human (representative of hominoids) is restricted only to its pedicle, greatly reducing its cross-sectional area. Loss of erector spinae mass is largely a byproduct of thoracic 'rigidification' caused by a substantial anterior projection of the column. (Reproduced with permission from Lovejoy 2005a. © LB Spurlock/MA McCollum.)

appeared in their newly terrestrial descendants (see Fig. 9.3). Apes evolved a special form of energy-absorptive gait called knuckle-walking (KW). Hominids became exclusively bipedal and thereby had to evolve novel energy-absorbing mechanisms in their hindlimbs (most terrestrial quadrupeds, including KW apes, can substantially ameliorate ground reaction with their forelimbs; Lovejoy & Latimer 1997).

It is a common misconception that the flexed-hip, flexed-knee bipedal posture of anthropoid apes derives from anatomical limitations in the structure of their hip joints. To the contrary, such positioning of the lower limb joints of non-human hominoids derives directly from their inability to achieve almost any degree of lumbar lordosis. Whereas the latter action is used to anteriorly relocate the center of mass of the head, arms, and trunk (HAT) over the point of ground support in humans, not being able to do so requires the simultaneous flexion of both hip and knee joints during bipedal posturing and locomotion in the great apes.

The human lower spine is remarkably mobile compared to that of the great apes because of several important anatomical features, including its greater length, a superoinferior shortening of the iliac blades so as to free up any contact with the lowest lumbar vertebra, and a dramatic alteration of the structure of the lumbar centra (Lovejoy 2005b). The latter involves a caudally progressive widening of the transverse distance separating the paired facet joints, and a progressive increase in the overall size of the lumbar centra. These changes in the facet joints permit greater imbrication (i.e. sliding) and thereby flexibility in the lower spine (Fig. 9.7), and allow even greater lordosis than would otherwise be possible in humans, had they been merely elongated by the addition of vertebrae (Latimer & Ward 1993).

Walking significant distances with a bent-hip/bent-knee (BHBK) gait is unquestionably fatiguing

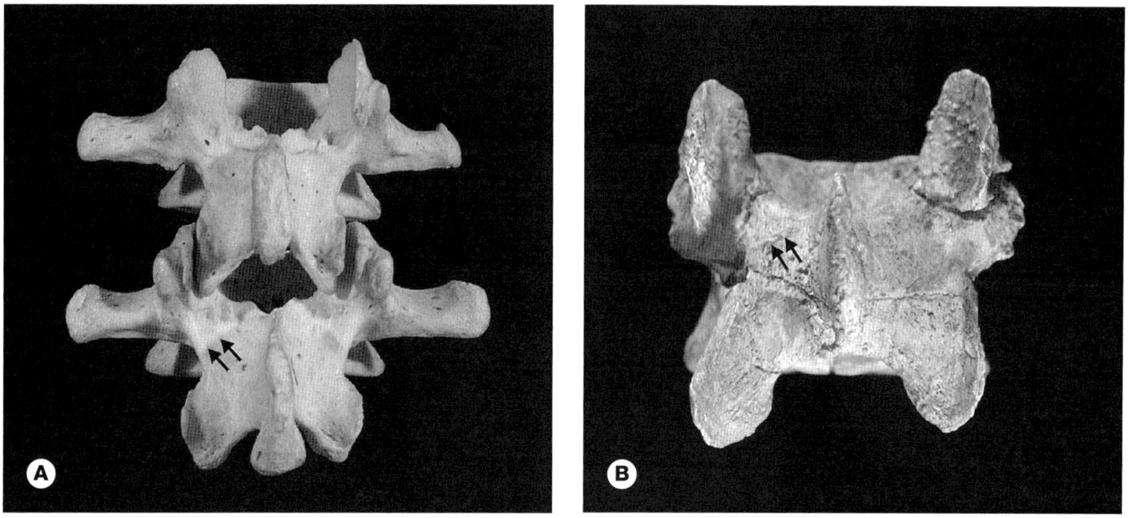

Fig. 9.7 Imbrication facets in (A) human and (B) AL-288-1 ('Lucy') lumbar vertebrae. Arrows on each L3 indicate the marginal limit of the area 'excavated' by contact with the zygapophyses of L2. As (Reprinted from Gaitand Posture, V21(1):95-112, Lovejoy CO: 'The natural history of human gait and posture': Part 2 Hip and Thigh © Elsevier BV.)

because of the relatively low lever advantage that accompanies these two joints when they cannot be placed in full extension (Carey & Crompton 2005). This leads to rapid muscle fatigue, which then reduces the ability to perform protective negative work and exposes lower limb joints to potential damage from mild to significant trauma that would otherwise be harmlessly ameliorated by eccentric contraction. Walking significant distances in a BHBK gait thus progressively exposes the entire lower limb to potential injury. Changes in lumbar spine configuration are therefore likely to have been among the *earliest* modifications to bipedality in ancestral hominids, and early hominids might have therefore virtually *never* walked with a BHBK gait. Evidence for this conclusion comes from the early hominid fossil record.

Although a number of isolated individual vertebrae and fragments of vertebrae have been recovered from *Au. afarensis* and other australopithecine species, four specimens are sufficiently complete to provide direct evidence about the nature of bipedality in ancestral hominids: STS-14 (Robinson 1972), STSW411, KNM-WT-17000 (Walker & Leakey 1993), and AL-288 (Johanson et al 1982). The first three of these allow a count to be made of the number of lumbars (although one, KNM-WT-17000, belongs to a descendant species, *Homo erectus*). Each displays six rather than five lumbar vertebrae (Robinson 1972, Rosenmanet al 2004, Sanders 1998, Walker & Leakey 1993). Inasmuch as only 5% of modern humans possess six lumbars, this is striking evidence of a unique form of early adaptation to bipedality that was apparently retained as late as one of its successive species, *H. erectus* (and of course, as just noted, still appears in a small percentage of modern humans).

The fourth specimen, AL-288, retains only a single lumbar but at the same time also preserves an intact sacrum. This allows a direct assessment of the spacing of its posterior facet joints (Fig. 9.8). As with humans, the transverse distance separating these joints is greater in the sacrum than in the lumbars above it (the AL-288 specimen is most likely a third lumbar). The recovery of the complete sacrum and complete innominate also permits a direct examination of their potential relationships between the pelvis and lumbar column. Such examination (Fig. 9.9) shows an absence of highly restrictive ligamentous relationships between the ilium and the (unrecovered) sixth lumbar. These details of spine anatomy in *Au. afarensis* and its descendant species highlight the special features of our lower spine.

The evolutionary basis of some modern spinal deficiencies

The australopithecine spine also differs from modern humans in that it largely lacks the progressive increase in the size of each lumbar centrum. In this regard it was still more like the lumbar spine of apes, in which all lumbar centra are of approximately

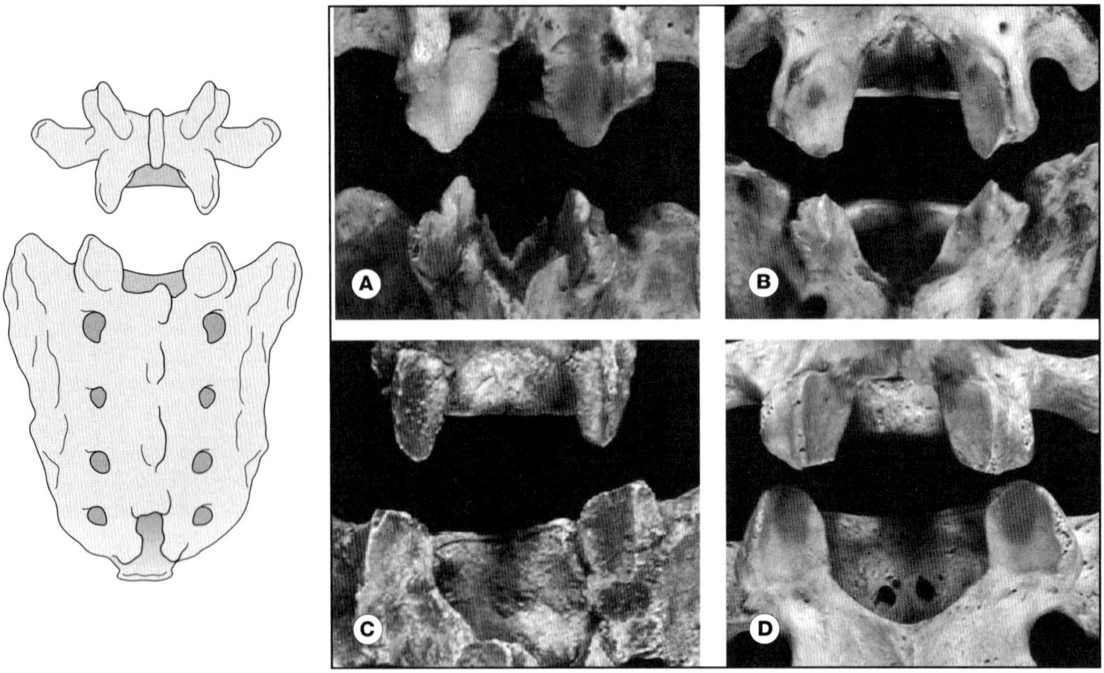

Fig. 9.8 Inferior to superior increasing size gradient within the lumbar facet joints. (A) Chimpanzee; (B) gorilla; (C) AL-288-1; (D) human. The cartoon shows the L3 of each specimen rotated 180° for this comparison (see also Fig. 9.9, L5 and L6). Note that the transverse distance separating the joint facets in the African apes is greater in their L3 than in their sacrum, whereas the reverse arrangement is present in the two hominids. As (Reprinted from Gaitand Posture, V21(1):95-112, Lovejoy CO: 'The natural history of human gait and posture': Part 2 Hip and Thigh © Elsevier BV.)

equal size. Thus modern humans have shortened our lumbar spines from six to five elements, and have also progressively increased the size of each centrum, such that the centrum of the first sacral is relatively enlarged in humans compared to those of australopithecines.

This change most likely results from difficulties brought about by invagination of our spine for increased rigidity (Lovejoy 2005b, Schultz 1930a, 1961). As noted earlier, this change caused the loss of a large portion of our erector spinae. Humans today therefore now suffer a rather perilous condition: an elongated, lordotic, lumbar spine that has only minimal erector spinae components with which it can be stabilized. It is little wonder that it is so frequently a source of injury and age-related trauma and degeneration.

As is well known, many such pathological changes derive from injury and degeneration of the lumbar intervertebral disks. The novel expansion of the size of human lumbar centra (especially the more caudal ones) has undoubtedly greatly improved the capacity of their annuli to resist torsional forces, because such expansion has greatly increased the second moments of their annuli about each vertebra's central (superoinferior) axis. In addition, the precarious region between our thorax and pelvis has also been somewhat reduced by elimination of one lumbar. Both changes represent improvements induced by natural selection acting on our ancestors in which spinal injuries must have been even more prevalent than they are today.

In fact, the spine of the KNM-WT-15000 *H. erectus* skeleton (which had six lumbars; see earlier) displays substantial evidence of scoliosis, including thoracic asymmetry, a unilateral rib facet on the clavicle, and possible premortem vertebral fracture (JC Ohman, BM Latimer, personal communications, and examination of original specimens by CO Lovejoy). Risk of scoliosis and erector spinae incompetence might have served as the most prominent selection factors favoring reduction in the length of the human lumbar column over the course of the Plio-Pleistocene.

It is of some further interest in this regard that idiopathic scoliosis is virtually unknown in any other primate except humans. Apes have so rigid a lumbar spine that scoliotic deviation, lacking an obvious developmental defect such as a wedged vertebra, is simply not possible. OWMs, while

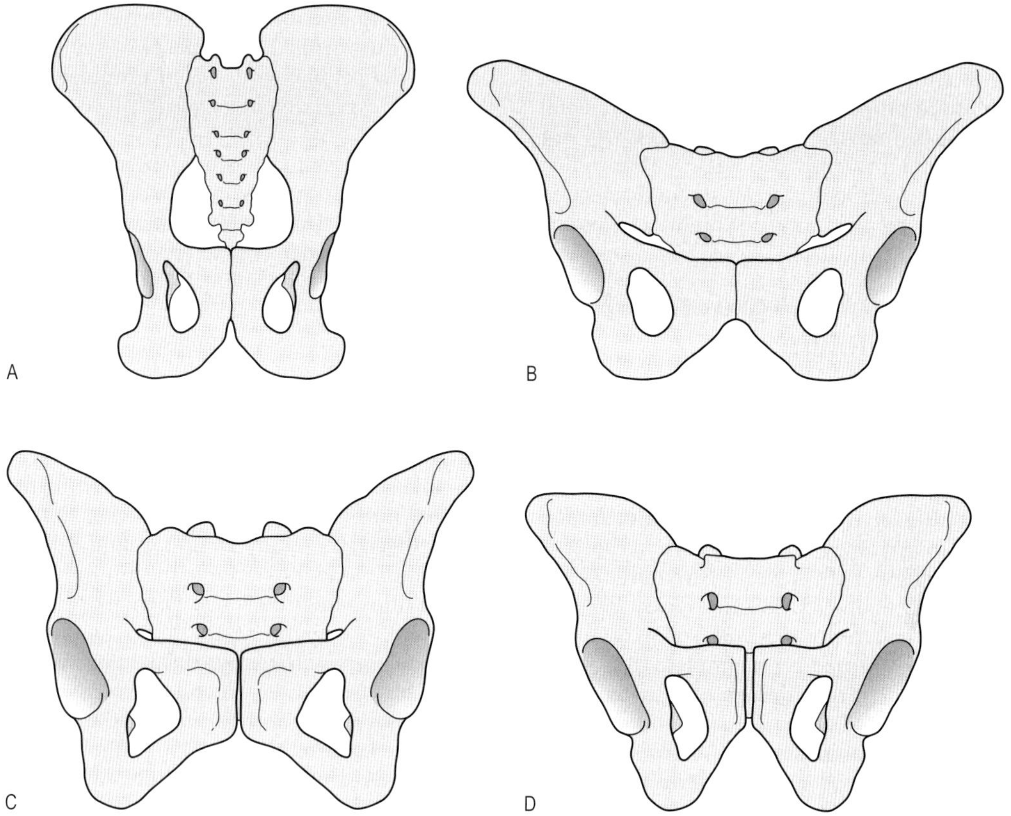

Fig. 9.9 Frontal projections of hominoid pelves. (A) Chimpanzee; (B) AL-288-1; (C) human female; (D) human male. Note the dramatic shortening of the hominid ilia and the absence of any dorsal projection that might 'entrap' their last lumbar (L5 in humans; L6 in *Au. afarensis*). (Reproduced with permission from Lovejoy 2005a. © LB Spurlock/MA McCollum.)

having a long lumbar spine, have such massive erector spinae that lumbar stabilization is easily maintained. Only humans have the dangerous combination of a long, mobile, lumbar spine, the requirement of a lordotic spine for locomotion, and a lack of a fully competent erector spinae. It is therefore possible that some idiopathic scoliosis might actually begin, imperceptibly, in the lumbar column and remain subclinical until modifications of the thorax are induced that then lead to increasing deformation as a downstream effect, thereby producing symptoms only after significant deficits. It is important in this regard that the author has never seen a case of scoliosis in any other primate; although the likelihood of survival to an age in which it could be recognized in a dry skeleton with this kind of deficit must be very low – yet it is clearly present in the single known complete *H. erectus* skeleton (KNM-WT-15000; see earlier).

It is also of some clinical relevance that a recent review of a large number of primate skeletons by Latimer (personal communication) reveals no cases of spondylolysis, another malady that apparently never occurs in apes or monkeys but which is quite common in humans (almost 5% of the human population; Hollinshead 1963). Latimer (personal communication) has argued that spondylolysis is more frequent in individuals in which the inferiorly progressive 'spread' of the lowest lumbar is less than those of normal, non-spondylolytic, spines (see above and Fig. 9.8), suggesting that the disorder is epigenetic and might derive from excessive propinquity of the neural arches during the initial development of lordosis during the early acquisition of bipedality in childhood.

However, the debilitating effects of spondylolysis (i.e. spondylolisthesis) have apparently occurred either only sporadically or not within an age period of significant survivorship (most individuals in earlier human populations rarely survived to an age in excess of 45 years; Lovejoy et al 1977) sufficient for selection to eliminate the disorder. The argument that spondylolysis was the primary selective force in favor of the inferiorly progressive spread of the lumbar zygapophyses (Latimer & Ward 1993, Lovejoy & Latimer 1997) is probably now null, as these are more properly viewed as a fundamental aspect of our novel lordosis (necessary for bipedality). It might simply be a negative byproduct of this important adaptation, against which selection has had little opportunity to favor alternative anatomical arrangements.

Evolutionary background of the human pelvis

Although a number of pelvic fragments have been found for australopithecines, two nearly complete innominates and sacra allow the best assessment of pelvic function in this genus: those of AL-288-1 and STS-14. They are remarkably similar in overall morphology and preserve a host of anatomical details. Both have also required some significant restoration (AL-288-1; Lovejoy 1979) or reconstruction and restoration (STS-14; Rosenman et al 1999) but the former is so complete that, given bilaterality, it can be regarded as a virtually intact specimen.

In addition to changes in the lumbar spine, the completely novel positioning of the hip joint and SIJ in the human lower limb also represents higher-order refinements of anatomical structure, and whereas the ability to completely extend the hip and knee made possible by spinal retroflexion would have greatly reduced fatigue during extended bouts of upright walking, ultimately fatigue could only be fully eliminated through the complete reorganization of muscle function that accompanies hominid upright walking, and in particular the development of the unique human abductor apparatus (Lovejoy 2005a).

In the shift from quadrupedal progression to bipedality, the activity of the hamstrings becomes primarily restricted to the control and deceleration of the limb in swing phase (along with an obvious variety of other postural duties) and the gluteus minimus and medius to pelvic stabilization during single support (they are no longer hip extensors) (Rose & Gamble 1994). The primary role of the gluteus maximus is no longer to be an extensor of the lower limb (except in anatomical laboratory courses) but rather to stabilize the trunk upon the lower limb, bracing the SIJ and preventing forward rotation of the head, arms, and trunk (HAT) at ground contact (Lovejoy 2005b). The quadriceps, along with the plantarflexors (with which their contraction must be synchronized so as to coordinate progressive elongation of the limb during the latter phases of stance phase), become the primary muscles of propulsion within the thigh, especially in running (Rose & Gamble 1994).

That these primary shifts in muscle function were already fully accomplished in *Au. afarensis* can be gleaned from study of various dimensions and morphological characters of AL-288-1. The introduction of substantial freedom in the lower spine (including the fact that the lumbar curve was effected with six vertebrae; Rosenman et al 2004) permitted retroflexion of the SIJs and thus a pelvic positioning not only close to that in humans but even more dramatically so. When the AL-288-1 pelvis is viewed from the lateral aspect (Fig. 9.10), it can be seen that all of the specialized features of modern humans have been achieved; that is, the primary vector of body weight, acting through the L6–S1 joint passes posterior to the hip joint, the lever arm of the hamstrings has been retroflexed and shortened, the course of the iliopsoas (acting as a hip flexor) is now to recurve back to its insertion on the lesser trochanter (thereby effecting a deep groove between the acetabulum and the iliopectineal eminence; Le Gros Clark 1955, 1978). The lordosis at the L6–S1 joint is approximately equal to that of *H. sapiens*.

These changes in iliac position place the anterior abductors into their human-like position for active pelvic balance during single support phase, i.e. one in which they can contract at or near their resting length, minimizing fatigue. This unique capacity of the hip joint in hominids to prevent pelvic 'drop' (positive Trendelenberg sign) has also gained significant mechanical advantage in australopithecine pelves by virtue of their having also acquired exceedingly long femoral necks. In fact, neck length in these specimens exceeds not only the neck length of other hominoids, but those of modern humans as well. It is thus not intermediate between apes and humans but is completely unique (Lovejoy 1974, 1978, Lovejoy et al 1973).

One of the most dramatic changes in the bony evidence surrounding hip function in australopithecines can be found in radiographic examination of their proximal femora. As shown in Fig. 9.11, the distribution of cortical bone in humans and apes differs dramatically (Lovejoy 1988, Lovejoy et al 1973). Whereas apes exhibit a complete ring of cortex at their neck/shaft juncture that resembles a diaphyseal cross-section, humans bear strong cortex only in the bottom portion of this interface, and normally lack any significant cortex in its

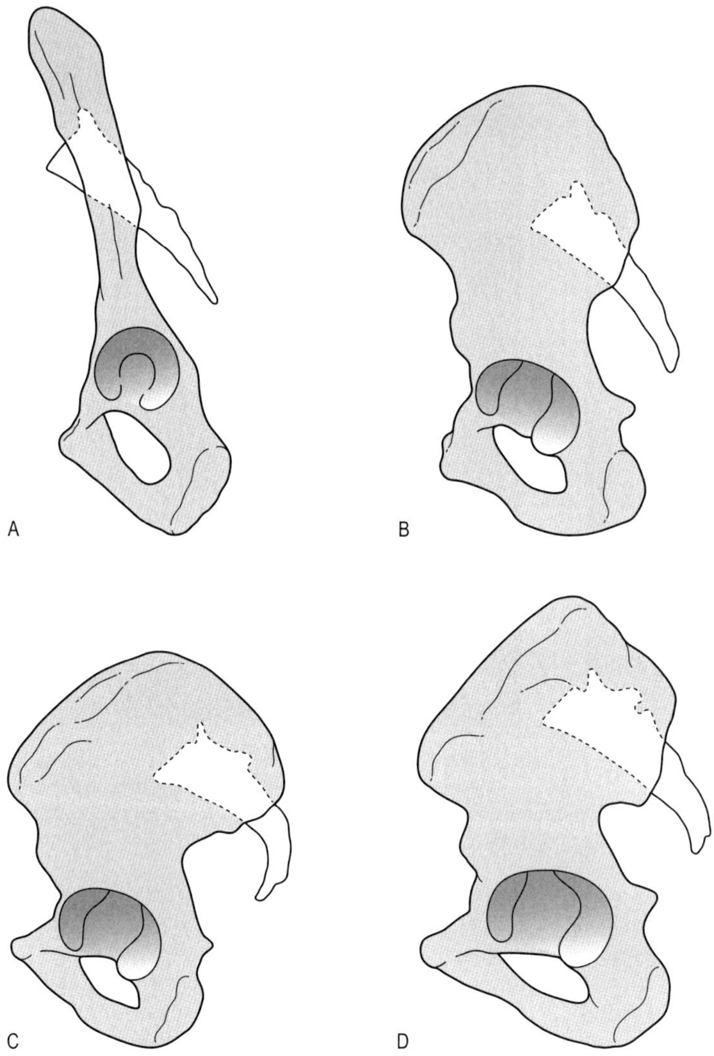

Fig. 9.10 Lateral projections of pelves shown in Fig. 9.9. Note the human-like angulated disposition of the facet(s) for the origin of the hamstrings (especially semimembranosus) in AL-288-1, unlike the single plane present in the chimpanzee. Also note the similar line of action of body mass acting on the sacral centrum in the two hominids. (Reproduced with permission from Lovejoy 2005a. © LB Spurlock MA/McCollum.)

upper portion. This is highly significant because the femoral neck is cantilevered whenever the limb is in stance phase and this distinct difference in cortical distribution signals very different hip joint loading in humans and apes.

An obvious mechanical explanation involves the human abductor apparatus. Because the primary abductors (the anterior gluteals) as well as the numerous 'auxiliary' ones (piriformis, the gemelli, and the obturators) together produce a strong horizontal component when contracted during single support, this component may be responsible for eliminating much of the tensile stress that emanates from the femoral neck's cantilevered condition during loading. As shown in Fig. 9.12, this creates a high compressive load in the lower part of the femoral neck and progressively reduces stress along an inferomedial to superolateral transect of the neck/shaft interface. As chimpanzees, which lack the abductor apparatus, almost certainly subject their femoral necks to less stereotyped loading than occurs in human walking and running, sufficient signal might be produced in the upper regions of their neck/shaft interfaces to encourage robust bone production during development, probably by progressive consolidation of trabeculae

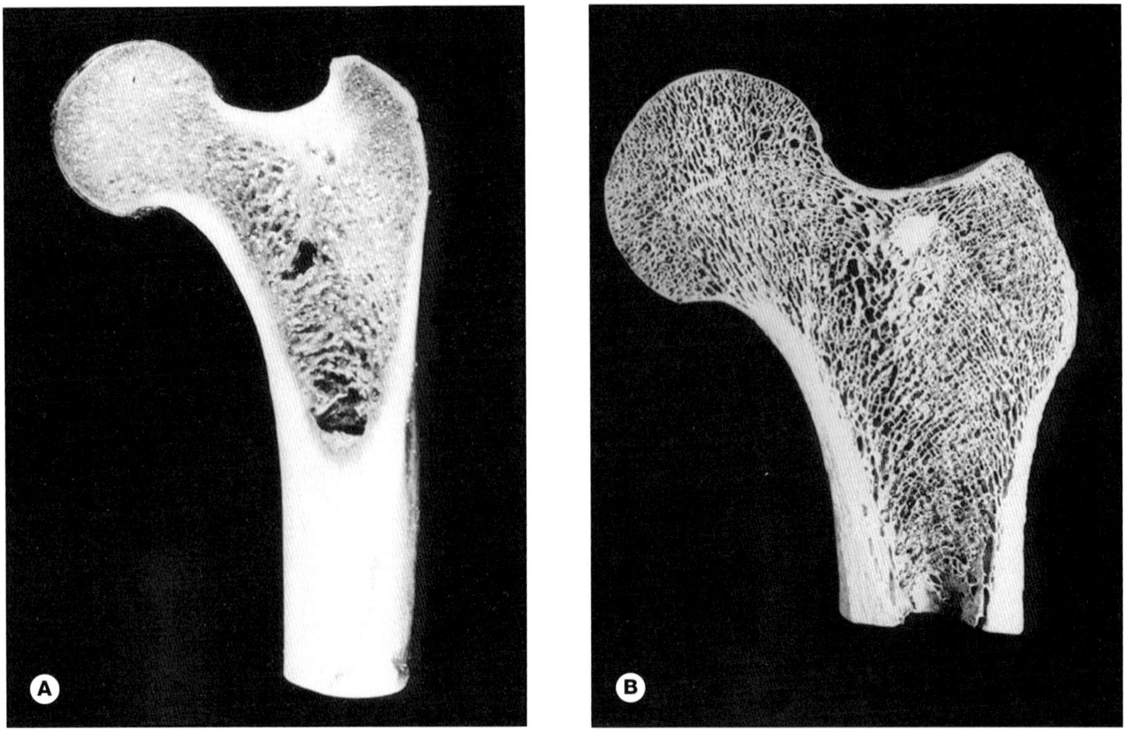

Fig. 9.11 Coronal sections of normal adult chimpanzee (left) and human (right) proximal femurs. Whereas the shaft cortex is approximately equal in the two specimens, there is almost no cortical bone in the superior portion of the human femoral neck, a normal finding. For further discussion see text. As (Reprinted from Gaitand Posture, V21(1):95-112, Lovejoy CO: 'The natural history of human gait and posture': Part 2 Hip and Thigh © Elsevier BV.)

left behind by the primary growth plates of the proximal femur. This results in their adult cortical cross sections having a 'shaft-like' appearance unlike those of modern humans.

An alternative explanation is that these differences in bone distribution do not emanate directly from differences in loading regimen but from possible differences in pattern formation. The proximal femoral epiphysis begins its 'life' as a single epiphysis and becomes separated into a head and greater trochanter only later in development. Prior to this separation, there is no opportunity for the deposition of superior subperiosteal cortex, as the entire proximal end remains subchondral. If the separation of the two growth plates became ontogenetically delayed in hominids as a consequence of substantial differences in growth patterning, then the superolateral aspect of the human femoral neck might experience a shorter period of independent growth prior to epiphyseal fusion, and thus less opportunity for subperiosteal acquisition of cortex.

Both explanations are consistent with recent confirmation of the loading patterns hypothesized to occur in the femoral necks of humans and chimpanzees. Kalmey & Lovejoy (2002) studied cartilage fiber orientation in the femoral necks of these two taxa. As predicted, the substantial cortex in the upper portion of chimpanzee femora was highly birefringent (indicative of tensile loading during deposition), whereas the inferior cortex of both taxa and human superior cortex (consistent with a compressive loading regimen) were much less so. These data do not resolve the conflict between the two etiologies, however, because the second is not dependent on loading pattern and would, in theory, obtain in any loading situation.

Satisfactory radiographs of proximal femora from *Au. afarensis* are rare (as they are for other early hominid fossils) because radiopaque matrix is often embedded in the specimens, making it difficult to visualize their internal structure. A dramatic exception is specimen MAK-VP-1/1, a nearly adult femur (the trochanters are fully fused and the head was partially fused but lost during fossilization) from the site of Maka (Clark et al 1984, Lovejoy et al 2002). This specimen, which dates from approximately 3.4 MYA, is completely free

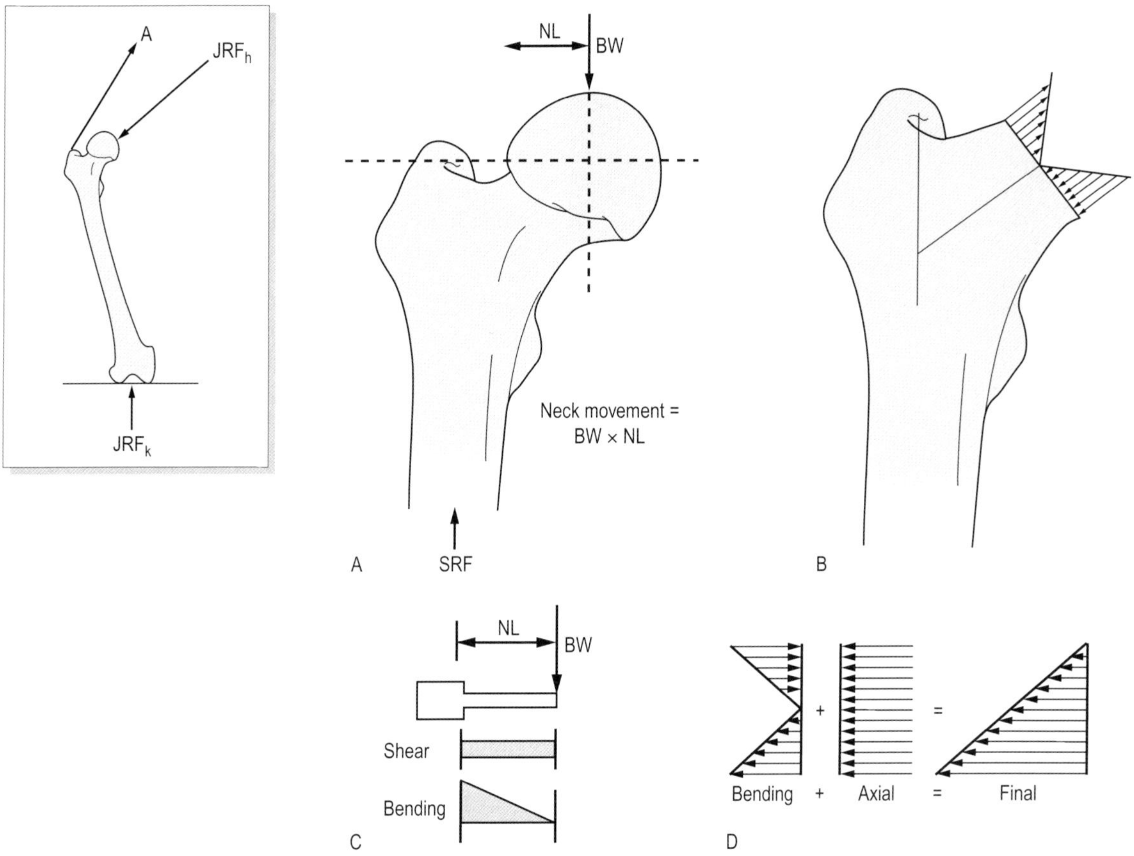

Fig. 9.12 Stress distribution in the human femur during single support. (A) Space diagram showing lines of action of body mass and shaft reaction; these two forces constitute a couple whose separation is NL (neck length), and generate stress as shown in (C). (B) Typical bending stress distribution generated from cantilevered conditions shown in (A). (D) Contraction of the abductors during single support (see inset) compresses the femoral neck. The addition of this stress to that also generated by bending yields the distribution shown here, with minimal tension at the top of the femoral neck and maximum compression at its bottom. Chimpanzees, which lack an effective abductor apparatus (and therefore display a Trendelenburg gait), apparently fail to generate sufficient neck compression to eliminate tension along the top of the femoral neck. This is consistent with collagen fiber orientation in humans and chimpanzees. A, abductor contraction force; BW, body weight; JRF_h, joint reaction force acting at hip; JRF_k, joint reaction force acting at knee; SRF, shaft reaction force. As (Reprinted from Gaitand Posture, V21(1):95-112, Lovejoy CO: 'The natural history of human gait and posture': Part 2 Hip and Thigh © Elsevier BV.)

of any included matrix. As a consequence, both CT and conventional radiography produce clear images of its internal structure (Fig. 9.13). There is a complete absence of cortical bone in the superolateral aspect of this specimen's neck, which serves as a marker of the presence of a human-like abductor apparatus.

The evolutionary basis of some modern pelvic deficiencies

The special histories of the human lumbar spine and pelvis have made them entirely unique among mammals, without any contemporary equivalents, and – importantly for clinical studies – without any potential animal models. The highly unusual and specialized human pelvis is certainly also subject to unique forms of pathology just as is our spine (see earlier). Most obvious is the excessive frequency of fracture of the femoral neck, with which there is pronounced morbidity.

This malady has an obvious evolutionary etiology. As humans age, the diversity of their physical activities declines precipitously and, other than simple everyday activities that involve limited load bearing, become largely restricted to walking. This has the effect of further increasing the femoral

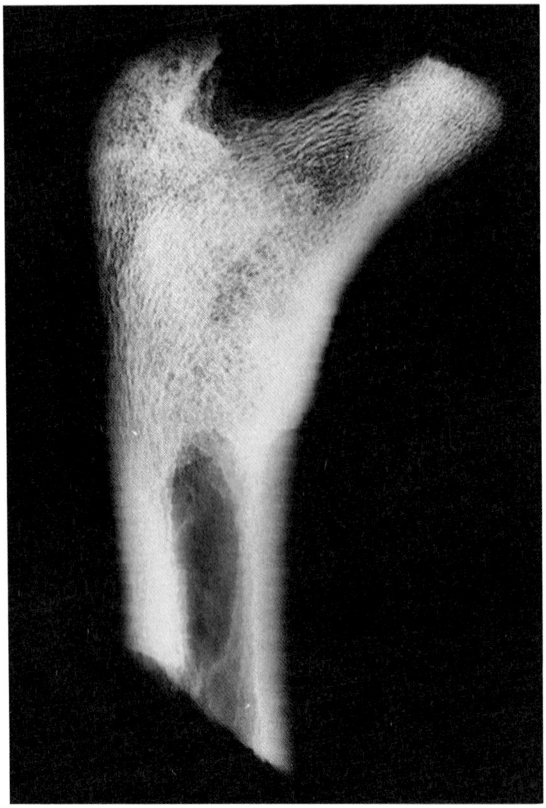

Fig. 9.13 Anteroposterior Faxitron (© Hewlett-Packard Corp.) X-ray of specimen MAK-VP-1/1 (the femoral head was lost before recovery of the specimen). There is no included matrix to hide trabecular structure and relationships. The specimen shows a virtual absence of superior neck trabeculae, typical of modern humans, and dramatic evidence of a highly evolved abductor apparatus. (Reproduced with permission from Lovejoy et al 2002.)

neck's stereotyped loading (restricting it only to stance phase), which can even further weaken, via osteoporosis, the already tenuous cortical bone in its superior portion. This is the conclusion of a recent extensive study of this problem, which the reader is encouraged to consult (Mayhew et al 2005).

Finally, another source of frequent pathology, and one central to the mission of this volume, is the special and unique structure of the human SIJ. Its structure also differs from that of apes, being substantially larger in area and form, but apparently not in histological structure and surface anatomy. These differences derive from its unique role in the human bipedality (Lovejoy & Latimer 1997, Lovejoy et al 1997). Its role in locomotion has become entirely unique for two reasons: the lordosis required for advantageous positioning of the HAT in humans, and the need for special forms of kinetic energy amelioration from heel strike to foot flat. Humans have no forelimb mechanisms to deal with the latter problem and have adapted to it in myriad ways (see Box 9.1, p. 144).

One of these revolves around the problem of trunk inertia and its control during the early phases of ground contact. Control of the HAT falls, *inter alia*, to eccentric contraction of the gluteus maximus (see earlier; Greenman 1990), which is among the factors that have caused it to become uniquely enlarged in hominids. Other related energy-dissipating devices are nutation and counternutation at the SIJ (Greenman 1990, and see Chapter 8), which passively stretch not only the joint's unusually extensive capsule, but other major ligaments, such as the sacrotuberous, as well (see Chapter 8). It is especially noteworthy that the human sacrotuberous ligament has undergone considerable hypertrophy compared to its counterpart in other primates. The SIJs role in human locomotion has become unique not only because we locomote only with our hindlimbs, but also because our thorax is entirely isolated from our pelvis by virtue of lumbar 're-elongation,' while at the same time lacking relatively strong erector spinae.

All of these factors have led directly to the special considerations and novel detailed adaptations within the human SIJ (see Chapter 8). There is no need to discuss these further here, as they are fully described in effective detail in Chapter 1 of this volume. The reader is therefore referred to that chapter for details of their various mechanical roles, which, like most of the traits described above, are entirely unique to humans by virtue of our exceptional evolutionary history (see also Chapter 8).

Summary

The human locomotor pattern is unique among both primates and mammals in general. It evolved early in human evolutionary history and is, at a minimum, four million years old. Our spine and pelvis differ radically in structure and function from those of even our closest relatives, the anthropoid apes, and the advanced degree of adaptation to bipedality in our ancient ancestors demonstrates that humans are well adapted to this unique form of locomotion. This being the case, it might at first seem odd that the special role of the hindlimb in human locomotion (*viz.* the requirement that it both propel the trunk as well as ameliorate ground reaction force at heel strike) continues to cause several common maladies that have not been eliminated by natural selection. These include: (1) idiopathic scoliosis, which is not observed in other primates – only in humans – and results from our unique combination of an elongated lumbar spine controlled by a minimally sized erector spinae; (2) spondylolysis (and spondylolisthesis), brought about by our uniquely elongated lumbar column and its attendant lordosis; (3) femoral neck fracture, which results from the failure of our stereotyped locomotor pattern to maintain sufficient cortex in the upper portion of the femoral neck; and (4) osteochondral pathology of the sacroiliac joint, a result of high loading induced by this joint's unique role of ameliorating ground reaction contact stress during upright ambulation, i.e. the effects of time and loading on excessive nutation and counternutation in this joint. The negative effects of each of these save the first is easily recognized as not normally occurring until after the average age at which reproduction ceases, and thus cannot be attributed to a lack of natural selection but only to recent advances in the human capacity to survive into prolonged adulthood.

Acknowledgements

I thank B Latimer, MA McCollum, R Meindl, SW Simpson, G Suwa, CV Ward and TD White for valuable discussions about the topics discussed here, MA McCollum for special help with illustrations, and L Spurlock for artwork. I also thank the Cleveland Museum of Natural History (Cleveland, Ohio), and the Royal Museum for Central Africa, Tervuren, Belgium for invaluable access to primate specimens, and curators L Jellema (CMNH) and W Wendelen (RMCA) for indispensable assistance.

References

Benton RS 1967 Morphological evidence for adaptations within the epaxial region of the primates. In: van der Hoeven F (ed) The baboon in medical research: volume II. University of Texas Press, Austin, TX, p201–216

Bramble DM, Lieberman DE 2004 Endurance running and the evolution of *Homo*. Nature 432:345–352

Brunet M, Guy F, Pilbeam D et al 2002 A new hominid from the upper miocene of Chad, Central Africa. Nature 418:145–151

Carey TS, Crompton RH 2005 The metabolic costs of 'bent-hip, bent-knee' walking in humans. J Hum Evol 48:25–44

Cartmill M, Milton K 1978 The lorisiform wrist joint and the evolution of 'brachiating' adaptations in the Hominoidea. Am J Phys Anthropol 47:249–272

Clark JD, Asfaw B, Assefa G et al 1984 Palaeoanthropological discoveries in the Middle Awash Valley, Ethiopia. Nature 307:423–428

Dart RA 1925 *Australopithecus africanus*: the man-ape of South Africa. Nature 115:195–199

Galik K, Senut B, Pickford M et al 2004 External and internal morphology of the BAR 1002'00 *Orrorin tugenensis* femur. Science 305:1450–1453

Gould SJ, Lewontin RC 1979 The spandrels of San Marco and the Panglossian paradigm: a critique of the adaptationist programme. Proc R Soc Lond (Biol) 205:147–164

Greenman PE 1990 Clinical aspects of sacroiliac function in walking. J Manual Med 6:354–359

Haile-Selassie Y, Asfaw B, White TD 2004 Hominid cranial remains from upper Pleistocene deposits at Aduma, Middle Awash, Ethiopia. Am J Phys Anthropol 123: 1–10

Hartman CG, Straus WL 1933 The anatomy of the rhesus monkey. Williams and Wilkins, Baltimore, MD

Hollinshead WH 1963 Functional anatomy of the limbs and back. WB Saunders, Philadelphia, PA

Johanson DC, Lovejoy CO, Kimbel WH et al 1982 Morphology of the Pliocene partial hominid skeleton (A.L. 288-1) from the Hadar formation, Ethiopia. Am J Phys Anthropol 57:403–452

Kalmey JK, Lovejoy CO 2002 Collagen fiber orientation in the femoral necks of apes and humans: do their histological structures reflect differences in locomotor loading? Bone 31:327–332

Kelley J 1997 Paleobiological and phylogenetic significance of life history in Miocene hominoids. In: Begun DR, Ward CV, Rose MD (eds) Function, phylogeny, and fossils: Miocene hominoid evolution and adaptations. Plenum Press, New York, p173–208

Latimer B, Ward CV 1993 The thoracic and lumbar vertebrae. In: Walker A, Leakey R (eds) The Nariokotome *Homo erectus* skeleton. Harvard University Press, Cambridge, MA, p266–293

Le Gros Clark WE 1955 The os innominatum of the recent pongidae with special reference to that of the Australopithecinae. Am J Phys Anthropol 13:19–27

Le Gros Clark WE 1978 The fossil evidence for human evolution. 3. University of Chicago Press, Chicago, IL

Lewis OJ 1974 The wrist articulations of the anthropoidea. In: Jenkins Jr FA (ed) Primate locomotion. Academic Press, New York, p143–170

Lovejoy CO 1974 The gait of australopithecines. Yearb Phys Anthropol 16:18–30

Lovejoy CO 1978 A biomechanical review of the locomotor diversity of early hominids. In: Jolly C (ed) Early hominids of Africa. Duckworth, London, p403–429

Lovejoy CO 1979 A reconstruction of the pelvis of A.L.-288-1 (Hadar Formation, Ethiopia). Am J Phys Anthropol 50:413

Lovejoy CO 1981 The origin of man. Science 211:341–350

Lovejoy CO 1988 Evolution of human walking. Sci Am 259:118–125

Lovejoy CO 2005a The natural history of human gait and posture. Part 1: spine and pelvis. Gait Posture 21:95–112

Lovejoy CO 2005b The natural history of human gait and posture. Part 2: hip and thigh. Gait Posture 21: 113–124

Lovejoy CO, Latimer B 1997 Evolutionary aspects of the human lumbosacral spine and their bearing on the function of the intervertebral and sacroiliac joints. In: Vleeming A et al (eds) Movement, stability, and low back pain: the essential role of the pelvis. Churchill Livingstone, London, p213–226

Lovejoy CO, Heiple KG, Burstein AH 1973 The gait of *Australopithecus*. Am J Phys Anthropol 38:757–780

Lovejoy CO, Meindl RS, Pryzbeck TR et al 1977 The palaeodemography of the Libben site, Ottowa County, Ohio. Science 198:291–293

Lovejoy CO, Meindl RS, Tague R, Latimer B 1997 The comparative senescent biology of the hominoid pelvis and its implications for the use of age-at-death indicators in the human skeleton. In: Paine RR (ed) Integrating archaeological demography: multidisciplinary approaches to prehistoric population. Southern Illinois University Press, Carbondale, IL

Lovejoy CO, Meindl RS, Ohman JC et al 2002 The Maka femur and its bearing on the antiquity of human walking: applying contemporary concepts of morphogenesis to the human fossil record. Am J Phys Anthropol 119: 97–133

Lovejoy CO, McCollum M, Reno PL, Rosenman BA 2003 Developmental biology and human evolution. Ann Rev Anthropol 32:85–109

MacLatchy L, Gebo D, Kityo R, Pilbeam D 2000 Postcranial functional morphology of *Morotopithecus bishopi*, with implications for the evolution of modern ape locomotion. J Hum Evol 39:159–183

Mayhew PM, Thomas CD, Clement JG et al 2005 Relation between age, femoral neck cortical stability, and hip fracture risk. Lancet 366:129–135

Moya-Sola S, Kohler M, Alba DM 2004 *Pierolapithecus catalaunicus*, a new middle Miocene great ape from Spain. Science 306:1339–1344

Nakatsukasa M, Ward CV, Walker A et al 2004 Tail loss in *Proconsul heseloni*. J Hum Evol 46:777–784

Ohman JC, Lovejoy CO, White TD 2005 Questions about Orrorin femur. Science 307:845

Pianka ER 1988 Evolutionary ecology (4th edn). Harper and Row, New York

Pickford M 2001 Discovery of earliest hominid remains. Science 291:986

Pilbeam D 2004 The anthropoid postcranial axial skeleton: comments on development, variation, and evolution. J Exp Zoo B Mol Dev Evol 302:241–267

Reno PL, McCollum MA, Lovejoy CO, Meindl RS 2000 Adaptationism and the anthropoid postcranium: selection does not govern the length of the radial neck. J Morphol 246:59–67

Robinson JT 1972 Early hominid posture and locomotion. University of Chicago Press, Chicago, IL

Rose J, Gamble JG 1994 Human walking. Williams & Wilkins, Baltimore, MD

Rosenman BA, Lovejoy CO, Spurlock LB 1999 A reconstruction of the STS-14 pelvis, and the obstetrics of *Australopithecus*. Am J Phys Anthropol 235:235

Rosenman BA, Lovejoy CO, McCollum MA 2002 Development of the vertebral column. In: Walker RA, Lovejoy CO, Bedford ME, Yee W (eds) Skeletal and developmental anatomy. FA Davis, Philadelphia, PA, p53–79

Rosenman BA, Heiple KF, Lovejoy CO 2004 Lumbar vertebral number in hominids and hominoids. J Morphol 260:323

Sanders WJ 1998 Comparative morphometric study of the australopithecine vertebral series Stw–H8/H41. J Hum Evol 34:249–302

Schultz AH 1930 The skeleton of the trunk and limbs of higher primates. Hum Biol 2:303–438

Schultz AH 1961 Vertebral column and thorax. Primatologia 5:1–66

Schultz AH, Straus WL 1945 The numbers of vertebrae in primates. Proc Natl Acad Sci 89:626

Sibley CJ, Ahlquist JE 1987 DNA hybridization evidence of hominoid phylogeny: Results from expanded data set. J Mol Evol 26:99–105

Stevens LS, Lovejoy CO 2004 Morphological variation in the hominoid vertebral column: Implications for the evolution of human locomotion. Am J Phys Anthropol 123:S38, 187–188

Walker A, Leakey RE 1993 The Nariokotome *Homo erectus* skeleton. Harvard University Press, Cambridge, MA

Ward CV, Walker A, Teaford MF, Odhiambo I 1993 Partial skeleton of *Proconsul nyanzae* from Mfangano Island, Kenya. Am J Phys Anthropol 90:77–112

Ward CV, Begun DR, Rose MD 1997 Function and phylogeny in Miocene hominoids. In: Begun DR, Ward CV, Rose MD (eds) Function, phylogeny, and fossils: Miocene hominoid evolution and adaptations. Plenum Press, New York, p1–12

Ward CV, Leakey MG, Walker A 2001 Morphology of *Australopithecus anamensis* from Kanapoi and Allia Bay, Kenya. J Hum Evol 41:255–368

White TD, Suwa G, Berhane A 1994 *Australopithecus ramidus*, a new species of early hominid from Aramis, Ethiopia. Nature 371:306–312

White TD, Suwa G, Asfaw B 1995 *Ardipithecus ramidus*, a new species of early hominid from Aramis, Ethiopia. Nature 375:88

Wood BA 1996 Human evolution. BioEssays 18:945–954

Young NM, MacLatchy L 2004 The phylogenetic position of *Morotopithecus*. J Hum Evol 46:163–184

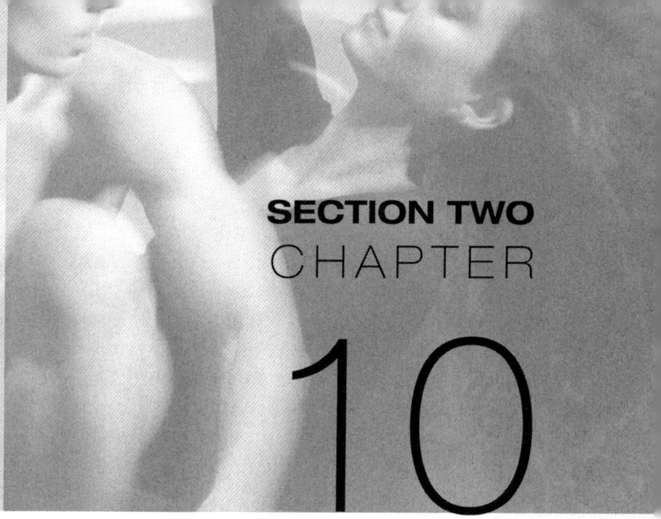

SECTION TWO
CHAPTER
10

Kinematic models and the human pelvis

A Huson

Introduction

This chapter deals with some kinematic concepts the author uses when modeling the human locomotor apparatus (Huson 1983, Huson et al 1989). Although most of our work focused on the lower extremity, and did not pay particular attention to the sacroiliac joint (SIJ), there is still a clear link with the approach and ideas of Vleeming's and Snijders' work (see Chapter 8).

In biomechanics, the human musculoskeletal system is often represented by a so-called multibody system comprising: (1) a number of rigid bodies (bones), which are connected to each other by (2) movable linkages (joints) and (3) force generators (muscles). This is, of course, an abstraction, a reduction of the complex reality. However, such an approach can enable us to unravel the complexity of particular mechanical relationships. An elegant example is Vleeming's and Snijders' explanation of the self-locking effect in the construction of the pelvis. Their model gives us an idea of the roles played by: (1) friction; (2) the position of contact surfaces between the bones; and (3) certain pelvic dimensions as parameters of pelvic shape in the functional task to keep the pelvic assembly together under a vertical static load.

The sacrum and the pelvic bones, connected to each other by the SIJ and the pubic symphysis, form what can be described as a closed kinematic chain. This chain contains only three links connected by three linkages. Had these linkages been simple hinges, the chain would have been in kinematic terms a rigid structure. However, due to the nature of the pelvis and its linkages, this is – in kinematic as well as in static terms – not the case, because the ring has a certain mobility or deformability instead. Many, if not all of the subsystems of the musculoskeletal system can be described as kinematic chains, either closed or open. Whereas the pelvis is structurally a closed chain, many of the other chains are open, and can be closed voluntarily. The general effect of such a closure leads to an increase of its kinematic constraints; in other words, it is a reduction of the chain's kinematic degrees of freedom of motion (DFOM). In more general terms, closure leads to a reduction of the chain's mobility, or to a gain in stability. Let us consider this effect in more detail.

Closed kinematic chains

Figure 10.1 shows a very simple model of the lower part of the human body, consisting of only the pelvis with the lower extremities and standing on a supporting base. In this case, the pelvis is conceived of as a single rigid piece. The pelvis, the thighs, the legs, and both feet, which are supposed to be firmly connected to the supporting floor by the combined effects of gravity and friction, form together a closed kinematic chain, containing six links. The linkages or joints in this model have been considerably simplified for modeling purposes. In this model, all the joints are reduced to simple hinge joints. For the time being, we assume that the muscles running in different directions around these joints are able to impose this reduction on the joints. Furthermore, in this model the feet are slightly abducted by exorotation of both legs at the hip joints. Notice that, in this position, only the knees are locked in full extension. The model can keep itself in an upright position while standing on a flat supporting surface without any external support. Moreover, it can keep its hips and ankles still in a midposition between full extension and flexion. Apparently, no muscles are needed to stabilize these joints other than those supposed to change the hips kinematically into hinges: another example of a self-locking effect. We have called this self-locking effect a muscle-saving principle because the chain can kinematically be stabilized with less muscular effort than would be expected from the total number of joints involved (Huson 1983). The next figures will explain this typical effect in more detail.

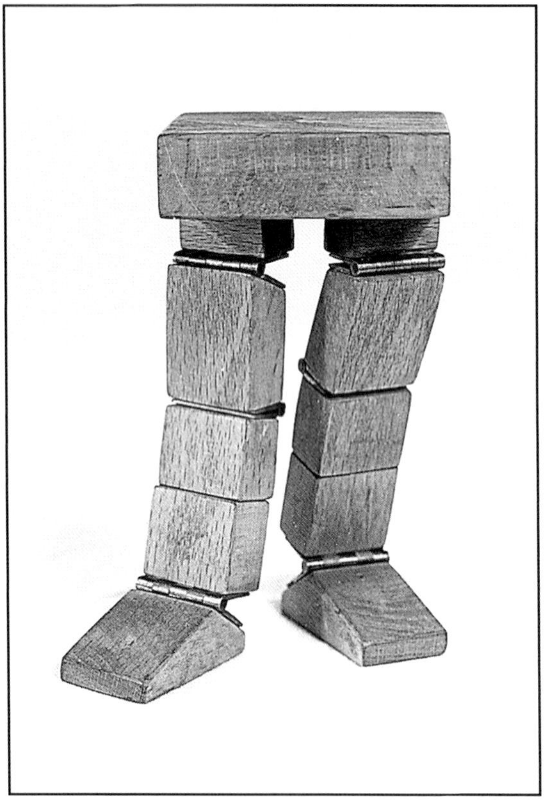

Fig. 10.1 A simple model of the lower part of the human body comprising the pelvis (the upper block as one of its six links), the thighs (two other links), the legs (again two links), and both feet (the feet, together with the floor, representing the sixth link). The purpose of the horizontal cleft dividing the legs into two parts will be clarified in Fig. 10.8. See text for further explanation.

Two-dimensional simple chains

Figure 10.2 shows an open kinematic chain comprising four links. It has one fixed or base link – indicated by the number 1 and recognizable by its hatching – and two arms – one of them containing two links (the right arm with the numbers 3 and 4)

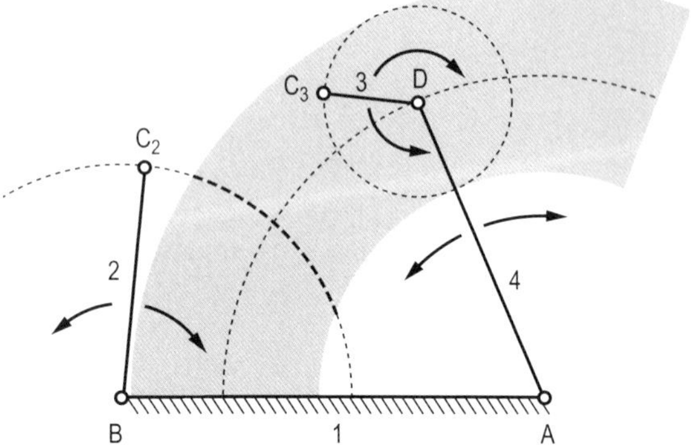

Fig. 10.2 A two-dimensional or planar four-bar chain. See text for further explanation.

and the other one having only one link (number 2 at the left-hand side). All of the linkages – A (between links 4 and 1), B (between links 2 and 1), and D (between links 3 and 4) – are simple hinges. Because their axes run parallel to each other and perpendicular to the plane of the drawing, this chain is called a two-dimensional or planar chain.

Its motions occur in a single plane or in a set of parallel planes, in which case the motions can be projected on a single plane. Point C_2 of the one-link arm can move along the circular path about B. Likewise, point D can move along a circular path with A as its center of rotation, whereas in the position of link 4, point C_3 can move along the circular path with D as its rotation center. However, as soon as link 4 is set free to rotate about A, point C_3 can move freely within the boundaries of the curved lightly shaded area. Consequently, links 2 and 4 have only one DFOM each, whereas link 3 has two.

After assembling the two arms by joining the points C_3 and C_2 into a new hinge, i.e. after closure of the chain, the kinematic conditions within the chain change dramatically. The newly formed hinge C can move only along the common circular path of both formerly open arms: the segment in bold of the circular path about B. Thus, link 3 has a limited freedom of one DFOM. It must be noted that in its closed configuration, the chain is provided with four hinges, one more than in its open condition. Together, they are good for four DFOM. Yet the actual kinematic freedom of all the links allows only one DFOM. This is because after closure both points C and D can move only along the circular paths about A and B in a particular combination, prescribed by the length of the connecting link 3. Apparently, three DFOM have disappeared after closure of the chain (see also the upper part of Fig. 10.4, below). Let us see what happens if we add one more link to the chain.

The upper part of Fig. 10.3 shows again an open chain, but in this case consisting of five links. This chain too has one fixed, or base link, number 1 (again recognizable by its hatching). However, in this chain both arms have two links each: numbers 2 and 3 at the left, and numbers 4 and 5 at the right. Consequently, both end links – 3 and 4 – can move with two DFOM within the boundaries of the two curved dark and lightly shaded areas.

As soon as the two arms are connected with each other by assembling D_3 and D_4 into a new hinge, the mobility of D in the now-closed chain is limited to the overlapping area only: the central non-shaded white area. This means that links 3 and 4 still have two DFOM each. However, in its closed configuration (the lower part of Fig. 10.3), the chain is provided with five hinges, representing in total five DFOM. Again, three DFOM have disappeared after closure of the chain. A similar reduction of three DFOM would occur if we added another link to the chain, resulting in a six-bar chain that has one link having three DFOM with respect to its reference link.

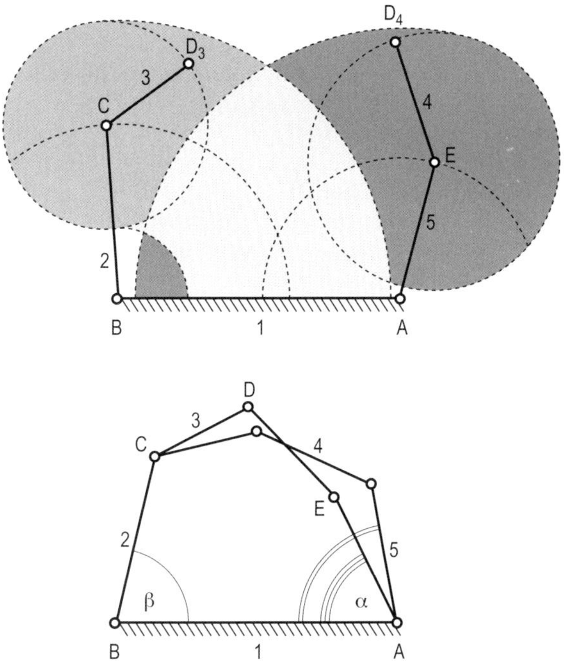

Fig. 10.3 The upper part shows a two-dimensional, five-bar chain in an open condition similar to the chain in Fig. 10.2. The lower part depicts a closed five-bar chain with two DFOM for point D. The position of the chain can be defined unequivocally by defining two variables, the angles α and β.

Compound closed chains

It is important to note that the four-bar chain, having only one DFOM, can be stabilized (immobilized) by stabilizing just one of its four hinges. However, if we add one more link to the chain, turning it into a five-bar chain, two joints have to be stabilized to immobilize all the other joints. As soon as we loosen one of these two stabilized joints, the chain has regained one DFOM, which means that, apart from the other as yet still immobilized joint, the other three joints can immediately move freely again.

Such an effect will also be seen under similar conditions if similar but longer chains are considered. The longer such a chain is, the more joints will be included in the increase of instability when one of its joints becomes disconnected or one of its links is broken. In other words, the muscle-saving principle suddenly loses its effect if the chain changes from the kinematic condition of zero DFOM to one or more DFOM.

If we consider the chain comprising the pelvis and both legs under the conditions of human walking, such sudden changes in its state of kinematic constraints occur physiologically at heel strike and toe-off. During each step cycle, the chain is alternately closed and opened twice, and as to be expected, it is exactly at these critical events that the main bursts of muscle activity occur (Morrenhof 1989).

Figure 10.4 shows two examples of a closed kinematic chain, the upper having only four links, the lower having six links, but now in two different configurations. The upper one is a simple-closed chain, like our four- and five-bar chains depicted in Figs 10.2 and 10.3. The lower chain, however, is a so-called compound-closed chain, having one link

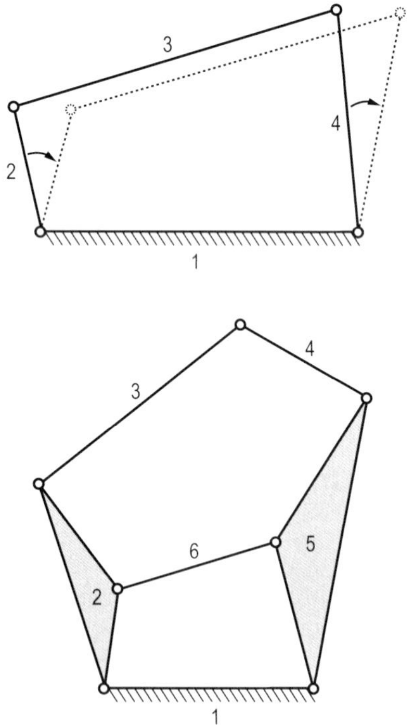

Fig. 10.4 Two different configurations of a closed, two-dimensional chain. The upper one has four links yielding one DFOM and is a simple chain. The lower one is a compound-closed chain and also has only one DFOM, even though it has seven linkages.

(number 6) as a cross-link between the two opposite triangular links 2 and 5. The simple chain has four hinges and its resulting kinematic freedom is one DFOM. This means a reduction, as we have seen, of three DFOM as a consequence of closure in a planar system. The compound chain, however, has seven hinges, yet a mobility of only one DFOM. It will move only according to a single prescribed and reproducible motion mode. Thus, reduction after closure in a compound configuration goes much further, as in this example apparently six DFOM have disappeared. Very long chains constructed as coupled compound configurations can produce even greater reductions.

Three-dimensional closed kinematic chains

In addition to the configuration characteristics such as compound closure, another boundary condition determines the extent to which the mobility of a particular kinematic chain will be reduced. If a simple closed chain is not a two-dimensional or planar chain, but a three-dimensional or spatial chain instead, closure of the chain in a simple configuration will produce a reduction of six DFOM, twice the reduction occurring after closure of a planar chain. In a spatial chain, hinge-like linkages have no parallel axes and these chains might even have ball and socket joints; in more general terms, they can have joints with more DFOM than simple hinges have. Their motions do not occur in single plane only but in space. Therefore they have to be described with respect to three orthogonal references axes. Figure 10.5 shows such a three-dimensional chain in two different positions.

In spatial configurations of closed kinematic chains, the reduction of its DFOM will also increase considerably when the chain has a compound configuration. Such three-dimensional, compound-closed kinematic chains occur in the complex skeletoligamentous system of the human body. A typical example is the carpal complex of the human wrist. Figure 10.6 shows a schematic representation of this complex. An estimation of the kinematic reduction incorporated in this system yields 20 to 30 DFOM, depending on certain assumptions concerning its kinematic features. This might illustrate why rupture of a single small ligament (e.g. an injury of the fibrous connection between lunatum and scaphoid, which is so hard to detect on a standard X-ray), or fracture of only one bone (e.g. the notorious scaphoid fracture), is

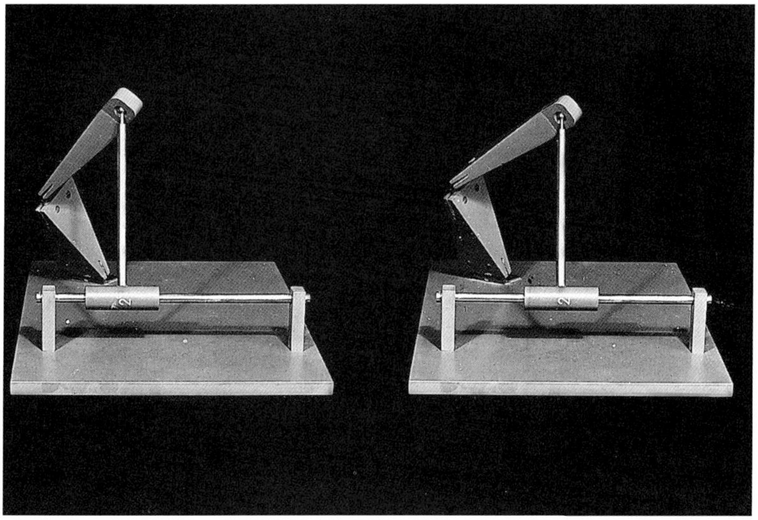

Fig. 10.5 Two different positions of a three-dimensional or spatial four-bar chain. The chain has only one DFOM, although its joints together represent seven DFOM: (2 × 1) + 3 + 2 = 7. The four joints comprise two hinges (the two lower joints of the long arm, visible in the background, each having one DFOM), one ball and socket joint (the upper joint of the long arm having three DFOM: three rotational modes), and one cylindrical joint (the joint in the foreground having two DFOM: one rotational and one translational mode).

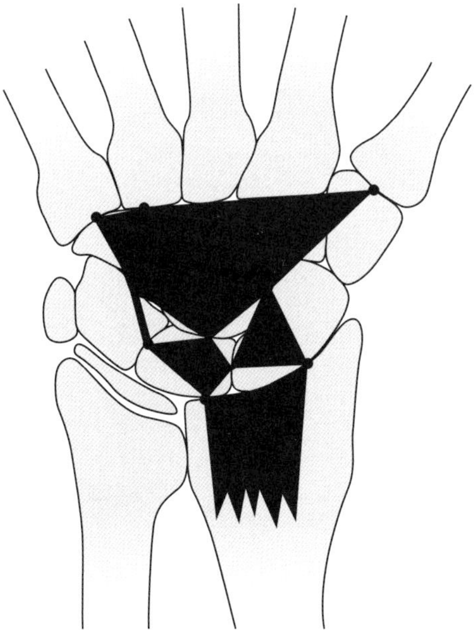

Fig. 10.6 Schematic representation of the carpus as a spatial, compound-closed kinematic chain. This example comprises only the following linkages: the radio-scaphoid joint, the radio-lunatum joint, the lunato-scaphoid joint, the lunato-triquetrum joint, the hamato-scaphoid joint, the hamato-lunatum joint, and the hamato-triquetrum joint.

such a fatal occurrence for the normal function of the carpal mechanism.

Tibial torsion: a kinematic constraint?

We will now return to the model consisting of pelvis, lower extremities, and floor because it demonstrates another interesting kinematic feature. Figure 10.7 shows a schematic representation of the model. The left-hand part of this figure illustrates that the model can be seen as an open box with six sides. These sides are connected to each other by a set of six hinges comprising two subsets of three parallel hinges. It is obvious that the upper side can move vertically up and down, simultaneously stretching or folding the sides of the box. Thus the upper lid of the box has one DFOM.

In the central figure, the box has been translated into our pelvis-with-lower-limbs model, showing similar kinematic features. According to the foregoing reasoning, this is a spatial, simple-closed kinematic chain with six hinges, and for this reason it should be subject to a reduction of six DFOM. Actually, this means that its kinematic condition should have yielded a mobility of zero DFOM: it should have been immobile! However, its actual kinematic condition produces, as we have seen from the example of the six-sided box, one DFOM. This

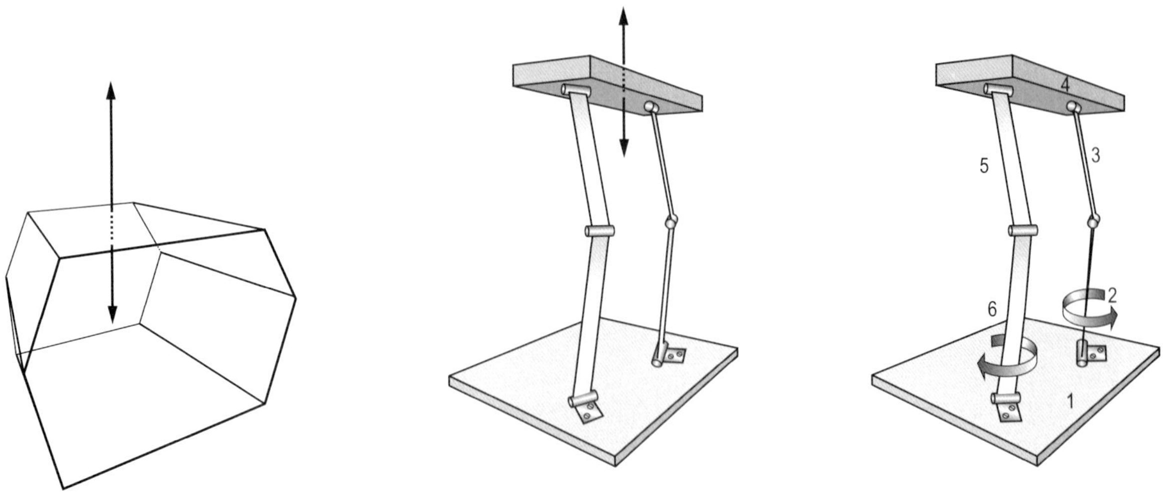

Fig. 10.7 Drawings of two different configurations of the model shown in Fig. 10.1 (central and right), together with their basic kinematic model (left).

is due to its particular kinematic feature of having two sets of three parallel hinge axes.

The figure at the right shows our pelvis-legs-and-feet model again, but in contrast to the central model this one is not able to move up and down: it does indeed have zero DFOM. The difference has to be sought in the torsion of the two bars that represent the lower legs. This torsion disturbs the parallel position of the hinge axes of knee and ankle. The chain has apparently acquired the kinematic features of a spatial chain, and this is sufficient to give a further reduction of the mobility of the closed chain. It is a well-established fact that tibial (external) torsion is a real anatomical characteristic of the human lower limb that develops during the first 10 years after birth (Lang & Wachsmuth 1972).

A physical representation of the model (Fig. 10.8) demonstrates this special kinematic effect. The model can stand upright (as did the model in Fig. 10.1) but now it is able to do so with flexed knees, while the hips and ankles are still in the midpositions of their motion ranges. Owing to the external torsion of the lower links (the tibial parts) of the legs, these joints apparently need no external stabilizing support to maintain their positions, like the situation demonstrated in Fig. 10.1. However, this configuration of the limbs and joints leads to another complication. To obtain full flat contact between the supporting surface and the feet, the model has to lean backwards. To prevent it from falling down backwards, the feet have to be fixed

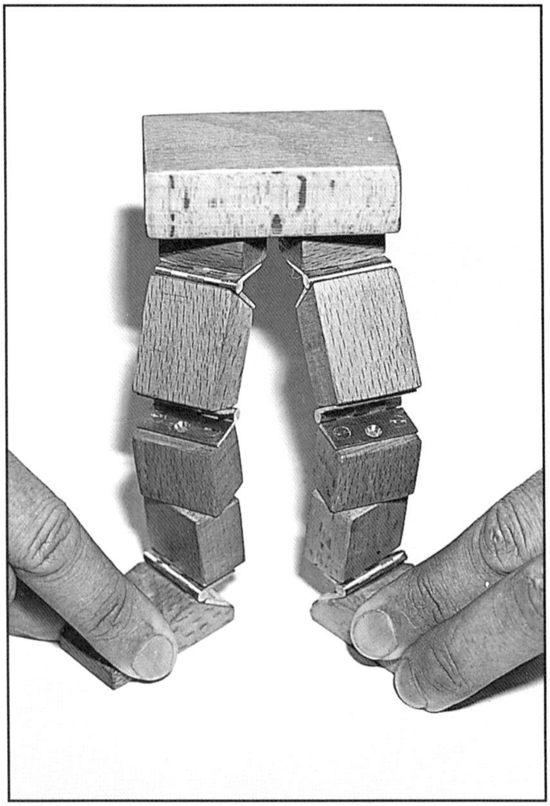

Fig. 10.8 The model from Fig. 10.7 in a physical representation.

to the floor, as can be seen in the figure. As soon as one hand is removed, the model collapses. Again, removing this external stabilization leads to the collapse of the model. Thus, under certain kinematic conditions, a particular anatomic feature, such as a tibial torsion, produces a kinematic boundary condition with a functional effect that concerns all the joints within the closed kinematic chain of pelvis and legs.

Apart from this contribution to 'self-locking', the tibial torsion has yet another functional effect. This effect became apparent in the backward-leaning posture of the model when both feet were placed in flat contact with the floor (Fig. 10.8). If we avoid this backward-leaning posture by holding the pelvic piece of the model vertically in line with its feet, the model assumes the posture shown in Fig. 10.9. In this figure, the model is brought into a vertical alignment of the pelvis and feet, while its knees are slightly abducted and flexed. In this position, however, the tibial torsion forces both feet into an everted, or pronated, position with respect to the floor. An additional abduction of the flexed knees to improve bilateral stabilization will further increase this effect. To bring the feet into firm contact with the ground, both feet must invert. Thus inversion seems to be an indispensable mechanism in the normal functional range of the lower extremities and not merely a useful capability of the foot to adapt its position to an uneven underground.

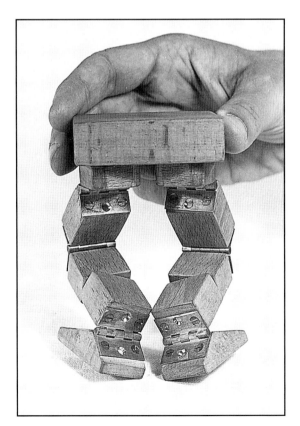

Fig. 10.9 The same model as in Fig. 10.8 from dorsal, but in this position the feet are everted. See text for further explanation.

A kinematic model for the tarsal motions

Inversion is effected by the tarsal mechanism of the foot, which again has the configuration of a spatial, closed kinematic chain with only one DFOM. As will be apparent from Fig. 10.10, which shows a kinematic model of the foot in two positions, inversion of the tarsus is a complex combination of different motions of the bones involved in the tarsal mechanism. When the foot is inverted by tilting over its lateral border, the accompanying adduction of the foot is blocked and has to be compensated for by an external rotation of the leg. The ankle mortice compels the talus into a similar and concurrent abduction, and the calcaneus follows this motion with a less extensive abduction and a slight inversion tilt. The abducting talar head forces the navicular together with the cuboid into an inversion added to the calcaneal inversion. Thus the forefoot supinates with respect to the hindfoot. This becomes visible as a heightening of the medial foot arch. In certain postures, as we saw in Fig. 10.9, inversion is an indispensable mechanism. Thus if the legs are used with flexed knees, the knee

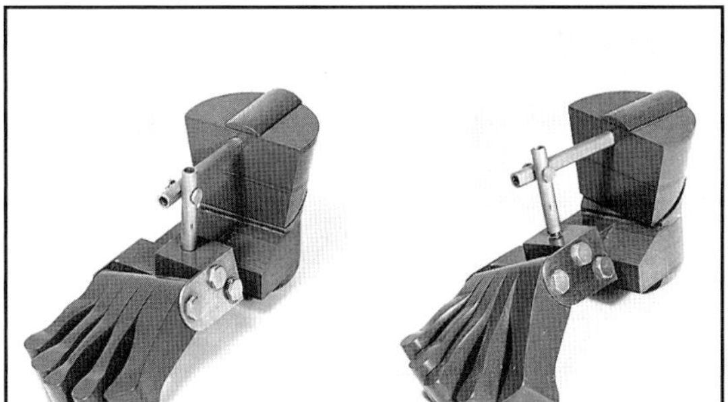

Fig. 10.10 A physical model of the foot comprising the tarsus and metatarsus. The tarsal part is represented as a spatial, closed kinematic, four-bar chain. At the left is the neutral position, at the right, the inversion position.

joints must provide for the possibility of meeting this requirement by allowing external and internal rotation in their flexed position to make the feet free for a compensating inversion (Huson 1991).

Final remarks and discussion

The examples shown all point to the fact that the human body comprises a great number of kinematic chains. Therefore, mobility and stability of the human body in terms of their kinematic DFOM is determined by the kinematic constraints of these chains. Such constraints can be imposed by muscles (active elements) and ligaments (passive elements). However, apart from these easily recognizable elements, there are, as we have seen, other determinants that are less self-evident. Such structural and/or configuration-dependent determinants are the:

- actual state of the chain: closed versus open
- composition of the chain: compound versus simple
- dimensionality of the chain: two- versus three-dimensional
- axial angularity, i.e. a special relationship between the axes of motion of the joints in the chain, such as parallelism or coaxiality.

So far, we have dealt only with the kinematic approach to modeling; forces have not been taken into consideration. A more complete picture of the conditions that determine mobility and stability requires a more comprehensive model, including the acting forces (see Chapter 8). Such a more comprehensive approach enables us to observe within the locomotor system mechanical effects acting at a distance in a musculoskeletal system, such as we have seen in our kinematic models (Bobbert & Van Ingen Schenau 1988). The ideas presented by Vleeming, Stoeckart and Snijders concerning the force streams and their anatomical findings give clear support to this point.

Summary

1. Changes in the kinematic condition of a particular closed articular chain in the human body have immediate effects on the kinematics of other joints.
2. These effects can be observed even at a great distance, thus affecting the kinematic behavior of the whole chain.
3. The model predicts that reduction of the stability of the SIJ (loosening of the joint) must lead to instability of other joints.
4. This is especially relevant since it is difficult to stabilize the loosened SIJ effectively and directly with the help of local muscles.

References

Bobbert MF, Van Ingen Schenau GJ 1988 Co-ordination in vertical jumping. Journal of Biomechanics 21:249–262

Huson A 1983 Morphology and technology. Acta Morphologica Neerlando-Scandinavica 21:69–81

Huson A 1991 Functional anatomy of the foot. In: Jahss MJ (ed) Disorders of the foot. Medical and surgical management, 2nd edn, vol. I, part II. WB Saunders, Philadelphia, pp 409–431

Huson A, Spoor CW, Verbout AJ 1989 A model of the human knee, derived from kinematic principles and its relevance for endoprosthesis design. Acta Morphologica Neerlando-Scandinavica 27:45–62

Lang J, Wachsmuth W 1972 Praktische Anatomie, vol. I, part IV. Springer, Berlin, p282

Morrenhof JW 1989 Stabilisation of the human hip-joint. A kinematical study. PhD thesis, Medical Faculty, University of Leiden, the Netherlands

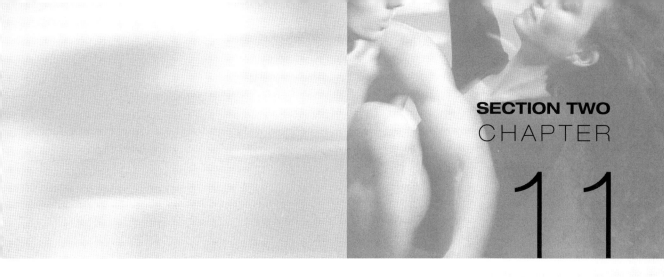

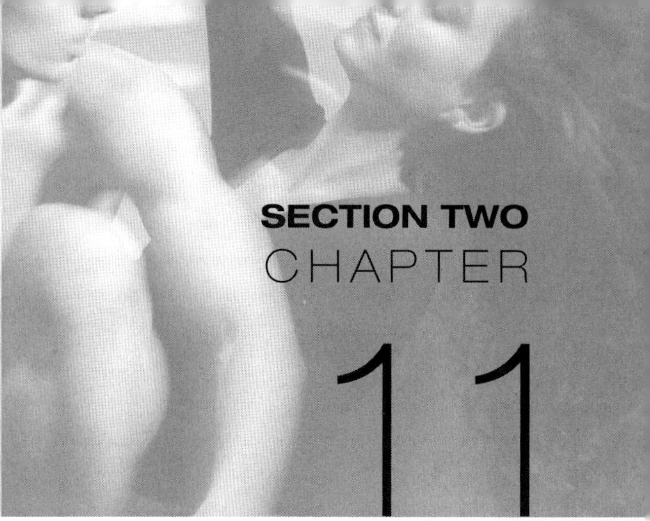

SECTION TWO
CHAPTER
11

How to use the spine, pelvis, and legs effectively in lifting

Michael A Adams and Patricia Dolan

Introduction

Recent advances in our understanding of back pain have shown that spinal pathology arises from interactions between genetic and environmental influences, and that subsequent pain and disability are strongly influenced by individual psycho-social factors, including personality. The detailed evidence, which has been reviewed in our recent book (Adams et al 2006) and in a review paper of the same name (Adams 2004), shows that a simple mechanistic or 'injury' model of back pain is no longer tenable. However, this does not mean that environmental considerations such as lifting technique are no longer important. On the contrary, it implies that lifting technique is even more important for some individuals than others, and the only practicable way of helping vulnerable individuals to protect their backs is to advise everyone involved in manual handling how to protect their backs. Consequently, the topic of how to lift weights properly is as important now as it ever was.

Poor manual handling technique is an important risk factor for back pain

Epidemiological and ergonomic studies confirm that workplace activities that load the spine severely are closely associated with back pain in general (Marras et al 1993), and with acute disc prolapse in particular (Kelsey et al 1984). It is therefore important to try to identify the 'best' way to lift – to indicate which technique or techniques minimize loading of vulnerable tissues in the spine. Some biomechanical analyses concentrate on one aspect of the problem, such as the shear force acting on the lumbar spine (Potvin et al 1991), or the activity of the back muscles (Dolan & Adams 1993), or leg muscles (Trafimow et al 1993). However, lifting is performed by the whole body and many structures can give rise to back pain including the intervertebral discs (Kuslich et al 1991, Schwarzer et al 1995b), apophyseal joints (Schwarzer et al 1995c), and sacroiliac joint (SIJ; Muche et al 2003, Schwarzer et al 1995a). Recommendations on how to lift must not disregard any one structure in favor of the others.

Lift with a straight back!

The need to include many anatomical structures makes the problem of lifting appear very complicated. A possible solution would be to construct a detailed mathematical model to cope with all of the complexity and then to choose some 'optimizing principle' (such as minimizing the shear or compressive force acting on L5–S1) to solve the equations and 'discover' the best way of lifting. Unfortunately, this approach requires many assumptions and approximations that would then be questioned if the final 'solution' offended common sense or preconceived opinion. A simpler and more humble approach is to assess the validity of advice on lifting that has stood the test of time. The most widespread and enduring advice is to 'lift with a straight back,' and there is evidence from photographs (Fig. 11.1) and radiographs (Cholewicki & McGill 1992) that many experienced weightlifters do exactly this. Consequently, a major theme of this chapter is to examine the implications of lifting with a straight back for all of the major structures involved in lifting, including the lumbar spine, pelvis, and legs.

Preview of this chapter

The section 'Mechanics of lifting' explains why heavy lifting can lead to high compressive and bending forces acting on the lumbar spine. It also suggests why it would be useful to try to employ the lumbodorsal fascia to assist in lifting. The 'Benefits of lifting with a straight back' are then explained in terms of load sharing between and within various spinal structures. This is followed by a discussion of how a straight back can facilitate the action of back muscles. The next two sections – 'Role of the lumbodorsal fascia in lifting' and 'Role

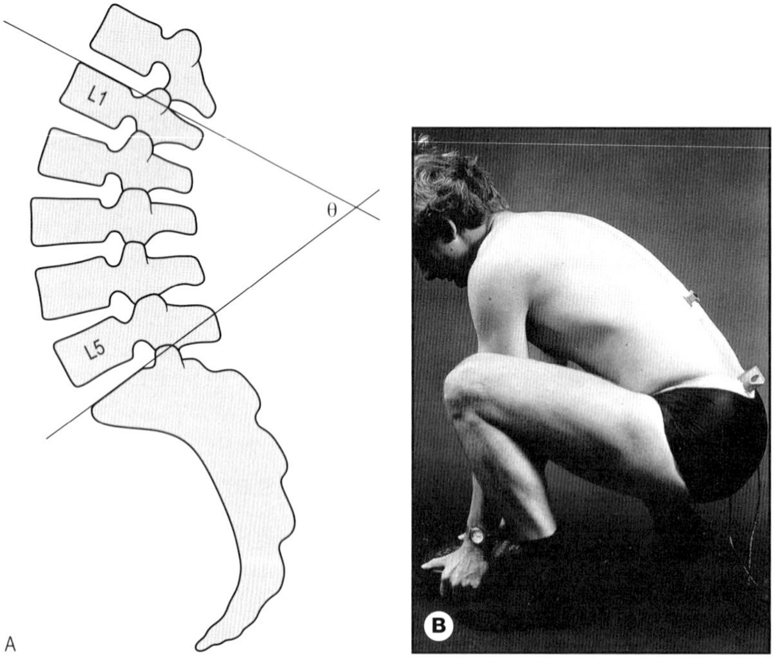

Fig. 11.1 (A) The curvature of a cadaver lumbar spine can be designated by the angle (θ) as defined in the figure. This curvature is increased in 'lordotic' postures such as standing erect, and reduced in 'straight back' (flexed) postures. (B) The lumbar and lower thoracic spine are approximately straight when objects are lifted from the ground.

of the legs in lifting' – widen the discussion of lifting to include these vital structures. Particular dangers associated with 'Twisting while lifting' and 'Time-dependent influences during lifting' are then considered. A note of realism is introduced by considering how both expert and novice lifters actually prefer to lift weights from the ground, and the practice of the experts is seen to be consistent with theoretical considerations. The final 'Discussion' and 'Conclusions' sections pull the evidence together in order to explain how to use the spine, pelvis, and legs effectively during lifting.

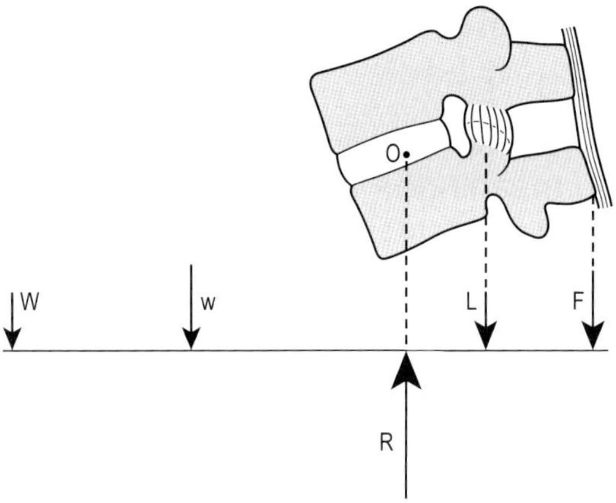

Fig. 11.2 During lifting, the spine pivots about a center of rotation (O) near the middle of each intervertebral disc. The forward bending moment arising from the weight lifted (W) and from upper body weight (w) must be balanced by the extensor moment generated by tensile structures lying posterior to O. Only two of these are shown: the lumbodorsal fascia (F) and the ligaments of the apophyseal joints (L). The ligaments act on a shorter lever arm than the fascia and so must exert a higher compressive 'penalty' on the disc. The lumbar back muscles lie between L and F. The resultant compressive force acting on the spine (R) is the sum total of these tensile and compressive forces.

Mechanics of lifting

Back muscles must generate high forces during weight lifting

During lifting movements, the upper body pivots about centers of rotation, which lie in the nucleus pulposus of each intervertebral disc (Pearcy & Bogduk 1988). Tensile forces in structures lying posterior to each pivot must generate an 'extensor moment' (a moment is a force multiplied by a distance) that opposes the 'flexor moment' due to the weight of the upper body and the object being lifted. Because the back muscles act on shorter lever arms than these weights, the forces generated by them must be correspondingly larger. During a very slow or static lift, when accelerating ('inertial') forces can be discounted, the extensor and flexor moments must balance (see Fig. 11.2). The influence of accelerations will be considered later.

Lifting is best done by muscles and fascia that act on big lever arms

The required extensor moment can be generated by tension in many structures, including the posterior annulus fibrosus, the ligaments of the neural arch, the erector spinae muscles, and the lumbodorsal fascia. As the extensor moment generated by each structure is equal to the tensile force acting in it multiplied by the lever arm between that structure and the center of rotation in the disc, it is apparent that some structures are better placed than others to assist in lifting: those that lie furthest from the pivot can generate a high extensor moment with only a small tensile force. This is advantageous, because these tensile forces all act to pull the vertebrae closer together and so compress the intervertebral disc. In general, the greater the lever arm, the greater the extensor moment for the same compressive 'penalty' on the disc (Fig. 11.2).

Stretching ligaments and fascia during lifting can save energy

Tension in elastic tissues such as ligaments and fascia can reduce the metabolic cost of lifting because 'strain energy' stored during forward bending can be recovered later when straightening up. The strain energy stored in each tissue is equal to the area under its force–deformation curve, and so is approximately proportional to the maximum stretching of the structure multiplied by the maximum tension acting in it. The lumbodorsal fascia is both strong and extensible and so has the capacity to store a great deal of strain energy. Grazing animals make great use of stored strain energy when lifting their head and neck from the ground, and humans involved in repetitive lifting do likewise.

The benefits of lifting with a straight back

Lumbar curvature is a convenient and meaningful way of quantifying spinal 'posture'

Lumbar curvature, as defined in Fig. 11.1A, is a convenient and meaningful measure of posture because it affects load sharing between various structures of the spine. First, it determines the relative orientation of adjacent lumbar vertebral bodies, and thereby affects the distribution of stress acting in the intervertebral discs. Second, it influences the distribution of compressive loading between the discs and the neural arch. Third, lumbar curvature affects tension in the intervertebral ligaments, particularly those of the neural arch.

As discussed in the Introduction, it has long been recognized that heavy weights should be lifted with a straight back, but what does a 'straight back' actually mean? The shape of the back during erect standing actually increases the spine's curves, rather than reduces them (Adams et al 1988), and standing upright involves considerable lumbar lordosis. Conversely, a fully flexed toe-touching posture reverses the lumbar curvature into a kyphosis. In between these extremes, a straight back can be achieved by moderate lumbar flexion combined with some thoracic extension, in order to flatten the curves naturally present in an unloaded cadaver spine (Adams & Dolan 1991, Dolan et al 1994a). As far as the lumbar spine is concerned, it is useful to contrast 'straight back' postures, which flatten the lumbar lordosis, and 'lordotic' (or 'erect') postures, which preserve or exaggerate it.

A straight back leads to even stress distributions within the intervertebral discs

The height of intervertebral discs (6–12 mm) is small compared to their anteroposterior diameter (30–45 mm), so small angulations of adjacent vertebral bodies in the sagittal plane greatly deform the annulus fibrosus in the vertical direction. For example, flexion of 10–12° can stretch the posterior annulus by 50% or more and compress the anterior annulus by approximately 30% (Adams & Hutton 1982). It is not surprising, therefore, that lumbar curvature has a profound effect on stress distributions within the disc. For example,

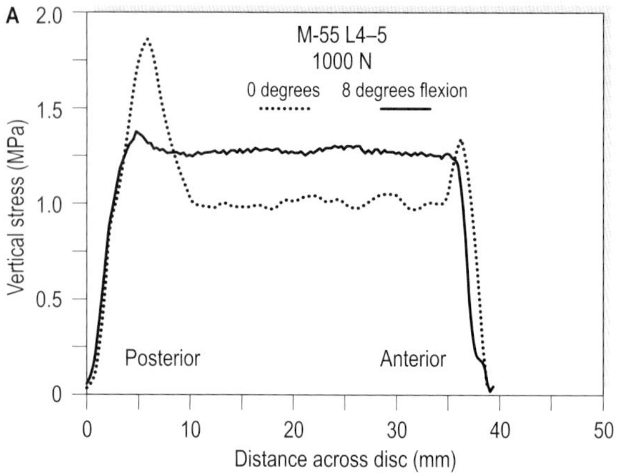

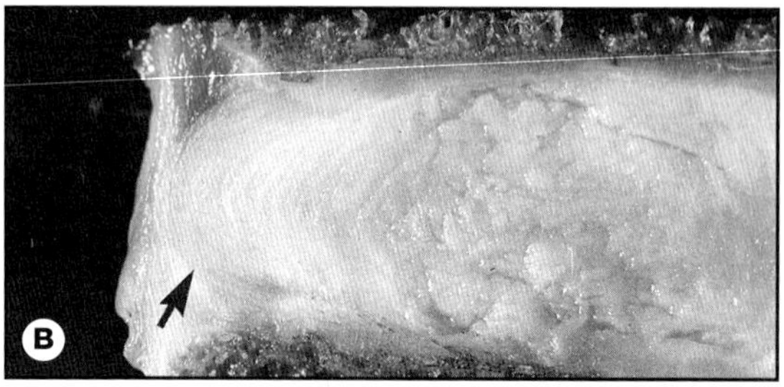

Fig. 11.3 (A) The distribution of vertical compressive stress across the midsagittal diameter of a typical L4–L5 intervertebral disc loaded with a compressive force of 1000 N (male, 55 years old, posterior on left). Lordotic postures ('0 deg.') are characterized by a stress peak in the posterior annulus. Moderate flexion removes this peak, but increases slightly the pressure in the nucleus pulposus. (B) A disc of similar age cut through in the midsagittal plane after sustained loading in simulated lordotic posture. (The anterior annulus is missing from this close-up.) Note the bulging of the lamellae in the posterior annulus (arrowed).

lordotic postures create concentrations of vertical compressive stress within the posterior annulus (Fig. 11.3), particularly following sustained 'creep' loading or following damage to an adjacent vertebra (Adams et al 2000b). Repetitive loading in lordotic posture can cause 'hairpin bend' deformations of lamellae within the posterior annulus, leading to posterior bulging of the disc (Adams et al 1988). Moderate flexion of lumbar motion segments brings the endplates approximately parallel, and equalizes compressive stress across the whole disc (Adams et al 1988), as shown in Fig. 11.3. Flexion right up to the elastic limit of the intervertebral ligaments can generate concentrations of compressive stress in the anterior annulus (Adams et al 1994b, McNally & Adams 1992) but these are rarely as high as similar concentrations in the posterior annulus and are unlikely to have significant adverse effects on what is the strongest and thickest region of most lumbar discs.

Spinal flexion and extension also influence tensile stresses within intervertebral discs. The outer posterior annulus resists flexion rather like a ligament (Adams et al 1994a) but its proximity to the center of rotation means that it generates only a small extensor moment and applies a very high compressive penalty to the rest of the disc. When stretched vertically, the posterior annulus fails at a stress of 9 MPa and a strain of 34% (Green et al 1993). The small resting length of the posterior annulus means that total stretch at failure is less than 3 mm, so there is little potential for energy storage. Even this potential will not normally be realized, because the intervertebral ligaments prevent the posterior annulus from being stretched to its elastic limit (Adams et al 1994a). In any case, the discs are not well suited to store energy because they are avascular, and therefore unable to dissipate that proportion of the stored energy which is lost as heat (hysteresis energy). Thermal damage to collagen and to cells might well be a problem in large, poorly vascularized skeletal tissues (Wilson & Goodship 1994). Flexion close to or beyond the normal physiological limit stretches and thins the posterior annulus to such an extent that the disc can prolapse posteriorly if it is subjected to a high compressive force at the same time (Adams & Hutton 1982, 1985). Posterior disc prolapse can occur even if the flexion angle is not extreme (Fig. 11.4), provided that the compressive force exceeds physiological limits (Adams et al 2000a). For these reasons, high tensile forces in the outer posterior annulus in full flexion do little to assist in the mechanics of lifting, and they could lead to thermal or physical damage to the tissue. Evidently, full lumbar flexion should be avoided during heavy lifting.

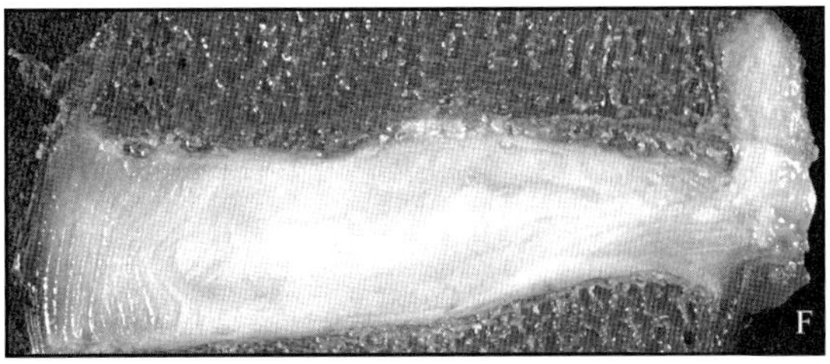

Fig. 11.4 Disc prolapse produced in a cadaveric specimen by high loading in compression and bending (male specimen, aged 40, L2–L3). In this case, the compressive force when prolapse occurred (9.8 kN) was supraphysiological, but the flexion angle (6°) was not. (Reproduced from Adams et al 2006, with permission of Churchill Livingstone, Edinburgh.)

A straight back unloads the apophyseal joints

Lordotic postures generate high contact stresses in the lower margins of the apophyseal joints and can cause extra-articular impingement of the inferior articular processes on the lamina below, especially following sustained loading and in elderly people with narrowed discs (Dunlop et al 1984, Pollintine et al 2004b). This reduces slightly the compressive stresses within the disc, especially in the nucleus pulposus (Adams et al 1994b). Only a few degrees of flexion are required to relieve the apophyseal joints of all axial loading (Adams & Hutton 1980, Pollintine et al 2004b) as shown in Fig. 11.5B.

A straight back stretches some intervertebral ligaments

Lumbar flexion generates tensile forces in the ligaments of the neural arch (Adams et al 1994b) and ligament tension increases the pressure in the center of the disc (Adams et al 1994b), as shown in Fig. 11.5A. Most intervertebral ligaments act on shorter lever arms than the back muscles (see Fig. 11.2), so the maximum extensor moment they can generate in full flexion is typically only 35 Nm, even though the combined tensile force in the ligaments may exceed 1–2 kN (Adams & Dolan 1991, Adams et al 1980). Evidently their modest ability to generate extensor moment is associated with a high compressive penalty on the discs, as discussed above. Furthermore, intervertebral ligaments are stretched by only 2–8 mm at the elastic limit (Adams et al 1980) so they are not important energy stores during lifting. Their main function appears to be to protect the disc from excessive bending (Adams et al 1994a) rather than to assist the back muscles during lifting.

A straight back has a high compressive strength

The compressive strength of motion segments positioned in moderate flexion appears to be particularly high (Hutton & Adams 1982), whereas more substantial flexion, to approximately 75% of the full range allowed by the intervertebral ligaments, causes motion segment strength to be similar to that found in lordosis (Adams et al 1994b). Evidently, the beneficial effect of an even stress

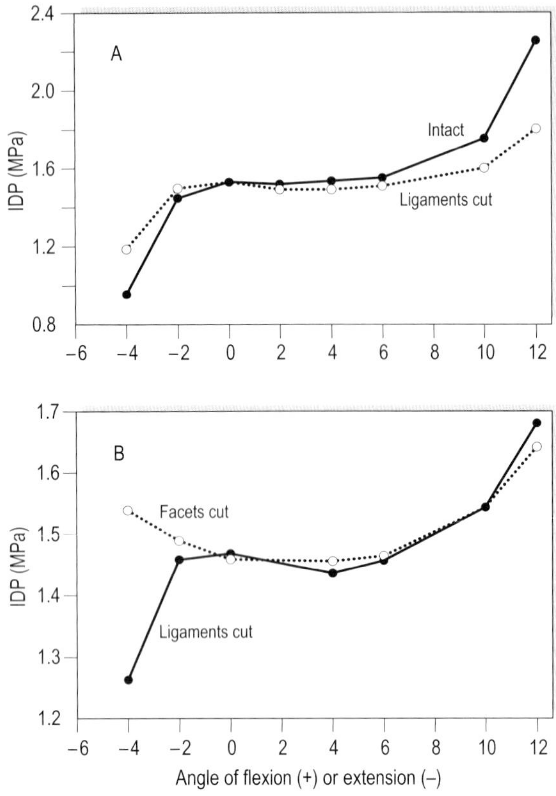

Fig. 11.5 Intradiscal pressure (IDP) measured in a cadaveric motion segment varies with the angle of flexion or extension, even though the applied compressive force is constant (2 kN). (A) Cutting the ligaments of the neural arch reduces IDP in flexion by removing ligament prestress. (B) Removing the bony surfaces of the apophyseal (facet) joints increases IDP in extension because the facets no longer resist part of the compressive force. (Reproduced with permission from Adams et al 2006.)

distribution in the disc in flexion is offset by a slight overall increase in magnitude and by the loss of any contribution from the neural arch to compressive load-bearing. Fully flexed or hyperflexed specimens appear to be weaker in compression (Adams & Hutton 1982, Granhed et al 1989), presumably because of the extra forces exerted on the disc by stretched ligaments (see Fig. 11.5A) and because the posterior annulus is stretched and thinned (Adams & Hutton 1982). In old and degenerated spines, intervertebral disc narrowing usually leads to the neural arch 'stress-shielding' the anterior regions of the vertebral body (Pollintine et al 2004a) so that this region of the vertebra becomes particularly weak and vulnerable to compressive failure when the spine is flexed. These results suggest that elderly people in particular should avoid fully flexing their thoracolumbar spine when lifting.

The evidence in this section indicates that the lumbar spine is best able to distribute high compressive loading when positioned in the moderately flexed ('flat back') posture. Lordotic postures generate stress concentrations in the posterior annulus and apophyseal joints, whereas full flexion increases the risk of injury to the discs, ligaments and vertebral bodies.

Action of the trunk muscles during lifting

Muscle lever arms and the influence of lumbar curvature

The center of the lumbar back extensor muscles lies approximately 6–8 cm posterior to the center of the discs (McGill & Norman 1987, McGill et al 1988), so they are better positioned to generate extensor moments than the intervertebral ligaments, which lie on smaller lever arms (Adams et al 1980). Some of this moment generation comes from stretching of noncontractile collagenous tissue within the muscle. Muscles of the thoracic spine are even better positioned because they are connected to the sacrum by a long tendon lying approximately 8.5 cm posterior to the center of the lumbar discs (McGill et al 1988). In full flexion, collagen fiber reorientation allows the back muscles to be stretched by 15–59% (Macintosh et al 1993). Note, however, that this stretching is measured relative to the upright standing position, in which the lumbar spine is slightly extended (Adams et al 1988) and the muscles correspondingly shortened relative to their resting position. The considerable strength of non-contractile tissues within the back muscles, combined with their great length and ability to be stretched, means that their energy storage capacity is high.

It has been suggested that lumbar flexion decreases the lever arms of the back muscles (Tveit et al 1994) but this could be an artifact of muscles being squashed when subjects try to adopt a flexed posture inside the confines of an MRI scanner. Certainly, this finding receives little support from a more comprehensive study performed on subjects in more natural but fully flexed postures (Bogduk et al 1992, Macintosh et al 1993). Full flexion reverses the forward shear force that the back muscles normally exert on the L5 vertebra (Macintosh et al 1993).

Stretched muscles can generate higher forces

Active force generation in muscle is generally highest at muscle lengths between 100 and 110% of resting length, because of optimal overlap between actin and myosin. Muscles that are stretched more than this can resist additional tensile forces because of tension in their collagenous tissues (fascia, epimysium, perimysium, and endomysium), which form a strong passive linkage between tendons. Fibers of the perimysium and endomysium generally run at an oblique angle to the muscle axis, and this angle diminishes when the muscle is stretched (Purslow 1989). Post-mortem rectus abdominis muscle can withstand tensile stresses of approximately 14 N/cm^2 once rigor mortis subsides (Katake 1961) so the typical 40 cm^2 cross-sectional area of the lumbar extensor muscles (McGill et al 1988) suggests that they, and their tendons, can withstand tensile forces of up to 560 N while remaining electrically inactive. This could be an underestimate, because different muscles have different proportions of collagenous fibers within them, and the back muscles might be expected to have a particularly high collagen content, and hence passive strength.

Antagonistic contraction of the back and abdominal muscles varies with posture

During manual handling tasks, back muscle activity is often accompanied by antagonistic contraction of the abdominal muscles which increases the stability of the trunk in general (Stokes et al 2000, van Dieen et al 2003) and the sacroiliac joints in particular (Richardson et al 2002). In flexed postures, where the spine is stabilized by tension in stretched passive tissues such as the lumbodorsal fascia and erector spinae aponeurosis, the need for stabilizing activity is small. Previous studies suggest that, in such circumstances, levels of abdominal muscle activity remain below 4% of those associated with a maximum voluntary contraction (Lavender et al 1994), and the associated increases in spinal compression are probably no more than 5–15% (Kingma et al 2001, Mannion et al 2000). When manual handling tasks are performed in upright or semi-upright postures, the level of cocontraction increases considerably, especially when the trunk is twisted, and this can increase spinal compression by as much as 45% (Granata & Marras 1995). The requirement for stabilizing muscle activity is also affected by preparedness and there is evidence that expectation of a loading event can cause co-activation of certain muscles in advance of the application of load (Hodges & Richardson 1997, Mannion et al 2000).

Role of the lumbodorsal fascia in lifting

The lumbodorsal fascia is very strong

The lumbodorsal fascia consists of several broad collagenous sheets, the strongest and most posterior of which overlies the erector spinae muscles (Vleeming et al 1995). Its precise mechanical function is disputed, but its strength is undeniable. Experiments on small tissue samples indicate that the posterior layer alone can resist 335 N in the caudocephalad direction (Tesh et al 1987). This probably underestimates its strength *in situ*, because the act of cutting out a small sample of tissue disrupts the collagen network and reduces tissue strength: experiments on small samples of annulus fibrosus suggest that they have only 44% of their strength in an intact disc (Adams & Green 1993). In effect, collagen fibers behave like the chopped fibers in fiberglass, in that their ability to reinforce the surrounding matrix is proportional to their length. If these results can be applied to the lumbodorsal fascia, then the posterior layer alone could resist a longitudinal force of 760 N. This figure does not include those fibers of the supraspinous ligament, which span more than one spinous process. Much of the supraspinous ligament passes from the upper lumbar spine to the sacrum with only loose attachments to the lower lumbar spinous processes, and it is barely distinguishable from the midline thickening of the lumbodorsal fascia. The 'untethered' portion might explain the apparent difference in strength of the 'supraspinous ligament' in motion segments from the lower and upper lumbar levels: this difference is approximately 450 N in old cadavers (Myklebust et al 1988), suggesting that the untethered portion of the supraspinous ligament might be at least this strong. In young individuals, it might be even stronger. Its mechanical role will be similar to that of the fascia, and their combined strength probably exceeds 1 kN.

The lumbodorsal fascia can generate large extensor moments with the lowest compressive penalty because it lies approximately 9 cm posterior to the center of the intervertebral discs (Tracy et al 1989). The maximum stretching of the lumbodorsal fascia in full flexion is approximately 30%, or

15 cm. If the fascia and supraspinous ligament do indeed have a combined strength of over 1 kN as suggested above, then it has the potential to store large amounts of strain energy.

Tension in the lumbodorsal fascia depends on lumbopelvic posture

Can flexing the lumbar spine generate substantial antiflexion forces in the passive tissues posterior to the spine? In an attempt to answer this question, we developed a technique for estimating the size of the antiflexion moment generated by passive (i.e. electrically silent) tissues in living people (Dolan et al 1994b). Healthy subjects adopted a stooped posture and pulled up with increasing force on a load cell attached to the ground (Fig. 11.6, upper). The lever arms shown in Fig. 11.6 were measured and the total antiflexion (extensor) moment was calculated from the load cell data and from the position of the upper body. Extensor moment was plotted against electromyographic (EMG) activity in the erector spinae muscles, recorded using skin-surface electrodes at the levels of T10 and L3. The relationship between extensor moment and EMG activity was linear, with an intercept on the extensor moment axis (Fig. 11.6, lower). This intercept – *I* – was a measure of the total extensor moment produced by the subject when the back muscles first began to contract: it is a direct measure of the extensor moment associated with passive tissues of the trunk. Each subject repeated their isometric pulls on the load cell while positioned in varying amounts of lumbar flexion, and the dependence of *I* on lumbar flexion is shown in Fig. 11.7. *I* rises rapidly to 100 Nm as the limit of lumbar flexion is approached, and does not fall below 20 Nm even when the back is upright. Clearly, at least 20 Nm of *I* is not attributable to stretched tissues posterior to the center of rotation, but the remaining 80 Nm probably is. Note that *I* includes the passive resistance of tissues present in a motion segment: this component is shown separately in Fig. 11.7 as *M*. Figure 11.7 answers the question posed above: lumbar flexion to 80% can indeed generate a considerable extensor moment

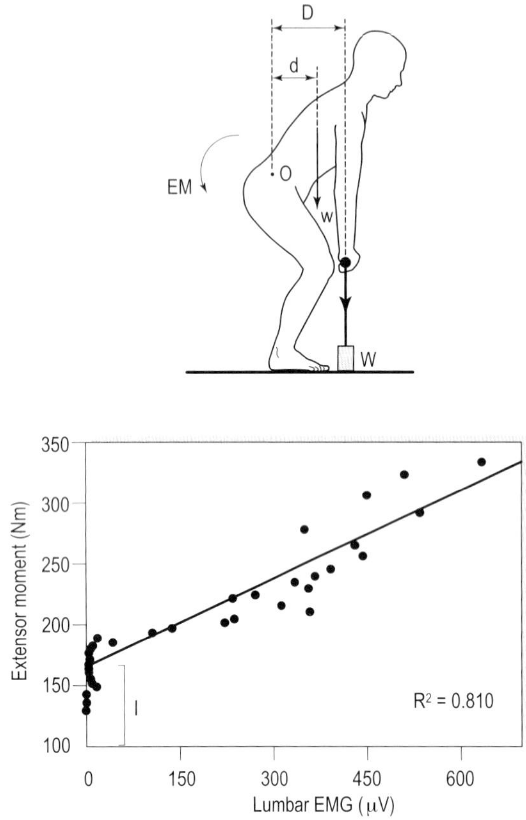

Fig. 11.6 (Upper) Subjects pulled up with increasing force on a load cell attached to the floor. The total extensor moment generated by active and passive tissues (EM) was calculated from the load cell force W, upper body weight w, and the lever arms D and d. (Lower) When extensor moment was plotted against the electromyographic activity of the back muscles, there was an intercept – *I* – which denotes a 'passive' extensor moment unrelated to back muscle activity. (Reproduced with permission from Dolan et al 1994b.)

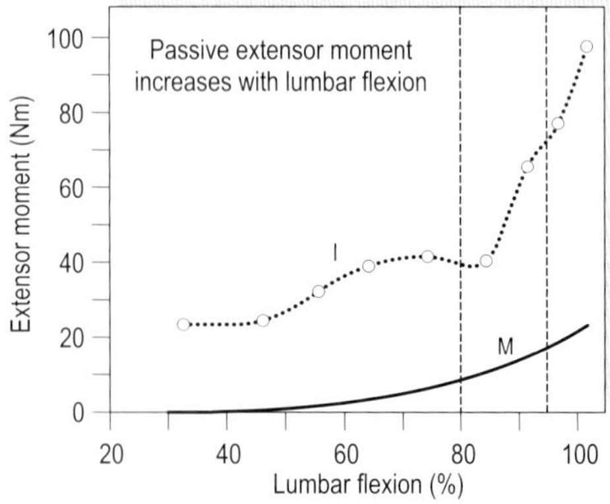

Fig. 11.7 The upper curve shows that the total 'passive' extensor moment (*I*) increases with lumbar flexion, where 100% flexion refers to the toe-touching posture in life (Dolan et al 1994b). During lifting, peak lumbar flexion is usually in the range shown by the dotted lines: in this range, only a small proportion of *I* is attributable to the intervertebral discs and ligaments. This component of *I* is denoted *M*. (Data from Adams & Dolan 1991.)

in passive tissues. Very little of this is attributable to the posterior annulus or intervertebral ligaments, which impose high compressive penalties on the discs, and most of it probably comes from the lumbodorsal fascia.

A flat back stretches the lumbodorsal fascia. Tension in the fascia then stabilizes the SIJs by pressing the opposing undulating surfaces closely together and increasing their resistance to shearing movements by the mechanism of 'force closure' (Vleeming et al 1990).

Muscles can help to tension the lumbodorsal fascia

Several muscles including the latissimus dorsi, gluteus maximus, transversus abdominis, and – to a lesser extent – the internal obliques have attachments to the lumbodorsal fascia, so active contraction of these muscles should increase tension in the fascia. The importance of such an effect in generating extensor moments during lifting has been the subject of much debate in recent years. As mentioned above, we have found that, in upright postures, where passive stretching of the lumbodorsal fascia is not a factor, extensor moments of approximately 20 Nm can be generated in the absence of any back muscle activity. Furthermore, in flexed postures, this passive extensor moment can increase further during an isometric pull, even though the back muscles remain electrically silent and the lumbar flexion angle is constant (see Fig. 11.6, lower). Skin-surface electrodes have a large pick-up area and electrical silence has been demonstrated in all of the muscles close to the lumbar and thoracic spine in flexed postures (Dolan et al 1994b, Gupta 2001). Therefore, muscles remote from the recording electrodes, which can apply tension to the lumbodorsal fascia, might be responsible for this extensor moment.

In theory, contraction of the abdominal muscles should exert a lateral pull on the lumbodorsal fascia which, because of the arrangement of collagen fibers in the fascia, could generate a longitudinal tension in this tissue (Barker et al 2004, Gracovetsky et al 1981). However, anatomically precise calculations suggest that extensor moments of no more than 6 Nm would be generated, even during a maximal contraction (Macintosh et al 1987). Latissimus dorsi also has the potential to pull strongly on the lumbodorsal fascia (Barker et al 2004), but EMG studies (Dolan et al 1994b, van Wingerden et al 2004) and a mathematical model (McGill & Norman 1988) suggest that they do not, at least during normal lifting movements that do not involve pulling of the weight towards the body. The gluteus maximus muscle is the largest, and possibly the most powerful, muscle in the body and also has extensive attachments to the lumbodorsal fascia, so this is the most likely candidate for tensioning this fascia when it is already stretched in a flat-back or flexed posture (van Wingerden et al 2004, Vleeming et al 1995). The abdominal muscles might then act mainly to prevent lateral contraction of the fascia and help to stabilize the spine in the frontal plane (Tesh et al 1987). The synchronous activation of muscles attached to the lumbodorsal fascia suggests that a stretched fascia might have a proprioceptive function that allows it to coordinate the activity of the major muscle groups attached to it. However, the finding that the passive extensor moment is substantially larger in flexed postures (Dolan et al 1994b) suggests that flexing the lumbar spine is probably the most effective way of employing the fascia to assist in heavy lifting.

Role of the legs in lifting

Bending the knees reduces bending stresses on the spine

High bending stresses play a major role in damaging intervertebral discs and ligaments, especially when high compressive forces are also present (Adams & Hutton 1982, Adams et al 2000a). Bending moments acting on the osteoligamentous lumbar spine during lifting can be quantified by comparing lumbar flexion movements *in vivo* with the bending stiffness properties of cadaveric lumbar spines (Adams & Dolan 1991). Results suggest that bending moments increase by approximately 100% when subjects fail to bend their knees, with peak bending moments rising to 14 Nm when picking up a pen and 21 Nm when lifting a 20 kg weight (Dolan et al 1994a).

Bending the knees is not always beneficial

Spinal compression, however, is *not* reduced by bending the knees. In fact, lifting with bent knees acts to *increase* the peak spinal compressive force on the lumbar spine compared with lifting with the knees straight. This effect was observed across a range of loads, in both men and women, and the average increase was 12% (Dolan et al 1994a). Evidently, lifting with bent knees reduces spinal bending at the expense of a slight increase in spinal compression. However, this may still be beneficial, because people who apply most bending to their spines during arduous laboratory lifting tasks are more likely to develop back pain subsequently (Mannion et al 1997). Bending the knees is not always practicable when heavy weights are lifted frequently, because quadriceps strength can then become a limiting factor, and subjects begin to extend their knees earlier and lift more with their backs (Schipplein et al 1990, Trafimow et al 1993).

Twisting while lifting

Twisting increases stress concentrations in the spine

In the lumbar spine, the orientation of the apophyseal joints restricts axial rotation to just 1–2° of movement to each side at each spinal level (Duncan & Ahmed 1991, Pearcy & Tibrewal 1984). This restriction might be less when the spine is also flexed, but the measurements in support of this hypothesis suffer from large skin-movement artifacts (Pearcy 1993) and there is other evidence that the increased anterior shear forces found in stooped postures actually reduce the already limited range of axial rotation even further (Gunzburg et al 1991). Nevertheless, it is widely believed that twisting while lifting is bad for the back, and Fig. 11.8A suggests why. Postures that are traditionally described as flexion plus axial rotation are really combinations of flexion and lateral bending, and lateral bending can indeed be harmful to the lumbar spine. The addition of lateral bending to flexion causes additional compression of the lateral annulus and apophyseal joint on the concave (ipsilateral) side, and additional stretching of the annulus and apophyseal joint capsule on the convex (contralateral) side (Fig. 11.8B). Increased compressive stresses have been measured in the posterolateral annulus of cadaveric specimens subjected to combined flexion and axial rotation (Steffen et al 1998) and it is the posterolateral annulus that usually exhibits maximum disc stresses (Edwards et al 2001) and which is the most common site of radial fissures.

Twisting reduces ligamentous protection for the disc

The supraspinous and interspinous ligaments protect the intervertebral disc in hyperflexion (Adams et al 1980, 1994a) but their location on

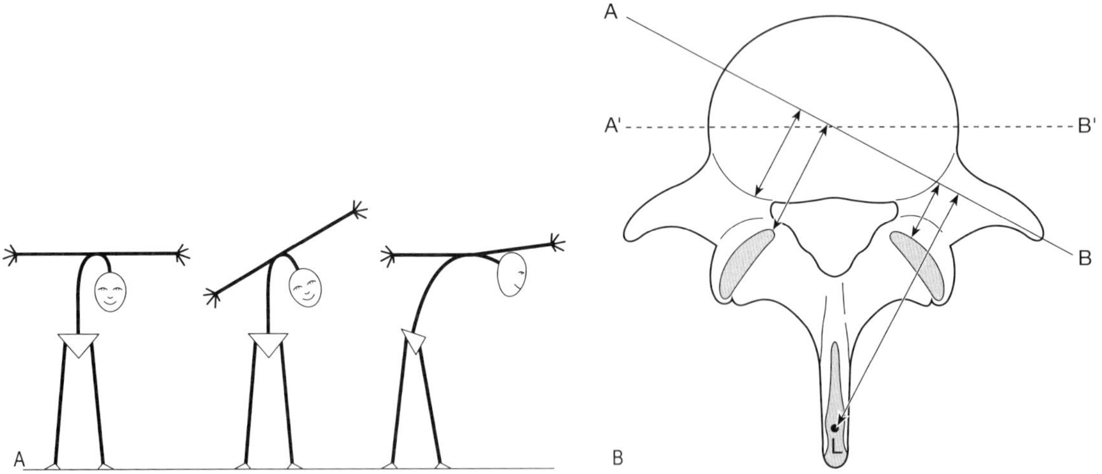

Fig. 11.8 The effects of twisting while lifting. (A) Bending directly forwards flexes the lumbar spine but if the lumbar spine is axially rotated at the same time then the upper body will be rotated as shown in the middle diagram. Adding lateral bending to forward flexion produces the asymmetrical bending shown on the right. This might also involve some coupled axial rotation, but axial rotation is not a primary movement. (B) Superior view of a lumbar vertebra. Bending forwards and to one side causes the oblique axis of bending (AB) to lie close to one apophyseal joint, but far from one posterolateral corner of the disc. The left posterolateral annulus will be stretched more than in normal flexion about A'B'. Furthermore, stretching of the interspinous/supraspinous ligament (L) will be reduced, so its function as a 'check' on forward bending is jeopardized. (Reproduced from Adams et al 2006, with permission of Churchill Livingstone, Edinburgh.)

the sagitthal midline of the vertebra means that they are not stretched by a component of lateral bending, even though the lateral bending generates additional compressive and tensile stresses in the lateral margins of the disc (Fig. 11.8B). In this way, a combination of forwards and lateral bending ('twisting while lifting') is particularly likely to injure the posterolateral margins of the lumbar discs.

Twisting affects spinal loading *in vivo*

Asymmetric movements are associated with increased back muscle activity on the side contralateral to the direction of twisting or lateral bending (Dolan et al 2001, Lavender et al 1992, Seroussi & Pope 1987, van Dieen 1996) and reduced activity on the ipsilateral side (Dolan et al 2001). Estimates of moments acting on the lumbosacral joint indicate that, when lifting weights from the ground, sagittal moments decrease with increasing trunk rotation (Dolan et al 2001). However, lateral flexion and rotational torques increase so that total net moment remains almost constant (Kingma et al 1998). These results suggest that twisting while lifting from the ground has little effect on spinal compressive loading, although the experimental techniques in these studies do not fully account for antagonistic activity from the abdominal muscles. Twisting while lifting does, however, increase peak bending moments acting on the osteoligamentous spine by up to 30% (Dolan et al 1994a), and twisting in more upright postures causes substantial cocontraction of abdominal muscles, increasing spinal compression by up to 45% (Granata & Marras 1995, Lavender et al 1992). These findings could explain why asymmetric lifting is an important risk factor for low back pain (Marras et al 1993).

Time-dependent influences in lifting

Viscoelastic effects *in vitro* influence load-sharing between discs and ligaments

Experiments on cadaveric spines have shown that repeated flexion causes the bending moment resisted by the osteoligamentous spine to fall by 17% after just 5 minutes (Adams & Dolan 1996). Similarly, 5 minutes of sustained flexion reduces the spine's resistance to bending by 42%. Most of this 'stress relaxation' is caused by fluid expulsion from stretched tissues, and the effect is greatest in the intervertebral ligaments because they are relatively thin, so that fluid can be expelled more easily from them than from the thicker intervertebral discs (Yahia et al 1991). As a result, the intervertebral discs resist a higher proportion of the bending moment acting on the spine after sustained bending.

Sustained compressive loading of the spine expels water from the intervertebral discs, increases slack in the annulus and intervertebral ligaments, and reduces the spine's resistance to bending by 40% in just 2 hours (Adams & Dolan 1996). The effect is particularly marked in the discs, which resist a smaller proportion of the bending moment acting on the spine after compressive creep. Conversely, a long period of unloading allows the discs to absorb water and resist bending more, with the result that disc prolapse becomes more likely (Adams et al 1987). These effects can explain why avoiding bending movements during the first few hours of each day reduces the risk of recurrent back pain (Snook et al 1998).

Rapid flexion movements performed in 0.5 seconds increase the spine's resistance to bending by 10–15% compared to slower movements performed over several seconds (Adams & Dolan 1996). This effect is mostly attributable to high internal resistance to rapid fluid movements in loaded tissues, and it suggests that rapid bending movements are more likely to injure discs and ligaments than slow movements up to the same flexion angle.

In combination, viscoelastic effects in cadaveric intervertebral discs and ligaments can profoundly influence how they resist bending. Rapid movements cause all passive tissues to resist more strongly, and resistance is concentrated in the intervertebral discs following sustained flexion, and before compressive creep loading. The next sections show how time-dependent effects influence spine mechanics in living people.

Rapid lifting movements increase spinal compression

Lifting weights rapidly from the ground requires the back muscles to generate higher extensor moments than slow lifting movements. This is because some of the extensor moment is used to accelerate the weight and upper body towards the upright position. Such 'dynamic' muscle forces typically increase peak spinal compression by 20–100% compared to quasistatic lifting, with the precise figure depending on the speed of movement (Buseck et al 1988, Dolan et al 1994a, Leskinen 1985, McGill & Norman 1985). Rapid lifting movements also cause the peaks of bending moment and compressive force to coincide (Dolan et al 1994a).

Muscle fatigue can increase bending stresses on the spine

The back muscles normally protect the underlying spine from excessive bending, but their protective action can be diminished during repetitive lifting if the back or leg muscles become fatigued and allow increased lumbar flexion (Dolan & Adams 1998, Potvin & Norman 1993, Trafimow et al 1993). Usually, peak bending moments *in vivo* remain below 40° of the values required to cause injury, even when muscles become fatigued, but in some individuals the threshold of fatigue damage accumulation may be exceeded (Dolan & Adams 1998). Muscle fatigue could therefore contribute to the risk of back injury during repetitive manual handling.

Repeated and sustained flexion can reduce muscle protection for the spine

Rapid forward bending movements of the spine cause the back muscles to contract vigorously in order to decelerate the upper body and prevent hyperflexion (Dolan & Adams 1993). This muscle activation might be at least partly reflex in nature (Fig. 11.9) through the action of muscle spindles and other types of mechanoreceptor found in spinal tissues (Holm et al 2002). Electrical stimulation of afferents in lumbar discs, capsules and ligaments seems to elicit reflex contraction of the multifidus and longissimus muscles (Indahl et al 1995, 1997, Solomonow et al 1998). Reflex activity of multifidus has also been demonstrated in anesthetized animals by stretching of the supraspinous ligament (Stubbs et al 1998) and by stimulation of nerves in the joint capsule of the sacroiliac joint (Indahl et al 1999). Prolonged or repetitive stretching of the supraspinous ligament causes the normal reflex activation of multifidus to diminish, and then disappear entirely (Solomonow et al 1999), and several hours of recovery time are required for the reflex to be fully restored (Solomonow et al 2000). Prolonged flexion causes creep stretching of spinal tissues in conscious humans (McGill & Brown

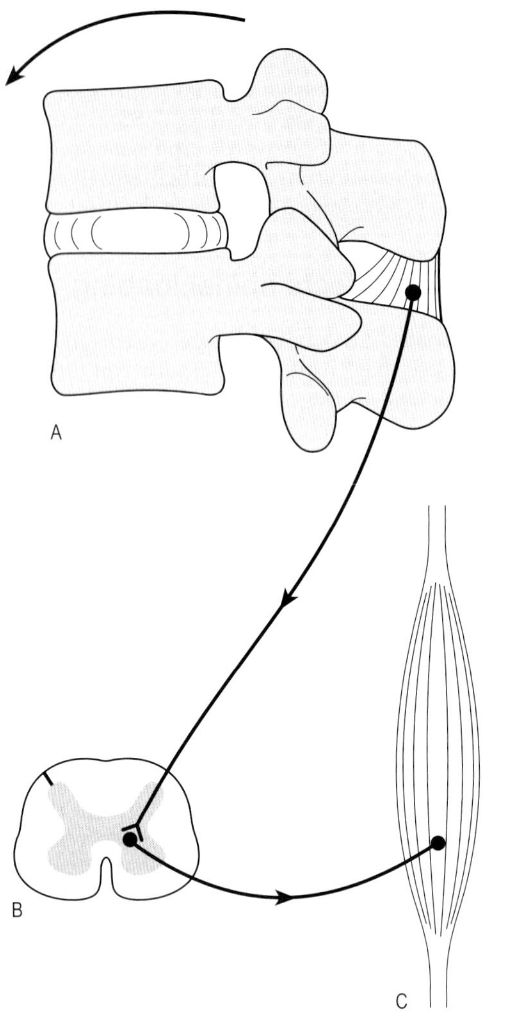

Fig. 11.9 In a spinal reflex, stimulation of receptors in a stretched muscle, ligament or tendon (A) sends a signal to the spinal cord (B), which sends a signal to the muscle (C). In this case, the muscle will contract to counter the initial stimulus. (Reproduced from Adams et al 2006, with permission of Churchill Livingstone, Edinburgh.)

1992) and creep-related uncoupling of tension and deformation may underlie the loss of spinal reflexes observed in the animal experiments. Any impairment of stretch reflexes will reduce the ability of the back muscles to protect the lumbar spine by contracting vigorously as the limit of flexion is approached (Fig. 11.10). In a recent study on living people (Dolan et al 2005) we found that activation of the erector spinae muscles during forward bending was delayed when creep was induced by sustained

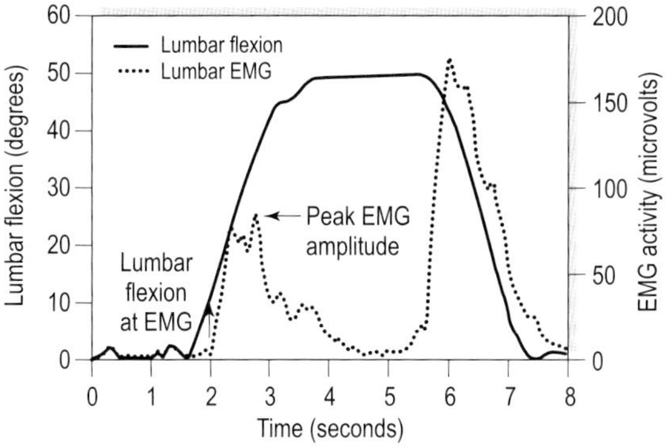

Fig. 11.10 Lumbar flexion and electromyographic (EMG) activity of the lumbar erector spinae, recorded from a subject performing a forward bending and lifting task. Note that EMG activity starts slightly after the initiation of lumbar flexion, and that peak activity occurs shortly before the lumbar spine reaches full flexion. Evidently, the back muscles decelerate the upper body during the flexion stage of movement, but then fall silent ('flexion relaxation') when the lumbar spine reaches static full flexion.

or repetitive spinal flexion, and that this was associated with impaired spinal proprioception. This mechanism may allow increased lumbar flexion during bending tasks, increasing the risk of bending injury to the lumbar spine.

Diurnal effects: lifting is more dangerous in the early morning

The increased water content of the intervertebral discs following a night's recumbency makes the spine stiffer in bending (Adams et al 1987). Much of this effect is lost within the first hour of rising (Dolan & Adams 2001, Krag et al 1990) but during this time the peak bending moment acting on the osteoligamentous spine during forward bending tasks is increased by more than 100% compared to later in the day (Dolan & Adams 2001). Evidently, reflex activation of the back muscles does not fully compensate for diurnal changes in spinal stiffness, suggesting that the small increase in disc height that occurs overnight is insufficient to have much influence on the activity of stretch receptors in spinal muscles, ligaments and tendons. Spinal flexion movements performed first thing in the morning might therefore increase the risk of bending injury to the intervertebral discs and ligaments. Conversely, avoiding lumbar flexion in the early morning reduces the recurrence of back pain (Snook et al 1998).

How do people try to lift in practice?

Elite weightlifters have been shown by videofluoroscopic analysis to flex their lumbar spine by a moderate amount during extreme lifting (Cholewicki & McGill 1992). It is pertinent to consider whether average people also lift with a straight back in the manner shown by the experts (and by the subject in Fig. 11.1). This is a confused topic because several authors have claimed that subjects 'maintained a normal lordosis' during lifting, even though accompanying photographs show that this is plainly not the case!

Objective dynamic measurements of lumbar curvature can be made *in vivo* using small goniometers attached to the skin surface overlying the L1 and S1 spinous processes. Such skin-surface measurements can correlate well with the angular movements of the underlying vertebrae (Adams et al 1986) and they show that people have a natural tendency to flex their lumbar spine during daily activities (Dolan et al 1988), especially when lifting (Adams & Dolan 1991, Dolan et al 1994a, 1994b). When asked to lift a 10 kg weight from the floor in a manner of their own choosing, most subjects bend their knees and flex their lumbar spine by 80–85% of its in vivo range between erect standing (0%) and full flexion (100%). Even when trained subjects tried their best to lift weights with a full lordosis, they averaged 57% lumbar flexion (Dolan et al 1994b). Lifting 10 kg from the floor with the knees straight usually requires 90–95% of lumbar flexion (Dolan et al 1994a, 1994b).

Comparisons between the ranges of movement observed in cadaveric spines and living people suggest that people do not flex right up to the elastic limit of their osteoligamentous lumbar spine, and that '100% flexion' *in vivo* means that lumbar motion segments are flexed approximately 70% of the way to their elastic limit (Adams & Dolan 1991). Further comparisons with the bending stiffness properties of lumbar motion segments indicate that '80% flexion' *in vivo* generates a bending moment on the osteoligamentous lumbar spine of only 8 Nm, which is approximately 14% of that required to cause the slightest detectable damage to a motion segment (Adams & Dolan 1991). For '100% flexion' *in vivo*, the equivalent bending moment is 21 Nm, which is 35% of that required to cause damage. Fatigue damage may possibly accumulate at 35% of the failure load, so it can be assumed that, for a living person, '80% flexion' is safe and 'moderate' whereas 100% might not be.

Discussion

The evidence presented above indicates that the lumbar spine is best able to resist high compressive forces when flexed by approximately 80% of the range between erect standing and full flexion. This 'flat back' posture is sufficient for passive tissues posterior to the spine (such as the lumbodorsal fascia) to generate substantial extensor moments. The tissues most involved act far from the center of rotation and so exert a small compressive penalty on the discs. They are also capable of storing a large amount of strain energy and so reduce the metabolic cost of lifting. Tension in the lumbodorsal fascia also helps to stabilize the SIJs because it forces the joint surfaces together (Vleeming et al 1995).

A flat back has other advantages and disadvantages (Adams et al 2006), some of which lie outside the scope of this review. Traditional advocacy of lordotic postures appears to be based on the fact that they reduce intradiscal pressure. However, we now know that this occurs because compressive force is transferred on to the posterior annulus and apophyseal joints, which are both innervated, without any compensatory increase in the spine's com-pressive strength (see above). Lordosis has also been advocated because it helps the back muscles to reduce anterior shear forces on the lower lumbar vertebrae (Macintosh et al 1993, Potvin et al 1991). The neural arch, however, can resist shear forces of approximately 2 kN (Cyron et al 1976), so this might not be of much consequence.

Although it appears advantageous to flatten the lumbar spine during lifting, it is undoubtedly important to avoid full flexion or hyperflexion because of the attendent risk of disc prolapse, and because of the time-dependent processes considered above which leave a bent back vulnerable to injury. Bending the knees and *attempting* to maintain a lordosis results in the lumbar spine being flexed by approximately 60–80% of its full range, which is just about right. Therefore the traditional advice to 'keep your back straight' or even 'preserve the hollow in your back' is probably good advice, even though it does not produce quite the effect that was intended. However, if the mechanics of lifting are to be understood and used to refine lifting technique, it is useful to distinguish between what people actually *do* and what they are *trying* to do.

Summary

1. Most people attempting to lift weights from the floor (in a laboratory) bend their knees, and flex their lumbar spine by approximately 80% of its full range between erect standing and touching the toes.
2. This moderately flexed or flat-back posture has several advantages: it evens up the distribution of compressive stress within the intervertebral discs; it substantially unloads the apophyseal joints; it maximizes back muscle strength; it allows stretched passive tissues such as the lumbodorsal fascia to assist in moment-generation, and to store strain energy, thereby reducing the metabolic cost of lifting; and it helps to stabilize the SIJ by the mechanism of force closure.
3. Bending the knees during lifting substantially reduces the peak bending stresses acting on the osteoligamentous lumbar spine. However, it can lead to slightly higher spinal compressive loading, and it requires the leg muscles to expend more energy by raising the upper body (and object to be lifted) against gravity.
4. 'Twisting while lifting' should be avoided. It involves components of lateral bending and axial rotation that serve to concentrate stresses in the posterolateral regions of the disc.
5. Lifting should be performed at a brisk pace, to minimize harmful 'creep' effects, but it should not be done so quickly that large muscle forces are required to decelerate the upper body.
6. Long periods of repetitive or sustained flexion should be avoided because they impair the ability of back muscles to protect the spine from hyperflexion.

References

Adams MA 2004 Biomechanics of back pain. Acupunct Med 22(4):178–188

Adams MA, Dolan P 1991 A technique for quantifying the bending moment acting on the lumbar spine in vivo. J Biomech 24(2):117–126

Adams MA, Dolan P 1996 Time-dependent changes in the lumbar spine's resistance to bending. Clin Biomech 11(4):194–200

Adams MA, Green TP 1993 Tensile properties of the annulus fibrosus. Part I The contribution of fibre-matrix interactions to tensile stiffness and strength. Eur Spine J 2:203–208

Adams MA, Hutton WC 1980 The effect of posture on the

role of the apophysial joints in resisting intervertebral compressive forces. J Bone Joint Surg [Br] 62(3):358–362
Adams MA, Hutton WC 1982 Prolapsed intervertebral disc. A hyperflexion injury. Spine 7(3):184–191
Adams MA, Hutton WC 1985 Gradual disc prolapse. Spine 10(6):524–531
Adams MA, Hutton WC, Stott JR 1980 The resistance to flexion of the lumbar intervertebral joint. Spine 5(3):245–253
Adams MA, Dolan P, Marx C, Hutton WC 1986 An electronic inclinometer technique for measuring lumbar curvature. Clin Biomech 1:130–134
Adams MA, Dolan P, Hutton WC 1987 Diurnal variations in the stresses on the lumbar spine. Spine 12(2): 130–137
Adams MA, Dolan P, Hutton WC 1988 The lumbar spine in backward bending. Spine 13(9):1019–1026
Adams MA, Green TP, Dolan P 1994a The strength in anterior bending of lumbar intervertebral discs. Spine 19(19):2197–2203
Adams MA, McNally DS, Chinn H, Dolan P 1994b Posture and the compressive strength of the lumbar spine. Clin Biomech 9:5–14
Adams MA, Freeman BJ, Morrison HP et al 2000a Mechanical initiation of intervertebral disc degeneration. Spine 25(13):1625–1636
Adams MA, May S, Freeman BJ et al 2000b Effects of backward bending on lumbar intervertebral discs. Relevance to physical therapy treatments for low back pain. Spine 25(4):431–437; discussion 438
Adams MA, Bogduk N, Burton K, Dolan P 2006 The biomechanics of back pain, 2nd edn. Churchill Livingstone, Edinburgh
Barker PJ, Briggs CA, Bogeski G 2004 Tensile transmission across the lumbar fasciae in unembalmed cadavers: effects of tension to various muscular attachments. Spine 29(2):129–138
Bogduk N, Macintosh JE, Pearcy MJ 1992 A universal model of the lumbar back muscles in the upright position. Spine 17(8):897–913
Buseck M, Schipplein OD, Andersson GB, Andriacchi TP 1988 Influence of dynamic factors and external loads on the moment at the lumbar spine in lifting. Spine 13(8):918–921
Cholewicki J, McGill SM 1992 Lumbar posterior ligament involvement during extremely heavy lifts estimated from fluoroscopic measurements. J Biomech 25(1):17–28
Cyron BM, Hutton WC, Troup JD 1976 Spondylolytic fractures. J Bone Joint Surg [Br] 58-B(4):462–466
Dolan P, Adams MA 1993 The relationship between EMG activity and extensor moment generation in the erector spinae muscles during bending and lifting activities. J Biomech 26(4–5):513–522
Dolan P, Adams MA 1998 Repetitive lifting tasks fatigue the back muscles and increase the bending moment acting on the lumbar spine. J Biomech 31(8):713–721
Dolan P, Adams MA 2001 Recent advances in lumbar spinal mechanics and their significance for modelling. Clin Biomech 16(Suppl 1):S8–S16
Dolan P, Adams MA, Hutton WC 1988 Commonly adopted postures and their effect on the lumbar spine. Spine 13(2):197–201
Dolan P, Earley M, Adams MA 1994a Bending and compressive stresses acting on the lumbar spine during lifting activities. J Biomech 27(10):1237–1248
Dolan P, Mannion AF, Adams MA 1994b Passive tissues help the back muscles to generate extensor moments during lifting. J Biomech 27(8):1077–1085
Dolan P, Kingma I, De Looze MP et al 2001 An EMG technique for measuring spinal loading during asymmetric lifting. Clin Biomech 16(Suppl 1):S17–24
Dolan P, Shandall S, Hodges K, Adams MA 2005 'Creep' in spinal tissues impairs spinal proprioception and delays activation of the back muscles. Presented to the Orthopaedic Research Society; Washington, USA, February
Duncan NA, Ahmed AM 1991 The role of axial rotation in the etiology of unilateral disc prolapse. An experimental and finite-element analysis. Spine 16(9):1089–1098
Dunlop RB, Adams MA, Hutton WC 1984 Disc space narrowing and the lumbar facet joints. J Bone Joint Surg [Br] 66(5):706–710
Edwards WT, Ordway NR, Zheng Y et al 2001 Peak stresses observed in the posterior lateral anulus. Spine 26(16):1753–1759
Gracovetsky S, Farfan HF, Lamy C 1981 The mechanism of the lumbar spine. Spine 6(3):249–262
Granata KP, Marras WS 1995 The influence of trunk muscle coactivity on dynamic spinal loads. Spine 20(8):913–919
Granhed H, Jonson R, Hansson T 1989 Mineral content and strength of lumbar vertebrae. A cadaver study. Acta Orthop Scand 60(1):105–109
Green TP, Adams MA, Dolan P 1993 Tensile properties of the annulus fibrosus. Part II Ultimate tensile strength and fatigue life. Eur Spine J 2:209–214
Gunzburg R, Hutton W, Fraser R 1991 Axial rotation of the lumbar spine and the effect of flexion. An in vitro and in vivo biomechanical study. Spine 16(1):22–28
Gupta A 2001 Analyses of myo-electrical silence of erectors spinae. J Biomech 34(4):491–496
Hodges PW, Richardson CA 1997 Relationship between limb movement speed and associated contraction of the trunk muscles. Ergonomics 40(11):1220–1230
Holm S, Indahl A, Solomonow M 2002 Sensorimotor control of the spine. J Electromyogr Kinesiol 12(3): 219–234
Hutton WC, Adams MA 1982 Can the lumbar spine be crushed in heavy lifting? Spine 7(6):586–590
Indahl A, Kaigle A, Reikeras O, Holm S 1995 Electromyographic response of the porcine multifidus musculature after nerve stimulation. Spine 20(24):2652–2658
Indahl A, Kaigle AM, Reikeras O, Holm SH 1997 Interaction between the porcine lumbar intervertebral disc, zygapophysial joints, and paraspinal muscles. Spine 22(24):2834–2840
Indahl A, Kaigle A, Reikeras O, Holm S 1999 Sacroiliac joint involvement in activation of the porcine spinal and gluteal musculature. J Spinal Disord 12(4):325–330

Katake K 1961 Studies on the strength of human skeletal muscles. J Kyoto Pref Med Univ 69:463–483

Kelsey JL, Githens PB, White AAD et al 1984 An epidemiologic study of lifting and twisting on the job and risk for acute prolapsed lumbar intervertebral disc. J Orthop Res 2(1):61–66

Kingma I, van Dieen JH, de Looze M et al 1998 Asymmetric low back loading in asymmetric lifting movements is not prevented by pelvic twist [see comments]. J Biomech 31(6):527–534

Kingma I, Baten CT, Dolan P et al 2001 Lumbar loading during lifting: a comparative study of three measurement techniques. J Electromyogr Kinesiol 11(5): 337–345

Krag MH, Cohen MC, Haugh LD, Pope MH 1990 Body height change during upright and recumbent posture. Spine 15(3):202–207

Kuslich SD, Ulstrom CL, Michael CJ 1991 The tissue origin of low back pain and sciatica: a report of pain response to tissue stimulation during operations on the lumbar spine using local anesthesia. Orthop Clin North Am 22(2):181–187

Lavender SA, Tsuang YH, Hafezi A et al 1992 Coactivation of the trunk muscles during asymmetric loading of the torso. Hum Factors 34(2):239–247

Lavender S, Trafimow J, Andersson GB et al 1994 Trunk muscle activation. The effects of torso flexion, moment direction, and moment magnitude. Spine 19(7):771–778

Leskinen TP 1985 Comparison of static and dynamic biomechanical models. Ergonomics 28(1):285–291

Macintosh JE, Bogduk N, Gracovetsky S 1987 The biomechanics of the thoracolumbar fascia. Clin Biomech 2:78–83

Macintosh JE, Bogduk N, Pearcy MJ 1993 The effects of flexion on the geometry and actions of the lumbar erector spinae. Spine 18(7):884–893

Mannion AF, Adams MA, Dolan P 1997 People who load their spines heavily during standard lifting tasks are more likely to develop low back pain. Presented to the International Society for the Study of the Lumbar Spine, Singapore, May 1997

Mannion AF, Adams MA, Dolan P 2000 Sudden and unexpected loading generates high forces on the lumbar spine. Spine 25(7):842–852

Marras WS, Lavender SA, Leurgans SE et al 1993 The role of dynamic three-dimensional trunk motion in occupationally-related low back disorders. The effects of workplace factors, trunk position, and trunk motion characteristics on risk of injury. Spine 18(5):617–628

McGill SM, Brown S 1992 Creep response of the lumbar spine to prolonged full flexion. Clin Biomech 7:43–46

McGill SM, Norman RW 1985 Dynamically and statically determined low back moments during lifting. J Biomech 18(12):877–885

McGill SM, Norman RW 1987 Effects of an anatomically detailed erector spinae model on L4/L5 disc compression and shear. J Biomech 20(6):591–600

McGill SM, Norman RW 1988 Potential of lumbodorsal fascia forces to generate back extension moments during squat lifts [see comments]. J Biomed Eng 10(4):312–318

McGill SM, Patt N, Norman RW 1988 Measurement of the trunk musculature of active males using CT scan radiography: implications for force and moment generating capacity about the L4/L5 joint. J Biomech 21(4):329–341

McNally DS, Adams MA 1992 Internal intervertebral disc mechanics as revealed by stress profilometry. Spine 17(1):66–73

Muche B, Bollow M, Francois RJ et al 2003 Anatomic structures involved in early- and late-stage sacroiliitis in spondylarthritis: a detailed analysis by contrast-enhanced magnetic resonance imaging. Arthritis Rheum 48(5):1374–1384

Myklebust JB, Pintar F, Yoganandan N et al 1988 Tensile strength of spinal ligaments. Spine 13(5):526–531

Pearcy MJ 1993 Twisting mobility of the human back in flexed postures. Spine 18(1):114–119

Pearcy MJ, Bogduk N 1988 Instantaneous axes of rotation of the lumbar intervertebral joints. Spine 13(9): 1033–1041

Pearcy MJ, Tibrewal SB 1984 Axial rotation and lateral bending in the normal lumbar spine measured by three-dimensional radiography. Spine 9(6):582–587

Pollintine P, Dolan P, Tobias JH, Adams MA 2004a Intervertebral disc degeneration can lead to 'stress-shielding' of the anterior vertebral body: a cause of osteoporotic vertebral fracture? Spine 29(7):774–782

Pollintine P, Przybyla A, Dolan P, Adams MA 2004b Neural arch load-bearing in old and degenerated spines. J Biomech 37:197–204

Potvin JR, Norman RW 1993 Quantification of erector spinae muscle fatigue during prolonged, dynamic lifting tasks. Eur J Appl Physiol Occup Physiol 67(6):554–562

Potvin JR, Norman RW, McGill SM 1991 Reduction in anterior shear forces on the L4/L5 disc by the lumbar musculature. Clin Biomech 6:88–96

Purslow PP 1989 Strain-induced reorientation of an intramuscular connective tissue network: implications for passive muscle elasticity. J Biomech 22(1):21–31

Richardson CA, Snijders CJ, Hides JA et al 2002 The relation between the transversus abdominis muscles, sacroiliac joint mechanics, and low back pain. Spine 27(4):399–405

Schipplein OD, Trafimow JH, Andersson GB, Andriacchi TP 1990 Relationship between moments at the L5/S1 level, hip and knee joint when lifting. J Biomech 23(9):907–912

Schwarzer AC, Aprill CN, Bogduk N 1995a The sacroiliac joint in chronic low back pain. Spine 20(1):31–37

Schwarzer AC, Aprill CN, Derby R et al 1995b The prevalence and clinical features of internal disc disruption in patients with chronic low back pain [see comments]. Spine 20(17):1878–1883

Schwarzer AC, Wang SC, Bogduk N et al 1995c Prevalence and clinical features of lumbar zygapophysial joint pain: a study in an Australian population with chronic low back pain. Ann Rheum Dis 54(2):100–106

Seroussi RE, Pope MH 1987 The relationship between trunk muscle electromyography and lifting moments in the sagittal and frontal planes. J Biomech 20(2):135–146

Snook SH, Webster BS, McGorry RW et al 1998 The reduction of chronic nonspecific low back pain through the control of early morning lumbar flexion. A randomized controlled trial. Spine 23(23):2601–2607

Solomonow M, Zhou BH, Harris M et al 1998 The ligamento-muscular stabilizing system of the spine. Spine 23(23):2552–2562

Solomonow M, Zhou BH, Baratta RV et al 1999 Biomechanics of increased exposure to lumbar injury caused by cyclic loading: Part 1. Loss of reflexive muscular stabilization. Spine 24(23):2426–2434

Solomonow M, Zhou BH, Baratta RV et al 2000 Biexponential recovery model of lumbar viscoelastic laxity and reflexive muscular activity after prolonged cyclic loading. Clin Biomech 15(3):167–175

Steffen T, Baramki HG, Rubin R et al 1998 Lumbar intradiscal pressure measured in the anterior and posterolateral annular regions during asymmetrical loading. Clin Biomech 13(7):495–505

Stokes IA, Gardner-Morse M, Henry SM, Badger GJ 2000 Decrease in trunk muscular response to perturbation with preactivation of lumbar spinal musculature. Spine 25(15):1957–1964

Stubbs M, Harris M, Solomonow M et al 1998 Ligamento-muscular protective reflex in the lumbar spine of the feline. J Electromyogr Kinesiol 8(4):197–204

Tesh KM, Dunn JS, Evans JH 1987 The abdominal muscles and vertebral stability. Spine 12(5):501–508

Tracy MF, Gibson MJ, Szypryt EP et al 1989 The geometry of the muscles of the lumbar spine determined by magnetic resonance imaging. Spine 14(2):186–193

Trafimow JH, Schipplein OD, Novak GJ, Andersson GB 1993 The effects of quadriceps fatigue on the technique of lifting. Spine 18(3):364–367

Tveit P, Daggfeldt K, Hetland S, Thorstensson A 1994 Erector spinae lever arm length variations with changes in spinal curvature. Spine 19(2):199–204

van Dieen JH 1996 Asymmetry of erector spinae muscle activity in twisted postures and consistency of muscle activation patterns across subjects. Spine 21(22): 2651–2661

van Dieen JH, Cholewicki J, Radebold A 2003 Trunk muscle recruitment patterns in patients with low back pain enhance the stability of the lumbar spine. Spine 28(8):834–841

van Wingerden JP, Vleeming A, Buyruk HM, Raissadat K 2004 Stabilization of the sacroiliac joint in vivo: verification of muscular contribution to force closure of the pelvis. Eur Spine J 13(3):199–205

Vleeming A, Volkers AC, Snijders CJ, Stoeckart R 1990 Relation between form and function in the sacroiliac joint. Part II: Biomechanical aspects. Spine 15(2):133–136

Vleeming A, Pool-Goudzwaard AL, Stoeckart R et al 1995 The posterior layer of the thoracolumbar fascia. Its function in load transfer from spine to legs. Spine 20(7):753–758

Wilson AM, Goodship AE 1994 Exercise-induced hyperthermia as a possible mechanism for tendon degeneration. J Biomech 27(7):899–905

Yahia LH, Audet J, Drouin G 1991 Rheological properties of the human lumbar spine ligaments. J Biomed Eng 13(5):399–406

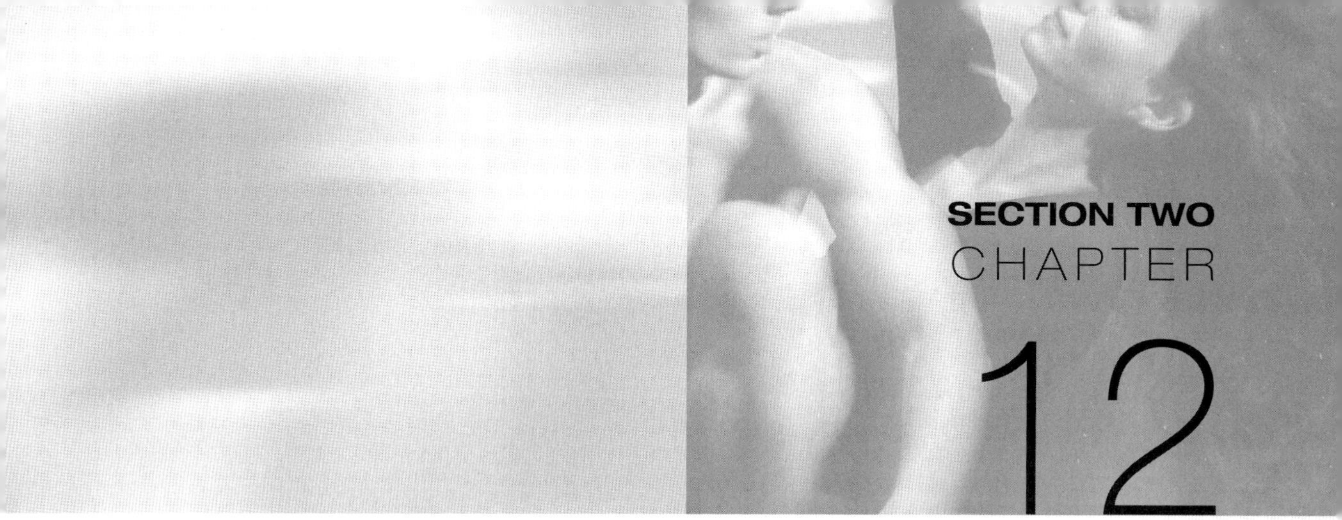

SECTION TWO

CHAPTER

12

Is the sacroiliac joint an evolved costovertebral joint?

Serge Gracovetsky

Introduction

The sacroiliac joint (SIJ) is receiving a considerable amount of attention and several competing ideas have been proposed to explain how the joint works and its role in locomotion. Yet – surprisingly – the literature does not demonstrate an overwhelming interest in understanding how the SIJ ended up the way it is. The purpose of this short chapter is to examine a limited amount of fossil record of vertebrates to get an appreciation as to how the SIJ might have evolved with time. As the fossil record is incomplete, some of the statements in this chapter might be somewhat speculative. The reader interested in a discussion on the comparative anatomy of man with respect to other primates and the evolution of the human pelvis from the hominid fossil record should consult Chapter 9. In that chapter, Lovejoy restricts his comments to specimens younger than 10 million years, whereas we considered specimens older than 100 million years.

Both dinosaurs and early mammals share a common ancestor. Although the dinosaurs are no longer with us, these animals had to solve the same basic locomotory problems as the mammals. Indeed, in both instances, these biological machines walked or ran on the surface of the earth under the influence of the planet's constant gravitational field.

The humble beginnings

It is generally agreed that the land was colonized by the early fish. Living in water reduces the apparent weight and fish had no reason to develop supporting limbs. Upon landing, the general configuration was that of an

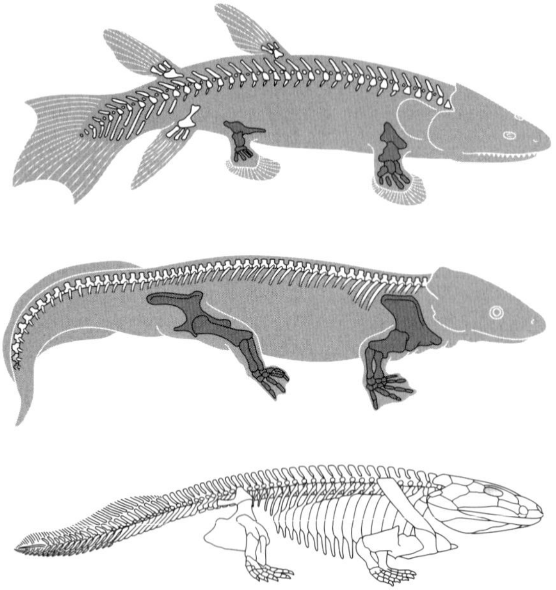

Fig. 12.1 (Top) Lobe-finned fish; (Middle) early amphibian; (Bottom) axial skeleton of the 360-million-year-old amphibian Ichthyostega (Schmalhausen 1968). Note the four scapulas that progressively began front/rear differentiation to adapt to land life (Stuttgart School District 2005). Note also that the Ichthyostega has limited ribs up to the sacral vertebrae.

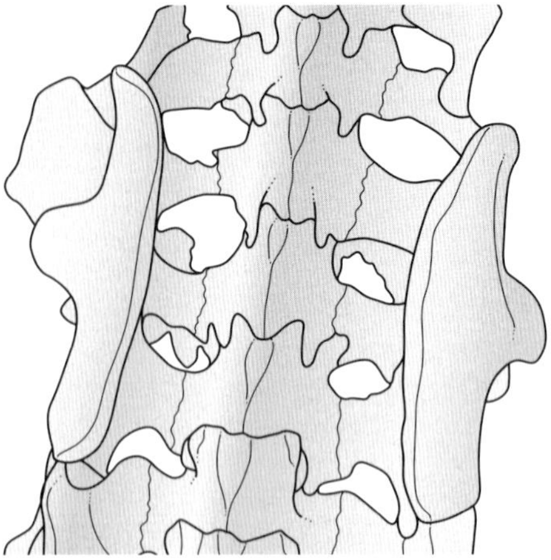

Fig. 12.3 Enlargement of the dorsal view of the axial skeleton of Thrinaxodon. Note the rib structure extending the transverse processes connecting the ilium to the spine. Jenkins (1971, p. 60 and 61) describes it as follows: 'Lumbar ribs are synostosed to the transverse processes along a serrated suture and the articulation is not loose… All five sacral ribs are fused to synapophyses. Not only are the capitular and tubercular facets confluent, as they are on lumbar ribs, but the capitular and tubercular processes also fuse and cannot be distinguished'. In other words, the ribs and the transverse processes are fused from the lumbar spine down. As far as the sacroiliac joint is concerned, the following description has been added: 'The remainder of the first sacral rib…contacts the medial surface of the ilium etc…'.

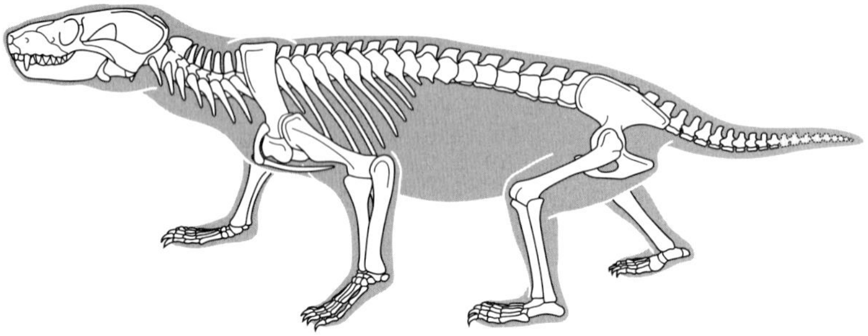

Fig. 12.2 Skeletal reconstruction of the 250-million-year-old African Cynodont *Thrinaxodon liorhimus*.

animal with a long rib cage and what is termed to be 'four' scapulas (Fig. 12.1).

The differentiation between the front and rear scapulas occurred in a few million years. The early amphibians already had a basic pelvic structure floating on shorter ribs. This is very apparent in the therapsids living some 250 million years ago; they were the precursors of the mammals (Figs 12.2 & 12.3).

A similar arrangement can be found in dinosaurs. For instance the well-preserved skeleton of Psittacosaurus demonstrates the relation between ilium, sacral ribs, transverse processes and the spine (Figs 12.4 & 12.5). The same arrangement could be found on much larger dinosaurs such as the Jingshanosaurus (Fig. 12.6).

The human side

The development of the human fetus follows the evolutionary steps of its ancestors. At term, the human fetus has a pelvic arrangement that reminds

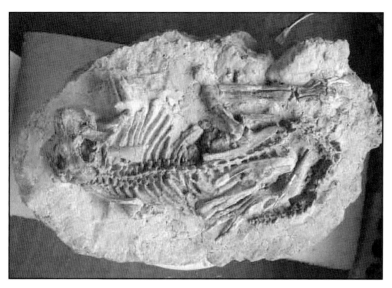

Fig. 12.4 Psittacosaurus (115 million years old) embedded in stone. The animal was the size of a 25 kg dog.

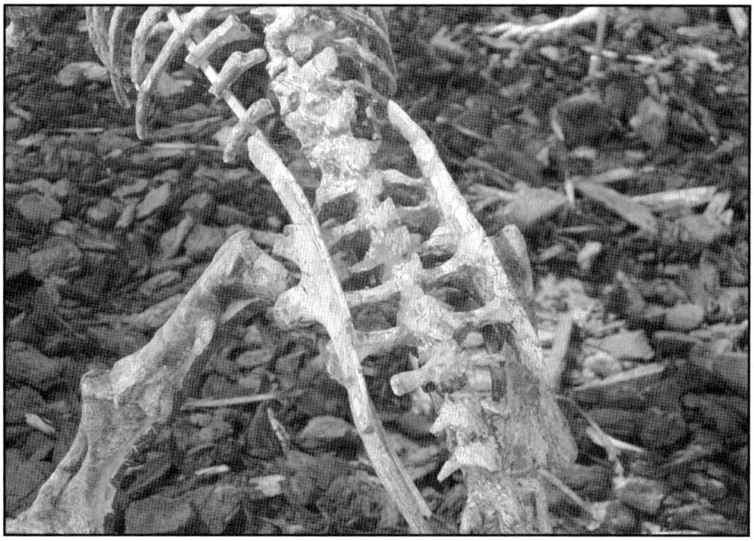

Fig. 12.5 Psittacosaurus reconstructed pelvic structure (Reproduced with permission from the Montreal Exhibition 2005).

of that of the early mammals (Fig. 12.7). For instance, the distinct (three) bones that constitute the Cynodont's pelvis (Fig. 12.8) can also be found in the human infant from birth to the mid-teen years. These three bones fuse when the child reaches 16 years of age.

The fossil evidence illustrated by Fig. 12.4 suggests that the SIJ is a modified costovertebral joint (see Chapter 19), more specifically the articular facet of the transverse process of the corresponding sacral vertebrae.

Each rib is resting in between two adjacent vertebrae and one transverse process. The ligaments holding the rib to the vertebrae are the upper part of the stellate ligament (from the anterior part of the superior vertebrae) and the lower part of the stellate ligament (from the anterior part of the inferior vertebra), which probably corresponds to

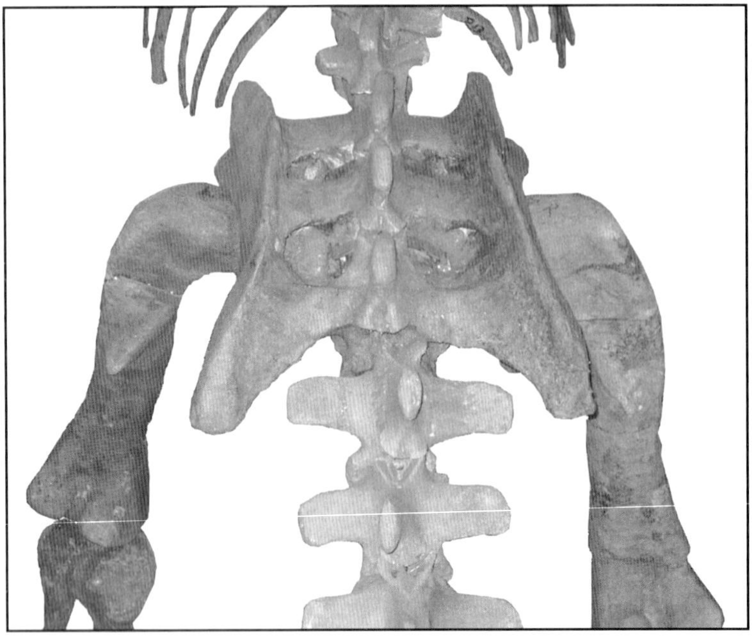

Fig. 12.6 Jingshanosaurus (Jurassic inferior). The animal is about 2 m high. The pelvis arrangement is similar to that of Psittacosaurus (Reproduced with permission from the Montreal Exhibition 2005).

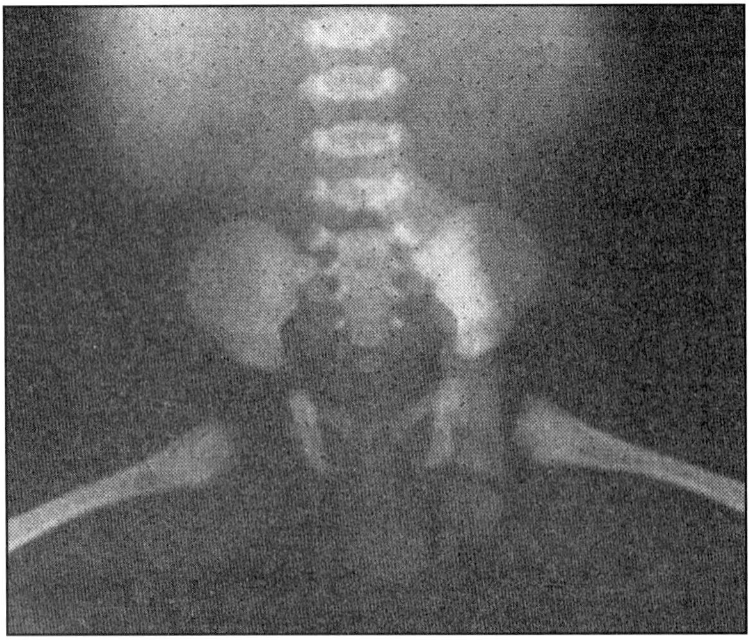

Fig. 12.7 Radiograph of full-term fetal skeleton. Notice the transverse processes (Reproduced with permission from Lockhart et al 1959).

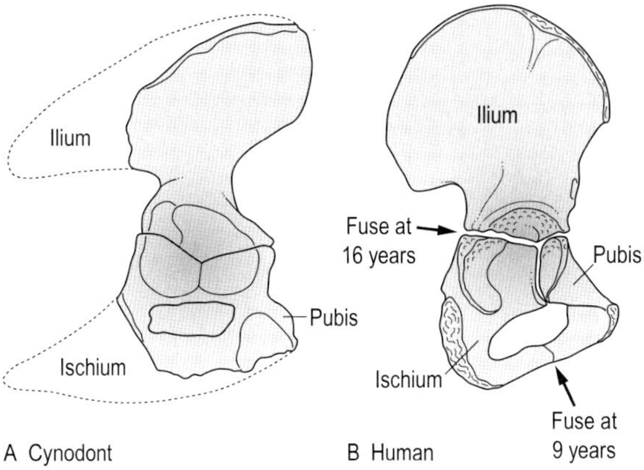

Fig. 12.8 The 250-million-year-old adult Cynodont primitive pelvis (A; Reproduced with permission from Jenkins 1971) is made of three distinct bones that become fused around 16 years of age in the human (B; Reproduced with permission from Lockhart et al 1959).

the anterior SI ligaments. Posteriorly and proximally, holding the rib to the two adjacent ligaments, is the interarticular ligament, which corresponds to the interosseous ligament that connects the sacrum to the ilium. That ligament is very deeply seated and very strong. It can be thought of as being an extension of the capsular ligaments of the facets that can be found higher up in the lumbar spine.

Note that the iliolumbar ligament linking the transverse process of L4 or L5 to the iliac crest can be compared with the posterior interosseous ligament. Indeed, the entire spinal anatomy from cervical vertebrae to pelvis can be made congruent.

The SIJ is a synovial joint like the other facets. The SIJ is a stable joint that has all the characteristics of the 'normal' facet joints of the thoracic spine, save for the restrictions in motion imposed by the tight fit of the ridge created by the projection of the transverse process into the innominate (see Chapter 19).

The available material demonstrates that the fusion of the ribs and transverse processes articulated on the ilium was nearly achieved some 250 million years ago. The proof that the pelvic girdle (pubis) evolved from the corresponding fused ribs was not evident in the specimen available to us at this time. A specimen that would demonstrate that aspect of rib transformation must be older than the 360-million-year-old Ichthyostega and we do not know if such a specimen has been found. Hence, the statement that the pelvis is also made of fused ribs must be considered to be a speculation at this time. We intend to visit museums of natural history in the hope that this 'smoking gun' has indeed been unearthed before.

Summary

The available fossil material is strongly consistent with the view that the SIJ is an evolved costovertebral joint. However, although many fossils had ribs going all the way to L5, we did not find an old enough specimen that would convincingly demonstrate that the pelvis is a set of fused modified ribs.

References

Jenkins F 1971 The postcranial skeleton of African cynodonts. Bulletin 36. Peabody Museum of Natural History, Yale University, New Haven, CT

Lockhart RD, Hamilton GF, Fyfe FW 1959 Anatomy of the human body. Faber and Faber, London

Montreal dinosaur exhibition at the Old Harbor 2005 June–October. Montreal, Canada

Schmalhausen LL 1968 The origin of terrestrial vertebrates. Academic Press, London

Stuttgart School District 2005 Massengale biology place. Online. Available: www.sps.k12.ar.us/massengale/vertebrate_notes.htm

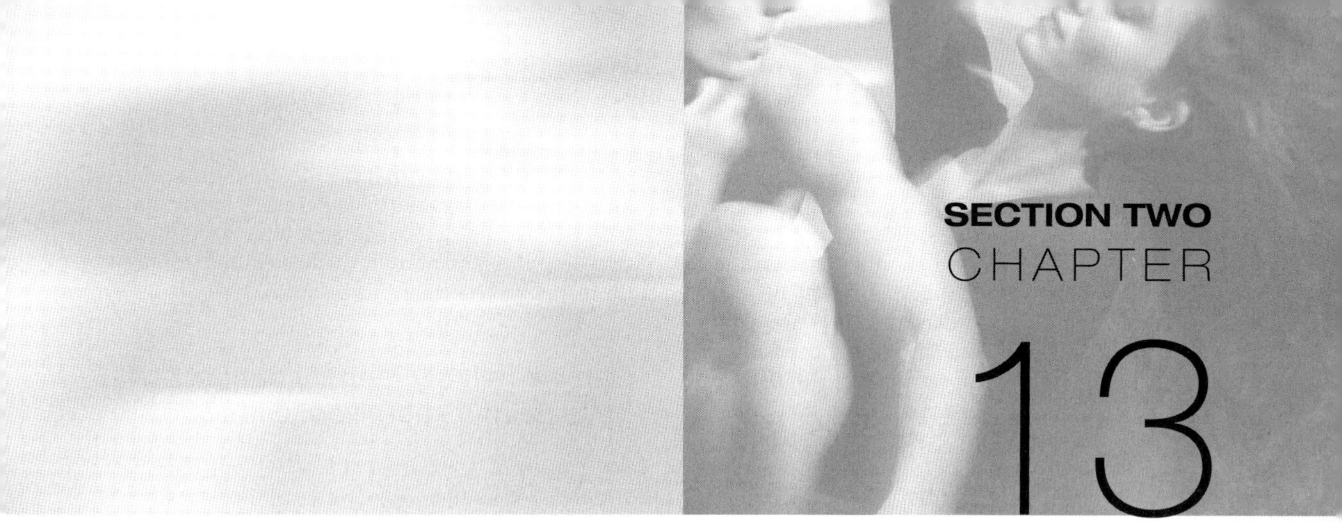

SECTION TWO
CHAPTER
13

The evolution of myths and facts regarding function and dysfunction of the pelvic girdle

Diane Lee

Introduction

The pelvic girdle is a source of mystery to many health practitioners and yet, amongst some, there is a long-held belief that it plays a significant role in low back pain. In the past, models for assessment and treatment of the pelvic girdle were taught by experienced clinicians whose protocols and techniques were accepted without scientific evidence of reliability or efficacy. Recently, some of these long-held beliefs have been challenged for their apparent lack of reliability, sensitivity, and specificity. This chapter outlines the evolution of some of these myths and what the recent research has revealed regarding them. In addition, some of the conclusions from this research will be challenged in the hope of preventing the perpetuation of more myths. The gap between what we *know* about the function of the pelvic girdle and what we *need to know* as clinicians treating pelvic girdle pain will be outlined and suggestions for future research offered.

Myths and Facts

Does the sacroiliac joint cause low back pain?

A commonly held myth is that pain in the pelvic girdle is merely referred from the lumbar spine (Cyriax 1954, Kirkaldy-Willis & Hill 1979). The question is, can the sacroiliac joint (SIJ) cause pain and, if so, where does this occur? This is important for establishing inclusion criteria for research pertaining to the pelvic girdle. Fortin et al (1994a, 1994b, 1999) investigated the location of pain that resulted when the SIJ in healthy subjects was irritated by being injected – under fluoroscopy – with sufficient contrast material to irritate the joint structures; this was followed by an anesthetic. The sensory changes (hyperesthesia and anesthesia) were mapped subsequent to each injection. From these studies, the SIJ is now known to cause pain approximately 10 cm caudally and 3 cm laterally from the posterior superior iliac spine (Fig. 13.1). Occasionally (two out of ten subjects) the pain referred into the posterolateral thigh to the superior aspect of the greater trochanter. Therefore, the SIJ is capable of producing *pelvic girdle pain* (between the iliac crest and the gluteal fold) and not low back pain. This pattern is known as 'Fortin's distribution of pain.' In 1995, Schwarzer et al investigated the prevalence of pain from the SIJ joint in a chronic-low-back-pain population. By injecting a local anesthetic via fluoroscopy into the SIJ and recording the pain-relieving response, they demonstrated that the SIJ can contribute to low back pain in 15–21% of the subjects studied. Would this percentage have been higher if the inclusion criteria had specified just pelvic girdle pain and not low back pain? Would this percentage have been higher if the capsule and ligaments of the SIJ had been considered in the pain production?

Vleeming et al (2002) confirmed that the long dorsal SIJ ligament is a significant pain generator in patients with pelvic girdle pain (sensitivity 76%). When the study was repeated with more specific inclusion criteria [severe pelvic girdle pain coupled with a positive posterior pelvic pain provocation test (Ostgaard et al 1994) and a positive active straight leg raise test (Mens et al 1999, 2001, 2002)], the sensitivity was 98%.

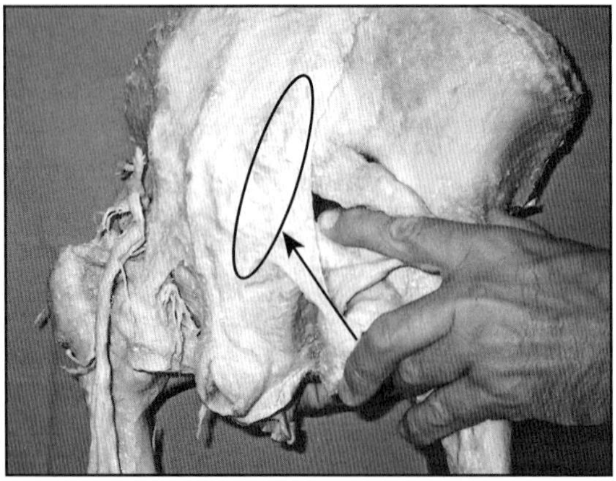

Fig. 13.1 The location of pain from an irritated sacroiliac joint (Fortin 1994a). (Reproduced with permission from Diane G. Lee Physiotherapist Corp ©.)

In short, we know that the SIJ and the associated ligaments are capable of generating pelvic girdle pain that is confined to the region between the iliac crest and the gluteal fold; this fact should be noted for inclusion criteria in future studies.

Can we reliably identify patients who have painful sacroiliac joints?

Several studies (Albert et al 2000, Carmichael 1987, Dreyfuss et al 1996, Herzog et al 1989, Laslett & Williams 1994, Maigne et al 1996, Ostgaard et al 1994, Potter & Rothstein 1985) have investigated the interexaminer reliability of pain provocation, position, and mobility tests for the pelvic girdle. Whereas the pain provocation tests have shown reliability (Albert et al 2000, Laslett & Williams 1994, Ostgaard et al 1994), the position and mobility tests have not.

Albert et al (2000) note that the low reliability of the position and mobility tests might be due to examiner bias and skill and propose that instead of abandoning these tests, we should seek to improve the skills of the examiners. They emphasize that a higher degree of standardization for all tests is required if interexaminer reliability is to occur.

With respect to sensitivity and specificity, Albert et al's (2000) study of 15 tests demonstrated high values for several tests. For the SIJ and the associated ligaments, the posterior pelvic pain provocation test (Ostgaard et al 1994), Faber test, and cranio-caudal glide scored well. For the pubic symphysis and the associated ligaments, palpation of the joint for tenderness and Trendelenburg's test scored well.

These findings differ from often quoted studies of Maigne et al (1996) and Dreyfuss et al (1996). In both of these studies, the investigators could not find any test (or medical history) that accurately predicted when pain was arising from the SIJ. In both of these studies, the SIJ was injected with an anesthetic block and the impact was correlated to the pain provocation tests. This procedure specifically studies the synovial portion of the SIJ and the thin anterior ligaments, and excludes the dorsal structures such as the interosseus and dorsal SIJ ligaments. To date, no anesthetic block studies have considered the role of the dorsal ligaments in the production of posterior pelvic girdle pain and no study has correlated these structures with the traditional pain provocation tests for the SIJ.

In conclusion, external pain provocation tests of the pelvic girdle are reliable, sensitive, and specific but cannot identify which structure is causing the pain. To date, the position and mobility tests for the SIJ and pubic symphysis have not shown reliability, although some question remains as to the standardization of the techniques investigated and skill level of the examiners.

Does the sacroiliac joint move?

A long-held myth has been that the SIJ is immobile except during pregnancy. Since the middle of the 19th century, both postmortem and *in vivo* studies have been done in an attempt to clarify the movements of the SIJs and the pubic symphysis and the axes about which these movements occur (Colachis et al 1963, Egund et al 1978, Jacob & Kissling 1995, Lavignolle et al 1983, Miller et al 1987, Sturesson et al 1989, 2000, Walheim & Selvik 1984, Weisl 1954, 1955). Of this research, the studies by Jacob & Kissling (1995) and Sturesson et al (1989, 2000) are of note.

Jacob & Kissling (1995) inserted Kirschner wires into the innominate bones and sacrum and then used Roentgen stereophotogrammetric analysis (RSA) to investigate mobility of the SIJ in healthy subjects during standing forward and backward bending, and left and right standing hip flexion. The average values for rotation and translation of the SIJ were low: 1.8° of rotation coupled with 0.7 mm of translation for the men and 1.9° of rotation coupled with 0.9 mm translation for the women. No statistical differences were noted for either age or gender.

Sturesson et al (1989, 2000) also used RSA to investigate mobility of the SIJ after the insertion of small tantalum balls into the sacrum and innominate bones. The subjects studied had been independently diagnosed by an orthopedic surgeon, chiropractor, and two physiotherapists as having a SIJ disorder. In this study, the investigators found a mean of 2.5° of innominate rotation (coupled with a mean of 0.7 mm of translation). This study considered the positional changes between the sacrum and the innominate in supine, prone with hyperextension of the left and then the right leg, standing, sitting with straight knees, and standing hip flexion. Of note is that this study found the same amplitude of motion in their unhealthy subjects as Jacob & Kissling (1995) found in their healthy group.

Thus, we can confidently say that yes, the SIJ moves; however, the question that arises is 'How significant is the amplitude of SIJ mobility in determining impaired function of the pelvic girdle?' This research suggests that amplitude of motion is not an indicator of function or dysfunction in the pelvic girdle.

Can we reliably detect motion at the sacroiliac joint?

Do we have reliable and practical tests for analyzing motion of the SIJ? As you might suspect, the answer is no, not yet. Carmichael (1987), Dreyfuss et al (1996), Herzog et al (1989), Potter & Rothstein (1985), Sturesson (1999), and several others have tried to demonstrate intra- and intertester reliability for many tests commonly used clinically to measure either position or motion of the SIJ. None of these studies was able to demonstrate reliability. There is considerable debate in the literature regarding the methods used, the subjects tested, the standardization of the technique, the skill of the tester, and the statistical analysis used to determine the results in these studies. For the most part, all of the tests investigated relied on active motion of the patient (standing forward bending, seated forward bending, Gillet or standing hip flexion test) and this can be a problem. Movement of a bone requires not only articular mobility but also activation of the muscular system; the pattern of motion produced reflects both the individual's motor control and joint mobility. Consider the patient with a complete tear of the rotator cuff of the shoulder. On active abduction of the arm, there is an apparent loss of motion; the arm can often only abduct to approximately 45°. However, on testing the passive mobility of the glenohumeral joint, full range of motion is noted. Thus, unless the subjects are screened for neuromuscular deficits (anatomical and motor control) there is no guarantee that they are actually performing the same quality/amplitude of motion each time they move! Sturesson et al's studies (1999, 2000) have clearly shown that the standing hip flexion test (Gillet) cannot be used to interpret the apparent motion (or lack thereof) of the SIJ. An active mobility test cannot conclusively determine the passive mobility of a joint.

In 1992, two specific, passive tests for evaluating mobility of the SIJ were proposed (Lee 1992, 2004; Figs 13.2 & 13.3). As the neutral zone of motion for all joints is greatest when the joint is in its loose-packed or resting position (Panjabi 1992a, 1992b), these passive mobility tests for the SIJ are done with the patient in supine lying to avoid any self-bracing or self-locking (Vleeming et al 1990a, 1990b). Essentially, these tests examine the ability

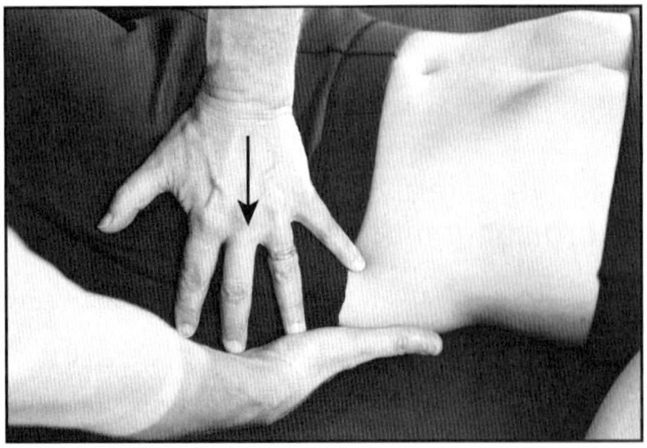

Fig. 13.2 This test examines the ability of the sacroiliac joint to resist an anteroposterior translation force. The arrow indicates the direction of force applied by the therapist's hand. (Reproduced with permission from Diane G. Lee Physiotherapist Corp ©.)

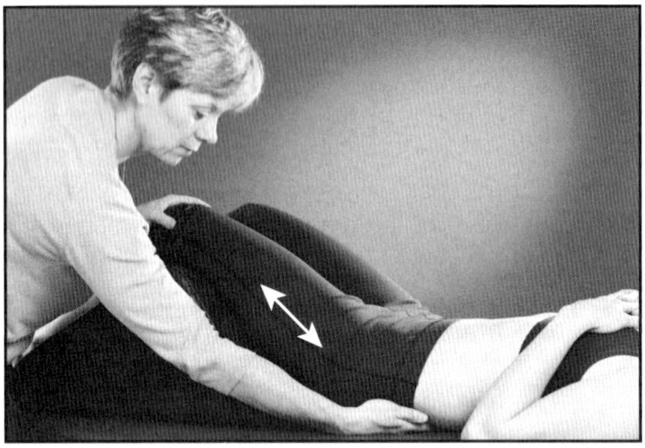

Fig. 13.3 This test examines the ability of the sacroiliac joint to resist a vertical translation force. The arrows indicate the resultant force on the innominate produced through 'pushing and pulling' the femur. (Reproduced with permission from Diane G. Lee Physiotherapist Corp ©.)

of the innominate to translate in the anteroposterior and craniocaudal planes relative to the sacrum. Although this motion is small, experienced clinicians are capable of feeling it. In 1995, a pilot project was conducted to determine if these tests could be reliable for measuring amplitude of motion at the SIJ. We failed, and I was astonished because – when allowed to use a clinical reasoning process and a complete subjective and objective examination of the patient – we usually agreed on the clinical diagnosis. What we failed to consider was the significant role that compression (force closure) has on articular mobility and the research that followed has helped to clarify why so many studies have failed to show reliability for both active and passive motion analysis of the SIJ.

In 1995, Buyruk et al (1995a) established that Doppler imaging of vibration (DIV) could be used to measure stiffness of the SIJ. A vibration of 200 Hz was applied to the innominate and the transference of this vibration was measured across the SIJ joint under different experimental conditions. This method could reliably detect when compression of the SIJ was artificially increased (screws placed across the joint and compression applied) or decreased (screws removed and the articular ligaments cut). The subjectivity of the human hand and eye could now be removed and the quantity of 'stiffness' measured *in vivo*.

In healthy subjects, both Buyruk et al (1995) and Damen (2002a) used the DIV method to show that, *in vivo*, stiffness of the SIJ is variable and therefore the range of motion between individuals is likely variable. In addition, both researchers found that stiffness of the left and right SIJ is symmetric in healthy subjects (the same on both sides), whereas in subjects with pelvic girdle pain asymmetry was found (one side was less or more stiff than the other) (Buyruk et al 1997, 1999, Damen et al 2001, 2002b). Therefore, in future reliability studies for motion analysis of the SIJ, focus should be on whether or not there is symmetry or asymmetry of motion. Less emphasis should be placed on the amplitude of motion (hypermobile, hypomobile).

Richardson et al (2002) and van Wingerden et al (2004) have also used the DIV method to confirm that activation of certain muscle groups can increase compression (stiffness) of the SIJ joint. Both the deep stabilizing (local) and muscle sling (global) systems (Bergmark 1989) were tested in these studies and although a few muscles were measured in each, it is impossible to know exactly which muscles were responsible for the increase in stiffness/compression.

In conclusion, we know that the SIJ joints are capable of a small amount of both angular (1–4°) and translatoric (1–3 mm) motion and that the amplitude of this motion is variable between subjects; however, within one subject it should be symmetric between sides. This research also suggests that any passive motion analysis of the SIJ joint needs to consider the:

- patient position at the time of testing: arms by the sides because an arms overhead position will passively tighten the anterior and posterior oblique muscle slings
- degree of resting tone in the myofascial systems.

With this in mind, future studies for motion analysis can be designed without these methodological flaws.

Current thoughts – a changing paradigm

Recent anatomical and biomechanical research has led to a clearer understanding of how load is transferred through the low back and pelvic girdle (Hodges & Richardson 1996, 1997, Hodges 1997, 2003b, Hodges et al 2001a, 2001b, 2001c, 2003, Hungerford 2003, Hungerford et al 2004, Mens et al 1999, Richardson et al 1999, Snijders et al 1993a, 1993b, Vleeming et al 1990a, 1990b, 1995, 1996). From this research, an integrated model based on function and not pain has evolved (Lee & Vleeming 1998) (Fig. 13.4).

As the joints of the pelvic girdle are mobile, stabilization is required if loads are to be transferred optimally. Stability (effective load transfer) is achieved when the passive, active, and control systems work together to approximate the joint surfaces at the time of loading. The amount of approximation required is variable and difficult to quantify since it depends on an individual's structure and the forces they need to control. Consequently, the ability to effectively transfer load through the pelvic girdle is dynamic and depends on optimal function of the bones, joints and ligaments (form closure) (Vleeming et al 1990a, 1990b), optimal function of the muscles and fascia (force closure) (Barker et al 2004, Hungerford 2003, Hungerford et el 2004, McGill 2002, O'Sullivan 2000, Richardson et al 2002, 2004, Vleeming et al 1995) and appropriate neural function (motor control, emotional state) (Hodges 1997, 2003b, Hodges et al 2001b, 2003, Holstege et al 1996, Hungerford 2003).

In the self-locked or close-packed position, the joint is under significant compression due to tension from the capsule and ligaments. The resultant compression increases the friction between the articular surfaces and facilitates the resistance to shear (Snijders et al 1993a, 1993b, Vleeming et al 1990b). The self-locked position for the SIJ is full nutation of the sacrum or posterior rotation of the innominate (van Wingerden et al 1993, Vleeming et al 1990a, 1990b). This position is therefore ideal for high loading tasks. Studies have shown (Hungerford et al 2004, Sturesson 1999, Sturesson et al 2000) that nutation of the sacrum occurs during forward/backward bending of the trunk and during standing hip flexion.

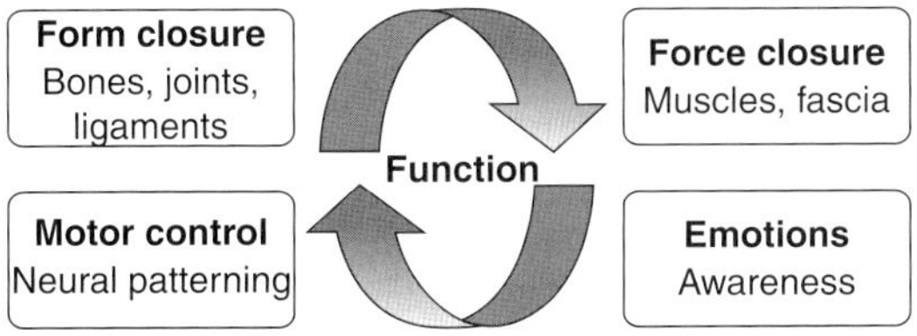

Fig. 13.4 The integrated model of function has four components: form closure (structure), force closure (forces produced by myofascial action), motor control (specific timing of muscle action/inaction during loading) and emotions.

In low-load situations (e.g. lying supine and raising one leg, standing, sitting and parts of the gait cycle), the joints of the pelvic girdle are not self-locked; the sacrum is suspended between the two innominate bones and stabilized by activation of both the local and global muscle systems. The amount of muscular activation required for stability depends on the forces being transferred and the individual's degree of form closure.

Research (Barbic et al 2003, Bø & Stein 1994, Constantinou & Govan 1982, Hodges 1997, 2003a, Hodges & Gandevia 2000a, 2000b, Hodges & Richardson 1997, Hungerford et al 2004, Moseley et al 2002, 2003, Sapsford et al 2001) has shown that, in health, the local system is anticipatory when the central nervous system can predict the timing of the load. In other words, these muscles should increase their activity *before* any loading or motion occurs. This anticipatory contraction prepares the joints of the lumbar spine (Hodges et al 2003) and pelvis (Richardson et al 2002) to receive the impending load and prevents excessive intersegmental and intrapelvic shearing regardless of the position of the joint. The articular compression and the resultant resistance to translation should occur prior to the onset of any movement. The timing of specific muscle contraction is critical for the effective transfer of loads through the pelvic girdle (Hodges 2003b). In addition, muscular strength and endurance is required (Hodges 2003b, McGill 2002) for all functional tasks. In both the assessment and treatment of patients with pelvic girdle pain, both motor control (sequencing and timing of muscle activation) and muscle capacity (strength and endurance) need to be addressed.

Thus, this research leads us to enquire about tests that examine an individual's functional status (ability to effectively transfer loads) as opposed to those that attempt to identify a pain generator.

Are there any reliable tests for measuring effective load transfer through the pelvic girdle?

The one leg standing test (Stork test, standing hip flexion test) examines the ability of the low back, pelvis and hip to transfer load unilaterally as well as for the pelvis to allow intrapelvic rotation (Hungerford 2003, 2004). The stability of the pelvic girdle on the weight-bearing side is assessed during standing hip flexion by noting any innominate motion (relative to the sacrum) as load is transferred to one leg (Fig. 13.5). The innominate should remain posteriorly rotated relative to the sacrum as weight is transferred onto the supporting leg. A positive test occurs when the innominate anteriorly rotates relative to the sacrum (Hungerford et al 2004). Intertester reliability studies for this test have been completed and good results were found (Hungerford, unpublished data); the sensitivity and specificity studies are being developed.

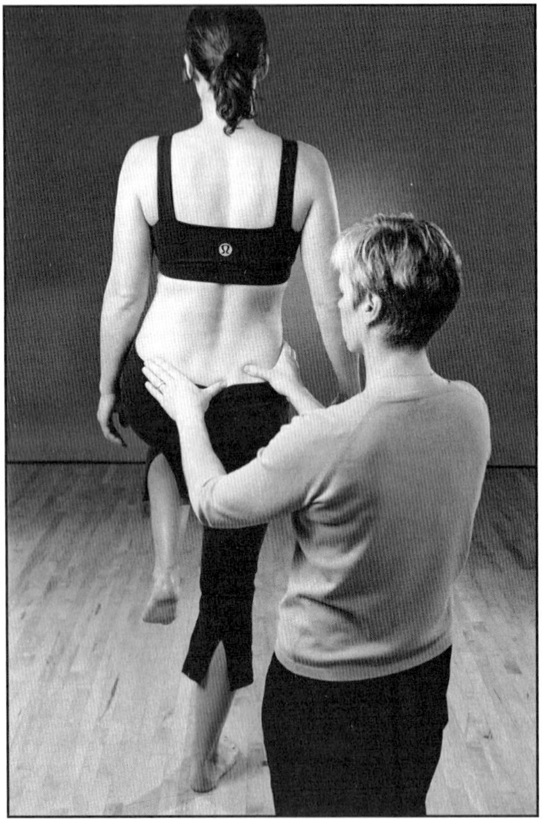

Fig. 13.5 Stability between the innominate and sacrum is palpated on the weight-bearing side. The innominate should remain posteriorly rotated relative to the sacrum. In patients with failed load transfer through the pelvic girdle the innominate anteriorly rotates. Further tests are required to differentiate the cause of the functional instability. (Reproduced with permission from Diane G. Lee Physiotherapist Corp ©.)

The supine active straight leg raise test (ASLR) has been validated as a clinical test for measuring effective load transfer between the trunk and lower limbs (Mens et al 1999, 2001, 2002) and is reliable, sensitive, and specific for pelvic girdle pain. When the lumbopelvic region is functioning optimally, the leg should rise effortlessly from the table and the pelvis should not move (flex, extend, laterally bend, or rotate) relative to the thorax and/or lower extremity. As the SIJ is in an unlocked or loose-packed position during this test, proper activation of both the local and global muscle systems are required. Several compensation strategies have been noted (Richardson et al 1999, 2004, Lee 2004) when stabilization of the lumbopelvic region is insufficient or inappropriately timed and the ASLR test can be used to identify these strategies (Fig. 13.6A). The application of compression to the pelvis has been shown (Mens et al 1999) to reduce the effort necessary to lift the leg for patients with pelvic girdle pain and instability. Varying the location of the compression force can assist the clinician to determine exactly where more compression is needed functionally to facilitate load transfer through the pelvic girdle (Lee 2004, Lee & Lee 2004) (Fig. 13.6B).

So far, the ASLR test is the only test which has withstood scientific scrutiny for the assessment of load transfer through the pelvic girdle; its primary function. Therefore it is still not possible to be totally evidence-based in clinical practice if 'evidence-based' means using only those tests that have withstood scientific scrutiny. However, what does 'evidence-based practice' truly mean? Sackett et al (2000) define it as the process of integrating the best research evidence available with both clinical expertise and patient values. Clinical expertise and the models that evolve from it are still necessary to bridge the gap between what we know scientifically and what we need to know practically to treat patients with pelvic girdle pain.

How effective are our treatment protocols?

To date, only one randomized controlled trial has considered the efficacy of a physiotherapeutic treatment program for pelvic girdle pain (Stuge et al 2004). The program was conducted on a subgroup of patients with pelvic girdle pain; those who experienced ongoing pain after pregnancy. The significant variable tested in this study was 'specific stabilizing exercises', which included exercises

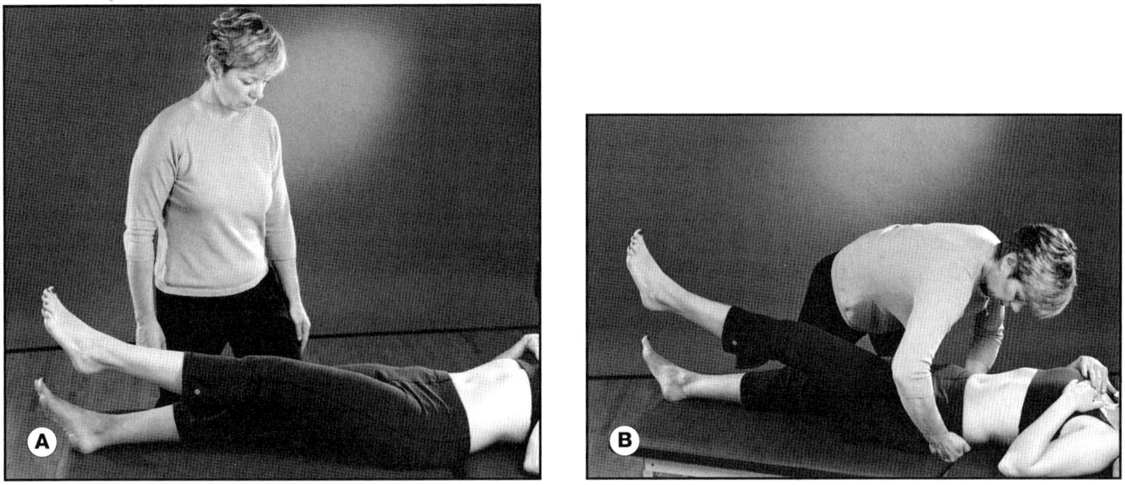

Fig. 13.6 (A) The active straight leg raise test in this subject reveals an abnormal pattern of thoracopelvic stabilization. The thorax is extending relative to the pelvic girdle and the pelvis is rotating relative to the elevating leg. The subject reports and the therapist observes that it takes considerably more effort to lift the left leg. (B) More compression of the posterior pelvic girdle is needed for optimal load transfer if compression posteriorly at the level of the PSISs facilitates elevation of the leg (effort is less). The pelvic girdle can be compressed in a variety of locations to assist in differential diagnosis and for exercise planning. (Reproduced with permission from Diane G. Lee Physiotherapist Corp ©.)

to retrain the local system (Richardson et al 1999) and global system slings (Vleeming et al 1990a). The program was individualized to each patient's specific needs and designed to minimize dropouts and maximize compliance. This program was shown to statistically produce significant improvements in pain intensity and disability and a higher quality of life for those involved.

The future

Recently, guidelines for the diagnosis and treatment of pelvic girdle pain were presented (Vleeming et al 2004). After an extensive review of the literature, this working group recognized the need for much more research in all areas pertaining to pelvic girdle pain (epidemiology, biomechanics, diagnostics) before any controlled trials of clinical outcomes can be done. We need to identify subgroups of patients with pelvic girdle pain according to specific impairments recognizing that all patients with pelvic girdle pain do not have the same impairments. We need to develop more diagnostic tests relevant to motion and load transfer for both the SIJ and the pubic symphysis and then to test them for reliability, sensitivity and specificity for pelvic girdle pain. A self-report questionnaire that specifically identifies those patients with failed load transfer through the pelvic girdle is required. Currently, all self-report scales pertain to the low back, not to the pelvic girdle.

When all of this is established, we will then have the ability to develop sound studies (randomized and controlled) to test the efficacy of treatment programs that are specific to each subgroup of impairment that leads to pelvic girdle pain. Until then, the best evidence-based treatment will be to use an integrated multimodal approach that considers the biomechanical, neuromuscular and emoional needs of the patient with pelvic girdle pain.

Summary

- **Do the sacroiliac joints cause low back pain?** No, the SIJs cause pelvic girdle pain, a fact not always considered in research in this area.
- **Can we reliably identify patients who have painful sacroiliac joints?** Yes, but not specifically which structure is causing their pain.
- **Does the sacroiliac joint move?** Yes, however the evidence suggests that amplitude of movement is not an indicator of function nor dysfunction.

- **Can we reliably detect motion at the sacroiliac joint?** There are many methodological problems with past reliability studies for testing mobility of the SIJ. Future studies should consider correlating manual findings against the current evidence obtained through the DIV method to determine the validity of the test and then follow this with reliability studies.
- **Are there any valid tests for measuring effective load transfer through the pelvic girdle?** Yes, the one leg standing test and the active straight leg raise test.
- **Can clinicians be evidence-based in clinical practice?** No, not yet, however we can be evidence-informed.
- **How effective are our treatment protocols?** Only one RCT has been done for pelvic girdle pain; this study has shown that we can be effective.

References

Albert H, Godskesen M, Westergaard J 2000 Evaluation of clinical tests used in classification procedures in pregnancy-related pelvic joint pain. European Spine 9:161–166

Barbic M, Kralj B, Cor A 2003 Compliance of the bladder neck supporting structures: importance of activity pattern of levator ani muscle and content of elastic fibers of endopelvic fascia. Neurourology and Urodynamics 22:269

Barker PJ, Briggs CA, Bogeski G 2004 Tensile transmission across the lumbar fascia in unembalmed cadavers. Spine 29(2):129

Bergmark A 1989 Stability of the lumbar spine. A study in mechanical engineering. Acta Orthopedica Scandinavica 230(60):20

Bø K, Stein R 1994 Needle EMG registration of striated urethral wall and pelvic floor muscle activity patterns during cough, Valsalva, abdominal, hip adductor, and gluteal muscles contractions in nulliparous healthy females. Neurourology and Urodynamics 13:35

Buyruk HM, Stam HJ, Snijders CJ et al 1995a The use of colour Doppler imaging for the assessment of sacroiliac joint stiffness: a study on embalmed human pelvises. European Journal of Radiology 21:112

Buyruk HM, Snijders CJ, Vleeming A et al 1995b The measurements of sacroiliac joint stiffness with colour Doppler imaging: a study on healthy subjects. European Journal of Radiology 21:117

Buyruk HM, Stam HJ, Snijders CJ et al 1997 Measurement of sacroiliac joint stiffness with color Doppler imaging and the importance of asymmetric stiffness in sacroiliac pathology. In: Vleeming A et al (eds) Movement, stability and low back pain. Churchill Livingstone, Edinburgh, p297

Buyruk HM, Stam HJ, Snijders CJ et al 1999 Measurement of sacroiliac joint stiffness in peripartum pelvic pain patients with Doppler imaging of vibrations (DIV). European Journal of Obstetrics and Gynecological Reproduction Biology 83(2):159

Carmichael JP 1987 Inter- and intra-examiner reliability of palpation for sacroiliac joint dysfunction. Journal of Manipulative Physical Therapy 10(4):164

Colachis SC, Worden RE, Bechtol CO, Strohm BR 1963 Movement of the sacroiliac joint in the adult male: a preliminary report. Archives of Physical Medicine and Rehabilitation 44:490

Constantinou CE, Govan DE 1982 Spatial distribution and timing of transmitted and reflexly generated urethral pressures in healthy women. Journal of Urology 127:964

Cyriax J 1954 Textbook of orthopaedic medicine. Cassell, London

Damen L, Buyruk HM, Guler-Uysal F et al 2001 Pelvic pain during pregnancy is associated with asymmetric laxity of the sacroiliac joints. Acta Obstetrica Gynecologica Scandinavica 80:1019

Damen L, Stijnen T, Roebroeck ME et al 2002a Reliability of sacroiliac joint laxity measurement with Doppler imaging of vibrations. Ultrasound in Medicine and Biology 28:407

Damen L, Buyruk HM, Guler-Uysal F et al 2002b Prognostic value of asymmetric laxity of the sacroiliac joints in pregnancy-related pelvic pain. Spine 27(24):2820

Dreyfuss P, Michaelsen M, Pauza D et al 1996 The value of history and physical examination in diagnosing sacroiliac joint pain. Spine 21:2594

Egund N, Olsson TH, Schmid H 1978 Movements in the sacro-iliac joints demonstrated with Roentgen stereo-photogrammetry. Acta Radiologica 19:833

Fortin JD, Dwyer A, West S, Pier J 1994a Sacroiliac joint pain referral patterns upon application of a new injection/arthrography technique. I: Asymptomatic volunteers. Spine 19(13):1475

Fortin JD, Dwyer A, Aprill C et al 1994b Sacroiliac joint pain referral patterns. II: Clinical evaluation. Spine 19(13):1483

Fortin JD, Kissling RO, O'Connor BL, Vilensky JA 1999 Sacroiliac joint innervation and pain. American Journal of Orthopedics December:687

Herzog W, Read L, Conway PJW et al 1989 Reliability of motion palpation procedures to detect sacroiliac joint fixations. Journal of Manipulative and Physical Therapy 12(2):86

Hodges PW 1997 Feedforward contraction of transversus abdominis is not influenced by the direction of arm movement. Experimental Brain Research 114:362

Hodges PW 2003a Neuromechanical control of the spine. PhD thesis. Karolinska Institutet, Stockholm, Sweden

Hodges PW 2003b Core stability exercise in chronic low back pain. Orthopaedic Clinics of North America 34:245

Hodges PW, Gandevia SC 2000a Changes in intra-abdominal pressure during postural and respiratory activation of the human diaphragm. Journal of Applied Physiology 89:967

Hodges PW, Gandevia SC 2000b Activation of the human diaphragm during a repetitive postural task. Journal of Physiology 522(1):165

Hodges PW, Richardson CA 1996 Inefficient muscular stabilization of the lumbar spine associated with low back pain: a motor control evaluation of transversus abdominis. Spine 21(22):2640

Hodges PW, Richardson CA 1997 Contraction of the abdominal muscles associated with movement of the lower limb. Physical Therapy 77:132

Hodges PW, Cresswell AG, Daggfeldt K, Thorstensson A 2001a In vivo measurement of the effect of intra-abdominal pressure on the human spine. Journal of Biomechanics 34:347

Hodges PW, Cresswell AG, Thorstensson A 2001b Perturbed upper limb movements cause short-latency postural responses in trunk muscles. Experimental Brain Research 138:243

Hodges PW, Heinjnen I, Gandevia SC 2001c Postural activity of the diaphragm is reduced in humans when respiratory demand increases. Journal of Physiology 537(3):999

Hodges PW, Kaigle Holm A, Holm S et al 2003 Intervertebral stiffness of the spine is increased by evoked contraction of transversus abdominis and the diaphragm: in vivo porcine studies. Spine 28(23):2594

Holstege G, Bandler R, Saper CB 1996 The emotional motor system. Elsevier Science, Amsterdam

Hungerford BA 2003 Evidence of altered lumbopelvic muscle recruitment in the presence of sacroiliac joint pain. Spine 28(14):1593

Hungerford BA, Gilleard W, Lee D 2004 Alteration of pelvic bone motion determined in subjects with posterior pelvic pain using skin markers. Clinical Biomechanics (19):456

Jacob HAC, Kissling RO 1995 The mobility of the sacroiliac joints in healthy volunteers between 20 and 50 years of age. Clinical Biomechanics 10(7):352

Kirkaldy-Willis WH, Hill RJ 1979 A more precise diagnosis for low back pain. Spine 4:102

Laslett M, Williams W 1994 The reliability of selected pain provocation tests for sacroiliac joint pathology. Spine 19(11):1243

Lavignolle B, Vital JM, Senegas J et al 1983 An approach to the functional anatomy of the sacroiliac joints in vivo. Anatomica Clinica 5:169

Lee DG 1992 Intra-articular versus extra-articular dysfunction of the sacroiliac joint – a method of differentiation. IFOMT Proceedings, Fifth International Conference. Vail, CO, p69

Lee DG 2004 The pelvic girdle, 3rd edn. Elsevier Science, Edinburgh

Lee DG, Lee LJ 2004 An integrated approach to the assessment and treatment of the lumbopelvic–hip region. Online. Available: www.dianelee.ca

Lee DG, Vleeming A 1998 Impaired load transfer through the pelvic girdle – a new model of altered neutral zone function. In: Proceedings from the Third Interdisciplinary World Congress on Low Back and Pelvic Pain. Vienna, Austria

Maigne JY, Aivaliklis A, Pfefer F 1996 Results of sacroiliac joint double block and value of sacroiliac pain provocation tests in 54 patients with low back pain. Spine 21:1889

McGill S 2002 Low back disorders – evidence-based prevention and rehabilitation. Human Kinetics, Canada

Mens JMA, Vleeming A, Snijders CJ et al 1999 The active straight leg raising test and mobility of the pelvic joints. European Spine 8:468

Mens JMA, Vleeming A, Snijders CJ et al 2001 Reliability and validity of the active straight leg raise test in posterior pelvic pain since pregnancy. Spine 26(10): 1167

Mens JMA, Vleeming A, Snijders CJ et al 2002 Validity of the active straight leg raise test for measuring disease severity in patients with posterior pelvic pain after pregnancy. Spine 27(2):196

Miller JAA, Schultz AB, Andersson GBJ 1987 Load-displacement behavior of sacro-iliac joints. Journal of Orthopedic Research 5:92

Moseley GL, Hodges PW, Gandevia SC 2002 Deep and superficial fibers of the lumbar multifidus muscle are differentially active during voluntary arm movements. Spine 27(2):E29

Moseley GL, Hodges PW, Gandevia SC 2003 External perturbation of the trunk in standing humans differentially activates components of the medial back muscles. Journal of Physiology 547(2):581

O'Sullivan P 2000 Lumbar segmental 'instability': clinical presentation and specific stabilizing exercise management. Manual Therapy 5(1):2

Östgaard HC, Zetherstrom G, Roos-Hansson E 1994 The posterior pelvic pain provocation test in pregnant women. European Spine Journal 3:258

Panjabi MM 1992a The stabilizing system of the spine. Part I: function, dysfunction, adaptation, and enhancement. Journal of Spinal Disorders 5(4):383

Panjabi MM 1992b The stabilizing system of the spine. Part II. Neutral zone and instability hypothesis. Journal of Spinal Disorders 5(4):390

Potter NA, Rothstein J 1985 Intertester reliability for selected clinical tests of the sacroiliac joint. Physical Therapy 65(11):1671

Richardson CA, Jull GA, Hodges PW, Hides JA 1999 Therapeutic exercise for spinal segmental stabilization in low back pain – scientific basis and clinical approach. Churchill Livingstone, Edinburgh

Richardson CA, Snijders CJ, Hides JA et al 2002 The relationship between the transversely oriented abdominal muscles, sacroiliac joint mechanics and low back pain. Spine 27(4):399

Richardson CA, Hodges PW, Hides JA 2004 Therapeutic exercise for lumbopelvic stabilization, 2nd edn. Churchill Livingstone, Edinburgh

Sackett DL, Straus S, Richardson WS, Rosenbuerg, Haynes RB 2000 Evidence-based medicine. How to practice and teach EBM. Elsevier Science, New York

Sapsford RR, Hodges PW, Richardson CA et al 2001 Co-activation of the abdominal and pelvic floor muscles during voluntary exercises. Neurourology and Urodynamics 20:31

Schwarzer AC, Aprill CN, Bogduk N 1995 The sacroiliac joint in chronic low back pain. Spine 20:31

Snijders CJ, Vleeming A, Stoeckart R 1993a Transfer of lumbosacral load to iliac bones and legs. 1: Biomechanics of self-bracing of the sacroiliac joints and its significance for treatment and exercise. Clinical Biomechanics 8:285

Snijders CJ, Vleeming A, Stoeckart R 1993b Transfer of lumbosacral load to iliac bones and legs. 2: Loading of the sacroiliac joints when lifting in a stooped posture. Clinical Biomechanics 8:295

Stuge B, Lærum E, Kirkesola G, Vøllestad N 2004 The efficacy of a treatment program focusing on specific stabilizing exercises for pelvic girdle pain after pregnancy. Spine 29(4):351

Sturesson B 1999 Load and movement of the sacroiliac joint. PhD thesis. Lund University, Sweden

Sturesson B, Selvik G, Udén A 1989 Movements of the sacroiliac joints: a Roentgen stereophotogrammetric analysis. Spine 14(2):162

Sturesson B, Udén A, Vleeming A 2000 A radiostereometric analysis of movements of the sacroiliac joints during the standing hip flexion test. Spine 25(3):364

van Wingerden JP, Vleeming A, Snijders CJ, Stoeckart R 1993 A functional–anatomical approach to the spine–pelvis mechanism: interaction between the biceps femoris muscle and the sacrotuberous ligament. European Spine Journal 2:140

van Wingerden JP, Vleeming A, Buyruk HM, Raissadat K 2004 Stabilization of the sacroiliac joint in vivo: verification of muscular contribution to force closure of the pelvis. European Spine Journal 13(3):199

Vleeming A, Stoeckart R, Volkers ACW, Snijders CJ 1990a Relation between form and function in the sacroiliac joint. 1: Clinical anatomical aspects. Spine 15(2):130

Vleeming A, Volkers ACW, Snijders CJ, Stoeckart R 1990b Relation between form and function in the sacroiliac joint. 2: Biomechanical aspects. Spine 15(2):133

Vleeming A, Pool-Goudzwaard AL, Stoeckart R et al 1995 The posterior layer of the thoracolumbar fascia: its function in load transfer from spine to legs. Spine 20:753

Vleeming A, Pool-Goudzwaard AL, Hammudoghlu D et al 1996 The function of the long dorsal sacroiliac ligament: its implication for understanding low back pain. Spine 21(5):556

Vleeming A, de Vries HJ, Mens JM, van Wingerden JP 2002 Possible role of the long dorsal sacroiliac ligament in women with peripartum pelvic pain. Acta Obstetrica Gynecologica Scandinavica 81(5):430

Vleeming A, Albert HB, Östgaard HC, Stuge B, Sturesson B 2004 European guidelines on the diagnosis and treatment of pelvic girdle pain. Proceedings of the Fifth Interdisciplinary World Congress on Low Back and Pelvic Pain. November 10–13, Melbourne, Australia, p6

Walheim GG, Selvik G 1984 Mobility of the pubic symphysis. Clinical Orthopaedics and Related Research 191:129

Weisl H 1954 The articular surfaces of the sacro-iliac joint and their relation to the movements of the sacrum. Acta Anatomica 22:1

Weisl H 1955 The movements of the sacro-iliac joint. Acta Anatomica 23:80

PART TWO

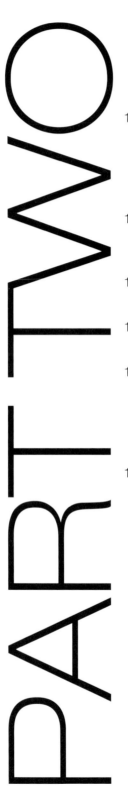

Insights in function and dysfunction of the lumbopelvic region

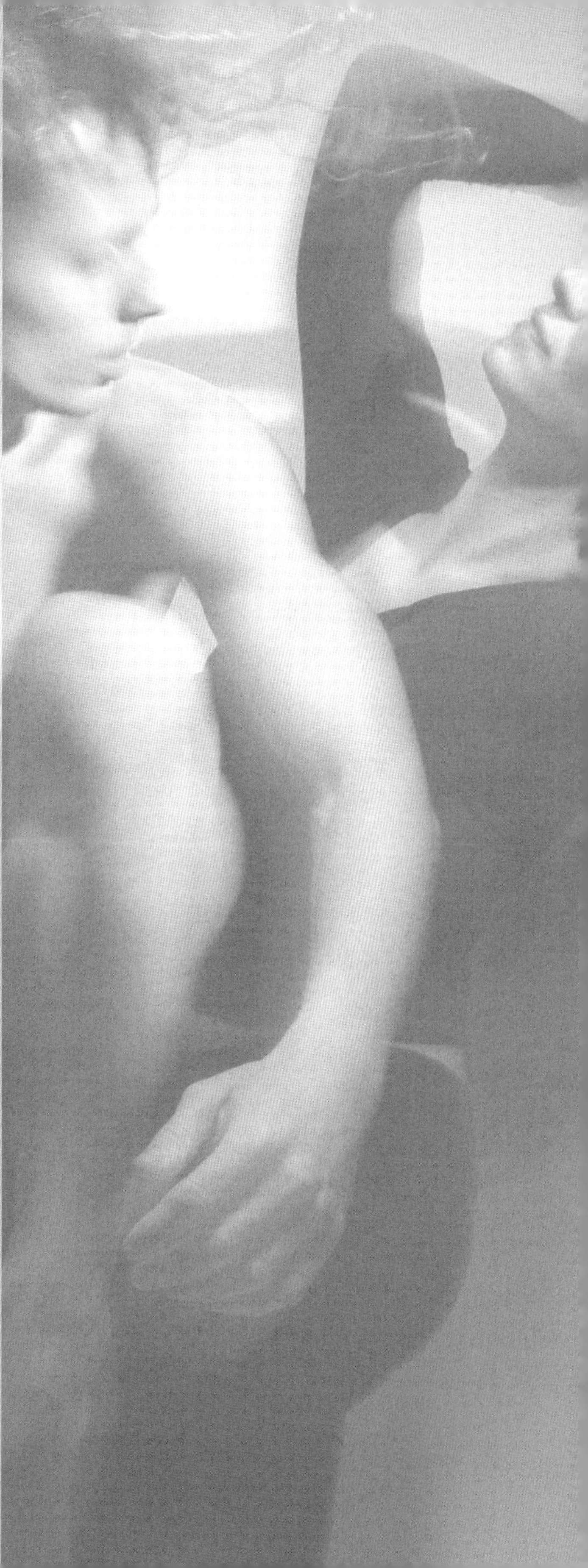

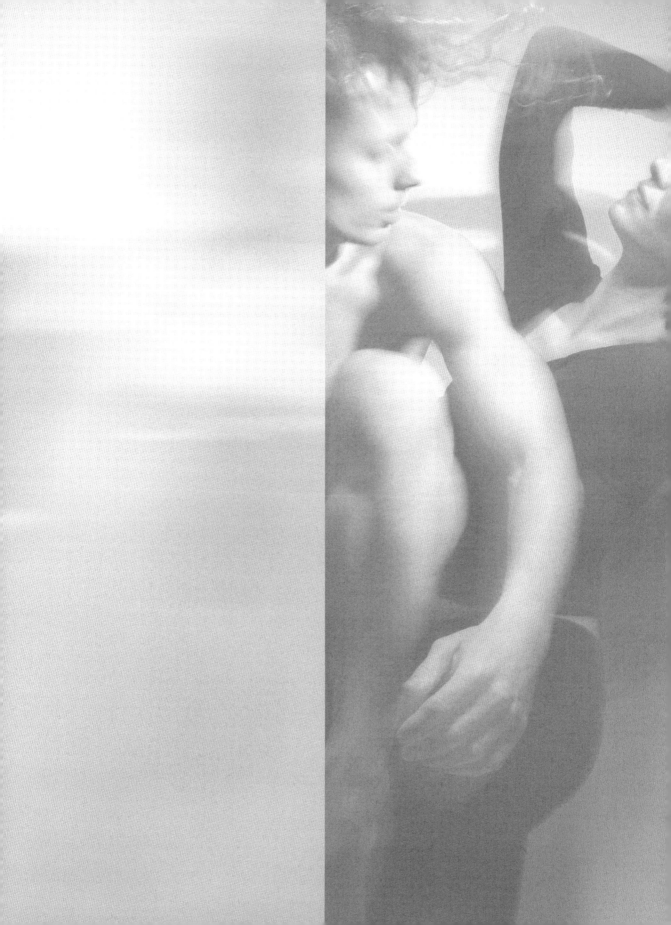

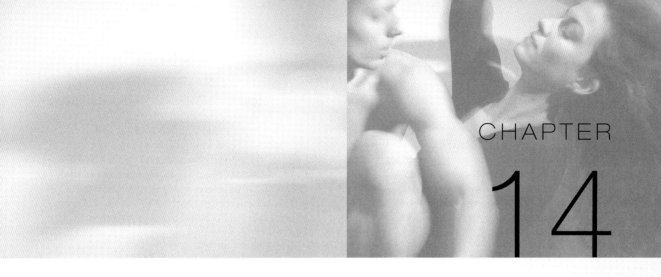

CHAPTER 14

Anatomical, biomechanical, and clinical perspectives on sacroiliac joints: an integrative synthesis of biodynamic mechanisms related to ankylosing spondylitis

Alfonse T Masi, Michael Benjamin and Andry Vleeming

Introduction

Bilateral sacroiliac joint (SIJ) involvement is a hallmark of ankylosing spondylitis (AS) (Khan 2002). The characteristic lesions typically progress from sacroiliitis to the quite unique intra-articular trabecular bony fusion (Dihlmann 1980, Resnick et al 1977). Less is known about the SIJ than other joints of clinical significance. This chapter reviews its essential functional anatomy, kinetics and kinematics, in relation to clinical and pathological features of AS.

Stability and mobility are instantaneously counteropposing states of the pelvis and SIJs (Vleeming et al 2004; see Chapter 8). An integrated structural and musculoligamentous model is presented to explain the requisite kinetic balance of stability and mobility. In the 'form-force' closure concept (Vleeming et al 1990a, 1990b), stability is partly achieved by the anatomical form and congruity of bones and their joints, and binding ligaments, and by the dynamically active muscular 'force-closure' mechanisms. Such a model is needed for efficient loading and bipedal mobility. The system requires optimal myofascial integrity and sufficiency, attuned by neuromotor control.

Mechanical muscle tone, or the intrinsic elasticity of the myofascial tissues, is an essential component in efficient neuromotor control mechanisms (Walsh 1992). Myofascial tone depends on its intrinsic, passive mechanical properties as well as active contraction forces. Axial musculo-ligamentous tonicity was recently proposed to vary constitutionally among individuals in the population as a polymorphic trait, and hypertonicity might predispose to AS (Masi & Walsh 2003). Thus, altered biomechanics is believed to play a role in AS. The models of 'form-force' closure (Vleeming et al 1990a, 1990b) and axial musculoligamentous hypertonicity (Masi & Walsh 2003) are mutually complementary concepts and help to explain a novel proposed physiopathogenesis of AS.

Persistently excessive compressional forces and stiffness of the spine, sacrum, and SIJs in AS could contribute to the earliest sacroiliac changes of osteitis (Ahlstrom et al 1990, Dihlmann 1980, Jurriaans & Friedman 1997, McGonagle et al 1998, and see Chapter 21) as well as progression to its latest stage lesion of intra-articular bony fusion (Dihlmann 1980, Resnick et al 1977, see Chapter 21). Concurrently, such altered kinetic forces could exert greater tensional strains on ligamentous and tendinous attachments at various bony sites on the sacrum and spine, leading to the characteristic enthesopathy lesions (Ball 1971, 1979, Benjamin & McGonagle 2001). Exaggerated spinal–pelvic force transfers could secondarily lead to excessive impacts and stresses being transmitted to lower extremity joints, and contribute to those typical involvements of AS (Khan 2002, Masi et al 2001).

The proposed biomechanical pathways in AS do not exclude other etiological or immunological mechanisms that might initiate the process or operate concurrently (McGonagle et al 2001). The validity of the proposed kinetic and kinematic concepts needs to be tested in controlled studies. Biomechanical functions at various anatomical sites and at different stages of AS need to be critically investigated, as reviewed in this chapter.

The normal structure of sacroiliac joints

Articular and osteoligamentous structures

In bipedal humans, the SIJs are highly specialized synovial joints that permit stable, yet flexible, support to the upper body (Bogduk 1997, Snijders et al 1993a, 1993b, Solonen 1957, Vleeming et al 1990a, 1990b, 1997; and see Chapter 8). The SIJ articular surfaces are not smooth but have interdigitating symmetrical grooves and ridges (Solonen 1957, Vleeming 1990, Vleeming et al 1990a, 1990b), which contribute to the highest coefficient of friction of any diarthrodial joint. This property enhances the stability of the joint against shearing (Vleeming 1990a, 1990b). The 'keystone-like' bony anatomy of the sacrum (Soames 1995) further contributes to stability within the pelvic ring. The bone is wider superiorly at its base than inferiorly, and wider anteriorly than posteriorly, permitting the sacrum to become 'wedged' cranially and dorsally into the ilia within the pelvic ring (Bogduk 1997, Lee 1999). This anatomical structure in humans is adapted to resist shearing from vertical compression (e.g. gravity) and anteriorly directed forces on the spine (Abitbol 1987, Aiello & Dean 1990a, 1990b).

The posterior interosseous ligaments of the SIJs are prominent. The joint space can become partly or completely obliterated, and they are sometimes classed as amphiarthroses (Gerlach & Lierse 1992), symphyses (Puhakka et al 2004), or syndesmoses (Soames 1995). 'Accessory SIJs' are described; these are extracapsular fibrocartilaginous articulations for biomechanical enhancement. Bakland & Hansen (1984) described an 'axial' SIJ, which is surrounded by the interosseous ligaments and lies dorsal to the main auricular shaped surface of the synovial SIJ. They called this articulation the 'axial part of the sacroiliac joint,' because of its supposed location at the axis for transverse sacroiliac rotary movements that lies here. The 'axial joint' has a larger convexity on its iliac side than the smaller concavity on its sacral side, but congruity might be improved somewhat by an iliac plate of fibrocartilage.

The SIJs act as important stress-relievers in the 'force–motion' relationships between the trunk and lower limbs (Lee 1999, Snijders et al 1993a, 1993b, Vleeming et al 1997; and see Chapter 8). They ensure that the pelvic girdle is not a solid ring of bone that could easily fracture under the great forces to which it might be subject, either from trauma (Adams et al 2002) or many bipedal functions (Lovejoy 1988). During gait, SIJs provide sufficient flexibility for the intrapelvic forces to be transferred effectively to and from the lumbar spine and lower extremities (Lee 1999, Lovejoy 1988, Snijders et al 1993a, 1993b, Vleeming et al 1997; and see Chapter 8). Typically, the SIJ is formed within sacral segments S1, S2, and S3, although inclusion of the complete S3 segment in the SIJ is not common for females. The bony anatomy is highly variable in size, shape, and contour among individuals (Bakland & Hansen 1984, Bellamy et al 1983, Bowen & Cassidy 1981, Sashin 1930, Schunke 1938, Solonen 1957). Also, the shape of the joint changes markedly from infancy to adulthood (Bowen & Cassidy 1981).

In the adult, the joint has an auricular or C-shaped or L-shaped configuration, which 'opens' posteriorly (Fig. 14.1). The SIJs lie obliquely at an angle to the sagittal plane (Bowen & Cassidy

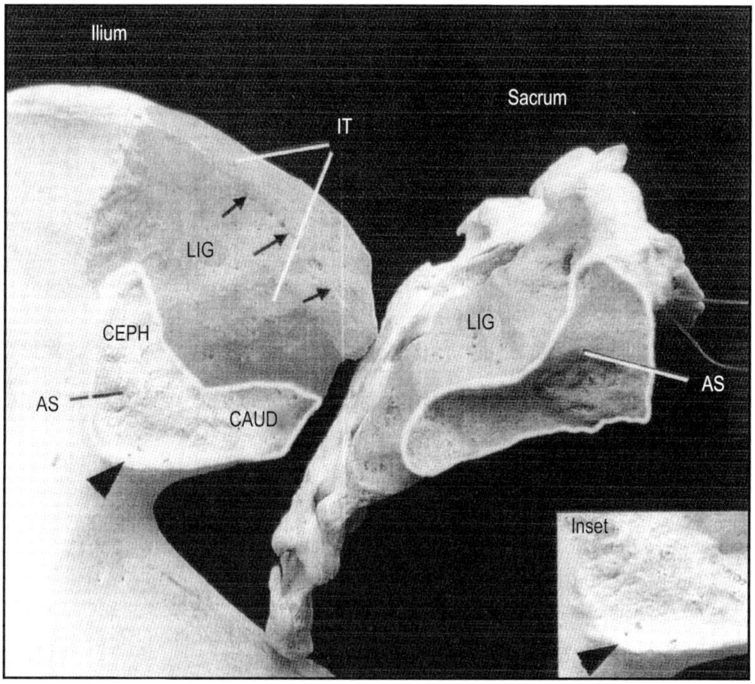

Fig. 14.1 The right sacroiliac joint is opened so that the opposing surfaces can be viewed simultaneously. The anterior (synovial) part of the joint has caudal (CAUD, nearly horizontal) and cephalad (CEPH, nearly vertical) arms that articulate in the intact skeleton. The topography of the articular surfaces (AS) is irregular but congruent, with slight convexity on the ilial side, and complementary concavity on the sacral side. Both auricular surfaces have numerous pits and surface roughenings and these are clearly visible in the inset. This is an enlargement of the iliac auricular surface – corresponding points on the two photographs are indicated by arrowheads. The more posterior part of the joint is shaded and is a syndesmosis. It provides extensive areas for ligamentous attachment (LIG), particularly the strong, interosseous ligament, which is attached to the region that lies at the center of an 'axial joint' – the pivotal point around which the sacrum rotates in nutational and counternutational movements. The erector spinae muscle is attached to the most posterior part of the iliac tuberosity (IT). A sharp ridge on the tuberosity (black arrows) demarcates the boundary between its muscular and ligamentous parts. Note the wedge shape of the sacrum, with the superior part of the bone, nearer the sacral promontory, being wider anteroposteriorly than the inferior part.

1981). In the standing position, the S1 part of the joint lies mainly vertical and its surface runs obliquely and sagittally from a craniolateral to a slightly caudomedial direction (with propeller-like contour) (Dijkstra et al 1989). The iliac tuberosity is situated dorsal to the auricular (synovial) surface of the SIJ, and anterior to the posterior iliac crest. It forms the iliac part of the 'axial sacroiliac joint' (Bakland & Hansen 1984), and extends dorsally to the posterior superior iliac spine (PSIS). The PSIS serves as an attachment for the strong, long dorsal sacroiliac ligament (LDSIL) or the 'long ligament' (Vleeming et al 1996, 2002).

Regarding the hypothesis that axial musculo-ligamentous hypertonicity might play a role in AS, the strong tendinous aponeurosis of the erector spinae (ES) muscle is closely linked to the sacrum and posterior superficial SIJ ligaments (McGill 1987, Vleeming et al 1996).

Kampen & Tillmann (1998) reported that the iliac joint surface is 'fibrocartilaginous' only in early childhood and that it becomes more hyaline with maturation. In the adult, the hyaline cartilage can reach 4 mm in thickness on the sacral surface of the joint, but does not exceed 1–2 mm on the iliac surface (Bowen & Cassidy 1981, Kampen & Tillmann 1998, Walker 1992); however, the iliac cartilage has a greater cell density (McLauchlan & Gardner 2002). Salsabili et al (1995) found that the sacral, but not the ilial, cartilage was thicker in females than males. The subchondral plate supporting the articular cartilage is thicker on the ilial than on the sacral aspect (Kampen & Tillman 1998, McLauchlan & Gardner 2002). The plate is most dense towards the cranial and caudal ends of the joint, and least dense near the center of the auricular surfaces (Putz & Muller-Gerbl 1992). The underlying cancellous bone is also denser on the iliac side (McLauchlan & Gardner 2002). The large sacrum and SIJs are believed to transfer axial forces laterally into the ilia and vice versa (Bogduk 1997). Initial sacroiliitis lesions of AS tend to occur earlier on the ilial side (Brower 1989, Dihlmann 1980, Muche et al 2003), which might be more susceptible to exaggerated compressive stresses than the sacral side with its thicker cartilage (see below).

The SIJ capsule closely follows its articular margins. In addition, the associated core ligaments (Fig. 14.2) are numerous and strong (Palastanga et al 1998), including the ventral, dorsal, and interosseous ligaments (Soames 1995). The last mentioned are most strongly developed and surround the 'axial sacroiliac joint' (Bakland & Hansen 1984). Short and long dorsal sacroiliac ligaments complement the interosseous ligaments (Vleeming et al 1996). The LDSIL, which originates from the PSIS, is the most superficially and dorsally located of the SIJ ligaments. It is easily palpable caudally, inferior to the PSIS, but is often missed because of its 'bone hard' firmness (Vleeming et al 1996). The LDSIL runs largely vertically downwards from the PSIS to the third and fourth transverse tubercles of the sacrum. This ligament particularly resists counter-nutation or the posterior movement of the sacrum relative to the ilium (Vleeming et al 1996).

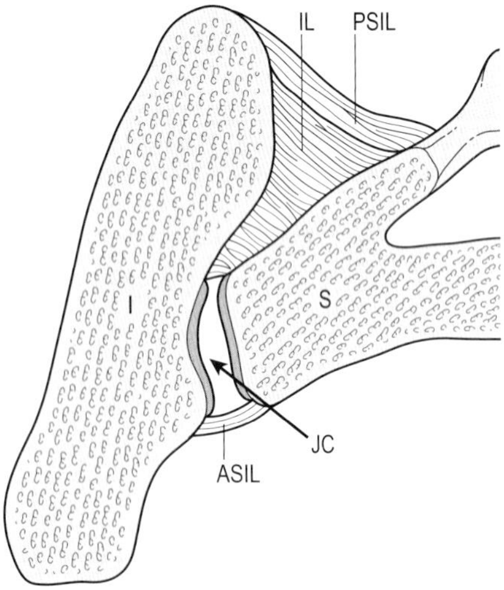

Fig. 14.2 Diagrammatic representation of a horizontal section through the sacroiliac joint. A distinction is shown between its anterior or ventral (synovial) part, in which an arrow points to the joint cavity (JC, the auricular part of the joint), and its more dorsal, posterior syndesmosis. The latter is characterized by the strong interosseous ligament (IL), which links the ilium (I) to the sacrum (S) and by the posterior superior iliac ligament (PSIL). The so-called 'axial joint' part is not visible because the transverse section is below the S1 level. An anterior superior iliac ligament (ASIL) joins the two bones in front of the synovial part of the joint.

The sacrotuberous, sacrospinous, and iliolumbar ligaments are strong accessory SIJ ligaments (Palastanga et al 1998). The iliolumbar ligaments are connected to both the dorsal and ventral sacroiliac transverse ligaments (Pool-Goudzwaard et al 2001). Notably, all of these ligaments serve for the attachment of muscle fibers either directly or indirectly, which thereby contribute dynamic support to the SIJ.

At this point, a statement on functional joint stability (or 'stiffness') is relevant to the proposed hypothesis on AS. Stability is the capacity of the system to return to its original static or dynamic state after a perturbation. Sufficient or adequate compression of the SIJs can be defined as the amount required to guarantee the necessary stability or stiffness for the particular demands of static or dynamic load transfer, at optimal utilization of energy (Vleeming et al 1990b, 2004; and see Chapter 8). Thus, stability *per se* is an instantaneous phenomenon (McGill et al 2003), and counteropposing to flexibility. Neither too little nor too much SIJ stability from either mechanical stiffness properties or force closure/compression is optimal (see below). Further research is needed on the influence of intrinsic mechanical properties (viscoelastic behaviors) of musculature, be it in isolated fiber types (Davis & Epstein 2003), natural locomotion (Dickinson et al 2000), stabilizing functions (Wagner & Blickhan 1999), or dynamic parameters of muscle (Thaller & Wagner 2004). Such challenging studies promise to clarify basic mechanical properties of muscle, and a possible role of intrinsic musculoligamentous tone or stiffness in AS (Masi & Walsh 2003, Masi et al 2003).

Innervation of the sacroiliac joints

The SIJs are richly innervated and have abundant nociceptors, but controversy exists on the spinal segments from which these nerves are derived. According to Grob et al (1995), the joint is innervated exclusively by the S1–S4 dorsal rami. In contrast, Ikeda (1991) suggests that ventral rami supply the anterior portion of the joint (upper part – L5; lower part – predominantly S2) and that dorsal rami supply the posterior portion (upper part – L5; lower part – from the sacral nerves) (see also Chapter 1).

The plexus formed from branches of the dorsal rami is complex. This network forms an intimate and poorly understood relationship with the overlying multifidus muscle and the surrounding dorsal SIJ ligaments. The medial divisions of the dorsal rami penetrate the sacral multifidus muscle, whereas the lateral divisions anastomose with each other within the multifidus compartment (Willard et al 1998). These lateral divisions exit multifidus by passing around and even through the LDSIL. As these nerves pass deep to the ligament, they flatten into a remarkably thin ribbon that contains a very delicate microvascular system for the dorsal rami (Willard et al 1998). The multifidi muscles are restricted superficially by the tight aponeurosis of the posterior layer of the thoracolumbar fascia (TLF), which is especially strongly developed and tight over the sacrum. The integrity of the delicate dorsal rami or plexus could be compromised by structural or functional changes of the LDSIL or multifidus. The anatomical arrangement could further predispose to such nerve injury in the setting of lumbosacral musculoligamentous hypertonicity. Other nerve entrapment mechanisms may occur. Alternatively, primary injury to the delicate nerves or microvascular system from inflammatory processes might secondarily activate axial muscles by altered nociceptor responsivity or neuromotor stimulation (Indahl et al 1999, 2001).

Pain induced experimentally by injection techniques into human SIJs radiates to the lower back, buttocks, and posterior thighs (Brower 1989, Fortin et al 1994a, 1994b). Nociceptors from the SIJs can sensitize the spinal cord and expand the normal anatomical pain patterns. Importantly, increased nociception might alter the normal pattern of muscle activation, and thus secondarily increase resting tension or tone (Wyke 1980). Indeed, an experimental study on pigs (Indahl et al 1999, 2001) revealed that stimulation of the SIJ within its ventral area initiated a muscular response predominately in the gluteus maximus and quadratus lumborum. However, in terms of the currently proposed hypotheses, stimulation directly under the dorsal capsule of the SIJ elicited a response predominately in the deep medial multifidus fascicles (Indahl et al 1999). Such neural pathways could potentially set up a cyclic response of: dorsal sacral enthesopathy → dorsal capsular nerve stimulation → multifidus hypertonicity → further dorsal sacral enthesopathic stresses. Wherever the process starts in the neuromotor control cycle, neural pathways might perpetuate multifidus hypertonicity. A better understanding of afferent nociceptors and reflex neuromotor pathways affecting the SIJ in normal subjects, and subjects with low back pain (LBP), will help to interpret the clinical patterns of pain and altered spinal muscular tone in AS (see below).

Kinetics and kinematics of the sacroiliac joints

Disturbed or excessive force transfers through the SIJs can cause exaggerated compressional, tensional, or torsional stresses on these joints, with altered transmission to the spine and lower limbs, resulting in deleterious tissue effects or pathoanatomical consequences (Nordin & Frankel 2001, Porterfield & DeRosa 1998). In contrast to excessive SIJ stiffness, a counteropposing condition of insufficient stability is believed to occur in the syndrome of pregnancy-related pelvic girdle pain (PGP). Insufficient and asymmetric compression of the SIJs was shown to occur in PGP (Damen et al 2002, Mens et al 1999, 2001, 2002). Non-optimal load transfers and clinical effects would be expected to occur from either the suspected excessive pelvic and SIJ stiffness (Lee & Vleeming 1998, Masi & Walsh 2003) or the documented insufficient pelvic girdle stability of PGP (Mens et al 2001).

Structural changes in the lower lumbar spine and SIJs are strongly influenced by mechanical forces associated with growth, maintaining an upright posture, and especially with bipedal gait (Abitbol 1987, Aiello & Dean 1990a, 1990b, Bellamy et al 1983, Boszczyk et al 2001a, Bowen & Cassidy 1981). Great compressional, rotational, and tensional forces are exerted on these joints (Bogduk 1997, Boszczyk et al 2001a), particularly at their ligamentous attachment sites (McGill et al 1987, Miller et al 1987) (see below). For example, pelvic girdle fractures can develop parallel to the line of the SIJs in aging persons with extra-articular fusion of these joints (Adams et al 2002).

The frequency of SIJ bony fusion with aging is variously estimated. According to Stewart (1984), 6% of male and 1.5% of female skeletons aged 50 years or older showed para-articular osteophytosis of SIJs, usually anteriorly. However, that type of extra-articular bony bridging involves ligamentous osteophytosis and is due to degenerative mechanisms. It must be differentiated from the distinctive intra-articular trabecular bony fusion of AS, found essentially only in the idiopathic form or that associated with inflammatory bowel disease (Bellamy et al 1983, Cohen et al 1967, Dihlmann 1980, Resnick et al 1975, 1977). Such intra-articular, trabecular fusion is rarely observed in older skeletal populations (Stewart 1984).

Mobility of the SIJs is mainly passive and occurs in all three major planes, normally limited to only a few degrees at most (Bogduk 1997, Sturesson et al 1989, 2000a, 2000b, Vleeming et al 1992, Weisl 1955).

No muscle moves the SIJs directly, but several can effect movements either through attachments on the innominate or by tensing the pelvic floor (Lee 2004). Various muscles, such as the rectus femoris, sartorius, iliacus, gluteus maximus, and the hamstrings have adequate lever arms to move the ilia relative to the sacrum. Also, the SIJ can be moved by muscles that generate tension along fascial lines that cross the joint (Lee 2004). Strains on the SIJ might also result from unbalanced forces acting on the ilia. Examples include increased unilateral pull through the erector spinae trunci and quadratus lumborum, and asymmetrical pull on the sacrum by the multifidus. The SIJs can be regarded as relatively stable, yet flexible, which is essential for efficient force transfers between the long lever structures of the body that are actively controlled in bipedalism, e.g. the spine and legs (Vleeming et al 1997; and see Chapter 8).

The SIJs are relatively flat (see Fig. 14.1) and are well suited to transfer the large axial and transverse bending forces required in bipedal gait (Snijders et al 1993a, 1993b). However, such flat joints would be especially subject to shear were they not sufficiently stabilized by force closure at a perpendicular vector to the articular surfaces (Lee 1999, Snijders et al 1993a, 1993b, Vleeming et al 1997; and see Chapter 8). Accordingly, in addition to the increased joint surface friction, further stability is provided to the SIJs by force closure, partly maintained by the posterior ligamentous mass (Lee 1999, Snijders et al 1993a, 1993b, Vleeming et al 1997; and see Chapter 8). Also, activation of multifidus ('pumping up') can tense the thoracolumbar fascia and effect stabilization of the posterior lumbosacral joints (Barker & Briggs 1999, Barker et al 2004, Lee 2004, Richardson et al 2002, Vleeming et al 1995). Other ligaments that stabilize the SIJs include the sacrotuberous and sacrospinous, which are partially connected and resist nutation or the forward flexion of the sacrum relative to the ilium (Vleeming et al 1996, 2002). Also mentioned, the LDSIL resists posterior extension of the sacrum relative to the ilium (counternutation) (Vleeming et al 1996).

Individual variations in normal SIJ mobility (Vleeming et al 1992) and stiffness (van Wingerden et al 2004) are less well appreciated than the considerable individual variability in its structure (Bakland & Hansen 1984, Bellamy et al 1983, Bowen & Cassidy 1981, Sashin 1930, Schunke 1938, Solonen 1957). Limited data indicate that SIJ surface area is somewhat greater in adult males than females (Ebraheim et al 2003), and this presumably reflects increased biomechanical loading in males. The reported average auricular surface area has varied from 10.7 cm^2 (Ebraheim et al 2003) to 14.2 cm^2 (Miller et al 1987), and 18 cm^2 (Sashin 1930), compared to a ligamentous area of 22.3 cm^2 (Miller et al 1987). The distance between the center of rotation of the SIJ and a vertical line drawn through the center of gravity of the trunk is greater in men than women, further indicating increased mechanical loading of the SIJ in males (Vleeming 1990). Lumbar isometric strength is also almost twice as great in males than females (Graves et al 1990), requiring greater load transfers through the SIJs of males, and consistent with their three-fold greater occurrence of AS (Masi 1992, Masi & Walsh 2003). Men are proposed to be built for greater strength and stability than women (Brooke 1924).

In both sexes, SIJ mobility decreases from birth to puberty, but then increases transiently in adult females to a peak around 25 years of age (Brooke 1924). In males, joint mobility remains low, especially in middle and old age. Pelvic ligamentous laxity is associated with pregnancy and the post-partum period (Ostgaard et al 1994), and is believed to contribute to PGP (Damen et al 2002, Mens et al 1999, 2001). However, the role of SIJ instability in other low back pain syndromes is controversial (Lee 2004; and see Chapter 8), as its structural or tissue sources are difficult to localize (Porterfield & De Rosa 1998).

The form and force closure model of pelvic function and kinematic pathways

A model to explain stability *vis-à-vis* flexibility requirements of the pelvis

Forces are efficiently transferred by normal joints and entheses (attachments of tendons, ligaments or joint capsules to bones), which balance the differing elastic moduli of the tissues being connected (Biermann 1957, Knese & Biermann 1958). Importantly, enthesial sites usually feature conjoint attachments, as the tendon of the long head of the biceps femoris sharing a connection with the sacrotuberous ligament on the ischial tuberosity (van Wingerden et al 1993). In turn, this enthesis shares a connection with the sacrospinous ligament (Soames 1995). Equally, a chain of fascial continuity links the iliotibial tract proximally with erector spinae and the lateral collateral ligament of the knee joint distally with the tendon of popliteus (Soames 1995). Such conjoint attachments contribute to a kinetic chain, which directly assists in load transfers from the spine and sacrum to the lower limbs (Vleeming et al 1996, 2002).

Importantly, stability and flexibility modes are simultaneously counteropposing states in the SIJs and place conflicting demands on its joint construction. Moment-to-moment efficient neuromotor control of force closure is required to reinforce the normal postural myofascial tone that helps counteract gravity forces (Hodges & Richardson 1997a, 1997b). Both normal postural tone and force closure provide the requisite dynamic pelvic and SIJ stability for movements and positioning, at efficient energy costs (Lee & Vleeming 1998; and see Chapter 8). Musculoligamentous tone (or prestressing) results from synergy between the myofascial tissues and its neuromotor control (Solomonow et al 2003). Muscles can compensate for loss of tension in the lower lumbar viscoelastic tissues during periods of static postures (Solomonow et al 2003). In turn, too little myofascial tone requires increased compensatory neuromotor activation, with resultant decreased precision of movements (Hodges & Richardson 1997a, 1997b, Hodges et al 1999, Layne et al 2001).

By contrast, hypertonicity generally inhibits ease of movements (Lee 2003, 2004), which we propose might occur in AS (Masi & Walsh 2003, Masi et al 2003, Viitanen 1999). Stiffness and elasticity are counteropposing physical properties ('mirror images'), which provide stability and flexibility, respectively. Inordinate stiffness at a locus in an anatomy chain (Myers 2001) diminishes force transfers and concentrates stresses at that point.

The bipedal posture that humans have adopted requires greater resistance to gravity and increased lumbopelvic compressional forces for the necessary stability, at the expense of mobility, than quadripedal existence (Abitbol 1987, 1989, 1995, Aiello & Dean 1990a, 1990b, Boszczyk et al 2001a, Lovejoy 1988). Human bipedal equilibrium stance is most efficient, with oxygen consumption being only 7% higher than in the lying position (Abitbol 1988). However, excess of either stability or flexibility of the SIJ would be disadvantageous for efficient movements and load transfers. The musculoligamentous force closure system permits efficient and large load transfers that could not be sustained by pelvic structures alone (Lee 1999, Snijders et al 1993a, 1993b, Vleeming et al 1997; and see Chapter 8). Additionally, the normal body prestressing provides the necessary postural tone demanded for gravitational forces (Gallasch & Kozlovskaya 1998).

Before actual movements take place, self-bracing or prestressing is essential in kinematic chains (Snijders et al 1993a, 1993b). A gain in stability must be achieved when either the levers are elongated or the requisite response time is shortened. This is accomplished by increasing the force closure (e.g. stiffening) of the system (Huson 1997). Such increase in stability necessarily leads to a corresponding reduction in the chain's mobility (Huson 1997). Few mentions have been made of the influences of individual variabilities in resting postural muscle tone on lumbopelvic stiffness (Hodges et al 2003, Lee 2004, Masi & Walsh 2003, Masi et al 2003, McGill et al 2003, van Wingerden et al 2004). This review calls attention to intrinsic axial musculoligamentous hypertonicity contributing to excessive lumbopelvic stiffness, and being a possible predisposing factor to AS (Masi & Walsh 2003, Masi et al 2003).

The pelvic closure model is a regional component within the integrated musculoligamentous kinematic systems in the body (Myers 2001). Such integrated kinematics can also be interpreted within broader macrostructural concepts of biotensegrity (Fuller et al 1975, Ingber 1998, 2003, Levin 1995, 2002). The biotensegrity model proposes networks of integrated musculoligamentous splinting (tensional) systems, reinforced by interspersed anatomical bony structures (compressional elements), as briefly outlined below.

Integrated pelvic musculoligamentous coupling systems

In bipedal gait, the SIJs are the 'hub' of forces transferred from the trunk to the ground and vice versa (Aiello & Dean 1990a, Bogduk 1997, Lovejoy 1998, Porterfield & DeRosa 1998, Vleeming et al 1997; and see Chapter 8). Importantly, when tissue tolerances are exceeded, forces that are inefficiently transferred, or not transferred at all, must be directly absorbed by the impacted tissues (Benjamin et al 2002, Lee 1999, Nordin & Frankel 2001, Vleeming et al 1997). Inefficient transfers increase risk of overload injury, either acutely, as in sports mishaps or trauma, or chronically, as in degenerative joint diseases or possibly in AS.

Normally, considerable compressional, rotational, and tensional forces are transferred effectively across the SIJs by virtue of the interconnected and coordinated regional musculoligamentous systems (Vleeming et al 1997; and see Chapter 8). Parts of these systems include the coupling of anterior abdominal and posterior deeper spinal musculoligamentous components (Fig. 14.3). Additionally, cross-bracing occurs in the more superficial oblique muscles of the back, e.g. latissimus dorsi and contralateral gluteus maximus, as well as in the thoracolumbar fascia (Lee 1999, 2004; Fig. 14.4). Each of these coupled, cross-bracing structures allows for both load transfers and synchronous splinting of the trunk, pelvis, and contralateral thighs. These splinting mechanisms create perpendicular compressional force vectors across the central SIJs and lumbar facet joints, which is relevant to an understanding of pathoanatomical pathways in AS.

The anterior oblique abdominal musculoligamentous system partially connects with the deep longitudinal spinal musculoligamentous systems via the transversus abdominis (TA) aponeurosis, providing stability to the trunk and lumbopelvis (Fig. 14.3). In turn, the deep posterior spinal longitudinal systems are themselves coupled via the strong aponeurosis of the erector spinae, which is partly connected to the sacrotuberous ligament and can even transfer forces to the biceps femoris (Vleeming et al 1996; Fig. 14.4). Dorsally and more

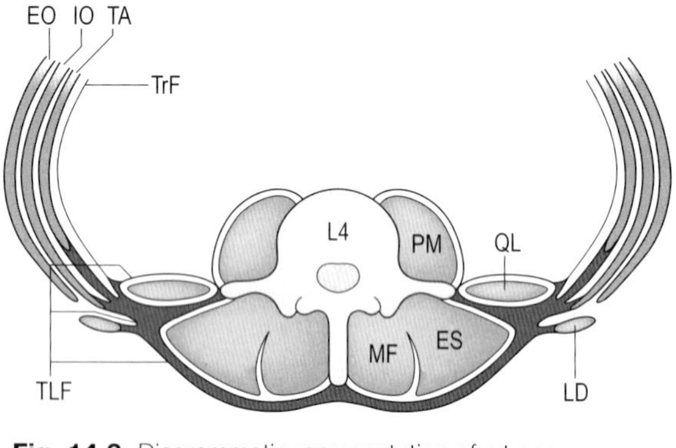

Fig. 14.3 Diagrammatic representation of a transverse hemi-section through the trunk at the level of the fourth lumbar vertebra (L4) to show the integration of the fascial networks of the spinal and abdominal muscles. Note how the three layers of the thoracolumbar fascia (TLF; i.e. anterior, middle and posterior, from above downwards in the figure) are continuous with the fasciae surrounding quadratus lumborum (QL) and psoas major (PM). The transversus abdominis aponeurosis connects to the thoracolumbar fascia, acting as a brace for the three flat muscles of the abdominal wall [transversus abdominis (TA), internal oblique (IO), external oblique (EO)]. The abdominal muscles are attached to the ribs above and to the pelvis below, enclosing the abdominal cavity and permitting 'hoop tension' support to the trunk, as in a pressurized vessel. The transversalis fascia (TrF) connects to the anterior layer of the TLF. ES, erector spinae; LD, latissimus dorsi; MF, multifidus. (Adapted from Barker et al 2004.)

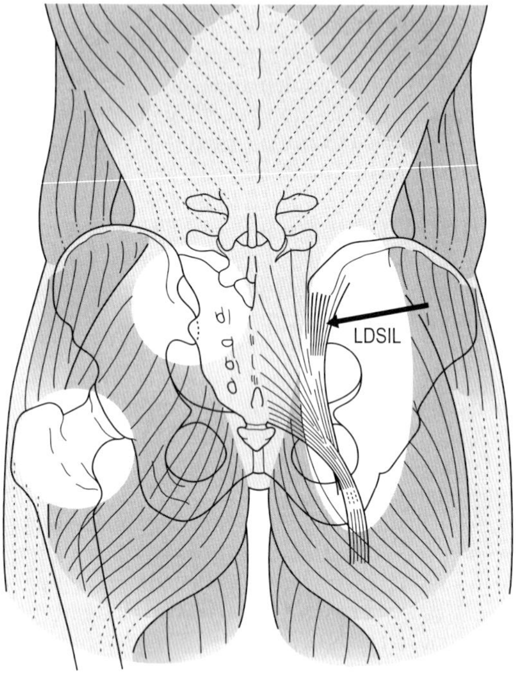

Fig 14.4 Posterior anatomical relations of the lumbopelvic region (after Vleeming et al 1995). On the left side the upper window shows the propeller-like configuration of the left surface of the sacroiliac joint (SIJ). The lower window on the left side shows the relation between posterior superficial muscles and how the pelvis is stabilized on the hip joint. On the right side, the window shows a connection between the hamstring tendons (particularly the biceps femoris tendon), and the sacrotuberous ligament that is regularly present. The arrow indicates the position of the long dorsal sacroiliac ligament (LDSIL). Note the location of the superficial lamina of the strong posterior layer of the thoracolumbar fascia (gray) over the lumbar and sacral region with attachments to both the latissimus dorsi and gluteus maximus muscles. This layer is particularly strongly developed over the sacrum. The strong aponeurotic sheath of erector spinae and multifidus is not depicted. The sacral part of the multifidus is encaged by both the aponeurosis and the posterior layer of the thoracolumbar fascia. The depicted sacrotuberous ligament has partial connections to the fascia and aponeurosis.

superficially, the latissimus dorsi is also partially coupled with the contralateral gluteus maximus via the lower posterior layer of the thoracolumbar fascia (Barker et al 2004, Bogduk & Macintosh 1984, Vleeming et al 1995; Fig. 14.4). These muscles also tend to be recruited in phasic fashion for particular activities (Mooney et al 2001). Additionally, the lateral (abductor) stabilizing system of the gluteus medius and minimus is coordinated (but not connected) with the contralateral limb adductors (Lee 1999, 2004).

Importantly, the reader should note that the hips can also be compressed from the coupling of the several musculoligamentous systems (Fig. 14.4), in addition to the highly developed abductor apparatus of bipedal humans (Kalmey & Lovejoy 2002). Such kinematic stresses might be accentuated in AS, and could relate in particular to the increased risk of hip disease in subjects with juvenile onsets (Masi et al 2001). The acetabulum is formed within the innominate by the junction of the ilium, ischium, and pubic bones, but does not fully ossify until the early twenties (Soames 1995). Such delayed ossification may lead to greater susceptibility to hip disease in juvenile AS, from excessive compressional stresses, than when disease onsets occur in mature adults (Masi et al 2001).

The principal areas of osteoligamentous support for the pelvic bone are the SIJ and the pubic symphysis, but biomechanical analyses show that the major part of load transfer is through its cortical shell (Dalstra & Huiskes 1995). Muscle forces have a stabilizing effect on the pelvic load transfer (Dalstra & Huiskes 1995). The pelvis requires stabilization for its own coordinated movements on the femurs as well as for controlled SIJ flexibility in various load transfers (Vleeming et al 1990a, 1990b, 1995). According to Bergmark (1989), the lower trunk, spine, and pelvis are stabilized by 'local' and 'global' systems of muscles engaged in the equilibrium of the lumbar spine (Figs 14.3 and 14.4). The global system consists of muscles with origins on the pelvis and insertions on the thoracic cage, which surround the abdominal cavity. The 'local' system of muscles has insertions or origins (or both) at lumbar vertebrae (Bergmark 1989). These so-called 'local' muscles are closer to the centers of rotation of the spinal elements and SIJs, than the more superficial 'global' external oblique slings, and exert higher compressive forces (Bergmark 1989).

The local muscles, including the deeper multifidus, have a biomechanical advantage in providing truncal stabilization via increased force closure/compression of spinal elements and the SIJs. As a rule, they activate before initiating gross movements of the spine or limbs (Hodges & Richardson 1997a, 1997b, Hodges et al 1999, Moseley et al 2002). Recent studies have shown that the SIJs are suboptimally braced when pelvic floor function fails (O'Sullivan et al 2002) or when transversus and multifidus have insufficient function (Richardson et al 2002) or lessened stiffness (van Wingerden et al 2004). Lumbopelvic muscle recruitment is also altered in the presence of low back or SIJ pain (Hungerford et al 2003, 2004, Richardson et al 2002).

Individual variability in pelvic stiffness – its rationale and quantitative assessment

The pelvis, including the sacrum, SIJs, innominate bones, and symphysis pubis, forms a closed ring of variable stiffness (Buyruk et al 1995, 1999, Mens et al 2001). Accordingly, requirements for pelvic stability can change momentarily, demanding greater stiffness at one instant but increased flexibility at another. The structural features that contribute to SIJ stability via 'form closure' include: (1) the configuration of the interfacing joint surfaces, including the dorsocranial 'wedging' of the sacrum into the ilia; (2) the complementary ridges and grooves of the articular surfaces of the SIJs and resultant high coefficient of friction; and (3) the integrity of the binding ligaments, which are among the strongest in the body (Snijders et al 1993a, 1993b, Vleeming 1990, Vleeming et al 1990). Beginning in puberty, the strength of pelvic ligaments is greater in men than women, and is especially reduced in women during pregnancy and labor (Solonen 1957).

Variable stiffness of SIJs was recorded in a subset of women with peripartum PGP (Buyruk et al 1999, Damen et al 2002, Mens et al 2001, 2002), by a method of color Doppler imaging of velocity (DIV; Buryuk et al 1995, 1999, Damen et al 2002, van Wingerden et al 2004). Notably, voluntary isometric contractions of various muscles that cross the pelvis, e.g. the erector spinae, gluteus maximus, and biceps femoris, were shown to increase SIJ stiffness by such a technique (van Wingerden et al 2004). Asymmetric laxity of the SIJs detected during pregnancy was predictive of moderate or severe PGP, suggesting a mechanical contribution (Damen et al 2002).

The DIV methodology is demanding (de Groot et al 2004) and had been used only in a minority subset of women with PGP who also had sufficiently high baseline SIJ laxity to detect variations in the oscillations. The observed variability in baseline DIV thresholds was attributed to possible differences in individualized resting muscle tone (van Wingerden et al 2004). The DIV technique and other clinical methods are being pursued to quantify the stability or flexibility of SIJs (Damen et al 2002, Hungerford et al 2003, O'Sullivan et al 2002, Richardson et al 2002).

Impairment of the active straight leg-raising (ASLR) test was also demonstrated in women with PGP (Mens et al 1997, 1999), and was attributed to insufficient pelvic girdle stabilization required for force transfers between the legs and spine (Mens et al 2002). In most cases, a positive ASLR test could be corrected by increased form closure (Mens et al 2001). A relation was found between impaired ASLR test and radiographic evidence of asymmetry of pelvic joints (Mens et al 1999).

Limited movements of the sacroiliac joints

Anterior flexion of the sacrum relative to the ilia or nutation is an anteroposterior rotatory movement about a transverse axis. Muscles, such as multifidus, inserting directly on the dorsal side of the sacrum, could help to nutate the sacrum (MacIntosh & Bogduk 1991). The transverse axis of anteroposterior rotation typically passes through the lower part of the iliac tuberosities (Egund et al 1978, Weisl 1955), just dorsosuperior to the synovial articulation. The strong sacrotuberous, and sacrospinous ligaments resist nutation (Sashin 1930, Vleeming 1990, Vleeming et al 1997; and see Chapter 8). To the contrary, the relatively superficial LDSIL resists posterior sacral flexion relative to the ilia or counternutation (Vleeming et al 1996). The vast interosseous sacroiliac ligament is the strongest of the SIJ-supporting ligaments and fills the space dorsal and cephalad to the synovial portion of the joint. It provides for major multidirectional structural stability (Lee 1999, 2004).

An alternative biomechanical concept proposed for low back support is that the sacrum and the spine are 'suspended' between the ilia by the strength of the interosseous ligaments (as in a 'hammock'; Levin 1995, 2002; also see Chapter 15). Under certain reduced-gravity circumstances, such a hypothesized suspension mechanism might apply to a greater degree, or possibly in springing quadrupeds (Alexander 1984), rather than in bipedal standing or human walking. Empirical data have not yet been provided to support the concept of functional suspension of the human spine under axial loads. Presumably, depending on loading patterns and the kinetic needs for greater stability versus flexibility, the 'closure' *vis-à-vis* 'suspension' models of the SIJ, respectively, could vary instantaneously to different degrees. Concepts of biotensegrity (Ingber 1998, 2003, Levin 1995, 2002; also see Chapter 15) and myofascial anatomy chains (Myers 2001) propose that stresses in the locomotor system can be dissipated through continuous tension in the musculoligamentous fascial systems plus interspersed compressional elements (Masi & Walsh 2003). Varying degrees of force closure are consistent with such a concept.

Different investigators have described rotational, gliding, anteroposterior, and vertical movements of SIJs (Bellamy et al 1983, Solonen 1957, Sturesson et al 2000a, 2000b, Weisl 1955). Rotation of the sacrum around its transverse axis at S2 is considered to be the main movement (e.g. nutation and counter-nutation; Bellamy et al 1983, Vleeming 1990). It has been estimated by radiographic techniques to be about ±2° (Sturesson et al 1989, 2000a, 2000b).

In the gait cycle, ground reaction force is transmitted up the leg at initial heel strike, and results in ipsilateral nutation (Lovejoy 1988, Vleeming et al 1997; and see Chapter 8). Following heel strike, through the midstance phase, the ipsilateral gluteus medius and contralateral leg adductors are conjointly activated, in order to stabilize the pelvic girdle laterally on the femoral head (Lovejoy 1988, Lee 1999, 2004). During the swing phase of the contralateral leg, the pelvis normally rotates axially as a unit, towards the weight-bearing limb, in a transverse plane around a vertical axis between the extremities (Aiello & Dean 1990a, Lovejoy 1988).

In normal gait, the center of gravity of the body shifts along a smooth sinusoidal curve, both vertically and laterally, no more than 5 cm (Aiello & Dean 1990a). If the pelvic girdle is either too mobile or too stiff, it becomes unable to efficiently transfer loads, and requires greater energy (Abitbol 1988, Aiello & Dean 1990a). If the pelvis becomes overly stiffened, displacements in the center of gravity become exaggerated. Consequently, greater kinetic forces and impacts must be absorbed within the attached structures and their tissues. Possibly, increased lumbopelvic stiffening contributes to the pathoanatomic lesions observed in the sacrum, spine, and lower limbs of AS (see below). When the osteoligamentous–muscular structures and systems are properly pretensed and coordinated, eccentric muscular activity during gait largely absorbs shock and attenuates forces (Lee 1999, 2004). Thus, proper osteoligamentous–muscular tensing (tone) and neuromotor control are both essential components in efficient movements and force transfers.

Pathoanatomical effects of altered biomechanical function

Physiological loading maintains the health of the musculoskeletal tissues (Benjamin et al 2002, Porterfield & De Rosa 1998, Silver et al 2003). Insufficient stimulation leads to underdevelopment or atrophy, whereas prolonged or excessive stresses can exceed tissue tolerances and cause injuries (Benjamin et al 2002). Repair of injured or inflamed tissues, with or without continuing insults, can result in compromised function, cellular, and matrix proliferation. Chronic injuries can progress to granulation tissue, calcification, or other tissue remodeling (Benjamin & McGonagle 2001, Benjamin et al 2002). Such progressive stages of healing repair occur with chronic degenerative and inflammatory conditions or excessive tissue overloading (see below).

Entheses and enthesopathies

Entheses are regions where a tendon, ligament, or joint capsule attaches to bone (Benjamin & McGonagle 2001). Disorders of entheses (e.g. enthesopathies) are commonly found in seronegative (rheumatoid factor negative) spondyloarthropathies, including AS. The spondyloarthropathies are articular conditions that affect spinal as well as peripheral joints in different degrees (Khan 2002). Fibrous entheses are tendinous or ligamentous attachments to bone, either directly or indirectly via the periosteum (Benjamin & McGonagle 2001, Benjamin et al 2002). Fibrocartilagenous entheses are more common than fibrous. The uncalcified fibrocartilage serves to dissipate bending forces on the soft tissue side of the enthesis. The much thinner zone of calcified fibrocartilage promotes anchorage to bone by increasing the surface area at that interface (Benjamin & McGonagle 2001, Benjamin et al 2002).

Fibrous entheses are usually associated with a thicker layer of cortical bone than are fibrocartilaginous entheses (Benjamin & McGonagle 2001, Benjamin et al 2002). The mechanical properties of enthesial bone are determined by numerous factors, including its trabecular patterning. Fibrocartilaginous entheses and their typically thin subchondral plate are associated with compressive as well as tensional loading.

If inflammation is involved in causing enthesopathies, the process is called 'enthesitis' (Benjamin & McGonagle 2001, Benjamin et al 2002). A wide variety of overuse or sporting injuries might not be inflammatory but instead due to overloading and microinjury or degenerative mechanisms. These conditions are more properly classified as 'enthesopathies' than 'enthesitis' (Benjamin & McGonagle 2001, Benjamin et al 2002). Enthesis-associated sites of lesions in AS and related spondyloarthropathies are well recognized in the spine and lower extremity joints (Benjamin & McGonagle 2001, McGonagle et al 1998, 2001, 2003). In AS, osteitis of subchondral bone has been identified in the SIJs prior to erosive or inflammatory synovitis change (Ahlstrom et al 1990, Dihlmann 1980, Jurriaans & Friedman 1997, McGonagle et al 1998). Altered biomechanics involving SIJs might contribute to the early osteitis lesions and secondarily to the inflammatory synovial involvement in AS (see below).

Controversy currently exists regarding primary mechanisms of enthesitis *vis-à-vis* sacroiliitis in AS. A school of thought (François et al 2000, Muche et al 2003) argues that enthesitis is not a key feature of early stages of sacroiliitis in AS. Indeed, synovial involvement is considered to be a more characteristic feature of early disease than is enthesitis (Muche et al 2003). Muche et al note that the dorsocaudal synovial region is the part of the joint that is most commonly involved in early disease (e.g. within durations up to 6 months). However, their data show an equal frequency (64%) of subchondral bone (osteitis) and synovial involvements dorsally in early diagnosed disease. An updated MRI characterization of the SIJs in AS is also described in Chapter 21. Further research is needed on the sequential evolution and mechanisms of osteitis *vis-à-vis* synovial lesions in the sacroiliitis of AS, and how these lesions might relate to enthesopathic pathways.

Forward lifting of moderately heavy loads (of 265 N) can result in extremely large forces (nearly 7 kN) on the extensor spinae, being directly transmitted to their relatively small attachment areas (entheses) at the dorsal sacroiliac region (McGill 1987). Chronically excessive musculoligamentous tensions might thereby induce microinjury at the dorsal SIJ entheses, which are frequent sites of early involvement in AS (Muche et al 2003). Excessive enthesial and compressional stresses might concur at the SIJs and activate innate inflammatory pathways in the synovial compartment (Masi & Walsh 2003, Zou et al 2002).

Tumor necrosis factor-alpha (TNF-α) is postulated to play a central role in the inflammatory processes of sacroiliitis in AS (Braun et al 1995, Zou et al 2002). Chronic injury, rather than actively acquired immunological pathways, might locally activate TNF-α in the SIJ (Masi & Walsh 2003, Zou et al 2002). Combined inflammatory and biomechanical mechanisms have been proposed as central to the onset of AS (McGonagle et al 2003) and require further investigation. Late-stage enthesopathy of the spine was studied in AS (Ball 1971, 1979) but the anatomical basis of early lesions in the SIJ is less clear and of critical importance (Benjamin & McGonagle 2001, McGonagle et al 2003). According to the MRI studies by Muche et al (2003), greater involvement was noted on the iliac (58%) than the sacral (48%) side of the joint in early disease, but not in late disease. The iliac site, with thinner chondral lining than the sacral surface, may be more prone to increased force transmissions.

Biomechanical mechanisms can be inferred from immunological specificity of tissues (Boszczyk et al 2001b, Paquin et al 1983). Also, the localization of particular lesional sites might suggest differences in degrees of compressional versus tensional stresses. For example, SIJ osteitis might result mainly from compressional (and impacting) forces versus enthesopathy lesions from sacrospinal tensional stresses on the ligamentous attachments to bone (Benjamin & McGonagle 2001). Immunohistochemical data on the molecular profile of entheses could provide helpful findings to support or refute current hypotheses (McGonagle et al 2003, Poole 1998).

A kinematic model of central sacroiliac joint compressional and vertebral tensional stresses in ankylosing spondylitis

The present review incorporates the new model of variable form and force closure of the pelvis (Mens et al 1999, O'Sullivan et al 2002, Snijders et al 1993a, 1993b, Sturesson et al 2000a, 2000b, Vleeming et al 1990a, 1990b, 1992, 1995, 1996). Whether the proposed hypertonicity in AS (Masi & Walsh 2003) is a primary constitutional trait or is secondary to other biomechanical, neuromotor, or nociceptor mechanisms is unknown and requires further research.

The current interpretation assumes that the SIJs are the 'hub' of force transfers between the spine and lower limbs (Porterfield & De Rosa 1998) and that the pelvic platform and SIJs are variably stabilized by form and force closure mechanisms (see above). This kinematic model is proposed to stimulate further research on biomechanical pathways in AS (McGonagle et al 2003). Other independent or complementary disease mechanisms (McGonagle et al 2001) are not excluded by the proposed concepts.

Structure–function relationships

In biology, form and shape adjust (and adapt) to physical forces: tension, compression, and shear (Thompson 1917). Bony protuberances, e.g. ridges, tubercles, and tuberosities, develop in response to muscle pull and thus to mechanical forces. Furthermore, trabecular alignment in cancellous bone reflects the principal direction of strain, according to Wolff's law (Thompson 1917). No data are presently available to critically determine if alterations in the trabecular patterns of the sacrum or ilia occur in early AS. However, in late stage, the trabecular bony fusion of the SIJs is distinctive of this disease. A major unresolved issue in AS is whether bony alterations can occur in the absence of preceding inflammation. The nature of the primary lesion of SIJs is presently highly contentious (Benjamin & McGonagle 2001).

Data are available on age-related changes in the articular cartilage of the human SIJ (Kampen & Tillman 1998, Vleeming et al 1992) but comparable information is not available for AS patients. The subchondral osteitis recognized in the SIJs of early AS patients by MRI is localized, particularly on the iliac and ventral side of the joint (Ahlstrom et al 1990, Jurriaans & Friedman 1997, McGonagle et al 1998). The cartilage is thinner on the iliac compared to the sacral side, and is less smooth (Vleeming et al 1990a). Radiographically, another condition, osteitis condensans ilii, shows osteitis lesions of the SIJ similar to early AS and also localizes to the inferior iliac side (de Bosset et al 1978, Dihlmann 1980, Olivieri et al 1990). This condition is not a form of spondyloarthropathy but occurs primarily in adult women and is often secondary to pelvic overloading during pregnancy. These comparisons might suggest that microtrauma could play a role in onset of SIJ disease and its localization. Unlike AS cases, patients with osteitis condensans ilii do not typically progress to erosions or joint space narrowing of less than 2 mm in an SIJ (Olivieri et al 1990).

Shear is greater on the iliac side of the joint, as the sacral aspect is loaded in a more perpendicular fashion (Bogduk 1997, Kampen & Tillman 1998). The ilial articular cartilage might be less specialized to transfer compressional loading than the sacral surface with its thicker layer (Kampen & Tillman 1998, Walker 1992). Certainly, a general correlation exists between functional loading on synovial joints and the thickness of their articular cartilage (Wong & Carter 2003). Also, a relation occurs between functional loading and development of symmetrical ridges and depressions of the auricular bone and cartilage of SIJs (Vleeming et al 1990a, 1992b).

The osteitis in AS might be analogous to compressional and impacting lesional mechanisms that have been suggested to cause bone edema of the knees in osteoarthritis (Felson et al 2003). In AS, however, the chronic central SIJ compression could also excessively immobilize and stabilize the joints, possibly explaining the unique evolution to end-stage intra-articular bony fusion.

The enthesitis process affecting the spine occurs mainly at ligamentous attachments, and accompanies the evolution of sacroiliitis (Ball 1971, 1979, Benjamin & McGonagle 2001). The spinal process was initially interpreted as an 'inflammatory enthesopathy,' in the landmark pathological study (Ball 1971). However, a subsequent report (Ball 1979), concluded that 'vertebral lesions are essentially due to trauma in a spine which for various reasons is susceptible to stress.'

One might suspect that sustained multifidus (Mf) hypertonicity could especially induce lumbosacral stress. Such hypertonicity could compress lumbar vertebrae as well as the SIJ, which are the typical sites of early AS involvements in adults. These muscles could also 'entrap' dorsal rami, which run an intricate course through the insertions on the sacrum (see above). The delicate rami also need to pass under or through the LDSIL. They innervate the SIJs, with direct or indirect consequences (Vleeming et al 1997, Willard et al 1998; and see Chapter 8). The multifidus plays a crucial role in stabilizing the SIJ due to its specific anatomy, inserting on the dorsal side of the sacrum and ilium (Bogduk 1997, MacIntosh & Bogduk 1986, 1991). Activation of this muscle has been demonstrated to stabilize the SIJs (Richardson et al 2002, van Wingerden et al 2004). The multifidus is also closely linked to the thoracolumbar fascia (Barker & Briggs 1999, Barker et al 2004; see Fig. 14.3), which is especially strongly developed, over the SIJ (Vleeming et al 1995). If hypertonicity of the erector spinae or Mf is documented in early AS, a primary mechanism would need to be distinguished from secondary activation, particularly of the Mf by posterior SIJ capsule provocation (Indahl et al 1999).

A further compounding factor in AS might be that bacterial antigens trigger immunologic or inflammatory reactions at sites of microtrauma (Benjamin & McGonagle 2001, McGonagle et al 2001, 2003, Rehakova et al 2000). Synergy between biomechanical and immune activation might be operating at localized lesional sites (Benjamin & McGonagle 2001).

Pathoanatomical evolution of lesions in ankylosing spondylitis

The features of persistence or progression of SIJ lesions are typical in AS, rather than remissions and repair (Brophy et al 2002). In adult-onset disease, AS manifestations usually begin in the SIJs and lumbosacral region and typically progress slowly up the spine, depending on the duration and severity. Such a pattern of disease progression is consistent with the relative magnitudes of force loading on the vertebral column, e.g. increasing loads at lower levels and being maximum at L5–S1 (Boszczyk et al 2001a, Lovejoy 1998).

The pathoanatomy of such distinctively progressing lesions might be conceived as a specialized tissue injury and repair process. During the evolution of this unique process, supportive stiffness of the involved structures persists, but elasticity, flexibility, and mobility functions fail, which are clinically characteristic of AS (Masi et al 2003, Viitanen 1999). Critical prospective studies, beginning at the earliest stages of AS or even prior to symptomatic onset among HLA-B27 susceptibles, e.g. first-degree relatives, are needed to test whether or not underlying axial musculoligamentous hypertonicity might predispose to such pathoanatomic processes.

Narrowing or obliteration of SIJ spaces has been commonly reported in paraplegics. However, complete bony fusion, as found in AS, is not well documented (Khan et al 1979, Wright et al 1965). Trunk mobility was proposed to be essential for maintaining SIJ integrity, and its absence in many paraplegics might compromise the structural integrity of the joint (Khan et al 1979). Whether or not excessive SIJ stabilization (compression/force closure) might similarly stress the joint requires investigation.

Lumbopelvic osteoarthritis might cause joint space narrowing and extra-articular osteophyte formation in SIJs of elderly people, but bilateral intra-articular bony fusion is rare (Stewart 1984). Such degenerative para-articular osteophytosis might immobilize SIJs and needs to be differentiated from the uncommon intra-articular ankylosis of AS (Dihlmann 1980, Resnick et al 1975, 1977). Intra-articular ankylosis of SIJs would be an exceptional finding in osteoarthritis, even in old age and with radiologically marked osteoarthrosis (Dijkstra et al 1989, Vleeming 1990). An orthopedic dictum is that compression and immobility are conducive to bony fusion (Levin S, personal communication), as can occur in the SIJs of AS. Also, enthesopathic calcification or osteophytes follow tensional stresses (Resnick D, personal communication), as occur in syndesmophytes of AS (Benjamin & McGonagle 2001).

Altered motor control of deeper core muscles, like the transversus abdominis, internal oblique, multifidus, diaphragmatic, and pelvic muscles, are believed to play an important role in back pain and support. These muscles exhibit anticipatory stabilizing ability, being activated just before gross movements (Hodges & Richardson 1997a, 1997b, Hodges et al 1999, O'Sullivan et al 2002, Richardson et al 2002). Either insufficient or excessive stiffening is believed to contribute to clinical consequences in the spine and pelvis (Lee 1999, 2004). However, specific mechanisms are not well defined. In AS, no information is available on anticipatory timing functions in early disease or on whether such alterations might play a role in the disorder.

The LDSIL has been demonstrated to be important in providing pelvic stability in women with peripartum PGP (Vleeming et al 1997, 2002). Such women show increased counternutation of the SIJ. They demonstrate tenderness on direct palpation over the LDSIL and are unable to perform the ASLR test normally, due to insufficient pelvic stability (Mens et al 1997). The ASLR test was demonstrated to be reliable in such women. Impairment was inferred to result from compromised integrity of load transfer between the lumbosacral spine and the lower limbs (Mens et al 2001). Such studies indicate that decreased SIJ stability in women might cause mechanical dysfunction. To the contrary, no data are available on functional testing or clinical sequelae of persons with excessive SIJ stiffness. Also, efficient tests, such as the ASLR, used to diagnose PGP, have not been critically and systematically applied to AS patients (Vleeming et al 2004).

Pathomechanical pathways of spinal symptoms and manifestations in ankylosing spondylitis

Essential clinical and course features of AS are summarized in Box 14.1, and are consistent with current pathoanatomical and biomechanical concepts of the lumbopelvis (De Rosa & Porterfield 1992, Porterfield & De Rosa 1998). Degrees of intensity of axial musculoligamentous force transfers in population subgroups parallel the age- and sex-specific risks for onset and course of AS (Masi 1992, Masi & Walsh 2003). Furthermore, course patterns of AS are individualized (Goodacre et al 1991), and radiologic progression also shows individualized variation (Brophy et al 2002). Such personalized host and clinical features suggest inherent variabilities of tissue tolerances to biomechanical failures. The disease course of AS is believed to be largely controlled by constitutional genetic factors (Doran et al 2003).

Typically, AS has an insidious onset of chronic back pain or stiffness in younger persons, which persists for at least 3 months, is associated with morning stiffness, and improves with physical activities (Calin et al 1977). These and the other features listed in Box 14.1 are consistent with chronic, physical lumbopelvic stiffness and thixotropic properties, e.g. reduced stiffness after movements (Masi & Walsh 2003). Excessive myofascial tone at rest or during inactivity might be contributing to the recognized patterns in AS. In contrast, most LBP is activity-related (Spitzer 1987) and typically initiated or exacerbated by postural movements that excessively load spinal tissues (De Rosa & Porterfield 1992).

Interpretation of low back symptomatology is complex and often requires precision diagnosis (Bogduk 1997, De Rosa & Porterfield 1992, Lee 1999, 2004, Lee & Vleeming 2005, Porterfield & De Rosa 1998). Many of the clinical or manual testing techniques (Kendall et al 1999) are not sufficiently reliable (Potter & Rothstein 1985, Waddell et al 1992). Thus, mechanistic judgments must be qualified at this time. Although ranges of lumbar flexion and extension movements in AS can be accurately measured (Williams et al 1993), further attention is needed to develop other standardized assessments of the lumbopelvis. Reliable clinical tests promise to provide relevant data on physical alterations in early AS, like the proposed European

Box 14.1

Pathomechanical indicators of symptoms and manifestations in ankylosing spondylitis

The following listing complements previously indicated distinguishing features of ankylosing spondylitis (AS; Masi & Walsh 2003):

- Population patterns of axial muscular forces mirror onset of age- and sex-specific risks of AS
- Subjective back stiffness often precedes or coincides with onset of back pains
- Initial pain can localize to sacral neurotomes but often involves higher spinal levels
- Disease course is persistent in mild cases or chronically progressive in the more active cases
- Individualized course patterns imply inherent risks and tolerances to tissue failures
- Inactivity magnifies spinal symptoms, suggesting a sustained force closure/compression
- Pain is typically worse at night, or upon arising, than after mobilizing and becoming active
- Unlike nerve impingements, symptoms are not typically positional- or movement-specific
- Uncomfortable movements are typically multiplanar, rather than being at 'barrier' positions
- Limitations of spinal mobility occur in all planes, and often involve chest exertions
- Slow deliberate spinal movements suggest true stiffness, rather than painful guarding alone
- Early objective firmness is noted in lumbar extensor muscles positioned in relaxed flexion
- Clinical history is consistent with chronic lumbopelvic stiffness (Calin et al 1977)

guidelines on low back pain, and especially the Working Group 4 guidelines dealing with pelvic girdle pain (Vleeming et al 2004; and see Chapter 8). The working group members recommended that the proposed diagnostic procedures for PGP be selectively applied to AS patients to determine whether the proposed tests are also valuable for AS patients.

Clinical and instrumented techniques to assess lumbar and sacroiliac joint stiffness in ankylosing spondylitis

Spinal stiffness is a core central symptom of AS in early disease, as important as pain, and often its predecessor (Bakker et al 1993, van der Heijde et al 1999). Stiffness is the counteropposing physical state of mobility, which is characteristically decreased in AS (Masi & Walsh 2003, Masi et al 2003, Viitanen 1999). Besides limitations in range of movement (Viitanen 1999), objective myofascial stiffness has not been frequently addressed in AS (Masi & Walsh 2003, Masi et al 2003). Controlled, functional manual assessments of the back should be further performed in AS (Levin & Stenstrom 2003), using standardized testing procedures (Vleeming et al 2005), which promise to provide new insights on biomechanical influences.

Reliable physical examination testing is needed for AS, analogous to that developed for SIJ pain in women. For example, the ASLR test (Mens et al 1997, 1999, 2002) verifies ability to transfer loads through the pelvis. The posterior pelvic pain provocation test (Ostgaard et al 1994) elicits and assesses posterior pelvic pain. The LDSIL test is a palpation technique to detect specific pain and tenderness in this ligament, which lies directly caudal to the PSIS (Vleeming et al 1996). It is expected that sustained increases of tension on this ligament will elicit tenderness when firmly palpated (Vleeming et al 1996, 2002). Further study is needed to differentiate which manual tests are sensitive and specific for excessive stability of AS *vis-à-vis* instability of PGP (Vleeming et al 2004; and see Chapter 8).

In unloaded, prone subjects, as when supported on an examination table, lumbar extensor muscles normally relax. In AS patients, systematic palpation for firmness or tautness of the erector spinae (ES) or multifidus at the level of L4, could help to assess the presence of axial myofascial hypertonicity (see Box 14.1). Positive findings should be distinguished as primary versus secondary alterations, and in relation to any associated LBP, tenderness, deformity, severity, and stage of disease. Significantly increased firmness of unloaded sacrospinal muscles in the earliest stages of AS might be a relatively specific finding versus other LBP patients, especially in the absence of associated pain or tenderness.

The bowstring sign of Jacques Forestier for early AS tests for palpably tensed or increased firmness of dorsolumbar muscles of the concave, ipsilateral side on passive mid-lateral inclination, which is opposite to relaxation in normals, as recently reviewed (Masi et al 2005). Further controlled research is needed of this sign in AS and other LBP patients.

Objective measurements of surface lumbar muscle stiffness or tone/compliance can be made using electronic device systems, e.g. a 'myotonometer' (Leonard et al 2003) or a 'hardness meter' (Ashina et al 1999, Sakai et al 1995). Also, good to excellent test–retest reliability was reported in a preliminary study on a new, hand-held 'Myoton-2' myometer in measurements of lower limb muscle visco-elastic stiffness (Bizzini & Mannion 2003). Such instrumentation promises to also be informative in AS, under rigorously controlled protocols and procedures to differentiate relaxed, EMG-silent versus activated status.

Lumbar spinal posterior–anterior stiffness can be accurately assessed using available electronic and mechanical instrumentation as well as strictly designed protocols (Chiradejnant et al 2003). Such noninvasive practical techniques have demonstrated a normal population distribution of posterior–anterior lumbar stiffness. Furthermore, a linear elastic component can be quantitated by mathematical modeling (Nicholson et al 2001). The latter property might reflect mainly axial musculoligamentous tonicity as opposed to other skin and soft tissue visco-elasticity. If the validity of measuring force-closure/compression of the SIJ with the DIV/oscillation method can be demonstrated (de Groot et al 2004), it too might help validate whether excessive joint stabilization occurs in AS patients.

Passive stiffness of the human lumbar torso can be quantitated (McGill et al 1994, Walsh 2003). Using a frictionless apparatus that allows the torso to 'float' on a bearing platform, stiffness in flexion/extension, lateral bending, and axial rotation can be measured (McGill et al 1994). A technique of rhythmic torques can measure physiological ranges of lower spinal muscular tonicity in axial rotation in seated position (Walsh 2003).

The musculoligamentous support system is biomechanically complex and greatly influenced by neuromotor control or reactivity (Hodges & Richardson 1997a, 1997b, Hodges et al 1999, 2003, O' Sullivan et al 2002, Porterfield & De Rosa 1998, Richardson et al 2002). Abnormalities of mobility and symptoms of pain or stiffness can result from varying degrees of: fascial–ligamentous alteration, degrees of intrinsic muscular tonicity, or sensitization of nociceptor mechanisms (Butler & Moseley 2003, Moseley et al 2002, 2003, Porterfield & De Rosa 1998).

Perhaps the most direct experimental method currently available to test the current hypothesis is direct measurement of the interstitial fluid pressure of the lumbar paraspinal muscles (Konno et al 1994, Styf 1987, 2004). Miniature transducer-tipped catheter techniques are accurate and practical on a controlled research basis, but have not yet been employed to study early AS patients (Konno et al 1994).

Clinical issues related to the kinetic concepts of ankylosing spondylitis

The dorsal sacrum and SIJ are the anatomical 'hub' of force transfers between the spine/lumbopelvis and legs (Porterfield & De Rosa 1998). Tissue failure at one level predisposes to extension of the stressful forces to adjacent levels in the axial kinematic chain, and leads to sequential injury processes. Hip involvement in AS, particularly in juvenile onset, can be contributed by excessive compressive mechanisms affecting the SIJ and pelvis stability (see Fig. 14.4), as reviewed above. The characteristic preponderance of lower, rather than upper, extremity joint involvement in AS can be contributed by excessive impacts from inefficient force transfers and exaggerated impacting. Sustained hypertonicity of multifidus might be suspected as one of the pathways that initiate increased force closure/compression of the SIJ, due to its specific anatomy.

The myotendinous systems of the body operate in an integrated fashion to provide efficient elastic energy stores in walking and running (Abitbol 1988, Alexander 1984, Lovejoy 1988, Novachek 1998). Hence, it would be practically impossible *in vivo* to separate the biomechanical functions of active contractile from passive fibrous tissues in a muscle–tendon (Walsh et al 1991), which is usually considered a functional unit. For example, a positive correlation between wrist joint hypermobility and resonant frequency of the forearm myofascial tissues has been observed in women (Walsh et al 1991).

Ligamentous laxity was reported to modulate the degree of axial manifestations in AS (Hordon & Bird 1988, Rovensky et al 2003, Viitanen 1999). Joint hypermobility is a common trait in the population, with an age- and sex-specific frequency distribution opposite to that of AS. Its prevalence is significantly greater in females than males and its incidence decreases during the juvenile years, opposite to AS. In a national UK study of female twins, hereditary factors (*circa* 70%) were shown to predominantly affect hypermobility (Hakim et al 2004). Thus, joint hypermobility and AS are both strongly determined by genetic factors. A relevant question is whether their comorbidities or co-occurrences are negatively correlated, as seems to be the case with AS and adolescent idiopathic scoliosis, a condition also associated with joint hypermobility (Masi et al 2003). Controlled clinical and genetic studies comparing these disorders promise to discriminate respective biomechanical alterations and tissue pathologies (Masi et al 2003).

Adaptive and evolutionary implications of axial musculoligamentous tonicity

In hominid evolution, empirical evidence suggests that thermoregulatory principles influenced body shape. Progressively wider bodies were found in populations from progressively colder climates (Ruff 1991). Also, local climatic conditions influenced evolution and distribution of human populations (Stringer 1995). Notably, HLA-B27 is strongly associated both with cold climates (Cavalli-Sforza et al 1994) and with AS (Khan 2002, Masi & Walsh 2003). Such relations suggest that adaptations in muscle-related thermogenesis might have occurred during human evolution in Arctic peoples (Bjerregaard & Young 1998, Fregly & Blatteis 1996). Human societies might have inhabited Arctic areas as long as 30 000 years ago (Pitulko et al 2004), rather than mainly migrating across the Bering land bridge, some 15 000 years ago. This longer existence in harsh, cold environments could have provided a longer interval for thermogenic adaptation and subsequent dispersion of the trait. Climatic selection was recently shown to influence mitochondrial DNA haplotype specificities (Mishmar et al 2003) and is correlated with differential efficiencies of energy metabolism (Ruiz-Pesini et al 2004). Studies on the energy balance and thermal efficiency of exercises of various muscle groups in persons with AS (or HLA-B27) versus controls would be relevant to the proposed concept. Preliminary data suggest that AS patients in labor occupations have lower serum lipids than matched controls (Masi & Walsh 2003), suggesting the possibility of increased energy expenditures related to axial musculoligamentous hypertonicity.

Paleoanthropologic data abundantly indicate that humans have undergone unique postcranial skeletal adaptive changes, in achieving energy-efficient, committed bipedal locomotion (Abitbol 1987, 1988, 1995, Aiello & Dean 1990a, 1990b, Lovejoy 1988, Novachek 1998). Muscular anatomy also adapted considerably, in response to the unique kinetic demands. Besides a fundamental response to gravity, postural muscle tone might additionally have provided adaptive advantages to thermal stresses. Such tonicity is proposed to be a polymorphic human trait and might contribute to clinical disorders, if the degree is either excessive (Masi & Walsh 2003) or insufficient (Masi et al 2003), and such hypothesis deserves critical investigation.

Summary

1. The form and force closure model of the pelvis was integrated with the recent concept of intrinsic axial myofascial hypertonicity in ankylosing spondylitis (AS) to explain the unique lesions of this disease in the sacroiliac joints (SIJs) and its vertebral enthesopathy.
2. Normal functional anatomy which permits balanced stability *vis-à-vis* mobility of the lumbopelvis in the erect human is reviewed, along with mechanisms of efficient load transfers between the trunk and extremities, that permit energy economies.
3. Optimal joint stiffness allows sufficient stability to control laxity and translations, but not an excess amount to inhibit mobility and efficient load transfers.
4. In AS, chronic axial myofascial hypertonicity is hypothesized to produce excess compressive closure of the pelvis and SIJs as well as increased tensional strains at vertebral attachment sites (enthesopathy), which are hallmark abnormalities in this disease.
5. Excessive axial myofascial stiffness could contribute to a preponderance of lower extremity arthropathy in AS, as well as increased risk of hip disease in juveniles.
6. The patterns of age- and sex-incidence risks of AS parallel myofascial maturation and axial muscular strength changes of the body

in development and aging. Specifically, AS predominates in males, begins in adolescence and early adulthood, and declines in middle and older ages, in contrast to degenerative disease of the spine.

7. Further controlled anatomical and biomechanical research in AS is needed for better understanding of the physiopathogenesis of this mysterious disease.

Acknowledgments

Support for this project was provided by the Department of Medicine, University of Illinois College of Medicine at Peoria, and a grant from the MTM Foundation. Sincere gratitude is expressed to Brooke Buchanan, Melissa Ginczycki, Danielle Hammond, Susan Jenkins, and Brittany Johnson for their outstanding contributions in the preparation of the manuscript, and to Doug Goessman for his expert graphic services.

References

Abitbol MM 1987 Evolution of the sacrum in hominoids. American Journal of Physical Anthropology 74:65–81

Abitbol MM 1988 Effect of posture and locomotion on energy expenditure. American Journal of Physical Anthropology 77:191–199

Abitbol MM 1989 Sacral curvature and supine posture. American Journal of Physical Anthropology 80:379–389

Abitbol MM 1995 Energy storage in the vertebral column. In: Vleeming A et al (eds) Second Interdisciplinary World Congress on Low Back Pain: the Integrated Function of the Lumbar Spine and Sacroiliac Joint, Part 1. San Diego, CA, p259–290

Adams MA, Bogduk N, Burton K et al 2002 The biomechanics of back pain. Churchill Livingstone: Edinburgh, p27

Ahlstrom H, Feltelius N, Nyman R et al 1990 Magnetic resonance imaging of sacroiliac joint inflammation. Arthritis and Rheumatism 33:1763–1769

Aiello L, Dean C 1990a Bipedal locomotion and the postcranial skeleton. In: Aiello L, Dean C (eds) An introduction to human evolutionary anatomy. Academic Press, London, p244–274

Aiello L, Dean C 1990b The hominoid pelvis. In: Aiello L, Dean C (eds) An introduction to human evolutionary anatomy. Academic Press, London, p429–456

Alexander RM 1984 Elastic energy stores in running vertebrates. American Zoologist 24:85–94

Ashina M, Bendtsen L, Jensen R et al 1999 Muscle hardness in patients with chronic tension-type headache: relation to actual headache state. Pain 79:201–205

Bakker C, Boers M, van der Linden S 1993 Measures to assess ankylosing spondylitis: taxonomy, review and recommendations. Journal of Rheumatology 20: 1724–1730

Bakland O, Hansen JH 1984 The 'axial sacroiliac joint.' Anatomia Clinica 6:29–36

Ball J 1971 Enthesopathy of rheumatoid and ankylosing spondylitis. Annals of the Rheumatic Diseases 30: 213–223

Ball J 1979 Articular pathology of ankylosing spondylitis. Clinical Orthopedics and Related Research 143:30–37

Barker PJ, Briggs CA 1999 Attachments of the posterior layer of lumbar fascia. Spine 24:1757–1764

Barker PJ, Briggs CA, Bogeski G 2004 Tensile transmission across the lumbar fasciae in unembalmed cadavers: effects of tension to various muscular attachments. Spine 29:129–138

Bellamy N, Park W, Rooney PJ 1983 What do we know about the sacroiliac joint? Seminars in Arthritis and Rheumatism 12:282–313

Benjamin M, McGonagle D 2001 The anatomical basis for disease localisation in seronegative spondyloarthropathy at entheses and related sites. Journal of Anatomy 199:503–526

Benjamin M, Kumai T, Milz S et al 2002 The skeletal attachment of tendons–tendon entheses. Comparative Biochemistry and Physiology. Part A, molecular and integrative physiology 133:931–945

Bergmark A 1989 Stability of the lumbar spine. A study in mechanical engineering. Acta Orthopaedica Scandinavica (suppl) 230:1–54

Biermann H 1957 Die knochenbildung im bereich periostaler-diaphysarer sehnen- und bandanstaze. [Ossification in the region of periosteal–diaphysial tendon and ligament insertion] Zeistschrift für Zellforschung und Mikroskopische Anatomie 46: 635–671

Bizzini M, Mannion AF 2003 Reliability of a new, hand-held device for assessing skeletal muscle stiffness. Clinical Biomechanics 18:459–461

Bjerregaard P, Young TK 1998 The circumpolar Inuit: health of a population in transition. Munksgaard, Copenhagen

Bogduk N 1997 Clinical anatomy of the lumbar spine and sacrum, 3rd edn. Churchill Livingstone, New York, p63–66, 177–185

Bogduk N, Macintosh JE 1984 The applied anatomy of the thoracolumbar fascia. Spine 9:164–170

Boszczyk BM, Boszczyk AA, Putz R 2001a Comparative and functional anatomy of the mammalian lumbar spine. The Anatomical Record 264:157–168

Boszczyk BM, Boszczyk AA, Putz R et al 2001b An immunohistochemical study of the dorsal capsule of the lumbar and thoracic facet joints. Spine 26:E338–E343

Bowen V, Cassidy JD 1981 Macroscopic and microscopic anatomy of the sacroiliac joint from embryonic life until the eighth decade. Spine 6:620–628

Braun J, Bollow M, Neure L et al 1995 Use of immunohistologic and *in situ* hybridization techniques in the

examination of sacroiliac joint biopsy specimens from patients with ankylosing spondylitis. Arthritis and Rheumatism 38:499–505
Brooke R 1924 The sacroiliac joint. Journal of Anatomy 58:299–305
Brophy S, Mackay K, Al-Saidi A et al 2002 The natural history of ankylosing spondylitis as defined by radiological progression. Journal of Rheumatology 29: 1236–1243
Brower AC 1989 Disorders of the sacroiliac joint. Surgical Rounds for Orthopedics 13:47–54
Butler DS, Moseley GL 2003 Explain pain. NOI Group Publications, Adelaide, Australia
Buyruk HM, Snijders CJ, Vleeming A et al 1995 The measurements of sacroiliac joint stiffness with colour Doppler imaging: a study on healthy subjects. European Journal of Radiology 21:117–121
Buyruk HM, Stam HJ, Snijders CJ et al 1999 Measurement of sacroiliac joint stiffness in peripartum pelvic pain patients with Doppler imaging of vibrations (DIV). European Journal of Obstetrics and Gynecological Reproduction Biology 83:159–163
Calin A, Porta J, Fries JF et al 1977 Clinical history as a screening test for ankylosing spondylitis. Journal of the American Medical Association 237(24):2613–2614
Cavalli-Sforza LL, Menozzi P, Piazza A 1994 The history and geography of human genes. Princeton University Press, Princeton, NJ, Table 2.13.2 p142–145; HLA-B27 geographic map p307, 308
Chiradejnant A, Maher CG, Latimer J 2003 Objective manual assessment of lumbar posteroanterior stiffness is now possible. Journal of Manipulative Physiological Therapeutics 26:34–39
Cohen AS, McNeill M, Calkins E et al 1967 The 'normal' sacroiliac joint: analysis of 88 sacroiliac roentgenograms. American Journal of Roentgenology 100:559–563
Dalstra M, Huiskes R 1995 Load transfer across the pelvic bone. Journal of Biomechanics 28:715–724
Damen L, Buyruk HM, Guler-Uysal F et al 2002 The prognostic value of asymmetric laxity of the sacroiliac joints in pregnancy-related pelvic pain. Spine 27: 2820–2824
Davis JS, Epstein ND 2003 Kinetic effects of fiber type on the two subcomponents of the Huxley–Simmons phase 2 in muscle. Biophysical Journal 85:390–401
de Bosset P, Gordon DA, Smythe HA et al 1978 Comparison of osteitis condensans ilii and ankylosing spondylitis in female patients: clinical, radiological and HLA-typing characteristics. Journal of Chronic Diseases 31:171–181
de Groot M, Spoor CW, Snijders CJ 2004 Critical notes on the technique of Doppler imaging of vibrations (DIV). Ultrasound in Medicine and Biology 30:363–367
De Rosa CP, Porterfield JA 1992 A physical therapy model for the treatment of low back pain. Physical Therapy 72:261–272
Dickinson MH, Farley CT, Full RJ et al 2000 How animals move: an integrative view. Science 288:100–106
Dihlmann W 1980 Diagnostic radiology of the sacroiliac joints. Georg Thieme Verlag, New York
Dijkstra PF, Vleeming A, Stoeckart R 1989 Complex motion tomography of the sacroiliac joint. An anatomical and roentgenological study. RoFo: Fortschritte auf dem Gebiete der Rontgenstrahlen und der Nuklearmedizin 150:635–642
Doran MF, Brophy S, Mackay K et al 2003 Predictors of longterm outcome in ankylosing spondylitis. Journal of Rheumatology 30:316–320
Ebraheim NA, Madsen TD, Xu R et al 2003 Dynamic changes in the contact area of the sacroiliac joint. Orthopedics 26:711–714
Egund N, Olsson TH, Schmid H et al 1978 Movements in the sacroiliac joints demonstrated with Roentgen stereophotogrammetry. Acta Radiologica: Diagnosis 19:833–846
Felson DT, McLaughlin S, Goggins J et al 2003 Bone marrow edema and its relation to progression of knee osteoarthritis. Annals of Internal Medicine 139: 330–336
Fortin JD, Dwyer AP, West S et al 1994a Sacroiliac joint pain referral maps upon application of a new injection/arthrography technique. Part I: Asymptomatic volunteers. Spine 19:1475–1482
Fortin JD, Aprill CN, Ponthieux B et al 1994b Sacroiliac joint pain referral patterns. Part II: Clinical evaluation. Spine 19:1483–1489
François RJ, Gardner DL, Degrave EJ et al 2000 Histopathologic evidence that sacroiliitis in ankylosing spondylitis is not merely enthesitis. Arthritis and Rheumatism 43:2011–2024
Fregly MJ, Blatteis CM 1996 (eds) Handbook of physiology. Section 4, environmental physiology, vols 1 and 2. Published for the American Physiological Society, Oxford University Press, New York
Fuller RB, Applewhite EJ, Loeb AL 1975 Synergetics: explorations in the geometry of thinking. Macmillan, New York, p 314–431
Gallasch E, Kozlovskaya IB 1998 Vibrografic signs of autonomous muscle tone studied in long term space missions. Acta Astronautica 43:101–106
Gerlach UJ, Lierse W 1992 Functional construction of the sacroiliac ligamentous apparatus. Acta Anatomica (Basel) 144:97–102
Goodacre JA, Mander M, Dick WC 1991 Patients with ankylosing spondylitis show individual patterns of variation in disease activity. British Journal of Rheumatology 30:336–338. Comment in: British Journal of Rheumatology 1992; 31:143–144
Graves JE, Pollock ML, Carpenter DM et al 1990 Quantitative assessment of full range-of-motion isometric lumbar extension strength. Spine 15:289–294
Grob KR, Neuhuber WL, Kissling RO 1995 Die innervation des sacroiliacalgelenkes beim menschen [Innervation of the sacroiliac joint of the human]. Zeitschrift für Rheumatologie 54:117–122
Hakim AJ, Cherkas LF, Grahame R et al 2004 The genetic epidemiology of joint hypermobility: a population study of female twins. Arthritis and Rheumatism 50:2640–2644

Hodges PW, Richardson CA 1997a Feedforward contraction of transversus abdominis is not influenced by the direction of arm movement. Experimental Brain Research 114:362–370

Hodges PW, Richardson CA 1997b Contraction of the abdominal muscles associated with movement of the lower limb. Physical Therapy 77:132–144

Hodges PW, Cresswell AG, Thorstensson A 1999 Preparatory trunk motion accompanies rapid upper limb movement. Experimental Brain Research 124:69–79

Hodges PW, Kaigle Holm A, Holm S et al 2003 Intervertebral stiffness of the spine is increased by evoked contraction of transversus abdominis and the diaphragm: in vivo porcine studies. Spine 28:2594–2601

Hordon LD, Bird HA 1988 Joint laxity and ankylosing spondylitis. British Journal of Rheumatology 27: 241–242 (Letter).

Hungerford B, Gilleard W, Hodges PW 2003 Evidence of altered lumbopelvic muscle recruitment in the presence of sacroiliac joint pain. Spine 28:1593–1600

Hungerford B, Gilleard W, Lee D 2004 Alteration of pelvic bone motion determined in subjects with posterior pelvic pain using skin markers. Clinical Biomechanics 19:456–464

Huson A 1997 Kinematic models and the human pelvis. In: Vleeming A et al (eds). Movement, stability and low back pain: the essential role of the pelvis. Churchill Livingstone, New York, p123–131

Ikeda R 1991 Innervation of the sacroiliac joint. Macroscopical and histological studies. Nippon Ika Daigaku Zasshi 58:587–596

Indahl A, Kaigle A, Reikeras O et al 1999 Sacroiliac joint involvement in activation of the porcine spinal and gluteal musculature. Journal of Spinal Disorders 12:325–330

Indahl A, Kaigle A, Reikeras O et al 2001 Pain and muscle reflexes of the sacroiliac joint. In: 4th interdisciplinary world congress on low back and pelvic pain: 'Moving from structure to function.' November 8–10, 2001, Montreal, Canada, p 134–136

Ingber DE 1998 The architecture of life. Scientific American 278 (1):48–57

Ingber DE 2003 Mechanobiology and diseases of mechanotransduction. Annals of Medicine 35:564–577

Jurriaans E, Friedman L 1997 CT and MRI of the sacroiliac joints. In: Vleeming A et al (eds) Movement, stability and low back pain: the essential role of the pelvis. Churchill Livingstone, New York, p347–367

Kalmey JK, Lovejoy CO 2002 Collagen fiber orientation in the femoral necks of apes and humans: do their histological structures reflect differences in locomotor loading? Bone 31:327–332

Kampen WU, Tillmann B 1998 Age-related changes in the articular cartilage of human sacroiliac joint. Anatomy and Embryology 198:505–513

Kendall FP, McCreary EK, Provance PG 1999 Muscles, testing and function: with posture and pain, 4th edn. Williams and Wilkins, Baltimore, MD

Khan MA 2002 Update on spondyloarthropathies. Annals of Internal Medicine 136:896–907

Khan MA, Kushner I, Freehafer AA 1979 Sacroiliac joint abnormalities in paraplegics. Annals of the Rheumatic Diseases 38:317–319

Knese KH, Biermann H 1958 Die knochenbildung an sehnen- und bandansatzen im bereich ursprunglich chondraler apophysen. Zeistchrift für Zellforschung und Mikroskopische Anatomie 49:142–187

Konno S, Kikuchi S, Nagaosa Y 1994 The relationship between intramuscular pressure of the paraspinal muscles and low back pain. Spine 19:2186–2189

Layne CS, Mulavara AP, McDonald PV et al 2001 The effect of long duration spaceflight on postural control during self-generated perturbations. Journal of Applied Physiology 90:997–1006

Lee DG 1999 The pelvic girdle: an approach to the examination and treatment of the lumbo-pelvic-hip region, 2nd edn. Churchill Livingstone, Edinburgh

Lee DG 2004 The pelvic girdle, 3rd edn. Churchill Livingstone, Edinburgh

Lee DG, Vleeming A 1998 Impaired load transfer through the pelvic girdle–a new model of altered neutral zone function. In: Vleeming A et al (eds). Proceedings of the Third Interdisciplinary World Congress on Low Back and Pelvic Pain. Vienna, Austria

Lee DG, Vleeming A 2005 The management of pelvic joint pain and dysfunction. In: Boyling J, Jull G (eds) Grieve's modern manual therapy, the vertebral column, 3rd edn. Churchill Livingstone, Edinburgh

Lee LJ 2003 Restoring force closure/motor control of the thorax. In: DG Lee (ed) The thorax – an integrated approach. Diane G. Lee Physiotherapist Corporation, Surrey, Canada. Online. Available:http://www.dianelee.ca

Leonard CT, Deshner WP, Romo JW et al 2003 Myotonometer intra- and interrater reliabilities. Archives of Physical Medicine and Rehabilitation 84:928–932

Levin SM 1995 The sacrum in three-dimensional space. Spine: State of the Art Reviews 9:381–388

Levin SM 2002 The tensegrity-truss as a model for spine mechanics: biotensegrity. Journal of Mechanics in Medicine and Biology 2(3-04):375–388

Levin U, Stenstrom CH 2003 Force and time recording for validating the sacroiliac distraction test. Clinical Biomechanics 18:821–826

Lovejoy CO 1988 Evolution of human walking. Scientific American 259(5):118–125

MacIntosh JE, Bogduk N 1986 The biomechanics of the lumbar multifidus. Clinical Biomechanics 1:205–213

MacIntosh JE, Bogduk N 1991 The attachments of the lumbar erector spinae. Spine 16:783–792

Masi AT 1992 Do sex hormones play a role in ankylosing spondylitis? Rheumatic Disease Clinics of North America 18:153–176

Masi AT, Walsh EG 2003 Ankylosing spondylitis: integrated clinical and physiological perspectives. Clinical and Experimental Rheumatology 21:1–8

Masi AT, King JR, Burgos-Vargas R 2001 Novel concepts of severity mechanisms in ankylosing spondylitis. Journal of Rheumatology 28:2151–2154

Masi AT, Dorsch JL, Cholewicki J 2003 Are adolescent idiopathic scoliosis and ankylosing spondylitis counter-opposing conditions? A hypothesis on biomechanical contributions predisposing to these spinal disorders. Clinical and Experimental Rheumatology 21:573–580

Masi AT, Sierakowski S, Kim JM 2005 Jacques Forestier's *vanished* bowstring sign in ankylosing spondylitis: a call to test its validity and possible relation to spinal myofascial hypertonicity. Clinical and Experimental Rheumatology 23:760–766

McGill SM 1987 A biomechanical perspective of sacro-iliac pain. Clinical Biomechanics 2:145–151

McGill SM, Seguin J, Bennett G 1994 Passive stiffness of the lumbar torso in flexion, extension, lateral bending, and axial rotation. Effect of belt wearing and breath holding. Spine 19:696–704

McGill SM, Grenier S, Kavcic N et al 2003 Coordination of muscle activity to assure stability of the lumbar spine. Journal of Electromyography and Kinesiology 13: 353–359

McGonagle D, Gibbon W, O'Connor P 1998 Characteristic magnetic resonance imaging (MRI) entheseal changes of knee synovitis in spondylarthropathy. Arthritis and Rheumatism 41:694–700

McGonagle D, Stockwin L, Isaacs J et al 2001 An enthesitis based model for the pathogenesis of spondyloarthropathy. Additive effects of microbial adjuvant and biomechanical factors at disease sites. Journal of Rheumatology 28:2155–2159

McGonagle D, Marzo-Ortega H, Benjamin M et al 2003 Report on the Second International Enthesitis Workshop. Arthritis and Rheumatism 48:896–905

McLauchlan GJ, Gardner DL 2002 Sacral and iliac articular cartilage thickness and cellularity: relationship to subchondral bone end-plate thickness and cancellous bone density. Rheumatology 41:375–380

Mens JMA, Vleeming A, Snijders CJ et al 1997 Active straight leg raising test: a clinical approach to the load transfer function of the pelvic girdle. In: Vleeming A et al (eds) Movement, stability and low back pain: the essential role of the pelvis. Churchill Livingstone, New York, p425–431

Mens JMA, Vleeming A, Snijders CJ et al 1999 The active straight leg raising test and mobility of the pelvic joints. European Spine Journal 8:468–473

Mens JMA, Vleeming A, Snijders CJ et al 2001 Reliability and validity of the active straight leg raise test in posterior pelvic pain since pregnancy. Spine 26:1167–1171

Mens JMA, Vleeming A, Snijders CJ et al 2002 Validity of the active straight leg raise test for measuring disease severity in patients with posterior pelvic pain after pregnancy. Spine 27:196–200

Miller JAA, Schultz AB, Andersson GBJ 1987 Load-displacement behavior of sacroiliac joints. Journal of Orthopaedic Research 5:92–101

Mishmar D, Ruiz-Pesini E, Golik P et al 2003 Natural selection shaped regional mtDNA variation in humans. Proceedings of the National Academy of Sciences of the United States of America 100:171–176

Mooney V, Pozos R, Vleeming A et al 2001 Exercise treatment for sacroiliac pain. Orthopedics 24:29–32

Moseley GL, Hodges PW, Gandevia SC 2002 Deep and superficial fibers of the lumbar multifidus muscle are differentially active during voluntary arm movements. Spine 27:E29–E36.

Moseley GL, Hodges PW, Gandevia SC 2003 External perturbation of the trunk in standing humans differentially activates components of the medial back muscles. Journal of Physiology 547:581–587

Muche B, Bollow M, Francois RJ et al 2003 Anatomic structures involved in early- and late-stage sacroiliitis in spondylarthritis: a detailed analysis by contrast-enhanced magnetic resonance imaging. Arthritis and Rheumatism 48:1374–1384

Myers TW 2001 Anatomy trains: myofascial meridians for manual and movement therapists. Churchill Livingstone, Edinburgh

Nicholson L, Maher C, Adams R et al 2001 Stiffness properties of the human lumbar spine: a lumped parameter model. Clinical Biomechanics 16:285–292

Nordin M, Frankel VH (eds) 2001 Basic biomechanics of the musculoskeletal system, 3rd edn. Lippincott Williams and Wilkins, Philadelphia, PA

Novachek TF 1998 The biomechanics of running. Gait and Posture 7:77–95

Olivieri I, Gemignani G, Camerini E et al 1990 Differential diagnosis between osteitis condensans ilii and sacroiliitis. Journal of Rheumatology 17:1504–1512

Östgaard HC, Zetherström GBJ, Roos-Hansson E 1994 The posterior pelvic pain provocation test in pregnant women. European Spine Journal 3:258–260

O'Sullivan PB, Beales DJ, Beetham JA et al 2002 Altered motor control strategies in subjects with sacroiliac joint pain during the active straight leg raise test. Spine 27: E1–E8

Palastanga N, Field D, Soames RW 1998 Anatomy and human movement: structure and function, 3rd edn. Butterworth Heinemann, Oxford, UK

Paquin JD, van der Rest M, Marie PJ et al 1983 Biochemical and morphologic studies of cartilage from the adult human sacroiliac joint. Arthritis and Rheumatism 26:887–895

Pitulko VV, Nikolsky PA, Girya EY et al 2004 The Yana RHS Site: humans in the arctic before the last glacial maximum. Science 303:52–56

Poole AR 1998 The histopathology of ankylosing spondylitis: are there unifying hypotheses? The American Journal of the Medical Sciences 316:228–233

Pool-Goudzwaard A, Kleinrensink GJ, Snijders CJ et al 2001 The sacroiliac part of the iliolumbar ligament. Journal of Anatomy 199:457–463

Porterfield JA, DeRosa C 1998 Mechanical low back pain: perspectives in functional anatomy, 2nd edn. WB Saunders, Philadelphia, PA

Potter NA, Rothstein JM 1985 Intertester reliability for selected clinical tests of the sacroiliac joint. Physical Therapy 65:1671–1675

Puhakka KB, Melsen F, Jurik AG et al 2004 MR imaging of

the normal sacroiliac joint with correlation to histology. Skeletal Radiology 33:15–28 [E-pub November 2003]

Putz R, Muller-Gerbl M 1992 Anatomic characteristics of the pelvic girdle. Unfallchirurg 95:164–167

Rehakova Z, Capkova J, Stepankova R et al 2000 Germ-free mice do not develop ankylosing enthesopathy, a spontaneous joint disease. Human Immunology 61:555–558

Resnick D, Niwayama G, Goergen TG 1975 Degenerative disease of the sacroiliac joint. Journal of Investigative Radiology 10:608–621

Resnick D, Niwayama G, Goergen TG 1977 Comparison of radiographic abnormalities of the sacroiliac joint in degenerative disease and ankylosing spondylitis. American Journal of Roentgenology 128:189–196

Richardson CA, Snijders CJ, Hides JA et al 2002 The relationship between the transversely oriented abdominal muscles, sacroiliac joint mechanics, and low back pain. Spine 27:399–405

Rovensky J, Zlnay M, Zlnay D 2003 Marfans syndrome and ankylosing spondylitis. Israel Medical Association Journal 5:153 (Letter)

Ruff CB 1991 Climate and body shape in hominid evolution. Journal of Human Evolution 21:81–105

Ruiz-Pesini E, Mishmar D, Brandon M et al 2004 Effects of purifying and adaptive selection on regional variation in human mtDNA. Science 303:223–226

Sakai F, Ebihara S, Akiyama M et al 1995 Pericranial muscle hardness in tension-type headache. A non-invasive measurement method and its clinical application. Brain 118:523–531

Salsabili N, Valojerdy MR, Hogg DA 1995 Variations in thickness of articular cartilage in the human sacroiliac joint. Clinical Anatomy 8:388–390

Sashin D 1930 A critical analysis of the anatomy and the pathologic changes in sacroiliac joints. Journal of Bone and Joint Surgery 12:891–910

Schunke GB 1938 The anatomy and development of the sacroiliac joint in man. The Anatomical Record 72: 313–331

Silver FH, DeVore D, Siperko LM 2003 Invited review: role of mechanophysiology in aging of ECM: effects of changes in mechanochemical transduction. Journal of Applied Physiology 95:2134–2141

Snijders CJ, Vleeming A, Stoeckart R 1993a Transfer of lumbosacral load to iliac bones and legs. Part I: Biomechanics of self-bracing of the sacroiliac joints and its significance for treatment and exercise. Clinical Biomechanics 8:285–294

Snijders CJ, Vleeming A, Stoeckart R 1993b Transfer of lumbosacral load to iliac bones and legs. Part II: Loading of the sacroiliac joints when lifting in a stooped posture. Clinical Biomechanics 8:295–301

Soames RW 1995 Skeletal system In: Bannister LH et al (eds) Gray's anatomy, 38th edn. Churchill Livingstone, Edinburgh, p425–900

Solomonow M, Baratta RV, Banks A et al 2003 Flexion-relaxation response to static lumbar flexion in males and females. Clinical Biomechanics 18:273–279

Solonen KA 1957 The sacroiliac joint in the light of anatomical, roentgenological and clinical studies. Acta Orthopaedica Scandinavica (suppl) 27:1–127

Spitzer WO 1987 Quebec task force on spinal disorders: scientific approach to the assessment and management of activity-related spinal disorders. Spine 12:S1–S58

Stewart TD 1984 Pathologic changes in aging sacroiliac joints. A study of dissecting room skeletons. Clinical Orthopedics and Related Research 183:188–196

Stringer CB 1995 The evolution and distribution of later Pleistocene human populations. In: Vrba ES et al (eds). Paleoclimate and evolution, with emphasis on human origins. Yale University Press, New Haven, CT, p524–531

Sturesson B, Selvik G, Udén A 1989 Movements of the sacroiliac joints. A roentgen stereophotogrammetric analysis. Spine 14:162–165

Sturesson B, Udén A, Vleeming A 2000a A radiostereometric analysis of the movements of the sacroiliac joints in the reciprocal straddle position. Spine 25:214–217

Sturesson B, Udén A, Vleeming A 2000b A radiostereometric analysis of movements of the sacroiliac joints during the standing hip flexion test. Spine 25:364–368

Styf J 1987 Pressure in the erector spinae muscle during exercise. Spine 12:675–679

Styf J 2004 Compartment syndromes: diagnosis, treatment, and complications. CRC Press, Boca Raton, FL, p1–8, p235–256, p257–282

Thaller S, Wagner H 2004 The relation between Hill's equation and individual muscle properties. Journal of Theoretical Biology 231:319–332

Thompson DW 1917 On growth and form. Cambridge University Press, Cambridge, UK

van der Heijde D, van der Linden S, Dougados M et al 1999 Ankylosing spondylitis: plenary discussion and results of voting on selection of domains and some specific instruments. Journal of Rheumatology 26:1003–1005

van Wingerden JP, Vleeming A, Snijders CJ et al 1993 A functional–anatomical approach to the spine–pelvis mechanism: interaction between the biceps femoris muscle and the sacrotuberous ligament. European Spine Journal 2:140–144

van Wingerden JP, Vleeming A, Buyruk HM et al 2004 Stabilization of the sacroiliac joint in vivo: verification of muscular contribution to force closure of the pelvis. European Spine Journal 13:199–205.

Viitanen JV 1999 Do pathological opposites cancel each other out? Do all patients with both hypermobility and spondyloarthropathy fulfill a criterion of any disease? Scandinavian Journal of Rheumatology 28:120–122

Vleeming A 1990 The sacroiliac joint. A clinical–anatomical, biomechanical and radiological study. Thesis, Erasmus University, Rotterdam

Vleeming A, Stoeckart R, Volkers ACW et al 1990a Relation between form and function in the sacroiliac joint. Part I: clinical anatomical aspects. Spine 15:130–132

Vleeming A, Volkers ACW, Snijders CJ et al 1990b Relation between form and function in the sacroiliac joint. Part II: biomechanical aspects. Spine 15:133–136

Vleeming A, van Wingerden JP, Dijkstra PF et al 1992 Mobility in the sacroiliac joints in the elderly: a kinematic and radiological study. Clinical Biomechanics 7:170–176

Vleeming A, Pool-Goudzwaard AL, Stoeckart R et al 1995 The posterior layer of the thoracolumbar fascia. Its function in load transfer from spine to legs. Spine 20:753–758

Vleeming A, Pool-Goudzwaard AL, Hammudoghlu D et al 1996 The function of the long dorsal sacroiliac ligament: its implication for understanding low back pain. Spine 21:556–562

Vleeming A, Snijders CJ, Stoeckart R et al 1997 The role of the sacroiliac joints in coupling between spine, pelvis, legs and arms. In: Vleeming A et al (eds) Movement, stability and low back pain: the essential role of the pelvis. Churchill Livingstone, New York, p53–71

Vleeming A, de Vries HJ, Mens JMA et al 2002 Possible role of the long dorsal sacroiliac ligament in women with peripartum pelvic pain. Acta Obstetricia et Gynecologica Scandinavica 81:430–436

Vleeming A, Albert H, Lee D et al 2004 A definition of joint stability. In: European COST guideline report, Working Group 4

Waddell G, Somerville D, Henderson I et al 1992 Objective clinical evaluation of physical impairment in chronic low back pain. Spine 17:617–628

Wagner H, Blickhan R 1999 Stabilizing function of skeletal muscles: an analytical investigation. Journal of Theoretical Biology 199:163–169

Walker JM 1992 The sacroiliac joint: a critical review. Physical Therapy 72:903–916

Walsh EG 1992 Muscles, masses, and motion: the physiology of normality, hypertonicity, spasticity, and rigidity. MacKeith Press, London

Walsh EG 2003 Axial rotation of the lower human spine by rhythmic torques automatically generated at the resonant frequency. Experimental Physiology 88: 305–308

Walsh EG, Lambert M, Wright GW et al 1991 Resonant frequency at the wrist in hypermobile women. Experimental Physiology 76:271–275

Weisl H 1955 The movements of the sacroiliac joint. Acta Anatomica 23:80–91

Willard FH, Carreiro JE, Manko W 1998 The long posterior interosseous ligament and the sacrococcygeal plexus. In: Vleeming A, Mooney V, Tilscher H , Dorman T, Snijders C J (eds) Third interdisciplinary world congress on low back and pelvic pain, Office of Continuing Medical Education, University of California, San Diego, CA

Williams R, Binkley J, Bloch R et al 1993 Reliability of the modified-modified Schöber and double inclinometer methods for measuring lumbar flexion and extension. Physical Therapy 73:26–37

Wong M, Carter DR 2003 Articular cartilage functional histomorphology and mechanobiology: a research perspective. Bone 33:1–13

Wright V, Catterall RD, Cook JB 1965 Bone and joint changes in paraplegic men. Annals of Rheumatic Diseases 24:419–431

Wyke B 1980 The neurology of low back pain. In: Jayson MIV (ed) The lumbar spine and back pain, 2nd edn. Pitman, London, p265–339

Zou JX, Braun J, Sieper J 2002 Immunological basis for the use of TNF alpha-blocking agents in ankylosing spondylitis and immunological changes during treatment. Clinical and Experimental Rheumatology:S34–S37

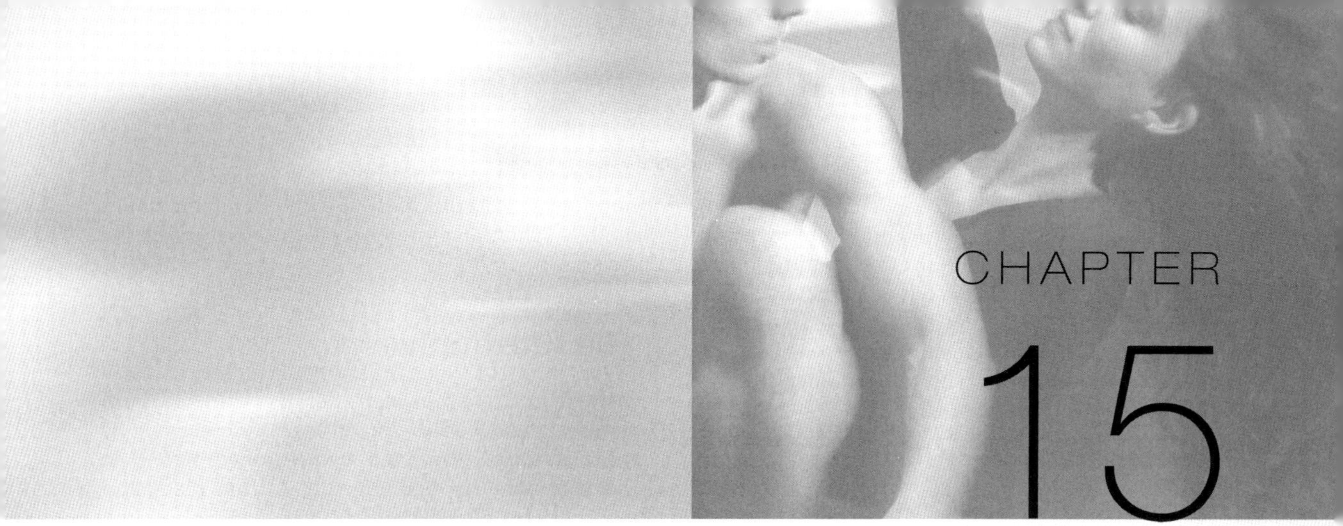

CHAPTER 15

A suspensory system for the sacrum in pelvic mechanics: biotensegrity

SM Levin

The paradigm

According to conventional wisdom, the human spine behaves as an architectural column or pillar and transfers the superincumbent weight through the sacrum, to the ilium, through the hips and down the lower extremities. The pillar holds the base in place with the pressing weight of gravity. In this model, the sacrum, as the base, locks into the pelvis, either as a wedge or by some other gravity-dependent closure.

In a tensegrity model as applied to biologic structures – biotensegrity – the bones of the skeleton are not considered a supporting column but compression elements enmeshed in the interstices of a highly organized tension network. The bones, including the sacrum, 'float' in this network much like the hub of a wire spoke cycle wheel suspended in its tension-spoke network.

The anomalies

Architectural pillars orient vertically and function only in a gravity field and are rigid, immobile, base heavy, and unidirectional. Pillars and columns resist compression forces well but need reinforcement when stressed by bending moments and shear. Stressed by internal shear, they are high-energy-consuming structures. Rigid Newtonian mechanical laws govern conventional columns. If biologic systems conformed to these laws, the human bony spine would bend with less than the weight of the head on top of it (Morris & Lucas 1964) and the vertebral bodies would crush under the leverage of a fly rod held in a hand. Animals larger than a lion would continually break their bones, and dinosaurs and mastodons larger than a present-day elephant would have been crushed under their own weight. Urinary bladders and pregnant uteri would burst when full and, with each heartbeat, arteries would lengthen enough to crowd the brain out of the skull (Gordon 1978).

Although it is a teleological conceit that the human spine acts as a column, phylogenetic and ontogenetic development of the human spine was not in the form of a column, but as some form of a beam. It would not be an ordinary beam – a rigid bar – but an extraordinary beam composed of rigid body segments connected by flexible connective tissue elements that floated the segments in space (Fielding et al 1976). During human gestational development and during the first year or so of life, when a child does no more than crawl, the human spine does not function as a column but as such a beam. In many postures the human spine does not function as a column or even a simple beam. When the spine is horizontal, as when crawling or swimming, the sacrum is not a base of a column but the connecting element that ties the articulated beam to the pelvic ring. Even when upright, the vertebral blocks are not fixed by the weight of the load above, as they would be in an architectural pillar. S-shaped curves can create intolerable loads and instability in a column, particularly if it is an articulated column that has flexible, near-frictionless joints, as does the spine. With each breath, the interconnected vertebrae translate, some forward, some backward. Whereas architectural columns bear loads from above, the human spine can accept loads from any direction with arms and legs cantilevered out in any way. The hallmark of a pillar is stability, but the hallmark of a spine is flexibility and movement. Movement of an articulated column, even along a horizontal, is more challenging than moving an upright Titan missile to its launch pad. The spine can bend forward so people can touch their toes and bend backward almost equally well. It can twist and bend simultaneously. It can perform intricately controlled movements in space, as in gymnastics, dance, aquatic diving, or basketball. The spine is flexible, mobile, functionally independent of gravity, and has property behavior inconsistent with an architectural column or beam.

In all studies, the spine, unlike columns and beams, is a low energy consumer. The individual components of the spine, and indeed the structure as a whole, behave non-linearly and do not conform to the standard linear Newtonian mechanical laws that govern columns and beams (Fox 1988, Panjabi & White 2001). In an attempt to make complex problems simple, bioengineers have converted non-linear complexities to linear mathematics models. This misrepresents the true nature of the structures.

The alternative

Instead of a column, consider the spine to be a series of rigid bodies, like a beaded chain. Just as the beads are connected by tensioned wires, so the vertebrae are tied together by the discs and soft tissues. The sacrum is the connecting link to the pelvis, but what locks the sacrum in place so that the spine is supported in all its functions? An omnidirectional mechanical system exists that can function in any posture and be capable of transferring considerable loads, coming from any direction, through the pelvis and to the lower extremities. Such a system must be consistent with evolutionary theory. It must also be structurally hierarchical so that in any instant in its ontological development it is mechanically functional and stable. (Embryos and fetuses do not fall apart either in or out of the womb.)

Kinematics

The kinematics of the pelvis must take into account mechanical laws that affect a free body in space. A rigid body in space is described as having six degrees of freedom of movement in a three-dimensional Cartesian coordinate system (Fig. 15.1). However, although in classical mechanics there are six degrees of freedom, others have considered that describing twelve degrees of freedom – six positive and six negative – might be more useful. This system seems suitable for describing the complex movements of the sacrum. Before we can discuss the dynamics of the sacrum or any other structure, we should understand the statics of that structure. How is the sacrum stabilized in its position in the body?

Statics

To fix in space a body that has twelve degrees of freedom, it seems logical that there need to be twelve restraints. Fuller (1975) proves this (Fig. 15.2). This principle is demonstrated in a wire-spoke bicycle wheel. A minimum of twelve tension spokes rigidly fixes the hub in space (anything more than twelve is a fail-safe mechanism) (Fig. 15.3). In a bicycle wheel, tension-loaded spokes transmit compressive loads from the frame and the ground. The hub remains suspended in its tension network and the compression loads distribute around the rim. The compression elements are discontinuous and behave in a counterintuitive way. Rather than becoming the primary support elements of the system, as they would be in a pillar or wagon wheel model, the compression elements become secondary to the tension support network. Fuller (1975) calls these structures 'tensegrity' structures, a contraction of 'tension integrity'. Tensegrity structures transmit loads through tension and compression only. Because they are fully triangulated, there are no bending moments in these structures, nor is there shear. The most frequently used model of the pelvis conceives of the sacrum as a 'keystone' of a Roman arch wedged between the wings of the ilia. Anatomists have long recognized that the sacrum hangs from the ilia by its ligaments (Grant 1952, Kapandji 1977) (Fig. 15.4). Dijkstra (see Chapter 20) and DonTigny (see Chapter 18) illustrate this anatomic configuration. Rather than being a 'keystone' in a Roman arch, the sacrum is the reverse of a keystone with the articular surfaces of the sacrum farther apart in front than they are behind, which would allow the sacrum to sink into the pelvis. It is as if the sacrum was hanging on the undersurface of a slippery rock face. The small ridges and rough surfaces described at the articular interface could not keep it from falling. Arches are unidirectional and depend on gravity to hold everything in place. The whole concept of an arch falls apart when a biped stands on one leg. The 'arch' becomes a cantilever with completely different mechanics than

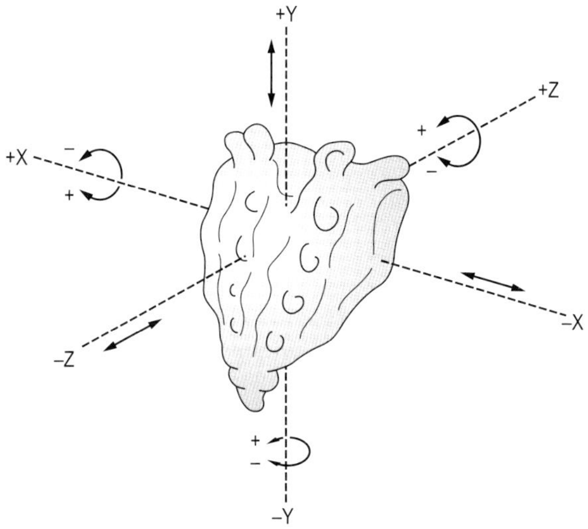

Fig. 15.1 The sacrum in a three-dimensional Cartesian coordinate system. A body can be described as rotating around the three axes, X, Y and Z, in one direction, positively (+), or the other, negatively (–). It also can be described as translating (+) or (–) in the XY, XZ, or YZ planes. A body free to move in any direction is characterized as having 12 degrees of freedom.

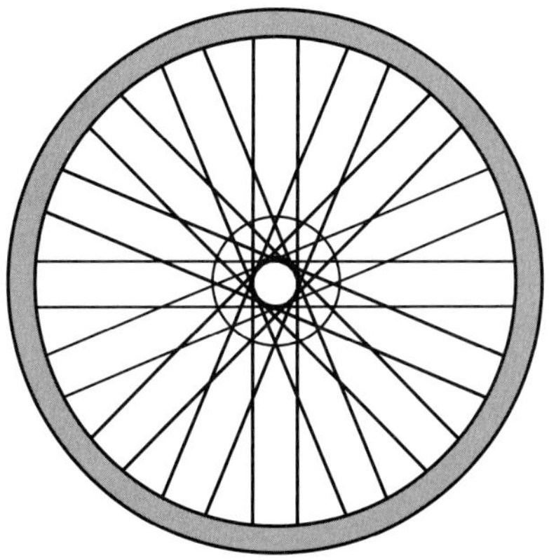

Fig. 15.3 A wire-spoke cycle wheel. The hub is rigidly fixed in a tension network. The compressive load applied to the hub by the weight of the load is transferred to the rim solely through tension. The load distributes evenly around the rim. The bicycle frame and its load hang from the hubs like a hammock between trees.

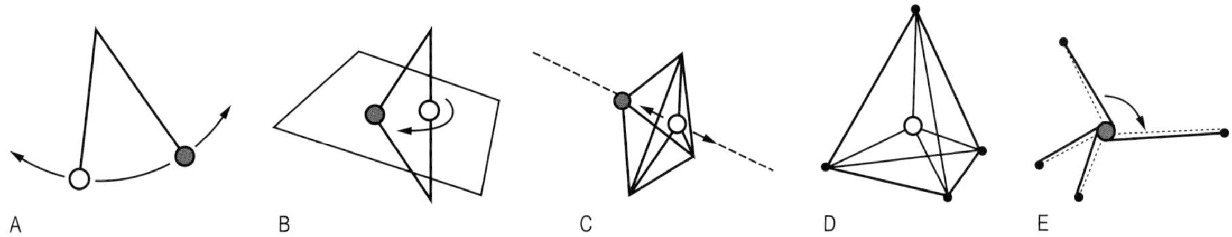

Fig. 15.2 Fixing a point in space. Four vectors of restraint define a minimum system in which a point is fixed in space (D). However, turbining is still possible (E). An additional eight restraints are needed to rigidly fix a point. (Adapted from Fuller 1975.)

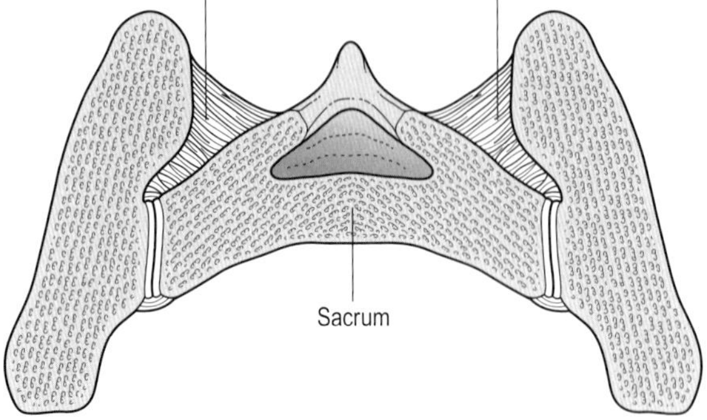

Fig. 15.4 The sacrum suspended from the ilia by the interosseous sacroiliac ligaments. (Adapted from Grant 1952, p 340.)

a weight-bearing arch. Form fit is not an option in a cantilever. Force fit will require exceedingly high friction and huge musculoligamentous forces that are, in addition to being exceedingly inefficient, not available in the pelvic constructs of vertebrates.

A ligamentous tension system for support and stability is consistent with the known anatomy. If we use a bicycle wheel tensegrity structure as our model for the pelvis, the pelvic ring would be the rim and the sacrum would be the hub of the pelvis. The many tension elements of ligaments and muscles attached to the sacrum stabilize it (Fig. 15.5). The sacrum suspends as a compression element within the musculoligamentous envelope and transfers its loads through that tension network. Even when a person stands on one leg, the sacrum sits within its tension network. This tension network provides omnidirectional structural stability, independent of gravity and hierarchical. The rim could distribute its load, rather than locally loading the forces at a point.

In a tensegrity system, the forces generated at the hip would not concentrate in the acetabulum but be efficiently distributed throughout the rim, the pelvic bones and soft tissue. The sacrum would remain suspended in its soft tissue envelope (Willard 1995; also see Chapter 1) and transmit the loads above and the forces below through the pelvic ligaments and muscles. Suspended in its tension network, it does not require gravity to hold it in place, as does a keystone model. The tensegrity-modeled sacrum functions right side up, upside down, or sideways. A tension-fixed sacrum works equally well for the upright or space-walking human, the horizontal horse, the flying bat, or the swimming otter. It is the most widely adaptable, and therefore the most likely, pelvic model.

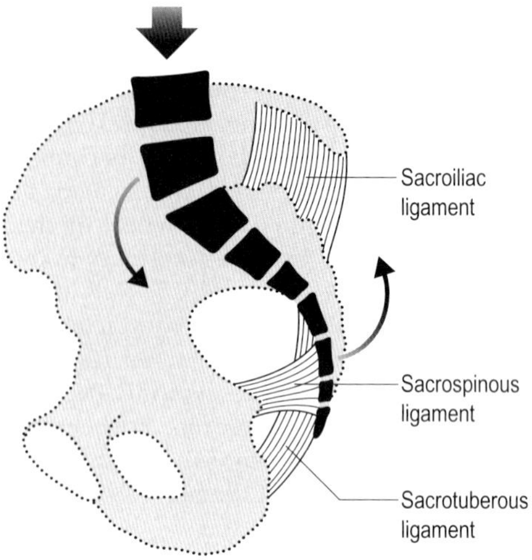

Fig. 15.5 The sacrum suspends in the pelvic ring by its many ligaments. Motion is restricted by the balanced tension of these ligaments.

Dynamics

As a hub suspended by its spokes, the tension system must have a dynamic balance of the tension structures. A load on the wheel hub does not change its relative position within the rim. If the tension of the spokes remains constant and the spokes do not distort, the hub does not move at all. Ligaments of the body, likewise, have a high tensile strength and do not distort much when loaded. Assuming a minimum of properly vectored restraints, as with the bicycle model, the sacrum cannot translate or rotate in any direction. It is fixed in position as is the hub of a wheel. Some of the restraints would have to be altered to allow pistoning or rotation to occur. However, if the sacrum moves in tandem with the other bones of the pelvis, so that the ligaments remain at the same length, tension-coupled movement patterns occur.

The body does have this coupled movement option available. It is present in the double tie bar hinge mechanism that is the model for the dynamics of knee movement (Dye 1987, Muller 1983). This type of movement occurs in the 'Jacob's ladder' (Fig. 15.6), an old children's toy. This is a series of tiles connected by crossed ribbons under tension. Flipping one of the tiles creates a controlled tumble. If the end tiles are held apart so that the entire structure is held in tension, the coupled tumbling can occur from top to bottom, bottom to top or sideways. This crossed ligament pattern, clearly

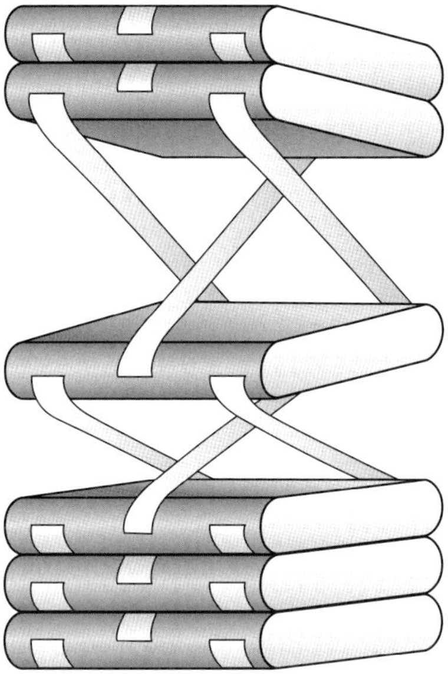

Fig 15.6 Jacob's ladder. Tilting a rigid tile at one end creates a controlled tumble of the other tiles by a crossed tie bar mechanism. The ties remain of the same length and tension throughout the movement.

evident in the knee, also exists in the spine, at the disc, ligament, and muscle level (Gracovetsky 1988, Kapandji 1977). It explains the coupled motion observed in the spine (White & Panjabi 1978). It is also evident in other joints, such as the capsular ligaments of the hip and the crossed patterns of ligaments and muscles of the back. This crossed tie bar pattern is present at the sacroiliac joints (SIJs) with the crossing patterns of the numerous muscles and soft tissues of the pelvis–spine–hip complex well described in several other chapters of this book. The crossed tie bar mechanism at the SIJ would account for the 'click-clack' phenomenon of the sacrum recognized by Snijders et al (1997). By rotating the ilia, as we do when we walk, the sacrum is forced to tumble and the movement transmits, Jacob's ladder-like, up the spine and to the limbs. Both the static and the dynamic mechanics of the pelvic structures are explained with tensegrity modeling.

The evolution of the structure

To fully understand pelvic mechanics and its integration in body mechanisms, it must be placed in its proper context. The tensegrity pelvic system is not creationist in design but is created by the physics of evolution (Fox 1988, Levin 1982, 1986,

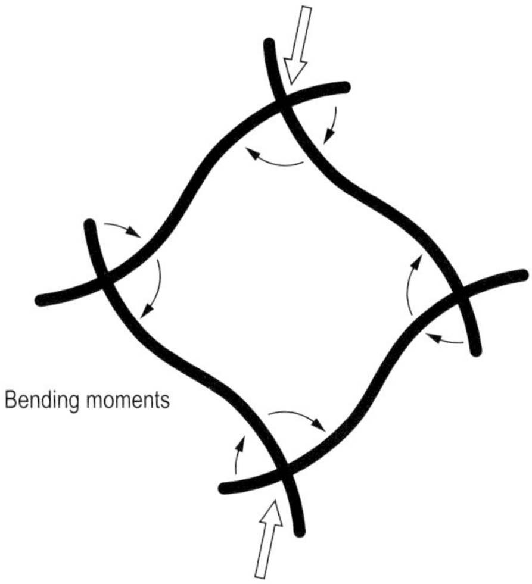

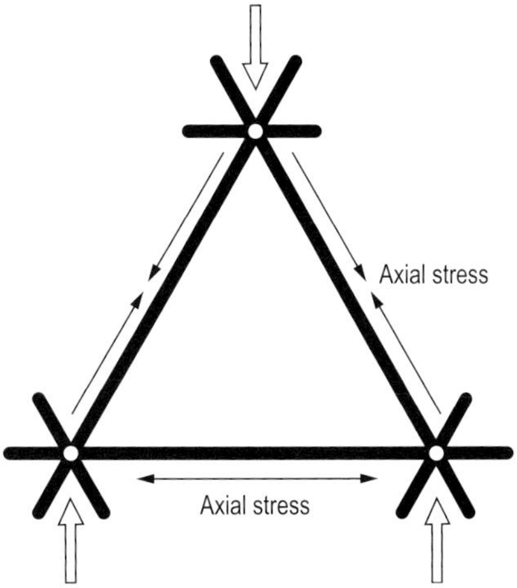

Fig. 15.7 Square frame structures are unstable and must have rigid joints to prevent collapse. Torque is created around these joints. Triangular frames are inherently stable, even with frictionless joints. The elements are under either tension or compression without any torque at the joints. (Adapted from Pearce 1978.)

Prigogine & Stengers 1984). For a biologic structure to exist as an entity it must be inherently stable and self-contained, not only when fully developed, but also at each instance of its existence. Only triangulated structures are inherently stable (Pearce 1978). Structures that are not fully triangulated have joints that must be rigidly fixed to keep from collapsing. These joints generate torque and bending moments and have high-energy requirements. Triangles are stable with flexible joints and have no torque or bending moments at the joints (Fig. 15.7). There are only tension and compression members in a triangle, so triangulated structures are low energy consumers. Because of their load distribution and high strength-to-weight ratios, engineers use truss systems made from triangles for constructing buildings and bridges. Intimately related to the laws of triangulation are the laws of closest packing (Pearce 1978). In a planar arrangement of structures, the space- and energy-efficient configuration is hexagonal closest packing, as in a beehive (Fig. 15.8). The laws of closest packing are the laws that apply to foams, colloids, and emulsions – the stuff of which biologic tissues are made (Perkowitz 2000). Thompson (1965) and later Gordon (1978), used truss systems to model biologic structures. As only trusses are stable when their joints are flexible, it follows that, if a structure has flexible joints and is stable, it must be triangulated. The mortar that holds biologic structures together is but slime. Stuck together by surface tension at the cellular level and loosely jointed at the organism level, biologic organisms must be hierarchical, fully triangulated constructs. Levin (2002) has described the evolution of the spine and skeletal system, from the cell (Ingber 2000) to the organism, as a hierarchical truss system with every body part structurally interdependent. The finite element, the building block of biologic tissue, appears to be the icosahedron (Levin 1986). The icosahedron is a regular solid with 20 triangular faces and 30 edges. Twelve vertices are created where three edges meet. Pressure on any point transmits along the 30 edges, some under tension, others under compression. It is possible to transfer all compression away from the outer edges by connecting opposite vertices of the icosahedron by compression rods. These rods do not pass through the center of the icosahedron but are eccentric and oddly angled; they hold the opposite corners away from each other. The outer shell of 30 edges is now entirely under tension, and the compression rods float within this tension shell like an endoskeleton (Fig. 15.9). A load applied to this structure causes a uniform increase in tension around all the edges and this distributes compression loads evenly to the six compression members. The mechanical properties of a tensegrity icosahedron are that they are omnidirectional structures, with the compression members and tension elements always maintaining their respective properties regardless of the direction of the applied load, just as the wire spokes of a bicycle wheel are always under tension and the hub is always being compressed. They can exist independent of gravity and are local load distributing. They have a unique structural property of behaving nonlinearly, as does the spine and its components, and most biologic tissue (Gordon 1988).

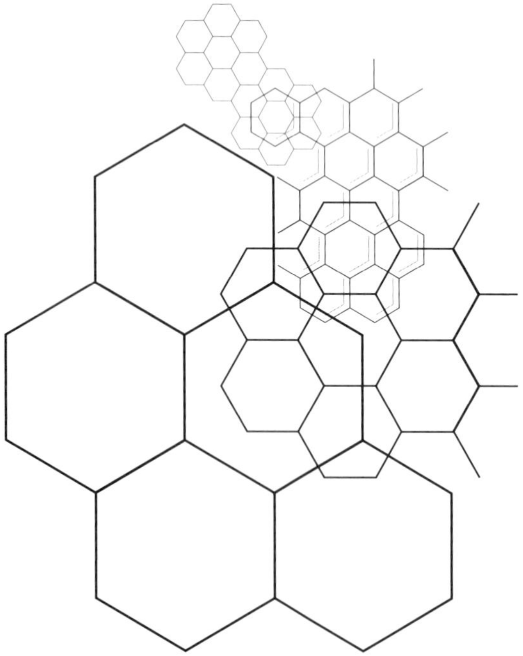

Fig. 15.8 Hierarchical closest packing of circles to hexagons.

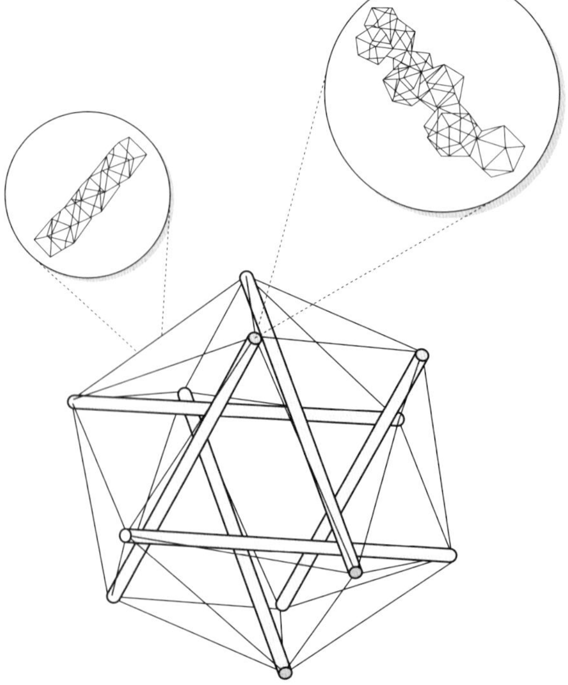

Fig. 15.9 A hierarchically constructed tensegrity icosahedron.

Fuller (1975) has shown that tensegrity icosahedra can link in an infinite array with any external form, as shown in Fig. 15.10. When linked, these structures can function as a single icosahedron in a hierarchical system. This model has been used to model endoskeletal structures, such as an upper extremity and spine (Levin 1990, 1997, 2002, 2005) with the bones functioning as the compression rods and the soft tissues as the tension elements. The concept that the musculoskeletal system is a continuous tension system is fully supported by Huijing et al's work on muscles and fascia (Huijing 1999, Huijing & Baan 2001a, 2001b), which has demonstrated that muscle is, in reality, one big organ functioning as a unit and all fascia are interconnected. This means that there would be no local loading of ligaments but that a load anywhere in the body is distributed throughout the fascial system. The structural model is represented by *The Needle*, a 20-meter tall tensegrity tower by Kenneth Snelson that sits in front of the Hirshhorn Museum in Washington, DC (Fig. 15.11).

If we apply these evolutionary structural concepts to the sacrum, we can see how the tensegrity sacropelvic model develops. The sacrum, fixed in space by the tension of its ligaments and fascial envelope, functions as the connecting link between the spine and upper (or forequarter) extremities, and the pelvis and lower (hindquarter) extremities. It evolved ontogenetically, directed not only by phylogenetic forces, but also by the physical forces of embryologic development (Thompson 1965, Wolff 1892). Carter (1991) theorizes that the mechanical forces *in utero* are the determinants of embryologic structure that, in turn, evolves to fetal and then newborn structure. From the physicalist and biomechanics viewpoint, as well as from Darwinian theory, the evolution of structure is an optimization problem (Fox 1988, Hildebrandt & Tromba 1984). At each step of development, the evolving structure optimizes so that it exists with the least amount of energy expenditure. At the cellular level, the internal structure of the cells, the microtubules, together with the cell wall, must

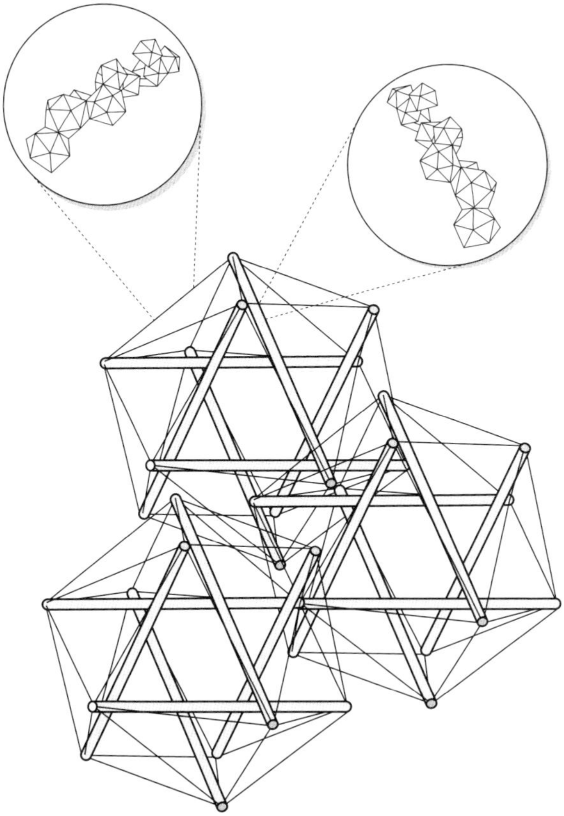

Fig. 15.10 An infinite array of tensegrity icosahedra. (Adapted from Fuller 1975.)

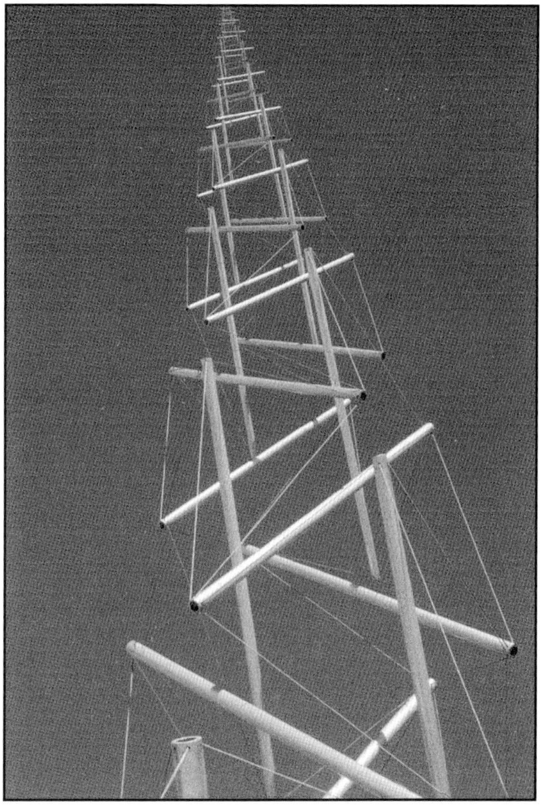

Fig. 15.11 *The Needle*. A 20-meter tall tensegrity tower. Hirshhorn Museum, Washington, DC.

resist the crushing forces of the surrounding milieu and the exploding forces of its internal metabolism. Following Wolff's law, the internal skeleton of the cell aligns itself in the most efficient way to resist those forces. Ingber and colleagues (Ingber & Jamieson 1985, Wang et al 1993) have shown that the internal microtubular skeletal structure of a cell is a tensegrity icosahedron. Other subcellular structures, such as viruses, cletherins, and endocysts, are icosahedra (de Duve 1984, Wildy & Home 1963). A hierarchical construction of an organism would use the same mechanical laws that build the most basic biologic structure and use it to generate the more complex organism. Not only is the beehive an icosahedron, but so is the bee's eye. Many other organelles and organisms look like and/or function as icosahedra (Levin 1982, 1986, 1990).

Following the concepts of Carter (1991), Wolff (1892), and Thompson (1965), a tensegrity-structured pelvis will build itself. Because the fetus develops upside down in a gravity-independent environment (like fish eggs in water), the pelvis develops as a tensegrity ring, which is the most efficient structure to do that job. It does not develop as a structure to resist superincumbent weight bearing. If it did, it would not function during its initial role in life of resisting *in utero* forces. The infant's pelvis would crush during delivery and the mother's pelvis would explode. A pelvis structured solely to bear weight on two legs would not serve the infant (nor the adult) well as it crawled on all fours. Ontogeny recapitulates phylogeny. The one-celled organism evolves as a series of stepwise mechanical accidents – which are consistent with physical laws and are the most energy efficient and most adaptable – into a complex, energy-efficient, symbiotic, multicelled organism. The different phyla get off the evolutionary ladder at different steps in the evolving process. To believe otherwise is to be a 'creationist' rather than a believer in Darwinian evolution. The development of a pelvis is not a 'design' but an evolutionary accident that worked in creating an energy-efficient, ambulating creature that could survive better in a gravity environment on land and could take advantage of the already evolved lungs that allowed breathing beyond the confines of the sea. It is the marvel of tensegrity structures that they are remarkably adaptable and can resist loads in a gravity-oriented environment equally well as they do when not affected by gravity (perhaps adding a few more trabeculae and ossifying some cartilage in accordance to Wolff's law). The pelvis is cancellous bone because the distributed loads require nothing more, nothing less. The ligaments are as strong as they need be to do what is required of them. Evolved to resist crushing forces from any direction, or exploding forces from within, the pelvis can adapt to unidirectional forces that are applied at two, three, or more points and distribute the load through the tension network of soft tissues that include local pelvic ligaments and extends throughout the entire fascial system (Huijing 1999, Huijing & Baan 2001a, 2001b) and compression network of bones.

Icosahedral tensegrity structures are self-organizing space frames that are hierarchical and evolutionary (Kroto 1988). They will build themselves, conforming to the laws of triangulation, closest packing, and, in biologic constructs, Wolff's Law. The pelvic wheel is a self-organizing structure that is part of a larger, fractal, space-frame, tensegrity construct with each part integrated into the whole. Simplicity and complexity intertwine in what Pearce (1978) calls 'minimum inventory, maximum diversity.'

Summary

Biologic structures, from subcellular to organism, are not constructed from rigid solids but from 'soft matter:' foams, colloids, and emulsions. The mechanics of soft matter differs from rigid solids in several ways (Perkowitz 2000). In biologic constructs, what has evolved, under the mechanical laws that apply to foam, is a system based on the tensegrity icosahedron, biotensegrity. This alternative approach to pelvic mechanics considers the pelvis part to be an integrated mechanical system based on the tensegrity icosahedron as its finite element. The sacrum is suspended in the interstices of the ligamentous structure like the hub of a wire bicycle wheel is suspended in the spokes. The ilia become part of the suspending 'rim.' This system can be used to model a static one-legged or two-legged stance, or the dynamic mechanical functions of the pelvis. Because of its ability to withstand omnidirectional forces, the tensegrity icosahedron is appropriate for modeling pelvic mechanics, from weight bearing to childbearing. Tensegrity structures are low-energy-requiring structures and, as such, are favored by natural selection. Because they are so adaptable and energy efficient, biotensegrity mechanics are also appropriate for modeling all biologic systems and subsystems at each stage of their development and whatever their eventual function.

References

Carter DR 1991 Musculoskeletal ontogeny, phylogeny, and functional adaptation. Journal of Biomechanics 24(suppl. 1):3–16

de Duve C 1984 A guided tour of the living cell. Scientific American Books, New York

Dye SF 1987 An evolutionary perspective of the knee. Journal of Bone and Joint Surgery 69-A:976–983

Fielding WJ, Burstein AH, Frankel VH 1976 The nuchal ligament. Spine 1(1):3–14

Fox RF 1988 Energy and the evolution of life. WH Freeman, New York

Fuller RB 1975 Synergetics. McMillian, New York, p314–431

Gordon JE 1978 Structures: or why things don't fall down. De Capa Press, New York

Gordon JE 1988 The science of structures and materials. WH Freeman, New York, p137–157

Gracovetsky S 1988 The spinal engine. Springer-Verlag, New York

Grant JCB 1952 A method of anatomy. Williams and Wilkins, Baltimore, MD

Hildebrandt S, Tromba A 1984 Mathematics and optimal form. Scientific American Books, New York

Huijing P 1999 Muscular force transmission: a unified, dual or multiple system? A review and some explorative experimental results. Archives of Physiology and Biochemistry 107(4):292–311

Huijing PA, Baan GC 2001a Extramuscular myofascial force transmission within the rat anterior tibial compartment: proximo-distal differences in muscle force. Acta Physiologica Scandinavica 173(3):297–311

Huijing PA, Baan GC 2001b Myofascial force transmission causes interaction between adjacent muscles and connective tissue: effects of blunt dissection and compartmental fasciotomy on length force characteristics of rat extensor digitorum longus muscle. Archives of Physiology and Biochemistry 109(2):97–109

Ingber DE 2000 The origin of cellular life. Bioessays 22(12):1160–1170

Ingber DE, Jamieson J 1985 Cells as tensegrity structures. Architectural regulation of histodifferentiation by physical forces transduced over basement membrane. Academic Press, New York

Kapandji IA 1977 The physiology of the joints [Trans. Honore LH]. Churchill Livingstone, Edinburgh

Kroto H 1988 Space, stars, C60, and soot. Science 242: 1139–1145

Levin SM 1982 Continuous tension, discontinuous compression, a model for biomechanical support of the body. Bulletin of Structural Integration, Rolf Institute, Bolder, CO, p31–33

Levin SM 1986 The icosahedron as the three-dimensional finite element in biomechanical support. In: Dillon JR (ed) Proceedings of the society of general systems research symposium on mental images, values and reality, 26–30 May. University of Philadelphia Society of General Systems Research, Philadelphia, pG14–26

Levin SM 1990 The space truss as a model for cervical spine mechanics – a systems science concept. In: Burns L (ed) Back pain – an international review. Kluwer Academic Publishers, Lancaster, Dordrecht, The Netherlands, p231–238

Levin SM 1997 Putting the shoulder to the wheel: a new biomechanical model for the shoulder girdle. Biomed Sci Instrum 33:412–7

Levin SM 2002 The tensegrity-truss as a model for spine mechanics. Journal of Mechanics in Medicine and Biology 2(3 & 4):375–388

Levin SM 2005 The scapula is a sesamoid bone. Journal of Biomechanics 38:1733–1734

Morris JM, Lucas DB 1964 Biomechanics of spinal bracing. Arizona Medicine 21:170–176

Muller W 1983 The knee. Form, function and ligament reconstruction. Springer, New York, p8–75

Panjabi MM, White AA 2001 Biomechanics in the musculoskeletal system. Churchill Livingstone, New York, p56–58

Pearce P 1978 Structure in nature as a strategy for design. MIT Press, Cambridge, MA

Perkowitz S 2000 Universal foam. Random House, New York, p16–19

Prigogine I, Stengers I 1984 Order out of chaos: man's new dialogue with nature. Bantam Books, London

Snijders CJ, Vleeming A, Stoeckart R et al 1997 Biomechanics of the interface between spine and pelvis in different postures. In: Stoeckart R (ed) Movement, stability and low back pain. Churchill Livingstone, Edinburgh, p103–114

Thompson D 1965 On growth and form. Cambridge University Press, London

Wang N, Butler JP, Ingber DE 1993 Mechanotransduction across the cell surface and through the cytoskeleton. Science 260(5111):1124–1127

White AA, Panjabi MM 1978 Clinical biomechanics of the spine. Lippincott, Philadelphia, PA, p1–57

Wildy P, Home RW 1963 Structure of animal virus particles. Progressive Medical Virology 5:1–42

Willard F 1995 The lumbosacral connection: the ligamentous structure of the low back and its relation to back pain. Rotterdam: ECO

Wolff J 1892 Das Gesetz der Transformation der Knocchen. Berlin: Hirschwald

CHAPTER 16

Why and how to optimize posture

Robert E Irvin

This chapter concerns basic and clinical science that reflects that the origin of most common, chronic pain is the chronic mechanical stressor that results from postural imperfection, whether to normal or abnormal extents. While proximate causes of acute and chronic pain can mediate this outcome, postural stressors – in concert with other stressors – provide the initial and ongoing conditions that predispose either to spontaneous onset of chronic pain or failure to recover from superimposed trauma. For this population, optimization of posture by the method described herein is routinely and enduringly followed by alleviation of 70–90% of chronic pain, according to this author.

Introduction

Approximately 85% of chronic lumbopelvic pain is mechanically mediated. The present chapter relates the great majority of such pain as a reversible effect of three mutually contrary and corresponding aspects.

1. *Imperfect posture*: a ubiquitous and chronic stressor as an origin (in contrast to proximate cause) of most noxious stimulae (Irvin 1997).
2. The *proximate causes* of most noxious stimulae include arthrodial inflammation, restriction of soft and segmental tissues, focal impingement, and misalignment of joint segments.
3. From this origin and these proximate causes there is variable perception of pain, which is attributable to corticolimbic, spinal, and peripheral sensitization (kindling) of the nervous system, which effect lowering of the sensory threshold for pain (Rome & Rome 2000).

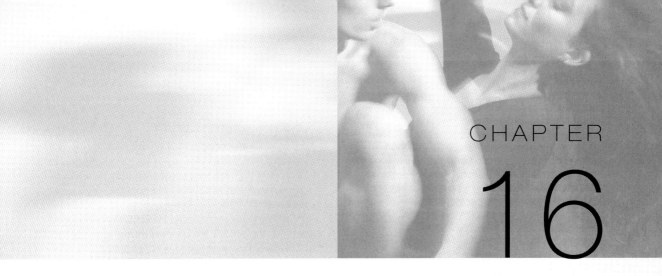

Treatment of these proximate causes of chronic pain yields temporary relief for most people. In contrast, enduring reduction of chronic pain throughout the body is routinely achieved by use of a heel lift to improve posture by leveling the (normally unlevel) sacral base (Hoffman & Hoffman 1994, Irvin 1986, 1998). This relief is attributable to reduction of the kindled state and proximate cause by reduction of the chronic postural stressor that is an unlevel pelvis.

Kindling occurs at any of three neurologic levels: corticolimbic, spinal, or peripheral. It induces a lasting set of neuroreceptive changes in response to noxious stimulae (Perlin et al 1993) and is, in effect, a form of gain control that complicates the correspondence between a given noxious stimulus and the resultant nociception by introducing an intermediate and immeasurable gain in the perception of pain.

Spinal kindling is similar to the chronically facilitated spinal segment described by Denslow et al (1947). Rome & Rome (2000) expand this concept to include the peripheral and corticolimbic portions of the nervous system.

This neurologic augmentation of chronic pain is termed 'limbically augmented pain syndrome' (LAPS). Rome & Rome (2000) relate that chronic stressors, which can be psychologic and cultural, can induce kindling. A third, ubiquitous and chronic stressor with the potential to induce kindling, and which is *not* discussed by Rome & Rome (2000), is postural stress. The Romes' theory of nocigenesis lends itself precisely to a schema that illustrates a role of posture as a chronic stressor, in addition to psychologic and cultural stressors, in the gain of chronic pain (Fig. 16.1).

A perplexing aspect of this picture, given the normal presence of imperfect posture, is the question of why do some people hurt whereas others do not? Other chronic stressors, such as psychologic and cultural influences, can come into play to effect the varied extents of kindling.

Given: (1) that treatment of proximate causes of chronic pain commonly yields temporary relief; and (2) the difficulty of modifying cultural and psychologic stressors, the most practical strategy for enduring relief of mechanically mediated pain is to include: (3) treatment aimed to optimize posture.

Description of manipulable posture

Optimal posture is that shape and attitude of the body, with respect to gravitation, having the greatest economy of stance and movement.

Posture is directly correspondent to three boundary conditions, i.e. three bodily aspects that, by virtue of their centrality to the postural systematics, directly regulate the overall geometry of the body (Figs 16.2 and 16.3). The three central boundaries of the geometric form of the postural system are:

1. The *center of gravitational interaction* is the feet and ankles, at the center of the equal and opposing vectors of weight and ground support (Figs 16.2, 16.4).

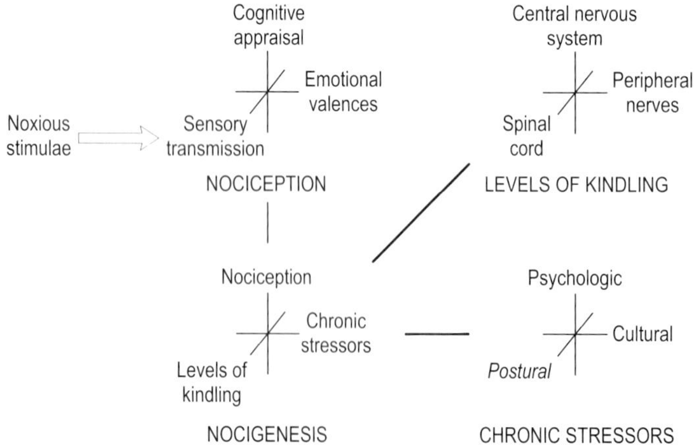

Fig. 16.1 A schematic of the genesis of pain (nocigenesis) whereby chronic stressors kindle the nervous system to increase the perception of pain (nociception) by the lowering of sensory threshold to positively affect chronic pain.

2. The *neurologic center* of posture is the CNS, which comprises motor efferents, sensory afferents, and consciousness. The CNS is usually proper in its activity and does not necessitate modification for the optimization of posture. The center of postural afferents is the postural control system, or the vestibular nucleus, and is itself comprised of the confluence of three afferents (Figs 16.2, 16.5):

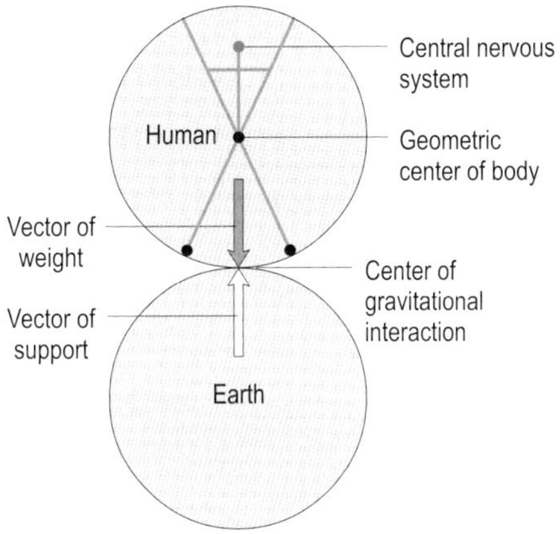

Fig. 16.2 A schematic of the three central boundaries of the postural system. These boundaries are the feet (center of gravitational interaction), the sacral base (geometric center), and the central nervous system.

   a. *abducent nerves*: regulate the lateral rectus of the eyes, tracking horizontal
   b. *vestibulocochlear nerves*: monitor the inner ear, tracking vertical
   c. *vestibulospinal tracts*: monitor the distribution of weight bearing across the articular surfaces of support.
3. The *geometric center* is the sacral base that is approximately equidistant from the outstretched tips of the toes and fingers (Figs 16.2, 16.6).

The geometric center of the human, illustrated in the Vitruvian man by Leonardo da Vinci, does not strictly follow the description by Vitruvius of the proportionate man, whereby the human figure is fully outstretched with both the feet and hands *extended* (Vitruvius *De Architura*). Instead, de Vinci depicts the feet as *flat*, rendering the geometric center the *navel*. When the feet are extended, true to Vitruvius' description, the approximate geometric center of man is the *sacral base*.

A schematic of the interactive fundamentals of the human postural system is shown in Fig. 16.7 (Irvin 1997). From this schema of the manipulable aspects of posture, coupled with the Romes' model of chronic nocigenesis (see Fig. 16.1), as such pain relates to chronic stressors, then the nature of mechanically mediated chronic pain can be understood. Using the following method

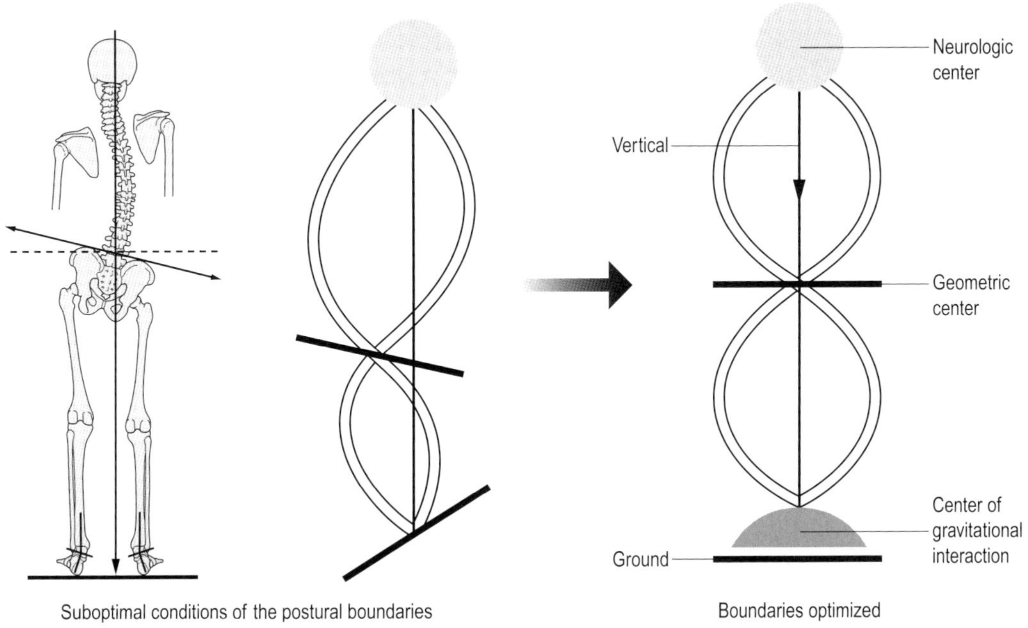

Fig. 16.3 When suboptimal conditions of the postural boundaries are optimized (arrow), the geometric symmetry of the body is general enhanced.

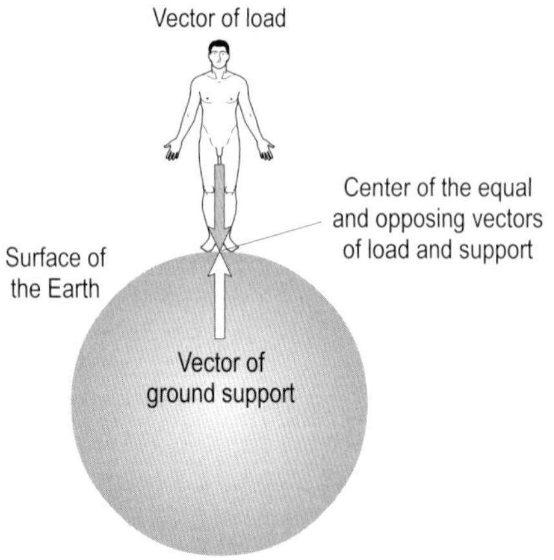

Fig. 16.4 The feet are central to the gravitational interaction of the equal and opposite vectors (arrows) of bodily weight and ground support.

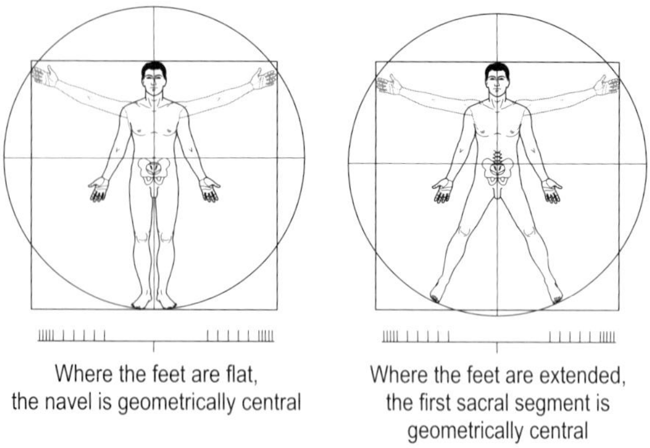

Where the feet are flat, the navel is geometrically central
Where the feet are extended, the first sacral segment is geometrically central

Fig. 16.6 Where the entirety of the outstretched body is considered, from the tips of the toes to the tips of the fingers, the approximate geometric center of posture is the sacral base.

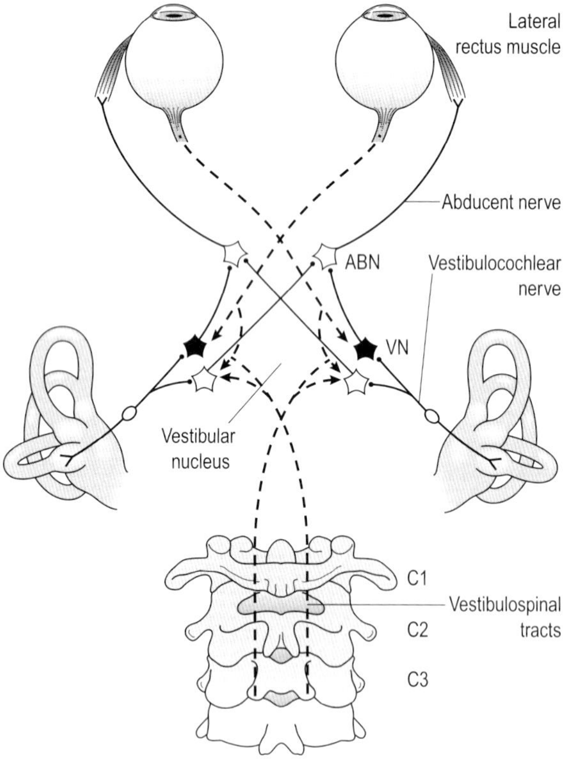

Fig. 16.5 The neurologic center of posture is the postural control center, which resides in the vestibular nucleus and is composed of the confluence of the vestibulospinal tracts, the vestibulocochlear nerves, and the abducent nerves.

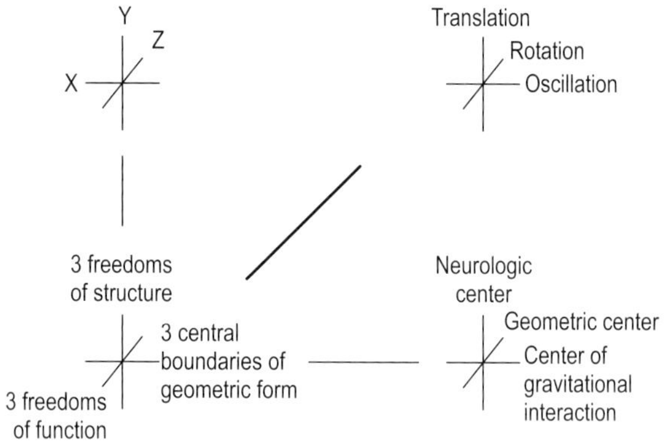

Fig. 16.7 A schematic of the human postural system. The structures function correspondingly within the boundary conditions of the geometric form of the body.

for optimization of posture, most mechanically mediated, chronic pain can be alleviated by correction of the postural stressor. Where necessary, this method for global reduction of postural stress can be used along with accepted methods for treatment of proximate causes of chronic pain, and sacral bar a greatly enhanced outcome over that by treatment of proximate causes alone can be expected.

Method for optimization of posture (10-step recovery from suboptimal posture)

1. Foot orthotics to restore arches and vertically align the ankles.

2. Radiography of the pelvic level in the coronal plane, standing.
3. Measurement of the pelvic level, standing.
4. Use of a heel lift to level the pelvis, standing.
5. External augmentation of the shoe to replace a thicker heel lift.
6. Delineation of the sacral angle and lumbar load in the sagittal plane, standing.
7. Use of a therapeutic posture to reduce lumbopelvic lordosis.
8. Radiography of the lumbopelvis in the coronal plane, seated, and use of an ischial lift to level the pelvis.
9. Manual manipulation to reduce arthrodial restriction and joint segmental misalignment.
10. Radiographic re-evaluation with lifts/foot orthotics in place.

1. Foot orthotics to restore the arches of the feet and vertically align the ankles

For most people, there is an extent of flatness of the arches (pes planus), with angularity of the ankles (pes valgus) (Fig. 16.8). These deformities relative to the postural ideal can be corrected by the precise use of individually crafted foot orthotics (Fig. 16.9).

The reader is to be alerted to the fact that the conventional use of orthotics is far short of their clinical potential. The root word for orthotic is *orthotata* (Greek), which means 'to correct or straighten.' Contemporary use of orthotics is to provide a measure of support with modest correction for the arches of the feet, far short of full correction.

Fitting the initial orthotics for full correction of pes planovalgus can result in too abrupt a correction, the stress of which can cause some patients such discomfort that they reject the orthotics. Standard practice is that patients stop at partial correction without later moving on to a more robust orthotic. A modest correction of the feet and ankles has the greatest benefit local to the orthotics, namely the feet, ankles, and knees. The greater is the extent of correction, the further upward is the symmetrization of the posture.

Towards a full correction, the initial orthotics are casted via a Styrofoam imprint of the feet collected in the upright stance so as to reflect the initial conditions of the feet, and these orthotics are subsequently augmented incrementally (biweekly or monthly) by an orthotist towards full correction of the feet and ankles (Irvin 1998). When the limits of augmentation of the initial orthotic are reached, a second set can be made that approximates full correction by making a plaster cast of the feet while not bearing weight and while the feet are held in the anatomic position. By this incremental correction under weighted and not-weight-bearing conditions, tolerance to full correction is high.

2. Radiography of the pelvic level in the coronal plane, standing

Measurement of the attitude of the base of the sacrum in the coronal plane while standing is by

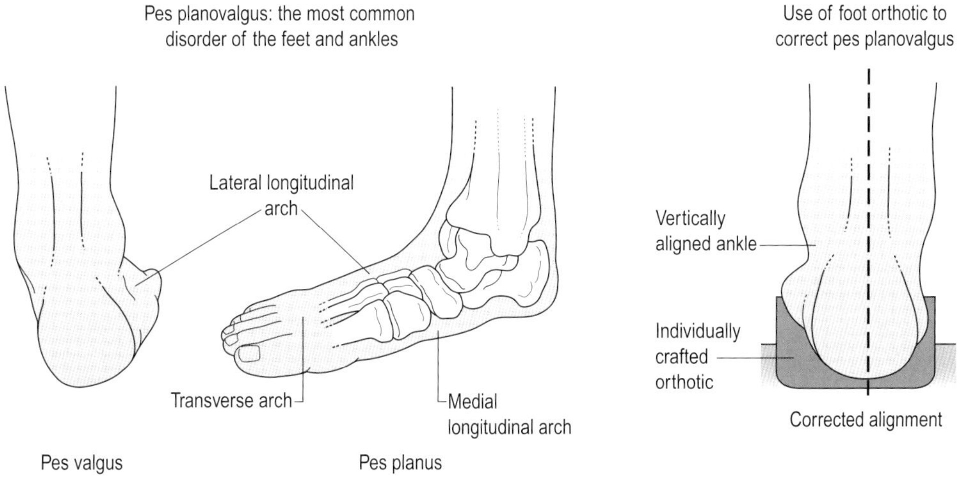

Fig. 16.8 The most common disorder of the feet and ankles is flatness of the arches of the feet (pes planus) and angularity of the ankle (pes valgus). By the precise shaping of a foot orthotic, the amplitudes of the arches of the feet can be optimized and the ankles rendered straight and vertically aligned.

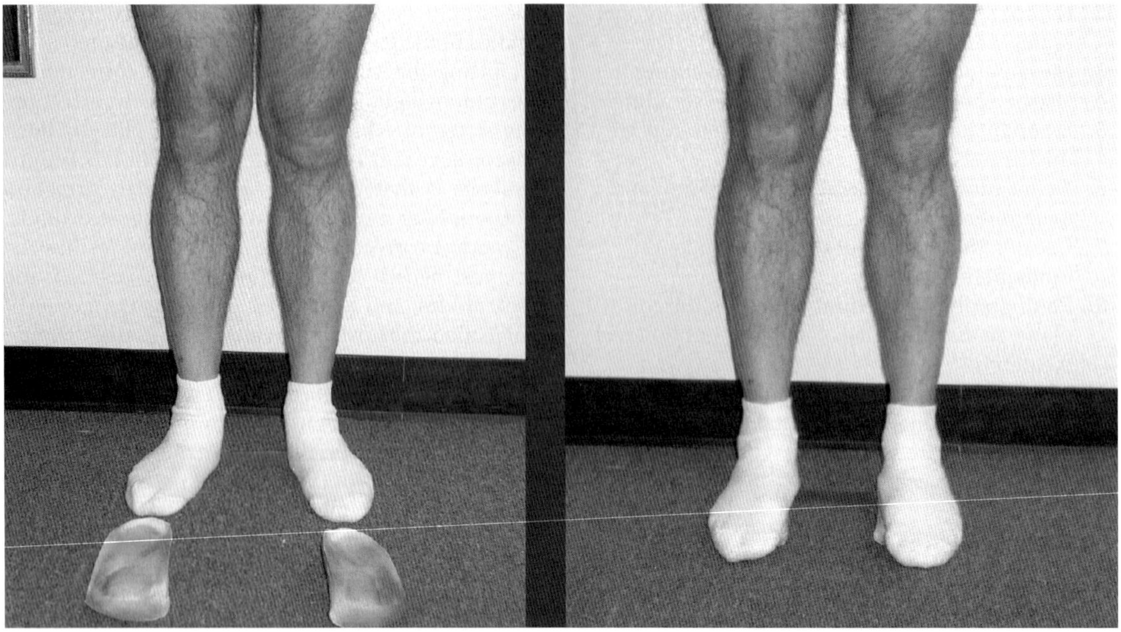

Fig. 16.9 Use of foot orthotics to correct pes planovalgus. (A) Pes planovalgus, with the orthotics positioned in front of the feet. (B) The feet standing on top of the orthotics, with the pes planovalgus corrected.

plain radiography. This is performed with the patient standing in the anatomic position.

On a minimum of two occasions throughout the course of treatment, the lumbar spine and pelvis are radiographed with the patient in the upright stance. This examination, termed a postural study (Denslow et al 1955, Loyd 1934), is initially performed without shoes unless the patient currently wears foot orthotics and/or a heel lift, in which case the initial study is performed with shoes on and these implements in place. On completion of the initial course of treatment aimed to correct the measured postural deficits, the patient is re-radiographed, with heel lift and/or foot orthotics, to evaluate response to treatment and measure residual postural deficit for further correction.

For the standing anteroposterior view in the coronal plane, the feet are parallel, positioned directly beneath the acetabulae, with the buttocks in direct contact with the plane of the film cassette. This contact minimizes possible pelvic rotation with respect to the vertical axis. The participant folds the arms across the chest with the hands on the shoulders in order to remove the arms from the visualized field.

Rectangular film, 35 × 43 cm, is supported vertically on a base that is horizontally controlled via a bubble level. A Quanta III intensifying screen is used with constant kilovoltage (kVp) technique. The focal-spot-to-film distance is 1.07 m, with the ray centered at the level of L5. For each view, approximately 0.12 rad is delivered to the midplane at 80kVp and 40 mAs.

3. Measurement of the pelvic level, standing

For most adults, the base of the sacrum viewed in the coronal plane is not level. For the average adult, unlevelness of the sacral base, standing, delineated by the method described below is 6.7 ± 1.0 mm (Irvin 1991). Unlevelness of ≤ 2 mm is present for 98% of adults and can be clinically significant. The lumbar spine tends to angle laterally, concave towards the high side of the sacral base, in order to maintain postural balance (Greenman 1979). Unlevelness of the pelvis can be reliably reduced by the use of a heel lift beneath the low side of the pelvis, and this reduction can be measured radiographically (Fann 2003, Irvin 1991).

Delineation of the sacral base is by drawing a line parallel to the transverse stratum of eburnation, thought to be a physiologic response to the compressive stress of weight bearing, in accord with Wolff's Law. This truly delineates the weight-bearing plane of the sacral base (F M Wilkins 1980, personal communication) (Fig. 16.10).

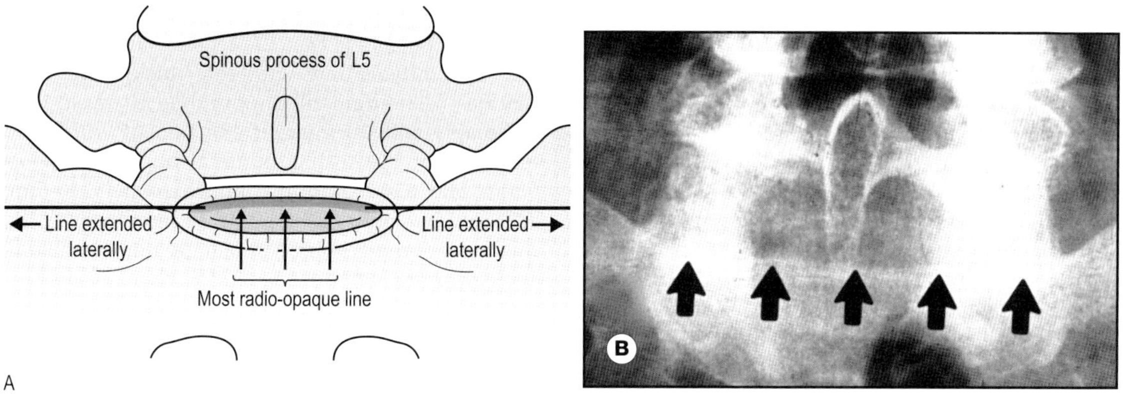

Fig. 16.10 (A) Line drawing of the radiographic reference for the delineation of the base of the sacrum that directly bears the load of the lumbar spine and is geometrically central to the overall skeletal frame. (B) A radiograph of the base of the sacrum (unlevel) with arrows that emphasize the transverse stratum of greatest radio-opacity that is the sacral base.

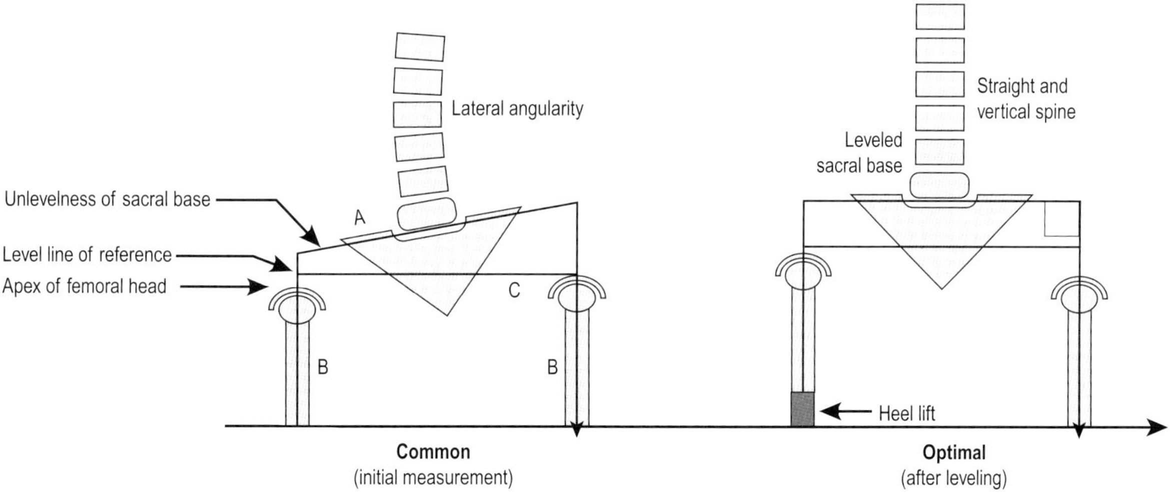

Fig. 16.11 Illustrated measurement of the pelvic level by postural radiography, and leveling of the pelvis by use of a heel lift.

The margin of error of unlevelness of the sacral base measured radiographically, on two occasions with a 1-year interval, is ±0.75 mm (Greenman 1979). For most subjects and operators, the measurement of the unlevelness of the transverse stratum of the sacral base is easily made. In approximately 10% of subjects, a clear delineation of this reference plane is somewhat difficult.

The film is supported in a film holder with its lower margin level (Fig. 16.11). The weight-bearing plane of the sacral base is delineated on the film by line A, which is drawn parallel to the transverse stratum of eburnation within the sacral base (see Fig. 16.11), and this line is extended as far laterally as are the femoral heads. For the standing study, two vertical lines (B) are drawn, one each through the femoral heads and these are extended upwards to intersect with line A. A horizontal line (C) is constructed from the lateral margin of the film at a level above the femoral heads and below line A, and this horizontal reference is extended to intersect the lines B. The vertical line segments (B), right and left, that span from the horizontal reference line C and sacral bar line A, are measured in millimeters and subtracted, the lesser from the greater. The difference is the millimeters of unlevelness of the sacral base with respect to the lateral position of the femora, for the reason that modification of the pelvic level is by a heel lift that acts on the pelvis via the femora.

The operator is cautioned against the use of any reference other than the transverse stratum of eburnation for delineation of the weight-bearing plane of the sacral base. There can be significant disagreement between unlevelness measured by the stratum of eburnation, as compared to unlevelness measured using as reference the alar notches, heights of the femoral heads, or the heights of the iliac crests (Dott et al 1994). This stratum of eburnation is recommended as reference for the plane of weight bearing over these other references for the reason that other references do not actually bear the spinal weight (Irvin 1991). Whereas other references for the pelvic level are easier to delineate, they do not directly bear the weight of the lumbar spine and are not the central boundary of posture.

4. Use of a heel lift to level the pelvis, standing

Sacral unlevelness when standing can be corrected by placement of a heel lift inside the shoe on the low side of the pelvis. The lift is composed of material that is not compressible under the stress of human weight, such as cork or rubber. As 2 mm can be clinically significant, for those patients with unlevelness of 2 mm, incorporate a 2 mm lift. For those patients with unlevelness > 3 mm, the thickness of the initial lift recommended by this author is 3 mm. An initial lift of thickness > 5 mm can be followed by transient discomfort of the musculoskeleton, secondary to the stress from accommodation to the altered posture.

Biweekly, the heel lift can safely be augmented in thickness by 2 mm. Addition of greater than 2 mm, or this addition more often than biweekly, can be followed by transient discomfort and for this reason is also not recommended by this author (Irvin 1991).

5. External augmentation of the shoe to replace a thicker heel lift

If the thickness of the heel lift exceeds the available space within the shoe, either the excess lift is added to the outer heel (by an orthotist or cobbler) or the vertical span of the contralateral heel is reduced (for women's shoes with high heels). For subjects with an augmentation of the heel greater than 8 mm, the thickness of the sole is also augmented so the difference between the augmented thickness of the heel and sole does not exceed 8 mm. This increase in thickness of the sole is intended to minimize the difference in pitch between the right and left shoes and thereby avoid secondary torsion of the pelvis about the vertical axis.

A practical limit to this rule regarding augmentation of the sole is that the tensile strength of the sole is commensurate with sole thickness. A sole that has been augmented more than 10 mm can be noticeably stiff during gait. For benefit within the tolerance of comfort, a minimal augmentation is 5 mm and a maximum is approximately 10 mm. This guide might have to be ignored where the thickness of the heel lift is much greater than usual, such as for an inch thickness (~26 mm).

6. Delineation of the sacral angle and lumbar load in the sagittal plane, standing

This measurement is an indication of the attitude of sacral support of the lumbar spine by the sacral base, and where the load from the weight of the lumbar spine passes through the sacral base in the sagittal plane. For the theoretically ideal posture in the sagittal plane, there is vertical alignment of the following points: the external meatus of the ear, the acromioclavicular joint, the midpoint of the body of L3, the anterior third of the sacral base, the greater trochanter, the lateral condyle of the knee, and the distal fibular head. Load of the sacral base can be represented by extension of the lumbosacral portion of this imaginary line constructed from the midpoint of the vertebral body of L3 and extended downward through the level of the sacral base (Fig. 16.12, frames A and B). Ideally, the load represented by this line passes through the anterior third of the sacral base. When lumbopelvic lordosis is present (Fig. 16.12, frame C), treatment is aimed to minimize the excessive sacral tilt, and position the superincumbent load of the lumbar spine over the sacral base (Fig. 16.12, frame D).

From the lateral and sagittal view, the attitude of the sacral base (the sacral angle) is measured by the modified method of Ferguson (1930), who studied pelvic tilt in cadavers radiographed in the lateral recumbent position. Greenman (1979) observes that for living subjects filmed in the upright stance, the normal angle is closer to 40° ±2°.

In the sagittal plane, measure the sacral angle by the modified method of Ferguson (1930):

1. Place a dot at the anterior and posterior margins of the sacral base.
2. A line (A) is drawn to connect these dots, and is extended posteriorly for a span of 7.5–10 cm (3–4 inches).
3. A horizontal line of reference (B), constructed from the lateral margin of the film, is drawn from the sacral promontory, and extended posteriorly for three to four inches.

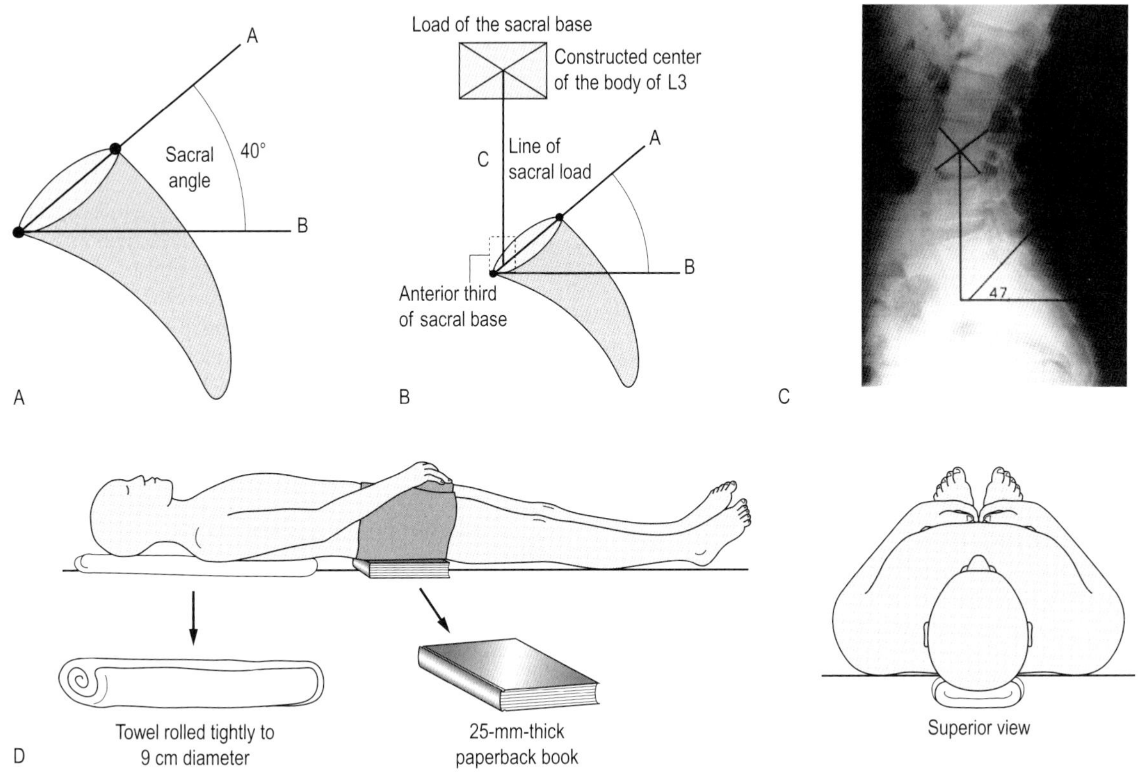

Fig. 16.12 (A) Line drawing of a sagittal view of the lumbopelvis to depict the attitude of the sacral base (line A) relative to horizontal (line B). (B) The line of sacral load by the lumbar spine (line C) on the sacral base. (C) Radiography of lumbopelvic lordosis, standing, with anteriorly displaced sacral load and increased sacral angle (47°) (lumbopelvic lordosis). (D) A therapeutic posture for the reduction of lumbopelvic lordosis (making use of a book and towel).

4. The angle between lines A and B is measured, and is referred to as the modified angle of Ferguson, or the sacral angle.

The method for delineation of the sacral load from the lumbar spine is as follows:

1. One dot is placed at each of the four corners of the vertebral body of L3.
2. Two diagonal lines are drawn to connect the four dots, intersecting at approximately the midpoint of the body of L3.
3. A vertical line (C) is drawn extended downward from the midpoint of L3 to the level of the anterior margin of the sacral base; this line indicates the placement of sacral load.

Suboptimal conditions of posture can alter the sacral level, angle, and load. Directly, unlevelness of the sacral base misloads structures in the coronal plane. Indirectly, postural imbalance that generates torque about one cardinal axis indirectly causes torque about all three cardinal axes by virtue of operational linkage. Torsion, or rotation, about two or more axes can result. An example is where pelvic obliquity can result in lumbopelvic lordosis.

Pes planovalgus also appears causative of lumbopelvic lordosis, for the reason that correction of the former is commonly followed by reduction of the latter. Unilateral pes valgus causes torsion of the pelvis about the vertical axis, with misloading in the transverse plane. Under condition of bilateral pes planovalgus, there is torque about the transverse axis of the pelvis, with tendency for pelvic torsion in the sagittal plane, favoring lumbopelvic lordosis. The line of sacral load can be displaced either anteriorly or posteriorly. Anterior displacement of the sacral load results in a shear stress at the lumbosacral junction as well as an anterior-ward torque about the transverse axis. Anterior displacement can be measured as millimeters of horizontal displacement of the vertical line of sacral load from the promontory of the sacral base.

Where there is posterior displacement of the line of sacral load, this line passes through the middle or posterior portion of the sacral base, or even posterior to the sacral base, measured as millimeters of horizontal span extending from the anterior margin of the sacral base to the vertical line of sacral load. Posterior displacement of sacral load shifts the load from the vertebral bodies and base of the sacrum toward the pedicles and intervertebral facets. These structures are less suitable for bearing load than are the bodies of the vertebrae and the first sacral segment, and this chronic misloading can result in facet degeneration that is mechanically mediated.

7. Use of a therapeutic posture to reduce lumbopelvic lordosis

Where pes planovalgus is being corrected by foot orthotics, the torsional pressure towards the lumbopelvis is correspondingly reduced. Reduction of lumbopelvic lordosis is further advanced by reduction of posterior lumbopelvic restriction that is reflective of the prior lordosis. This reduction of postural bias can be done by the daily practice of a therapeutic posture configured to reduce thoracolumbopelvic restriction in the sagittal plane.

Throughout the course of postural correction, and especially for those patients with lumbopelvic lordosis, a therapeutic posture (see Fig. 16.12, frame D) is practiced daily at home to reduce resistance of the torso and lumbopelvis to postural correction, to accelerate relief of pain, to reduce excess sacral tilt and displacement of sacral load, and to minimize possible transitional discomforts consequent to the stress of postural correction. The susceptibility for some patients to have a temporary increase in discomfort towards the conclusion of postural optimization is greatly reduced for those who practice this posture throughout the course of treatment. Patients recline daily for 20 min in a relaxed, supine position on a carpeted floor with a towel rolled tightly to a diameter of approximately 9 cm and placed lengthwise on the floor beneath the thoracic spine, extending from the level of T12 to beyond the occiput. A paperback book, approximately 25 mm (1 inch) thick, is placed directly beneath the sacrum. A hardback book can temporarily cause mild numbness across the dorsum of the sacrum.

This posture can reduce lordosis of the lumbopelvis, and kyphosis of the thorax. When the course of postural optimization is completed, continued practice of this posture is optional for relief from daily postural stress, but is not necessary to maintain the achieved reduction of lumbopelvic lordosis, so long as the prescribed heel lift and/or foot orthotics are used routinely.

8. Radiography of the lumbopelvis in the coronal plane, seated, and use of an ischial lift to level the pelvis

For the seated stance, the patient sits on a rectangular box so as to render both the hips and knees at a 90° angle. The thighs are abducted about 40° from the midline to remove the femurs from the line of sight of the ischia on the film. The tube is positioned with the ray centered at L5, and the arms cross the chest with the hands on the opposite shoulders.

For the seated view (Fig. 16.13), the technique for measurement of the attitude of the sacral base is identical to that for the standing view, with the exception that the vertical lines are constructed so as to pass through the lowermost angle of the ischia, rather than through the apices of the femora. This is for reason that the seated sacral unlevelness is to be corrected by placement of an ischial lift beneath the angle of the ischia on the low side of the pelvis.

Sacral unlevelness while seated can be corrected in increments up to 5 mm monthly, until the unlevelness initially measured has been replaced by the ischial lift, composed of rubber or cork, in the three seats most often used (in the automobile, the favorite chair at home, and the chair used at work), positioned beneath the angle of the ischium on the low side of the pelvis.

9. Manual manipulation to reduce arthrodial restriction and misalignment

At the time of the introduction of the lift, and with each augmentation of thickness, the soft tissues and joints of the subjects are examined for restriction from the physiologic range of motion. Where such resistance is identified, this restriction is reduced by manual manipulation, improving function and reducing resistance to increase in postural symmetry. This activity is performed for an average of 20 minutes per session. This cycle is repeated biweekly until the thickness of the lift is equal to the number of millimeters of sacral unlevelness initially measured.

10. Radiographic re-evaluation with lifts/foot orthotics in place

Two weeks after the final increase in lift thickness, the patient is radiographed a second time, standing, with the heel lift/foot orthotics inside the shoe while standing and the ischial lift under the ischium while

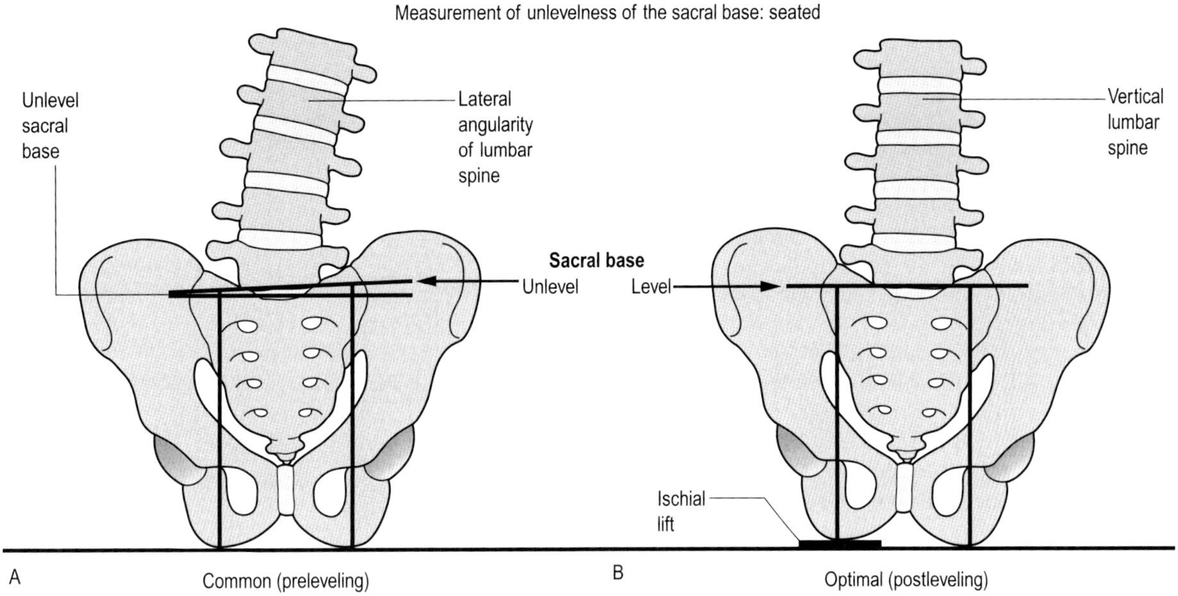

Fig. 16.13 A diagram of the measurement of unlevelness of the base of the sacrum radiographed (A) while seated on a firm, flat, and horizontal surface, and (B) while standing in the anatomic position. Note that the bilateral lines of vertical reference pass through the angle of the ischia where seated, but through the apex of the femoral heads when standing, in accord with the later position of the ischial and heel lifts used to correct unlevelness.

seated. From this second film, the measurements are repeated and compared with the initial films for improvement, and residual sacral unlevelness/ sacral tilt/ displacement of sacral load, if present, is noted for further correction.

Where the initial films demonstrate pelvic obliquity with lumbopelvic lordosis, the follow-up study typically reflects reduction of lumbopelvic lordosis with reduction of sacral unlevelness that is significantly less than the thickness of the heel lift. This disparity between the initial unlevelness, the lift thickness, and the subsequent reduction of pelvic unlevelness is reflective of: (1) the effect of the foot orthotics to straighten the unequal angularity of the ankles; and (2) revelation of sacral unlevelness not fully measurable under conditions of the initially increased sacral tilt.

Overdose of heel lift

A clinical example of excessive 'dose' of heel lift was the case of a 52-year-old patient with chronic and idiopathic pain of the low back. Postural radiography revealed an 11 mm unlevelness of the sacral base, with 13° of lateral angularity of the lumbar spine. The patient was told of this unlevelness and initially given a 3 mm heel lift. Later that same day she increased her lift to the full 11 mm. Ten days later she reported that her low back pain was much better but that she was experiencing new discomforts in multiple regions of the musculoskeleton. Repeat of the postural radiography showed a level sacral base and reduction of the lateral bend of the lumbar spine from 13° to 2°. The new discomforts were attributed to the stress of abrupt reduction of the lumbopelvic obliquity. Pleased with her radiographic improvement, she opted to continue with the lift at the full thickness and to ride out the subsequent discomforts.

The multiregional discomforts gradually worsened over the next several weeks such that by the third week after the introduction of the lift she was unable to stand and required a wheelchair for transportation. It was 5 weeks after the introduction of the lift before she fully recovered her level of function and comfort that was typical prior to the lift, and, by the end of the sixth week, she reported an overall and marked improvement of her original pains as well as alleviation of the pain that developed after the excessive advancement of lift thickness. Although this case is extreme, it demonstrates that a risk of abrupt and full leveling of the sacral base from 11 mm of unlevelness is possibly debilitating pain, albeit temporary.

Clinical outcomes

Use of a heel lift to level the sacral base, in concert with manual manipulation to reduce arthrodial restriction and misalignment, yields enduring alleviation of >70% of the number of regions with mechanically mediated chronic pain (Irvin 1997, 1998) (Fig. 16.14).

Anecdotally, when the feet and ankles are also optimized and the seated pelvis leveled, the number of regions with such pain is, in my experience, enduringly relieved by ≥90%.

For those with ≤20 degrees of lateral angularity of the lumbar spine, the degree of lateral angularity is reduced by an average of 30% (Irvin 1991). Anecdotally, for those with lateral angularity of 35 degrees or less, with unlevelness of up to 45 mm,

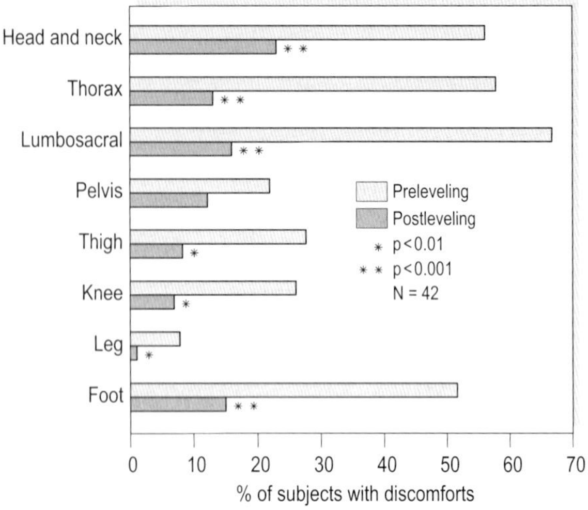

Fig. 16.14 Graphic effect on multiregional, chronic pains for an adult population by the use of a heel lift to level the sacral base. More than 70% of the regions with chronic pain are alleviated.

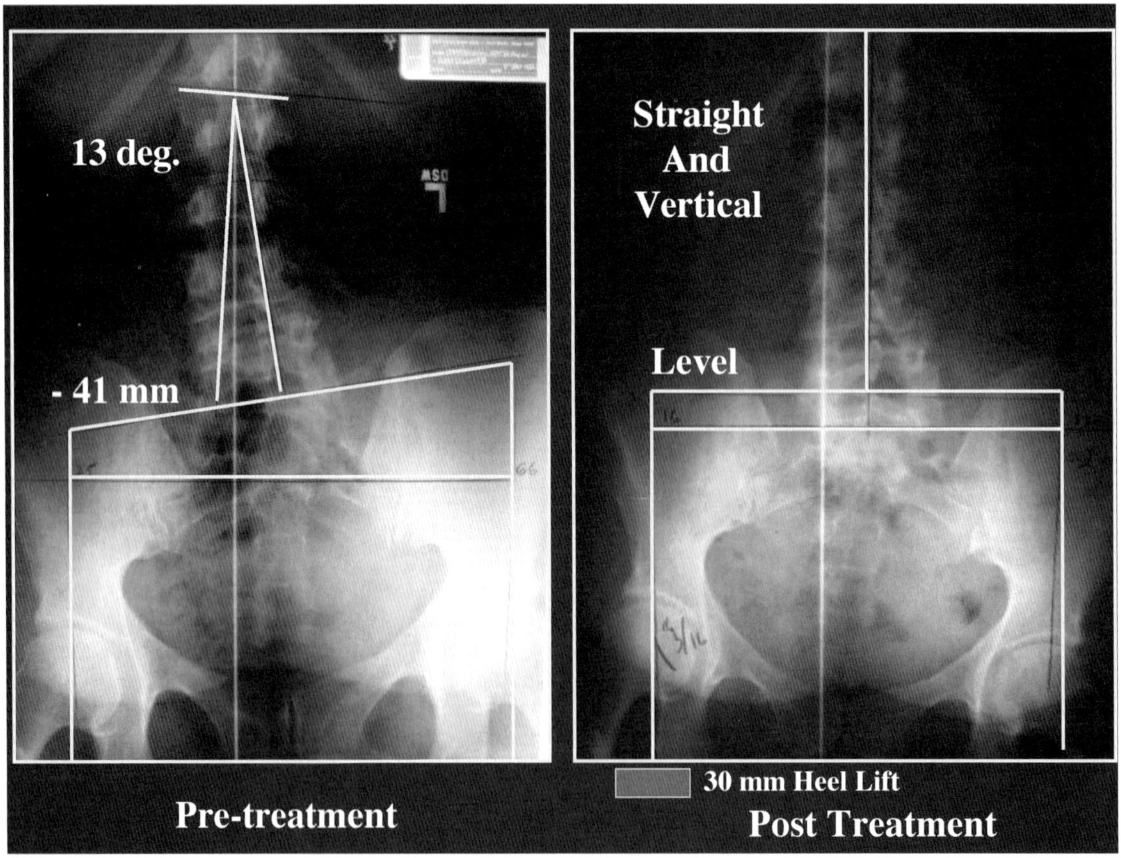

Fig. 16.15 For a 53-year-old female with 13° of lumbar scoliosis, leveling the sacral base is followed by full correction of lumbar scoliosis.

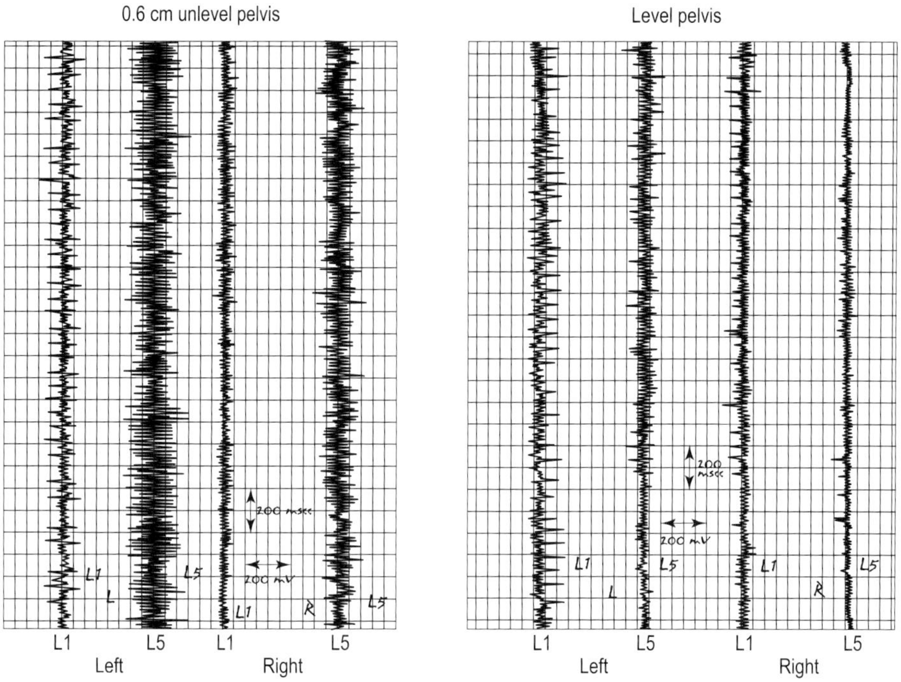

Fig. 16.16 Transcutaneous electromyography of the paralumbar musculature collected at the levels of L1 and L5 while standing, for an unlevel pelvis, pretreatment, and a level pelvis, post treatment. Pelvic leveling is followed by marked reduction and symmetrization of electrical activity.

this angularity is reduced as much or more than 30% when the sacral base is leveled (Fig. 16.15).

The activity of the paralumbar motor neurons for the standing lumbopelvis with normal [6.25 mm (1/4 inch)] pelvic unlevelness is markedly greater and asymmetric, right to left, compared to the activity of the same lumbopelvis when leveled by a 7-mm heel lift (Barker & Irvin 1986, Irvin 1998) (Fig. 16.16). These findings reflect the increase in economy of the upright stance that is posturally balanced (Kappler 1982).

Summary

Most chronic pain is mediated by mechanical stress. This chapter features posture as normally being imbalanced and consequently the primary source of mechanical stress.

The method for postural optimization by the precise use of orthotics is described. Experimental outcomes for partial optimization of posture by use of a heel lift to level the standing pelvis are enduring alleviation of > 70% of mechanically mediated chronic pain, and reduction of idiopathic lumbar scoliosis by 30%. Anecdotally, when: (1) foot orthotics are used to fully correct flattened arches of the feet and vertically align the ankles; (2) heel lift is used to level the pelvis, standing; and (3) ischial lift is used to level the pelvis, seated, then > 90% of common, chronic pain is enduringly alleviated according to this author.

Conclusion: that postural imbalance is the origin of the majority of mechanically mediated chronic musculoskeletal pain. Where standard therapeutics for proximate causes of chronic pain are broadened to include improvement or optimization of posture, far better outcomes can be expected than otherwise.

References

Barker DJ, Irvin RE 1986 Electromyographic responses to osteopathic manipulative treatment and structural balancing. Journal of the American Osteopathic Association 86:605–122

Denslow JS, Korr I, Krems A 1947 Quantitative studies of chronic facilitation in human motorneuron pools. American Journal of Physiology 150:229–238

Denslow JS, Chase JA, Gutensohn OR et al 1955 Methods

in taking and interpreting weight bearing x-ray films. Journal of the American Osteopathic Association 54:663–670

Dott GA, Hart CL, McKay C 1994 Predictability of sacral base unlevelness based on iliac crest measurements. Journal of the American Osteopathic Association 5:383

Fann AV 2003 Validation of postural radiographs as a way to measure change in pelvic obliquity. Archives of Physical Medicine and Rehabilitation 84(1):75–78

Greenman PE 1979 Lift therapy: use and abuse. Journal of the American Osteopathic Association 79:238–250

Hoffman K, Hoffman L 1994 Effects of adding sacral base leveling to osteopathic manipulative treatment of back pain: a pilot study. Journal of the American Osteopathic Association 3:217–322

Irvin RE 1986 Postural balancing; a regimen for the routine reversal of chronic somatic dysfunction. Journal of the American Osteopathic Association 86:608

Irvin RE 1991 Reduction of lumbar scoliosis by the use of heel lift to level the sacral base. Journal of the American Osteopathic Association 911:34–44

Irvin RE 1997 Sub-optimal posture; the origin of the majority of musculoskeletal pain of the musculoskeletal system. In: Vleeming A et al (eds) Movement, instability and low back pain. Edinburgh: Churchill Livingstone, p133–155

Irvin RE 1998 The origin and relief of common pain. Journal of the Back and Musculoskeletal Rehabilitation 11:89–130

Kappler RE 1982 Postural balance and motion patterns. Journal of the American Osteopathic Association 81:598–606

Loyd P 1934 Roentgenographic postural examination of the lumbar spine and pelvis. Read before the College of Osteopathic Surgeons. Manipulative treatment of back pain: a pilot study. Journal of the American Osteopathic Association 3:217–222

Perlin JB, Gerwin CM, Panchision DM et al 1993 Kindling produces long-lasting and selective changes in gene expression of hippocampal neurons. Proceedings of the National Academy of Sciences USA 90:1741–1745

Rome PR, Rome JD 2000 Limbically augmented pain syndrome (LAPS): kindling, corticolimbic sensitization, and the convergence of affective and sensory symptoms in chronic pain disorders. Pain Medicine 1(1):7–23

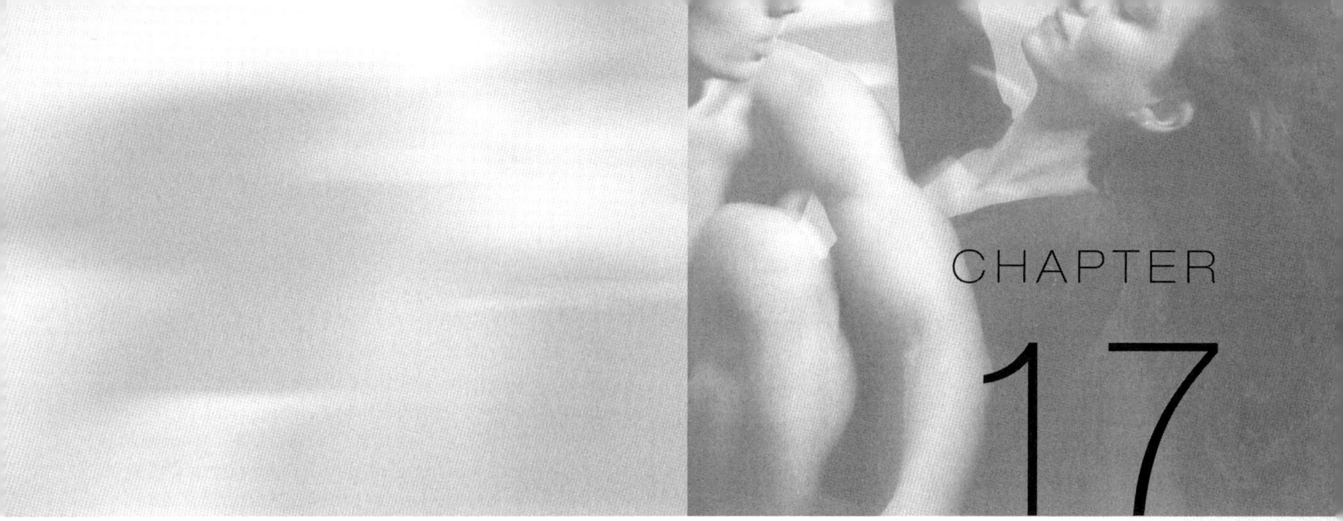

CHAPTER 17

Gait style as an etiology to lower back pain

Howard J Dananberg

Introduction

Lower back pain is a worldwide phenomenon. Despite its prevalence, there is much disagreement as to any specific underlying cause. What is known is that lumbosacral lesions visible on X-ray, MRI, CT scans, etc. can often exist in healthy subjects without symptoms of lower back pain. If classic markers for back pain exist in asymptomatic subjects, does their existence in symptomatic patients actually denote a cause and effect relationship? The answer most likely involves the complex interaction between actual pathologic entities within the spine coupled with the mechanical stresses applied to these same spinal structures on a daily basis. Whereas lifting and twisting injuries can and do cause back pain, simple acts such as reaching over or bending minimally can precipitate an acute lower-back disabling event. If the act of simply bending can promote an acute lower back episode, does this really represent *the* injury, or instead is it the final maneuver in a long period of lumbar stress? One overlooked stress to the back – but one truly present on a daily basis – is gait style. Any single step would never produce sufficient mechanical stress to cause injury. Over sufficient time, however, the tens of millions of steps taken can represent a repetitive strain injury (RSI) and, as such, be an underlying cause and/or perpetuating factor in the lower back symptom process.

What is well known about lower back pain is the recurrent nature of the disorder. A previously published study found a 71% recurrence in symptoms within 12 months of an initial acute lower back pain (LBP) episode (Von Korff et al 1993). If gait style does represent a true RSI, then treatment should have a very positive effect on recurrence of symptoms.

In 1999, a study involving 32 subjects previously deemed at medical endpoint LBP was published (Dananberg & Guiliano 1999). It involved treating gait style with custom foot orthotics (CFO) objectively fabricated by in-shoe pressure testing apparatus. Of the original 32 subjects, 32 were followed for 3 months, and 23 for between 12 and 24 months. The study used the Quebec Back Pain Disability Scale (QBPDS) questionnaire, which contains 20 questions involving activities of daily living. Each is scored 0–5, with 0 being easily possible, and 5 being impossible due to pain. Some subjects did not answer all questions, so mean pain score is determined by totaling the responses and dividing by the number of questions answered. Pain scores can then be compared or averaged across groups of subjects. Each patient in the Dananberg & Guiliano study completed the QBPDS questionnaire before the onset of treatment, again at 3 months, and then at the conclusion. Results were compared to the original QBPDS paper published in *Spine* (Kopec et al 1995). After 3 months of standard lower back care, subjects in the QBPDS study showed a drop from 2.40 to 2.02 in pain levels. The gait study group showed a drop from 2.42 to 1.71. At the average follow-up time of 13.9 months, the gait study group had a pain level of 1.73. In other words, once the pain level receded, it did not rebound for a time period exceeding 1 year. Considering that 84% of the subjects in the gait study of medical endpoint subjects showed significant improvement, gait style should be considered during the lower back patient evaluation.

The mechanics of gait

When the ancestors of our human species became bipedal millions of years ago, they needed an ambulation system that would function in a highly efficient fashion over long distances. Upright human walking is that efficient system. To appreciate its mechanics, some prior misconceptions must first be addressed.

It has been theorized that walking is the process in which muscles fire, creating force moments across joints, which in turn drive the weight-bearing limb to push the body forward (Inman 1981). This view cannot be supported by either logic or currently available information on muscle function. Muscles in the weight-bearing limb predominantly function eccentrically (Winter & Scott 1991). Eccentric contraction represents the resistance to motion. Although this is highly efficient (1.5–6.0 times that of concentric contraction or muscle shortening; Abbott 1952), it cannot create the 'push' required for walking. When concentric contraction finally occurs in the gastrocnemius, for example, both the knee and hip have already begun to flex forward. This would equate to the concept of pushing rope! Flexible systems cannot be effectively driven in this manner. Therefore, another model must be used to understand the mechanics of human walking.

The human body can be viewed as a perpetual motion gait machine. The pendular actions of arms and legs act reciprocally, storing potential energy and returning kinetic energy in the process. These actions are visible as counter-rotations between the pelvic and shoulder girdles. Storage occurs in the ligamentous, muscular, and tendinous structures of the lower back (Dorman 1995). The cross-connections between the ipsilateral latissimus dorsi and contralateral gluteus maximus muscle via the fascia thoracolumbocalis are ideally suited to this storage capacity. Each step prepares for the next one; the effect is to create a forward-directed rotation on the pelvic hemisphere as it coordinates with the limb that is about to begin the swing phase motion (Gracovetsky 1987).

During walking, there are periods of both single and double limb support (Fig. 17.1). Substantial forward motion can only occur in the approximately 400 ms of single support phase. As the weight-bearing limb supports the body, the contralateral limb acts to *pull* the center of mass forward (Claeys 1983). Essentially, the swinging limb lifts the center of body mass (CoM) storing potential energy in the process. Once the CoM reaches its apex during the mid-single-support period, it begins to be pulled back to earth by gravity. The potential energy stored during the initial phase, is now returned as kinetic energy. This action of the CoM falling forward, acts to thrust the trailing, weight-bearing limb against the ground. This produces a reactive longitudinal ground shear force on the supporting surface. The ground does not move, so the individual advances.

Eccentric muscular contraction that is present during the single support phase serves to support the weight-bearing limb against the forces described above.

For the gait scenario as described to function and permit the torso to remain erect, the lower extremity must function in elegant coordination with the upper body. It is the ability of the hip joint and foot/ankle complex to permit forward motion while simultaneously managing internal and external limb rotation. As the body passes over the weight-bearing foot (right limb viewed from the right side), the hip joint

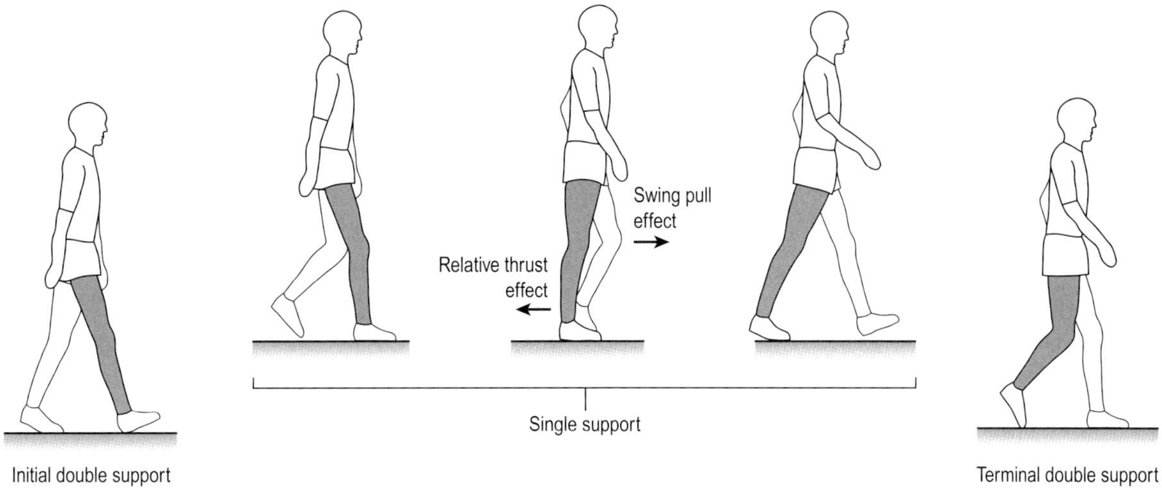

Fig. 17.1 Single and double support phases of gait

permits a clockwise rotation in synchronization with foot level sagittal plane rotation (heel lift) and external rotation accommodation (supination). This permits the torso to remain erect as the leg and thigh extend under it. The foot's triplanar motion permits efficient advancement beyond a fixed point (Fig. 17.2). Should either the foot or hip joint malfunction, the efficiency of the walking process can be negatively impacted.

Rotation of the hip joint is simple to visualize. It is a ball and socket joint that permits sagittal plane extension during the single support phase. The foot, however, comprises 26 joints, which rotate in a complex yet interdependent manner. It must coordinate the effect of lower extremity internal rotation that is coordinated with and takes place with the impact forces present at heel strike (pronation). It must then reverse the pronation direction of motion by midstep and begin supination, as it accommodates lower extremity external rotation caused by pelvic motion created by the contralateral swing limb. All the while, it must simultaneously stabilize itself to forces that can reach multiples of body weight prior to toeoff, while permitting the entire body to pass over it. This final event, sagittal plane pivot, requires that the foot maintain a portion of its structure in ground contact while the remainder of the foot passes directly over the fixed portion. These actions are repeated at least 2500 times per day, all within the time span of approximately 600–750 ms.

The ability of the foot to permit the body to advance forward over it is a complicated action. There are three separate sites at which this pivotal response occurs (Dananberg 1995, Perry 1992).

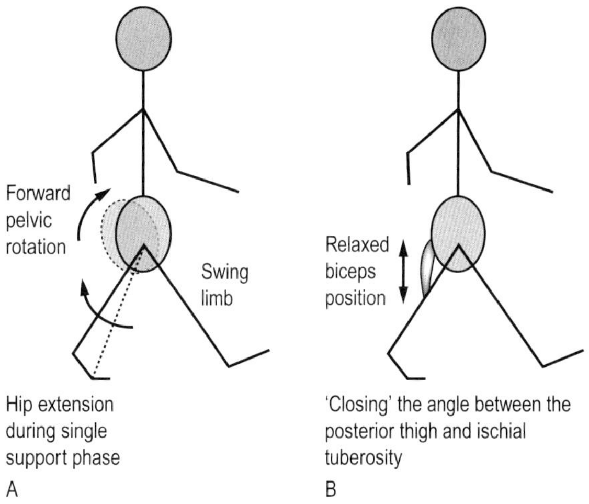

Fig 17.2 The coordination of hip extension, forward pelvic rotation, and biceps relaxation.

The initial location is the inferior, rounded undersurface of the calcaneus. This motion is completed following heel strike, once the forefoot touches the floor. With the heel and forefoot in contact with the ground, the ankle becomes the next site of rotation. It passively dorsiflexes as the pull of the swing limb advances the center of mass over it (Perry 1992). Dorsiflexion of the ankle is an intricate movement. The dome of the talus is shaped as a truncated pyramid, wider anteriorly than posteriorly. Therefore, as dorsiflexion occurs, the ankle joint must expand to accept the widening surface of the talar dome. This expansion is dependent on a translation motion of the fibula. It moves upward and laterally, reorienting the fibers of the syndosmosis that connect it to the tibia. Not only does this permit continued dorsiflexion, but it also appears to store energy that will be used for ankle reversal into plantar flexion later in the step. The above two actions occur in a period of less than 200 ms.

The final pivotal 'hurdle' occurs in the second half of the single support phase. This represents the peak reactive ground thrust periods during the final 200 ms of one-leg support and further co-ordinates with the greatest forces concurrently being applied. As the foot must act as both a shock absorber at heel strike and then reverse to be a rigid platform for propulsion at this time, a system must be present to regulate these events sequentially and establish a stable structure from a flexible one. As this occurs, it must continue to permit the body to advance forward directly over it. This dual function (propulsion/stability) has been shown to be dependent on the proper function of the first metatarsophalangeal (MTP) joint, the final pivotal site. In 1954, the British research physician J H Hicks proposed such a mechanism in the *Journal of Anatomy*. As recently as 1995, his concepts have been proven most accurate (Thordarson 1995).

This action, known as the windlass effect, is a purely mechanical (and therefore non-muscular) response. It uses the plantar aponeurosis as a tension band, altering its tightness as required by body and foot position. The plantar aponeurosis originates from the base of the calcaneus and inserts into the base of the proximal phalanx of the great toe (as well as providing smaller fibers to the lesser digits). As the MTP joint dorsiflexes to permit heel lift, the large, drum-like shape of the first metatarsal head–sesamoid bone complex serves as a mechanically advantaged cam, tightening the aponeurosis between the heel and toes. As the aponeurosis tightens, it secondarily close-packs the calcaneal cuboid joint on the lateral column of the foot (Bojsen-Møller 1979). In other words, the same movement that permits the body to pivot over the planted foot simultaneously stabilizes it to the stresses that are cyclically applied (Fig. 17.3).

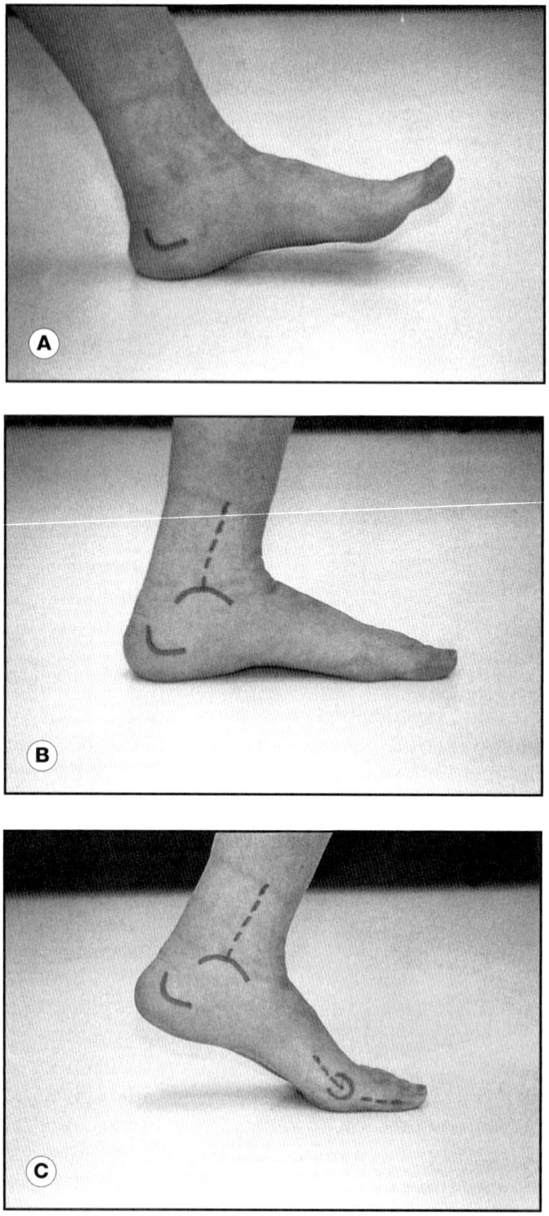

Fig. 17.3 (A) At heel strike, the round underside of the calcaneus serves as the initial pivotal site. (B) Once foot flat is achieved, sagittal motion is now accommodated by the ankle joint via dorsiflexion. (C) At heel lift, ankle motion reverses to plantarflexion as the metatarsophalangeal (MTP) joint provides for the balance of the required sagittal plane motion.

The swing phase terminates with heel strike, and the entire process reverses, the trailing limb beginning its transition to swing movement. The passage from the stance to swing represents a mechanical challenge. It requires taking the 10.5 kg limb from an 'at rest' position to a full-speed, swing motion in 100 ms. The greater the efficiency in this transformation, the less the muscular input required.

The ability to create efficient swing phase is a direct function of: (1) the ability of the hip flexor muscles to function; (2) the action of the spinal engine to store and return energy for pelvic rotation; and (3) the ability of the limb to create 'pre-swing' motion necessary to accelerate the limb prior to actual toeoff (Dananberg 2001). During single support phase, the weight-bearing limb extends from under the torso. This limb will extend up to the end of single support. With opposite heel strike, the trailing limb reverses direction and, from the extended position, begins its pre-swing forward flexion motion. The knee and hip 'give way' forward as the limb accelerates forward prior to toeoff. At toeoff, the pelvis is being rotated via the spinal engine while the hip flexors act to 'perpetuate' the already flexing limb into its forward swinging motion.

Foot level sagittal plane motion restriction

The efficiency of the human gait system is dependent on the simple process of being able to advance the center of body mass over the weight-bearing foot as described above. However, restriction in this process was described initially in the 1980s (Dananberg 1986). Loss of motion at the foot level during the gait cycle, at the time when the proximal aspects of the body create the forces for forward motion, cause an aberration in the efficiency of this mechanism. Power created for forward motion must then be dissipated. It is this process that is fundamental in understanding the cause and effect relationship of gait to chronic lower back symptoms.

The three sites of pivotal function at the foot were mentioned earlier. The round underside of the calcaneus with – essentially – 'no moving parts', rarely fails to provide its initial pivotal action. The ankle and first MTP joints, however, are complex in their movements and, either singly or combined, can act to block normal progression.

Ankle equinus, or failure to achieve 10° of dorsiflexion while loaded, is a common pathomechanical entity. It has been shown to be an etiologic source of foot and postural pain in patients diagnosed as having it (Root et al 1977). Techniques of stretching the Achilles tendon and triceps surae complex, ankle manipulations, and even surgical intervention for lengthening have been conceived as methods to negate this pathomechanical influence. In and of itself, however, it would not impede forward progress provided that the last pivotal site, the first MTP joint, initiated its dorsiflexion motion early enough in the stance phase. It is the ability of the first MTP joint to react to the pull of the body over it that ultimately dictates the ability to advance the body over the bearing foot.

Degenerative joint disease of the hip is well known. A characteristic gait style develops when sagittal plane motion is restricted at the hip due to arthritic changes. Interestingly, the fundamental gait style visible in the presence of sagittal plane foot restriction can be quite similar to that seen from hip degeneration. As both the hip and foot sagittal rotation is required for the torso to remain upright during the single support phase of the gait cycle, restriction to either can result in postural changes and lumbar stress during walking (Fig. 17.4).

Functional hallux limitus

Functional hallux limitus (Fhl) represents a complete locking of the primary sagittal plane pivotal site, the first MTP joint, strictly during all or portions of the single support phase of the gait cycle. This is true despite the fact that full range of motion

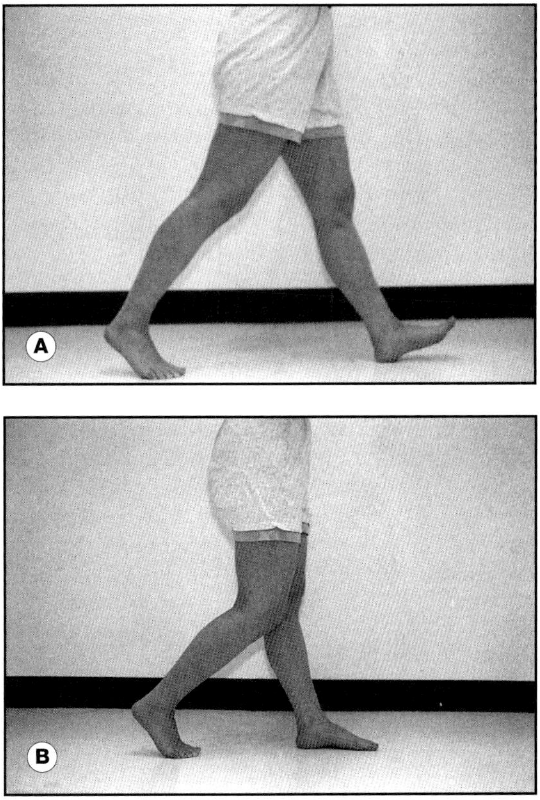

Fig 17.4 (A) At the end of single support phase, the weight-bearing (trailing) limb reaches the peak amount of extension at the hip joint. The knee is fully extended and the foot has lifted off the support surface via motion at the metatarsophalangeal (MTP) joints. (B) During double support, the trailing leg 'gives way,' flexing and accelerating forward in preparation for toeoff and subsequent swing phase.

occurs in the non-weight-bearing examination. As such, it is an entity that represents a paradox between those findings present during clinical examination and those found during function (gait). This contradiction defines Fhl. The functional abilities present during non-weight-bearing physical examination concerning range of motion are the opposite of those found during walking. Its capacity to permit forward advancement while simultaneously creating close-packed alignment never materializes. The manifestations of its presence are most often visible at alternative sites that act to compensate for the failure of this joint to provide the motion necessary for forward progression. Clinically, and in true Fhl, the patient will rarely if ever exhibit symptoms of pain or swelling associated with this joint. The relationship between Fhl and more proximal postural symptoms has therefore not been readily apparent (Dananberg 1986, 1993a, 1993b, Wernick & Dananberg 1988) (Fig. 17.5).

Recognizing that these sagittal plane motions exist, then the logical sequence of progression would dictate that foot level restrictions would lead to more proximal restriction as well. In 2001, a paper was presented at the fourth world congress on lower back pain that detailed this process (Dananberg 2001). It retrospectively reviewed hip joint range of motion on 20 subjects walking before and after intervention with custom foot orthotics. It demonstrated a 50% increase in hip joint extension by the conclusion of single support phase as a result of the functional changes brought about by the custom foot orthotic. As sagittal plane restriction was the essence of the foot orthotic treatment process, its impact on the more proximal structures was quite significant with a measurable increase in hip extension present by the conclusion of single support phase.

The effect of limited hip extension

When Fhl is present, the most evident marker is its effect on hip extension. During normal gait, the hip joint will extend approximately 15° by the end of single support phase. This action: (1) permits the torso to remain erect; (2) allows for thrust against the support surface; (3) positions the limb appropriately in a position from which it can be lifted for the next swing phase; and (4) 'closes the angle' between the posterior aspect of the weight-bearing leg and the posterior aspect of the ischial tuberosity. Each of these is significant in understanding the process of lower back pain.

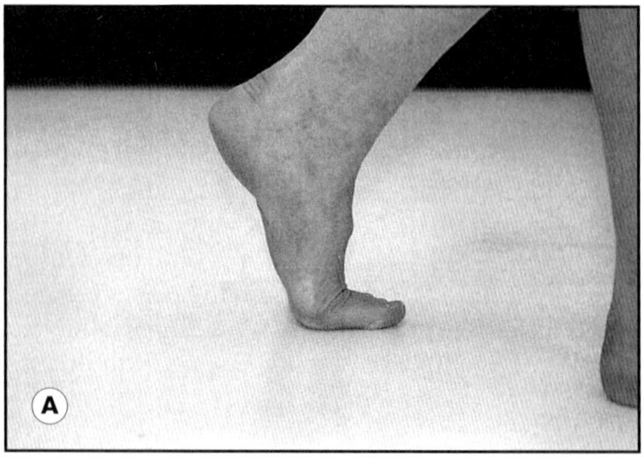

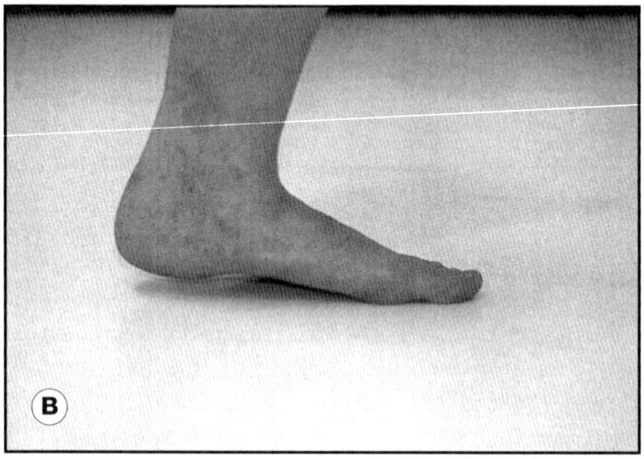

Fig. 17.5 (A) Normal range of motion (ROM) of the first metatarsophalangeal (MTP) joint when viewed in a double support stance position. (B) During the second half of the single support phase of the same foot, note the inability of the first MTP joint to exhibit any ROM. This paradox, that ROM of motion, while available in some positions, fails to occur during single support, defines functional hallux limitus (Fhl).

Facilitating an erect torso

As the thigh extends from under the torso, the rotary motion at the hip permits the lumbar spine to remain upright. Should hip motion abruptly stop, lumbar flexion occurs that creates disc compression as well as muscular overuse.

Undergoing extension for thrust

The extension of the leg and thigh permit the body efficiently to use the process of energy return to create forward motion. Failure of this motion then requires additional muscular input, resulting in fatigue.

Positioning the limb to initiate swing phase

The process for efficiently initiating the swing phase was described earlier. Should the thigh fail to extend adequately, this entire mechanism fails. As the limb to be lifted weighs 15% of body weight, it therefore represents a significant load on the iliopsoas structure. When the iliopsoas fires but the femur is fixed, Kapandji (1974) has shown that the lumbar spine will side-bend and rotate. These pathomechanical actions will shear intervertebral discs and create an environment that has been shown to induce intervertebral disc herniation. Iliopsoas overuse will also produce both back and groin pain associated with this pathomechanical process.

'Closing the angle' between the weight-bearing leg and ischial tuberosity

The ability of the pelvis to rotate forward during single support was shown earlier to be related to the relaxed biceps femoris. Should hip extension fail to develop, the angle between the posterior thigh and the ischial tuberosity will instead 'open.' Torso flexion replaces hip extension, further exacerbating the situation. This will create tension in the biceps and, when sufficient, will cause Golgi tendon response and biceps firing. It will then force a premature halt of pelvic forward rotation, and if torso flexion is sufficient, pelvic rotation will reverse to an anterior-to-posterior movement. This action will create tightening of the sacrotuberous ligament as the reversal of motion creates a sacral counternutation. Motion necessary for pre-swing is prematurely exhausted, thus affecting the preload motion to initiate the next swing phase.

Patients with lower back pain as a rule exhibit tight hamstrings. This underlying mechanism should be noted, as the standard treatment of stretching the hamstrings will not alter the mechanics that bring about the tightness (Fig. 17.6).

The accommodation of lateral trunk bending

When full extension of the weight-bearing limb ceases, the ability to create the following swing phase efficiently is lost. Obvious overuse to the iliopsoas results but additional mechanisms are available to assist in developing the next swing phase motion.

A universal accommodation to this appears as the lateral trunk bend. Patients will routinely bend from the ipsilateral restricted side to the contralateral side at ipsilateral toeoff. This motion is generally created by two muscle groups: the contralateral quadratus lumborum and contralateral gluteus maximus/iliotibial band complex. When activated, these structures create a lateral trunk-bending

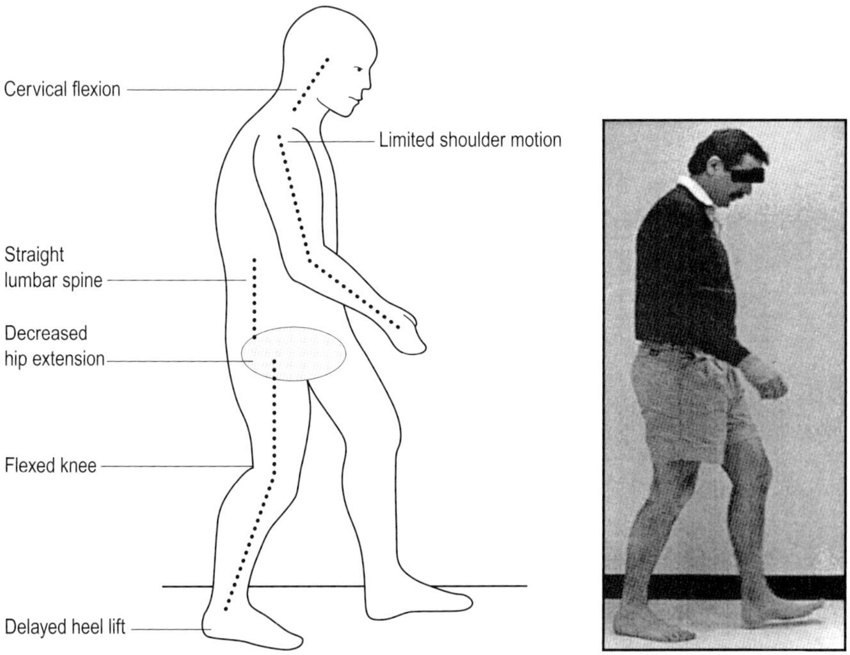

Fig. 17.6 Flexion compensation for functional hallux limitus (Fhl).

motion that 'drags' the trailing limb into the swing phase. Several pain patterns can be created by this mechanism: pain in the quadratus lumborum between the twelfth rib and iliac crest; greater trochanteric bursitis; lateral knee pain; and, owing to the quadratus lumborum's partial insertion into the iliolumbar ligament, disc compression pain related to rotation of the fifth lumbar vertebra (Dananberg 1993b).

Identifying Fhl

Aside from the visualization of Fhl during gait, there are two examination techniques for static recognition of this pathomechanical entity. The first involves the patient in the seated position. For the right foot, the examiner places his or her right thumb directly under the first metatarsal head. A plantar-to-dorsal force is exerted. Then, with the left thumb placed on the underside of the great toe interphalangeal joint, a dorsiflexion force is placed on the toe. Failure to achieve 20–25° of dorsiflexion prior to resistance indicates Fhl.

The other method involves the patient standing. With the weight shifted predominately to the side to be examined, the examiner attempts to dorsiflex the great toe on the first metatarsal. A failure to raise the toe indicates Fhl (Fig. 17.7).

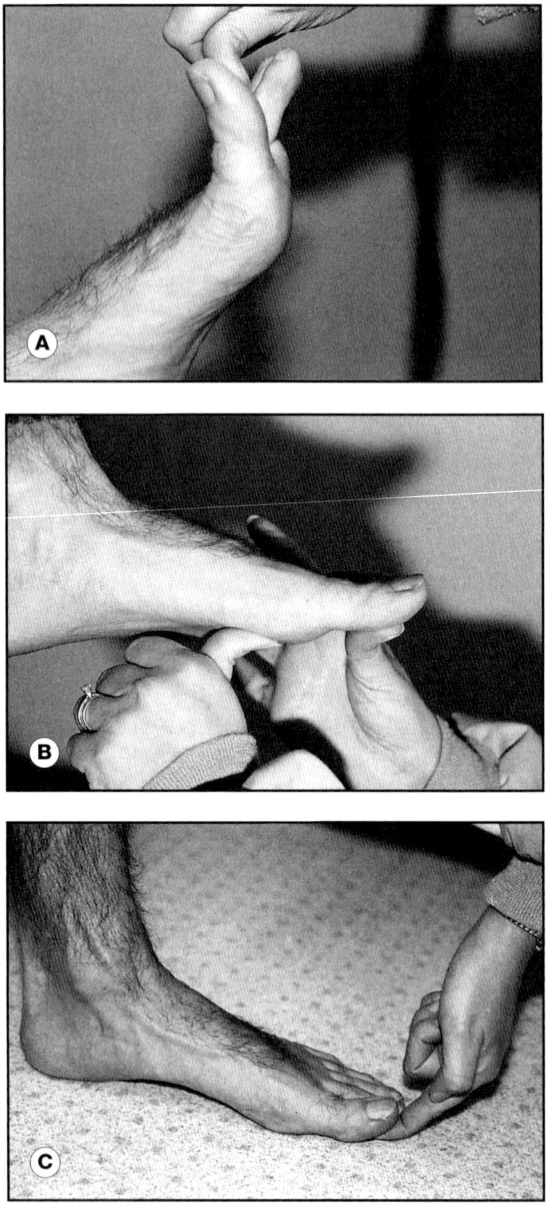

Fig 17.7 (A) In the non-weight-bearing analysis, range of motion (ROM) of the first metatarsophalangeal (MTP) joint is available and normal. (B) When examined with pressure of the clinician's thumb under the 1st metatarsal head while simultaneously attempting to dorsiflex the hallux, range of motion is not available. This test is diagnostic of functional hallux limitus (Fhl).

Treatment options for Fhl

As Fhl is a functional disorder, treatment must promote normal motion at the first MTP joint during the period in the gait cycle when this motion is required. Simply training and/or stretching muscle groups will not adequately address this problem. Just as eyeglasses can correct a functional visual disturbance, so can functional, custom-made foot orthotic devices be effective in dealing with chronic postural complaints based on subtle gait disturbance.

There are several aspects to custom foot orthotic fabrication, including: (1) impression taking and (2) selecting appropriate material and prescription for design (the prescribing of foot orthotics is a subject that is well beyond the limits of this chapter).

Impression taking

Impressions for custom foot orthotics can be done in several ways. The traditional podiatric approach is either prone or supine, neutral position plaster of Paris casting. This takes considerable experience to accurately capture the proper alignment features of the individual foot being treated. Step-in foam boxes can be used but these often distort foot position during the semi-weight-bearing impression process.

Newer methods now exist for optical scans of the foot. This converts the foot to a digital image, which can then be reproduced at the orthotic laboratory for device fabrication.

Selecting appropriate material

Foot orthotics have four basic features: the shell, the post, the top cover, and the extension. Various materials are now available from which to construct the foot orthotic shell. The shell of the device conforms to the patient's foot, usually extending from the back of the heel to just proximal to the metatarsal heads. This distal endpoint is very important, and should never extend to under the metatarsal heads as this would negatively affect the function of the foot. The posts are devices under the heel and forefoot that are used to cant the device depending on foot morphology and function. These are extremely important aspects to the orthotics function. The top cover is either padded or unpadded. It can be made of leather or vinyl, but some full length foam devices do not require this feature. Extensions are the section from the metatarsal heads to the toes. It can be padded, firm, or have various cutouts (depressions) to manage foot segment loading. Each of the components can be made of a variety of materials that can affect the function of the device.

Shells: rigid, semi-rigid, flexible

Depending on the flexibility of the foot, fairly rigid materials might be required to maintain adequate control of lax foot segments. For this purpose, carbon fiber of various thickness, polydur, and the thicker versions of polypropylene or polynylon may be used. The general rule for these materials is that the thicker they are, the stiffer they are. Care should be taken to ensure that these devices will fit inside a shoe once fabricated.

When the foot is less mobile than normal, and requires positioning combined with cushioning to promote improved function, the foam type devices or more flexible subortholene or polynylons are very helpful.

Posts

These are cants on the bottom side of the orthotic, and are designed to redirect forces applied to the foot during gait. A different posting configuration is possible to influence the forefoot independent of the rearfoot, and depends on various morphologic and functional attributes. These posts can be made of stryrene–butadiene rubber (SBR) of varying densities, or in some casts, from extremely rigid methyl methacrylate. On occasion, these can also be of soft material, to encourage motion when little exists. In addition, heel lifts are often added to the posting material, accommodating leg length differences of 3–5 mm.

Extensions

These can be made of different materials, density, and thickness combinations, and with different intents. Softer materials under the first metatarsal head (not first MTP joint) can be very helpful in plantarflexing the metatarsal head and preventing the development of Fhl. The use of firmer materials under the toes can also help in more stubborn cases of Fhl, but dorsiflexing the digits and relatively plantarflexing the metatarsal heads to improve function.

Prefabs

The use of podiatric-type custom foot orthotics requires a true expertise. Many brands of pre-fabricated devices, however, offer the nonpodiatrist an opportunity for a trial procedure to see if gait is negatively influencing lower back pain. If properly modified with heel lifts and first metatarsal head cutouts, patients can often see how they will fare before continuing with a more costly custom-made device.

Observational gait analysis for lower back assessment

Although this chapter cannot begin to do justice to gait analysis for the chronic back pain patient, some specific features are often easily visible and these should be included in the back examination assessment:

- Unequal arm swing: this is a very common accommodation to leg length discrepancy. Subjects most often exhibit greater arm swing on the shorter lower limb side. Use of small incremental lifts to level the pelvis are advisable when this phenomenon is visible.
- Delayed heel lift: the timing of heel lift is a highly significant aspect of efficient gait. In a normal gait cycle, the heel of the weight-bearing side should lift off the support surface prior to the opposite, swing limb's heel making contact. Failure to lift the heel during single support phase will result in limited hip

extension and its subsequent sequealae. Should only one side demonstrate this characteristic, then leg length discrepancy probably exists along with Fhl.
- Lateral trunk bending: patients whose torso sways left and right excessively during the gait cycle are exhibiting a lateral trunk bend. This can cause excessive overuse to the lateral trochanteric bursa, iliotibial band, and quadratus lumborum. These sites are almost always located on the shorter side of the body, so usually match well with excessive arm swing.
- Excessively pronated feet: feet that stand in an abducted position and low arch appearance often require custom foot orthotic management. These can be complex and should be referred for appropriate podiatric management.

Summary

Viewing either recurrent acute or chronic lower back pain as a functional disorder is an advance in the current treatment process. The subtle alterations in an individual's gait when repeated over millions of cycles create overuse-type symptoms in the structures of the lumbosacral spine. The functional disorder can create abnormalities that, over sufficient time, become visible on either computerized tomography or magnetic resonance imaging. Just as often, however, the structures of the lumbosacral spine can be quite normal in appearance yet be painful in response to the cyclic stress placed upon them. The abnormal gait process causes repeated strain on the lower back by destabilizing the natural support mechanics at specific times in the gait cycle. This results is a series of mechanical inefficiencies that culminate in the failure to competently initiate the swing phase of motion. As each limb weighs 15% of body weight, the stress load of lifting this limb improperly can be enormous (over 20 tons per day). The cumulative burden of 'dragging a limb' into the swing phase can create the non-specific-type symptoms that are so common in the lower back pain population. These include:

- myogenic overuse symptoms of the iliopsoas group, quadratus lumborum, and gluteus maximus–iliotibial band complex
- structural symptoms at the origin of the iliopsoas (lumbar spine), insertion of the quadratus lumborum (L5 – via iliolumbar ligament), and sacrum via anatomic connection of the biceps femoris/sacrotuberous ligament.

The dysfunction of the foot plays a major role in preventing the body from passing over it efficiently during gait. The compensatory motions (listed below) are visible in the structures proximal to the foot, and can be thought of as 'gait markers' in observing the recurrent acute/chronic lower back pain patient:

- forward head position – cervical flexion
- straight lumbar spine – torso flexion
- decreased hip extension during single support phase
- flexed knee in midstance
- failure of heel lift during single support phase – visible foot pronation.

As these can all be manifestations of asymptomatic functional aberrations from the foot's pivotal sites, examination of the biomechanics of the foot is essential in this patient population. When foot mechanics, Fhl, leg length discrepancy, and the overall style of walking are addressed as primary stress-creating mechanisms with properly fabricated custom foot orthotics, significant improvement in 84% of long-term, chronic lower back pain patients can be expected according to this author.

References

Abbott BC 1952 The physiological cost of negative work. Journal of Physiology 117:380–390

Bojsen-Møller F 1979 Calcaneocuboid joint and stability of the longitudinal arch of the foot at high and low gear push off. Journal of Anatomy 129(1):165–176

Claeys R 1983 The analysis of ground reaction forces in pathologic gait. International Orthopaedics 7:113–119

Dananberg HJ 1986 Functional hallux limitus and its effect on normal ambulation. Journal of Current Podiatric Medicine, April

Dananberg HJ 1993a Gait style as an etiology to chronic postural pain. Part I: Functional hallux limitus. Journal of the American Podiatric Medical Association 83(8):433–441

Dananberg HJ 1993b Gait style as an etiology to chronic postural pain. Part II: The postural compensatory process. Journal of the American Podiatric Medical Association 83(11):615–624

Dananberg HJ 1995 Lower extremity mechanics and their effect on lumbosacral function. Spine Review 9(2): 389–405

Dananberg HJ 2001 Gait style and its relevance in the management of chronic lower back pain. In: Vleeming A et al (eds) Proceedings of the Fourth Interdisciplinary World Congress Of Low Back and Pelvic Pain. 8–10 November. ECO, Rotterdam, p225–230

Dananberg HJ, Guiliano M 1999 Chronic lower back pain and its response to custom foot orthoses. Journal of the American Podiatric Medical Association 89:109–117

Dorman T 1995 Elastic energy of the pelvis. Spine Review 9(2):365–379
Gracovetsky S 1987 The spinal engine. Springer-Verlag, Vienna
Hicks JH 1954 The mechanics of the foot. Part II: The plantar aponeurosis and the arch. Journal of Anatomy 88:25–30
Inman V 1981 Human walking. Williams & Wilkins, Baltimore, MD
Kapandji I A 1974 The physiology of the joints, vol. 3, The trunk and vertebral column, 2nd edn. Churchill Livingstone, Edinburgh
Kopec JA, Esdaile JM, Abrahamowicz M et al 1995 The Quebec Back Pain Disability Scale: measurement properties. Spine 20:473
Perry J 1992 Gait analysis: normal and pathologic function. Slack, Thorofare, NJ
Root M, Weed J, Orien W 1977 Abnormal and normal function of the foot. Clinical Biomechanics Corp., Los Angeles, CA
Thordarson DB 1995 Dynamic support of the human longitudinal arch. Clinical Orthopedics and Related Research 316:165–172
Von Korff, M, Deyo RA, Cherkin D et al 1993 Back pain in primary care: outcome in 1 year. Spine 19:855
Wernick J, Dananberg HJ 1988 Secondary active retrograde pronation as the ideology to overuse injuries in podiatry tracts. Data Trace Medical Publishers, Baltimore, MD
Winter DA, Scott S 1991 Technique for interpretation of electromyography for concentric and eccentric contractions in gait. Journal of Electromyography and Kinesiology 1(4):263–269

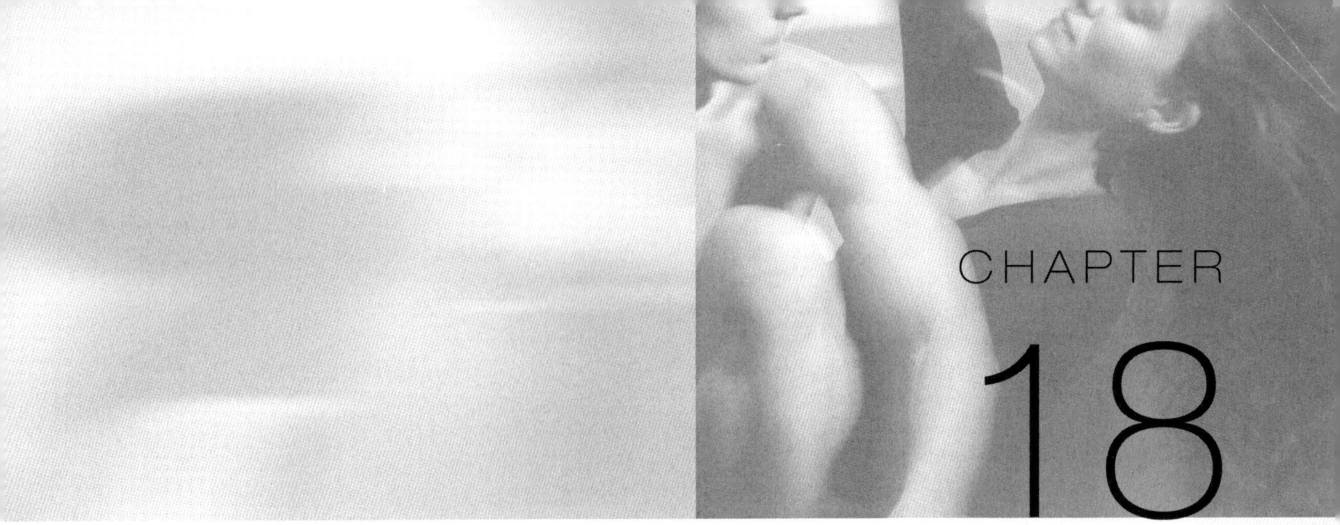

CHAPTER 18

A detailed and critical biomechanical analysis of the sacroiliac joints and relevant kinesiology: the implications for lumbopelvic function and dysfunction

Richard L DonTigny

Introduction

One day in 1964 I treated a young woman with idiopathic low back pain (LBP) syndrome. She got essentially no relief from her treatment but called me the next day, asked to cancel her next treatment and told me she was free of pain. I asked her what she had done to relieve the pain as I had not been able to help her. She hesitated for a moment and then told me she had fallen from her tractor. I realized that she had a reversible biomechanical problem that was cured by a happy accident and that if I could determine the nature of that problem I should be able to resolve it in the clinic with less traumatic methods.

I had some idea that it might be in the sacroiliac joint (SIJ) and began a personal investigation into the cause of LBP. By 1965 I had developed a method of treatment that allowed me to have at least 80% of all my patients with LBP essentially free of pain immediately following a simple manual correction of a perceived subluxation in anterior rotation. Although the condition could recur, it could be controlled with appropriate corrective exercises and prevented by simply supporting the anterior pelvis with the abdominal muscles when leaning forward to lift, bend, or lower.

This method was so effective that I felt I had a professional obligation to share it with my colleagues. It took 8 years to get published the first time and usually 4 to 5 years for each succeeding publication as I gradually improved my methods and my biomechanics.

In 1982 White suggested:

> *It may well be that idiopathic backache will be found to be caused by some condition that is a subtle variation from normal. Otherwise, we probably would have found the cause already. If back pain were caused by a highly*

unusual condition, then fewer people would suffer from this disorder.

White was correct. I have described a commonly overlooked, measurable, reversible, biomechanical lesion of the SIJ as this subtle variation from normal (DonTigny 1990). *Apparently, not only does every patient with LBP have essentially the same problem, varying in degree and chronicity, but they essentially all respond to the same corrective method.* Now I can have over 90% of all patients with low back pain free of pain within minutes and if you do what I did, with practice, you will get the same results.

The purposes of this chapter are threefold. The first is to do a detailed analysis and present a revised biomechanical model of pelvic mechanics and the self-bracing principle. The second is to describe movement and function of the SIJ on the asymmetric pelvis. The third is to delineate the pathomechanics of the SIJ and its associated conditions.

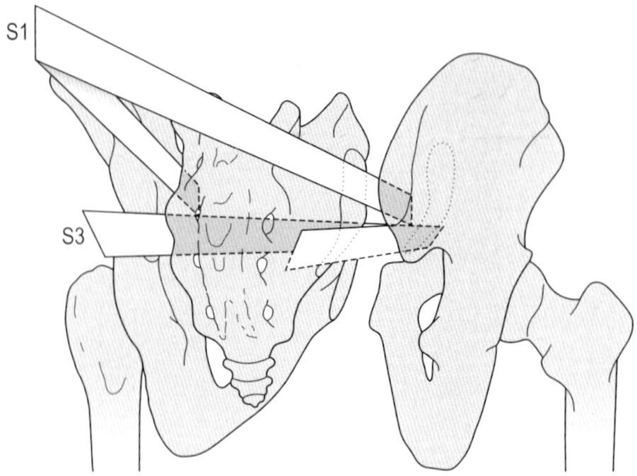

Fig. 18.1 Angulations of the S1 and S3 surfaces of the sacroiliac joints (SIJs). Unrestricted loading of the body of the sacrum would tend to decrease friction at both S1 and S3.

Structure, movement, and ligamentous loading

Movements of the innominate bones and the sacrum are only somewhat interdependent. With flexion of the lumbar spine there is a tendency toward a ventral inclination or nutation of the sacrum on the stabilized innominate bones. With extension, dorsal inclination or contranutation occurs, probably on a transverse axis through the joint. Weisl (1953) found that the sacrum descends between the innominate bones with superincumbent weight loading when moving from a supine to an erect posture. This movement is in accord with Erhard & Bowling (1977), who stated that for all practical purposes the only motions permitted are gliding in a ventral and caudal direction and return to the resting position. The variation in the angular configuration of the joint surfaces allows this movement (Fig. 18.1) (DonTigny 1994).

Ligamentous influence and functional mechanics

Structurally, the sacrum is suspended from the ilia by the dense posterior interosseous ligaments and functions as the reverse of a keystone by hanging more deeply between the ilia with increased loading. The posterior superior iliac spines (PSIS) converge slightly with increased weight loading on the sacrum. Vukicevic et al (1991) found that the joints do not approximate with weight loading as long as the posterior interosseous ligaments are intact. This indicates that loading of the posterior interosseous ligaments will separate the surfaces of the SIJs. If the sacrum functioned as a keystone, the joint surfaces would approximate and the PSISs would diverge. The superincumbent weight is transferred from the sacrum through the posterior interosseous ligaments to the innominate bones and not through the SIJs, which, in my opinion, are essentially non-weight-bearing.

Superincumbent weight loading on the sacrum causes it to incline ventrally (nutate), creating a primary loading stress on the posterior interosseous ligaments (PIL). Movement is limited because the PIL are short. This causes the caudal end of the sacrum to move posteriorly creating a counterbalancing tensile stress on the sacrotuberous (ST) and sacrospinous (SS) ligaments probably equal to the primary loading force. These balanced tensile forces result in a force couple and a tendency to rotate around a transverse axis created by and perpendicular to the force couple (Fig. 18.2) (DonTigny 1994). Force couples absorb, balance and redirect various forces such as linear velocity, linear acceleration, angular acceleration, linear momentum, angular momentum, the rate of change of momentum, force and moment of force (Fig. 18.3) (DonTigny 1994).

If these forces are balanced bilaterally on the sacrum, a force-dependent transverse axis is established through the sacrum, but not necessarily through the joints. *Because the primary loading is on the PIL and the secondary loading is on the ST and SS ligaments, the axis of rotation must be between these*

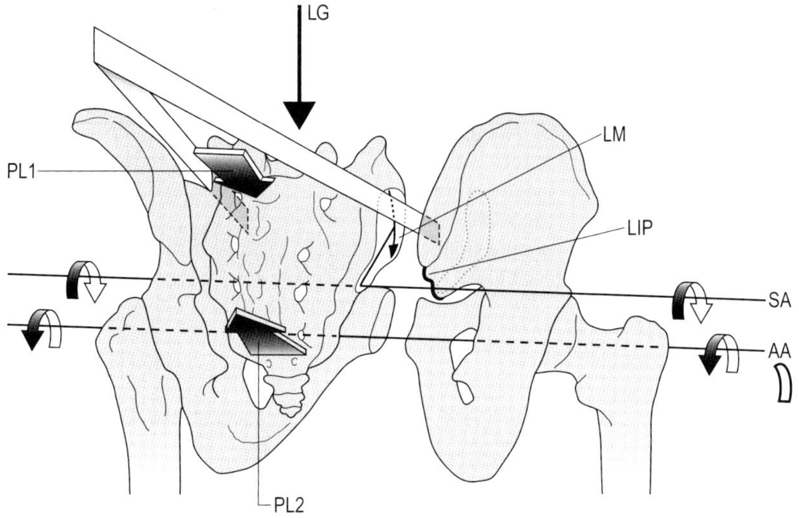

Fig. 18.2 The superincumbent weight indicated by the line of gravity (LG) puts a primary loading stress (PL1) on the posterior interosseous and the iliolumbar ligaments and a secondary loading stress (PL2) on the sacrotuberous and the sacrospinous ligaments. A force couple is formed between the primary and secondary loading forces with an axis of rotation between them. The loading movement (LM) is on the sacral axis (SA). A secondary loading occurs on the acetabular axis (AA) (see Fig. 18.4). A bony ilial lip (LIP) over S3 sacral forces the sacral axis and prevents any movement in posterior rotation of the innominate bone on the sacrum.

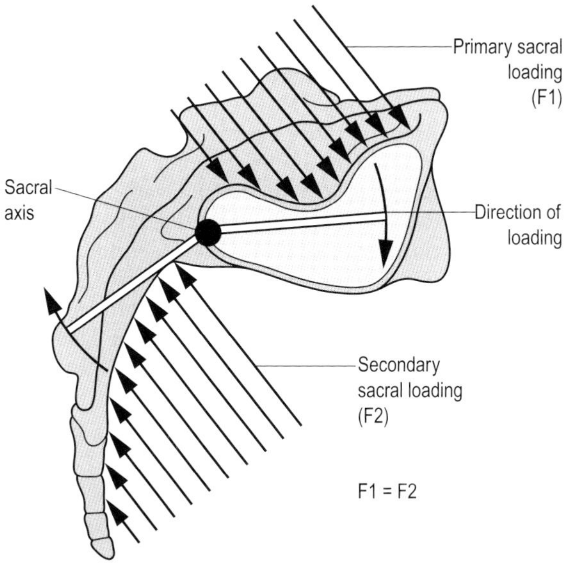

Fig. 18.3 Two equal and parallel forces acting in opposite directions define the sacral axis. If the forces are spread the force dependent axis is more narrowly defined. (Reproduced with permission from DonTigny 2004.)

two sets of ligaments at the most posterior aspect of the S3 segment of the SIJ immediately anterior to the posterior inferior iliac spine (see Fig. 18.2) This axis should probably be considered as being an axis for sacral rotation rather than an axis for the sacroiliac joint per se. This loading only loads and positions the joint for normal movement and function.

Self-bracing revisited and revised

When the sacrum is loaded everything changes. Vleeming et al (1990a) described self-bracing of the SIJ as a result of force closure and form closure. With primary loading, the angle of the S1 sacral segment moves downward on the adjacent joint surface of the ilia and separates from that segment slightly, preventing both form or force closure (DonTigny 2005a). The line of gravity is anterior to the joints but posterior to the acetabula. This causes a posterior rotation of the innominate bones on the sacrum that, in turn, creates a secondary loading on the sacroiliac ligaments. The secondary loading further tightens the ST ligaments and the PIL causing the sacrum to extend dorsally on the sacral axis, decreasing shear at the lumbosacral joints and creating a secondary, balancing force couple (Fig. 18.4). Note the top and bottom views of this bilateral double couple (Fig. 18.5). Even though it looks as if the relatively broad angulations of the S1 sacral segments are held snugly against the corresponding S1 ilial segments to create a form closure, these forces are all in balance, serve to maintain the ilial convexities in the sacral concavities, and maintain that balanced tension on these ligaments to prepare them for normal function. As the primary anterior loading force is equal to the primary posterior loading force and the secondary loading forces balance both of these forces, the force of joint closure is probably nil. It appears that neither form nor force closure occurs with static loading except perhaps at the extreme of posterior pelvic rotation. The bony transverse axis serves as a fulcrum and prevents any significant form or force closure.

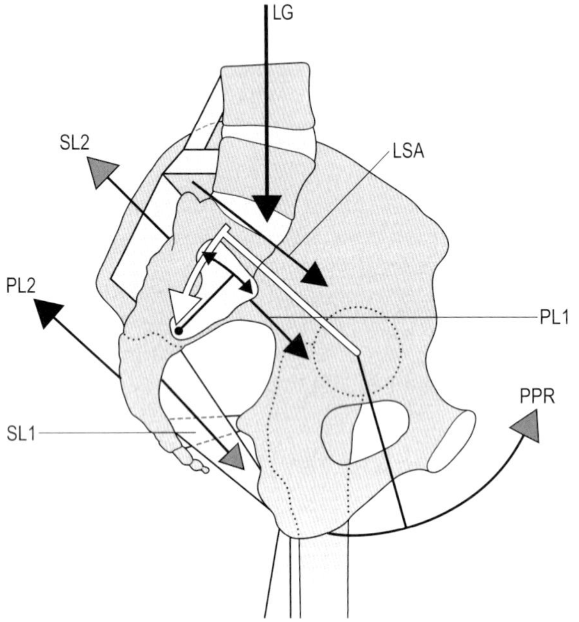

Fig. 18.4 The double couple. The simultaneous sequential loading of the pelvis, with the line of gravity (LG) posterior to the acetabula, causes a posterior pelvic rotation (PPR) on an acetabular axis. It is this PPR that reverses the ventral sacral inclination, putting a balancing force on the primary loading stress (PL1) and secondary loading stress (PL2) and in effect creating a secondary balancing force couple (SL1 and SL2). The sacroiliac joint (SIJ) moves downward relative to the acetabula, the sacrum is extended, the lumbar lordosis is flattened, the lumbosacral angle (LSA) is decreased, and shear is decreased on the lumbosacral joint. (Reproduced with permission from DonTigny 2004.)

Joint closure is balanced and totally dependent on the line of gravity being posterior to the acetabula. The SIJs are vulnerable to dysfunction with any shift in the line of gravity anterior to the acetabula such as is caused when lifting, bending or lowering. This anterior shift would cause the innominate bones to rotate anteriorly on an acetabular axis, loosening the force couple, decreasing friction, and result in a partial dislocation (subluxation) of the innominates cephalad and laterally on the sacrum (DonTigny 1973, 1979, 1985, 1990, 1993, 1994, 1999, 2004, 2005a, 2005b).

Movement and function on the asymmetric pelvis

During normal ambulation, when taking a step, the innominate on the side of loading rotates posteriorly and the innominate on the side of the trailing leg rotates anteriorly, on an axis through the symphysis pubis. In response to this movement the sacrum flexes laterally and rotates (Pitkin & Pheasant 1936).

Demonstration

This sacral movement is easy to demonstrate. While sitting, palpate the tip of your coccyx and translate your left leg forward and your right back, to create an asymmetric pelvis, rocking on the ischial tuberosities (Fig. 18.6). Feel the sacrum flex right and left to create an oblique axis of rotation when you translate your legs. Note especially how your trunk is caused to twist toward the side of the posteriorly rotated innominate bone. Now hold the right thigh back and the left forward and flex your trunk down toward the right. Feel the coccyx move posteriorly when the sacrum flexes anteriorly as it moves on the oblique axis. Palpate the sacral origin of the gluteus maximus on the right as you extend your trunk and feel how it pulls the sacrum downward on the innominate to assist the ST ligament.

The oblique axis

I used a full-size model of a pelvis with the sacrum held tightly against both innominates with strong elastic to simulate normal movement. Rotating the innominate on the side of loading (right) posteriorly and the innominate of the side of the trailing leg anteriorly, the sacrum was carried downward on

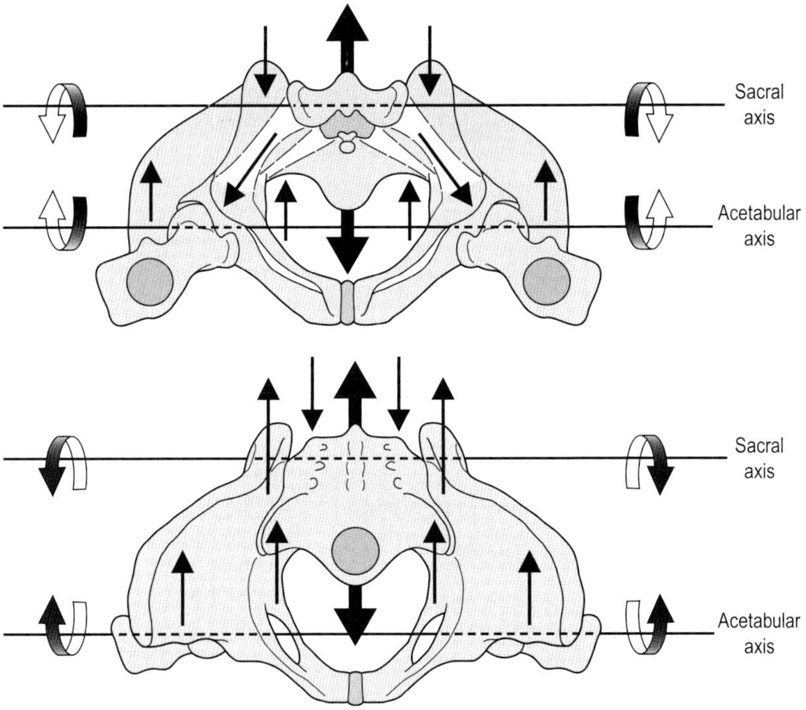

Fig. 18.5 The bilateral double couple. Primary forces (large arrows) and secondary forces (small arrows) are shown in these top and bottom views of the double force couple. Note how the posterior rotation of the innominate bones pulls the sacrum posteriorly with the posterior interosseous ligaments. The primary loading force is still present, although probably diminished and no form or force closure is evident. (Reproduced with permission from DonTigny 2004.)

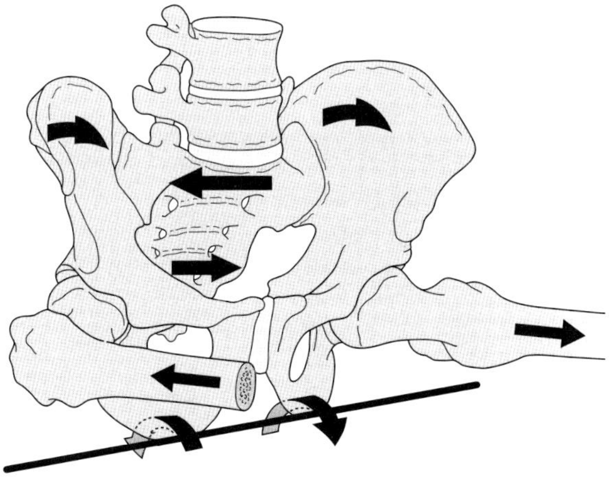

Fig. 18.6 Translating the right leg posteriorly and the left anteriorly creates an asymmetric pelvis and causes the sacrum to incline toward the side of loading to create a force-dependent oblique sacral axis. Rotation occurs with forward trunk flexion on that oblique axis. (Reproduced with permission from DonTigny 2004.)

the side of loading, and upward on the contralateral side. *In vivo,* this lateral sacral flexion is probably caused by the PIL. The joint is approximated at S1 on the right and at S3 on the left (Fig. 18.7) *causing both a form and a force closure only at those specific points.*

A force-dependent oblique axis of rotation is formed. As the superincumbent weight is on the anterior sacrum the joint is opened at S1 on the left and at S3 on the right causing a functional destabilization of the joint. As the line of gravity is anterior to the SIJ this functional destabilization causes the sacrum to open and move anteriorly at S1 on the left and posteriorly at S3 on the right. It moves on that oblique axis to drive rotation of the spine (Fig. 18.8). Apparently, the dense posterior interosseous ligaments cause the same effect *in vivo* as in the previous demonstration (see Fig. 18.6). The amount of rotation that occurs is directly related to and varies with the amount of asymmetry that takes place. The longer the stride, the greater the asymmetry and the greater are the lateral sacral flexion and rotation. *The lateral sacral flexion and rotation precedes loading and drives the spine to rotate to ease the loading force on that side.*

When the sacrum is flexed obliquely increasing lumbar lordosis a considerable force is required to extend the sacrum back to the erect position when the pelvis is symmetrical at the single support phase of normal gait. This is accomplished when the sacral origin of the gluteus maximus muscle functions to extend the sacrum and the piriformis muscle pulls it laterally to symmetry (Fig. 18.9). *These two muscles work together to support the function of the ST and SS ligaments and should probably be considered the prime movers of the SIJ.*

Sacral flexion and rotation is repeated each step and causes an oscillation of the sacrum (Pierrynowski et al 1988) with an increase in lumbar lordosis and the spinal curves from the sacrum cephalad. The spinal curves recover when the pelvis is again symmetrical at the single support phase (Fig. 18.10). This rhythmic sacrocranial vertebral oscillation was measured by Thorstensson et al (1984) in treadmill studies and found to be about 2–2.5 cm at L3 and 1–1.5 cm at C7. The spine acts as a decreasing waveform to damp this oscillation in order to keep the head stable while ambulating. It appears to function as a biologic image-stabilizing system (DonTigny 2004, 2005a). The posterior movement of the spine just prior to symmetry at single support then facilitates the hip flexors in the forward propulsion of the trailing leg.

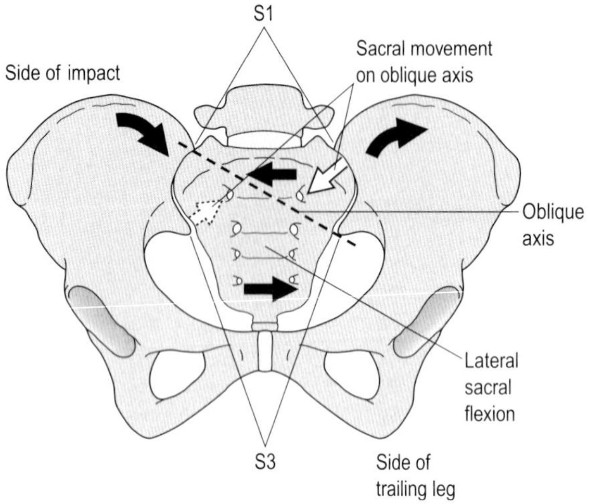

Fig. 18.7 Posterior rotation (right) and anterior rotation (left) demonstrating joint closure at S1 (right) and at S3 (left) to create an oblique axis (OA). A functional destabilization occurs at S1 (left) and S3 (right), allowing the joint to open and move on that oblique axis. (Reproduced with permission from DonTigny 2004.)

Pathomechanics and the subluxation at S3

When standing, the pelvis is symmetrical, the sacrum is loaded and the ligaments are in balance. No muscle power is necessary to maintain the position

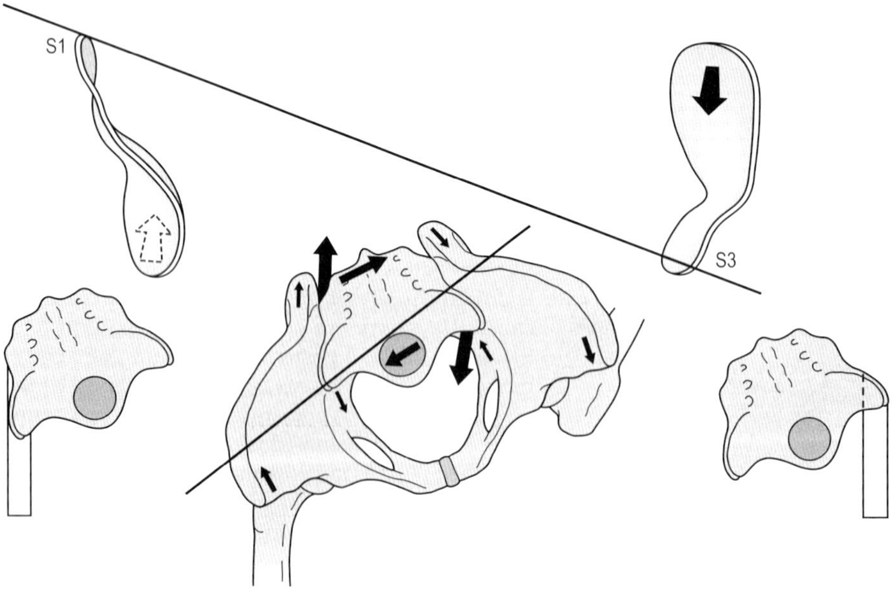

Fig. 18.8 Cranial view of the pelvis demonstrating the probable movement on the oblique axis. (Reproduced with permission from DonTigny 2004.)

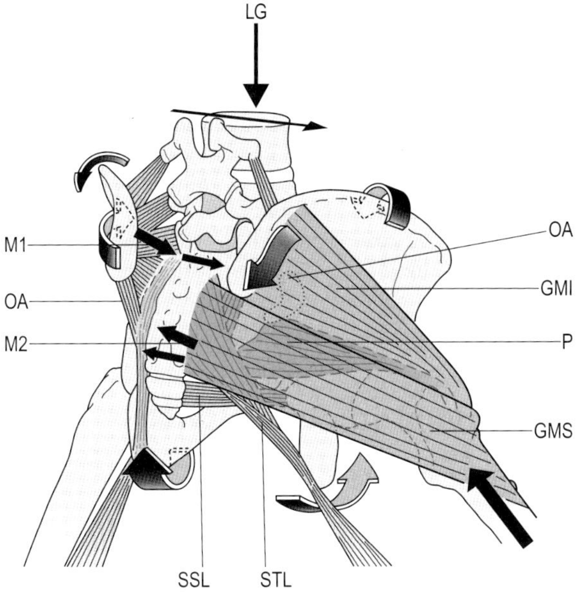

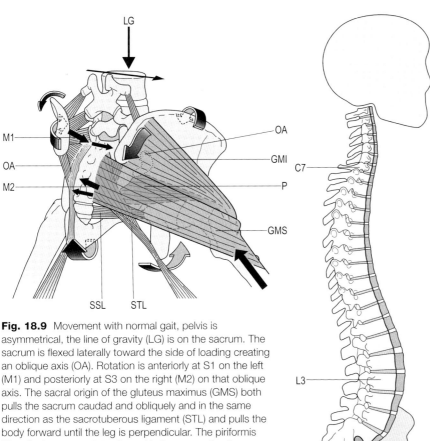

Fig. 18.9 Movement with normal gait, pelvis is asymmetrical, the line of gravity (LG) is on the sacrum. The sacrum is flexed laterally toward the side of loading creating an oblique axis (OA). Rotation is anteriorly at S1 on the left (M1) and posteriorly at S3 on the right (M2) on that oblique axis. The sacral origin of the gluteus maximus (GMS) both pulls the sacrum caudad and obliquely and in the same direction as the sacrotuberous ligament (STL) and pulls the body forward until the leg is perpendicular. The piriformis (P) pulls the sacrum laterally and in the same direction as the sacrospinous ligament (SSL). The ilial origin of the gluteus maximus (GMI) sequentially undergoes an eccentric contraction to decrease loading on the contralateral side with the next step. (Reproduced with permission from DonTigny 2004.)

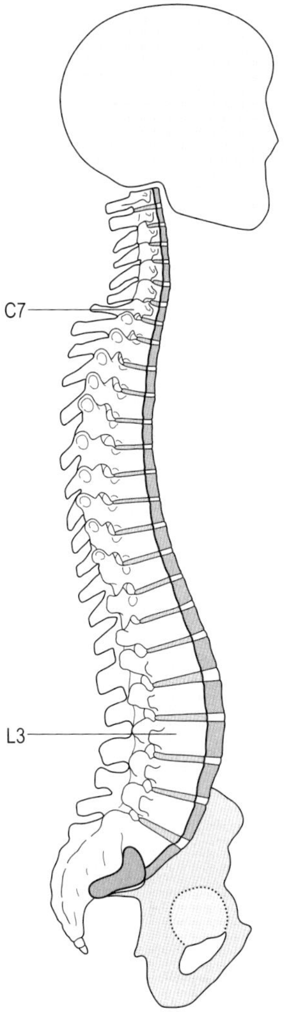

Fig. 18.10 The lateral sacral flexion and rotation during normal gait creates a rhythmic sacrocranial vertebral oscillation. The gray area indicates the approximate amount of vertebral movement caused by the sacral movement. Thorstensson et al (1984) measured this in treadmill studies to be 1–1.5 cm at C7 and 2–2.5 cm at L3. The spine appears to function as a decreasing waveform to damp this oscillation and control head movement. (Reproduced with permission from DonTigny 2004.)

of posterior pelvic rotation. When leaning forward to lift, bend or lower the line of gravity moves anteriorly to the acetabula and the innominates will rotate anteriorly on an acetabular axis.

The most critical support necessary to maintain self-bracing when leaning forward is a strong voluntary contraction by the abdominal muscles (Fig. 18.11) (DonTigny 1979). Specifically, the rectus abdominis and the abdominal oblique muscles work with the sacral origin of the gluteus maximus and the piriformis muscles to maintain the self-bracing position of the pelvis in this position. The transverse abdominis muscle has been described as assisting in self-bracing, but that is likely minimal at best. Other than having a stiffening action on the spine, the transverse abdominis muscle has little effect on the secondary loading forces.

McGill (2001) stated:

Richardson's group developed a therapy program designed to re-educate the motor system to activate the transverse abdominis in a normal way with low back pain patients. Hollowing was developed as a motor re-education exercise and not necessarily to be recommended to patients who require enhanced stability for performance of the activities of daily living, which has been

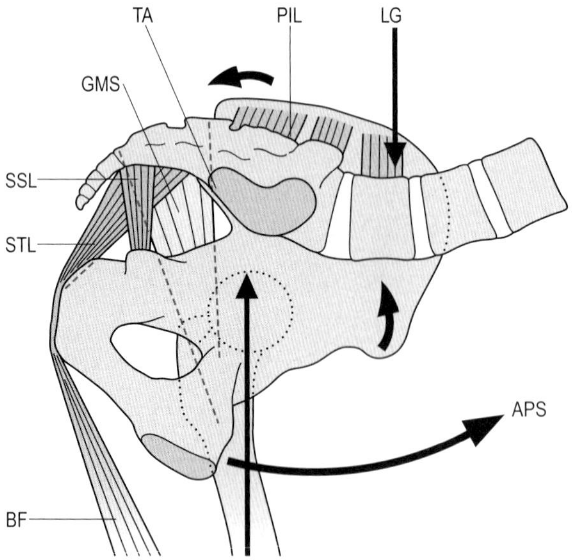

Fig. 18.11 Maintenance of the self-bracing position as the line of gravity (LG) moves anteriorly. Gravity maintains tension on the posterior interosseous ligaments (PIL). Anterior pelvic support (APS) from the rectus abdominis and the abdominal obliques maintains tension on the sacrospinous (SSL) and sacrotuberous (STL) ligaments and is essential to preserve function while leaning forward to perform any task. The sacral origin of the gluteus maximus muscle (GMS) stabilizes the sacrum. The transverse sacral axis (TA) is approximately at the distal aspect of the S3 sacral segment. The biceps femoris (BF) helps to stabilize the pelvis.

misinterpreted by some practitioners. Rather abdominal bracing, that activates the three layers of the abdominal wall with no 'drawing in' is much more effective at enhancing spine stability.

Vleeming et al (1990a, 1990b) have stated that in erect standing the gluteus maximus and the piriformis muscles act to increase self-bracing. However, acting bilaterally they would tend to pull the distal sacrum anteriorly, which would *decrease* tension in the ST ligament, disable the secondary loading and decrease self-bracing. When leaning forward to perform any task the sacral origin of the gluteus maximus and the piriformis muscles stabilize the sacrum. Any shift in the line of gravity anterior to the acetabula so as to cause an anterior rotation of the innominate bones on the sacrum on an acetabular axis would cause a pathological release of the self-bracing position. The force couple is disabled. The force-dependent axis of rotation is disabled and the innominates will rotate anteriorly on an *acetabular axis* and result in a movement cephalad and laterally on the sacrum. The stabilizing force from the gluteus maximus and the piriformis muscles would tend to pull the innominates posteriorly at the acetabula enhancing this anterior rotation resulting in a subluxation of the joint at the S3 segment (Fig. 18.12). Fixation occurs with the ilial convexities riding up and out of the sacral concavities, displacing the transverse sacral axis at S3 and spreading the joint. The anterior innominate rotation appears to loosen the PIL so some movement is still possible at the S1 segment.

Associated conditions

As the innominates rotate cephalad and laterally on the sacrum they stretch the superficial long posterior and the short posterior SI ligaments (DonTigny 1993, 2005b, Shuman 1953, Vleeming et al 1995). Primary painful points occur medial and distal to the PSIS at the attachments of the long and short posterior SI ligaments and at the posterior inferior iliac spine (PIIS). This dysfunction causes a separation of the sacral origin of the piriformis muscle from its secondary origin at the roof of the greater sciatic notch. *These painful points are all extra-articular and not affected by injections into the SIJ.* The sacral origin of the gluteus maximus muscle is also separated from its ilial origin just distal to the PSISs and the iliacus muscle is separated from its origin on the iliac fossa from a small secondary origin on the sacrum. The gluteal separation may cause pain on a line from the PSIS to the trochanter and may cause a trochanteric bursitis and pain down the iliotibial band.

The force couple is disabled causing an increase in loading forces and resulting in increased pain to the joints of the pelvis, pain up the back and down the legs. This might be mistaken for a fibromyalgia or fibromyositis. The increased loading may also cause microfractures of the subchondral bone, roughening of the joint surfaces and result in a destructive arthritis of the hip. Many patients having hip replacement surgery have had a long history of LBP on the ipsilateral side.

As the innominates rotate cephalad they take the tension off of the iliolumbar ligaments (ILL) destabilizing L4–L5 and L5–S1 and increasing shear and torsion shear to the disk (DonTigny 1994). This is probably the cause of degenerative disc disease and was investigated and verified by Pool-Goudzwaard et al (1998) who stated that this explains why the prevalence of herniations at the

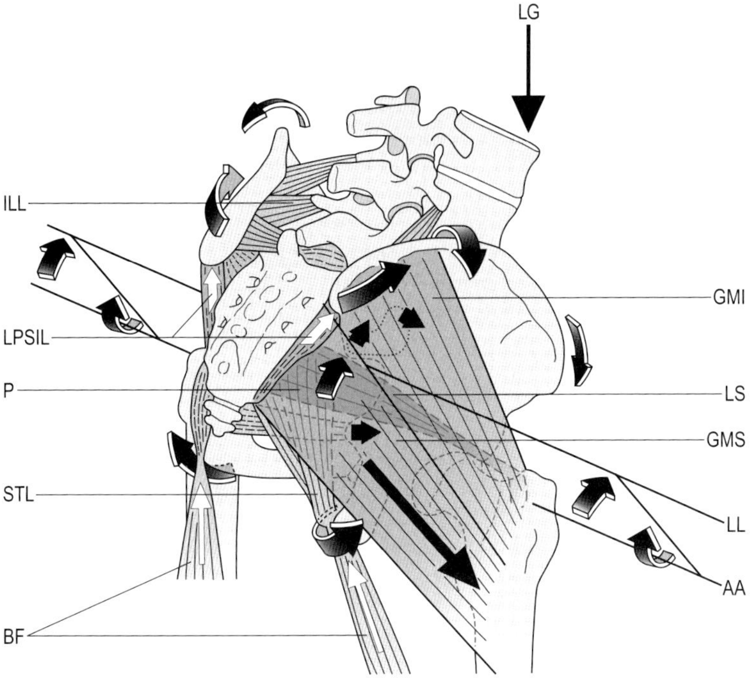

Fig. 18.12 As the line of gravity (LG) moves anteriorly to the acetabular axis (AA), the innominate will rotate anteriorly on the AA, loosening the sacrotuberous ligament (STL) and disabling the secondary loading forces causing a failure of the force couple with a resultant pathologic release of self-bracing. This stretches the superficial long posterior SI ligaments (LPSIL) and loosens the iliolumbar ligaments (ILL) destabilizing L4–L5 and L5–S1. The ilial origin of the gluteus maximus (GMI) is separated from the sacral origin (GMS) of a line of separation (LS) distal to the posterior superior iliac spines (PSISs). The sacral origin of the piriformis (P) is separated from its secondary origin at the roof of the greater sciatic notch. The primary stress on the sacroiliac joint (SIJ) is on the line of lift (LL) at the point of the transverse axis at the posterior inferior iliac spine. With the rotation the SIJs rise up over the acetabula causing the legs to appear longer and stretching the biceps femoris (BF). (Reproduced with permission from DonTigny 2004.)

level of L4–L5 and L5–S1 are higher than other segments in the lumbar spine. With the cephalad movement, the SIJs move over the acetabula causing the legs to appear longer when comparing the malleoli in the midline. The biceps femoris muscle is stretched and may cause a recurvatum of the knees. Its attachment to the lateral capsule of the knee might interfere with normal patellar tracking.

Anteriorly the psoas muscles are stretched as are the spinal nerves. The dorsal roots are more susceptible to stretch than the motor roots so numbness and paresthesias might occur. Total mechanical block comes at 15% elongation (Sunderland & Bradley 1971). Stretching the psoas muscles to relieve tight hip flexors is counter-productive because the stretch also increases the anterior rotation. Correcting the dysfunction will reverse the stretch on the psoas muscle.

With increased severity the joint capsule may be disrupted. Fortin (1995) reported rents in the anterior capsule at the S1 segment and in the posterior capsule at the S3 segment. He further found contrast media surrounding the L5 nerve root and within the body of the psoas muscle. He suggested that the extravasation of inflammatory mediators from a dysfunctional SIJ to adjacent neural tissues might explain the radicular complaints of some patients. These leaking rents might also cause cysts to form on the SIJ.

Dorman et al (1995) found an inhibition of the gluteus medius muscle when the innominate was held in anterior rotation. Dannanberg (1997) found an inhibition of the peroneus longus muscle with SIJ dysfunction (SIJD) that caused a functional hallux limitus.

Abdominal pain at Baer's point can be mis-diagnosed as appendicitis or ovarian pain. This point has been described as being on a line from the umbilicus to the anterior superior iliac spine (ASIS), 5 cm from the umbilicus and its relief by correction of SIJD (Mennell 1952). Norman (1968) reported relieving this lower abdominal pain with injections into the SIJ. This cause of lower abdominal pain is commonly overlooked. I remember a 30-year-old woman with a 4-year history of LBP and abdominal pain. She had both ovaries removed without relief. She was free of both the LBP and the abdominal pain immediately following correction of the SIJ.

The asymmetric pelvis may distort tension on the pelvic floor and result in symptoms that may be diagnosed as coccygodynia, levator ani syndrome, proctalgia fugax, or tension myalgia of the pelvic floor (Travell & Simons 1992). In 2001, I had a physical therapist in one of my workshops who teaches incontinence training in Hong Kong. She e-mailed me several weeks later and told me that after correction of the SIJ many patients no longer needed the training.

The asymmetric pelvis with an apparent long leg can cause a lumbar scoliosis with a convexity on the contralateral side. This can occur in prepubertal children without pain. Asymmetric weight bearing can cause asymmetric development in the spine.

Correction and confirmation

I have found that SIJD is essentially always caused by an anterior rotation of the innominate bones cephalad and laterally on the sacrum with a pathological release of the self-bracing position. Correction is simply the restoration of the position of self-bracing by manually rotating each innominate bone so as to cause it to move caudad and medially on the sacrum. This can be done with a direct rotation, by grasping the innominate bone and rotating it; a traction correction, pulling the leg at about a 45° angle of PSLR (passive straight leg raising); or by a strong isometric contraction (Fig. 18.13). The patient can be taught to self-correct either with a direct corrective stretch (Fig. 18.14) or with an isometric contraction (Fig. 18.15).

The leg length will always appear to shorten with correction. Sometimes the patient will have a short leg on the more painful side but this is merely a secondary shift of the S1 segment on the pathological S3 axis as the ilial convexity of that segment seeks the sacral concavity. *This is clinically*

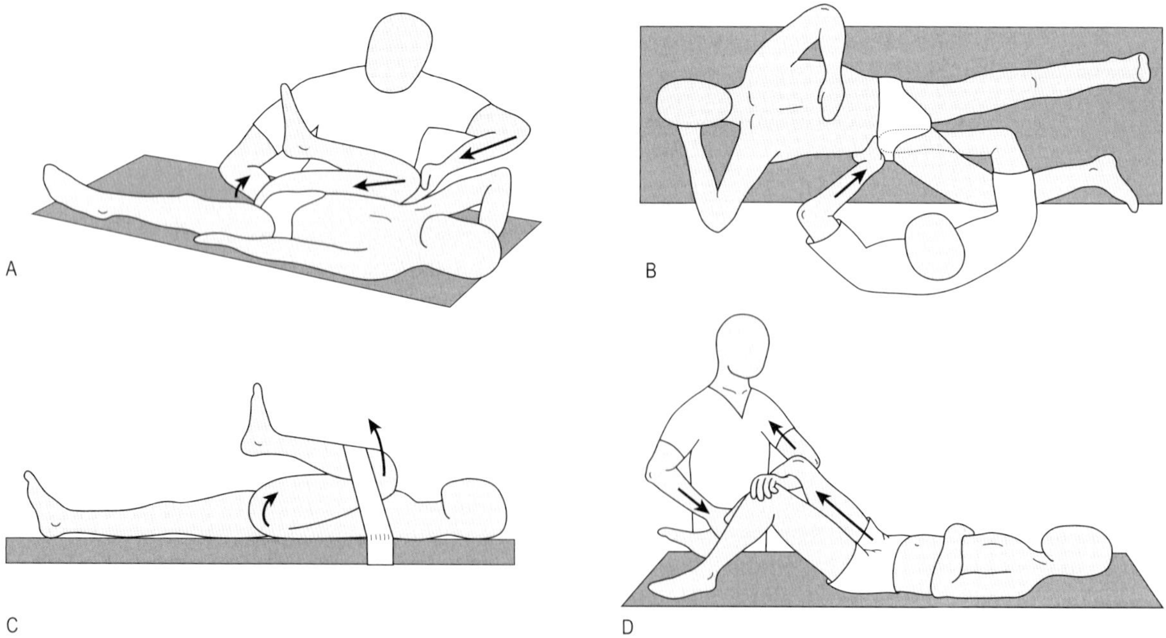

Fig. 18.13 Various methods of manual correction of dysfunction to restore self-bracing. (A) Using the leg as a lever. Take knee into axilla. (B) Direct mobilization to cause the posterior superior iliac spines (PSISs) to move caudally and medially on the sacrum. One hand is under the ischial tuberosity and the other on the very back part of the iliac crest. (C) Isometric hip extension against a strap (Swart 1923). Push knee hard against resistance, manual or belt. (D) Using the contralateral knee as a fulcrum while distracting the thigh and pelvis with the forearm just enough pressure is put on the lower leg with the other hand to keep the knee from extending. This is a very effective method of correction, simple and painless.

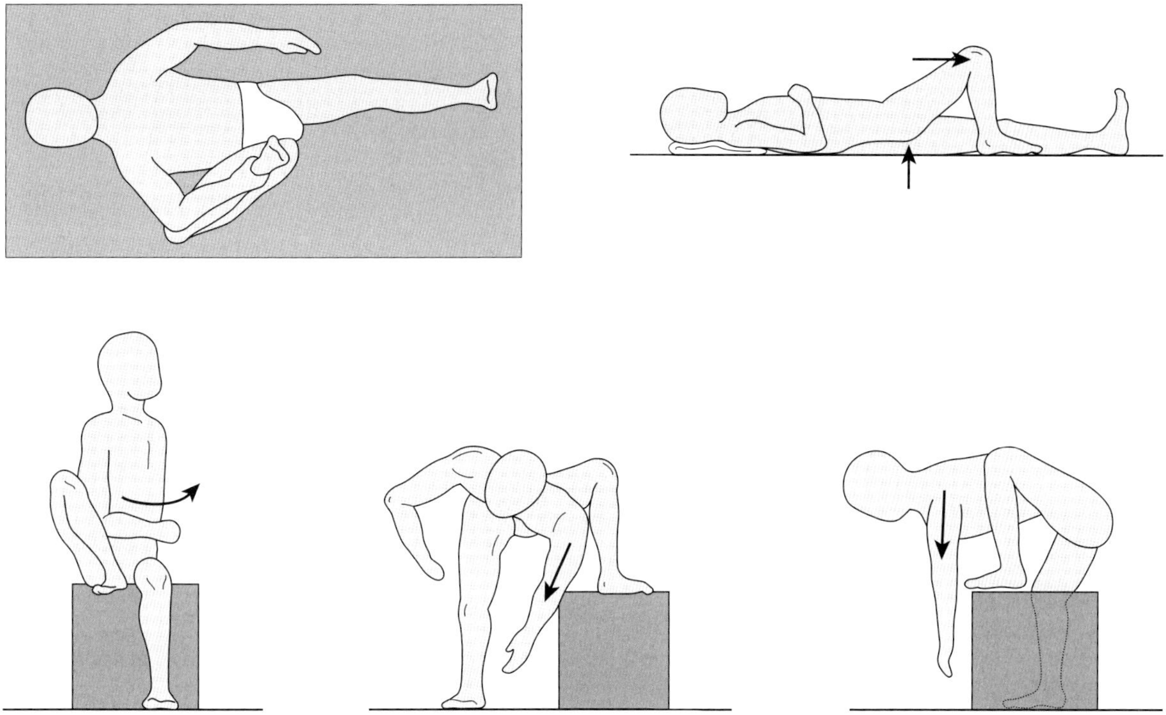

Fig. 18.14 Restoration of the self-bracing position using a direct stretch can be carried out while sitting, standing or lying.

insignificant and the SIJ must be treated the same on both sides. With correction, the long leg will get shorter and the short leg will get shorter yet. The joint is very tight and acts like a stuck drawer; you must correct one side and then the other, five or six times on each side, alternating each time and checking the leg length, not until the legs are equal but until the legs no longer appear to shorten. It is both interesting and enlightening to pull on a long leg or on a short leg and watch it shorten. Heel lifts are counterproductive as they only level the sacral base without correcting the dysfunction.

Prevention of dysfunction is by supporting the pelvis with the primary abdominal muscles when leaning forward. The unstable joint can be helped with a lumbosacral support, put on while lying supine and after a correction has been made. Proliferant injections into the long posterior sacroiliac ligaments will help to stabilize the unstable SIJ. Early prolotherapy may be advantageous in preventing the chronic problem.

While assisting in the evaluation of chronic LBP patients I found I was unable to fully correct a few of the patients who had all of the SIJ ligaments proliferated. Presently, I am under the opinion that proliferation into all of the SI ligaments can tighten these ligaments, hold the joint in the subluxed position, and prevent correction. It also appears to me that proliferation into the iliolumbar ligament may tighten that ligament and prevent correction. Wait until the SIJ is stable first and then, if necessary, prolo the iliolumbar. In the event of an unstable back rather than surgical fixation of the SIJ it is probably critical to preserve function, probably by reinforcing the long posterior SI ligaments. Excess rigidity may cause systems failures. If the SIJ is so unstable as to make fixation necessary, it should always be fixated in the corrected, self-bracing position.

Frequency of occurrence

In a study of 1000 consecutive cases of ILBPS (idiopathic low back pain syndrome), Shaw (1992) found a dysfunction of the sacroiliac joints in 98% and treated it aggressively. He also found a relationship of the SIJ to the discs as his surgical incidence for herniated discs dropped dramatically to 0.2%. His results were so stunning that few believed him. I have also found that the vast majority of LPB patients have SIJD and nearly all patients diagnosed with degenerative disc disease

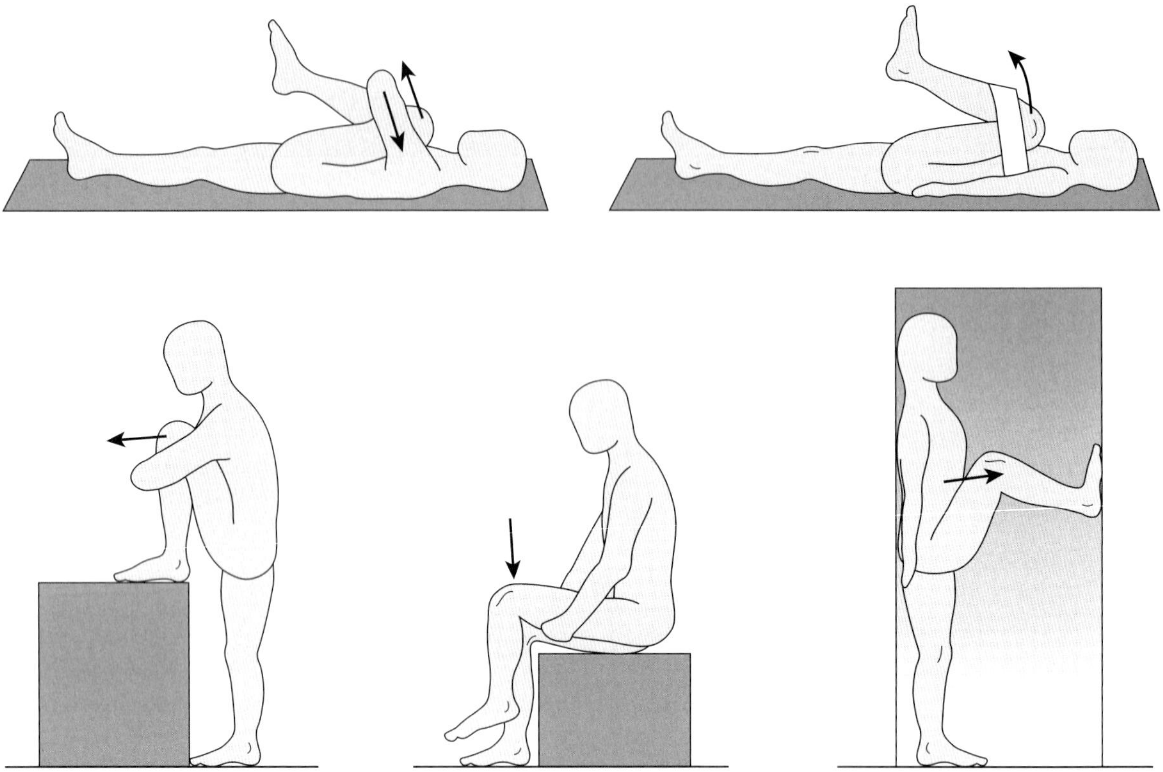

Fig. 18.15 Muscle energy techniques can be used in a variety of positions.

also have SIJD. Many patients with low levels of LBP but with hip disease or seemingly unrelated knee pain or patellar tracking abnormalities should also be evaluated for SIJD. Correct the SIJ first and then reassess.

Summary

1. The lumbosacroiliac complex appears to function as a self-compensating force coupled with a moment of force that serves as a force-dependent transverse axis of rotation through the posterior aspect of the SIJ. These force couples increase joint stability through a principle of self-bracing, which allows for the storage and release of energy and serves to balance forces of gravity, weight-loading, inertia, rotation, and acceleration and deceleration.
2. A pathological release of self-bracing may occur if the abdominal muscles fail to support the anterior pelvis when leaning forward. The innominate bones then subluxate on the sacrum on an acetabular axis, with fixation. The resulting lesion can mimic disc degeneration or might give the impression of a multifactorial etiology and prevents normal function of the force couple.
3. Treatment of SIJD is the restoration of the self-bracing position through the manual correction of the innominate bones caudad and medially on the sacrum. The legs always appear to shorten with this correction. Prevention of SIJD is by stabilizing the anterior pelvis with an active contraction of the abdominal muscles to maintain self-bracing, especially when leaning forward.
4. The most likely underlying cause of idiopathic low back pain is this subtle, measurable, reversible, biomechanical lesion. It is a commonly overlooked variation from normal, is easily corrected, and can be prevented with proper exercise. A thorough examination of the

SIJs must always be included in the evaluation of low back pain.

5. Research of low back pain that does not include the appropriate biomechanics or uses inappropriate biomechanical models will result in inappropriate findings, the inappropriate interpretation of evidence, inappropriate treatment and will delay recovery.

References

Dannanberg HJ 1997 Lower back pain as a gait-related repetitive motion injury. In: Vleeming A et al (eds) Movement, stability and low back pain: the essential role of the pelvis. Churchill Livingstone, London, p253–267

DonTigny RL 1973 Evaluation, manipulation and management of anterior dysfunction of the sacroiliac joint. The D.O. 14:215–226

DonTigny RL 1979 Dysfunction of the sacroiliac joint and its treatment. Journal of Orthopedics and Sports Physical Therapy 1:23–35

DonTigny RL 1985 Function and pathomechanics of the sacroiliac joint. Physical Therapy 65:35–44

DonTigny RL 1990 Anterior dysfunction of the sacroiliac joint as a major factor in the etiology of idiopathic low back pain syndrome. Physical Therapy 70:250–265

DonTigny RL 1993 Mechanics and treatment of the sacroiliac joint. Journal of Manual and Manipulative Therapy 1:3–12

DonTigny RL 1994 Function of the lumbosacroiliac complex as a self-compensating force couple with variable force-dependent transverse axis of rotation: A theoretical analysis. Journal of Manual and Manipulative Therapy 2:87–93

DonTigny RL 1999 Critical analysis of the sequence and extent of the result of the pathological failure of self-bracing of the sacroiliac joint. Journal of Manual and Manipulative Therapy 7:173–181 published concurrently in the Journal of Orthopaedic Medicine 2000; 22:16–23

DonTigny RL 2004 Pelvic dynamics and the S3 subluxation of the sacroiliac joint. CD-ROM. DonTigny, Havre, MT

DonTigny RL 2005a Critical analysis of the functional dynamics of the sacroiliac joints as they pertain to normal gait. Journal of Orthopaedic Medicine 27:3–10

DonTigny RL 2005b Pathology of the sacroiliac joint and its effect on normal gait. Journal of Orthopaedic Medicine 27:61–69

Dorman TA, Brierly S, Fray J, Pappani K 1995 Muscles and pelvic clutch: hip adductor inhibition in anterior rotation of the ilium. Journal of Manual and Manipulative Therapy 3:85–90

Erhard R, Bowling R 1977 The recognition of the pelvic component of low back and sciatic pain. Bulletin of Orthopaedic Section, American Physical Therapy Association 2(3):4–15

Fortin JD 1995 Sacroiliac joint injection and arthrography with imaging correlation. In: Lennard TA (ed) Physiatric procedures. Hanley & Belfus, Philadelphia. Reprinted in Vleeming A et al (eds) Secondary Interdisciplinary World Congress on Low Back Pain. San Diego, CA. 9–11 November. ECO, Rotterdam, p533–544

McGill S 2001 Achieving spine stability: Blending engineering and clinical approaches. In Vleeming A et al (eds) Fourth Interdisciplinary World Congress on Low Back and Pelvis Pain. 8–10 November, Montreal, Canada, p203–211

Mennell JB 1952 The science and art of joint manipulation: The spinal column. J & A Churchill Ltd, London, vol 2, p90

Norman GF 1968 Sacroiliac disease and its relationship to lower abdominal pain. American Journal of Surgery 116:54–56

Pierrynowski MR, Schroeder BC Garrity CB 1988 Three-dimensional sacroiliac motion during locomotion in asymptomatic male and female subjects. Presented at the 5th Canadian Society of Biomechanics, Ottawa, Canada, August

Pitkin HC, Pheasant HC 1936 Sacroarthrogentic tetalgia. Journal of Bone and Joint Surgery (US) 18:365–373

Pool-Goudzwaard AL, Hoek van Dijke G, Vleeming A et al 1998 The iliolumbar ligament influence on the coupling of the sacroiliac joint and the L5–S1 segment. In: Vleeming A et al (eds) The Third Interdisciplinary World Congress on Low Back and Pelvic Pain. 19–21 November, Vienna, Austria, p313–315

Shaw JL 1992 The role of the sacroiliac joint as a cause of low back pain and dysfunction. In: Vleeming A et al (eds) The First Interdisciplinary World Congress on Low Back Pain and its Relation to the Sacroiliac Joint. San Diego, CA, 5–6 November, p67–80

Shuman D 1953 Technic for treating instability of the joints by sclerotherapy. Osteopathic Profession, May 1953

Sunderland S, Bradley KC 1971 Stress–strain phenomena in human spinal nerve roots. Brain 95:120

Swart J 1923 Osteopathic strap technique. Joseph Swart Publisher, Kansas City, KS, p15

Thorstensson A, Nilson J, Carlson H, Zomlefer MR 1984 Trunk movements in human locomotion. Acta Physiologic Scandinavica 121:9–22

Travell JG, Simons DG 1992 Myofascial pain and dysfunction: a trigger point manual (vol II). Williams & Wilkins, Baltimore, MD, p110–113

Vleeming A, Stoeckart R, Volkers ACW, Snijders CJ 1990a Relation between form and function in the sacroiliac joint. 1: clinical anatomical aspects. Spine 15:130–132

Vleeming A, Stoeckart R, Volkers, ACW, Snijders CJ 1990b Relation between form and function in the sacroiliac joint. 2: biomechanical aspects. Spine 15(2):133–136

Vleeming A, Pool-Goudzwaard AL, Hammudoglu D et al 1995 The function of the long dorsal sacroiliac ligament: its implication for understanding low back pain. In: Vleeming A et al (eds) Second Interdisciplinary World Congress on Low Back Pain. San Diego, CA, 9–11 November. ECO, Rotterdam, p125–137

Vukicevic S, Marusic A, Stavljenic A et al 1991 Holographic analysis of the human pelvis. Spine 16:209–214

Weisl H 1953 The relation of movement to structure in the sacroiliac joint. PhD Thesis, University of Manchester, UK

White AA 1982 Introduction. In White AA, Gordon SL (eds) American Academy of Orthopaedic Surgeons Symposium on Idiopathic Low Back Pain. St Louis, MO. CV Mosby, St Louis, p2

CHAPTER 19

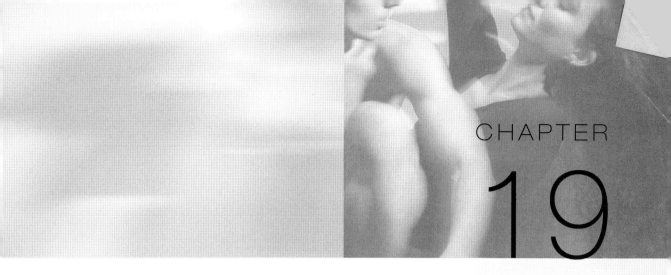

Stability or controlled instability?

Serge Gracovetsky

Introduction

The theory of the spinal engine (Gracovetsky 1988) explains how the primitive spinal motion of our fish ancestors remains the basis for human gait. The theory did not explain the contribution of the sacroiliac joint (SIJ) in the force transmission system linking the spine to the ground.

With two exceptions (Bogduk 1997, DonTigny 2004), all current proposals intending to clarify the role of the SIJ are hinged around the belief that the SIJ is 'essentially flat,' save for some irregularities increasing joint friction. The hypothesis that the SIJ was 'flat' required the invention of a complicated theory of force and form closure to stabilize the 'flat' SIJ and prevent it from falling apart under the load of the structures above S1. In that respect, the design of the SIJ seems faulty and contrary to evolutionary pressures. Which begs the question: why didn't we evolve with a stable SIJ?

There is a sense of *déjà vu*. During the 1970s, many gurus suggested that lordosis was an aberration that will be corrected in time. The spine *had* to become straight to accommodate the Swedish spinal compression theory of the time. The fact that monkeys already had a flat spine (Farfan 1978) did not register. Clearly, a better explanation for lordosis was needed and provided.

The anatomical features of the SIJ were noted and reported by many as a rough surface with high friction. The fact that no other role was assigned to the very peculiar SIJ topology seemed strange to me since it implies that the SIJ would be unnecessarily complicated, in perfect contradiction with my understanding of evolution. And so during the Christmas 2004 holidays, I took several pelvises and began to slice them to examine their SIJs and verify the 'flatness' and 'roughness' hypotheses. Sure enough, the SIJs were not flat but warped like a propeller with a significant ridge. That ridge is not a random design to increase roughness but a facet that perfectly locks the innominates into place. The dense ligaments across the SIJ guarantee that everything fits and stays together. No shear needs to be transmitted across a high friction SIJ since the forces are channeled as compressive forces across a facet joint, which is the best utilization of bony material.

And then it occurred to me that, because the sacrum is made of fused vertebrae, the pelvis corresponds to fused ribs, and that the SIJ might be thought of as being a modified costovertebral joint: the innominates articulate themselves on the fused transverse processes of the sacral vertebrae; the posterior interosseous ligament (PIL) is equivalent to the posterior costotransverse ligament (PCTL); the iliolumbar ligament can be seen as either a detached PIL or a form of PCTL, etc. In other words, the spine does not stop at L5. It goes all the way to the acetabulum. It has kept its anatomy with it, save for some modifications.

That is a satisfactory concept from an evolutionary standpoint. When our fish ancestors came to land, they had to evolve fins into limbs connected to the spine through the rib cage. Two complementary designs were kept; the shoulder system permitting force transfer and breathing; and the pelvis that did not have the breathing requirement. This arrangement can be found in all their vertebrates' descendants.

Suddenly, the knowledge acquired by studying the spinal engine could be extended to the SIJ as well. This methodology includes the current issues of stability, which do not give due consideration to the viscoelastic nature of collagen.

This chapter re-examines the generally accepted concepts of stability as it applies to the musculoskeletal system and more particularly to the spine/pelvis complex, and proposes a new solution to an old problem.

Stability and biomechanics

The musculoskeletal system of the vertebrate is essentially an unstable structure stabilized by the CNS. How this is done was investigated using tools from engineering textbooks (McGill 2001). But engineers are concerned by machines made of reasonably homogeneous material that does not deform appreciably with time. The problem is that we are made of viscoelastic materials that do deform with time, and it is not clear to what extent the hypotheses underlying these engineering stability theories are appropriate for viscoelastic structures.

In addition the current concepts of musculoskeletal stability are developed without considering the advantages of being an unstable structure stabilized by a complex control system.

The theory of stability

Essentially, all stability theories rely on a principle of energy minimization. A system will reach a stable position if the energy stored in the system is as low as can be. Consequently, the system remains at one location or on a specific trajectory because any deviation from that optimum position requires more energy.

The classical example given to illustrate the existence of a stable position is shown in Fig. 19.1. The ball rolls and stops at a position corresponding to the minimum potential energy. It can do that because there are energy walls that constraint the ball to one position, and deviating from that 'stable' position means climbing the potential energy wall.

There are a number of difficulties with this simplistic approach. For instance, moving from one stable position to the next should be a succession of battles against energy walls (Fig. 19.1B). But we know that moving around does not imply a continuous climbing in and out of energy walls. Our movements are fluid. That alone should alert us that this type of stability representation, appropriate

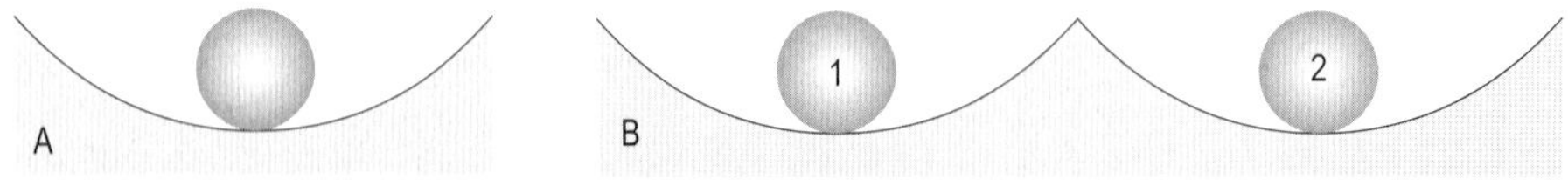

Fig. 19.1 (A) Standard representation of stability. (B) To move from position 1 to position 2 requires climbing an energy wall.

for many engineering problems, requires some modifications.

To circumvent the energy wall constraints, in the 1970s it was proposed that the joints could have a 'neutral' zone within which they can move without effort. But such a system might become unstable since motion is possible without energy constraints. There is no reason for the ball to stay at any particular place in the neutral zone (Fig. 19.2 left).

It was also proposed that the width of the neutral zone was related to the stability of the joint (Fig. 19.2). These conclusions were drawn from cadaver experiments and mathematical models on which an extensive amount of damage had to be inflicted to the joint before an unstable response was obtained. So far, the neutral zone argument has remained academic.

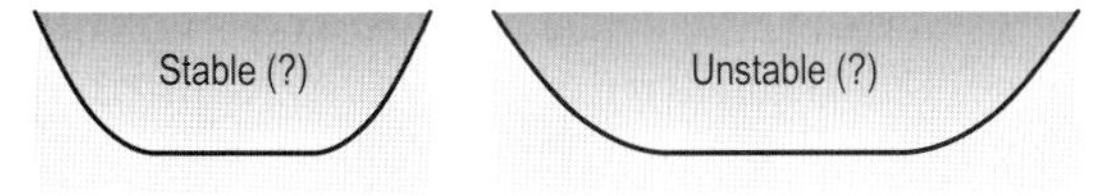

Fig. 19.2 The link between the width of the neutral zone and normal function has not been proven.

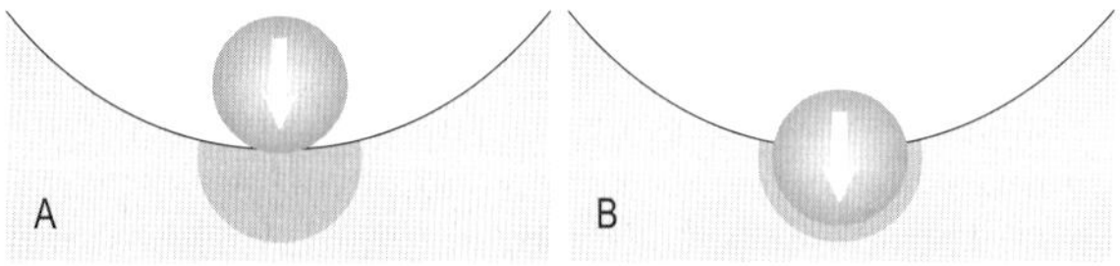

Fig. 19.3 Tissues deform under stress. When the ball stops (left) and remains motionless, the viscoelastic tissues underneath will deform and the ball will 'sink' into the tissues (right).

In addition, the link between anatomical perfection and function was debunked circa 1995 by the work of Boos et al (1995) who demonstrated that 75% of asymptomatic people had damage to the intervertebral joints, including disc herniation.

There is another problem with the application of classical stability to viscoelastic systems. Even if a 'stable' position existed, it could not be kept for long. Because biological materials are viscoelastic, they will deform as soon as a stress is applied (Fig. 19.3).

The viscoelastic structures

The resulting deformation will presumably trigger pain, and pain forces the CNS to unload the overstressed material, generally collagen. For instance, during the lifting of a heavy load, it is impossible to stop the movement and freeze because the collagenous lumbodorsal fascia would creep, disable itself, and force the back muscles to take up a level of load they could not sustain. The lift is aborted. Hence a position cannot be maintained and stabilized if it results in a substantial deformation of the viscoelastic structures.

The stability of a viscoelastic system can only be thought of as a collection of related positions that are very rapidly adopted and modified by the CNS. Posture is not static. Posture is a dynamic concept. The apparent steadiness of the erect stance is misleading. The 'steady' erect stance is maintained by cycling through a sequence of different but closely related postures.

The continuous loading and unloading of collagen requires the CNS to rapidly redirect forces. It has been known for quite some time that many combinations of muscles and ligaments correspond to any given posture. A 'steady' erect stance can be kept because the musculoskeletal system oscillates from one combination to the next in such a way that no structure ends up being continuously loaded. This helps explain why rehabilitation cannot be achieved by working on one exercise only and why a wide variety of exercises must be taught.

The redundancy of the musculature was described by the mathematical wizards of the 1970s who were confronted by models that demanded a rationale for using one combination of muscle and ligaments rather than another. Hence the idea of assigning a cost to each possible combination of muscles and picking the configuration that will result in the lowest cost. The buzzword was 'optimization theory.' For instance, one can decide that the 'best' configuration would be that which will minimize the compression at L5–S1. However, two problems were conveniently cast aside. First, the 'cost' of a configuration was arbitrary (say, compression at L5). Second, whatever the definition chosen for the cost, the model will always generate one unique solution, which runs contrary to the viscoelastic nature of the system. The resulting calculations were essentially used to publish papers to lengthen the authors' curriculum vitae.

Collagen and time constant

It could be argued that the need to switch from one muscular combination to the next is determined by the properties of collagen. In a series of studies in Sweden, Kazarian (1968) realized that collagen has a complex time-dependent response to loading. The most important factor for the purpose of this discussion is the fact that collagen has at least two time constants. One of them is about 20 minutes and another one of about 1/3 of a second.

Sleeping is a good example of the impact of the 20-minute time constant of collagen. Sleeping removes active muscular control from posture. The gravitational field applies a low level of forces and deforms the relaxed viscoelastic body. The 20-minute time constant determines the length of time during which we can remain motionless while slowly deforming our joints in the gravitational field. When collagen stretches too much, the deformation of a joint becomes too large, pain wakes up the CNS to flip over to a different posture. In so doing, the deformed collagen is unloaded, and a different structure becomes loaded. The cycle repeats until the night is over. The same principle applies when we are awake. During high loading conditions, the 1/3 of a second time constant becomes predominant, collagen deforms rapidly and posture must be corrected rapidly and continuously. This is why the lifting of heavy loads must be accomplished at speed to finish the movement before the lumbodorsal fascia's collagen overstretches even if the resulting acceleration on the load penalizes the lifter.

Posture is an average

The posture we strive to keep is the result of an oscillation between different combinations of muscles and ligaments. Rehabilitation means exercising each oscillation mode by using different training protocols. This oscillation is also necessary from a sensory perspective because the response of a neuron depends upon the rate of change of the excitation. A constant excitation ends up degrading sensory information. Not a particularly good idea for an unstable structure in a relentless gravitational field.

Unlike machines that work best under continuous loading, viscoelastic biomechanical machines do not like uniformity. The heart pulses do not deliver a constant pressure; if they did, the arteries will stretch and burst. Biomedical material demands to be impulse loaded. For instance, the spine needs to be impulse loaded during gait, and the well-intentioned strategy of cushioning soles may be somewhat misguided.

Why is instability an evolutionary advantage?

Interestingly, engineers purposely construct unstable machines. The modern jet fighter is one of them. This machine can be flown because dozens of computers force the unstable machine into a stable flight. Why not design a stable fighter in the first place? Survival is the short answer: a stable jet fighter might not be agile enough to escape an incoming missile. It takes less time to execute a maneuver by letting go an unstable machine instead of forcing a stable fighter into an evasive maneuver at a considerable energy cost.

Death will remove the genes of stable but slower systems from the pool of available descendants. If instability brings faster response and a better chance at avoiding predators, then instability will prevail over time. This is an evolutionary advantage in the Darwinian sense, and to keep that advantage, the problem is not to seek to stabilize at all cost an inherently unstable structure but to learn to control its instability.

But there is a price to pay for any mistake. Because the musculoskeletal system is inherently unstable, the loss of control might bring considerable damage to the unstable viscoelastic structure.

Application to lordosis control and gait

The need to avoid continuous loading of structures implies the existence of several strategies during gait. The spine must be in equilibrium and the sum of all torques must be zeroed at each intervertebral joint. For instance, at L4–L5, the external forces (load lifted, etc.) impose a clockwise moment that must be balanced by the counterclockwise action of muscles and ligaments (Fig. 19.4A,B).

These characteristic curves suggest that the distribution of forces supported by the spine can be modified by either changing the trunk flexion, or the lordosis, or both (Figs 19.5 and 19.6). As no one structure is continuously loaded, walking can be done for a long time.

It can be shown that every combination of muscle and ligament corresponds to minimizing and equalizing stress at all intervertebral joints. A corollary to that statement is that the minimization of stress is equivalent to a minimization of energy. In other words, the best gait posture results in using the minimum amount of food (energy minimization).

There is a safety factor built in; the CNS will not permit the stress to exceed $^2/_3$ of the ultimate (Gracovetsky 1988, p 167). This surprising finding was obtained by comparing the ultimate strength of disc and ligament at rupture in cadaver experiments with the calculations of what was actually being

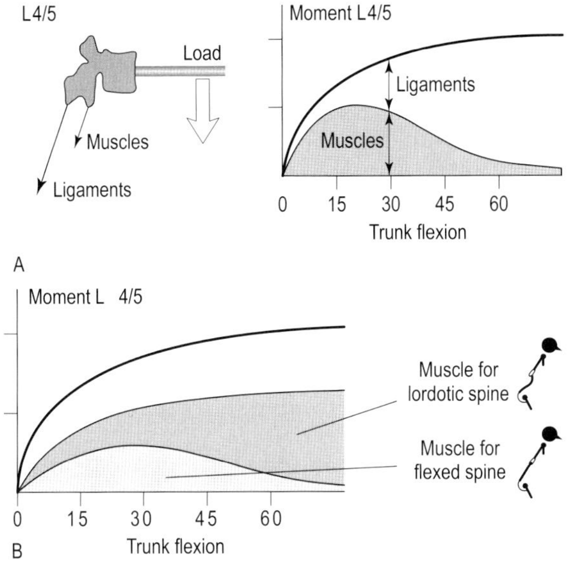

Fig. 19.4 (A) An external load is balanced by the action of the muscles and ligaments. The contribution of muscles and ligaments to balance the load at the L4–L5 level varies with the angle of forward flexion. In this illustration, the muscles are the erector spinae and they relax when the lumbodorsal fascia is sufficiently tight. (B) The muscle contribution is a function of both the angle of trunk flexion and the amount of lordosis. The lordotic spine prevents the posterior ligamentous system (PLS) from stretching and supporting the load. The muscles must work harder. A flexed spine permits the PLS to take up most of the load and the muscle relaxation phenomenon is observed.

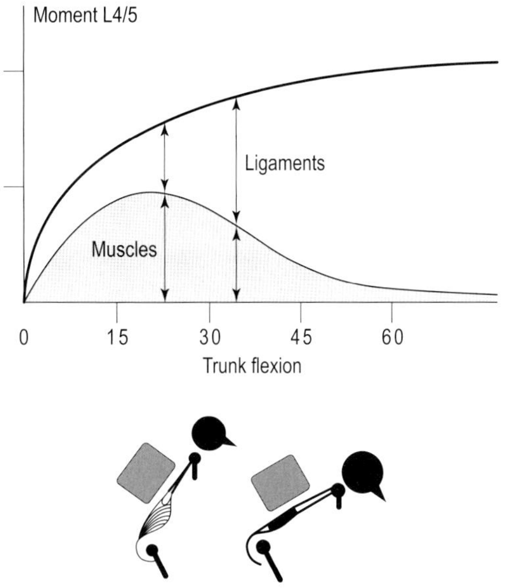

Fig. 19.5 Trunk flexion: during gait, the lordosis is modified at each step as the trunk flexion oscillates. The net result is that the distribution of forces going through the muscles and ligaments is also modified at each step.

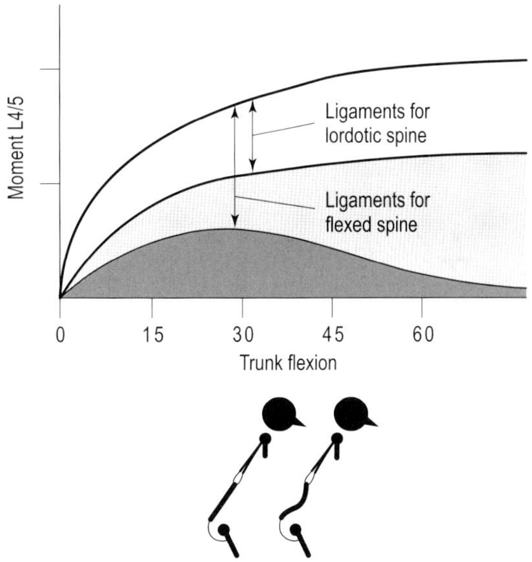

Fig. 19.6 Pelvic tilt: tilting the pelvis changes the distribution of forces between muscles and ligaments. The flexed spine has a greater part of its forces directed through the ligament system. As before, no structure ends up being continuously loaded.

done. The $^2/_3$ limit determines the maximum load that can be lifted safely. It is not clear why the CNS keeps such an important margin of safety. The $^1/_3$ reserve would explain why people under extreme fear seem to have the ability to do 'superhuman' tasks. What might be happening is that the safety factor that is normally preventing anyone from exceeding $^2/_3$ of his/her limit can be defeated if survival itself is at stake. This also explains why power lifters do not voluntarily flex their spine to the maximum possible, even if the best theoretical lifting posture is a maximally flexed spine. Indeed, the best theoretical limit leaves no margin for safety in case something goes wrong and hence the stability of the spine cannot be guaranteed. In practical terms, no intervertebral joint will be permitted to rotate more that $^2/_3$ of their respective physiological maximum since exceeding that limit increases the risk of destabilizing the spine, a predicted feature confirmed by numerous observations (McGill 2001).

This stability feature is also very pre-eminent in the cervical spine. Theoretically, the cervical spine of jet fighter pilots ought to survive close to 80 *g* of axial acceleration during ejection. However, the highest load that a pilot survived (many times!) was 47 *g* during live human experiments in 1948 by Colonel Stapp in New Mexico. Yet pilots can damage their cervical spine at ejection rates as low as 15 *g*. It would appear that a feedback loop triggers a muscle relaxation when the load exceeds a threshold in order to protect the spine by unloading. This reflex works well for power lifters, who have the option of releasing the barbell and letting it go, thereby immediately unloading their spine. A pilot being ejected does not have the option of unloading the cervical spine during ejection. Once the rocket has been fired, the pilot has to go through the entire motion, at the risk of critically injuring the neck (Helleur et al 1984).

The coupled motion of the spine

In 1985, it was proposed that the spine resonates in the gravitational field and forces the counter-rotation of pelvis and shoulders (Gracovetsky 1988). This theory is predicated on the existence of the coupled motion, a basic property of matter first discovered by Lovett in 1903. Lovett determined that if a rod bent in one plane (lordosis) is forced to bend into another plane (lateral bending) then the rod will induce an axial torque. This phenomenon was quantified in detail by Panjabi & White (1995). Note that this coupled motion is reversible; some types of sport exploit this feature (Table 19.1) (Gracovetsky 2004).

The following considerations might be useful for the rehabilitation therapist or the coaching of athletes to maximize the output of the spine without exceeding its limits.

Table 19.1 The three possible combinations of two motions that induce a third one

Type of coupling	Activity
Lordosis with lateral bending induces axial rotation	Baseball pitcher
Lordosis with axial rotation induces lateral bending	Cricket bowler
Lateral bending with axial rotation induces lordosis	Fosbury flop

Controlling the coupled motion of the spine

The cadaver experiments of Panjabi & White and others did not reveal the entire story behind the coupled motion of the spine because the spine is not a simple rod and no active musculature controls the facet joints. It can be shown that properly controlled facet joints may suppress or even reverse the coupled motion of a simple rod. This is illustrated in Fig. 19.7, which demonstrates that an important parameter for the stability of the spine is the control of the position of the center of rotation of each vertebra. For the same lateral bending and lordosis, the induced torque can be clockwise (Fig. 19.7B), counterclockwise (Fig. 19.7C), or neutral (Fig. 19.7E). In addition, bracing the spine is possible by locking up both facets (Fig. 19.7D).

Gait is a dynamic situation requiring a continuous adjustment of the position of the center of rotation to properly drive the pelvis. Spinal control is assured by the proper synchronization of the facets as the heel strike pulse entering the pelvis travels up the spine and initiates the counter rotation of spine and pelvis. The center of rotation of each intervertebral joint follows a cyclic path to insure that each facet contacts at the appropriate time (Fig. 19.8).

All the above spinal motion would be useless if it were not to result in some form of locomotion. The fish's body converts directly the lateral bend of the spine into a pressure wave acting on the water. For the vertebrate on land, the pelvis and the legs amplifying the pelvic motion must deliver that spinal motion to the ground and propel the animal forward. How this is done requires an appreciation of the functional anatomy of the pelvis and sacrum.

A second look at the sacroiliac joint

The evolutionary record suggests that locomotion was first achieved by the motion of the spine. The legs came after as an improvement, not as a substitute. For a variety of reasons, the paraspinal muscles do not have the necessary power to sustain high-velocity human gait, and more energy from the hip extensors must be fed to the spinal machinery. The mechanism by which the muscular energy liberated by the hip extensors reaches the spine requires the presence of a gravitational field as temporary energy storage. The energy recovered at heel strike ends up as a pulse at the acetabulum

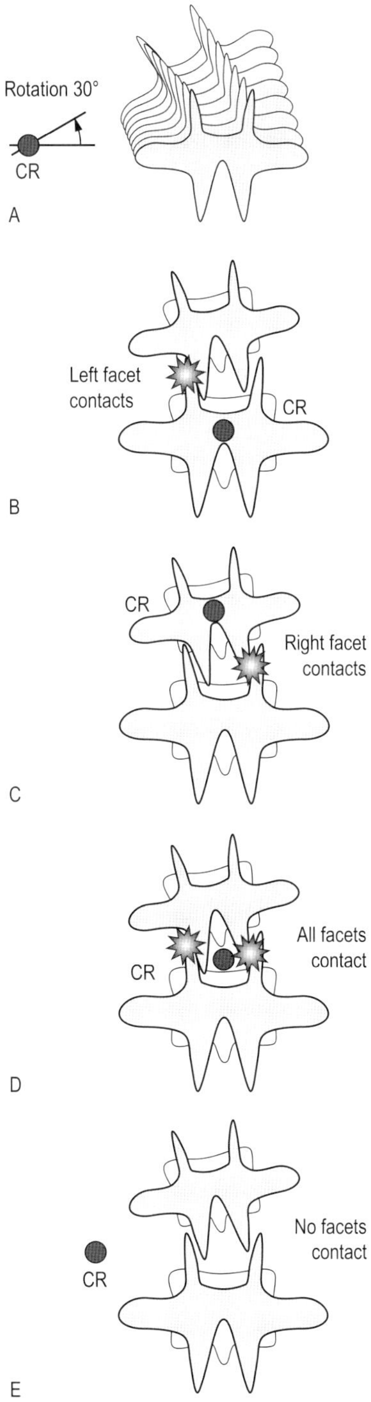

Fig. 19.7 (A) Definition of the center of rotation (CR). The vertebra is rotated counterclockwise by 30°. (B, C, D, and E) All are displayed for 10° of counterclockwise rotation. The only difference between the pictures is in the position of the center of rotation (black dot). (B) When the CR is below the disc, the left facet contacts. This would occur before left heel strike during gait, or while grabbing an object with the right hand and pulling across the chest. (C) When the CR is above the disc, the right facet contacts. This would occur during gait as the spine derotates to return to the erect stance after left heel push off, or while grabbing an object with the right hand and pulling straight. (D) When the CR is at the center of the disc, both left and right facet contact simultaneously. This is a bracing position for the spine to enhance stability. (E) When the CR is on the left of the spine, neither facet contacts.

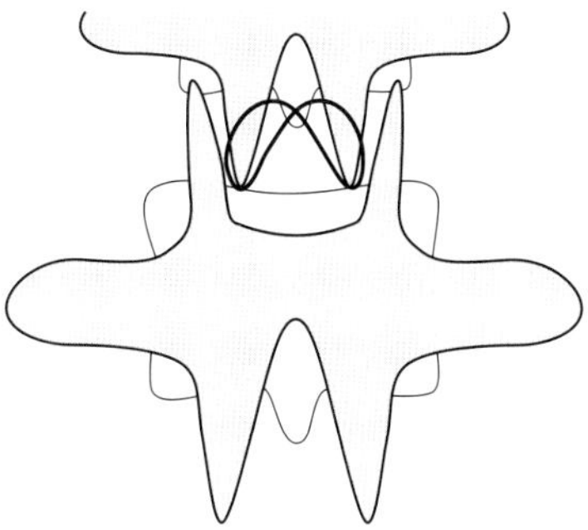

Fig. 19.8 During gait, the need to transfer torque through the facets imposes a specific path for the cyclic motion of the center of rotation (black curved line).

which is transmitted all the way up through the SIJ (Gracovetsky 2001).

The detail of the transfer of forces across the interface of the SIJ is quite complex. The current description of the SIJ considers the joint to be flat, which means that motion between pelvis and sacrum is possible. The irregularities of the SIJ surfaces, which have been noted by many over the years, have been invariably described as quasi-random and necessary to increase the friction of the SIJ (Weisl 1954).

To explain how the SIJ could function, and how the loads of the sacrum can be transferred to the legs through the SIJ, it is proposed that the noted irregularities of the SIJ surfaces would provide some type of form closure that must be complemented by a mechanism (force closure) for pressing the two sides of the SIJ together (Fig. 19.9) (Vleeming et al 1990). Proof of the existence of such a mechanism in the living has yet to be supplied, despite many attempts (van Wingerden et al 2004).

There are several fundamental objections to the current theories describing the function of the SIJ:

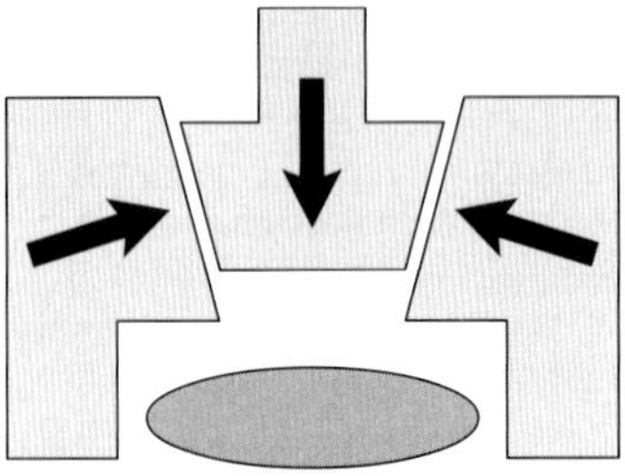

Fig. 19.9 The current theory proposes that the sacroiliac joint (SIJ) is flat and can slide if it were not for a lateral force maintaining the SIJ closed. The piriformis muscle would be a candidate for supplying the closure force. Collagen across the SIJ would also help as long as no creeping occurs.

Objection 1: Suppose that the form/force closure theory is true and that the SIJ is indeed 'flat.' Then muscle and/or ligament forces must be present at all times across the SIJ to balance the gravitational forces. As collagen is viscoelastic, it cannot be permanently loaded without creeping. If creeping occurs in the absence of muscle action then the SIJ opens up, its surfaces slip past each other and the joint subluxates. To prevent subluxation, muscles must therefore fire at all times to protect the 'flat' SIJ. This continuous muscle firing however has not been observed. Basmadjian (1979) noted very little electromyographic (EMG) activity during low-speed gait, and when resting in the erect stance, the EMG is essentially silent. In addition, firing a muscle requires energy. If such an energy-inefficient process could be avoided by a change in anatomy, then a better design should have evolved. Hence, the force/form closure theory must be revised and/or the flatness hypothesis of the SIJ must be reconsidered.

Objection 2: Is rooted in the anatomy itself. First, the SIJ has a double facet orientation. This precludes any kind of displacement proposed by the form/force closure theory advocates. At the S1 level, the angulation is backward by about 40°. At the S1 level it is forward by about 10° (Fig. 19.10). This reversal in angulation from S1 to S3 definitely precludes sliding motion. The SIJ surfaces cannot slip past each other without severe dislocation of the joint. Rather, the warped surfaces force the joint to exhibit a complex rotational movement not unlike that of the lumbar facets, and to appreciate that motion we need to determine where the centers of rotation are.

Objection 3: The irregular surfaces of the SIJ are not random but highly organized. This can be demonstrated by slicing a pelvis (Fig. 19.11). The major anatomical feature that seems to have been

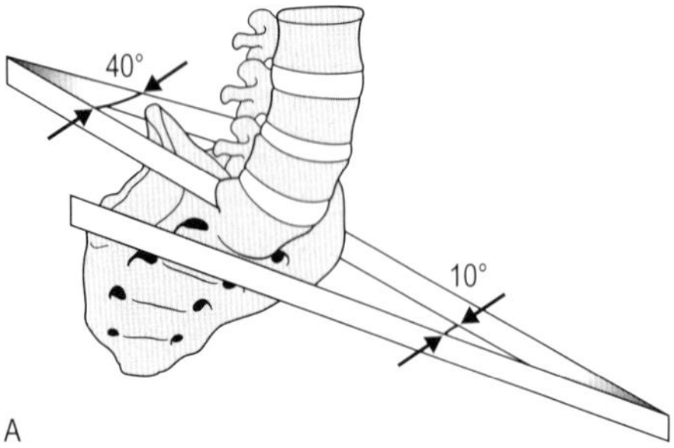

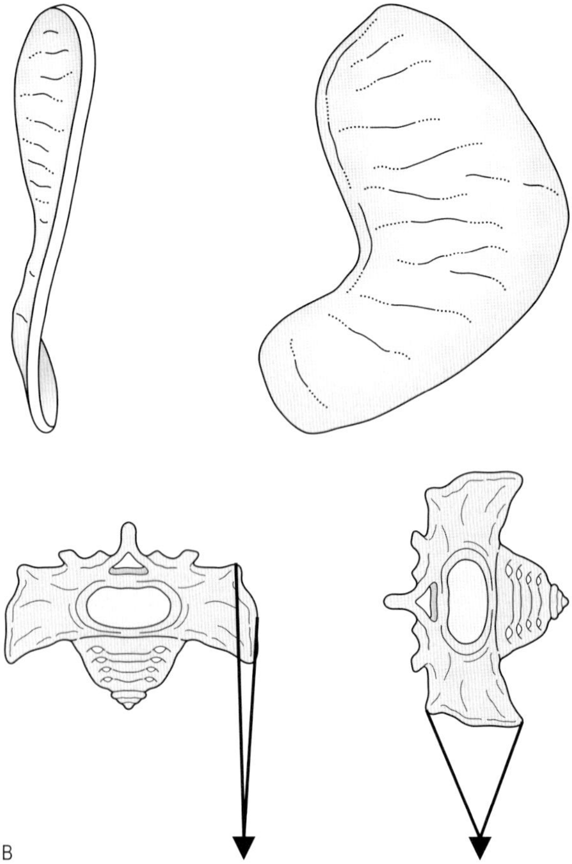

Fig. 19.10 (A) The orientation of the SIJ at the S1 and S3 levels changes significantly from about 10° forward to about 40° backward. The data of two independent studies can be found in Solonen (1957) and Dijkstra et al (1992). (B) The SIJ is a warped surface that cannot slide up and down. The sturdy ligaments holding sacrum and innominate will make that motion very difficult. Hence the need for any kind of supplemental force closure is not obvious on that consideration alone. The orientation of the surfaces is illustrated with respect to the top view of the sacrum.

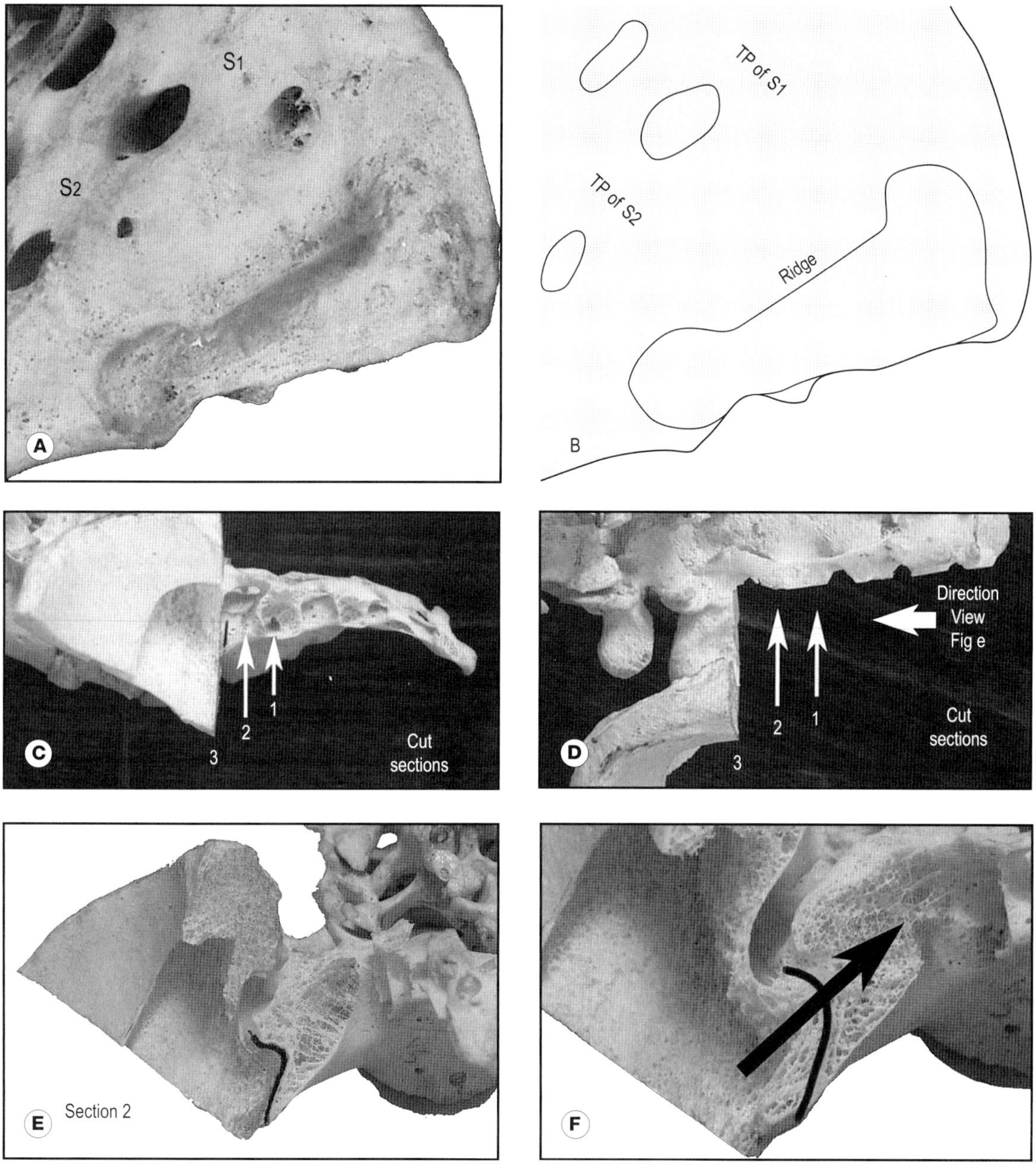

Fig. 19.11 (A) View of the SG ridge. (B) Schematic showing the position of the SG ridge with respect to the S1 and S2 transverse processes (TP). Note that the ridge is centered between the TP, an arrangement similar to that of the ribs at the thoracic spine level. (C) Side view of position of the cuts performed to illustrate the cross section of the SIJ. (D) Top view of position of the cuts performed to extract the cross section of the SIJ. Note the horizontal arrow indicating the orientation of the view illustrated in Fig. 19.11E, F. (E) Cross-section at level of cut 2. View from the back as indicated by the horizontal arrow in Fig. 19.11D. (F) Close-up of Fig. 19.11E. Proposed path for force transmission across the ridge. That force transmission vector is aligned with the acetabulum.

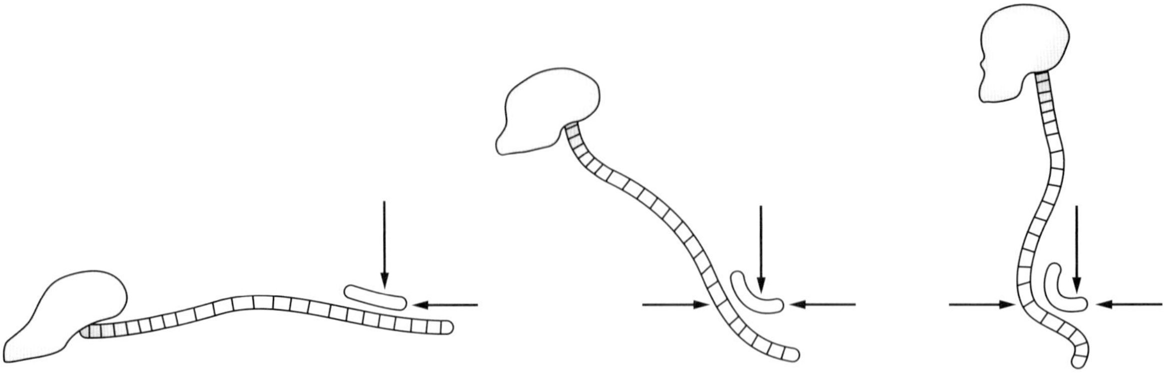

Fig. 19.12 The orientation of the ridge of the sacroiliac joint (SIJ) remains horizontal across the species from the quadruped to the primate to man (Delmas 1950). Note that the gravitational field remains perpendicular to the SIJ ridge.

overlooked is the presence of a ridge, which I will call the SG ridge. There is no question that the topology of the SIJ surfaces demonstrates the presence of a ridge (the SG ridge), which locks up directly inside the crease of the elbow of the SIJ on the innominate side. Each SG ridge is made of two fused facets at the tip of the fused transverse processes of S1 and S2. The curved shape of the human SIJ represents the inferior facet that locks into the SG ridge. This is a situation where the 'inferior' facet wraps around the superior facet to prevent any dislocation. The pounding of the legs via the acetabulum would be enough to dislocate the SIJ if it were not anatomically locked up and wrapped to maintain mechanical integrity across the joint. This design is not unique to humans. The inferior facets of the lumbar spine of mountain goats wraps around the corresponding superior facets presumably to stabilize the animal during its perilous jumps.

The orientation of the part of the SIJ supporting the ridge remains horizontal across the species (Fig. 19.12). This arrangement suggests that the ridge is responsible for supporting the sacrum over the innominates and that the primate orientation of the ridge would not permit a permanent erect stance because it would result in a slanted ridge that would be susceptible to shear. Hence it can be speculated that *Homo sapiens* had to evolve a ridge substantially perpendicular to the main axis of the spine before a truly bipedal stance could be maintained. Note also that the quadruped shoulder arrangement results also in forces being transmitted to the ribs and to the spine via the costovertebral joints.

It is generally accepted that the sacrum is made of fused vertebrae. It is perhaps less obvious that the pelvis might be constructed from the fused ribs corresponding to the sacral vertebrae. With that representation, the SIJ appears to be similar to the joint between ribs and vertebrae at the thoracic level. We propose that the SIJ is a modified costovertebral joint, more specifically the articular facet of the transverse process of the corresponding sacral vertebrae (Fig. 19.13).

Each rib rests in between two adjacent vertebrae and one transverse process. The ligaments holding the rib to the vertebrae are the upper part of the stellate ligament (from the anterior part of the superior vertebrae) and the lower part of the stellate ligament (from the anterior part of the inferior vertebra) which probably corresponds to the anterior SI ligaments. Posteriorly and proximally, holding the rib to the two adjacent ligaments is the interarticular ligament which corresponds to the interosseous ligament that connects the sacrum to the ilium. That ligament is very deeply seated and very strong. It can be thought of as being an extension of the capsular ligaments of the facets that can be found higher up in the lumbar spine.

Note that the iliolumbar ligament linking the transverse process of L4 or L5 to the iliac crest can be compared with the posterior interosseous ligament (Fig. 19.14). Indeed, the entire spinal anatomy from cervical to pelvis can be made congruent.

The SIJ is a synovial joint, like the other facets. The SIJ is a stable joint that has all the characteristics of the 'normal' facet joints of the thoracic spine, save for the restrictions in motion imposed by the tight fit of the SG ridge. In this regard, it is not helpful to mentally separate the sacrum and the innominates from the spine and the ribs, both in terms of name and function. The full spine goes from atlas all the way down to the acetabulum. The nomenclature

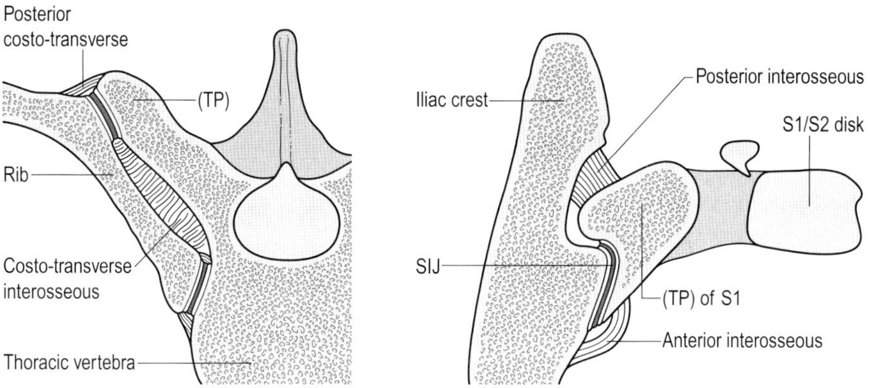

Fig. 19.13 Comparison of the anatomy of the junction of the thoracic vertebra (left) and the rib with the junction between the sacrum and the innominates (right). The posterior costotransverse ligament is mapped on to the posterior interosseous ligament, and the costotransverse interosseous ligament is mapped onto the anterior interosseous (sometimes called the anterior sacroiliac) ligament. Note that the cut across the sacrum is at the S1–S2 disc level. SIJ, sacroiliac joint; TP, transverse process.

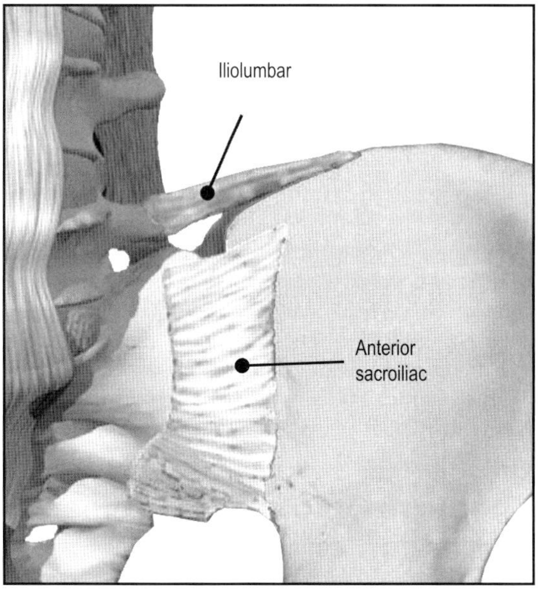

Fig. 19.14 The iliolumbar ligament can be seen as either part of the anterior (or ventral) sacroiliac ligament or as part of the posterior interosseous ligament. The attachment of the iliolumbar onto the iliac crest suggests that it behaves more like the anterior sacroiliac ligament.

used by anatomists sometimes obscures the function of the spine because it introduces artificial divisions between units that have similar function, or which have been modified and adapted through evolution.

The impact that is delivered to the acetabulum during gait is directly transferred to the SIJ facets and then all the way up to the spine. A cursory examination of the honeycomb structure that lies behind the SG ridge demonstrates that the bony cells are highly organized along a specific pattern that betrays the path of forces that must be transmitted across the SIJ (Fig. 19.15).

If the so-called irregular surfaces of the high-friction SIJ are the main force transmission paths, then one would expect a dense network of bony cells behind the walls; this is not the case. The bone is laid out at the SG ridge interface, precisely where one would expect to find continuity in the force transmission system based on solid bone compression and not shear along a much weaker SIJ line.

Controlling the pelvis using the sacroiliac joint

Having laid out the anatomical facts, I now propose to examine how the system might respond to gait. It is generally stated that the sacrum is literally hanging on its ligaments. This representation is incorrect because viscoelastic collagen subjected to continuous loading will creep. The SG ridge takes on the permanent component of the vertical load, and the ligaments and/or muscles take on any rapidly changing complementary force that would tend to open up the SIJ. The peculiar arrangement of the SIJ permits limited movement (Sturesson 2000) around the SG ridge, resulting in a rotation around two main axes within the constraints of the facets of the SIJ. This mechanism is similar to

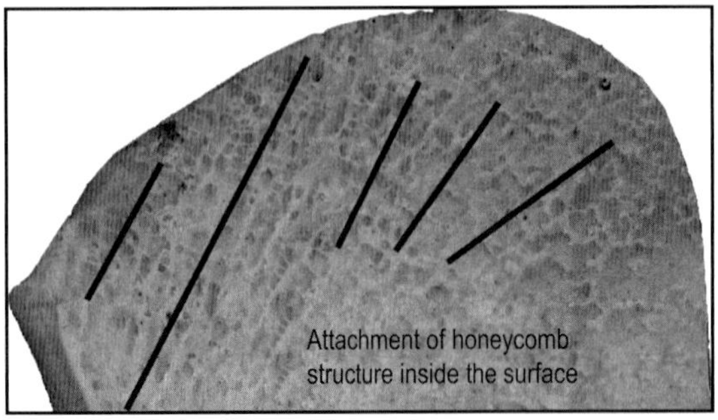

Fig. 19.15 This is a small portion of the inside of the ventral part of the innominate. The honeycomb structure of the bone has been removed leaving only the part of the honeycomb that is attached to the inside wall of the innominate. Note the clear orientation of the structure that betrays the lines of forces that must be channeled through the bone.

what is permitted by the lumbar spine facets, which enhance the coupled motion of the intervertebral joint. Hence the SIJ also exhibits a coupled motion of smaller magnitude, but greater force.

The articular surfaces at S1 and S3 define two axes of rotation. The pelvis motion will be determined by which axis is active during gait. The determination of what facet of the SIJ will be in contact depends on the spinal lordosis. In this regard, the division of the spinal column into cervical, thoracic, lumbar, and sacrum is not helpful because it presumes a different function for each segment. The clinician ought to think of the spine as an assembly of joints with either two or four facets (fused – two by two) starting at the acetabulum. It is known that ankylosing spondylitis starts at the SIJ and moves upwards. Perhaps we ought to reconsider the role of the SIJ as an integral part of the spine in the generation of LBP, a position advocated over the last 30 years by DonTigny (2004), who has designed a technique for rehabilitating LBP patients by first resolving the SIJ complaints (see Chapter 18).

Controlling the coupled motion of the pelvis

The coupled motion of the spine does not stop at the L5–S1 interface, simply because the spine does not stop there. The spine goes all the way to the sacral area and the well- known coupled motion of the spine extends to the pelvis/sacrum interface as well. The SIJ complexity permits generation and transfer of torque by an appropriate control of the center of rotation affecting the role of the SIJ in a way very similar to that of the spine above L5. The reader is encouraged to read DonTigny's contribution in Chapter 18 of this book.

In my view, the SG ridge acts as a fulcrum transferring most of the vertical forces across the SIJ. In addition, that ridge ensures the axial rotation of the pelvis by a mechanism similar to that of the facets of the lumbar spine. But the propeller shape of the SIJ allows the pelvis an additional movement (nutation) around the SG ridge and hence the need to control the relative motion of the innominates around the sacrum outside the coronal plane. The articulations at S1 and S3 permit the pelvis to cant and rotate anteriorly and posteriorly. The strong ligaments across the SIJ insure that once the innominates rotates anteriorly or posteriorly, they will return to their neutral position. One possible hypothesis for pelvic motion during gait is illustrated in Fig. 19.16.

The oscillations between the contacting facets at S1 and S3 can be made to function as illustrated in Fig. 19.17.

Hence, we propose that the relative movements of the sacrum and innominates and their consequences on the pelvic motion can be summarized in Table 19.2.

The situation during gait is somewhat more complex. The facets S1 and S3 on opposing innominates contact simultaneously and permit rotational control of the acetabulum, whereas the transfer of vertical loads is done through the SG ridge (Fig. 19.18). The complete and detailed explanation of this mechanism is beyond the scope of this chapter and has been published elsewhere (DonTigny 2004).

The position of the sacroiliac joint's center of rotation

The motion of the SIJ was studied by many using both cadavers and live subjects. In general, the studies have shown that the relative motion of the sacrum over either innominate is small (a few degrees) with the exception of Smidt (1995) claiming values ten times greater. Using stereophotogrammetry, Egund (1978) calculated that the position of the center of rotation of the SIJ is located at a point 50 mm posterior to the SIJ, in apparent conflict with the suggestions in Fig. 19.16.

There is no evidence showing that the quasistatic methodology used by Egund to calculate the position of the center of rotation can be extrapolated for gait studies. There is a very good reason for this:

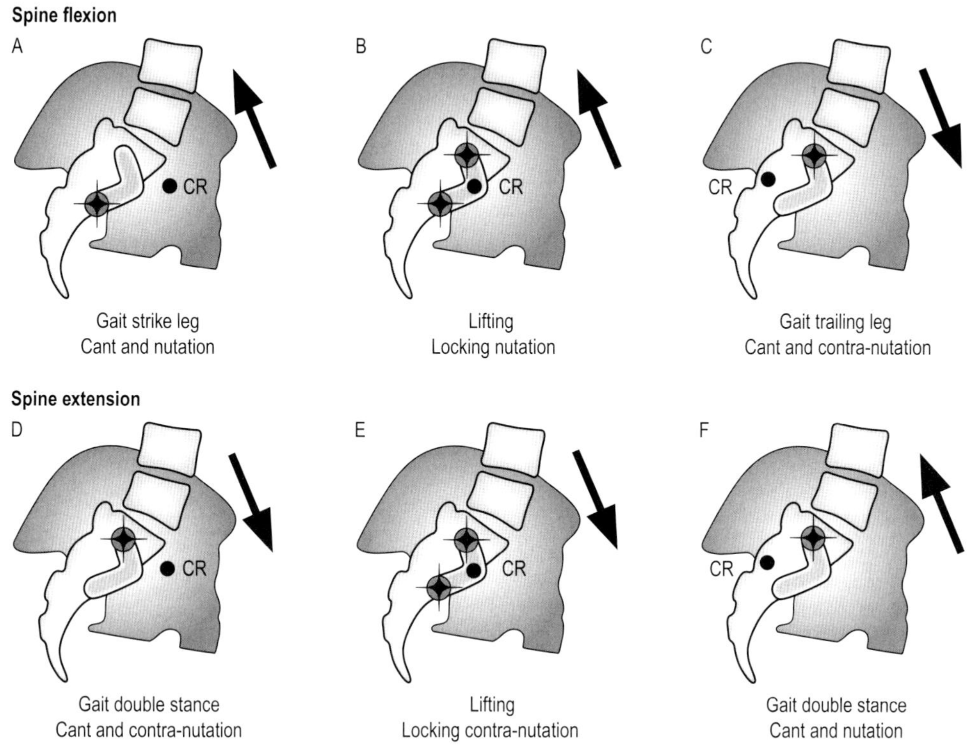

Fig. 19.16 There are six possible combinations of spinal motion and basic position of the center of rotation (CR = black dot). For spinal flexion, the center of rotation can be located either forward (A), inside (B), or behind (C) the sacroiliac joint (SIJ). For spinal extension, the same combinations are used (D, E, and F). Note that lifting a heavy load is possible regardless of the spinal lordosis because pelvis locking can be achieved while the spine is either flexed or extended (B + E). The counter motion of the innominates during gait is achieved by either the combination (A + C) or that of (D + F).

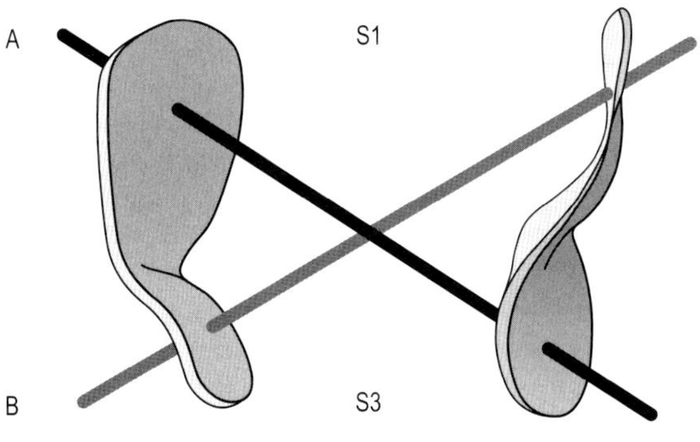

Fig. 19.17 The opposing facets at S1 and S3 contact simultaneously in an oscillating pattern between the two configurations (A) and (B) at each stride.

By the time the radiograph is taken, the collagen has stretched beyond its $^1/_3$ of a second time constant and hence the configuration cannot represent the dynamics of gait. In addition, an equally valid and arbitrary mathematical approach could place the center of rotation anywhere in the plane, including at all positions indicated in Fig. 19.16. Indeed, the determination of the motion of the SIJ in a plane using two radiographs requires solving one equation with two unknowns; an impossible task. To reduce the infinite number of solutions to a single one, it is customary to arbitrarily set a translation vector to zero and assign all movements to a hypothetical rotation [see Gracovetsky (1988) p 161–164 for a complete discussion of this issue, which is beyond the scope of this chapter].

The standard procedure for calculation of the center of rotation has serious clinical consequences that might explain why using the 50 mm value of Egund has led to surprising conclusions.

The motion of the SIJ is notoriously difficult to study *in vivo* and until better tools are designed, the details of the SIJ's movements will entail an unavoidable speculative component. Accordingly, the fact that there are no contradictions between the proposed description of the SIJ's motion and the current experimental knowledge does not prove that our proposal is correct. As usual, time will tell

Table 19.2 The motion of the innominate versus that of the sacrum is a function of the contacting facets combination (S1 alone, S3 alone, or S1 and S3). For instance, when S1 alone contacts during flexion, the sacrum cants while the innominate (on which the S1 facet is located) counternutates

Spine motion	S1	S3	S1 and S3
Flexion	Counternutation	Nutation	Nutation
Extension	Counternutation	Nutation	Counternutation
Result	Sacrum cants	Sacrum cants	Sacroiliac joint locked

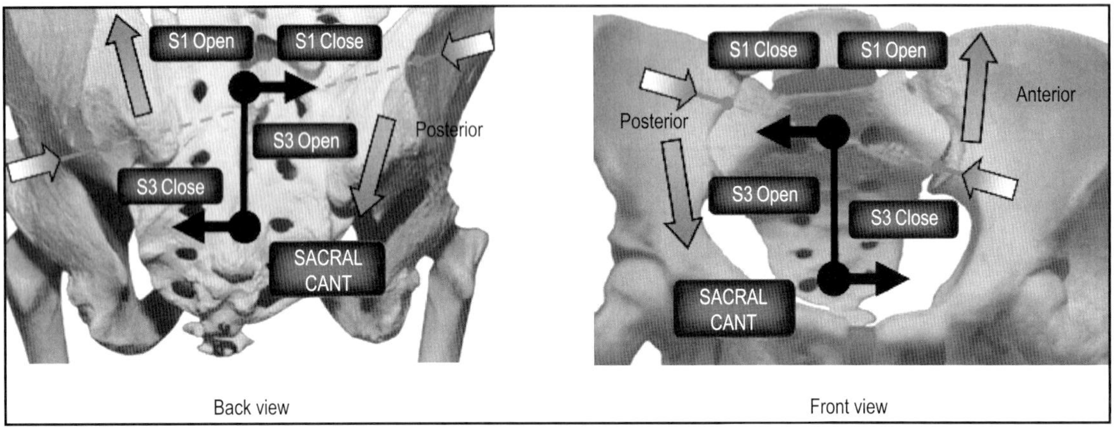

Fig. 19.18 Left and right: right heel strike. The right S1 and left S3 are closed. The right innominate has rotated posteriorly to maximize the advance of the right leg. The sacrum cants clockwise on the back view and counterclockwise on the left view. (Adapted from DonTigny 2005.)

and the reader should consider the ideas expressed in Fig. 19.16 as a platform for opening up a new direction for debate rather than a definite answer.

Where do we go from there?

The purpose of this work is to understand not only how we function but how we came to function that way. Our species is the end product of a long optimization process. Function drives the anatomy, and not the other way around. The fundamental hypothesis of this work is that locomotion within our energy niche is the driving force behind our anatomical design. Recent advances in decoding the human genome will permit an unprecedented access to our heritage and perhaps determine what the real function of the spine is. Indeed, restoring the function of the injured patient implies knowing what that normal function is, something which is still the subject of speculation.

If history is any guide, the ideas expressed in this chapter will trigger a considerable amount of unsolicited criticism. I hope some of this work will survive the mandatory peer review process and perhaps launch new students in directions we cannot even imagine today. As a member of the university community, encouraging progress through research is very rewarding.

The topics for investigation are many. First, I would review the anatomy of the SIJ from a functional perspective without any bias. Second, I would simulate the interaction between the ridge and the S1 and S3 facets to appreciate the possible locus of the instantaneous centers of rotation of the SIJ's movement during gait or even simple sagittal lifting. Understanding normal gait demands to know how the acetabulum orients its force vector: the shape of the neck of the femur is a good place to start. I would also give a very hard look at the shape of the innominate. Bone reacts to stress, and the arch of the iliac crest is a clue as to what is transferred through the SIJ.

Stability at minimum energy cost is essentially a collagen issue, and the forces that shaped us cannot be left out of the equation. I believe that sooner or later we will end up being confronted with the need to understand the relation between the viscoelastic properties of collagen and the gravitational constant of the planet. The constancy of the gravitational field across the Earth was instrumental in permitting our species to migrate away from its African birthplace.

The interested reader can contact me at gracovetsky@videotron.ca.

Summary

1. The spine and its surrounding structure are fundamentally unstable. The evolutionary advantage of instability seems to have been lost in the studies of the stability of the musculoskeletal system.
2. The standard representation of stability in use in the current literature is valid for homogeneous time-invariant material. The viscoelastic nature of biomechanical material precludes a straightforward application of these engineering concepts.
3. The sacrum is made of fused vertebrae and transverse processes, the pelvis is made of fused ribs and the sacroiliac joint is a modified costovertebral joint. Many ligamentous structures holding the SIJ together can be derived from the corresponding thoracocostal anatomy.
4. There exists a ridge at the tip of the transverse processes of S1 and S2 that locks into a corresponding shape in the innominates. That ridge transfers the vertical loads, leaving the SIJ relatively free to rotate around that hinge.
5. The SIJ is not flat; it is warped, and its surfaces cannot slip past each other. The ligaments across the SIJ are very strong and the geometry of the joint is such that there is no need for any kind of significant additional force closure to keep it together.
6. The control of the spine during gait and other activities depends upon the position of the center of rotation of adjacent vertebrae. The same concept can be applied to the SIJ which is an integral part of the force transmission system of the spine.
7. Our spinal machinery resonates in the constant gravitational field of the earth. Changing the 9.81 m/s^2 gravitational constant (on the moon or during long space flight) will detune the spinal machinery because the collagen will be either too stiff or too lax. There must be a fundamental relationship between the viscoelastic properties of collagen and the gravitational field value.

References

Basmadjian J 1979 Muscle alive: their function revealed by electromyography. Williams and Wilkins, Baltimore, MD

Bogduk N 1997 Clinical anatomy of the lumbar spine and sacrum, 3rd edn. Churchill Livingstone, Edinburgh

Boos N, Rieder R, Schade V et al 1995 The diagnostic accuracy of magnetic resonance imaging, work perception, and psychosocial factors in identifying symptomatic disc herniations. Spine 20(24):2613–2625

Delmas A 1950 Jonction sacro iliaque et statique du corps. Rev Rhumat 17(9):475–481

Dijkstra PF, Vleeming A, Stoeckart R 1992 Complex motion tomography of the sacroiliac joint. Clin Biomech 7:170–176

DonTigny RL 2004 Pelvic dynamics and the S3 subluxation of the sacroiliac joint. CD-ROM. DonTigny, Havre, MT

DonTigny RL 2005 Critical analysis of the functional dynamics of the sacroiliac joints as they pertain to normal gait. J Orthop Med 27(1):3–9

Egund N, Olsson TH, Schmid H, Selvik G 1978 Movements in the sacroiliac joints demonstrated with roentgen stereophotogrammetry. Acta Radio Diagn 19:833–846

Farfan HF 1978 The biomechanical advantage of lordosis and hip extension for upright activity. Man as compared with other anthropoids. Spine 3:336–324

Gracovetsky S 1988 The spinal engine. Springer-Verlag, New York

Gracovetsky S 2001 Analysis and interpretation of gait in relation to lumbopelvic function. In Vleeming A et al (eds) Proceedings of the Fourth Interdisciplinary World Congress on Low Back and Pelvic Pain, Montreal Canada. ECO, Rotterdam, p45–63

Gracovetsky S 2004 ECT conference, Antwerp. CD-ROM with 287 slides and notations. Available from: gracovetsky@videotron.ca

Helleur C, Gracovetsky S, Farfan H 1984 Tolerance of the human cervical spine to high acceleration: a modelling approach. Aviation, Space and Environmental Medicine 55:903–909

Kazarian L 1968 Acta Orth Scand (suppl)

Lovett AW 1903 A contribution to the study of the mechanics of the spine. Am J Anat 2:457–462

McGill S 2001 Achieving spine stability: Blending engineering and clinical approaches. In Vleeming A et al (eds) Fourth Interdisciplinary World Congress on Low Back and Pelvis Pain, 8–10 November. Montreal, Canada, p203–211

Panjabi M, White A 1995 Clinical biomechanics of the spine, 2nd edn. Lippincott, Philadelphia, PA

Smidt GL, McQuade K, Wei S, Barakatt E 1995 Sacroiliac kinematics for reciprocal straddle positions. Spine 20:1047–1054

Solonen KA 1957 The sacroiliac joint in the light of anatomical, roentgenological and clinical studies. Acta Orthopaedica Scandinavica 27 (suppl):4–127

Sturesson B, Udén A, Vleeming A 2000 A radiostereometric analysis of the movements of the sacroiliac joints in the reciprocal straddle position. Spine 25:214–217

van Wingerden JP, Vleeming A, Buyruk HM, Raissadat KL 2004 Stabilization of the sacroiliac joint in vivo: verification of muscular contribution to force closure of the pelvis. Eur Spine J 13(3):199–205

Vleeming A, Volkers AC, Snijders CJ, Stoeckart R 1990 Relationship between form and function in the SI joint, part II. Spine 15:133–136

Weisl H 1954 The articular surfaces of the sacroiliac joint and their relation to the movements of the sacrum. Acta Anatom (Basel) 22:1–14

PART THREE

Section One

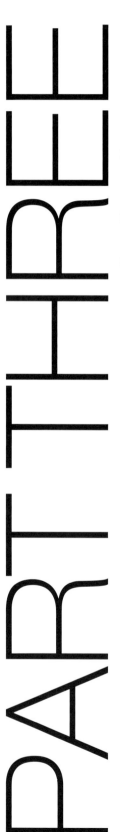

Diagnostic methods: Visualization in relation to pelvic dysfunction

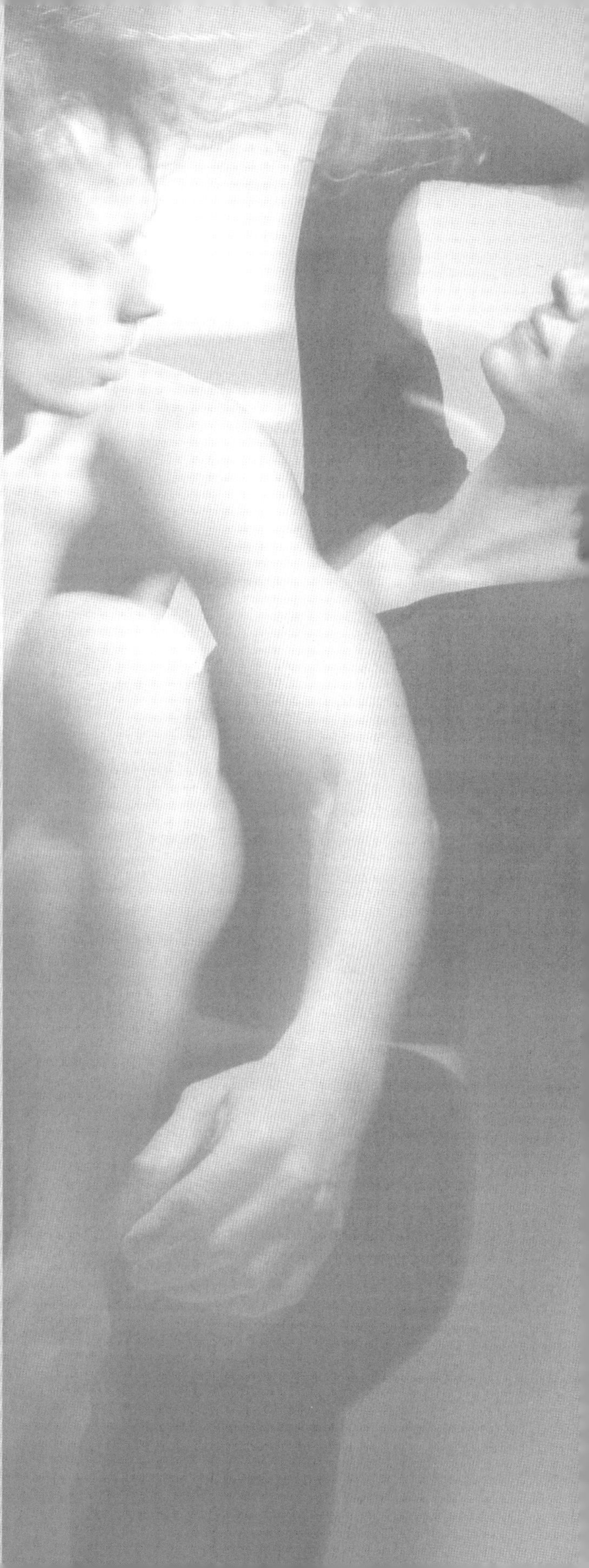

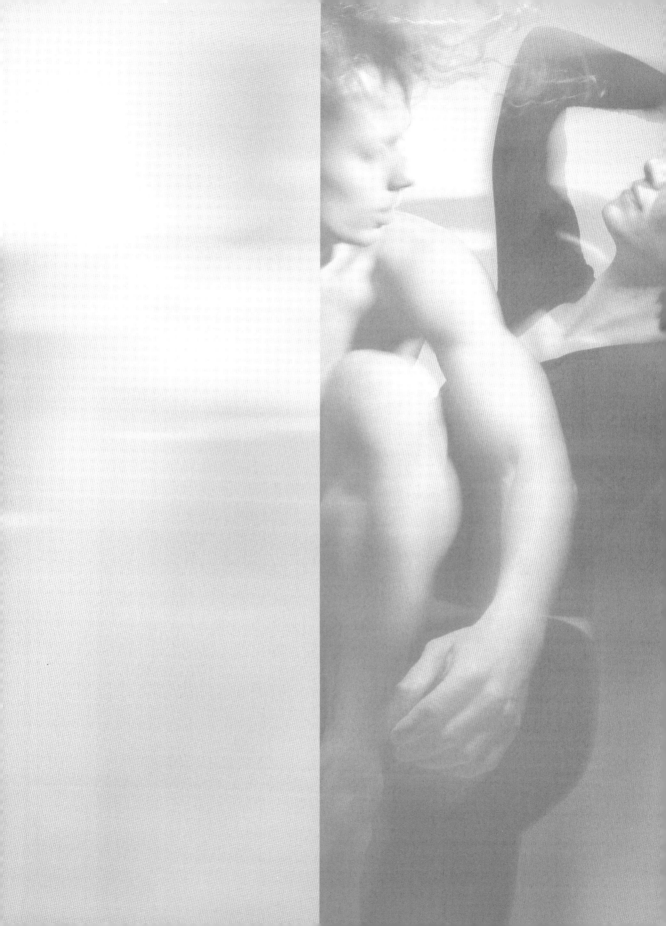

SECTION ONE

CHAPTER 20

Basic problems in the visualization of the sacroiliac joint

PF Dijkstra

The X-ray is a shadow of reality.

Introduction

Plain X-rays of the sacroiliac joints (SIJs) are often difficult to 'read'. A thorough understanding of the anatomy of the SIJ, and knowledge of how these images are made, is needed if we are to rebuild in our minds the flat image into a three-dimensional image. To enable understanding of X-rays of the SIJ, this chapter describes the process that produces the final image, and discusses the problems inherent in interpreting the radiologic anatomy. Some pathologic conditions of the SIJ will be shown.

Radiologic anatomy

X-ray absorption

The photons of X-ray radiation are more or less absorbed in our body. In general, there are four different groups of body constituents in terms of radiation: air, fat, water, and bone. Air (as in the lungs or gut) has a low absorption value; bone has the highest absorption value, depending on its calcium content.

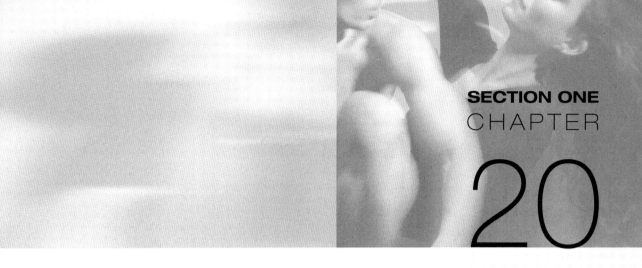

This differentiation allows us to 'see' the different parts of the body. Low absorption implies that many photons reach the photographic plate behind the body. That spot becomes black. Intermediate absorption gives shades of gray (as in body fat and muscles), and with high absorption, few photons reach the photographic plate, which remains white. There are several technical solutions to obtain a good image; these, however, will not be discussed here.

Projection of the object

There will always be a distortion of the object in the projection on the photographic plate. The X-ray tube can be seen as a point source from which the radiation leaves the tube as a fan beam in the direction of the object and the photographic plate. The further away from the tube, the broader the beam becomes. This means that on the edge of the beam, the enlargement of the object's projection will be greater than in the center (Fig. 20.1). Furthermore, parts of the object close to the tube will be projected larger than parts close to the photographic plate. Therefore, international rules exist to produce X-ray pictures. The more complicated the structure of the object, the more difficult to understand the final X-ray image. Knowledge of the density (amount of radiation absorption) and the normal anatomic features of the object is a prerequisite to finding pathological structures.

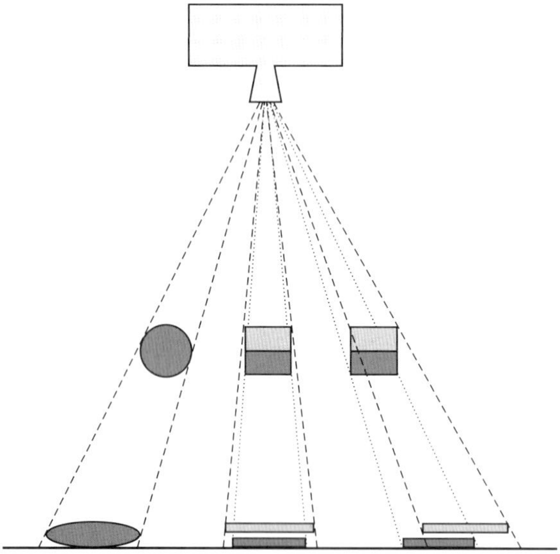

Fig. 20.1 The place of the object in the X-ray beam determines the object's projection. In the central ray (A), the top and bottom of the square are projected on top of each other, but the top is slightly larger than the bottom. At the right (B), top and bottom are shifted. The sphere on the left (C) is projected as an oval structure.

Imaging techniques

Plain X-ray

Plain X-rays should be used to get an overview of the sacrum and SIJ. We do not discuss the lateral view of the sacrum because it is not a helpful technique in investigating the SIJ. Several projections are possible but anteroposterior (AP) and 25° cranial angulated views are the most informative (Dijkstra 1993). Oblique views should not be used: they look nice but, by superimposing the front and back of the SIJ, they will hide more detail than they reveal (see Fig. 20.3 below).

Tomography

This technique produces an image as a slice of the body of 2–5 mm thick. Because of the construction of the X-ray machine, these slices are in the coronal, oblique, or sagittal plane, depending on the position of the patient. Axial slices are usually difficult or impossible to make. This is in contrast to computerized tomography (CT), in which only axial slices can be made. The new spiral CT machines are able to reconstruct all imaging planes. Tomography is carried out using a multidirectional movement of the X-ray tube. This means a spiral or hypocycloidal movement of 25°; all other movements are insufficient for the SIJ. Both types of multidirectional movement have their pros and cons; when aware of the ghost images of the system, there is no problem. It is essential with tomography that the part of the joint under investigation is tangential to the movement of the X-ray tube. In a complicated joint such as the SIJ, one has to be careful to position the patient in the right way. The greatest problem when reading tomograms is the ghost images; these are, in fact, quite easy to interpret when one has a thorough knowledge of the normal anatomy and an understanding of the tomographic process (Firooznia et al 1984).

Computerized tomography

CT should be carried out using a 2 mm slice thickness, with a 5 mm interval and a high-definition filter. The angulation of the gantry is not important, being merely a question of taste, but slice thickness and filter are very important. In my experience, a window of 1600 and level of 400 with a high (software) filter are very satisfactory.

It is not true that CT makes things easier: the pictures are just as difficult to read and to interpret as images obtained by other techniques. However, because of the high contrast in CT pictures, one is inclined to see more pathology. The borders of the joints are sharper, but the natural inclinations of the SIJs in the picture might fool one into thinking that erosions are present. Further discussion of CT scanning can be found in Chapter 21.

Magnetic resonance imaging

Magnetic resonance imaging (MRI) gives very promising results, and might eventually take over from most other imaging techniques. Up to now, the resolution of the images has been unsatisfactory with respect to small details in the SIJ cartilage.

MRI is very useful in the search for septic arthritis and is the only technique that can pinpoint the pathologic areas in bone and soft tissues.

Isotope studies

The possibility for discriminating between different diseases on the basis of isotope activity in the SIJ is very poor. In general, not more can be said than that some disease process is going on. It can be helpful in septic arthritis (leukocyte scan), when the origin of the disease is not clear, but in that case MRI is far more conclusive.

Choice

Plain X-rays are always taken to get an overview of the patient's problems. Which other techniques are used depends on the sort of pathology anticipated. In the Old World, as opposed to the Americas, tomography is still largely used, although it is being more and more replaced by CT. In septic arthritis, MRI should be used. In spondylarthropathy, CT and tomography can be used.

In cases of trauma, the technique depends on the status of the patient, but CT is the method of choice. Because the patient usually has several iron plates in the bones and is difficult to handle, it is easier to carry out tomography, with less disturbance in the picture. Because of the metal artifacts, CT scanning is usually not possible.

Radiologic anatomy of the SIJ

The angulation of the joints is measured with respect to the sagittal plain. S1 has an angulation of 20–25° lateral; S2 usually has an angulation of 10–15° lateral; S3 has a more or less sagittal angulation (0–5° medial; Fig. 20.2A,B). S1 is broader than S3 (Dijkstra et al 1989, Solonen 1957, Vleeming et al 1992).

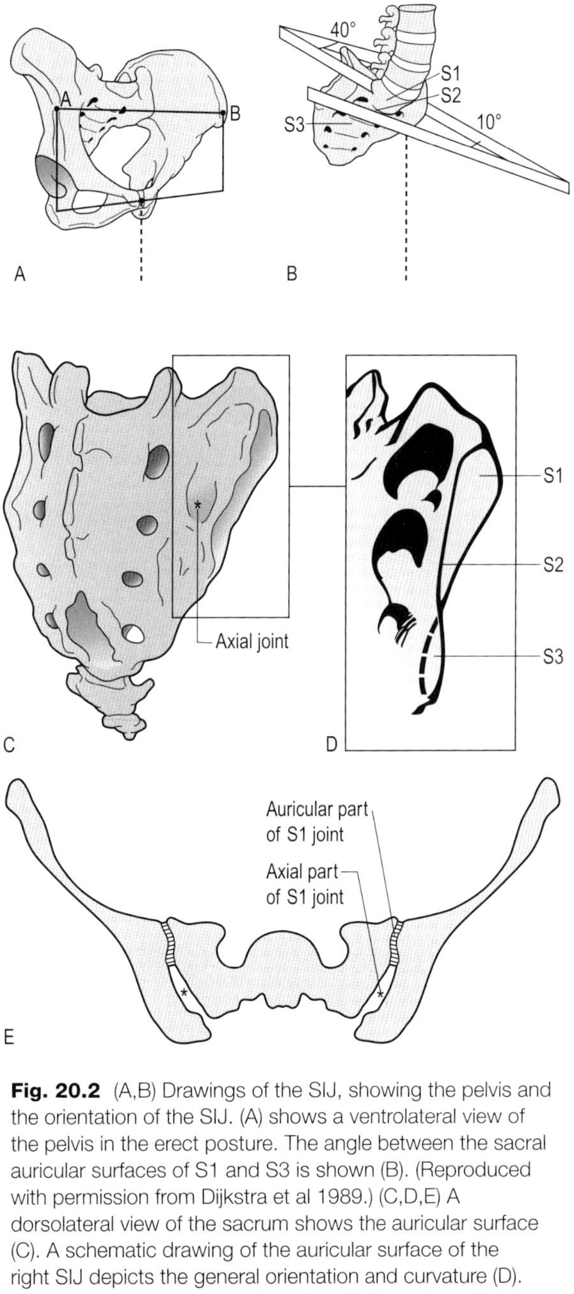

Fig. 20.2 (A,B) Drawings of the SIJ, showing the pelvis and the orientation of the SIJ. (A) shows a ventrolateral view of the pelvis in the erect posture. The angle between the sacral auricular surfaces of S1 and S3 is shown (B). (Reproduced with permission from Dijkstra et al 1989.) (C,D,E) A dorsolateral view of the sacrum shows the auricular surface (C). A schematic drawing of the auricular surface of the right SIJ depicts the general orientation and curvature (D). (E) shows a transverse section of the SIJ just above the ventral superior iliac spine and through the first pelvic sacral foramina. The hatched areas refer to the cartilage-covered auricular surface. The site of the axial joint, posterior to the auricular joint, is indicated by an asterisk.

Thus the joint has a double curvature: dorsoventral and craniocaudal. Obviously, in no single projection can all parts of the joint be viewed tangentially (Fig. 20.2C,D,E). With X-rays, we see a sharp edge only when it is perpendicular to our viewing direction; it is one of the problems specifically encountered in the SIJ. Fig. 20.3 shows the different projections that are obtained when the supine patient is turned from right to left. As a mental exercise, understanding these projections is the first step necessary to be able to diagnose malformations or disease of the SIJ.

The general direction of the SIJ joint from posterior to ventral is about 25°. Thus, if the patient is prone and the X-ray is taken in a posteroanterior direction, the joints seem to be covered in their entire length. This is the same when the joint is seen in the ventrodorsal direction with the patient turned 25°; this is called the oblique SIJ position. An oblique view seems nice, but it is a superimposition of all parts of the joint. To understand this more clearly, we have used a cadaver SIJ sawn into 5 mm slices. Figure 20.4 shows that the back and the front of one slice are quite different. In practice, the 25° cranial

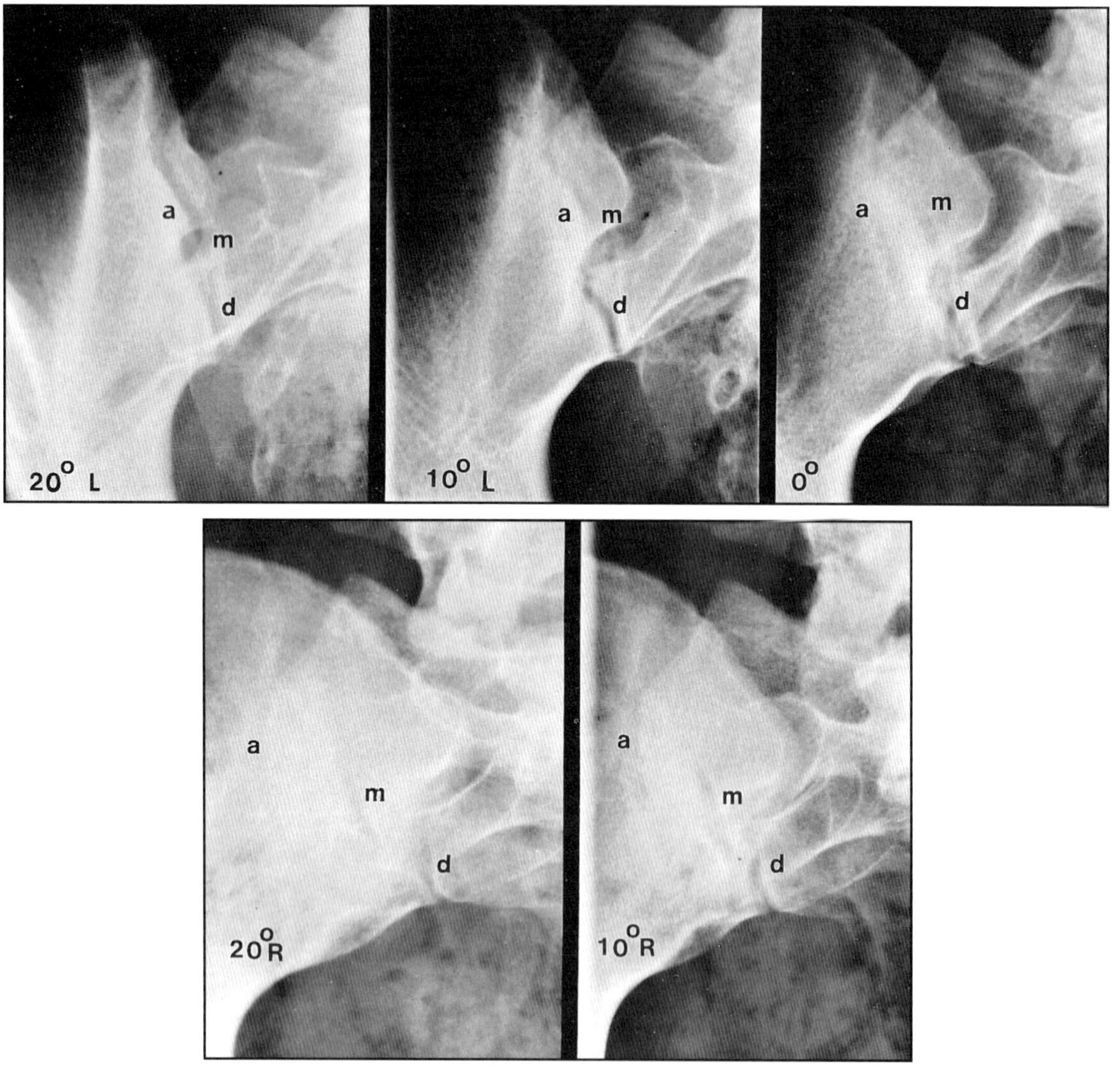

Fig. 20.3 The right sacroiliac joint (SIJ) seen from different angles in AP projection, from 20° left to 20° right in 10° steps. The ventral (a), middle (m) and posterior (d) parts of the joint are seen. In the 20° left directed projection, all parts are superimposed. This projection is a simulation of a posteroanterior projection or an anteroposterior projection with the patient turned 25° to the left, called the oblique position.

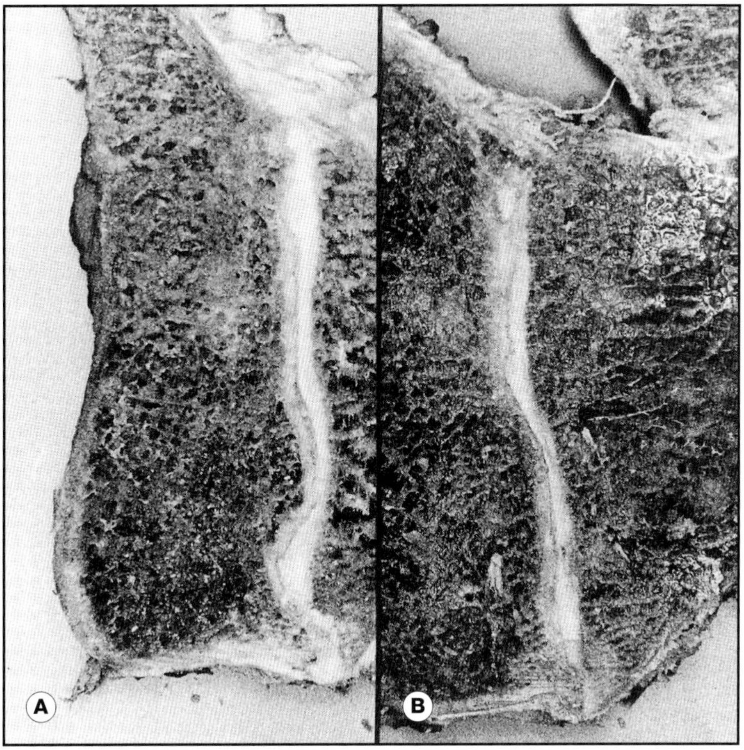

Fig. 20.4 Front (A) and back (B) of the same anatomic slice of a sacroiliac joint (SIJ). Note the difference in configuration of the joint, notwithstanding a slice thickness of only 5 mm. This gives an impression of how difficult it is to show all parts of the SIJ on X-ray: most parts of the joint are hidden in a plain X-ray. (Reproduced with permission from Dijkstra et al 1989.)

angled AP view gives the information to decide on further investigation.

In daily practice, the projections of the SIJ are those used for the lumbar spine, the pelvis, and the 25° cranial angled AP view. In CT scanning, transverse (Fig. 20.2C,D,E) or angulated transverse planes are used, but plain X-rays are taken in the coronal plane. Bearing in mind that the SIJ has a double curvature, we see in plain X-rays both the edges of the posterior and ventral parts of the joint as well as the middle part.

As an example, Fig. 20.5 shows a normal SIJ: Fig. 20.5A is the caudal part of the lumbar spine view, whereas Fig. 20.5B is a cranial angulated AP view. It is only in the second view that we can see the middle part of the joint. The posterior and the ventrolateral part of the joint are well seen in both views. Obviously, different projections influence the perception of the joint (Dijkstra 1993).

Figure 20.6 introduces tomography as a means of evaluating the SIJ. The plain X-ray in Fig. 20.6A shows a superimposed projection of segments of the joint. Tomography of the posterior part of the joint (Fig. 20.6B) shows left–right asymmetry and a hook-like projection near the axial part of the joint located dorsal of the auricular part (see Fig. 20.2E). The ventral part of the joint is well seen in Fig. 20.6C, and here we also see a persistent epiphysis in the joint. The epiphyses of the SIJ usually close at about 16 years of age; because of their projection, they can be a source of confusion.

Congenital variations

There are many congenital variations. The sacrum can be more or less absent, which is usually accompanied by partial absence of the uterus and/or ureter and kidney. In several of the patients presented here, congenital variations are present, for example transitional vertebra (see Figs 20.7, 20.8 and 20.10, below), asymmetry (see Fig. 20.7 below) and persistent division between sacral segments (see Fig. 20.7 below), and also persistent epiphyses (Fig. 20.6). The axial part of the SIJ (see Fig. 20.2E) can have a complex form and can give a confusing shadow (Fig. 20.6B). A nonclosure of the spinous process of L5 and S1 is sometimes associated with

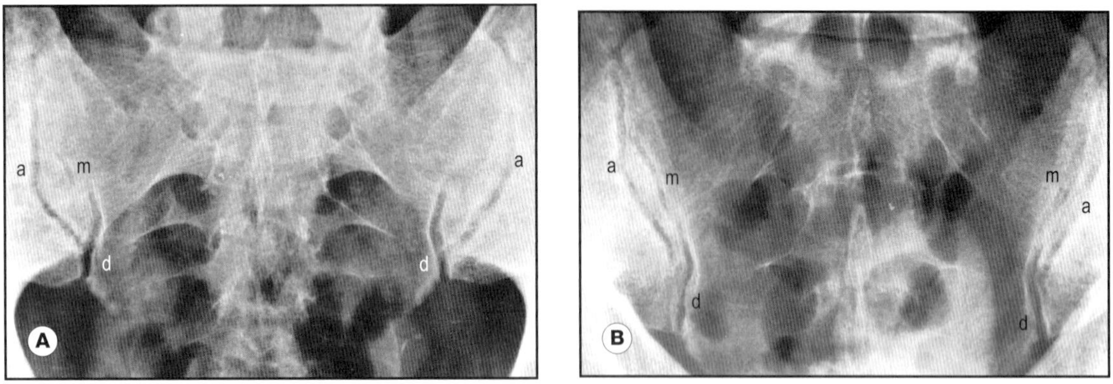

Fig. 20.5 A normal sacroiliac joint (SIJ) in two anteroposterior (AP) projections. a, ventral; m, middle; d, posterior parts of the joint. (A) The caudal part of a lumbar spine view. The SIJs are seen in the same projection as the lateral square in Fig. 20.1. The posterior part of S3 is more accentuated, and the middle part of the joint is usually not seen. (B) Cranial angulated AP view. The SIJs are in the center of the X-ray beam. Because the ventral and middle parts of the joint are closer to the X-ray tube, they are projected more to the lateral of the X-ray. The middle part of the joint is more easily seen.

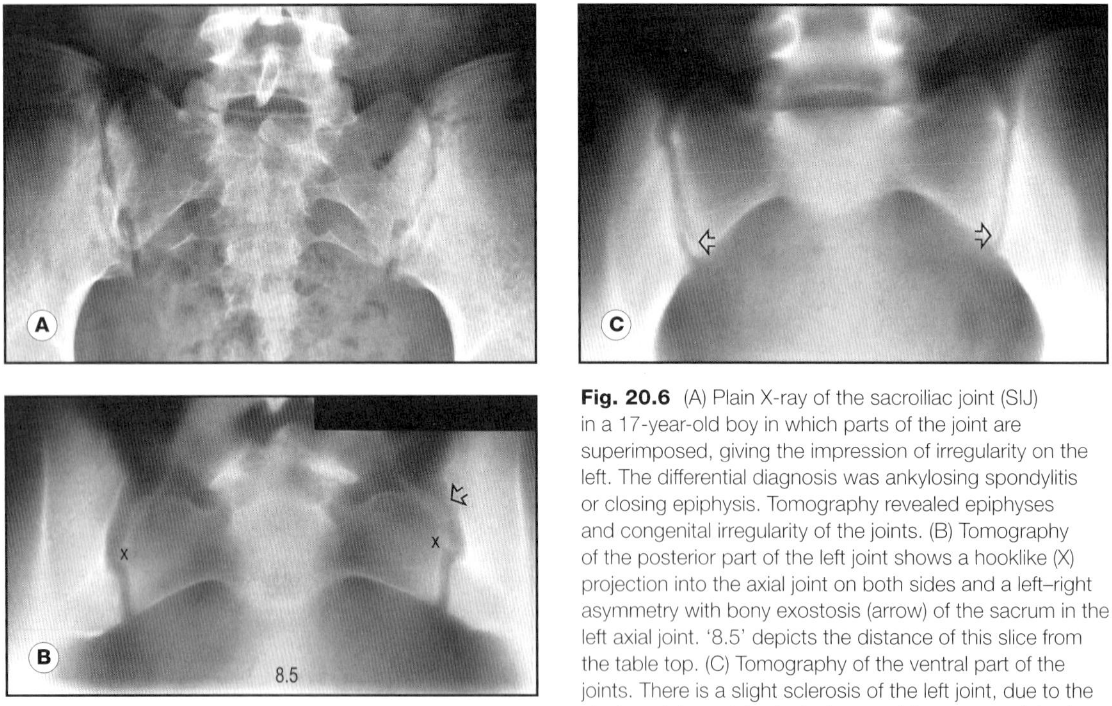

Fig. 20.6 (A) Plain X-ray of the sacroiliac joint (SIJ) in a 17-year-old boy in which parts of the joint are superimposed, giving the impression of irregularity on the left. The differential diagnosis was ankylosing spondylitis or closing epiphysis. Tomography revealed epiphyses and congenital irregularity of the joints. (B) Tomography of the posterior part of the left joint shows a hooklike (X) projection into the axial joint on both sides and a left–right asymmetry with bony exostosis (arrow) of the sacrum in the left axial joint. '8.5' depicts the distance of this slice from the table top. (C) Tomography of the ventral part of the joints. There is a slight sclerosis of the left joint, due to the closing of the epiphysis. In the caudal area, an epiphysis (arrows) is seen in the sacrum, especially on the right side.

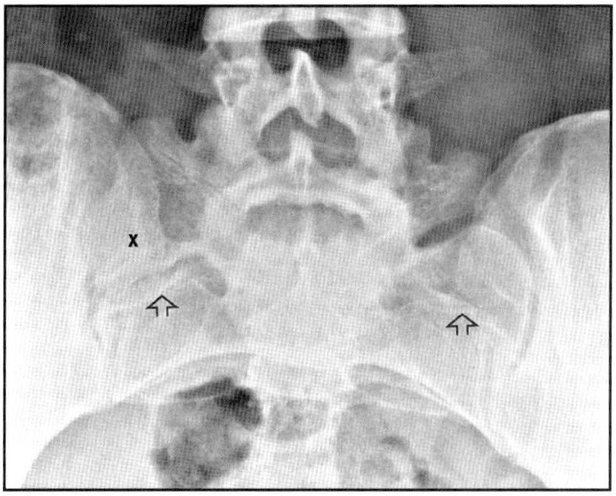

Fig. 20.7 A sacroiliac joint (SIJ) with congenital variations. There is a persistent S1–S2 division (arrows) and a fusion of the transverse process of L5 with S1 at the right side (X). The S1 on the left is more rounded and smaller than usual. (Reproduced with permission from Dijkstra 1993.)

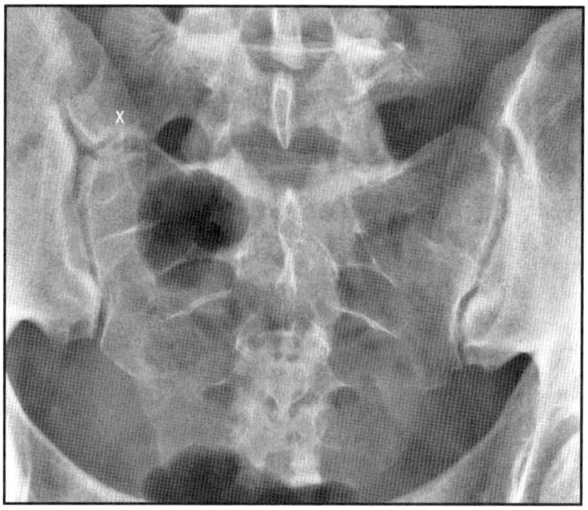

Fig. 20.8 A transitional vertebra L5–S1 is a congenital variation. There is a broad transverse process of L5 on the right, forming a joint with S1 (X). (Reproduced with permission from Dijkstra 1993.)

spina bifida, but in most people this variation is without clinical symptoms.

Symmetry

The SIJs often show left–right asymmetry. Many unnecessary X-rays can be avoided with some knowledge of this phenomenon. Figure 20.7 shows a persistent S1–S2 joint on both sides, and also a left–right asymmetry. The left SIJ is somewhat smaller than the right. At the right side of this SIJ, there is also a fusion of the transverse process of L5 with S1.

Transitional vertebra

The first sacral vertebra can be more or less fused with the fifth lumbar vertebra. This fusion is mostly asymmetric (Figs 20.7 and 20.8), but symmetric fusion can occur. There can be a joint between the transverse process of L5 and the body of S1 (Fig. 20.8 and see Fig. 20.10 below). These transitional vertebrae can be found in about 20% of those in whom L5–S1 is visible on X-ray.

Diseases of the sacroiliac joint

Osteoarthritis (arthrosis)

Osteoarthritis is usually a disease of the elderly but in the SIJ it can be found even at a young age. The ventral ligaments, especially, calcify. The transitional vertebrae also have a tendency to become involved in osteoarthritis. In young adults, a localized form of osteoarthritis can be found in the form of iliitis condensans, occurring more often in women than in men. There is an oval area of bony sclerosis on the iliac side of the SIJ, with sclerotic margins of the SIJ, often with subchondral cysts. In Fig. 20.9 the iliitis condensans is located in the caudal area of the SIJ. The plain X-ray is difficult to evaluate, but the tomography reveals the true nature of this ailment.

Figure 20.10 shows a bony bridge in the ventral ligament of the SIJ and osteoarthritis of the transitional vertebra L5–S1. As in this case, other parts of the SIJ are often not involved.

Osteoarthritis can be mistaken for ankylosing spondylitis. In the patient seen in Fig. 20.11, the AP view shows complete ankylosis of the right SIJ; the frontal tomogram is not of much help either. However, the oblique tomogram shows a narrowed but otherwise normal joint. This oblique tomogram is an example of a tailored investigation of the SIJ. By choosing a direction of the tomogram deliberately tangential to the joint, much more information can be obtained. By its nature, the tomogram will blur nontangential joint surfaces. Therefore we routinely perform oblique tomograms in areas where a nontangential joint surface can be expected.

Very severe osteoarthritis is seen on the CT of the patient depicted in Fig. 20.12. The ventral SIJ ligaments are thickened into bony bridges, the joint surfaces show sclerosis, and intraluminal bony

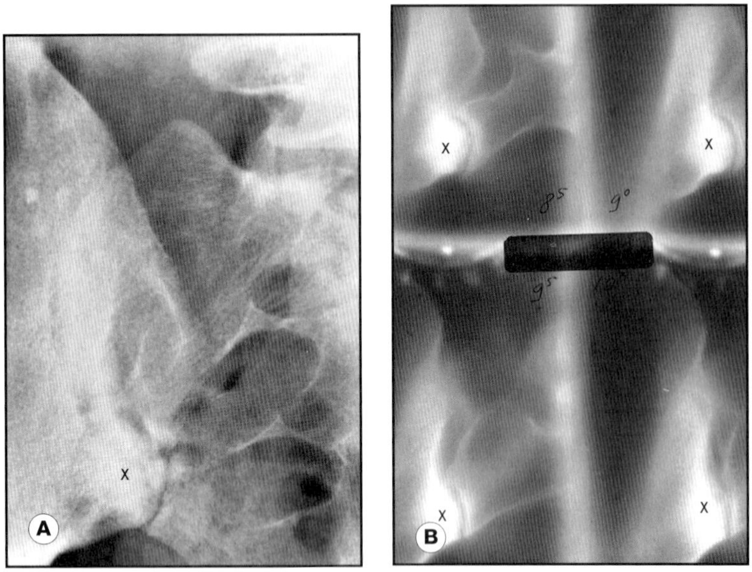

Fig. 20.9 Iliitis condensans. (A) Plain X-ray of the right sacroiliac joint (SIJ) with irregular and sclerosing changes in S3 (X). This type of sclerosis of the ilium can cause confusing plain X-rays. (B) Tomography of the posterior parts of the same SIJ. There is sclerosis of the ilium (X), with subchondral cysts and slight sclerosis of the sacrum, but normal joint width. The numbers 8.5 to 10 denote the distance from the table top.

bridges are seen. This case shows that intraluminal bony bridges do not exclusively occur in ankylosing spondylitis, as this patient had no clinical signs of ankylosing spondylitis.

Trauma

In pelvic trauma, it is often difficult to delineate fractures of the SIJ. CT is the first choice in those cases, but when external and internal fixation are necessary to stabilize the fractures, only tomography is useful. In Fig. 20.13 the SIJs show multiple fractures, as do the pubic bones. There are, of course, ghost images of the metal plates, but they do not prevent diagnosis.

Ankylosing spondylitis

Erosions, intraluminal bony bridges, and often ankylosis of the SIJ can be seen in ankylosing spondylitis. Most often (Dihlman 1982), sclerosis, erosions, and irregular joints are seen (Fig. 20.14).

In a young patient with low back pain, ankylosing spondylitis must be considered as a possible diagnosis. However, the majority of these patients do not show the full clinical picture, and a plain X-ray is much too often used as proof of the disease. We have therefore investigated the X-rays and clinical data of 56 consecutive patients referred to our clinic with suspected ankylosing spondylitis (Dijkstra et al 1989). Based on plain X-rays, 8.3% were normal and 26.3% showed sacroiliitis, the others were nondiagnostic but were said to have 'probable arthritis.' Based on frontal tomography, more sacroiliitis was found, but it did not alter many of the diagnoses. Oblique tomography, tailored to the curvature of the joints, gave surprising results. Now 43% of the joints appeared to be normal (see Fig. 20.11) and 36% showed sacroiliitis. The others showed features of congenital alteration and slight osteoarthritis. The importance of these observations is that they could be confirmed by clinical diagnosis. Making the correct diagnosis is especially important in cases of ankylosing spondylitis, because the wrong diagnosis can be devastating: no life insurance, no mortgage, and often no job. Much time in our clinic is now spent in altering the diagnosis given to these patients elsewhere, based on the criteria presented above.

Miscellaneous

Chondrocalcinosis is a disease of the elderly. Calcified cartilage can sometimes be seen in the

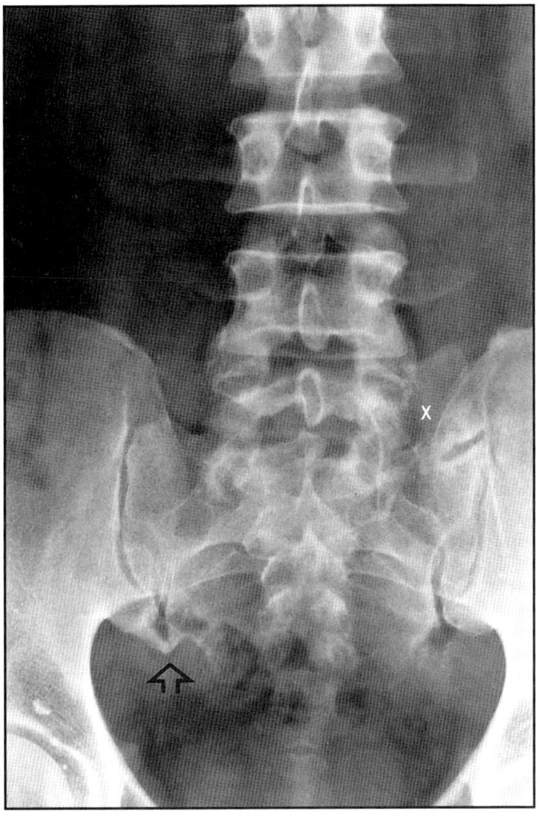

Fig. 20.10 Osteoarthritis of the right sacroiliac joint (SIJ) and left L5–S1 transitional vertebra (X). The figure shows a bony bridge in the ventral S1 ligament (arrow) and a transitional vertebra L5–S1 on the left, with sclerosis of the joint.

SIJ (Fig. 20.15). Whether this is clinically important is not known, as no systematic investigation has been carried out on this joint.

Hyperparathyroidism is seen in patients with severe kidney disease. In a clinical setting, this disease is not unexpected, but it can also be found without warning in the SIJ. It is the task of the radiologist to produce a reasonable differential diagnosis for these cases. Figure 20.16 shows a patient with kidney disease with severe destruction of the SIJ and osteolysis of the pubic symphysis.

Summary

1. It is essential to understand the normal plain X-ray.
2. Emphasis is placed on the use of (oblique) tomography tailored to the curvature of the SIJ. Otherwise, CT scanning has to be used. With spiral CT the situation might change, provided this technique becomes more sophisticated.
3. MRI is the technique for the future but is still difficult to handle for the SIJ. It is superior in bacterial arthritis and tumorous conditions.

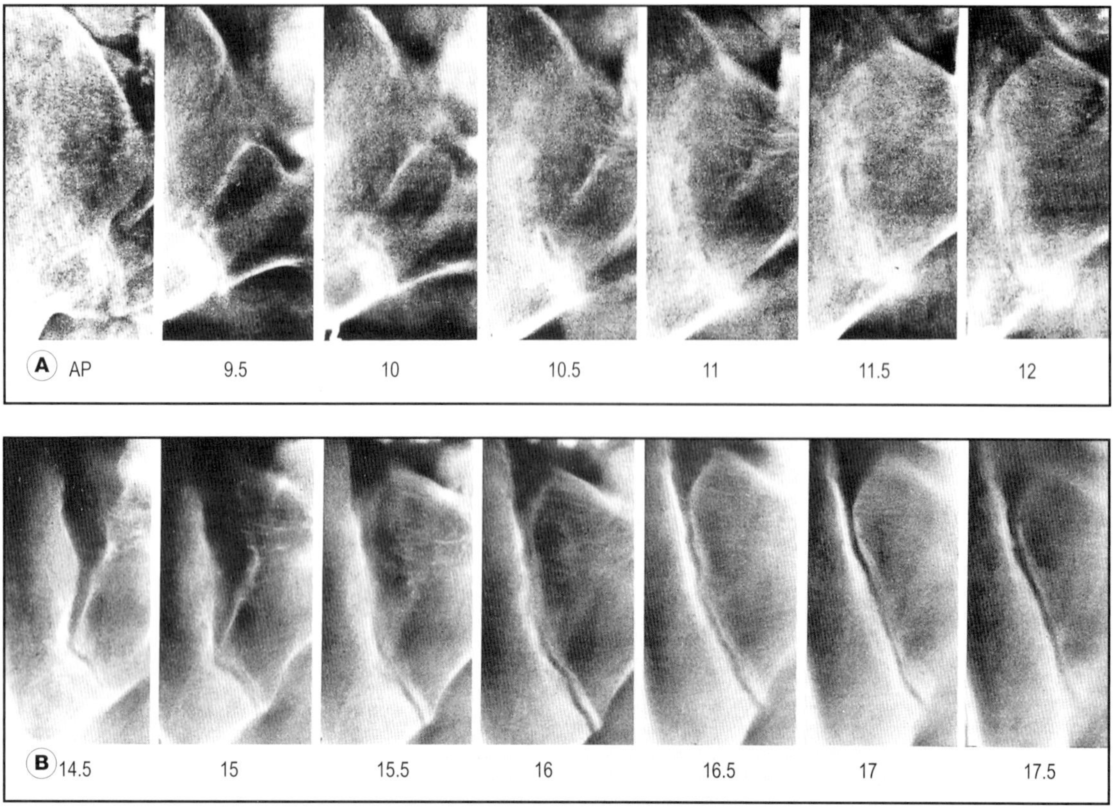

Fig. 20.11 Osteoarthritis of the sacroiliac joint (SIJ). (A) Ankylosing spondylitis is often wrongly diagnosed in cases of osteoarthritis. In this patient, the plain X-ray (AP) shows barely discernable SIJ. Frontal tomography (slices 9.5 to 12) shows sclerosis of the joint margins and irregular joints, as in this patient the tomography is no longer tangential to the direction of the joint. (B) In this oblique tomography (slices 14.5 to 17.5), the middle and ventral parts of the joints appear small, but without erosions, and with slight sclerotic borders as found in osteoarthritis. (Reproduced with permission from Dijkstra et al 1989.)

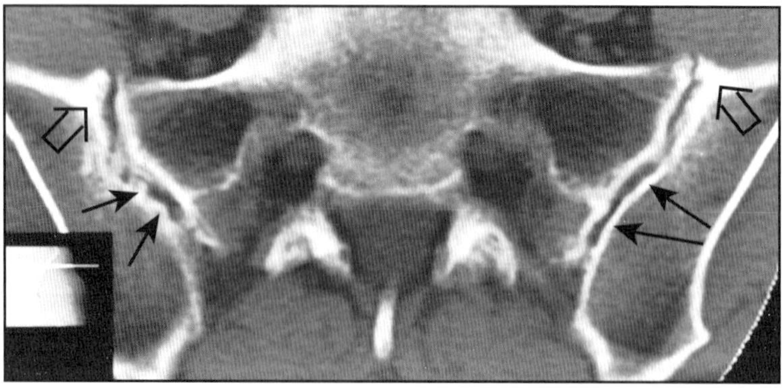

Fig. 20.12 Osteoarthritis with CT. In this patient (CT at the level of S2), severe sclerosis of the ventral sacroiliac joint (SIJ) ligaments and the joint margins was found. Even bony ankylosis (arrows) can be found.

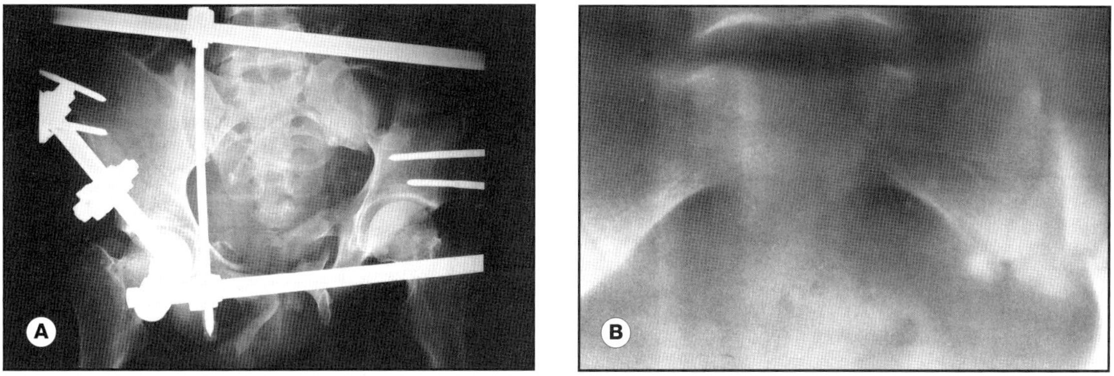

Fig. 20.13 (A) Severe pelvic trauma, stabilized with iron rods, can be difficult to X-ray. The precise extent of the fractures in the sacroiliac joint (SIJ) and pubic bones are difficult to establish in this severely traumatized patient. (B) In this patient, tomography shows severe luxation fractures of the left SIJ. Only mild ghost images of the iron rods are seen. Only the left SIJ is shown.

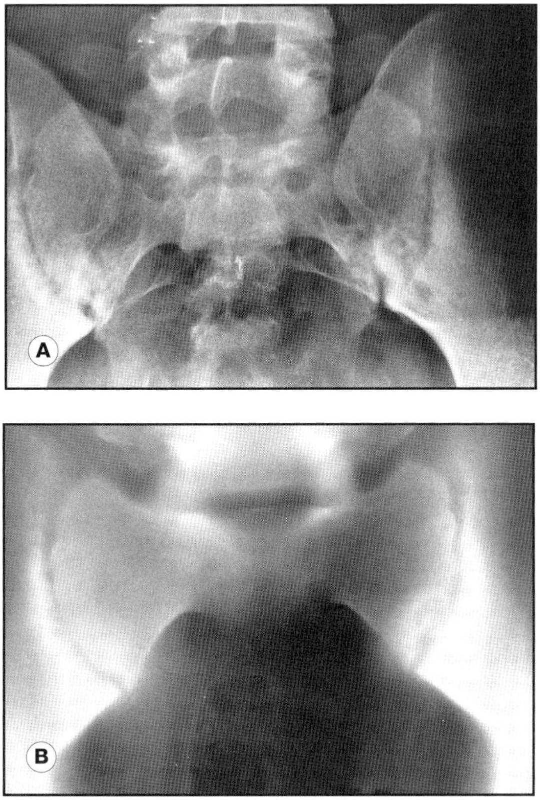

Fig. 20.14 Ankylosing spondylitis in a patient with Crohn's disease. (A) On X-ray, there are irregular joints with sclerotic borders and probably signs of ankylosis on the left side. (B) Tomography of the ventral part of the same sacroiliac joint (SIJ). Erosions and sclerosis are clearly seen, but no ankylosis. The 'ankylosis' seen was, in fact, a superimposition of parts of the joint.

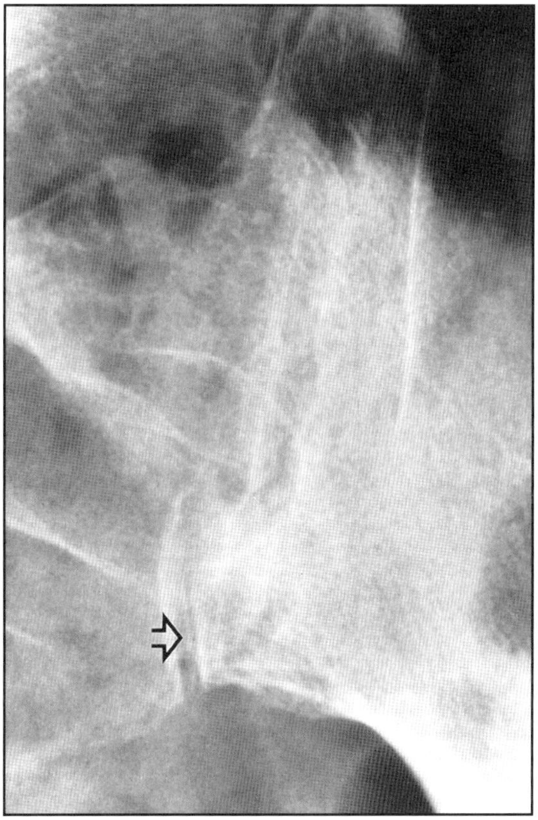

Fig. 20.15 Chondrocalcinosis can be found in any joint but is often not recognized in the sacroiliac joint (SIJ). The faint sclerotic line (arrow) in the left SIJ is calcification in the superficial layer of the iliac cartilage.

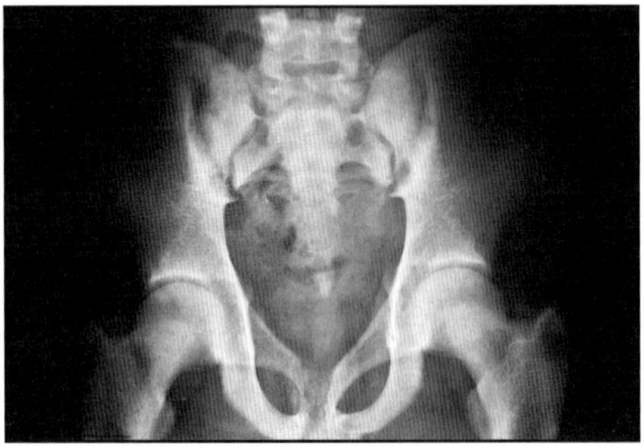

Fig. 20.16 Erosions and joint destruction in the sacroiliac joint (SIJ) and pubic symphysis due to secondary hyperparathyroidism in a patient with kidney disease.

References

Dihlman W 1982 Gelenke-Wirbelverbindungen. Klinische Radiologie. Thieme, Stuttgart

Dijkstra PF 1993 Radiology of the normal S. I. joint. Journal of Manual and Manipulative Therapy 1:87–94

Dijkstra PF, Vleeming A, Stoeckart R 1989 Complex motion tomography of the sacroiliac joint. An anatomical and roentgenologic study. Fortschritte auf dem Gebiete der Röntgenstralen 150:635–642

Firooznia HC, Golimbu C, Rofii M et al 1984 Computer tomography of the sacroiliac joints: comparison with complex motion tomography. Journal of Computed Tomography 8:31–34

Solonen KA 1957 The sacroiliac joint in the light of anatomical, roentgenological and clinical studies. Acta Orthopaedica Scandinavica 27 (suppl):4–127

Vleeming A, van Wingerden JP, Dijkstra PF et al 1992 Mobility in the S.I. joints in the elderly: a kinematic and radiologic study. Clinical Biomechanics 7:170–176

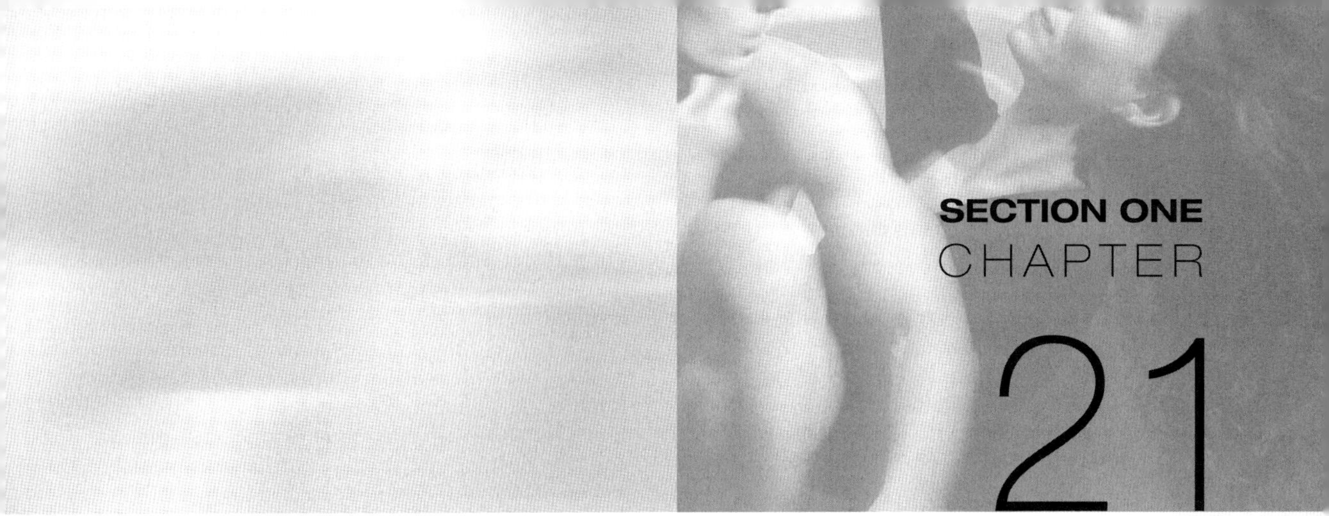

SECTION ONE CHAPTER 21

CT and MRI of the sacroiliac joints

John MD O'Neill and Erik Jurriaans

Introduction

The most common indication for imaging the sacroiliac joints (SIJs) is for the investigation of inflammatory low back pain in patients thought to have sacroiliitis (SII). The presence of inflammation within the SIJs, unilateral or bilateral, is an important criterion in the diagnosis of seronegative spondyloarthropathies (SNS) – a group of chronic autoimmune inflammatory joint diseases predominantly affecting the axial skeleton and often accompanied by peripheral arthritis. Ankylosing spondylitis (AS) is the prototype of the SNS, which also include psoriatic arthritis, reactive arthritis, arthritis associated with inflammatory bowel disease and undifferentiated spondyloarthropathies (Dougados et al 1991).

The onset of inflammatory low back pain in these patients is often insidious, with periods of relapse and remittance that often lead to a delay in clinical diagnosis. Using ankylosing spondylitis as our model for SNS, it has been demonstrated that there is a significant delay in the diagnosis from onset of symptoms. Feldtkeller et al (2000) found a mean delay in diagnosis of 8.9 years from the patient's initial onset of symptoms. This delay in diagnosis has a significant negative impact on the clinical and economic status of the patient (Carette et al 1983, Ward 2002). It is essential, therefore, for patient well-being – and particularly since the advent of treatment options with anti-tumor necrosis factor (anti-TNF) agents – that SII is diagnosed early in the course of the disease.

Imaging of the SIJ has a primary role in the diagnosis of SII and is an integral component of the modified New York criteria (van der Linden 1984). By contrast, the European Spondylarthropathy Study Group (Dougados et al 1991) relies predominantly on clinical assessment of inflammatory back pain; radiographic analysis is not essential for the diagnosis. In routine clinical practice, radiographic imaging has become an integral part of the investigation of patients with suspected SII.

Although plain X-rays remain the first and most widespread imaging modality employed in the investigation of SII, studies have shown that CT (Battafarano et al 1993, Fam et al 1985, Lawson et al 1982, Yu et al 1998) and MRI (Battafarano et al 1993, Docherty et al 1992, Murphey et al 1991, Puhakka et al 2004, Yu et al 1998) demonstrate improved sensitivity and specificity for the diagnosis of SII. Unfortunately, the determination of the exact sensitivities and specificities of these imaging modalities is severely hindered by the absence of a 'gold standard' investigation. Other imaging techniques used to diagnose SII include scintigraphy and ultrasound. Conventional tomography was employed prior to the use of cross-sectional imaging.

This chapter reviews the normal anatomy of the SIJs, including variance and pitfalls, CT and MRI technique, and indications for imaging the SIJs. In addition, we will review comparative studies of these different imaging modalities in the diagnosis of SII.

Normal anatomy sacroiliac joints

While it has long been recognized that the SIJs are a complex articulation, the description of the anatomy of the SIJs has undergone considerable revision recently. Traditionally, the SIJs were considered to consist of a smaller posterosuperior ligamentous compartment and a larger anteroinferior synovial compartment. More recent research by Puhakka et al (2004) has stimulated a debate on whether the articulation is best classified as a symphysis rather than a synovial joint. A complete description of the anatomy of the SIJ is beyond the scope of this chapter and is covered elsewhere in this book (see Chapter 14). A brief summary relevant to CT and MRI follows.

The articular margins of the sacrum and iliac bones are irregular with interdigitations, which limit mobility and enhance the strength of these joints (Resnick 2002). The articular surface of the sacrum is C- or L-shaped, opening dorsally. There are irregular bony pits dorsal to the articular surface at the site of ligamentous attachment, the dorsal syndesmosis. In the past, the articular surface of the sacrum was considered to be covered by a thick layer of hyaline cartilage and the ilium by a thinner layer of fibrocartilage. Recent evidence suggests that the periphery of the cartilage, with the exception of the distal third of the iliac cartilage, blends with the stabilizing ligaments as in a symphysis and forms a wide margin of fibrocartilage (Puhakka et al 2004). Cartilage at the center of all joints was hyaline with fibrocartilage only at the periphery. Kampen & Tillmann (1998) demonstrated that the iliac joint surface in childhood is fibrocartilaginous and later develops into hyaline cartilage. Previously, a synovial membrane was described lining a fibrous capsule that attached to the margins of the adjacent surfaces of the sacrum and ilium (Resnick 2002). In their correlation of MRI and histological findings, Puhakka et al (2004) found only a small synovial recess at the ventral aspect of the distal third of the ilium. A larger synovial lining was not identified. In light of the above histological analysis, Puhakka et al (2004) conclude that the SIJs are best described as a symphysis with characteristics of a synovial joint being restricted to the ventral aspect of the distal cartilaginous portion at the iliac side only.

Because of the oblique orientation of the SIJs on the frontal radiograph, there is considerable overlap of the joints on plain radiography. Cross-sectional imaging using either CT or MRI is necessary to image in detail the complex anatomy. The normal SIJ can demonstrate considerable variability, particularly with increasing age (Vogler et al 1984). Six anatomical variants have been observed in a review of 534 patients undergoing pelvic CT for indications other than disease of the SIJs (Prassopoulos et al 1999). These include accessory joints (19%), 'iliosacral complex' (6%), bipartite iliac bony plate (4%), crescent-like iliac bony plate (4%), semicircular defects at the sacral or iliac side (3%), and ossification centers (1%). Under the age of 30 years, the SIJs are usually symmetric in appearance. Asymmetry is identified in 77% of subjects over the age of 30 years and in 87% of subjects over the age of 40 years. The width of the normal SIJ varies from 2 to 5 mm (Lawson et al 1982, Vogler et al 1984). Certain findings commonly thought to indicate SII can be seen in normal subjects. These include nonuniform iliac sclerosis, focal joint space narrowing in patients over the age of 30 years, and ill-defined areas of subchondral sclerosis, particularly on the iliac side. These findings were seen in 83%, 74%, and 67% of normal subjects, respectively (Vogler et al 1984). Therefore, these CT findings are not reliable indicators of SII. The same article does identify findings that are uncommon in normal subjects and thought to be good indicators of SII. These include increased subchondral sclerosis in subjects under the age of 40 years, bilateral or unilateral joint space of less than 2 mm, erosions, and intra-articular ankylosis (Fig. 21.1). These findings were found in only 11%, 2%, 0%, 2%, and 0% of normal subjects, respectively. Therefore, these findings are regarded as good discriminators for the diagnosis of SII. A more recent study by Faflia et al (1998) suggests that a higher prevalence of asymmetric non-uniform joint space narrowing, ill-defined subchondral sclerosis and ankylosis was observed in women, obese and multiparous females than in age-matched males, and individuals of normal weight and nonmultiparous respectively.

The normal appearance of the SIJs as seen on MRI has been described by several authors (Ahlstrom et al 1990, Bollow et al 1995, 1997, Docherty et al 1992, Murphey et al 1991, Puhakka et al 2004, Wittram & Whitehouse 1995). The normal cartilage is well visualized as a zone of intermediate signal intensity on both T1 and T2 weighting bounded on either side by low signal intensity cortex of the adjacent sacrum and ilium. The adjacent cortical bone is well defined. The combined cartilage has a maximum thickness of 4 to 5 mm and is slightly thinner anteriorly and inferiorly (Murphey et al 1991). It is not possible to differentiate hyaline and fibrous cartilage or sacral and iliac cartilage by signal intensity although occasionally a signal void may be seen separating iliac and sacral cartilage, likely due to a vacuum phenomenon (Puhakka et al 2004). On T1FS (T1 fat-saturated), the cartilage is of intermediate to high signal intensity. Following the suppression of the high fat signal, the altered gray scale of the T1FS sequence improves visualization of the cartilage and adjacent cortical bone and is therefore superior to T1 sequences in assessing what has been previously considered to represent the synovial compartment (Wittram & Whitehouse 1995). In a study of patients with clinical evidence of SI, as well as a group of normal controls, Docherty et al (1992) found that proton-density (PD)-weighted images offered the best visualization of the cartilage. T1FS images were not assessed in this study. In keeping with the findings of Wittram & Whitehouse (1995), we have found the T1FS sequences best in imaging the articular cartilage. Standard T1 sequences are, however, invaluable in assessing the subchondral bone marrow and, in particular, in differentiating between subchondral sclerosis and fat which both appear as low signal on T1FS.

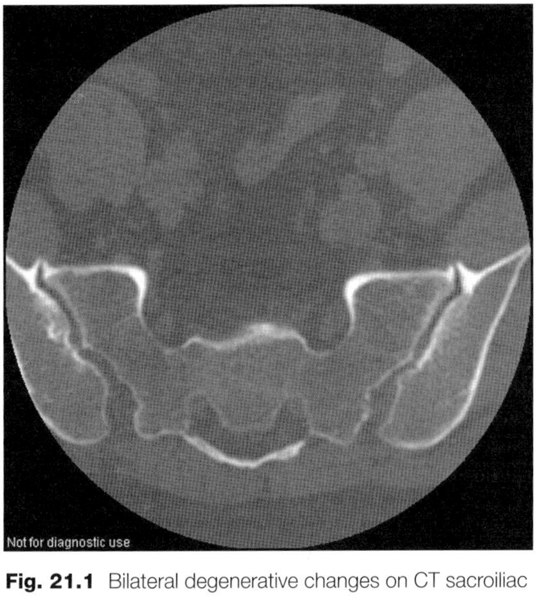

Fig. 21.1 Bilateral degenerative changes on CT sacroiliac joints (SIJs) in a 40-year-male patient. Axial CT reveals bilateral anterior osteophytosis, subchondral sclerosis and vacuum phenomenom. No erosions are identified.

Cortical erosions and subchondral sclerosis were not identified in a study of normal patients (Wittram & Whitehouse 1995) and in another study (Puhakka et al 2004), subchondral sclerosis does not exceed 1.5 mm in width in normal volunteers. A partial volume artifact between the anteroinferior synovial compartment of the SIJs and the posterosuperior ligamentous compartment should not be mistaken for an erosion (Wittram & Whitehouse 1995). In addition, prominent sacral irregularities and marrow defects at the attachment of the interosseous ligaments, termed insertion pits, can be seen in normal subjects (Murphey et al 1991). The characteristic site of the above described findings, the intact signal void of the adjacent cortical bone and the presence of fat within the ligamentous compartment, readily identified on a combination of T1 and T1FS sequences, resolves any potential dilemma. Anatomical variants such as an accessory articular facet of the SIJs are easily identified by MRI (Wittram & Whitehouse 1995). Most of the previous MRI descriptions of the normal SIJs utilized the oblique coronal plane. More recent evidence suggests that the above variants and potential pitfalls can be more readily appreciated by MRI in the oblique axial plane (Puhakka et al 2003).

In general, the adjacent bone marrow has a homogeneous intermediate signal intensity on T1. In adults, the subchondral bone may have heterogeneous signal due to nonuniform fatty replacement of hematopoietic bone marrow

(Levine et al 1994, Puhakka et al 2003). A patchy distribution of fat within the subchondral bone marrow was found in some normal patients and is of no significance in the absence of cortical erosions or subchondral sclerosis (Wittram & Whitehouse 1995). On fast short tau inversion recovery (Fast STIR) images, a well-defined para-articular band of subchondral high signal may be identified in normal patients (Wittram & Whitehouse 1995) and this should not be mistaken for subchondral edema, which is less well defined and more diffuse.

CT technique

There has been a significant change in CT technology since the first edition of this book. Multi-detector CT (MDCT) is now widely available and has rapidly become the norm. With this change, volume acquisition has replaced conventional techniques particularly those involving non-contiguous cuts that we described previously (Friedman et al 1993). Furthermore, MDCT using fine cuts produces an isotropic data set. This means that the image voxels acquired by high-resolution MDCT are equal in size in all dimensions (isotropic) and can be reformatted in orthogonal and oblique planes with no loss of image quality (Fig. 21.2). Both conventional CT and MDCT can be undertaken in the axial, coronal, or oblique coronal planes and then reformatted in other planes. With MDCT and the use of finer axial cuts comes the risk of an increase in radiation burden to the patient. Image acquisition in the semicoronal plane has been shown to reduce total effective dose in both female and male patients when compared to direct axial cuts (Jurik et al 2002). The coronal or semicoronal plane reduces direct exposure to the ovaries in female patients and also reduces the number of slices acquired when compared to the direct axial plane. Using a phantom to assess radiation dose, Jurik et al (2002) demonstrated a reduction of total effective dose by semicoronal CT by a factor of 2.5 when compared to conventional anteroposterior (AP) radiographs in female patients. Therefore, scanning in the semicoronal or coronal planes is preferred, particularly in young patients (Jurik et al 2002, Oudjhane et al 1993). A bolster or pillow can be placed under the patient's lumbar spine to increase the lumbar lordosis. This, combined with maximum gantry angulation, allows for direct coronal or steep oblique coronal imaging in most patients. In the older patients with limited mobility and loss of lumbar lordosis, direct axial image acquisition may be required. While modern MDCT scanners can acquire slices as thin as 0.625 mm, this is generally not necessary and we usually acquire the data set using 2.5 mm slice thickness reconstructed to 1.25 mm, which allows for high-resolution imaging.

MRI technique

A variety of MRI techniques have been described in imaging the SIJs. In general, the SIJs are scanned in the oblique coronal or semicoronal plane (coronal to the SIJs). The importance of the oblique axial plane in the MRI assessment of the SIJs has recently been emphasized (Puhakka et al 2003). Additional true axial images may also be acquired.

In general, our protocol includes 4-mm thick cuts with a 0.5-mm interspace on the oblique coronal images and a 1-mm interspace on axial images. A spinal quadrature surface coil is used. T1-weighted images without and with fat saturation, as well as short tau inversion recovery (STIR) sequences, are routine. The rationale for the sequence selection is discussed later in this chapter. As the vast majority of our studies are undertaken for the investigation of possible sacroiliitis or to assess response to treatment, T1 fat-saturated images are always obtained before and after the administration of intravenous gadolinium diethylenetriamine pentaacetic acid (Gd-DTPA).

We also obtain the post-gadolinium fat-saturated T1-weighted images in the oblique axial plane as well as fast spin echo fat-saturated proton density weighted (PDW) oblique axial images. Fast spin echo fat-saturated T2-weighted and fast multiplanar inversion recovery (FMPIR) sequences have also been used in assessing the SIJs. We have not found these additional sequences helpful and this has been confirmed by a recent study demonstrating no additional benefit from T2-weighted images (Puhakka et al 2003). We are currently performing a retrospective study comparing STIR sequence with post-gadolinium fat-saturated T1-weighted. Preliminary data suggest that gadolinium enhancement is not required in all cases.

Following the administration of intravenous gadolinium, the enhancement pattern can be quantified using delayed T1 fat-saturated images or a dynamic spoiled gradient echo (SPGR) sequence. A region of interest (ROI) can be drawn over a region of the cartilaginous compartment or subchondral bone and its signal intensity measured before, during and after the intravenous bolus of gadolinium. The

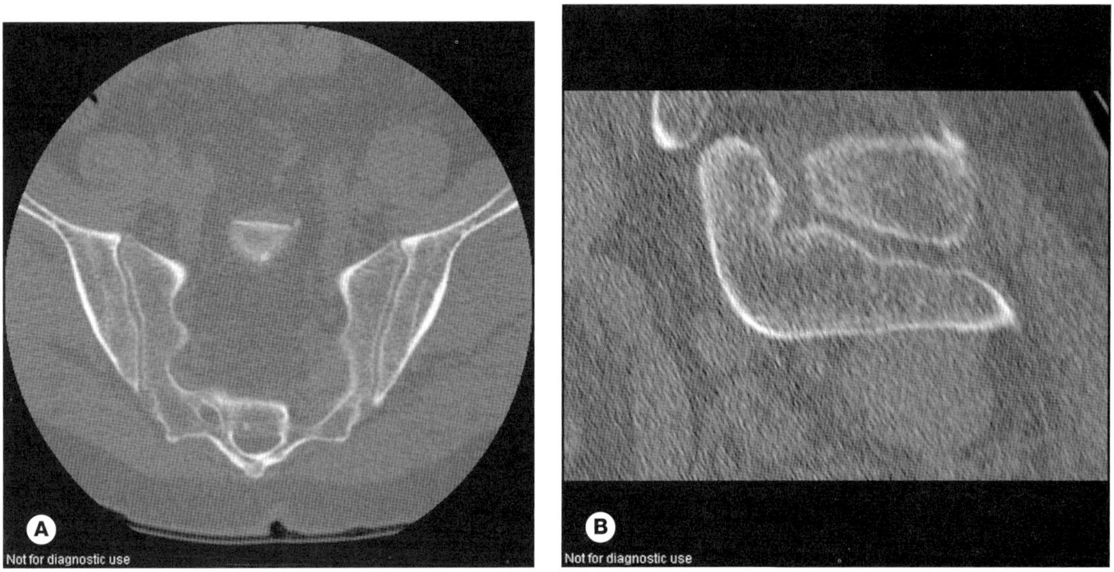

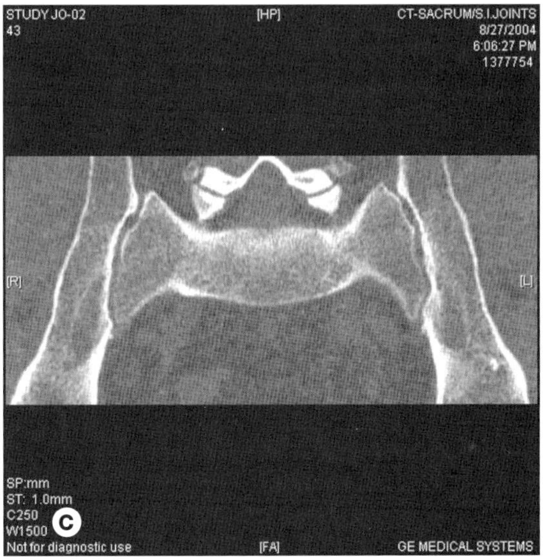

Fig. 21.2 Normal CT sacroiliac joints in a 25-year-old female; semicoronal acquisition with (A) axial (B) sagittal, and (C) coronal reconstruction demonstrate superb anatomical resolution. Note normal joint space, well-defined cortical outline without significant subchondral sclerosis.

increase in signal intensity can then be calculated and expressed as an enhancement factor (F_{enh}) (Bollow et al 1995, Braun et al 1994, Wittram & Whitehouse 1995):

$$F_{enh}\% = \frac{(SI_{max} - SI_o) \times 100}{SI_o}$$

where SI_o = signal intensity pre-gadolinium and SI_{max} = maximum signal intensity post-gadolinium.

Using a dynamic sequence, an enhancement gradient (G_{enh}) can be calculated (Bollow et al 1995, Braun et al 1994):

$$G_{enh}\%/\text{minute} = \frac{(SI_{max} - SI_o) \times 100}{SI_o \times T_{max}}$$

where T_{max} = the time interval from injection of gadolinium to SI_{max}.

Contrast enhancement of the normal SIJ is controversial. While enhancement of the supposed synovial compartment in normal subjects has been described (Braun et al 1994, Wittram & Whitehouse 1995), a larger series demonstrated no enhancement (Bollow et al 1995, Puhakka et al 2003) of the cartilaginous joint compartment and suggests that enhancement might be overcalled on oblique coronal images due to partial volume artifact with the adjacent vascular ligamentous compartment of the joint. The joint space of the syndesmosis has an abundance of enhancing vessels that can be readily identified on the oblique axial images. Therefore, it is recommended that enhancement seen on the oblique coronal images should only be called if it is confirmed on oblique axial images (Puhakka et al 2003).

In a study comparing plain radiography, CT, and MRI, Puhakka et al (2003) also assessed commonly used MRI sequences and recommend the following imaging protocol: semicoronal T1 and semicoronal and semiaxial STIR sequences are undertaken routinely. If these are normal, no further imaging is recommended. If these sequences are abnormal, semicoronal T1 fat-saturated sequences before and after intravenous gadolinium are recommended. To this, they subsequently added an oblique axial T1 fat-saturated following gadolinium in order to avoid the pitfalls described above (Puhakka et al 2003). Other authors advocate the use of intravenous gadolinium-enhanced MRI in the assessment of SII routinely. This topic is discussed later in this chapter.

The referring clinician needs to be aware of certain contraindications to MRI. These include cardiac pacemakers, cochlear implants, and ferromagnetic intracranial or intraorbital surgical clips or foreign bodies. Certain types of hardware elsewhere also are contraindicated. It is best to discuss possible contraindications with your MRI center. With the advent of short-bore MR scanners, claustrophobia is less of a problem but appropriate sedation is still required in some patients.

Imaging sacroiliac joints

A number of different imaging techniques are used in the diagnosis of SII. These include plain radiographs, conventional tomography, scintigraphy, ultrasound, CT, and MRI. Imaging allows for objective evidence of SII.

There are a number of possible indications for imaging of SIJs outside clinical trials; these are outlined in Box 21.1. Each potential indication should be reviewed in conjunction with the patient's presenting clinical history, current and previous investigations. Imaging should in routine clinical practice be performed only if it is going to affect the patient's diagnosis and/or management. Since the advent of anti-TNF agents in the treatment of AS, indications 3, 4, and 5 (Box 21.1) may have a role to play in the patient's clinical management. Further clinical trials are warranted for investigation of cross-sectional imaging with respect to these latter indications.

Box 21.1

Indications for imaging the sacroiliac joints

1. Investigation of inflammatory low back pain
2. Integral component in the diagnosis of ankylosing spondylitis
3. Assess extent of acute inflammatory changes in patients with sacroiliitis
4. Assess chronic changes in patients with sacroiliitis and degenerative osteoarthritis
5. Assess response to treatment if there is clinical uncertainty
6. Investigation of other primary pathologies including septic arthritis, trauma, insufficiency fractures, benign and malignant tumors
7. Image-guided therapy (joint injections)

Indications and the type of imaging employed in clinical trials are usually different from clinical practice. van der Heijde et al (2005a) described a set of recommendations on the conduction of clinical trials in AS. They identified six topics on which to focus including scope of the disease, definition of claims, assessment of signs and symptoms, assessment of function, structural damage and trial design. They recommend trial eligibility criteria to those who have evidence of SII on plain radiographs using the modified New York criteria. The Amor criteria and the criteria of the European Spondylarthropathy Study Group are also accepted with the amendment that radiographic SII should be present. The use of CT and MRI as part of the trial design was contentious, as there are no internationally accepted criteria for the grading of SII with these imaging techniques. CT and MRI, however, will identify patients with SII prior to plain radiographic evidence and, in addition, could improve the understanding of SII and is therefore recommended. We would refer the reader to the article by van der Heijde et al (2005a) for more detailed discussion of this topic.

This chapter deals predominantly with the role of CT and MRI imaging but it is appropriate that we review briefly the role of other imaging modalities.

Plain radiography

Plain radiography has played an important role in the investigation of SII and is an integral part in the diagnosis of AS (van der Linden et al 1984). The anatomy of the SIJ, due to its oblique nature and overlap of the sacral and iliac components (Forrester 1990), has led to significant inter- and intraobserver variations particularly in the interpretation of early SII (Hollingsworth et al 1983, Taylor et al 1991, Yazici et al 1987). Differentiation of these early changes from normal subjects has also proved difficult (Cohen et al 1968). This differentiation from normal patients is particularly problematic in women and in older age groups in whom early degenerative changes may simulate early SII. Plain radiographs of the SIJ can be performed as a dedicated AP study of the pelvis, which has been shown to be as sensitive as detailed oblique projections (Battistone et al 1998). Other studies have demonstrated that prone position does not provide significant change in the diagnosis when compared with the AP study (Robbins & Morse 1996). In addition, the AP study will have the advantage of including the hip joints, which may be a source of symptoms. Given the above limitations, plain radiography still has a primary role in the investigation of SII and should be performed as the initial imaging modality.

Conventional tomography

Although more sensitive than plain radiographs (De Smet et al 1982) it is associated with high radiation exposure in comparison with plain radiographs and has been replaced by cross-sectional imaging including CT and MRI.

Ultrasound

Ultrasound may have a potential role in imaging in several different areas. The first is its potential to assess the laxity of the SIJ that may have a role to play in patients with low back pain (Buyruk et al 1995). This may be a promising technique in the future but at present it requires more research (de Groot et al 2004). Color and duplex Doppler ultrasound has been used in the evaluation of active SII (Arslan et al 1999). This study assessed patients with active SII, osteoarthritis, and normal volunteers, and evaluated the posterior portion of the SIJs with color Doppler sonography. Vascularization around the posterior portion of SIJs and resistive index of detected arteries were evaluated and demonstrated increased vascularization with decreased resistive indices in this portion of SIJ in patients with active SII. A recent study (Klauser et al 2005) evaluated the use of ultrasound contrast agents for color Doppler ultrasound against MRI and found it to have a high negative predictive value for the detection of active SII. Again further research is warranted to assess what role ultrasound will play in the investigation of SII.

Nuclear medicine

Scintigraphy is a commonly used modality in the investigation of SII in clinical practice. It is very sensitive in the detection of early articular inflammatory change but is nonspecific. Radionuclide normally accumulates at the SIJs and the differentiation of normal uptake and early SII can be difficult. Quantitative analysis (Peh et al 1997) of the SIJs has proven more sensitive in this regard. There are limitations, however, due to the wide range of variation in quantitative evaluation in the normal population. Other factors including age and prominent first sacral spine may all cause difficulties. Scintigraphy has the advantage of demonstrating areas of increased bone turnover in sites other than the SIJs. Innac (2005) demonstrated poor sensitivity of quantitative scintigraphy when compared with MRI in symptomatic spondyloarthropathy patients with early disease on plain radiography.

CT

CT is excellent in demonstrating the anatomy of the SIJs and with modern equipment allows high-resolution axial acquisition with coronal and sagittal reconstruction. Modern comparative studies between plain radiographs and CT (Puhakka et al 2003, Yu et al 1998) have demonstrated marked advantage of CT in the delineation of chronic changes including erosions, subchondral sclerosis, ankylosis, and fat-replacement bone marrow (Figs 21.3, 21.4). CT has the advantage that it can demonstrate new bone formation at entheses (Puhakka et al 2003) that are not visualized on MRI. CT does not offer evaluation of acute inflammatory changes that can be delineated on MRI (these will be outlined later in this chapter) and CT involves the use of ionizing radiation. This can be limited by the use of semicoronal CT acquisition (Jurick et al 2002), as outlined in the section on CT technique earlier in the chapter.

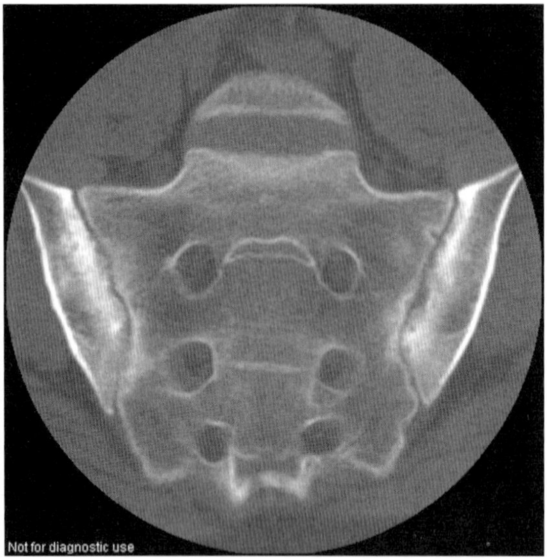

Fig. 21.3 Bilateral sacroiliitis (SII) in a 34-year-old male patient being investigated for a 2-year history of inflammatory low back pain who has a clinical suspicion of SII. Axial CT demonstrates bilateral SII, which is relatively symmetrical with early loss of joint space, subchondral sclerosis, marked erosions and poor definition of the cortical outline.

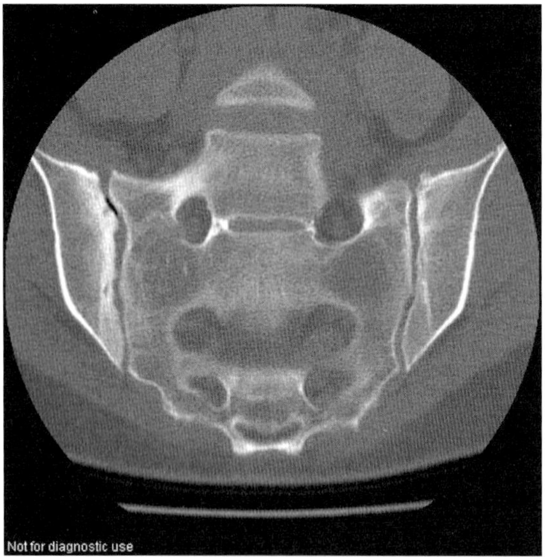

Fig. 21.4 Psoriatic spondyloarthropathy in a 42-year-old female patient who presented with inflammatory low back pain and a history of psoriasis. Semicoronal CT demonstrates unilateral sacroiliitis (SII) with right-sided SII as delineated by early loss of joint space, subchondral sclerosis predominantly of the iliac side joint with loss of cortical definition and subtle erosions. The left sacroiliac joint has minimal early degenerative changes with a subtle vacuum phenomenon and no features of SII.

CT and MRI in alternate SIJ pathology

CT is useful in diagnosing SIJ infection and may identify unilateral changes suggesting the diagnosis. Review of the examination on soft-tissue windows is essential lest soft-tissue abnormalities be missed. Changes involving the SIJ include widening of the joint cleft with erosions, thinning of the periarticular fatty-tissue layer, increase in size of adjacent muscles and abscess formation (Bankoff et al 1984, Sandrasegaran et al 1994).

CT may appear normal in the early course of the disease. Therefore, in the relevant clinical setting, more sensitive imaging modalities in the acute phase including radionuclide bone scan or MRI should be employed (Abbott & Carty 1993, Haliloglu et al 1994, Stürzenbecher et al 2000). Stürzenbecher et al (2000), in a study of eleven patients with unilateral septic SII, identified anterior and/or posterior subperiosteal and transcapsular infiltrations of juxta-articular muscle layers as characteristics of septic SII on MRI and this could be used to differentiate septic arthritis from SII in spondyloarthropathy. Fluoroscopic or CT-guided joint aspiration can also be beneficial in confirming the diagnosis and may be crucial in planning appropriate antimicrobial therapy.

CT and MRI may be invaluable in assessing and staging tumors at or about the SIJ. Bone destruction and soft tissue masses can be readily identified. The differentiation between benign and malignant bone lesions is usually possible.

Schwarzer et al (1995) have found CT useful following SIJ arthrography. In their investigation of a group of patients with chronic low back pain, they found a weak but statistically significant association between ventral capsular tears of the SIJ and relief of pain upon anesthetizing the joint. The extent and site of the capsular tears were well shown on CT, as were diverticulae of the capsule. The significance of these findings and the role of CT sacroiliac (SI) arthrography remain to be determined.

CT has a well-established role in the management of patients with pelvic trauma. It is the preferred imaging modality for assessing bone injury. While a correct pathoanatomic classification of pelvic fractures can be obtained by plain X-ray, CT provides additional information regarding acetabular fractures, involvement of the posterior pelvic ring, intra-articular fracture fragments, and fractures of the femoral head.

Finally, CT and MRI may be invaluable in the

diagnosis of insufficiency fractures. These fractures most commonly occur in elderly females with osteoporosis. The osteopenia makes assessment of plain X-rays difficult. The diagnosis can be confirmed by CT, which demonstrates patchy sclerosis, often with fissure-like fractures and no associated soft tissue mass (Fig. 21.5) (Rogers 1992). The absence of an associated mass makes it possible to differentiate an insufficiency fracture from a metastatic lesion, which is often a clinical dilemma in these patients (Rogers 1992).

Magnetic resonance imaging

In the first description of MRI in SII, Ahlstrom et al (1990) found striking changes in the subchondral bone marrow. They demonstrated the sensitivity of MRI to be similar to that of CT or conventional radiography, and emphasized the unique ability of MRI to demonstrate abnormalities in subchondral bone and periarticular bone marrow. They concluded that the early inflammatory changes in SII are likely to occur in the subchondral structures of the SIJ. This study opened the door for the potential use of MRI in the investigation of SII and thereafter a multitude of studies confirmed their initial finding and supported the development of MRI in the diagnosis and management of patients with SII. A brief overview of some of the important MRI studies will follow.

Wittram et al (1996), in a study of fifteen patients with definite SII, five equivocal patients and five controls, investigated the use of fat-suppressed contrast-enhanced MRI. The study demonstrated abnormal enhancement patterns on T1 fat-saturated sequences that corresponded to regions of abnormal high-signal intensity on fast STIR images in subchondral marrow in all cases. The high signal intensity on STIR is consistent with edema secondary to active inflammation (Battafarano et al 1993). STIR images suppress fat signal and are very sensitive in identifying increasing water content in inflammation and thus bone marrow edema (Fig. 21.6). It should be noted that bone marrow edema does not occur solely in active SII but may also be seen in degenerative changes which is described by Modic et al (1988) in their review of bone marrow adjacent to degenerative disc disease.

Oostveen et al (1999) investigated the diagnostic use of MRI in the early detection of SII in 25 HLA-B27-positive patients with inflammatory low back pain with less than or equal to grade two unilateral SII on conventional radiography, using the modified New York criteria. Baseline radiography and MRI were performed on entry into study and plain radiograph follow-up at three years. This was the first prospective longitudinal study to assess the diagnostic role of MRI in patients without definite radiographic SII in HLA-B27, plus patients with inflammatory low back pain and without

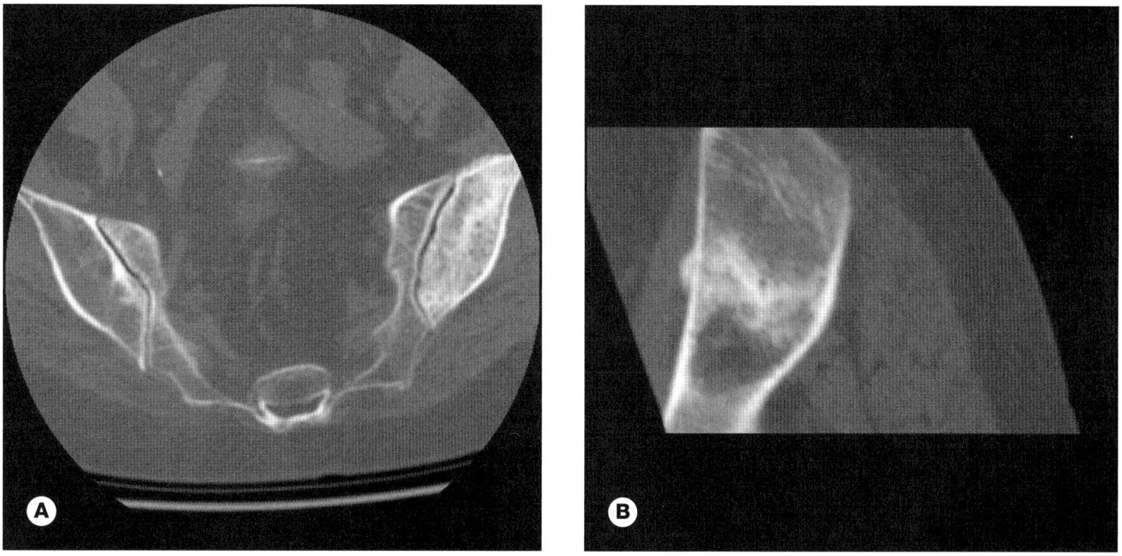

Fig. 21.5 Sacral insufficiency fracture in a 76-year-old female patient who presented with back pain and a history of pancreatic carcinoma. The image is from a CT of the abdomen and pelvis and demonstrates an insufficiency fracture of the left sacrum.

initial definite radiographic evidence of SII. On entering the study, MRI with clinical findings suggested definite diagnosis of AS in 16 patients, with two patients identified on radiography with unilateral grade 3 SII changes. Plain radiography at 3 years allowed a definite diagnosis of AS in 10 of the remaining 22 patients. It should be noted that the MRI used in this study was without gadolinium enhancement. The data do confirm significant findings of SII on MRI earlier than identified with plain radiographs.

Blum et al (1996) studied 44 consecutive patients with plain radiographs, quantitative sacroiliac scintigraphy, and MRI for active SII. MRI was the most sensitive (95%) compared to quantitative scintigraphy (48%) and conventional radiography (19%) for detection and confirmation of active SII. The study also demonstrates, in conjunction with that previously demonstrated by Shichikawa et al (1985), that subchondral osteitis was a consistent early histological change in AS. MRI was found to be highly sensitive in detecting subchondral bone marrow changes in the active stage and also at resolution. In addition, this study demonstrated good interobserver and intraobserver agreement for MRI findings.

Bollow et al (2000) compared the results of immunohistological analysis of CT-guided sacro-

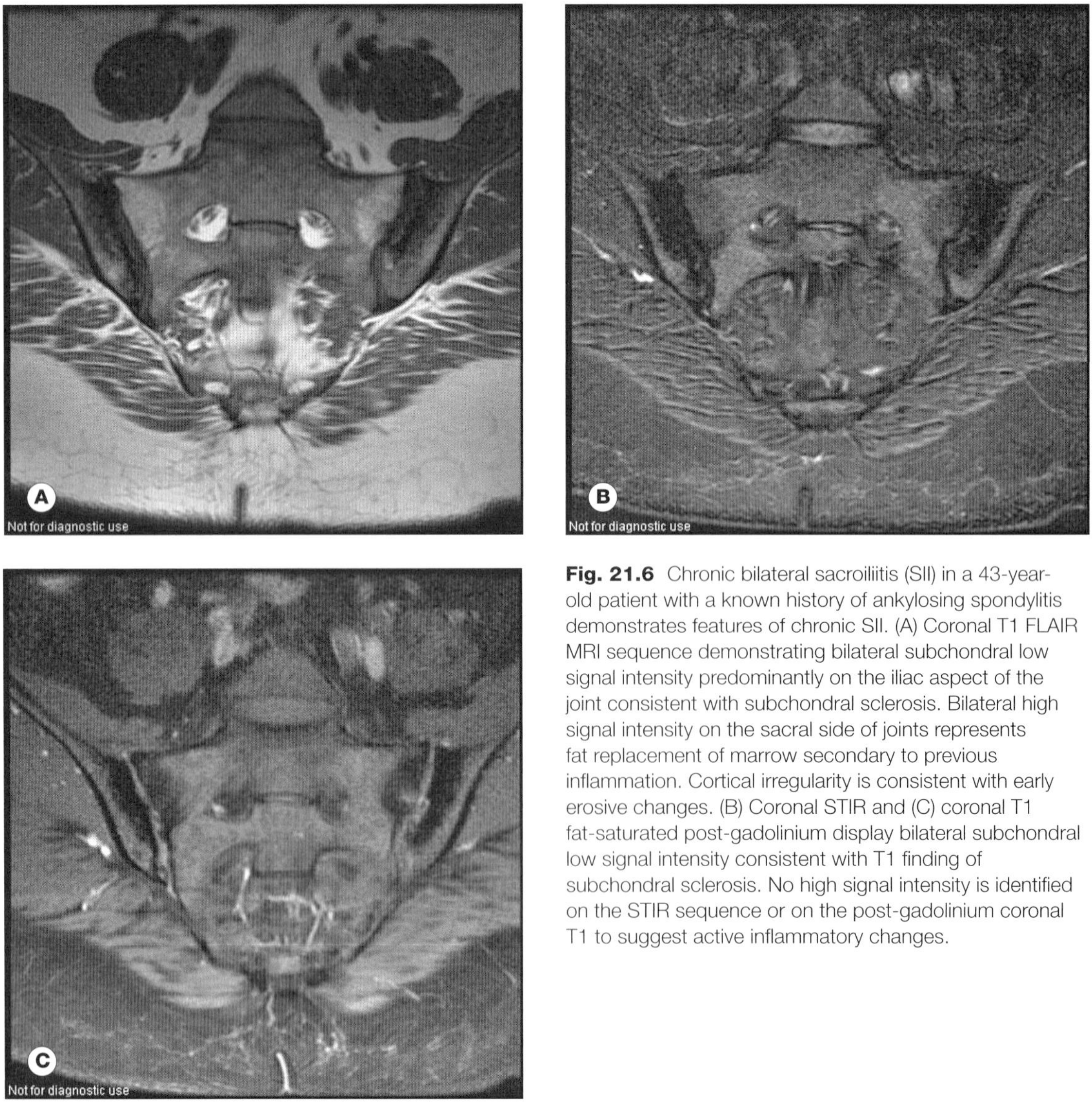

Fig. 21.6 Chronic bilateral sacroiliitis (SII) in a 43-year-old patient with a known history of ankylosing spondylitis demonstrates features of chronic SII. (A) Coronal T1 FLAIR MRI sequence demonstrating bilateral subchondral low signal intensity predominantly on the iliac aspect of the joint consistent with subchondral sclerosis. Bilateral high signal intensity on the sacral side of joints represents fat replacement of marrow secondary to previous inflammation. Cortical irregularity is consistent with early erosive changes. (B) Coronal STIR and (C) coronal T1 fat-saturated post-gadolinium display bilateral subchondral low signal intensity consistent with T1 finding of subchondral sclerosis. No high signal intensity is identified on the STIR sequence or on the post-gadolinium coronal T1 to suggest active inflammatory changes.

iliac biopsies with the degree of enhancement in SIJs on dynamic MRI. The study confirmed that T cells and macrophages are the predominant cells in early spondyloarthropathy and that the degree of cellularity correlates with the enhancement seen with dynamic gadolinium enhanced MRI. The cellularity supports the hypothesis of a foreign or self-antigen immune response in spondyloarthropathy. The exact foreign or self-antigens still need to be elucidated. The MRI imaging sequences in this study also included STIR imaging, which is very sensitive in the detection of edema and inflammation, although small areas of inflammation may be missed. In addition, STIR does not allow quantification of inflammatory activity. Although it is noted in the study that there were shortcomings in the small sample size of the study and the biopsy samples and difficulty in localization of the material obtained, this study is nevertheless significant in its findings as described above.

Muche et al (2003) assessed the anatomical structures in early and late-stage SII in patients with spondyloarthritis using contrast-enhanced MRI. This study evaluated 93 patients with spondyloarthritis and inflammatory back pain with plain radiographs and MRI, including gadolinium contrast-enhanced sequences. The SIJs were divided into nine individual components including the ventral and caudal joint capsule, cavum, subchondral bone, bone marrow, ligament enthesis, and ligaments. The sacral and iliac sides of the joint were separately evaluated. The patients involved in the study group were composed primarily of AS and undifferentiated spondyloarthropathy. The study demonstrated that SII was more often bilateral in AS (84%) than in undifferentiated spondyloarthropathy (48%). Inflammatory changes were found in a mean of 4.7 regions per joint, 4.5 regions in early disease and 5.2 regions in late disease with involvement of the iliac aspect of the joint more frequent than sacral side in early disease (58% versus 48%) compared with that in late disease (58% versus 63%). It is interesting to note that within this study, the dorsocaudal synovial aspect of the joint and bone marrow were both involved in early disease and that entheses and ligaments were more frequently involved in late stage. HLA-B27-positive patients were more prone to entheseal involvement than HLA-B27-negative patients. In this study, the STIR technique was unable to detect joint cavum inflammation as depicted by the gadolinium-enhanced sequences. As in the above studies, this is in agreement with dynamic gadolinium-enhanced MRI as the most sensitive indicator of acute inflammatory changes within the joint and that it is reasonable to accept this as the 'gold standard.' The subchondrium was involved in early disease more often than late disease and in the dorsal component of the joint versus the ventral joint component. There was no clear evidence that the subchondrium was the primary initial site of disease in view of the increased involvement of the dorsocaudal aspects of the synovial joint and adjacent bone marrow. This study suggests that early disease begins in the synovium; however this remains unresolved in the current literature. Underlying pathogenesis and the role of biodynamic mechanisms in spondylitis are outlined in greater detail in other chapters within this book (see Chapter 14).

The MISS initiative (MRI Imaging in Seronegative Spondyloarthropathy) is an international multicenter group currently developing a scoring system for SII and spinal disease and studying the use of MRI as an outcome measure (van der Heijde et al 2002). To further develop MRI applications for clinical trials in AS, the ASAS/OMERACT working group was formed as a follow-up initiative from MISS. This working group is a collaborative initiative of rheumatologists and musculoskeletal radiologists. Its working goal is to develop MRI as a measurement instrument and to have one valid scoring system in the assessment of AS (van der Heijde et al 2005b).

There is no accepted international staging for MRI findings in SII. The staging proposed by Bollow et al (1996) and Braun et al (2000) is commonly used. This grading system is divided into an activity index and a chronicity index. The activity index is subdivided into three grades – X, A, and B – which are differentiated by degree of enhancement on dynamic contrast-enhanced MRI. Grade X is less than 25% enhancement and considered normal enhancement without evidence of active SII; grade A is between 25 and 75% enhancement and indicative of moderate SII, and, finally, grade B is greater than 70% enhancement and indicative of severe SII. The chronicity index has five grades, with grade 0 indicating no chronic changes and grade 1 circumscribed accumulation of fat in the bone marrow and/or circumscribed subchondral sclerosis and/or less than or equal to two erosions. Grade 2 has normal joint space with similar features as in Grade 1 but greater than two erosions (see Fig. 21.6). Grade 3 has pseudodilatation of the joint with a minor degree of partial ankylosis, severe subchondral sclerosis and generalized bone marrow fat accumulation. Grade 4, the final grade has definite ankylosis involving greater than 25% of the joint (Fig. 21.7).

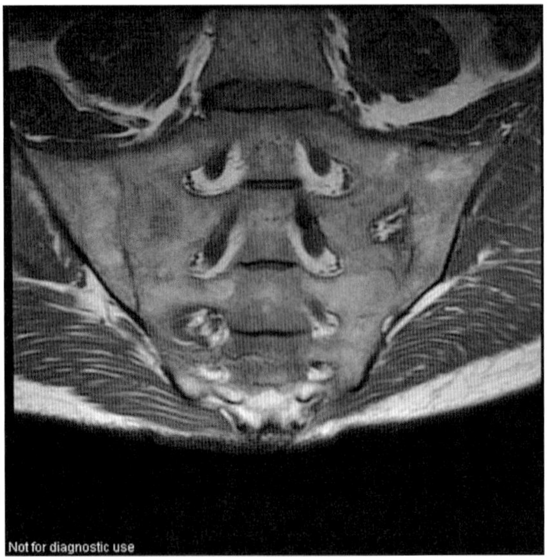

Fig. 21.7 MRI of bilateral sacroiliac joint ankylosis in a patient with chronic ankylosing spondylitis. Coronal T1 FLAIR MRI demonstrates obliteration of the joint space secondary to ankylosis of the left sacroiliac joint with incomplete ankylosis of the right sacroiliac joint. Coronal STIR and post-gadolinium T1 FLAIR sequences (not shown) demonstrated no features to suggest active inflammatory changes.

Hermann et al (2004) have proposed a less time-consuming semi-quantitative assessment for visual determination of disease activity on STIR and/or postcontrast T1 fat-saturated sequences (Fig. 21.8). SPARCC (Spondyloarthritis Research Consortium of Canada) is an alternative proposed grading system (Maksymowych et al 2005) that does not require contrast and limits the number of SIJ images requiring assessment. The SIJ is divided into quadrants and lesions are assessed for depth and intensity. Landewe et al (2005) and the ASAS/ OMERACT working group assessed several scoring methods in the evaluation of inflammatory activity and structural damage, including the recently proposed SPARCC scoring system and concluded (van der Heijde et al 2005b) that there was too little information on reliability and sensitivity to change to rank available methods. They recommended the development of a validation protocol by consensus and asked developers of scoring systems to apply this protocol. Current work is ongoing in the development of an international grading system that will be available for use in both clinical studies and in individual patient management.

Summary

The wide availability of conventional radiography and the marked cost advantage makes it the screening examination of choice in the investigation of SII. The main disadvantages of conventional X-rays are the lack of sensitivity in detecting early SII, the false positive rate, and the use of ionizing radiation. Furthermore, inter- and intraobserver variation in the interpretation of these examinations is high. When plain X-rays reveal definite evidence of SII, further investigation should be assessed on an individual patient basis.

Indications for MRI would include those with normal or equivocal plain radiographic findings. This is particularly important as MRI is significantly more sensitive than other imaging modalities in the early assessment of SII. In addition, patients who demonstrate positive findings on plain radiographs should also be considered for MRI if there is a clinical suspicion of active inflammation as this may have an effect on patients' treatment, e.g. anti-TNF treatment and assessment of response. In patients who are unresponsive to treatment regimes and there is ongoing clinical uncertainty, MRI may be beneficial in assessing whether there is ongoing inflammatory change. This is best performed with dynamic contrast-enhanced MRI to differentiate active inflammation from residual edema. In individual patient management, STIR is sensitive in demonstrating active SII although may underestimate the degree of inflammation particularly with respect to synovial involvement. Further study directly comparing dynamic contrast-enhanced MRI versus STIR MRI in the management of individual patients is required. MRI lacks ionizing radiation that is particularly advantageous in imaging of patients requiring sequential studies, female and young patients. Future research and the development of an international grading system for SII are underway.

Treatment of patients with AS was previously limited to nonsteroidal, anti-inflammatory drugs (NSAIDs) and physiotherapy. There is increasing evidence that anti-TNF therapy is efficacious in spondyloarthropathy (Brandt et al 2004, Braun et al 2002, Rudwaleit et al 2005, van den Bosch et al 2002). The Assessment in Ankylosing Spondylitis Working Group (ASAS) has reported an international consensus statement for the use of anti-TNF agents in patients with AS (Braun et al 2003) and has recently published its first update (Braun et al 2005). This consensus statement did not set guidelines for definite MRI evaluation of these patients due to

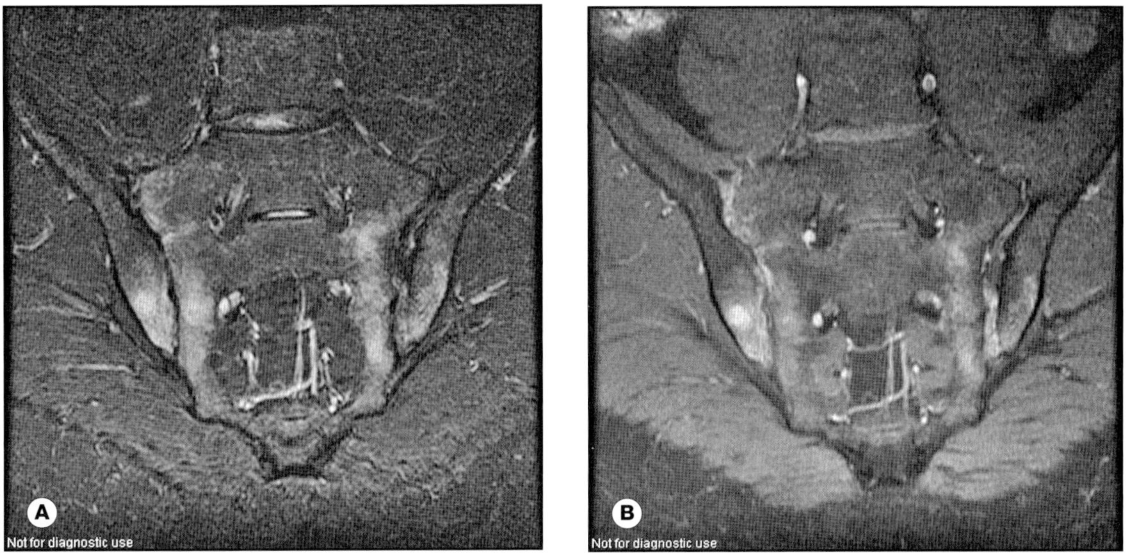

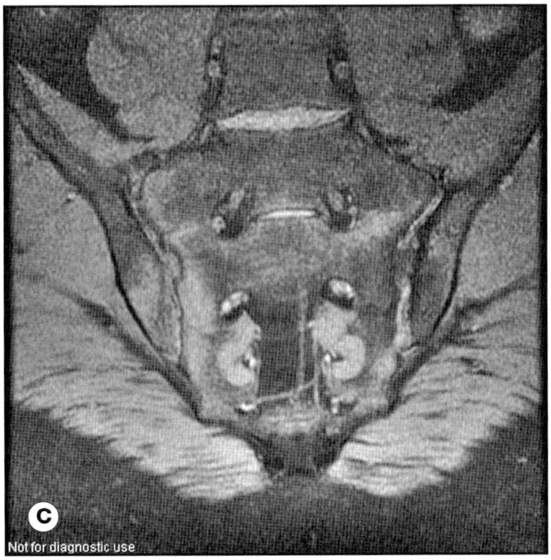

Fig. 21.8 MRI of active bilateral sacroiliitis (SII) in a 24-year-old male patient who presented with inflammatory low back pain. (A) Coronal STIR MRI demonstrates bilateral relatively symmetrical subchondral high signal intensity, bilateral moderate loss of joint space with early erosive changes and subtle increased signal intensity in the left sacroiliac joint of joint effusion or synovial proliferation. STIR cannot differentiate between the latter which requires gadolinium enhancement. (B) Coronal T1 fat-saturated post-gadolinium demonstrates bilateral enhancement within the joint space, consistent with synovial proliferation, bilateral enhancement of subchondral regions, loss of joint space, right greater than left with loss of cortical definition and subtle cortical erosions. (C) Coronal T1 fat-saturated pre-gadolinium confirms areas of increased signal on post-gadolinium study is true enhancement.

the fact that MRI is not widely available, not yet standardized, and due to its inherent cost. They do, however, suggest that the disease can be followed by MRI, CT, or plain radiographs. Further research on anti-TNF agents in patients with SII, and the role of MRI in the assessment of these patients before, during, and after therapy is required. Diagnosing AS early, prior to the development of structural radiographic changes will, in the authors' opinion and that of Rudwaleit & Sieper (2005), require changes to the diagnostic and classification criteria to include MRI which has the ability of assessing acute inflammatory changes early in the course of the disease.

The last decade has seen significant advances in the imaging of patients with SII and new hope for its treatment. The significant ongoing research that is taking place on an international basis will hopefully provide a better understanding of the underlying pathogenesis of the spondyloarthropathies and its optimum imaging, management and treatment.

References

Abbott GT, Carty H 1993 Pyogenic sacroiliitis, the missed diagnosis? British Journal of Radiology 66:120–122

Ahlstrom H, Feltelius N, Nyman R, Hallgren R 1990 Magnetic resonance imaging of sacroiliac joint inflammation. Arthritis and Rheumatism 33(12):1763–1769

Arslan H, Sakarya ME, Adak B et al 1999 Duplex and colour Doppler sonographic findings in active sacroiliitis. American Journal of Roentgenology 173(3):677–680

Bankoff MS, Sarno RC, Carter BL 1984 CT scanning in septic sacroiliac arthritis or periarticular osteomyelitis. Computed Radiology 8:165–170

Battafarano DF, West SG, Rak KM, et al 1993 Comparison of bone scan, computer tomography and magnetic resonance imaging in the diagnosis of active sacroiliitis. Seminars in Arthritis and Rheumatism 23(3):161–176

Battistone M, Manaster BJ, Reda DJ et al 1998 Radiographic diagnosis of sacroiliitis – are sacroiliac views really better? Journal of Rheumatology 25:2395–2401

Blum U, Buitrago-Tellez C, Mundinger A et al 1996 Magnetic resonance imaging for detection of active sacroiliitis – a prospective study comparing conventional radiography, scintigraphy and contrast-enhanced MRI. Journal of Rheumatology 23:2107–2115

Bollow M, Braun J, Hamm B et al 1995 Early sacroiliitis in patients with spondyloarthropathy: evaluation with dynamic gadolinium-enhanced MR imaging. Radiology 194(2):529–536

Bollow M, Braun J, Kannenberg J et al 1997 Normal morphology of SIJs in children: magnetic resonance studies related to age and sex. Skeletal Radiology 26:697–704

Bollow M, Fischer T, Reisshauer H et al 2000 Quantitative analysis of sacroiliac biopsies in spondyloarthropathies: T-cells and macrophages predominate in early and active sacroiliitis – cellularity correlates with a degree of enhancement detected by magnetic resonance imaging. Annals of Rheumatic Diseases 59:135–140

Brandt J, Khariouzov A, Listing G et al 2004 Successful short term treatment of patients with severe undifferentiated spondyloarthritis with anti-tumor necrosis factor-alpha fusion receptor protein etanercept. Journal of Rheumatology 31:531–538

Braun J, Bollow M, Eggens U et al 1994 Use of dynamic magnetic resonance imaging with fast imaging in the detection of early and advanced sacroiliitis in spondylarthropathy patients. Arthritis and Rheumatology 37(7):1039–45

Braun J, Sieper J, Bollow M 2000 Imaging of sacroiliitis. Clinical Rheumatology 19:51–57

Braun J, Brandt J, Listing G et al 2002 Treatment of active ankylosing spondylitis with infliximab; a randomized controlled multicentre trial. The Lancet 359:1187–1193

Braun J, Pham T, Sieper J et al 2003 International ASAS consensus statement for the use of anti-tumour necrosis factor in patients with ankylosing spondylitis. Annals of Rheumatic Disease 62:817–824

Braun J, Davis J, Dougados M et al 2005 First update of the International ASAS consensus statement for the use of anti-tumour necrosis factor in patients with ankylosing spondylitis. Annals Rheumatic Disease August 11 [e-pub ahead of print]

Buyruk HM, Snijders CJ, Vleeming A et al 1995 The measurements of sacroiliac joint stiffness with colour Doppler imaging: a study of healthy subjects. European Journal of Radiology 21:117–121

Cohen AS, McNeill JM, Calkins E et al 1968 The normal sacroiliac joint analysis of eighty-eight sacroiliac roentgenograms. American Journal of Roentgenology 100:559/563

de Groot M, Spoor C, Snijders C 2004 Critical notes on the technique of Doppler imaging of vibrations (DIV). Ultrasound in Medicine and Biology 30(3):363–367

de Smet AA, Gardner JD, Lindsley HP et al 1982 Tomography for evaluation of sacroiliitis. American Journal of Roentgenology 139(3):577–581

Docherty P, Mitchell MJ, MacMillan L et al 1992 Magnetic resonance imaging in the detection of sacroiliitis. Journal of Rheumatology 19:393–401

Dougados M, van der Linden S, Juhlin R et al 1991 The European Spondylarthropathy Study Group. Preliminary criteria for the classification of spondyloarthropathy. Arthritis & Rheumatology 34:1218–1227

Faflia CP, Prassopoulos PK, Daskalogiannaki ME et al 1998 Variation in the appearance of the normal sacroiliac joint on pelvic CT. Clinical Radiology 53(10):742–746

Fam A G, Rubenstein J D, Chin-Sang H et al 1985 Computed tomography in the diagnosis of early ankylosing spondylitis. Arthritis and Rheumatism 28(8): 930–937

Feldtkeller E, Bruckel J, Khan MA 2000 Scientific contributions of ankylosing spondylitis patient advocacy groups. Current Opinion in Rheumatology 12:239–247

Forrester DM 1990 Imaging of the sacroiliac joints. Radiological Clinics of North America 28(5):1055–1072

Friedman L, Silberberg PJ, Rainbow A, et al 1993 A limited low-dose computed tomography protocol to examine the sacroiliac joints. Canadian Association of Radiologists Journal 44(4):267–272

Haliloglu M, Kleiman MB, Siddiqui AR, Cohen MD 1994 Osteomyelitis and pyogenic infection of the sacroiliac joint. Pediatric Radiology 24:333–335

Hermann KG, Braun J, Fischer T et al 2004 Magnetic resonance imaging of sacroiliitis; anatomy, histological pathology, and MR morphology in grading. Radiologe 44:217–228

Hollingsworth PN, Cheah PS, Dawkins RL et al 1983 Observer variation in grading sacroiliac radiographs in HLA-B27 positive individuals. General Rheumatology 10:247–254

Inanc N, Atagündüz P, Sen F 2005 The investigation of sacroiliitis with different imaging techniques in spondyloarthropathies Rheumatology International 25(8):591–594

Jurik AG, Hansen J, Puhakka KB 2002 Effective radiation dose from spiral CT of sacroiliac joints in comparison with axial CT and conventional radiography. European Radiology 12:2820–2825

Kampen WU, Tillmann B 1998 Age-related changes in the articular cartilage of human sacroiliac joint. Anatomy and Embryology 198:505–513

Klauser A, Halpern EJ, Frauscher F et al 2005 Inflammatory low back pain: high negative predictive value of contrast-enhanced color Doppler ultrasound in the detection of inflamed sacroiliac joints. Arthritis and Rheumatism 53(3):440–444

Landewe R, Hermann K, van der Heijde D et al 2005 Scoring sacroiliac joints by magnetic resonance imging. A multiple reader reliability experiment. The Journal of Rheumatology 32(10):2050–2055.

Lawson T, Foley W, Carrera G, et al 1982 The sacroiliac joints: anatomic, plain roentgenographic, and computed tomographic analysis. Journal of Computer Assisted Tomography 6:307–314

Levine CD, Schweitzer ME, Ehrlich SM 1994 Pelvic marrow in adults. Skeletal Radiology 23(5):343–347

Maksymowych W, Inman R, Salonen D 2005 Spondyloarthritis Research Consortium of Canada magnetic resonance imaging index for assessment of sacroiliac joint inflammation in ankylosing spondylitis. Arthritis & Rheumatism 53(5):703–709

Modic MT, Steinberg PM, Ross JS et al 1988 Degenerative disk disease; assessment of changes in vertebral bone marrow with MR imaging. Radiology 166:193–199

Muche B, Bollow M, Francois RJ et al 2003 Anatomic structures identified in early and late stage sacroiliitis and spondyloarthritis. A detailed analysis by contrast-enhanced magnetic resonance imaging. Arthritis and Rheumatism 48(5):1374–1384

Murphey MD, Wetzel LH, Bramble JM et al 1991 Sacroiliitis: MR imaging findings. Radiology 180:239–244

Oostveen J, Prevo R, den Boer J et al 1999 Early detection of sacroiliitis on magnetic resonance imaging and subsequent development of sacroiliitis on plain radiography. A prospective, longitudinal study. Journal of Rheumatology 26:1953–1958

Oudjhane K, Azouz EM, Hughes S et al 1993 Computed tomography of the sacroiliac joints in children. Canadian Association Radiologists Journal 44(4):313–314

Peh WC, Ho WY, Luk KD 1997 Applications of bone scintigraphy in ankylosing spondylitis. Clinical Imaging 21:54–62

Prassopoulos PK, Faflia CP, Voloudaki AE et al 1999 Sacroiliac joints: anatomical variants on CT. Journal of Computer Assisted Tomography 23:323–327

Puhakka KB, Jurik AG, Egund N et al 2003 Imaging of sacroiliitis in early seronegative spondylarthropathy. Acta Radiologica 44:218–229

Puhakka KB, Melsen F, Jurik AG et al 2004 MR imaging of the normal sacroiliac joint with correlation to histology. Skeletal Radiology 33:15–28

Resnick D 2002 AS. In: Resnick D (ed) Diagnosis of bone and joint disorders, 4th edn. WB Saunders, Philadelphia, PA, p1023–1081

Robbins SE, Morse MH 1996 Is the acquisition of a separate view of the sacroiliac joints in the prone position justified in patients with back pain? Clinical Radiology 51:637–638

Rogers LF 1992 Radiology of skeletal trauma, 2nd edn. Churchill Livingstone, New York

Rudwaleit M, Sieper J 2005 Infliximab for the treatment of ankylosing spondylitis. Expert Opinon on Biolgic Therapy 5(8):1095–1099

Rudwaleit M, Khan M, Sieper J 2005 The challenge of diagnosis and classification in early ankylosing spondylitis. Arthritis and Rheumatism 52(4):1000–1008

Sandrasegaran K, Saifuddin A, Coral A et al 1994 Magnetic resonance imaging of septic sacroiliitis. Skeletal Radiology 23:289–292

Schwarzer AC, Aprill CN, Bogduk N 1995 The sacroiliac joint in chronic low back pain. Spine 20(1):31–37

Shichikawa K, Tsujimoto M, Nishioka J et al 1985 Histopathology of early sacroiliitis and enthesitis in ankylosing spondylitis. In: Ziff M, Cohen SB (eds) Advances in inflammation research. Vol. 9 The spondyloarthropathies. Raven Press, New York, p15–24

Stürzenbecher A, Braun J, Paris S et al 2000 MR imaging of septic sacroiliitis. Skeletal Radiology 29:439–446

van den Bosch F, Kruithof E, Baeten D et al 2002 Randomized double blind comparison of chimeric monoclonal antibody to tumour necrosis factor infliximab versus placebo in active spondyloarthropathy. Arthritis and Rheumatology 46:755–765

van der Heijde D, Braun J, McGonagle D 2002 Treatment trials in ankylosing spondylitis: Current and future considerations. Annuals of Rheumatic Diseases 61: iii24–iii32

van der Heijde D, Dougados M, Davis J et al 2005a Assessment in ankylosing spondylitis. Spondylitis International Working Group/Spondylitis Association of America recommendations for conducting clinical trials in ankylosing spondylitis. Arthritis and Rheumatism 52:386–394

van der Heijde D, Landewe R, Hermann K et al 2005b Application of the OMERACT filter to scoring methods for magnetic resonance imaging of the sacroiliac joints and the spine. Recommendations for a research agenda at Omeract 7. The Journal of Rheumatology 32(10): 2042–2047

van der Linden S, Valkenburg HA, Cats A 1984 Evaluation of diagnostic criteria for ankylosing spondylitis. A proposal for modification of the New York criteria. Arthritis and Rheumatism 27(4):361–368

Vogler JB 3rd, Brown WH, Helms CA et al 1984 The normal sacroiliac joint: a CT study of asymptomatic patients. Radiology 151(2):433–437

Ward MM 2002 Functional disability predicts total costs in patients with ankylosing spondylitis. Arthritis Rheumatology 46:223–231

Wittram C, Whitehouse GH 1995 Normal variation in the magnetic resonance imaging appearances of the sacroiliac joints: pitfalls in the diagnosis of sacroiliitis. Clinical Radiology 50(6):371–376

Wittram C, Whitehouse GH, Bucknall RC 1996 Fat-suppressed contrast-enhanced MR imaging in the assessment of sacroiliitis. Clinical Radiology 51: 554–558

Yazici H, Turunc M, Ozdogan H et al 1987 Observer variation in grading sacroiliac radiographs might be a cause of 'sacroiliitis' reported in certain disease states. Annals of the Rheumatic Diseases 46:139–145

Yu W, Feng F, Dion E et al 1998 Comparison of radiography, computed tomography and magnetic resonance imaging in the detection of sacroiliitis accompanying AS. Skeletal Radiology 27:311–320

SECTION ONE
CHAPTER
22

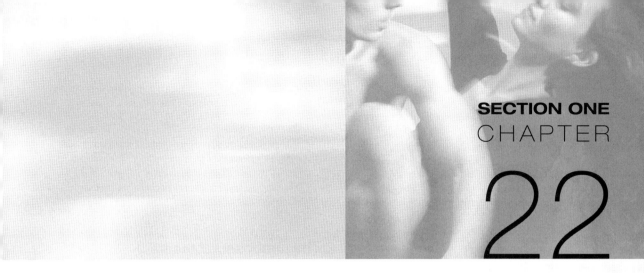

Visualization of pelvic biomechanical dysfunction

T Ravin

Introduction

Radiography and imaging of the lumbosacral spine for evaluation of biomechanical dysfunctions are more important now than ever. Since the beginning of the twentieth century, radiologists have tried to identify bony and soft tissue alterations that might help to explain the cause of low back pain on images of the spine. Over the years, many useful observations were forgotten or misplaced as technology changed our capabilities to image the pelvis and spine. The relentless pursuit of the 'disc' as a cause for back pain diverted radiographers and clinicians away from assessing images that could help to identify the functional causes of the pain.

There is now a renewed interest in spinal imaging, with an emphasis on functional assessment. Imaging makes it possible to diagnose several congenital and acquired biomechanical dysfunctions that significantly impact on treatment. The clinician interested in identifying the cause of low back pain can find considerable support in the careful evaluation of images. This chapter reviews some of the more important congenital abnormalities that affect low back and pelvic function, such as the unlevel sacral base, mixed lumbosacral joint orientation, steep lumbosacral angle, and a high L5 vertebral body. There are also some important acquired problems that can create low back and pelvic pain. These include mechanical joint dysfunctions that cause a short curve scoliosis, pubic dysfunctions, sacral torsions, coccygeal displacements, and ligamentous laxity that allows retrospondylolisthesis. The impact of gravity on our posture can be evaluated radiographically as changes in spinal position.

The treatment of low back and pelvic pain with manipulation, postural training, and injection therapy is increasing the importance of images in the assessment of the lumbosacral spine. Standing lumbar spine films are returning to their rightful position as benchmark studies in the evaluation of low back pain.

Technique

Plain film imaging of the lumbosacral spine should be taken standing. The basic examination consists of an anteroposterior (AP) film of the lumbar spine and pelvis, and a lateral film of the lumbosacral spine. The feet are shoulder width apart and the weight is equally distributed between the two legs. Lateral X-rays in flexion and extension are also useful. These images can, in some cases, define the nature of mechanical joint dysfunctions. The film of the pelvis should be taken so that the central ray of the beam, or where the cross-hairs point, is at the L4 level. This will reveal a good view of most of the structures of the lumbar spine and pelvis as well as a view of the femoral head, coccyx, and symphysis pubis. On the lateral lumbar film, the patient should be positioned so that the horizontal beam is at L4 and the vertical beam is centered on the spine. In the lateral view, the technique should be adjusted so that good detail of the lumbosacral junction, coccyx, and symphysis pubis can be well visualized. The third set of films, which might occasionally be obtained, is the oblique films for the evaluation of spondylolisthesis.

Congenital abnormalities and mechanical dysfunctions

The relationship between congenital abnormalities and mechanical dysfunctions is perhaps the single most important reason to image the spine. The reported incidence of clinically significant congenital abnormalities ranges from a maximum of 50% (Ferguson 1934) to a minimum of 6% (Frymoyer 1984). In the first decades of the twentieth century, O'Reilly, Ferguson, Mitchell, and others began to notice the relationship between congenital abnormalities and low back pain (Mitchell 1934, O'Reilly 1921). They observed that several common abnormalities, particularly those of the lumbosacral joints, were frequently associated with low back pain. These radiographic observations and their clinical corollaries became separated over the years. Now, at the start of the twenty-first century, with a rising interest in nonsurgical care of the back and renewed interest in functional assessment, it is again time to read these gems of clinical imaging literature. For example, in 1934 Ferguson wrote:

> *Our spines were developed for the four-footed position and are not yet adapted to the erect, so mechanical weakness at the lumbosacral area is usual rather than exceptional. We must consider the lumbosacral area not as normal or abnormal but as mechanically sound or mechanically unsound.*

The lumbosacral facets

The relationship between congenital alignment of articular surfaces and mechanical dysfunctions is best demonstrated at the lumbosacral junction. The clinical impression that lumbosacral joint asymmetry might be associated with a higher incidence of low back pain has some basis in fact and dates back to the early part of the twentieth century.

The normal lumbosacral facet joint is in the coronal plane (Van Schaik 1985) (Fig. 22.1). If the lumbosacral joints are more sagittal in nature, there will be greater stress on both the ligaments anteriorly and the lamina posteriorly (Sharma et al 1995) (Fig. 22.2). A sagittal facet orientation significantly increases the stress on the iliolumbar ligaments because in this joint orientation only these ligaments can resist lumbar flexion.

X-rays of the lumbosacral spine reveal many variations of the lumbosacral joints, including inclined, rudimentary, irregular, and defective joints (Jonsson et all 1989). Asymmetric lumbosacral joints, one being coronal and one sagittal, are some of the most common abnormalities in the low back (Fig. 22.3). This situation is a functional disaster and it is easy to envision how this situation could lead to a mechanical joint dysfunction. For example, if an individual has this lumbosacral facet alignment and lifts from the side, there will be the real possibility that one of the joints will malfunction. There is good reason for carrying out plain-film imaging of the lumbar spine for assessment of joint orientation, as it can be helpful in explaining persistent complaints of pain (Farfan 1967). Ferguson concluded that 'practically every person with a severe degree of asymmetry of these facets has symptoms referable to the lower part of the back.'

The high L5 vertebra

The presence of an L5 vertebra that is high, relative to the iliac crest, can also be a cause of low back pain. The increased length of the lumbar ligament

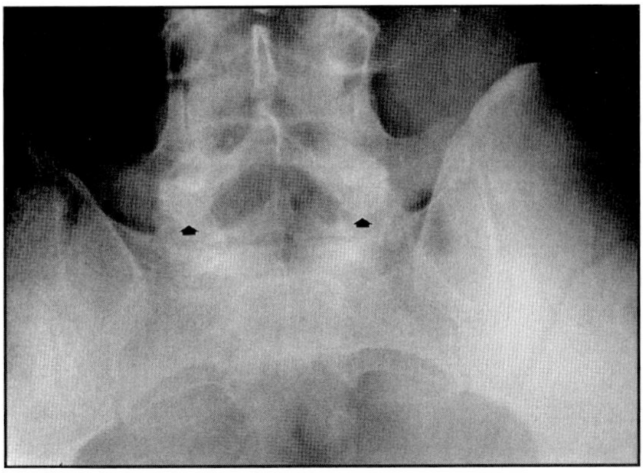

Fig. 22.1 The normal lumbosacral facets should have a coronal orientation (closed arrows). The orientation allows for flexion, extension, and some side-bending, but little rotation.

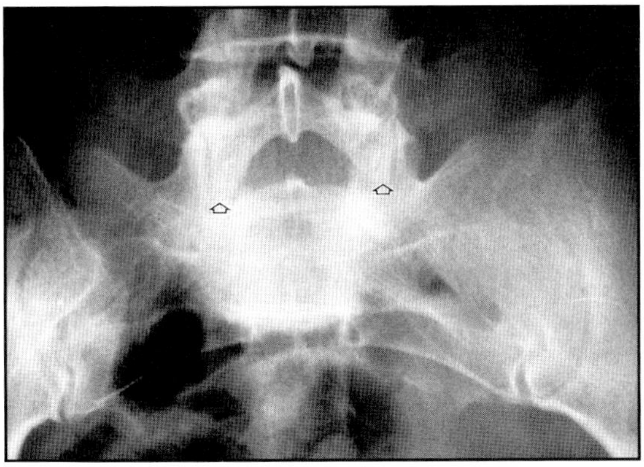

Fig. 22.2 Lumbosacral joints that are in the sagittal plane allow for excessive movement and are inherently unstable (open arrows). This orientation creates strain in almost all the soft tissue structures adjacent to the lumbosacral junction, particularly the ligaments.

in this anatomic variation increases its vulnerability to ligamentous strain when resisting nutation of the sacrum or flexion of the lumbar spine. Fig. 22.4 shows how this looks on the AP film of the pelvis. This congenital problem is not a frequent finding, but when present, is often associated with low back pain that will respond nicely to both prolotherapy (Klein et al 1993) and postural corrections (Kuchera & Jungman 1986).

Leg length and the unlevel sacral base

The importance of unequal leg lengths on mechanical dysfunctions and back pain has waxed and

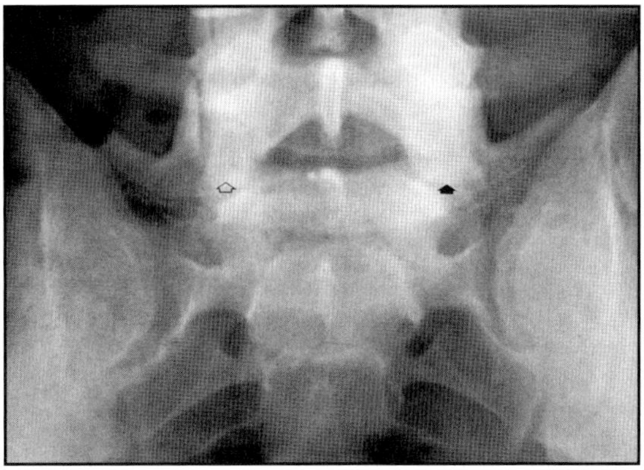

Fig. 22.3 The lumbosacral junction commonly has facets of different orientation: one joint has a coronal orientation (closed arrow) and the other is in a more sagittal plane (open arrow).

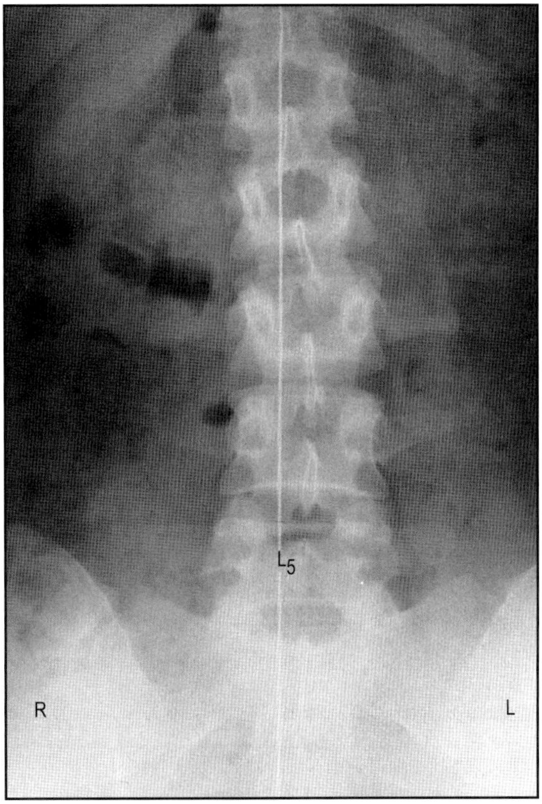

Fig. 22.4 The 'high L5 vertebra" is an important congenital variant. In this figure, notice that the transverse processes of the L5 vertebra are separated by a considerable distance form the medial side of the hip bones. The iliolumbar ligament spans this space. The white vertical line is a true vertical wire.

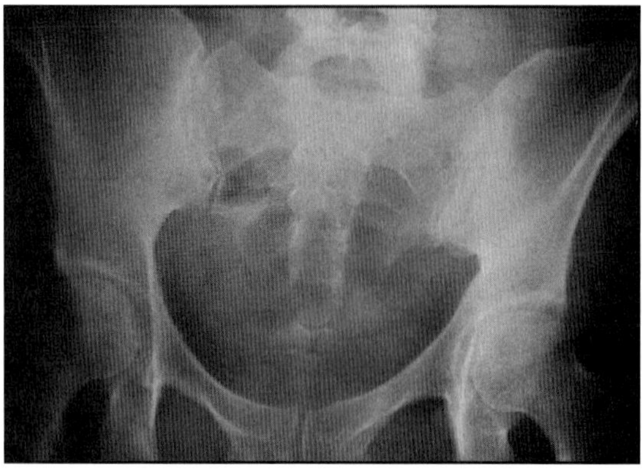

Fig. 22.5 Is the sacral base level? It is important to assess this on the standing AP pelvis film (see text).

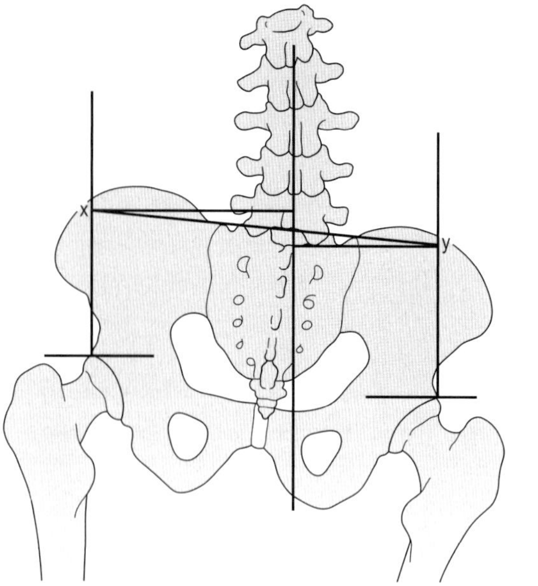

Fig. 22.6 Calculation of degree of sacral base inclination. First, find the lateral sacral notches, draw a connecting line and extend it across the innominate bones: line x–y. Draw two vertical lines from the apex of the femoral heads to meet the x–y line representing the sacral base inclination. Next, draw two horizontal lines across the film that intersects the sacral baseline at the femoral heads. The amount of foot lift necessary to correct the sacral base inclination is the distance in millimeters between these solid lines in the midline.

waned for nearly one hundred years (Kerr 1913). The height of the ankle and the length of the tibia and femur are just a part of this abnormality. The size of the ipsilateral hip bone and the sacral ala also affect what really matters. 'Is the sacral base level?' (Kappler 1983) is the real question. It is not unusual to find all of the structures in one of the rear quarters slightly smaller, so that leg length will be only one of the components of the unlevel sacral base. The impact of this anomaly on mechanical dysfunctions of the back seems to be directly related to the degree of tilt of the sacral base (Denslow 1983) (Fig. 22.5). The unlevel sacral base creates sacroiliac joint (SIJ) dysfunctions in the pelvis, such as sacral shears and torsions, and in the axial skeleton with the creation of long- and short-curve scoliosis (Kuchera 1995b; see also Chapter 9).

The next question is, 'Does an unlevel sacral base and treatment with foot lifts alter low back pain?' The results of this type of treatment have been unpredictable. Several authors have pointed out that in some individuals the treatment of leg length differences is an effective, simple, and inexpensive way to decrease low back pain (Heilig 1983). The mechanical correction of the unlevel sacral base can be carried out using 'foot lifts.' Fig. 22.6 illustrates how to calculate the amount of lift necessary to achieve a level sacral base.

An unlevel sacral base needs and demands a corrective curve in order to keep the eyes level with the horizon. These corrections often occur at the level of the lumbosacral junction and L4. If the sacrum is unlevel to one side, there will be a compensatory side-bending and rotation of L4 or L5 relative to S1, which will help to correct the sacral base tilt. As one can see from Fig. 22.7, identifying the side-bending and rotation is often not as difficult radiographically as one would imagine.

Ferguson's angle

The lumbosacral junction is uniquely individual and, when assessed on lateral radiography, contains considerable information about lumbar spine function. The angle created by a line that is horizontal and the cephalad surface of the first sacral vertebra is known as 'Ferguson's angle.' It is seldom measured but it is worth the effort. In 1934, Ferguson documented that this angle changed between standing and supine imaging (Fig. 22.8). He noted that the sacrum moved with gravitational stress and, in individuals with painful backs, that this movement was paradoxical. The fact that the angle became less when standing in patients with painful low backs has been clinically confirmed many times by individuals using the Levator (Jungmann 1992), an orthotic that aids the spine in resisting gravitational strain. The normal horizontal lumbosacral angle is about 42°. If the angle is greater than 52°, the sheer stresses at the lumbosacral junction become significant (Frisch 1994). Steep angles combined with abnormal lumbosacral joints are functionally unstable and significantly increase facet joint forces.

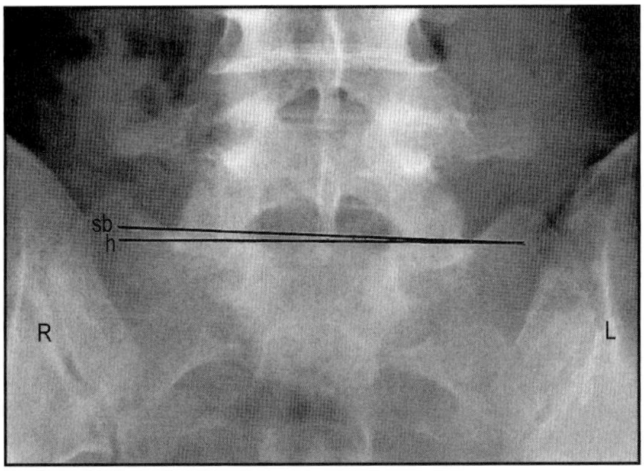

Fig. 22.7 In this figure, the sacral base inclines to the left (black line sb, line h being the horizontal). Notice that the L5 vertebra appears to be side-bent to the right. This compensatory right side-bending of L5 effectively straightens the lumbar spine and there will be little remaining scoliosis. In this situation, the L5 vertebra will not function in a completely normal manner as some of its normal ranges of motion are used to correct the unleveled sacral base.

Frymoyer (1984) noted that some of these abnormalities are often present in individuals who do not have any back pain at all and that these radiographic findings cannot be used to predict the presence of back pain. Clinical experience in treating the painful back, however, has shown that the finding of congenital abnormalities and sacral base unleveling on X-ray films often influences treatment protocols.

Somatic joint dysfunctions

The lumbar spine and pelvis are the most manipulated regions in the body. The presence of acquired somatic joint dysfunctions, created by trauma and ligament laxity, are often demonstrated in lumbosacral spine X-rays. X-rays can aid the clinician in identifying manipulable lesions. Radiographic description of the lesions should follow palpatory findings. The position of the lumbar vertebrae noted on physical examination can be described using the guidelines of Greenman (1995).

The current convention of describing vertebral motion is either from the perspective of the position in which the segment is stuck in or by the restrictive motion of the segment. Therefore, a segment that is backward bent (extended), right rotated and right side-bent has restriction of motion in forward bending (flexion), left side-bending and left rotation. Table 22.1 summarizes the changes. In radiography

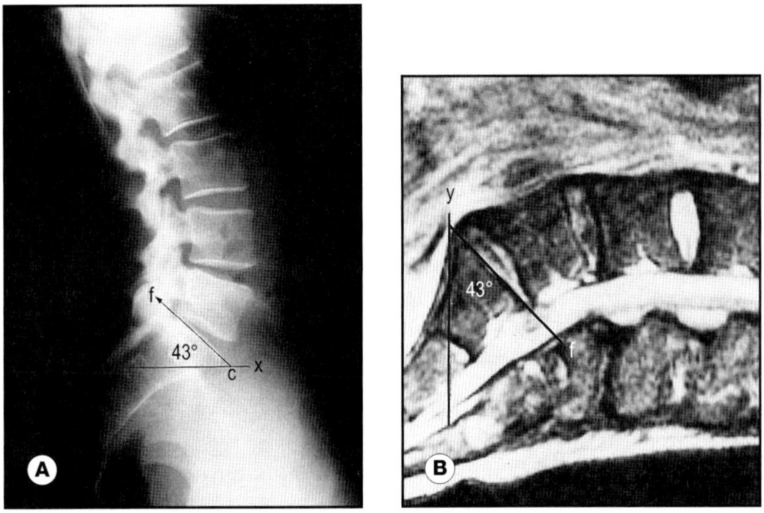

Fig. 22.8 Ferguson's angle changes between lying and standing and is not a static angle. It can, in fact, help to establish the presence of low back pain. In the normal individual, the angle should increase between lying supine and standing. In the standing image (A), line x is horizontal. In the supine image, line y is true vertical (B). This is an MRI image, which is one way to get a supine measurement of Ferguson's angle. The lines f are drawn along the cephalad surface of S1 in both images. This patient is abnormal because the angle did not increase between the supine and standing images.

Table 22.1 Vertebral motion

	Position	Motion restriction
L4 on L5	Extended	Flexion
	Left side-bent	Right side-bending
	Right rotated	Left rotation
	Left side-bent	Right side-bending

of the spine, the position description is the only one that can be used.

Bones

The radiographic evaluation of the pelvis and lumbar spine for somatic joint dysfunctions has remained a challenge since osteopaths and chiropractors began evaluating these structures in the early 1900s. The difficulty has been the correlation of the physical examination of a specific mechanical joint dysfunction with a specific radiographic finding. This has been and will remain a challenge to both the hand and the eye.

Mechanical dysfunctions of the pelvis and lumbar spine can generate numerous radiographic findings. The persistently side-bent and rotated lumbar vertebra – 'the short-curve scoliosis' – is often seen on both plain-film and computer-aided images. Side-bending is easy to see on radiography because the transverse processes are closer together on one side than the other (Fig. 22.9). Side-bending often comes with rotation, either towards or away from the side of the side-bending, as these spinal joint movements are coupled together. Due to the orientation of the zygapophyseal joints at L4–L5, which are nearly sagittal, there is limited rotation, but there will be a noticeable amount of side-bending.

Lateral flexion and extension views demonstrate movement of the lumbar vertebrae in the sagittal plane. These views allow the complete description of vertebral functional restrictions (Fig. 22.10). In the clinic, the specific manipulation needed to correct the problem should be determined by palpatory findings rather than radiographic ones. Clinically, the upper lumbar vertebrae are frequently involved in mechanical dysfunctions probably related to the attachments of the psoas muscles. These muscles can both extend and flex the upper lumbar vertebrae, but when in spasm they tend to cause extension.

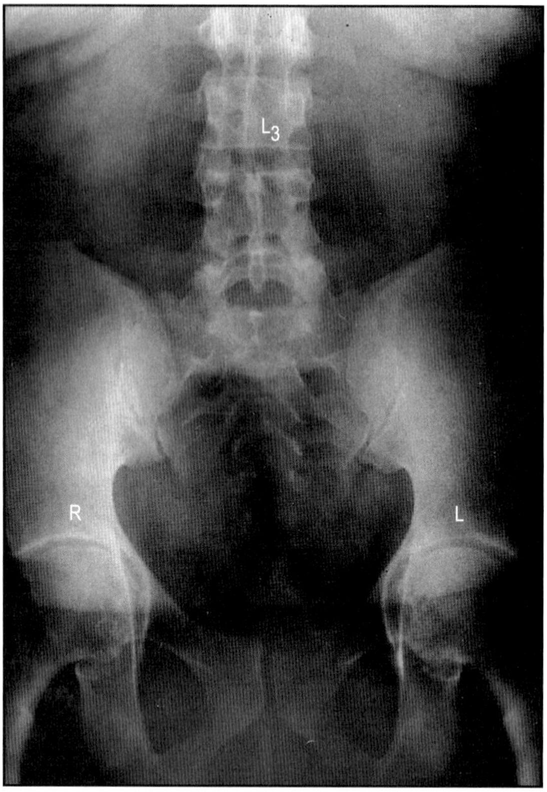

Fig. 22.9 'Short-curve scoliosis' in the AP projections is often a sign of mechanical dysfunction. In this lumbar spine, L3 is side-bent to the left and slightly rotated to the left. Notice that the L3–L4 disc space tapers to the left. In the lumbar spine, there is relatively more side-bending than rotation because of the sagittal orientation of the facets.

Ligaments

Ligamentous laxity allows increased motion of the lumbar vertebrae on each other. This finding can be identified on lateral films. Anatomic studies show that ligamentous laxity of the supraspinous, interspinous, and even facet joint capsules need to be present for spondylolisthesis to occur. The presence of ligamentous laxity is best demonstrated on the extension films, where the retrospondylolisthesis can be easily identified (Putto & Tallroth 1990). The radiographic changes range from subtle in neutral to considerable anterior spondylolisthesis on flexion films and obvious retrospondylolisthesis on extension films. Significant anterior spondylolisthesis is considered by some to be a reason for spinal fusion.

Figure 22.11 is an example of the retrospondylolisthesis. This abnormal movement can lead to

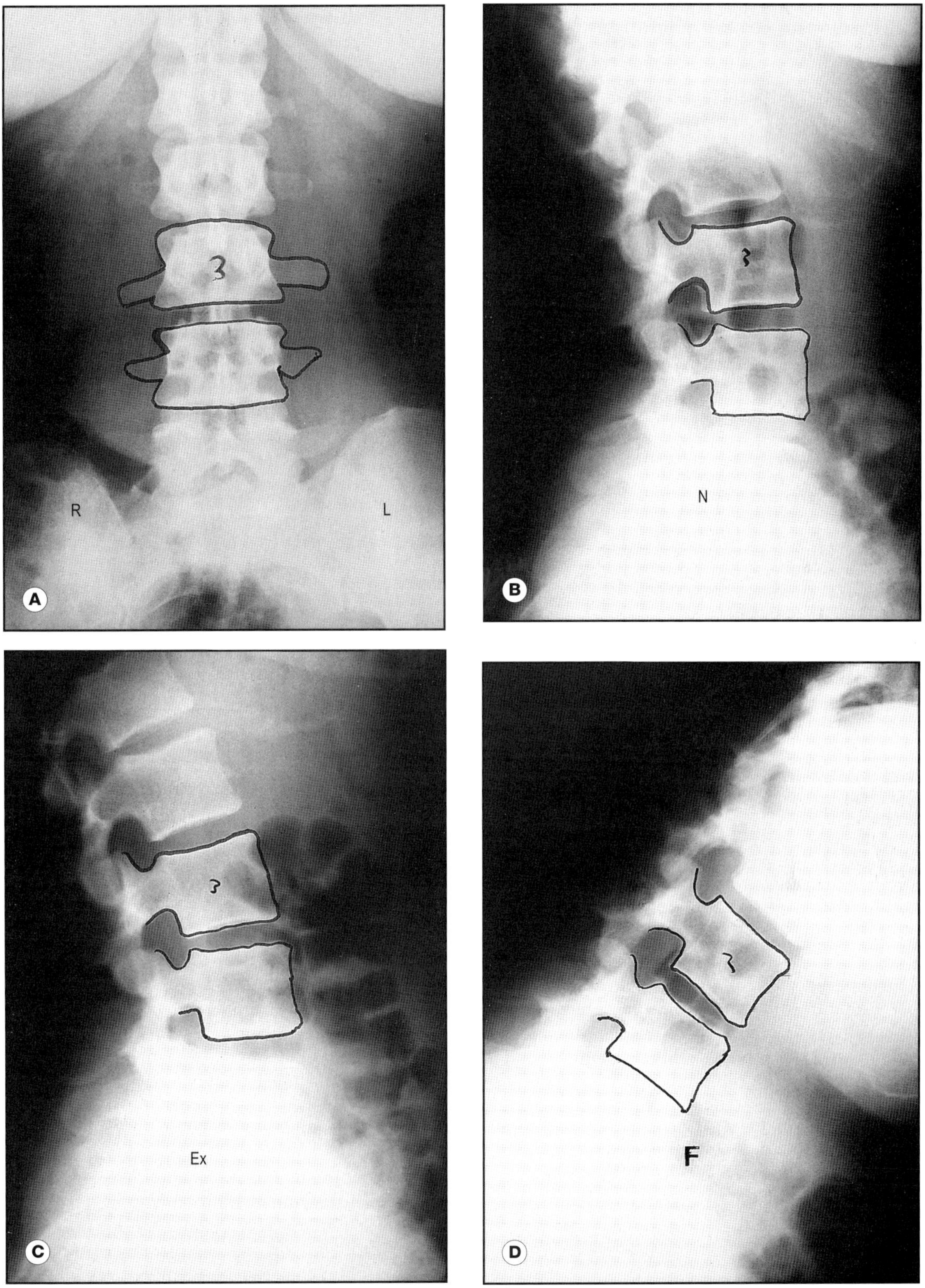

Fig. 22.10 This panel illustrates the presence of a mechanical joint dysfunction of L3. The L3 and L4 lumbar vertebrae are outlined in order to illustrate the vertebral motion. (A) An AP radiograph. (B) A standing lateral pelvis and lumbar spine in neutral (N). (C) In extension (Ex). (D) In flexion (F). Notice that the L3–L4 disc space does not appear to increase in size or shape when the patient tries to extend. This is because the L3 vertebra is already extended and cannot extend further. The L3 vertebra can still move into flexion so that when the patient bends forward, the L3 vertebra moves and makes the disc space nearly normal looking. This vertebral body is extended, side-bent right, and slightly rotated right.

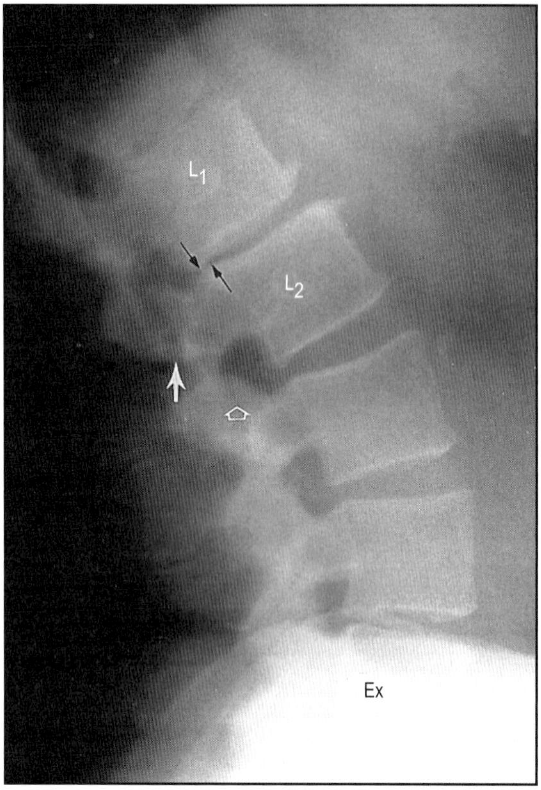

Fig. 22.11 Retrospondylolisthesis requires ligamentous laxity of almost all the ligaments surrounding the vertebra. This lateral lumbar spine was taken with the patient in extension. The white arrow points to the gap in the zygapophyseal joints at the L1–L2 level. Notice that this joint space is much larger than the joint space at L2–L3 (white arrowhead). The black closed arrows point to the posterior displacement of the L1 vertebral body. Notice the degenerative disc disease of the L1–L2 disc space.

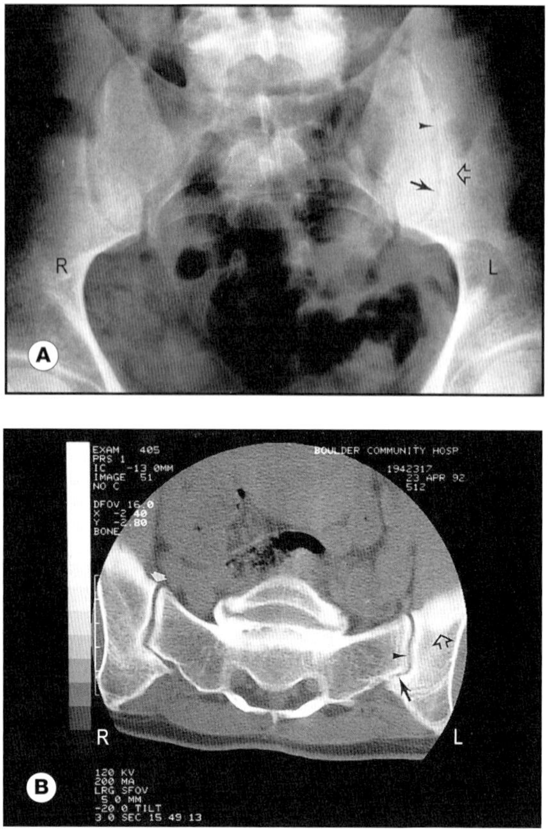

Fig. 22.12 Degenerative SI joint disease creates numerous radiographic changes. In panel (A), a standing MRI, the degenerative joint disease is manifest as a narrowed joint space (black arrowhead), irregular joint contours (black arrow), and marginal osteophyte formation (white arrow). Note the left sacral rotation on this MRI.

spinal nerve root compression, cause pain, alter nerve root function, and be misinterpreted as disc disease (Garfin et al 1995). The disc disease that accompanies the spondylolisthesis changes is often more obvious radiographically than is the spondylolisthesis itself. The static and horizontal magnetic resonance imaging (MRI) or computerized tomography (CT) images are often relied upon to explain back pain, but they seldom demonstrate the functional causes of lumbar and pelvic pain.

Joints

Degenerative joint disease of the SIJs seen on radiographic images is not usually thought of as reflecting mechanical dysfunction. The presence of periarticular osteophytes, subarticular sclerosis, or osteitis condensans and joint space narrowing are, however, good indicators of abnormal joint mechanics (Dilhmann 1980, Dreyfuss 1994) (Fig. 22.12). The developing consensus is that these findings represent the presence of mechanical joint dysfunctions and ligamentous laxity. These findings on all forms of imaging should be clues that mechanical dysfunctions might be present and are excellent documentation when correlated with the clinical findings (Greenman 1992).

Sacral torsion is the one major somatic dysfunction of the sacrum that can be identified on MRI/CT scanning. This is an osteopathic descriptive term and can be thought of as a sacrum that has rotated about an oblique or diagonal axis. This twisting is sometimes called 'asymlocation' (Dorman & Ravin

1991). It is possible because of the unique nature of the SIJs and the lumbosacral junction. The basic model of spinal mechanics leads us to believe that side-bending and rotation are integral parts of spinal and sacral motion. The normal sacrum lying horizontal in a gantry should be nearly parallel with the floor.

If there is a side-bent lesion anywhere in the spine, the most likely place for this spinal twist to be exhibited is at the level of the vertebra involved. However, it can occasionally manifest as rotation at either end of the spine – the sacrum or the atlas. This process is documented in the 'spinal engine' (Gracovetsky 1988). The sacral twisting component is often evident in MRI/CT scans. Normal patients without mechanical joint dysfunctions have a straight spine but if there are vertebral somatic joint dysfunctions that are side-bent and rotated, there will be some scoliosis of the spine. This curve or 'kink' in the spine will create a twisting that will travel to the sacrum.

The visualized twisting of the sacrum is not created by malposition of the patient by the technician but by mechanical dysfunction in the spine. If the sacral torsion is mechanically corrected by forcing the sacrum into horizontal, the patient will quickly become uncomfortable because the spine will be forced to side-bend and the imaging table will not allow the patient to do so.

Sacral torsion is clinically quite common in individuals with back pain, and the MRI/CT will quite often demonstrate some degree of sacral torsion. At present, the normal range of sacral torsion seen on MRI/CT is unknown, but the gross changes noted on many scans would clearly be abnormal (Fig. 22.13).

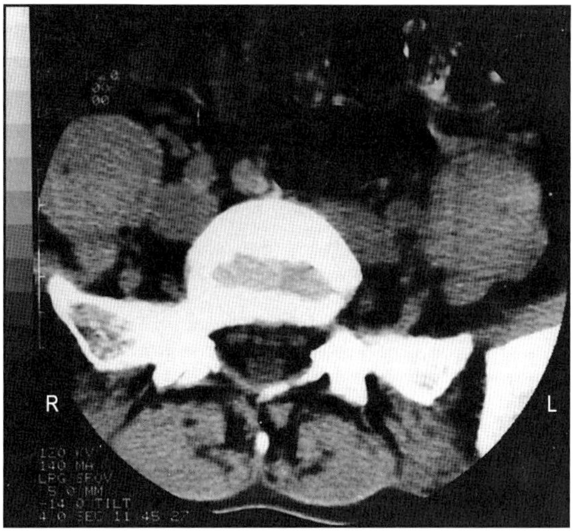

Fig. 22.13 This CT demonstrates significant left rotation of the sacrum. This much rotation is another finding of abnormal spinal joint mechanics.

Muscles

Somatic joints dysfunctions and ligamentous laxity alter the stresses on the muscles of the low back and pelvis. The gluteal and erector spinae muscles develop abnormal firing patterns in an attempt to stabilize the spine (McGill et al 2003). Initially, the muscles become bigger and stronger but, as the stress continues, the tendons develop enthesopathy (Palesy 1997). The enthesopathy causes inhibited firing of the muscles leading to atrophy and eventually fatty infiltration (Hodges & Moseley 2003). Research shows that paraspinal muscle tendinosis and enthesopathy could be a common cause of low back pain (Benjamin & McGonagle 2001).

MRI and ultrasound are used to image enthesopathy of the patellar, Achilles and extensor carpi ulnaris tendons. In these structures, abnormal signals have a variety of patterns that allow the differentiation of normal from abnormal tendon tissue (Towers et al 2003). In the pelvic and lumbar spine, identifying the actual sites of erector spinae and gluteal tendinosis is difficult but the secondary findings of muscle atrophy and fatty infiltration are not hard to find. In the case of low back pain without obvious disc or joint disease, ligamentous laxity or somatic joint dysfunctions should be considered a cause of lumbar muscle atrophy and fatty infiltration (Fig. 22.14).

Symphysis pubis

Mechanical dysfunction of the symphysis pubis is a common clinical diagnosis and can frequently be identified radiographically. The relationship of the pubes is critical in the clinical diagnosis and treatment of mechanical dysfunctions of the pelvis. Innominate up-slips, down-slips, and rotations are easily identified clinically. They can, and do, create radiographic changes in the joint space (Fig. 22.15). Evaluation of the symphysis pubis on AP pelvic images can aid in the documentation of displacement and is of considerable help to the treating clinician. It is crucial that these images are obtained standing. The three bones and three joints of the pelvis work in unison; dysfunction of one joint leads to instability in the entire structure, just as in the uncoupling of one angle in a triangle.

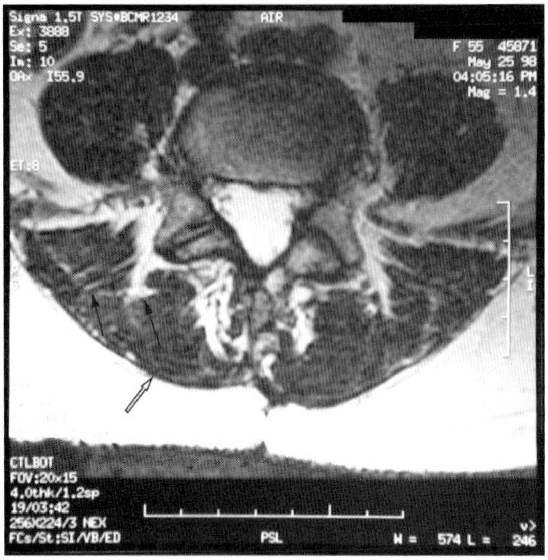

Fig. 22.14 Muscle atrophy (open arrow) and fatty infiltration (closed arrows) can be the result of reflex inhibition caused by tendinosis of the erector spinae muscles. These findings in the patient with low back pain but unremarkable discs and joints suggest the presence of lumbar and pelvic ligamentous laxity or somatic joint dysfunctions causing the tendinosis.

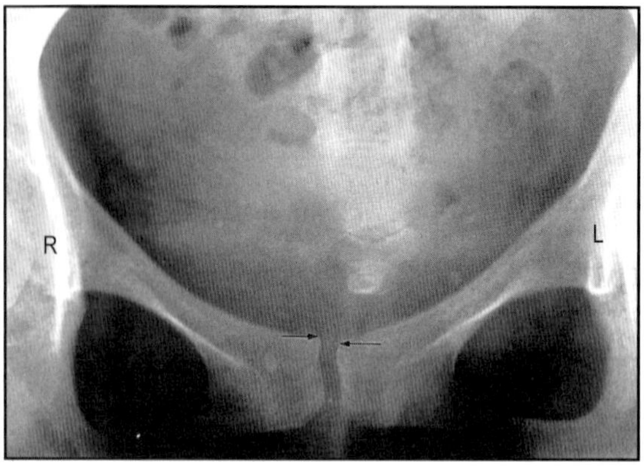

Fig. 22.15 Pubic dysfunctions occur when there is hip bone dysfunction. The black arrows point to the malalignment of the pubes on this standing AP pelvis. Notice the bony sclerosis of the left pubic bone, which reflects the early changes of osteitis involving the pubes.

That is why treatment of pelvic dysfunctions often begins with treatment of the pubes.

The radiographic manifestation of mechanical dysfunctions of the symphysis pubis is simply a malalignment of the two bones. This finding is sometimes considered to be positional but is most often the result of a true mechanical dysfunction of the pelvis. These pubic displacements, when combined with SIJ degenerative joint disease, are further evidence of the presence of pelvic mechanical dysfunction (see Fig. 22.15).

Coccyx

This small bone is often ignored on imaging but is a vital link between the bony pelvis and the soft tissues of the pelvic floor. The coccyx is directly attached to the sacrotuberous ligaments (Barral 1988) and to the dural sac by the filum terminale. It is also the posterior bony anchor of the pelvic floor muscles. Mechanical dysfunctions of this small bone can impact directly on the axial skeleton by way of the dura. It can create visceral dysfunctions by straining all the muscles and ligamentous structures of the pelvic floor. The coccyx is a vulnerable structure in many thin individuals, particularly those without gluteal muscle mass. Some individuals can literally be sitting on one of the most critical bones in the body. The coccyx is usually forced into excessive flexion and the somatic joint dysfunctions create symptoms that include low back pain, headaches, and even incontinence in females.

Mechanical displacements of this bone are often clinically hard to identify and frequently overlooked, so their radiographic demonstration is particularly helpful (Fig. 22.16). Plain film imaging is one of the best ways to identify displacements (see also Chapter 30).

Pelvic index and weight-bearing axis

Measurements of the pelvic index and the weight-bearing axis are helpful in defining how an individual is coping with the effects of gravity. The ideal posture is one in which gravitational force is directed along the structures adapted for weight bearing. This normal situation requires a minimum of energy for its maintenance. As the alignment of these structures changes with poor or abnormal posture, the gravitational force is redirected and creates additional stress on the muscles, tendons, and ligaments. The importance of gravitational stress on the bony, musculotendinous, and ligamentous structures of the lumbosacral junction is reflected in changes that can be measured on lateral films. These films reflect changes in posture created by the constant and underestimated stress of gravity. The ability of the musculoligamentous structures to maintain effectively both static and dynamic

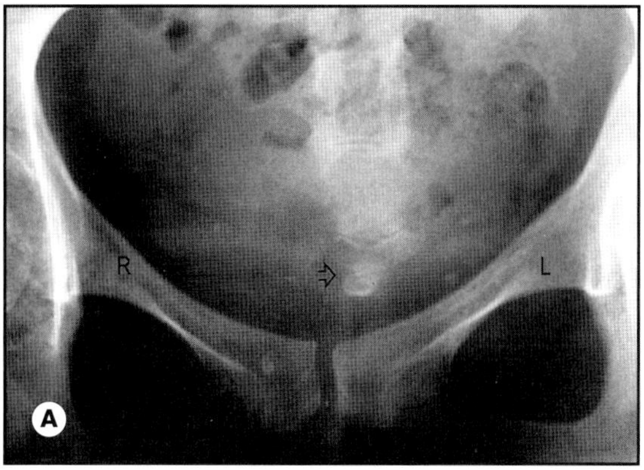

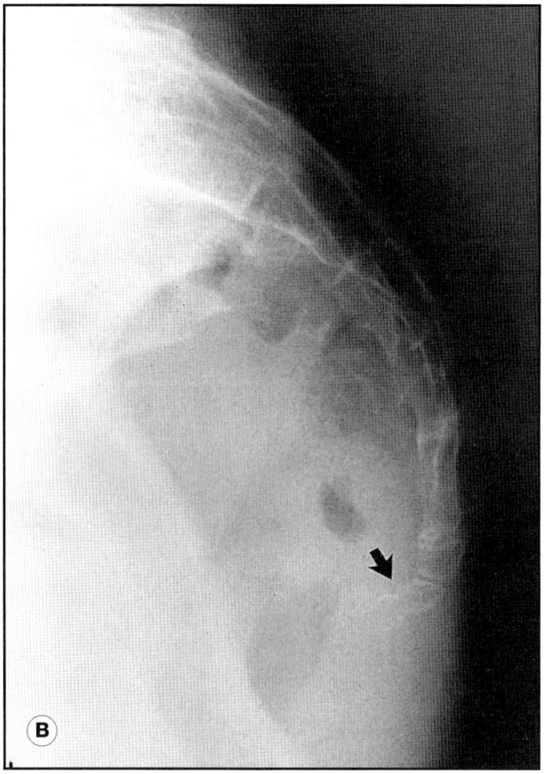

Fig. 22.16 The coccyx is easily seen on the AO pelvis films (A). However, it may be hard to identify on the lateral film (B). It is usually forced into abnormal flexion (black closed arrow) and in this case side-bent to the right (open arrow in A).

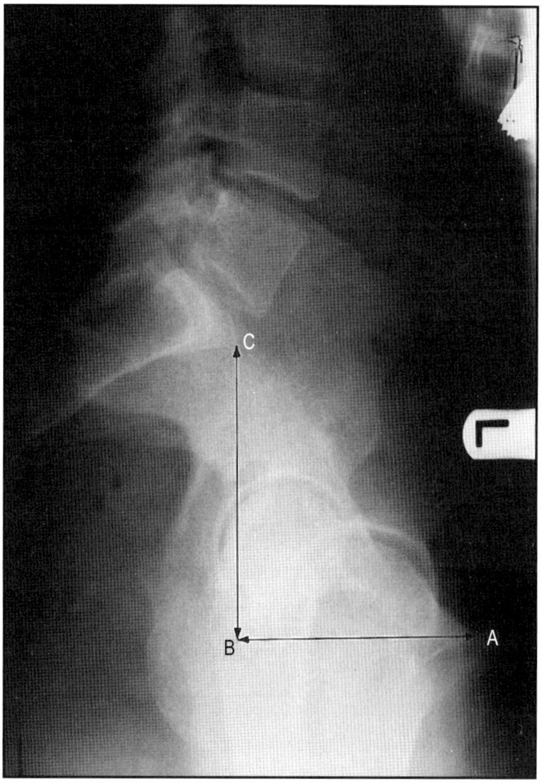

Fig. 22.17 The pelvic index is calculated by first finding point A, which is the crest of the pubes. Then find point C, which is at the sacral promontory. Draw a horizontal line from point A across the film, and then a vertical line from point C downwards until it intersects the horizontal line, which is point B. The pelvic index is the width in millimeters of line A–B divided by the length in millimeters of line B–C.

stability in the face of gravity can be estimated with the calculation of the pelvic index.

The pelvic index is a valuable measurement for the objective evaluation of the relative position of the sacrum with respect to the innominate bones. The importance of this measurement as a gauge of gravitational stress was first proposed by Jungmann in 1963. Changes in this index correlated with increasing age suggest that these alterations might be the result of gravitational strain. These measurements are obtained from the lateral lumbar–pelvic X-ray and can be helpful in identifying individuals whose bad posture is one of the primary causes of their back pain. This index can assess increased myofascial ligamentous strain created by bad posture (Janda 1986). The use of this index is currently increasing in the clinical setting as it also can aid in the identification of the muscle imbalances described as the 'Unterkreuz' by Janda (Kuchera 1995a) (Fig. 22.17).

The lateral image also contains information about the weight-bearing axis. This line is calculated by drawing a vertical line through the midpoint of the L3 vertebral body. This provides information regarding the sagittal plane balance of the individual (Fig. 22.18). This theoretical line passes through the external auditory canal, the lateral head of the humerus, the anterior body of L3, the head of the femur, the anterior third of the sacrum, and the lateral malleolus. This 'ideal' alignment requires a minimum of energy expenditure by the postural muscles. Displacement of this line anteriorly or posteriorly significantly increases muscle energy expenditure and ligamentous strain, particularly in the regions of the neck and pelvis.

The importance of calculating the pelvic index and the weight-bearing axis for diagnosis and therapy is further developed in Chapter 39, and the reader is encouraged to integrate this chapter.

Summary

There are many reasons to image the lumbar spine and pelvis for biomechanical dysfunctions. Several important congenital abnormalities can influence the stability of the lumbosacral spine:

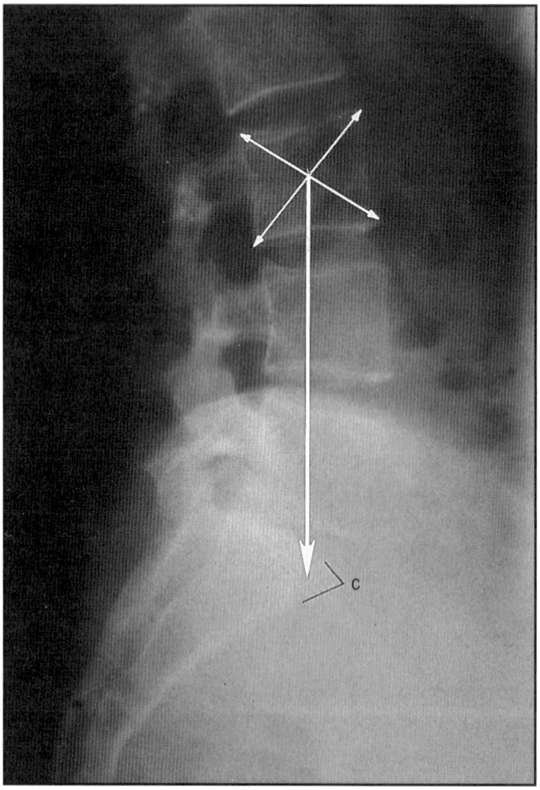

Fig. 22.18 The gravitational line should pass through the middle of the L3 vertebra and in front of the sacral promontory (point c in this figure). In this patient, the weight-bearing line is abnormal because it is posterior to the sacral promontory.

- Imaging demonstrates the orientation of the lumbosacral facets. The normal coronal facets are associated with fewer clinical problems than are facets of other orientations. Congenital anomalies of the facets are commonly associated with clinical problems.
- The presence of an unlevel sacral base demonstrated on the AP pelvic film can explain the resistance of a mechanical joint dysfunction to manipulation. The correction of the unlevel sacral base can be determined by measurements made from the X-rays.
- Ferguson's angle, often thought of as a static measure, is really a dynamic angle; the angle will be smaller in the painful back.
- The presence of a 'high L5' can explain persistent iliolumbar ligamentous pain. This radiographic finding implies a long iliolumbar ligament and one that might respond to prolotherapy.

Lumbosacral spine radiography can also reveal the presence of acquired biomechanical dysfunctions:

- 'The short-curve scoliosis' created by a side-bent and rotated lumbar vertebra. These are frequent findings on all types of images of the spine. These biomechanical dysfunctions are common causes of back, pelvic, and leg pain. The identification by imaging is important, as the treatment may depend on this form of documentation of their presence.
- The presence of a malaligned symphysis pubis. The radiographic signs are clear and can help to explain persistent lumbosacral instability.
- SIJs showing changes of degenerative disease may reflect the presence of longstanding mechanical dysfunction. The recognition of degenerative joint disease can be of considerable aid to the clinician struggling with an 'unstable back' by directing him or her to the primary cause.
- Atrophy and fatty infiltration of the paraspinal muscles of the lumbar spine and pelvis in the absence of disc and joint pathology but low back pain suggests the presence of spinal ligamentous instability and somatic joint dysfunctions.
- A coccyx in an excessively flexed position noted on X-ray can help to explain pelvic and low back pain that seems to have 'no explanation.'
- Sacral torsion or rotation and degenerative joint disease on computerized imaging can identify mechanical dysfunctions and the presence of longstanding instability.

- The pelvic index and the weight-bearing line that are calculated from the standing lateral images can explain how gravity affects biomechanical stability.

As our clinical understanding of the biomechanics of the lumbar spine and pelvis increases, we are forced to review these areas of imaging. Observations of mechanical dysfunctions collected over the last century are now finding a new place in contemporary spinal diagnostic and therapeutic literature. The past emphasis on imaging the discs and the SIJs without integrating congenital and acquired dysfunctions is passing, as this book reveals.

References

Barral JP 1988 Visceral manipulation. Eastland Press, Seattle, WA

Benjamin M, McGonagle D 2001 The anatomical basis for disease localization in seronegtative spondyloarthropathy at entheses and related sites. Journal of Anatomy 199:503–526

Denslow JS 1983 Mechanical stresses in the human lumbar spine and pelvis. In: Peterson B (ed) Postural balance and imbalance. American Academy of Osteopathy, Indianapolis, IN, p144–151

Dilhmann W 1980 Diagnostic radiology of the sacroiliac joints. Georg Thieme Verlag, New York

Dorman TA, Ravin TH 1991 Diagnosis and injection techniques in orthopedic medicine. Williams & Wilkins, Baltimore, MD

Dreyfuss P 1994 The sacroiliac joint: a review. International Spinal Injection Society 2:22–58

Farfan HF 1967 The relationship of facet orientation to intervertebral disc failure. Canadian Journal of Surgery 10:179–185

Ferguson AB 1934 The clinical and roentgenographic interpretation of lumbosacral anomalies. Radiology 22: 548–588

Frisch H 1994 Systematic musculoskeletal examination. Springer-Verlag, New York

Frymoyer JW 1984 Spine radiographs in patients with low-back pain. Journal of Bone and Joint Surgery (US) 66:1048–1055

Garfin SR, Rydevid B, Lind B 1995 Spinal nerve root compression. Spine 20:1810–1820

Gracovetsky S 1988 The spinal engine. Springer-Verlag, New York

Greenman PE 1992 Sacroiliac dysfunction in the failed low back pain syndrome. In: Vleeming A et al (eds) First Interdisciplinary World Congress on Low Back Pain and its Relation to the Sacroiliac Joint. 9–11 November, San Diego, CA, p329–352

Greenman PE 1995 Principles of manual medicine, 2nd edn. Williams & Wilkins, Baltimore, MD

Hodges PW, Moseley GL 2003 Pain and motor control of the lumbopelvic region: effect and possible mechanisms. Journal of Electromyography and Kinesiology 13: 361–370

Janda V 1986 Muscle weakness and inhibition (pseudoparesis) in back pain syndromes. In: Grieve GP (ed) Modern manual therapy of the vertebral column. Churchill Livingstone, Edinburgh, p113–118

Jonsson B, Stromquist B, Egund N 1989 Anomalous lumbosacral articulations and low-back pain evaluation and treatment. Spine 14:831–834

Jungmann M 1992 The Jungmann concept and technique of anti-gravity leverage, 2nd edn. Institute für Gravitational Strain Pathology, Rangley, ME

Kappler RE 1983 Postural balance and motion patterns. In: Peterson B (ed) Postural balance and imbalance. American Academy of Osteopathy, Indianapolis, IN, p6–12

Kerr HE 1913 Observations on anatomical short leg in a series of patients presenting themselves for treatment of low-back pain. Journal of the American Osteopathic Association 42:437–440

Klein RG, Eek BC, DeLong BW, Mooney V 1993 A randomized double-blind trial of dextrose-glycerine-phenol injections for chronic low back pain. Journal of Spinal Disorders 6: 23–33

Kuchera ML 1995a Gravitational strain pathophysiology and 'Unterkreuz' syndrome. Manuelle Medizin 33(2):56

Kuchera ML 1995b Prolotherapy in the lumbar spine and pelvis. Spine: State of the Art Reviews 9 (2):463–490

Kuchera ML, Jungmann M 1986 Inclusion of levator orthotics device in the management of refractive low back pain patients. Journal of American Osteopathic Association 86:673–678

McGill SM, Grenier S, Kavcic N, Cholewicki J 2003 Coordination of muscle activity to assure stability of the lumbar spine. Journal of Electromyography and Kinesiology 13:353–359

Mitchell GAG 1934 The lumbosacral junction. Journal of Bone and Joint Surgery (US) 16:233–254

O'Reilly A 1921 Backache and anatomical variations of the lumbosacral region. Journal of Orthopedic Surgery 3:171–187

Palesy PD 1997 Tendon and ligament insertions – a possible source of musculoskeletal pain. J Craniomandibular Practice 15:194–202

Putto E, Tallroth K 1990 Extension–flexion radiographs for motion studies of the lumbar spine – a comparison of two methods. Spine 15:107–110

Sharma M, Langrana NA, Rodrequez J 1995 Role of ligaments and facets in lumbar spine stability. Spine 20: 887–900

Towers JD, Russ EV, Golla SK 2003 Biomechanics of tendons and tendon failure. Seminars in Musculoskeletal Radiology 10:59–66

Van Schaik JPJ 1985 The orientation of laminae and facet joints in the lower lumbar spine. Spine 10:59–63

PART THREE

Section Two

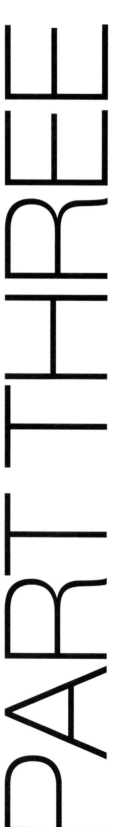

Diagnostic methods: The pelvic girdle

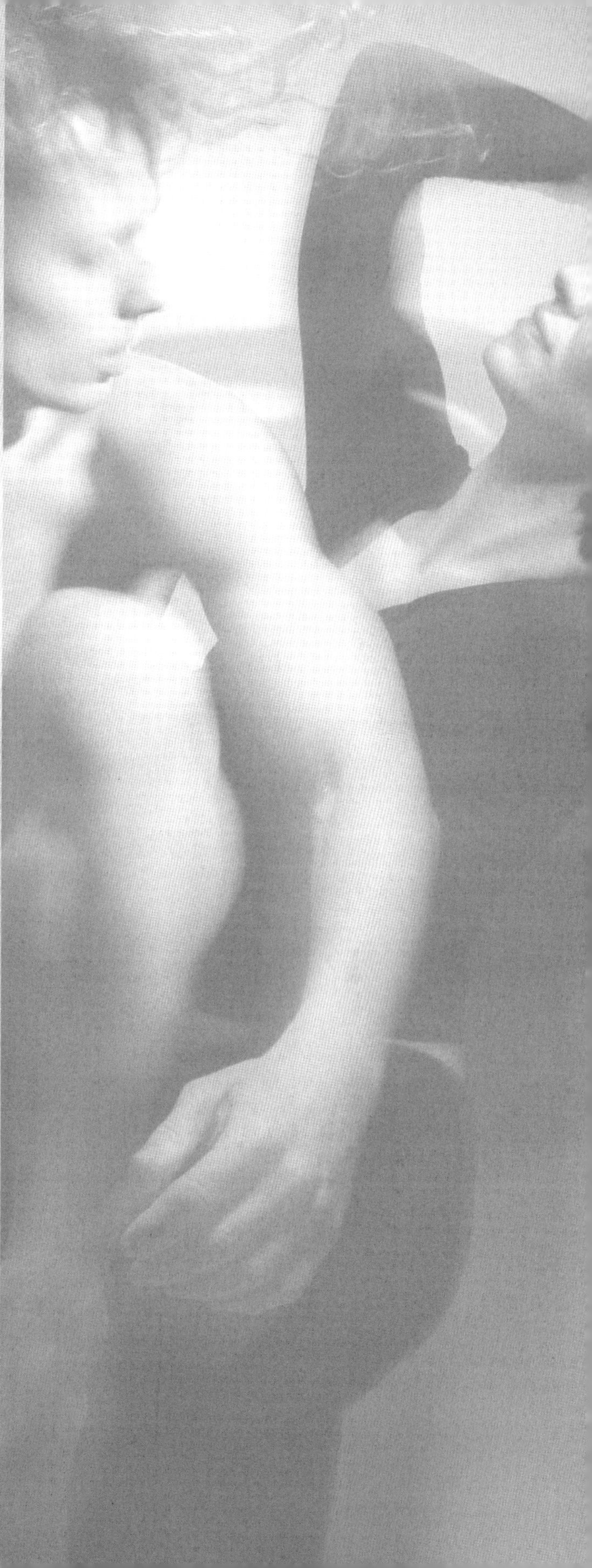

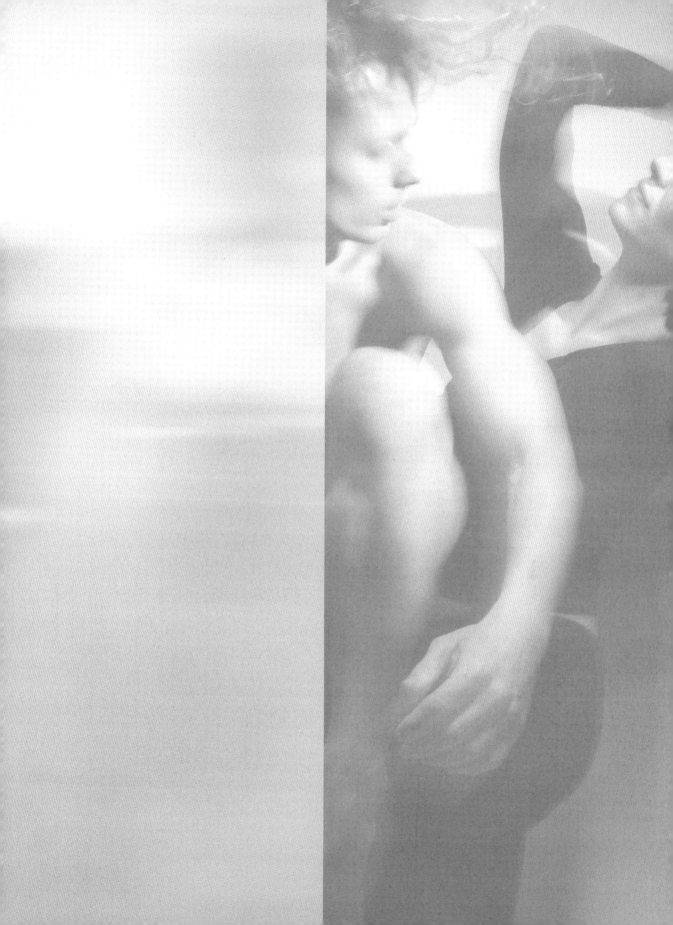

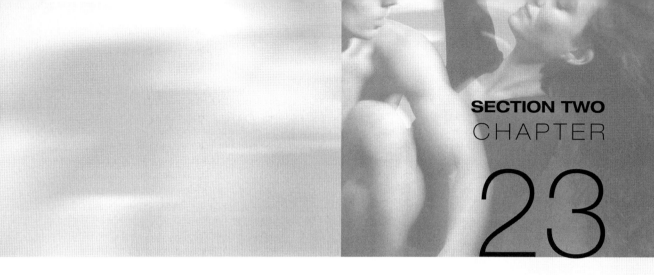

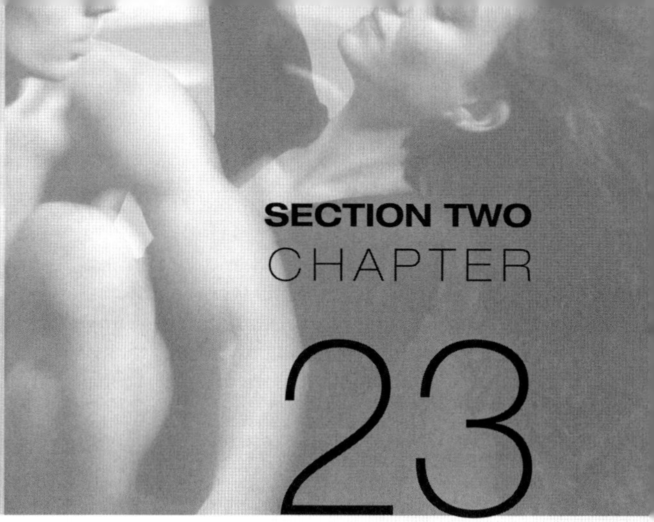

SECTION TWO
CHAPTER

23

Movement of the sacroiliac joint with special reference to the effect of load

Bengt Sturesson

Introduction

Postmortem studies have been performed since the middle of the nineteenth century to analyze movements in the sacroiliac joints (SIJs). Miller et al (1987) and Vleeming et al (1992) have demonstrated load displacement behavior on cadavers.

Weisl (1955) used lateral roentgenograms to perform studies on movements of living subjects. He noted 6-mm displacement between endpoints, but the error of measurement was calculated to be 3 mm. Colachis et al (1963) performed a study with rods in the iliac bones and reported 5 mm of translation but no other results. Selvik (1974) described a roentgen stereophotogrammetric analysis (RSA) by which it was possible to measure movements in all three dimensions. With this technique Egund et al (1978) demonstrated a maximal rotation of 2°.

Grieve (1983) used a stereophotogrammetric method analyzing movements of skin markers positioned on the posterior superior iliac spines and the sacrum. She calculated the difference in millimeters of movement between standing and standing with one leg in flexion. The average movement was estimated to be about 10 mm between the positions. The error of measurement was not calculated but it was stated that 'skin is not totally adherent to the underlying structures'.

Current *in vivo* studies

Three different techniques for analyzing *in vivo* SIJ movements have been used. Sturesson et al (1989, 1999a, 2000a, 2000b) and Tullberg et al (1998) used the RSA technique described by Selvik (1974). The investigations are discussed below.

Kissling & Jacob (1995) performed a study with Kirschner rods in both ilia and sacrum on healthy volunteers. Measurements were made in standing, anteflexion, and retroflexion of the lumbar spine. The study showed an average total rotation in the SIJ between standing erect on both feet and one-legged stance of about 2° (range 0.4–4.3°) and no significant differences were observed with regard to sex, age, or parturition.

Surprisingly, Smidt et al (1995) showed – with a stereophotogrammetric analysis of skin markers in the reciprocal straddle position – a movement much greater than any of the other modern studies reviewed: 'The mean composite oblique–sagittal sacroiliac motion which occurred between the right and left straddle position was 9 degrees.' The greatest error of measurement in this technique is the calculation of the bony landmarks. However, the authors rejected data with a difference of more than 5 mm compared to the neutral standing position. The error of the method is not quite clear.

Roentgen stereophotogrammetric analysis

Selvik introduced RSA in Lund, Sweden, in 1972, and presented it further in his thesis entitled *A roentgen stereophotogrammetric method for the study of the kinematics of the skeletal system* (Lund 1974). RSA is a computerized system for exact radiographic localization of landmarks in the human body.

Technique for sacroiliac motion analysis

Tantalum balls with a diameter of 0.8 mm are implanted into the pelvic bones, using an instrument with a cannula and a spring-piston-release mechanism-striker system (Aronsen 1974) that presses the ball into place. At least three, but usually between four and six, tantalum balls are placed geometrically well spread into each ilium and into the sacrum.

Two roentgen tubes are needed in the roentgen room. Optimal requirements are two ceiling-suspended telescopic units with exposure synchronization. The roentgen films are placed in parallel in a calibration cage with a frame containing tantalum balls. The relationship between the markers and the foci is established at the roentgen examination. This allows for free movements of the object. In the set-up used it is possible to make horizontal and vertical exposures, and the object can move freely in front of the roentgen films as long as it is positioned at the cross-over point of the roentgen beams (Fig. 23.1).

In the studies by Sturesson et al (1989, 1999a, 2000a, 2000b) the patients were examined in eleven different positions in the different studies. The following positions were used: (1) supine; (2) prone with hyperextension of the left leg; (3) prone with hyperextension of the right leg; (4) standing; (5) sitting with straight knees; (6) standing with the left hip maximally flexed; (7) standing with the right hip maximally flexed; (8) standing in the straddle position with the left hip maximally flexed; (9) standing in the straddle position with the right hip maximally flexed; (10) supine with an external Hoffman–Slätis frame; (11) standing with an external Hoffman–Slätis frame. In Tullberg et al's (1998) study the patients were examined in standing before and after treatment.

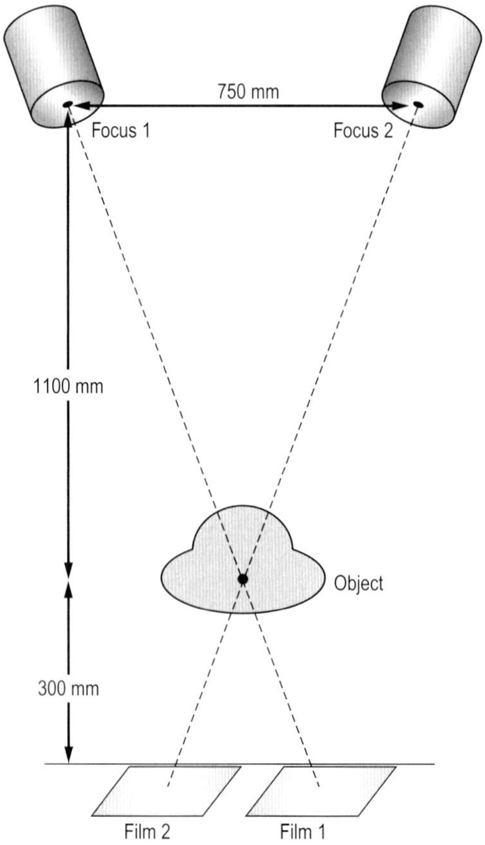

Fig. 23.1 The positions of roentgen tubes, object and roentgen films

Correct positioning of the patient is mandatory to achieve measurable radiographs. For example, if the lower limb is superimposed on the pelvis, the markers cannot be distinctly visualized. For this reason, only a few measurable examinations were made in the sitting position. When analyzing the position with the hip maximally flexed it was necessary to first maximally flex the hip and after that rotate the leg away from the radiation beams. A similar procedure was used when analyzing the films in the study of the effect of the external fixator. In some patients the steel rods of the Hoffmann–Slätis frame obscured the markers.

The sacrum was defined as the fixed segment and the movements were described as rotation around and translation along the three orthogonal axes, as illustrated in Fig. 23.2. The rotation around the helical axis was also analyzed. The movements given are for the center of gravity of the markers in each iliac bone. The mean error for rotation and translation was 0.1–0.2° and 0.1 mm, respectively.

Patient population of the RSA studies

In total, 41 patients (34 women 19–45 years of age, and 7 men aged 18–45 years) were included in the RSA studies by Sturesson et al (1989, 1999a, 2000a, 2000b). The studies were focused on various issues but the basic movement analysis was used in all studies to make the groups in the different studies comparable in a wider perspective. In all, 21 patients had unilateral sacroiliac pain and 20 patients had bilateral symptoms. The studies by Tullberg et al (1998) comprised 10 patients.

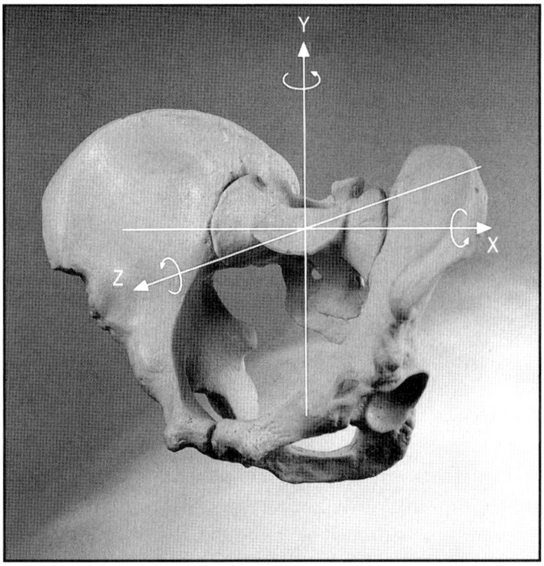

Fig. 23.2 The pelvis with the rotational axes.

Movement analysis

Supine to standing

In the supine position the load on the SIJ is less than in the standing position, when the weight of the upper body is transmitted through the SIJ. Consequently the sacrum was shown to rotate forwards relative to the ilia (nutation) when standing up from a supine position. As shown in Table 23.1, the rotation was equal on both sides, and the mean rotation was 1.3° around the helical axis. Although the rotation was rather small, more than 90% of the movement occurred around the X-axis. The mean rotation around the sagittal axis (Z) and the rotation around the longitudinal axis (Y) were close to zero. The range reflects in some cases a widening in the posterior part of the SIJ and in other cases a closing movement (Y-axis). The widening or closing pattern is also seen around the Z-axis, but to a lesser degree. Probably these movements around the Y- and Z-axes reflect the wide variation in the anatomy of the SIJ (Solonen 1957). The movements around the X-axis and the helical axis did not show statistical differences, thus it can be said that the innominates move around the sacrum as a unit or the sacrum moves symmetrically between the ilia.

Supine to sitting

Compared with the movement pattern from supine to standing, the movement from supine to sitting, both around the helical and the X-axis shows an increase of about 25%. However, the most interesting observation is a small but constant inward movement of the iliac crests, noted as positive values around the Z-axis for the left side and negative values for the right (Table 23.2).

Standing to prone with hyperextension

The largest movement in the SIJ was found between the 'standing to prone with hyperextension' positions (Tables 23.3 and 23.4). In the 'prone position with hyperextension' the load on the SIJ is low and in contrast to the other positions, the movement

Table 23.1 Movements of the SIJs when changing from supine to standing (degrees and mm)

Rotation around the...	Joint	*N*	Mean	SD	Range
X-axis	Left	40	−1.1	0.5	−2.3 to 0.0
	Right	41	−1.2	0.5	−2.5 to −0.2
Y-axis	Left	37	0.1	0.6	−1.0 to 2.0
	Right	38	0.3	0.3	−0.2 to 0.9
Z-axis	Left	37	0.0	0.3	−1.0 to 0.5
	Right	38	0.0	0.3	−0.4 to 1.0
Helical axis	Left	36	1.3	0.5	0.2 to 2.3
	Right	37	1.3	0.6	0.4 to 2.6
Translation	Left	31	0.5	0.3	0.1 to 1.5
	Right	32	0.4	0.3	−0.1 to 1.3

N = number of joints.

Table 23.2 Movements of the SIJs when changing from supine to sitting with straight legs (degrees and mm)

Rotation around the...	Joint	*N*	Mean	SD	Range
X-axis	Left	11	−1.4	0.6	−2.2 to 0.4
	Right	11	−1.4	0.6	−2.5 to 0.6
Y-axis	Left	11	0.1	0.4	0.6 to 1.1
	Right	11	0.4	0.4	−0.4 to 1.1
Z-axis	Left	11	0.5	0.2	0.2 to 0.8
	Right	11	−0.3	0.2	−0.7 to 0
Helical axis	Left	11	1.5	0.6	0.7 to 2.3
	Right	11	1.6	0.6	0.8 to 2.6
Translation	Left	11	0.5	0.4	0.1 to 1.2
	Right	11	0.5	0.1	0.4 to 0.8

N = number of joints.

showed a significant difference between the provoked and the nonprovoked side. The difference (mean) was 0.34° around the helical axis ($P < 0.0001$, paired *t*-test). Although the mean was close to zero, the range of movement around the Y-axis on the provoked side was also greater compared to that on the non-provoked side. The asymmetry in the SIJ probably enlarges the magnitude of the movement around the Y-axis at the end of the physiologic movement although the force is put around the X-axis.

Standing to standing with one hip maximally flexed

The standing flexion test, or 'rücklauf,' was a commonly used diagnostic test for sacroiliac pain. However, it showed low reliability (Potter & Rothstein 1985, Sturesson et al 1999b) and low reproducibility (McCombe et al 1989). In all, 22 patients considered to have sacroiliac pain were analyzed with RSA (Sturesson et al 2000a). The results showed very small movements in the

Table 23.3 Movement of the SIJ when changing position from standing to prone with the left leg hyperextended (degrees and mm)

Rotation around the...	Joint	*N*	Mean	SD	Range
X-axis	Left	30	1.9	0.9	–0.5 to 3.9
	Right	30	1.7	0.7	0.4 to 3.4
Y-axis	Left	30	–0.1	0.7	–1.3 to 2.4
	Right	29	–0.1	0.6	–2.0 to 1.2
Z-axis	Left	30	–0.2	0.3	–0.9 to 0.3
	Right	30	–0.1	0.8	–1.0 to 0.5
Helical axis	Left	30	2.1	0.7	0.9 to 3.9
	Right	29	1.8	0.5	0.6 to 4.0
Translation	Left	23	0.7	0.4	0.3 to 1.8
	Right	23	0.5	0.5	–0.5 to 1.6

N = number of joints.

Table 23.4 Movement of the SIJ when changing position from standing to prone with the right leg hyperextended (degrees and mm)

Rotation around the...	Joint	*N*	Mean	SD	Range
X-axis	Left	29	1.6	0.7	0.6 to 3.1
	Right	30	1.9	0.7	0.2 to 3.6
Y-axis	Left	29	–0.4	0.5	–1.2 to 1.1
	Right	30	–0.3	0.7	–1.2 to 2.0
Z-axis	Left	29	–0.1	0.3	–0.7 to 0.6
	Right	30	0.1	0.4	–0.8 to 0.8
Helical axis	Left	29	1.8	0.6	0.7 to 3.2
	Right	30	2.1	0.7	0.6 to 3.8
Translation	Left	23	0.6	0.3	0.2 to 1.6
	Right	25	0.6	0.5	–0.3 to 1.6

N = number of joints.

SIJ both on the provoked and the nonprovoked side (Tables 23.5 and 23.6). The small movements registered support the theory of form and force closure in the SIJ (Vleeming 1990a, 1990b). The self-locking mechanism when the pelvis is loaded in a one-leg standing position probably obstructs the movements in the sacroiliac joints.

Standing in the straddle position

Smidt et al (1995, 1997) reported in their studies large movements, between 9° and 36° in the SIJ using the sustained reciprocal straddle position. To re-evaluate these results, six women with longstanding (3 to 9 years) lumbopelvic pain after pregnancy were analyzed with RSA in the reciprocal straddle position (Tables 23.7 and 23.8). The data show that a reciprocal movement could be demonstrated in the SIJ in the reciprocal straddle position. However, the movements are tenfold smaller than reported in the studies by Smidt et al (1995, 1997). These data also indicate that there could be a reciprocal movement in the sacroiliac joints in walking, even though this movement would be much less because a normal gait consists of much shorter steps than the test situation, and includes no sustained stance.

Table 23.5 Movement of the SIJ when changing from standing on both feet to standing with the left hip maximally flexed (degrees and mm)

Rotation around the...	Joint	*N*	Mean	SD	Range
X-axis	Left	21	–0.2	0.4	–1.0 to 0.5
	Right	20	–0.2	0.4	–1.4 to 0.2
Y-axis	Left	21	0.2	0.4	–0.7 to 0.8
	Right	20	–0.1	0.4	–0.8 to 0.5
Z-axis	Left	21	0.2	0.3	–0.3 to 0.9
	Right	20	0.1	0.3	–0.4 to 0.8
Helical axis	Left	21	0.6	0.4	0.2 to 1.4
	Right	20	0.6	0.4	0.2 to 1.8
Translation along the helical axis	Left	21	0.3	0.2	0.1 to 1.0
	Right	20	0.3	0.4	0.0 to 2.2

N = number of joints.

Table 23.6 Movement of the SIJ when changing from standing on both feet to standing with the right hip maximally flexed (degrees and mm)

Rotation around the...	Joint	*N*	Mean	SD	Range
X-axis	Left	20	–0.1	0.5	–1.0 to 0.7
	Right	22	–0.2	0.3	–0.7 to 0.2
Y-axis	Left	20	0.0	0.5	–1.1 to 1.8
	Right	22	–0.2	0.5	–1.0 to 0.9
Z-axis	Left	20	0.1	0.4	–0.3 to 1.2
	Right	22	–0.2	0.3	–0.8 to 0.5
Helical axis	Left	20	0.7	0.5	0.1 to 1.8
	Right	22	0.7	0.3	0.2 to 1.2
Translation along helical axis	Left	20	0.3	0.2	0.0 to 0.7
	Right	22	0.3	0.2	0.0 to 0.8

N = number of joints.

This reciprocal movement could also explain the 'catching' of the leg in pregnant women (Sturesson et al 1997).

The effect of an external Hoffman–Slätis frame

External fixation with a Hoffman–Slätis frame indeed reduces SIJ mobility (Table 23.9). The SIJ movements were analyzed (Sturesson et al 1999a) in ten patients with RSA in supine and standing positions, preoperatively and postoperatively with the external fixator applied. Eight patients could be used for the statistical analysis and the median reduction in rotation was 55% on the left side and 63% on the right side around the helical axes, and 74% around the X-axes on the left side and 66% on the right side. Already when the external frame was tightened, an anterior rotation of the sacrum was observed. Together with the reduction in movement in the SIJ, this anterior rotation of the sacrum into a more stable position corresponds well to the principles of form and force closure introduced by Vleeming et al (1990b).

Table 23.7 Movements of the sacroiliac joints when alternating the straddle position from standing with the left hip maximally extended and the right hip maximally flexed, to standing with the right hip maximally extended and the left hip maximally flexed (the sacrum is the fixed segment) (degrees)

Rotation around the...	Joint	*N*	Mean	Range
X-axis	Left	6	−1.0	−0.3 to −1.6
	Right	6	0.9	0.8 to 1.1
Y-axis	Left	6	0.3	−0.8 to 1.0
	Right	6	0.4	0.2 to 0.8
Z-axis	Left	6	−0.5	−1.4 to 0.0
	Right	6	−0.4	−1.0 to 0.0
Helical axis	Left	6	1.3	0.7 to 2.1
	Right	6	1.2	0.9 to 1.3

N = number of joints.

Table 23.8 Movements of the innominates when alternating the straddle position from standing with the left hip maximally extended and the right hip maximally flexed, to standing with the right hip maximally extended and the left hip maximally flexed (the left ilium is selected as the fixed segment) (degrees)

Rotation around the...	*N*	Mean	Range
X-axis	6	1.9	1.3 to 2.4
Y-axis	6	0.2	−0.5 to 1.6
Z-axis	6	0.1	−0.2 to 0.4

N = number of joints.

The effect of manipulation

Tullberg et al (1998) studied the effect of manipulation. The patients were examined both clinically and with RSA before and after the manipulation. In none of the 10 patients did manipulation alter the position of the sacrum in relation to the ileum, defined by RSA. Positional test results changed from positive before manipulation to normal after.

Men versus women

The mean mobility of the SIJ for men is about 40% smaller than the movement registered for women between the positions 'supine to standing' (X-axis

Table 23.9 The difference in movement between supine and standing, with or without the external frame applied. The values around the transverse (X) and the helical (H) axes on the left and right side are presented. (Wilcoxon Sign rank test)

	N	Median	Range	*P*-value
Without frame X left	8	−1.2	−0.5 to −2.3	0.02
With frame X left	8	−0.5	−0.2 to −1.6	
Without frame H left	8	1.3	0.8 to 2.3	0.03
With frame H left	8	0.6	0.3 to 1.7	
Without frame X right	8	−1.1	−0.4 to −2.4	0.02
With frame X right	8	−0.4	−0.1 to −0.7	
Without frame H right	8	1.4	0.8 to 2.5	0.1
With frame H right	8	0.4	0.3 to 1.9	

N = number of joints.

Table 23.10 Movements of the sacroiliac joints around the X-axis and helical axis when changing from supine to standing position, split by sex (degrees)

Rotation around the...	Sex	*N*	Mean	Range
X-axis	Male	12	–0.7	–0.1 to –1.2
	Female	55	–1.3	0.0 to –2.4
Helical axis	Male	10	0.7	0.2 to 1.3
	Female	52	1.4	0.6 to 2.5

N = number of joints.

Table 23.11 Movements of the sacroiliac joints around the X-axis and helical axis when changing from supine to standing position, in patients with unilateral respectively bilateral symptoms (degrees)

Rotation around the...		*N*	Mean	Range
X-axis	Unilateral	41	–1.0	0 to –2.0
	Bilateral	40	–1.4	–0.6 to –2.5
Helical axis	Unilateral	35	1.2	0.2 to 2.2
	Bilateral	40	1.5	0.7 to 2.6

N = number of joints.

$P = 0.0002$; helical axis $P < 0.0001$ unpaired *t*-test; Table 23.10). Between the positions 'standing' and 'prone with hyperextension' the mean difference between men and women was about 30%.

Age

With age, there was no decrease in total mobility. In fact, there was a statistically significant increase with age between 'supine to sitting' ($r = 0.7$, $n = 11$, $P < 0.05$) and 'standing to prone with hyperextension' ($r = 0.6$, $n = 15$, $P < 0.01$ regression analysis).

Hypermobility

Interestingly, the movements in patients with bilateral symptoms ($n = 20$) were larger than those in the group with unilateral symptoms. In 'supine to standing' the mean rotation was 1.4° around the X-axis and 1.5° around the helical axis in the group with bilateral symptoms, and 1.1° and 1.2°, respectively, in the group with unilateral symptoms (X-axis $P = 0.0045$; helical axis $P = 0.0238$ unpaired *t*-test; Table 23.11).

Among the patients with unilateral symptoms, the mean mobility around both the X- and helical axes of the symptomatic joints was equal to the mobility of the asymptomatic joints. The standard deviations were about the same for symptomatic and asymptomatic joints.

Discussion

The first implantation of tantalum markers in patients occurred in 1973. In 1990 it was calculated that 2000 patients had been investigated using about 20 000 tantalum balls. Nowadays, about 50 000 tantalum balls have been implanted in 5000 patients, mostly in Sweden but also in the Netherlands and USA.

RSA has taken the role as the gold standard in determining mobility in orthopedic research concerning growth, small movements in joints and tendons, and in micromotion of arthroplasties. The error of the method is so small that hardly any other technique can compete in terms of precision. As with all methods, it has its drawbacks, for example, the procedure is time-consuming. Furthermore, there is a need for technical skill in all the different steps, and for the support of an engineer with knowledge of kinematic analysis (KINLAB, KINERR, X-RAY 90). Because of the radiation dose, RSA cannot be used on volunteers. The dose-equivalent of radiation in patients examined with 8 to 10 double exposures on the pelvic bones varied between 2.3 and 7.2 mSv (Sturesson et al 1989). This is equal to the radiation dose of an ordinary plain roentgenogram of the lower back and pelvis.

As far as the SIJ is concerned, the identical movements of symptomatic and asymptomatic joints show that RSA cannot identify a SIJ dysfunction. However, we have shown that there are probably small differences in mobility between patients with unilateral and with bilateral symptoms (see Table 23.11). It might be that patients with unilateral symptoms and those with bilateral symptoms reflect groups with a different etiology. Good evidence is lacking but it can be postulated that pain in patients with unilateral symptoms primarily is caused by trauma or reactive arthritis. In patients with bilateral symptoms the cause could be overload, for example after pregnancy, especially among women with relatively larger SIJ mobility. The SIJs are probably comparable with other joints and hypermobility is likely to involve a subgroup of individuals in the upper range of the normal distribution of mobility.

Standing on both legs as well as standing on one leg with the other leg flexed implies load on the SIJ. When standing on one leg not only does the load of the body weight act on the SIJ but so too do the stabilizing muscles around the pelvis. Thus the load is more than doubled as compared to standing on both legs. That means that the lateral forces on the SIJ must increase to withstand the increased load and to balance the entire pelvis as well as to stabilize the SIJ.

Kissling & Jacob (1995), using Kirschner wires in both ilia and sacrum, obtained similar results with stereophotogrammetry as were found with the RSA. The main advantage of their technique is the lack of radiation. However, the procedures and analyzing technique appear to be more complicated for the patients. Furthermore, the sacral bone is rather thin in the central part and it is difficult to get a good grip for the Kirschner wires. They can be placed in the lateral part of the sacrum but there they will be influenced by the large dorsal sacroiliac ligaments, thus affecting the accuracy.

Noninvasive techniques using different types of skin marker probably measure a complex motion, involving also the connective tissue and skin. In themselves, they cannot reflect real SIJ motion, but if compared with data obtained with the RSA or 'Kirschner wire technique' they can be of value in showing for example reduced mobility.

Summary

- RSA is a technique for measuring small SIJ movements with a high accuracy and specificity. The results probably reflect real SIJ movements. Another invasive technique using Kirschner wires shows a similar pattern of movement in the SIJ.
- The SIJ movements are small and normally distributed.
- SIJ mobility in men is on average 30–40% less than in women.
- Small differences in SIJ movements occur between patients with unilateral and patients with bilateral pain.
- No significant differences occur in mobility between symptomatic and asymptomatic joints in patients with unilateral symptoms.
- The RSA studies reveal no indications of hypo- or hypermobility.
- Manipulation does not alter the position of the SIJ.
- The movements of the SIJ are reduced by muscular force.
- The movements of the SIJ are reduced by increased load.
- The movements in the SIJ can be reduced by an external Hoffman–Slätis frame.
- The movements in the SIJ in the straddle position show a reciprocal pattern.
- The movements in the SIJ are greater in the less loaded situation compared to the loaded situation.
- For clinical use as yet no technique measuring mobility can be recommended because it cannot reveal a SIJ disorder. RSA and other mobility measuring techniques can be recommended for further research concerning SIJ biomechanics.

References

Aronson AS, Holst L, Selvik G 1974 An instrument for insertion of radiopaque bone markers. Radiology 113:733–734

Colachis SC Jr, Worden RE, Brechtol CO, Strohm BR 1963 Movement of the sacroiliac joint in the adult male: A preliminary report. Arch Phys Med Rehabil 44:490–498

Egund N, Olsson TH, Schmid H, Selvik G 1978 Movements in the sacroiliac joints demonstrated with roentgen stereophotogrammetry. Acta Radiol Diagn 19:833–846

Grieve EFM 1983 Mechanical dysfunction of the sacroiliac joint. Int Rehab Med 5:46–52

KINLAB, KINERR, X-ray 90; RSA BioMedical Innovations AB, Box 1450, S-901 24 Umeå, Sweden

Kissling RO, Jacob HAC 1995 The mobility of the sacro-iliac joint in healthy subjects. In: Vleeming A et al (eds) Second Interdisciplinary World Congress on Low Back Pain: the Integrated Function of the Lumbar Spine and Sacroiliac Joints, p411–422

McCombe PF, Fairbank JCT, Cockersole BC, Pynsent PB 1989 Reproducibility of physical signs in low-back pain. Spine 14:908–918

Miller JAA, Schultz AB, Andersson GBJ 1987 Load-displacement behaviour of sacro-iliac joints. J Orthop Res 5:92–101

Potter NA, Rothstein JM 1985 Intertester reliability for selected clinical tests of the sacroiliac joint. Phys Ther 11:1671–1675

Selvik G 1974 A roentgen stereophotogrammetric method for the study of the kinematics of the skeletal system. AV-centralen, Lund, Sweden. [Reprinted 1989.] Acta Orth Scand 60 (suppl):232

Smidt GL, McQuade K, Wei S-H, Barakatt E 1995 Sacroiliac kinematics for reciprocal straddle positions. Spine 20:1047–1054

Smidt GL, Wei S-H, McQuade K et al 1997 Sacroiliac motion for extreme hip positions. Spine 22:2073–2082

Solonen KA 1957 The sacroiliac joint in the light of anatomical, roentgenological and clinical studies. Acta Orthop Scand 27 (suppl):4–127

Sturesson B, Selvik G, Udén A 1989 Movements of the sacroiliac joints. A roentgen stereophotogrammetric analysis. Spine 14:162–165.

Sturesson B, Udén G, Udén A 1997 Pain pattern in pregnancy and 'catching' of the leg in pregnant women with posterior pelvic pain. Spine 22:1880–1891

Sturesson B, Udén A, Önsten I 1999a Can an external frame fixation reduce the movements in the sacroiliac joints? A radiostereometric analysis of 10 patients. Acta Orthop Scand 70(1):42–46

Sturesson B, Ekeblom A, Rylander G, Nelson NE 1999b A reliability study of diagnostic tests for sacroiliac joint dysfunction. In thesis Load and movement of the sacroiliac joint LUMEDW/MEDOM-1040-SE, pp. 29–34

Sturesson B, Udén A, Vleeming A 2000a A radiostereometric analysis of movements of the sacroiliac joints during the standing hip flexion test. Spine 25(3):364–368

Sturesson B, Udén A, Vleeming A 2000b A radiostereometric analysis of the movements of the sacroiliac joints in the reciprocal straddle position. Spine 25(2): 214–217

Tullberg T, Blomberg S, Branth B, Johnson R 1998 Manipulation does not alter the position of the sacroiliac joint. A roentgen stereophotogrammetric analysis. Spine 23(10):1124–1128

Vleeming A, Stoeckart R, Volkers ACW, Snijders CJ 1990a Relation between form and function in the sacroiliac joint. 1: Clinical anatomical aspects. Spine 15:130–132

Vleeming A, Volkers ACW, Snijders CJ, Stoeckart R 1990b Relation between form and function in the sacroiliac joint. 2: Biomechanical aspects. Spine 15(2):133–136

Vleeming A, van Wingerden JP, Dijkstra PF et al 1992 Mobility in the sacroiliac joints in the elderly: a kinematic and radiological study. Clin Biomech 7:170–176

Weisl H 1955 The movements of the sacro-iliac joint. Acta Anat 23:80–91

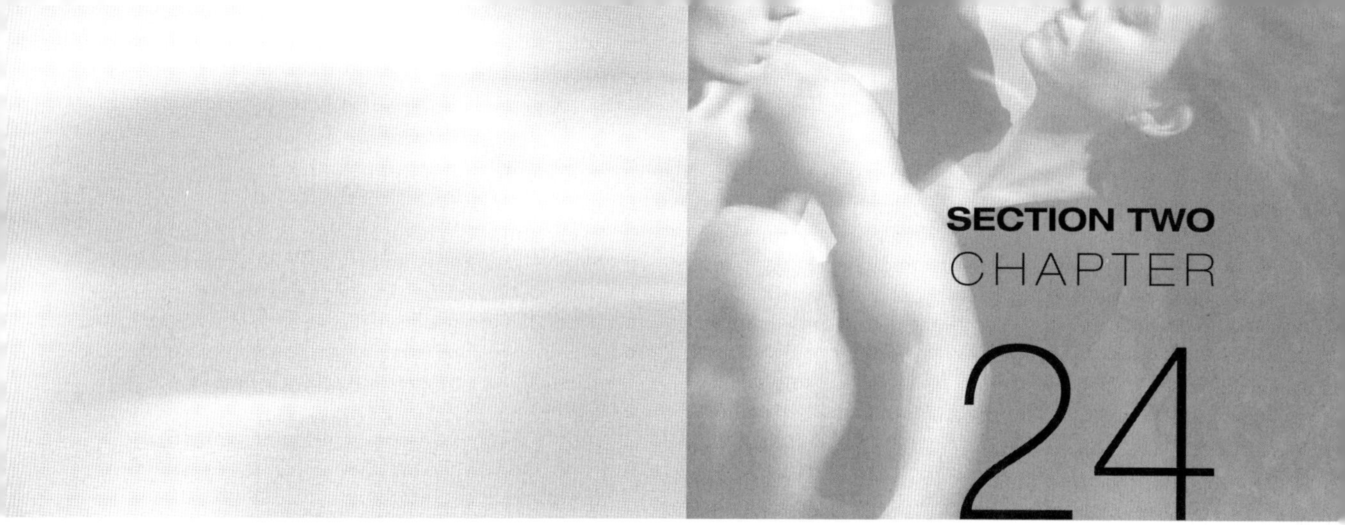

SECTION TWO
CHAPTER 24

What is pelvic girdle pain?

HC Östgaard

Introduction

Pelvic pain is a well-known problem that has been documented during pregnancy since the time of Hippocrates. It was believed that the pelvis expanded during the first pregnancy and remained permanently enlarged throughout life. In the sixteenth century, it was maintained that delivery was possible only because of enormous yielding of the female pelvis. At the end of the nineteenth century, Cantin (1899) found palpable evidence of movement of the pubic symphysis among all but 2% of 500 women late in pregnancy. He believed that increased motion in the pelvic joints was a problem in itself. He also believed that it was the most common and most overlooked problem in pregnancy.

Several authors have described pelvic pain in modern times (Albert et al 2001, 2002, Berg 1988, Farbrot 1952, Fast et al 1987, Kristiansson et al 1996, Larsen et al 1999, MacLennan et al 1986, Mantle et al 1997, Östgaard et al 1994a, Wu et al 2004). Increased motion in the symphysis pubis during pregnancy has been illustrated on X-rays from the eighth week in normal pregnancies (Genell 1949), by ultrasound during delivery (Bjorklund et al 1996), and during load-bearing post partum (Mens et al 1996), so there is no correlation between the increase in symphyseal motion and pelvic pain. Therefore, increased motion in the pelvic joints is not the main problem. However, there is scientific evidence that motion in the pelvic joints is poorly controlled and that activity and coordination in the large stabilizing muscles around the sacroiliac joints (SIJs) are disturbed among patients with pelvic girdle pain (Hungerford et al 2003, O'Sullivan et al 2002). Furthermore, asymmetric stiffness of the SIJ is more often found among patients with pelvic girdle pain (Damen et al 2001).

Despite the development of imaging techniques, including computerized tomography (CT), magnetic resonance tomography (MRT), ultrasound, and scintigraphy, most patients with pelvic pain have normal findings, indicating that the pain is not derived primarily from the skeleton and that there are no major soft-tissue changes. So, in line with what is known from unspecific lumbar back problems, pain in the pelvis is most likely to emanate from the large, stabilizing muscles around the pelvis. Therefore, we have to rely mainly on a thorough clinical examination and a good history when diagnosing pelvic pain.

Earlier studies have shown that it is important to separate pelvic pain from lumbar back pain during pregnancy (Endresen 1995, Kristiansson et al 1996, Östgaard et al 1991a, 1994a, 1996, Wu et al 2004). To emphasize the fact that this type of pain is not derived from the viscera inside the pelvis, but more likely from the muscles, ligaments, and joint capsules, the term 'pelvic girdle pain' was introduced. The two types of pain should be treated differently, because standard treatment of the lumbar muscles can increase pain in the pelvic girdle (Dumas et al 1995b).

Definition

Pelvic girdle pain (PGP) is a specific form of low back pain, which can occur separately or together with lumbar back pain. PGP generally arises in relation to pregnancy, more rarely after trauma or arthritis. Pain is experienced between the posterior iliac crest and the gluteal fold, particularly in the vicinity of the SIJ. The pain can radiate into the posterior thigh and can occur in conjunction with pain in the symphysis. The endurance capacity for standing, walking, and sitting is diminished and turning over in bed is difficult and painful. The diagnosis of PGP can be reached only after exclusion of lumbar causes. The pain and functional disturbances in relation to PGP must be reproducible by specific clinical tests.

Epidemiology

The incidence of PGP varies in different studies because different definitions of the diagnosis have been used and because different selections of patients have been made (Wu et al 2004). The true incidence of PGP in a general population is not known, but in two studies (Petersen et al 2004, Schwarzer et al 1995) it was estimated that a substantial portion of patients with nonspecific low back pain had some type of pelvic pain.

Many authors have attempted to describe the incidence and prevalence of PGP in pregnancy. However, obtaining a clear picture is difficult because the reported incidences of PGP and low back pain are not always separated in the literature, where incidence ranges between 4% and 76.4% (Wu et al 2004).

PGP is frequent among pregnant women and a few well-performed studies using modern definitions (Albert et al 2002, Berg et al 1988, Kristiansson et al 1996, Larsen et al 1999, Östgaard et al 1991a, 1994a) found that 20% of all pregnant women had PGP during pregnancy. Fortunately, the majority of women recover shortly after delivery but some (5–7%; Östgaard & Andersson 1992, Schwarzer et al 1995) with pain during pregnancy do not get well after delivery. These women often encounter little understanding when they seek medical advice for their pain. They are often misunderstood and treated as psychosomatic cases. Sometimes pain from the lumbar region of the back is confused with pain from the posterior pelvis, or vice versa. Therefore, unspecified treatment for back pain in pregnant women often fails (Dumas et al 1995a, 1995b).

Pain intensity has been reported to average 4.3 on a 0–10 visual analogue scale, with large variations and maximum pain intensity around the thirtieth week of pregnancy (Östgaard et al 1991a).

Diagnosing pelvic girdle pain

The patient will present a typical history with certain characteristics. Furthermore, pain and function impairment can be identified by a few well-defined, scientifically evaluated clinical tests.

History

- Pain in the posterior part of the pelvis, distal and lateral to the L5 (preferably illustrated on a pain drawing).
- The endurance capacity for standing, walking and sitting is reduced.
- Pronounced difficulty when turning over in bed.
- Free motion in hips and spine, no radiation below the knee.

Clinical tests

The posterior pelvic pain provocation test

The posterior pelvic pain provocation (4P) test is useful in identifying pelvic girdle pain. It is performed with the patient supine and her hip flexed to 90°. When the femur is gently pressed posteriorly by the examiner, simultaneously stabilizing the patient's pelvis, the test is said to be positive when the woman feels pain that she recognizes in her posterior pelvis (Östgaard et al 1994a, 1994b) (Figs 24.1 and 24.2). The test is not known to be specific for any anatomic structure but it does help to identify women with posterior pelvic pain. Evaluation of the test has shown that in this aspect the test has a specificity of 80% and a sensitivity of 81% (Östgaard et al 1994b). Patients with well-defined lumbar back pain diagnoses, herniated discs for example, will not have a positive test response (author's comment).

The Gaenslen test

The patient, lying supine, flexes the knee and hip at the side to be examined, the thigh being pressed against the abdomen with the aid of both the patient's hands clasped around the flexed knee.

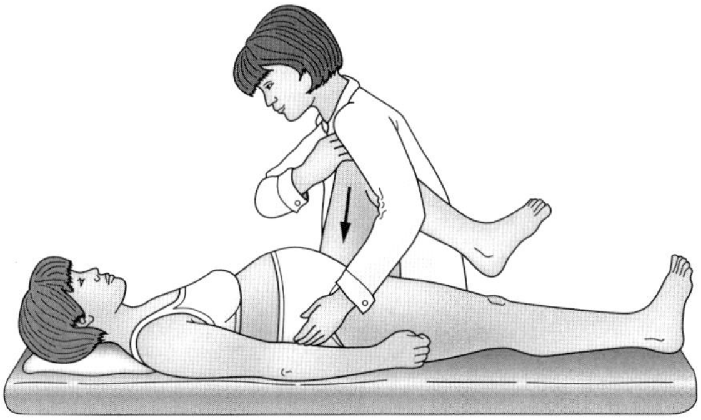

Fig. 24.1 The posterior pelvic pain provocation test.

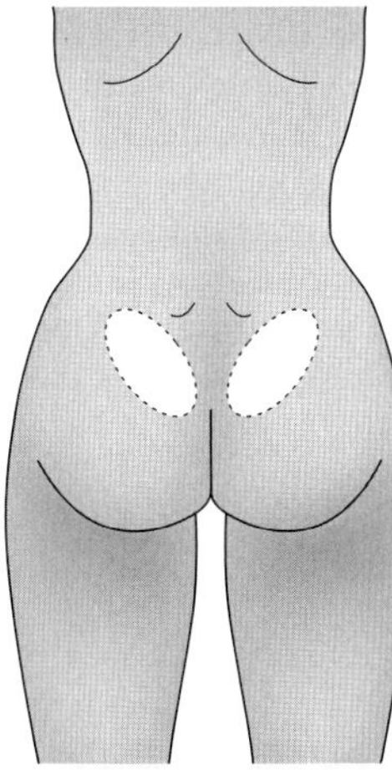

Fig. 24.2 Pain should be experienced here at provocation.

The patient is then moved to the side of the table and the opposite thigh is slowly hyperextended by the examiner with gradually increasing force by pressure of the examiner's hand on the top of the knee. With the opposite hand, the examiner assists the patient in fixing the lumbar spine and pelvis by pressure over the patient's clasped hands. The test is positive if the patient experiences pain. Gaenslen described this test in 1927 as a test for lumbosacral disease, but in the case of no lumbosacral disease, the test will provoke pain on the tested side in the pelvic girdle in patients with PGP (Albert et al 2000) (Fig. 24.3).

Long dorsal ligament test

The patient lies prone or – if pregnant – on her side, and is tested for tenderness on bilateral palpation of the long dorsal ligaments of the sacroiliac joints, directly under the caudal part of the posterior superior iliac spine. A skilled examiner scores the pain on a scale from: no pain = 0; mild = 1; moderate = 2; unbearable pain = 3. Both sides are added so that the sum score ranges from 0 to 6. The test has been studied only on postpartum women. Sensitivity for women with PGP was 76%, with higher sensitivity for women with serious pain (Vleeming et al 2002) (Fig. 24.4).

Patrick's faber test

The patient lies supine. One leg is flexed, abducted, and externally rotated (*faber*, abbreviation of flexion abduction and external rotation) so that the heel rests on the opposite knee. If pain is felt in the SIJ or in the symphysis the test is considered positive. HT Patrick (1860–1938) described this test for coxarthrosis, but in the case of a normal hip joint the test will provoke pain on the tested side among patients with PGP (Albert et al 2002) (Fig. 24.5).

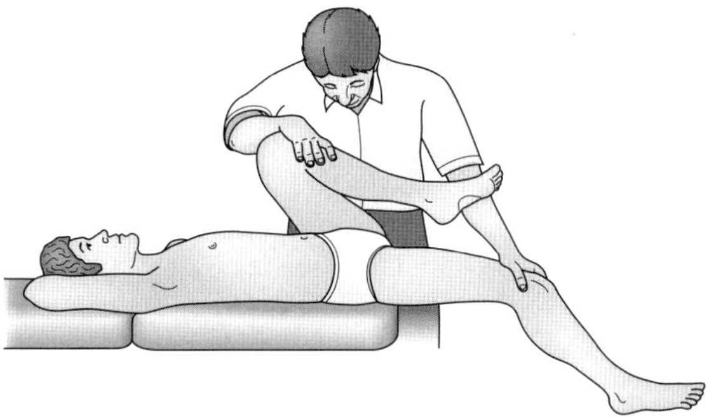

Fig. 24.3 The Gaenslen test.

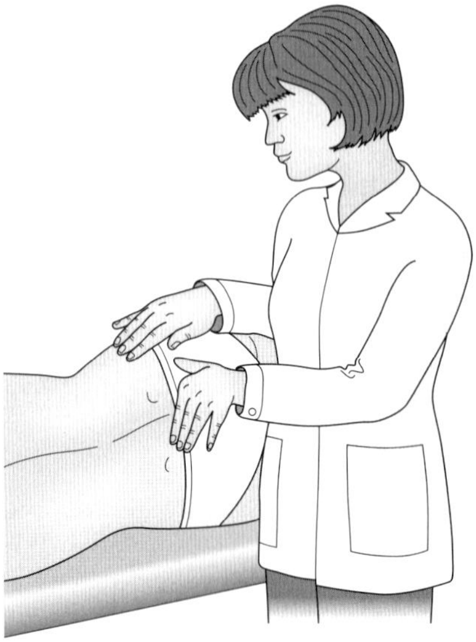

Fig. 24.4 The long dorsal ligament test.

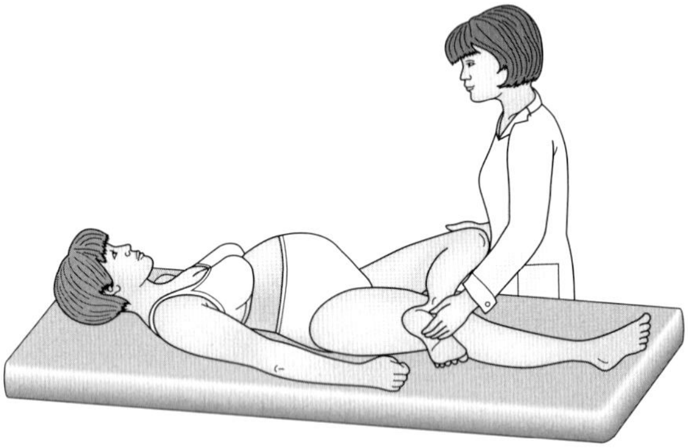

Fig. 24.5 Patrick's faber test.

Modified Trendelenburg test

The patient stands on one leg, flexes the other at 90° in hip and knee. If pain is experienced in the symphysis the test is positive (Albert et al 2000) (Fig. 24.6).

Active straight leg raise test

The test is functional and is performed with the patient in a supine position with straight leg and feet 20 cm apart. The test is performed after the instruction: 'Try to raise your legs, one after the other, above the couch for 20 cm without bending the knee'. The patient is asked to score impairment on a 6-point scale: not difficult at all = 0; minimally difficult = 1; somewhat difficult/difficult = 2; fairly difficult = 3; very difficult = 4; unable to do = 5.

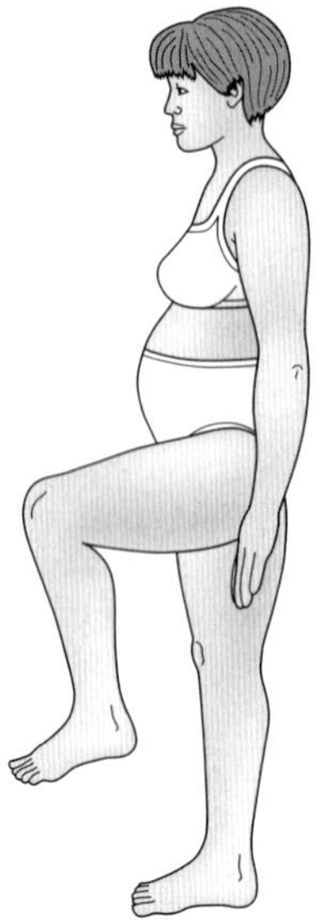

Fig. 24.6 The modified Trendelenburg test.

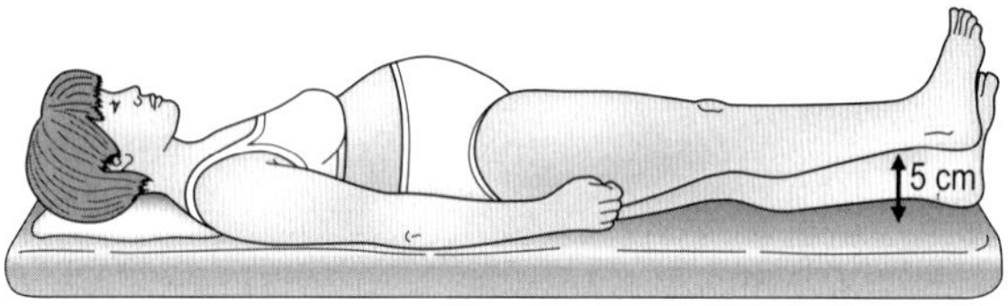

Fig. 24.7 The active straight leg raise test.

The scores on both sides are added, so that the sum score ranges from 0 to 10 (Mens et al 1999, 2002) (Fig. 24.7).

Pain drawings

Pain drawings are useful when back pain in a nonpregnant population is classified (Ransford et al 1975); they are also a great help among patients with PGP (Sturesson et al 1997). Patients can fill in these pain drawings before the consultation. The markings are in different areas for lumbar pain and PGP (Fig. 24.8). Furthermore, pain drawings will help to identify patients with non-physiologic pain patterns.

Development of pain

When using the above-mentioned criteria, the two types of pain will be distributed in incidence during pregnancy as shown in Fig. 24.9 (Norén et al 2002) and will respond to different physiotherapy

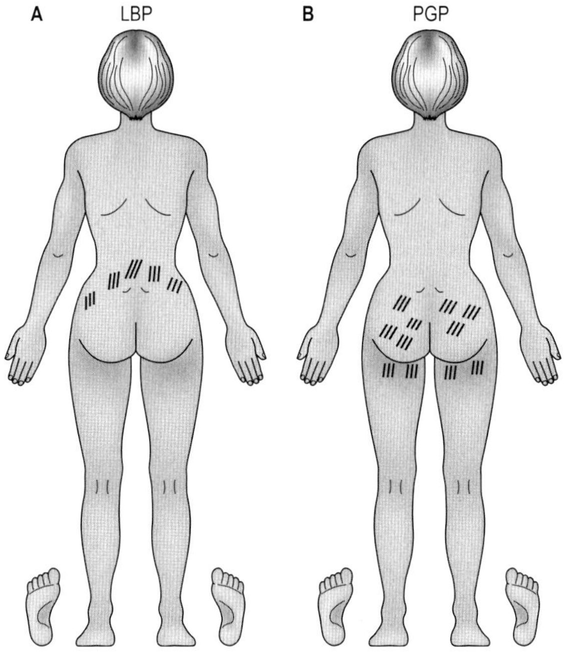

Fig. 24.8 Pain drawings of lumbar back pain (A) and pelvic girdle pain (B).

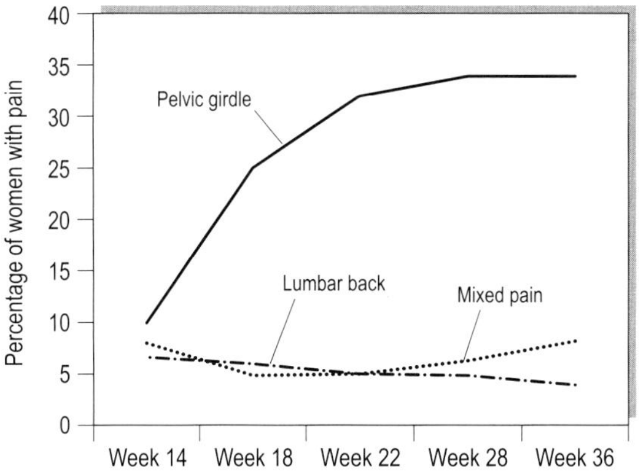

Fig. 24.9 Incidences of lumbar back pain, pelvic girdle pain, and mixed pain during pregnancy.

(Östgaard et al 1994a). About 10% of the women will have symptoms from the pelvis as well as from the lumbar back (Östgaard et al 1994a). The majority of these women will have had a lumbar back pain problem for a long time and have developed PGP later. Pain intensity is higher among patients with PGP. After pregnancy, pain in the lumbar back is the more intense. Furthermore, after delivery, women with PGP will improve more than women with lumbar pain (Östgaard et al 1996).

Box 24.1

Summary of characteristics for lumbar back and pelvic girdle pain

Lumbar back pain

- Often a history of lumbar back pain
- A pain drawing with markings cranial to the sacrum
- Pain and decreased range of motion in the lumbar spine
- Pain on palpation of the erector spine muscle
- A negative posterior pelvic pain provocation test

Pelvic girdle pain

- Debut of pain in relation to pregnancy, trauma or inflammatory joint disease
- Pain drawings with markings in the gluteal area
- Time- and weight-bearing-related pain
- Pain-free intervals with sudden attacks
- A free range of motion in the hips and spine and no nerve root syndrome
- Pain and difficulty when turning over in bed
- A positive posterior pelvic pain provocation test

After delivery

In the majority of women, PGP disappears within 3 months of delivery (Östgaard & Andersson 1992, Schwarzer et al 1995). However, some women develop chronic pain, which will persist even after the pelvic ligaments have regained their normal tension. These women should be referred to a physiotherapist for specific training of the muscles of the pelvis, abdomen, and back. It is important that the pelvic muscles are attended to firstly in order to control the movements in the pelvic joints, and only thereafter should training of the back muscles be initiated (Dumas et al 1995a, 1995b). This rehabilitation is slow, 6–12 months, and always includes periods of serious relapse, which is very discouraging. It is important that the women are informed about this at the beginning of rehabilitation (author's comment).

A small group of women with PGP recover shortly after delivery and return to a physically demanding daily life, only to experience severe PGP some months later. Unfortunately, this is a bad omen. These women can be difficult to treat and their rehabilitation can extend over several years. The treatment program is the same, but it should start at a very low level and increase very slowly, with careful observation of relapses. To avoid this problem, it should be emphasized that after delivery, although PGP has disappeared, strenuous work should be avoided for at least 6 months if a woman has suffered from that condition during pregnancy. There is a strong correlation between high pain intensity during pregnancy and persisting problems after delivery (Östgaard & Andersson 1992, Östgaard et al 1996).

Painkillers seldom have any substantial effect and are best avoided during pregnancy and breast-feeding. Among women who have been treated correctly during pregnancy, we have not seen severe prolonged postpartum problems. It should therefore be possible to avoid these persisting pain problems in the future (author's comment).

Women with pain during pregnancy often worry about their own future, harming the fetus, and their ability to take care of their newborn child being so disabled. However, there is evidence that problems with the child or the delivery itself in no way correlate with lumbar or pelvic girdle pain suffered during pregnancy (Östgaard et al 1991b). Furthermore, the pain normally reduces substantially after delivery, often within a few days, so taking care of the newborn baby is seldom a great problem.

In looking for an explanation for PGP, oral contraception is often mentioned. However, two studies (Bjorklund et al 2000, Östgaard et al 1991b) show that no such correlation exists. This indicates that all women can use oral contraception before and after pregnancy, from an orthopedic point of view.

Because pregnancy-induced hormonal changes are a prerequisite for PGP, speculations about breast-feeding have arisen. Breastfeeding is supposed to change normal hormone levels and block ovulation to prevent a new early pregnancy. This might have an impact on the ligaments of the pelvis and thus on pain. One study (Östgaard & Andersson 1992) shows no correlation between breastfeeding and regression of lumbar or pelvic pain after pregnancy, so having PGP is not a reason to stop breastfeeding. Furthermore, it is not logical to believe that breastfeeding, with its blocking effect on ovulation, should increase pregnancy-induced problems.

If more children are planned, one can speculate about the timing of the next pregnancy. There is no study on this issue, but even severe PGP often disappears within 1 year, provided that treatment is correct. Therefore PGP should not be the limiting factor when timing the next pregnancy. On the contrary, women well educated in the locomotor problems of pregnancy do not have to wait until all symptoms have disappeared before becoming pregnant again. In most cases, increased awareness of symptoms and early treatment will be sufficient. Lumbar back pain is little affected by a new pregnancy.

The question about vaginal delivery for women with pelvic girdle or lumbar pain is often raised. However, pregnancy in itself is the main reason for developing PGP, not delivery, so PGP is not an indication for Cesarean section, and lumbar pain is not affected by delivery. Therefore neither of these conditions should determine the way of delivery.

In some centers, chronic PGP is treated by fusion of the SIJs. This is, in my opinion, seldom necessary.

Anatomic pain localization

There are no studies on which structures are responsible for pain in patients with PGP; this is also the case with nonspecified lumbar back pain. However, coordination and exercise of the stabilizing muscles of the pelvic girdle, as well as a pelvic belt, help relieve pain and will eventually often cure the condition. It is therefore logical to conclude that uncontrolled, but not necessarily increased, motion in the SIJs resulting in extreme positions and in tense joint capsules and ligaments, instead of well-controlled muscular dynamic stabilized joints might create pain in joint capsules and ligaments. That pain in itself might create a reflex isometric contraction of the same stabilizing muscles of the pelvic girdle, and muscles working static instead of dynamic are painful and insufficient. A vicious circle is created and might go on indefinitely if left untreated. This theory might explain why the pain provocation tests work, and is in line with the functional observations among patients with PGP. However, it remains speculative because there are no studies on the subject.

The model

One model for taking care of pregnant women with back or pelvic pain is as follows. At her first visit to the midwife or obstetrician, the pregnant woman should be informed about possible future back and pelvic problems and where to get help, as well as the usual obstetric topics. A physiotherapist with a special interest in pregnancy problems is often preferable in this discussion. Helping a pregnant woman with such problems calls for teamwork because no obstetrician, midwife, or physiotherapist alone possesses all the necessary interdisciplinary knowledge. Whenever back pain occurs, the woman should have a thorough back and pelvic assessment and the problem should be identified as being lumbar back, PGP, or a combination of the two. An educational and training program should be developed with individual variations depending on the type of pain, and on demands from work and daily life. It has been shown that changes in ergonomics at the workplace are useful in reducing pain even during pregnancy (Östgaard et al 1994a). If needed, a pelvic belt should be provided. Initially, it is important that women are given at least one individual consultation with the physiotherapist, but later on they might join fitness classes for pregnant women with the same pain type. However, some 15% of the women change from one pain type to another during pregnancy, and they should also change their training (Östgaard et al 1994a). Furthermore, some women might get worse and have to return to individual therapy for a time.

Summary

1. Patients with any type of back pain should be identified as early as possible and enrolled in a special program according to pain, be it back or pelvic girdle.
2. Back pain in relation to pregnancy should always be divided into two types, depending on the pattern of pain: pain in the lumbar area, and pain in the pelvic girdle.
3. Differentiation into the two types of pain can be made by means of a short history taking and a simple back and pelvis examination, including the specific pelvic pain provocation tests.
4. The two groups of women should be provided with individual information about their specific condition, and a program for muscle training and relaxation should be developed accordingly.
5. Women with combined pelvic and lumbar problems must be treated for pelvic problems first and only later, when the pelvic girdle is under control, for lumbar back problems.
6. The program must respect individual needs at home and at work, and any change in pain pattern should be assessed and followed by changes in the program.
7. A pelvic belt is recommended for women with PGP.
8. The prescription of abundant rest as the only treatment will do few patients any good but will complicate rehabilitation because of general muscle wasting.
9. In case of pregnancy, PGP should disappear spontaneously within 3 months. If it does not, the woman should consult a physiotherapist with special insight in pelvic girdle treatment to avoid a chronic pain condition.
10. After delivery attention is often focused on the newborn, and the problems for the mother are either easily missed or are expected to disappear spontaneously along with other problems of pregnancy. Although newborn babies are fascinating, more attention should be paid to the mothers; they might not be as well as they pretend.

References

Albert H, Godskesen M, Westergaard J 2000 Evaluation of clinical tests used in classification procedures in pregnancy-related pelvic joint pain. Eur Spine J 9: 161–166

Albert H, Godskesen M, Westergaard J 2001 Prognosis in four syndromes of pregnancy-related pelvic pain. Acta Obstet Gynecol Scand 80: 505–510

Albert HB, Godskesen M, Westergaard JG 2002 Incidence of four syndromes of pregnancy-related pelvic joint pain. Spine 27:2831–2834

Berg G, Hammar M, Möller-Nielsen J et al 1988 Low back pain during pregnancy. Obstetrics and Gynecology 71:71–74

Bjorklund K, Bergström S, Lindgren PG, Ulmsten U 1996 Ultrasonographic measurement of the symphysis pubis: a potential method of studying symphysiolysis in pregnancy. Gynecol Obstet Invest 42:151–153

Bjorklund K, Nordstrom ML, Odlind V 2000 Combined oral contraceptives do not increase the risk of back and pelvic pain during pregnancy or after delivery. Acta Obstet Gynecol Scand 79:979–983

Cantin L 1899 Relouchement des symphysies et artralgies pelviennes d'origne gravidique. Thesis, Paris

Damen L, Buyruk HM, Guler-Uysal F et al 2001 Pelvic pain during pregnancy is associated with asymmetric laxity of the sacroiliac joints. Acta Obstet Gynecol Scand 80:1019–1024

Dumas G, Reid JG, Wolfe LA, McGrath MJ 1995a Exercise, posture, and back pain during pregnancy. 1: exercise and posture. Clin Biomech 10:98–103

Dumas G, Reid JG, Wolfe LA, McGrath MJ 1995b Exercise, posture, and back pain during pregnancy. 2: exercise and back pain. Clin Biomech 10:104–109

Endresen E 1995 Pelvic pain and low back pain in pregnant women. An epidemiological study. Scand J Rheumatol 24:135–141

Farbrot E 1952 The relationship of the effect and pain of pregnancy to the anatomy of the pelvis. Acta Radiologica 38:403–417

Fast A, Shapiro D, Ducommun J et al 1987 Low back pain in pregnancy. Spine 12: 368–371

Genell S 1949 Studies on insufficiencia pelvis (gravidarum et puerparum). Acta Obstetricia et Gynecologica Scandinavica 25:1–39

Hungerford B, Gilleard W, Hodges PW 2003 Evidence of altered lumbo-pelvic muscle recruitment in the presence of sacroiliac joint pain. Spine 28:1593–1600

Kristiansson P, Svärsudd K, von Schoultz B 1996 Back pain during pregnancy. Spine 21:702–709

Larsen EC, Wilken-Jensen C, Hansen A et al 1999 Symptom-giving pelvic girdle relsxation in pregnancy. I: Prevalence and risk factors. Acta Obstet Gynecol Scand 78(2):105–110

MacLennan AH, Nicolson R, Green RC, Bath M 1986 Serum relaxin and pelvic pain in pregnancy. Lancet ii:243–245

Mantle MJ, Greenwood RM, Curry HLF 1977 Backache in pregnancy. Rheumatol Rehab 16:95–101

Mens JMA, Vleeming A, Stoeckart R et al 1996 Understanding peripartum pelvic pain: implications of a patient survey. Spine 21:1303–1369

Mens JMA, Vleeming A, Stam HJ et al 1999 The active straight leg raise test and mobility of the pelvic joints. Eur Spine J 8:468–473

Mens JMA, Vleeming A, Stam HJ et al 2002 Validity of the active straight leg raise test for measuring disease severity in patients with posterior pelvic pain after pregnancy. Spine 27(2):196–200

O'Sullivan P, Beales D, Beetham J et al 2002 Altered motor control strategies in subjects with sacro-iliac joint pain during the active straight-leg raise test. Spine 27(1): E1–E8

Östgaard HC, Andersson GBJ 1992 Low back pain post partum. Spine 17: 53–55

Östgaard HC, Andersson GBJ, Karisson K 1991a Prevalence of back pain in pregnancy. Spine 16: 49–52

Östgaard HC, Wennergren M, Andersson GBJ 1991b The impact of low back and pelvic pain on the pregnancy outcome. Acta Obst Gynecol Scand 70:21–24

Östgaard HC, Zetherström G, Roos-Hansson E 1994a Reduction of back and posterior pelvic pain in relation to pregnancy. Spine 19:894–900

Östgaard HC, Zetherström G, Roos-Hansson E 1994b The posterior pelvic pain provocation test in pregnant women. Eur Spine J 3:258–260

Östgaard HC, Zetherström G, Roos-Hansson E 1996 Regression of back and posterior pelvic pain after pregnancy. Spine 21:2777–2780

Petersen T, Olsen S, Laslett M et al 2004 Inter-tester reliability of a new diagnostic classification system for patients with non-specific low back pain. Aust J Physiother 50:85–94

Ransford AO, Douglas C, Mooney V 1975 The pain drawing as an aid to the psychologic evaluation of patients with low back pain. Spine 1:127–134

Schwarzer AC, Aprill CN, Bogduk N 1995 The sacroiliac joint in chronic low back pain. Spine 20:31–37

Snijders CJ, Saroo JM, Snijder JGN, Hoedt HT 1976 Change in form of the spine as a consequence of pregnancy. Digest of the 11th International Conference on Medical and Biological Engineering. Ottawa, Ontario, p670–671

Sturesson B, Udén G, Udén A 1997 Pain pattern in pregnancy and 'catching ' of the leg in pregnant women with posterior pelvic pain. Spine 22:1880–1883

Vleeming A, de Vries HJ, Mens JM, van Wingerden JP 2002 Possible role of the long dorsal sacroiliac ligament in women with peripartum pelvic pain. Acta Obstet Gynecol Scand 81:430–436

Wu W, Meijer OG, Uegaki K et al 2004 Pregnancy-related pelvic girdle pain I. Eur Spine J 13:575–589

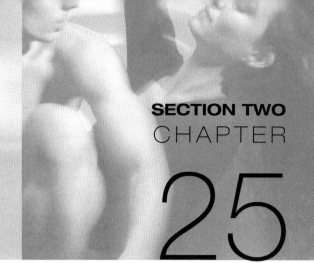

SECTION TWO
CHAPTER
25

The pattern of intrapelvic motion and lumbopelvic muscle recruitment alters in the presence of pelvic girdle pain

Barbara Hungerford and Wendy Gilleard

OUTLINE

This chapter is a compilation of research that investigated the patterns of intrapelvic motion and lumbopelvic muscle recruitment in healthy subjects and subjects with pelvic girdle pain (PGP). Motion of the pelvic bones in subjects with PGP and clinically assessed pelvic dysfunction was compared to pelvic bone motion in healthy subjects. The movements described are relative movements of the pelvic bones, as is palpable by the clinician, rather than sacroiliac joint motion.

Evaluation of lumbopelvic muscle recruitment for a single-leg support task was performed concurrently with the motion analysis to provide further insight into the mechanisms of pelvic stability during load transfer through the pelvis. Altered recruitment of transversus abdominis and lumbar multifidus muscles was found in the presence of PGP, as has been found previously in the lumbar spine. This research has increased our understanding of the changes that occur in the presence of PGP, and provided insight into methods by which failed load transfer through the lumbopelvic region can be assessed clinically. Furthermore, it has provided a basis from which future research can investigate the clinical relevance of alterations in motion and muscle recruitment, and the most effective mechanisms to assist return of normal function.

Introduction

The sacroiliac joint (SIJ) is a known source of low back pain and PGP (Fortin et al 1994, Schwarzer et al 1995). However, our understanding of in-vivo biomechanics of intrapelvic motion and the patterns of muscle recruitment required to maintain lumbopelvic stability during weight-bearing activities is limited. Similarly, there has been little comparison between the healthy population and PGP patients to determine if the patterns of intrapelvic motion and muscle recruitment in the lumbopelvic region vary when pain or dysfunction is present.

A small amount of motion occurs at the SIJ and the pubic symphysis during movements of the trunk and lower limbs (Jacob & Kissling 1995, Walheim & Selvick 1984). During weight-bearing activities such as standing, walking, and sitting, however, a primary function of the pelvis, and of the lumbar spine, is to transfer the loads generated by body weight and gravity to the lower limbs (Snijders et al 1993). How well this load is managed dictates the efficacy of function. The articular surfaces of the SIJ are relatively flat, and aligned close to the vertical plane (Snijders et al 1993). Flat joint surfaces are optimal for transference of loads, although the alignment of the SIJ makes it vulnerable to vertical shear loads, including gravitational force (Snijders et al 1998). The ligamentous structures that surround the SIJ and pubic symphysis create tensile and compressive forces across the joints that limit the available range of intrapelvic motion (Willard 1997). The viscoelastic properties of these ligaments, however, show a tendency for creep under prolonged loading (Vleeming et al 1992). Consequently, during weight-bearing activities, stabilization of intrapelvic motion is required for optimal transference of loads between the spine and the lower limbs (Snijders et al 1993, Vleeming et al 1990). Panjabi (1992) has stated that stability is achieved when the passive, active, and motor control systems work together. A balance is created between compression or approximation of joint surfaces, which is created by ligaments and muscles, and tension on the surrounding myofascial structures to allow stability during movement. The amount of approximation required is variable and is dependent on an individual's structure (form closure) and the forces they need to control (force closure). The ability to effectively transfer load through the pelvis therefore depends on:

1. Optimal function of the bones, joints and ligaments (Vleeming et al 1989a, 1990).
2. Optimal function of the muscles and fascia (Richardson et al 2002, Snijders et al 1998, Vleeming et al 1995a, 1995b).
3. Appropriate neural function (Hodges & Richardson 1997a).

The biomechanics of intrapelvic motion and stabilization of the pelvic girdle

For every joint, there is a position called the self-braced (close-packed) position in which there is maximum congruence of the articular surfaces and maximum ligamentous tension. In this position, the joint is under significant compression and the ability to resist shear forces is enhanced by tensioning of the passive structures and increased friction between the articular surfaces (Snijders et al 1993, Vleeming et al 1990). The self-braced position of the SIJ is nutation of the sacrum or relative posterior rotation of the innominate (Vleeming et al 1989a). Sturesson et al (2000) showed that nutation of the sacrum occurs bilaterally whenever the lumbopelvic spine is loaded vertically (sitting, standing). Counternutation of the sacrum, or anterior rotation of the innominate, is thought to be a relatively less stable position for the SIJ (Vleeming et al 1995b). The long dorsal ligament becomes taut during counternutation, however tension in other ligaments such as sacrotuberous and interosseous ligaments decreases (Vleeming et al 1996).

Muscle recruitment and lumbopelvic stability

The contribution of muscle force to stabilization of intrapelvic motion is dependent on the optimal control of the nervous system (Lee & Vleeming 2000). Little is known, however, about the timing of muscle activation in the lumbopelvic region in order to stabilize intrapelvic motion during vertical loading. Stability of intersegmental lumbar motion is maintained by a variety of strategies controlled by the CNS, which modulates the timing and pattern of muscle recruitment according to the demands placed on the lumbar spine (Hodges 2000). Deep trunk muscles, including transversus abdominis (TrA), multifidus, and lower fibers of obliquus internus abdominis (OI), activate prior to limb or trunk motion, and exhibit patterns of cocontraction, to increase spinal stiffness and limit intersegmental motion (Hodges & Richardson 1997a, 1997b, Moseley et al 2002). They might also assist stabilization of intrapelvic motion as compressive forces across the pubic symphysis are increased by activation of OI and adductor longus, while activation of OI, TrA, gluteus maximus, lattissimus dorsi, and the lumbar erector spinae increase compressive forces across the SIJ (Mooney et al 1997, Richardson et al 2002, Snijders et al 1998).

Initiation of a movement task such as standing onto the right leg requires that weight is first shifted to the left thereby increasing the vertical force required to transfer the center of mass across onto the right supporting leg (Rogers & Pai 1990). Displacement of body mass is preceded and accompanied by muscle activation to provide postural support for load transfer to the new single-leg support configuration. Hodges & Richardson (1997b) found early activation of TrA, OI, obliquus externus abdominis, and multifidus prior to limb motion. The authors hypothesize that a similar pattern of preactivation of TrA, OI, multifidus, pelvic floor, and gluteus maximus muscles prior to load transfer might induce posterior rotation of the innominate relative to the sacrum on the side of the supporting leg, thereby increasing tension onto the posterior SI ligaments and posterior layer of the thoracolumbar fascia, as discussed by Vleeming et al (1995a, 1995b). The increased ligament tension and associated increase in SIJ compression would result in increased SIJ stiffness prior to load transfer through the pelvis (Richardson et al 2002, Willard 1997).

The impact of posterior pelvic girdle pain

The SIJs and the posterior SIJ ligaments are a known source of posterior pelvic girdle pain (PPGP), although the relationship between pain and the patterning of pelvic motion remains unclear (Fortin et al 1994, Vleeming et al 2002). Jacob & Kissling (1995) noted that in the presence of SIJ symptoms, the amplitude of SIJ motion about a coronal axis increased during hip flexion in one subject. Mens et al (1999) also reported increased amplitude of anterior rotation of the innominate in posterior pelvic pain patients. Sturesson et al (2000) reported no difference in the amplitude or pattern of either angular or translational motion of the innominates when the left and right SIJs were compared in subjects with PPGP. Sturesson et al (2000) made no comparison to asymptomatic subjects. Buyruk et al (1999) and Damen et al (2002) showed that stiffness of the SIJ is asymmetric in subjects with PGP and that asymmetrical stiffness of the SIJs is prognostic for pelvic impairment and pain. It is presently unknown if PPGP alters the patterning of bone motion within the pelvis, or the patterning of lumbopelvic muscle recruitment during a weight-bearing activity.

Clinical assessment of pelvic girdle function

The supine active straight leg raise test (ASLR; Mens et al 2001) has been validated as a clinical test for measuring effective load transfer between the trunk and lower limbs. When the lumbopelvic region is functioning optimally, the leg should rise effortlessly from the table (effort graded from 0 to 5; Mens et al 1999). A correlation has been shown between positive ASLR findings and posterior pelvic pain (Mens et al 1999; O'Sullivan et al 2002). Similarly, Damen et al (2001) and Buyruk et al (1999) showed that the ASLR is positive in the presence of asymmetric stiffness of the SIJ. Healthy individuals, in comparison, have symmetrical stiffness values (Damen 2002). Another means of clinically evaluating the ability to maintain stability during load transfer through the lumbopelvic region is provided by the Stork test on the side of single-leg support (Fig. 25.1B). The ability of therapists to distinguish whether the innominate remained in its self-braced position of posterior rotation relative to sacral nutation, or not, has been shown to have good reliability (Hungerford et al 2006). However, the validity of this test is still under investigation. The research suggests that altered pelvic stabilization strategies might create asymmetry of SIJ stiffness and altered patterning of pelvic motion during load transfer (Damen et al 2001, Lee 2004, Mens et al 1999).

The aim of this study was to determine the three-dimensional pattern of pelvic bone motion occurring in subjects determined to have PPGP and impaired pelvic stabilization strategies during weight-bearing and non-weight-bearing components of a standing hip flexion movement. These results were compared to controls with clinically assessed normal pelvic stabilization and pelvic motion patterns. The pattern of recruitment of seven trunk and hip muscles was obtained simultaneously to provide further insight into stabilization strategies in the lumbopelvic region. It was hypothesized that the pattern of innominate bone motion and lumbopelvic muscle recruitment would alter in subjects with PPGP during both components of the movement trial.

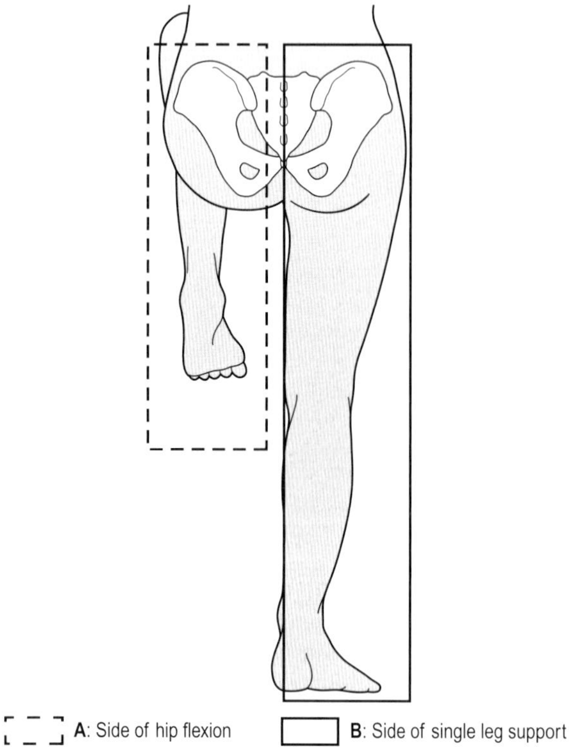

Fig. 25.1 The stork test. (A) Side of hip flexion. (B) Side of single-leg support.

Materials and methods

Subjects

Impaired pelvic stabilization and posterior pelvic girdle pain group

Fourteen male subjects with pain in the posterior pelvic/SI region, and a mean (range) age, height and weight of 32.7 (24–47) years, 176.8 (168–184) cm, and 77.0 (71–90) kg, volunteered for the study. The criteria for inclusion in this study were:

- Each subject in the PPGP group reported unilateral pain over the posterior pelvic/SI region (Fortin et al 1994) for more than 2 months, and no pain above the lumbosacral junction. The pain was consistently and predictably aggravated by activities that vertically loaded the pelvis (walking, standing or sitting).
- Positive results on the side of posterior pelvic pain in clinical tests for impaired lumbopelvic stabilization. These tests included:
  - Active straight leg raise test (Mens et al 1999, 2001): a positive test was indicated when the pelvis failed to remain in neutral alignment, and the subject reported difficulty or inability to elevate a straight leg in supine. The perceived difference of effort, or pain aggravation was scaled from 0 (not difficult to raise leg) to 5 (unable to perform ASLR).
  - Standing hip flexion test (Mitchell, 1995): during a left standing hip flexion, or Stork test (Fig. 25.1), the subject stands on their right leg and flexes the left hip towards 90°. The left innominate should posteriorly rotate relative to the sacrum (Jacob & Kissling 1995). A positive test was indicated when superior motion of the posterior superior iliac spine (PSIS) was palpated relative to the sacrum.
  - Passive joint glide test (Lee 2004): this test was used clinically to apply the research of Buyruk et al (1999) and Damen et al (2002) and to evaluate motion in the neutral zone of the SIJ. Panjabi (1992) noted that joints have nonlinear load–displacement curves and that the size of the neutral zone could increase with injury, articular degeneration, and/or weakness of the stabilizing musculature and that this is a more sensitive indicator than angular range of motion for detecting instability. All symptomatic subjects demonstrated asymmetric stiffness of the SIJ when the innominate was glided relative to the sacrum.

As the reliability and predictive ability of the standing hip flexion and passive joint glide tests remains uncertain (Carmichael 1987, Vincent-Smith & Gibbons 1999), all clinical tests were required to be positive on the side of pain, in conjunction with the ASLR test, for inclusion in the PPGP subject group. Subjects were excluded from the study if they could not flex each hip to 90° without pain, if they had undergone spinal surgery, or displayed overt neurological signs such as sensory paresthesia or motor paresis.

Control group

The PPGP group was age- and height-matched to a control group of 14 males with a mean (range) age, height, and weight of 33.5 (22–50) years, 176.0 (168–183) cm, and 72.5 (61–85) kg, respectively. The control subjects had no history of low back pain in the last 12 months, no history of congenital lumbar or pelvic anomalies, and tested negative to the ASLR, standing hip flexion and passive joint glide tests. Subjects were excluded if no palpable motion between the PSIS and S2 spinous process was observed during hip flexion in standing, or if they experienced pain during the clinical assessment.

All subjects were assessed by the same experienced physiotherapist to maintain continuity. Informed consent was given by each subject prior to participation in the study, and all rights of the subjects were protected. The study was approved by the institutional Human Ethics Committee.

Procedure

Fifteen lightweight, highly reflective, 15-mm diameter balls were used to define the bony landmarks of each innominate, both femoral segments, and the sacrum. The pelvic bony landmarks were chosen for their closeness to the skin surface with minimal overlying fascia, and because they reflected palpation points commonly used by therapists. Each innominate and femoral segment was therefore defined by three markers placed on identified bony landmarks while a three-armed triangular wand with a single marker attached to each arm was applied to the sacral spinous process of S2 (Hungerford et al 2004). All markers were applied to the skin while the subjects were standing.

Recordings of electromyographic (EMG) activity were made simultaneously to motion analysis using pairs of Ag/AgCl surface electrodes. The seven electrode sites were: (1) adductor longus (adductors); (2) long head of bicep femoris (biceps femoris); (3) tensor fascia latae (TFL); (4) gluteus medius; (5) gluteus maximus; (6) lumbar multifidus; and (7) lower fibers of OI, in the center of the triangle formed by a horizontal line between the anterior superior iliac spine of the innominate and the umbilicus, midline, and the inguinal ligament. A detailed description of electrode placement and materials has been described previously (Hungerford et al 2003).

Force platform data (960 Hz) were used to determine initiation of motion as body mass was transferred onto the supporting leg during hip flexion in standing and the initial time of single-leg support. The vertical ground reaction force data provided a means of determining whether trunk or hip musculature was activated prior to initiation of motion, and gave a common point for comparison of the temporal relationship of muscle activation between controls and subjects with PPGP (Hungerford et al 2003).

A six-camera Expert Vision Motion Analysis (Eva)™ Hi Res.6.0 System (Motion Analysis Corporation, CA, USA) was used to video (60 Hz) the subject motion. Measurements of a known angle showed the six-camera Eva™ system to be accurate to 0.25°. Following practice trials, data from one quiet standing trial were collected. The subject then performed five left and five right standing hip flexion trials. For example, during a left standing hip flexion trial the subject was asked to stand on his right leg, and flex his left hip and knee toward 90° hip flexion, then lower the foot back down. EMG data were recorded from the seven trunk and hip muscles simultaneously with motion analysis on the side of single-leg support.

Data analysis

The Eva™ motion analysis system was used to track the three-dimensional trajectories of each marker over time. These trajectories were then imported into Kintrak™ (Motion Analysis Corporation, CA, USA) which provided the three-dimensional angular rotation, and translation, of each innominate relative to the sacral segment throughout each trial, in respect to neutral position from the quiet standing trial. The axes of the innominate segment originated at each respective PSIS, and the sacral axes intercepted at the S2 spinous process (Fig. 25.2). Calculation of the angular kinematics has been described previously (Hungerford et al 2004). Kintrak™ subsequently determined relative angular and translational motion of each bone segment. Hip joint motion was determined by computing the motion of the femur, as defined by linking the three femoral markers, in relation to ipsilateral innominate motion. The hip joint center was determined using the equation provided by Tylkowski et al (1982).

The temporal relationship between initiation of motion and onset of EMG activity for all muscles was determined on the side of the supporting leg during flexion of the hip. Onset of EMG activity was expressed relative to the initiation of motion. Onsets prior to the initiation of motion were given a negative value. Onsets were compared between sides and between groups. EMG amplitude during 50-ms epochs before and after initiation of motion was also calculated to compare muscle recruitment patterns between groups.

All angular and translational motion was determined at maximum coronal axis motion of the innominate, relative to the sacrum, during hip flexion. The mean onset of EMG between groups and between sides was also calculated, and in order to determine if there was a significant difference. Two-tailed paired Student *t*-tests assuming unequal variance (Domholdt 1993) were performed for

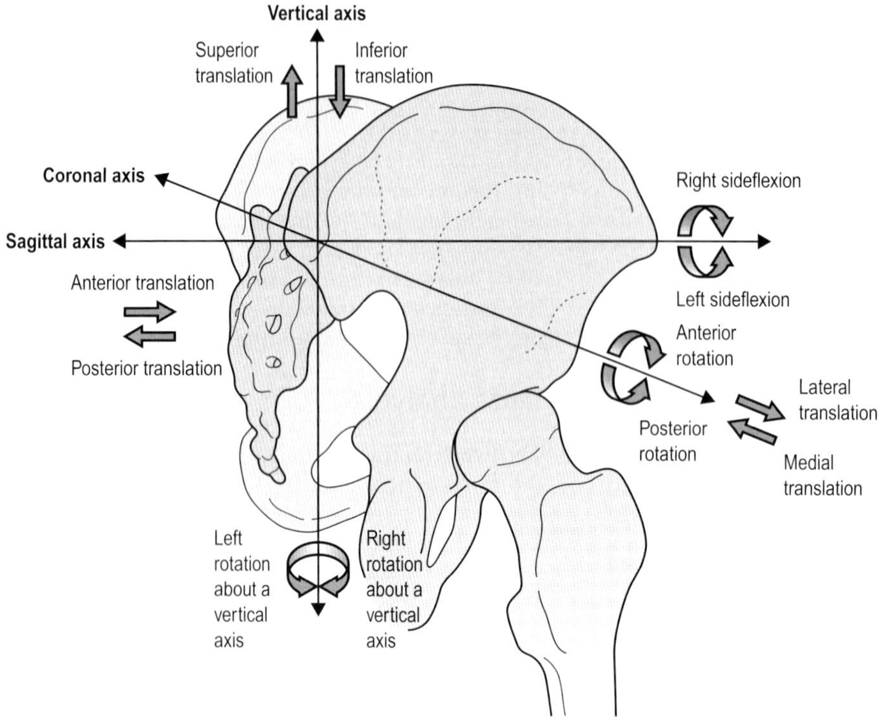

Fig. 25.2 The three axes of angular and translational motion of the innominate relative to the sacral segment. Note the axis of the innominate is centered at the PSIS. (Reproduced with permission from © AMTA P/L.)

all variables between the left and right side in the control group, and between the symptomatic side and the asymptomatic side in the PPGP group. To determine if there was a significant alteration to the mean angular and translational intrapelvic motion measured between the control subjects and the PPGP group, independent groups two-tailed Student *t*-tests assuming unequal variance (Domholdt 1993) were performed for all variables. Further graphical comparisons of coronal axis motion on the side of single-leg support were performed for each subject in the PPGP group. Two times the standard error of mean (SE) motion for each subject was determined and plotted. As the mean ±2 SE is approximately equal to the 95% confidence interval (Sim & Reid 1999), determination of no overlay of each subject's data was defined as a significant difference (Fig. 25.3).

Results

Intrapelvic motion

A noninvasive motion analysis system using skin-mounted markers was chosen to acquire the kinematic data of pelvic bone motion during a standing hip flexion movement for ethical reasons. Errors in determining the range of motion are likely to occur with an optoelectronic system due to skin marker motion relative to underlying bony landmarks (Maslen & Ackland 1994). Good to excellent reliability between trials has been reported for angular and translational motion reported using the reported motion analysis protocol (Gilleard 1999), however, the authors recognize that the movements noted reflect motion of the innominates, sacrum, and femurs in conjunction with overlying skin, and therefore the main emphasis of this study was to investigate the *patterns* of bone motion rather than the *range* of motion.

Intrapelvic motion on the side of hip flexion during a standing hip flexion movement

The angular and translational motions of the left and right innominates, during left and right standing hip flexion movements are summarized in Tables 25.1, 25.2, and 25.3. In the control subjects, standing hip flexion (Table 25.1A) produced posterior rotation of the non-weight-bearing innominate relative to the sacral segment. On the side of hip flexion, maximum

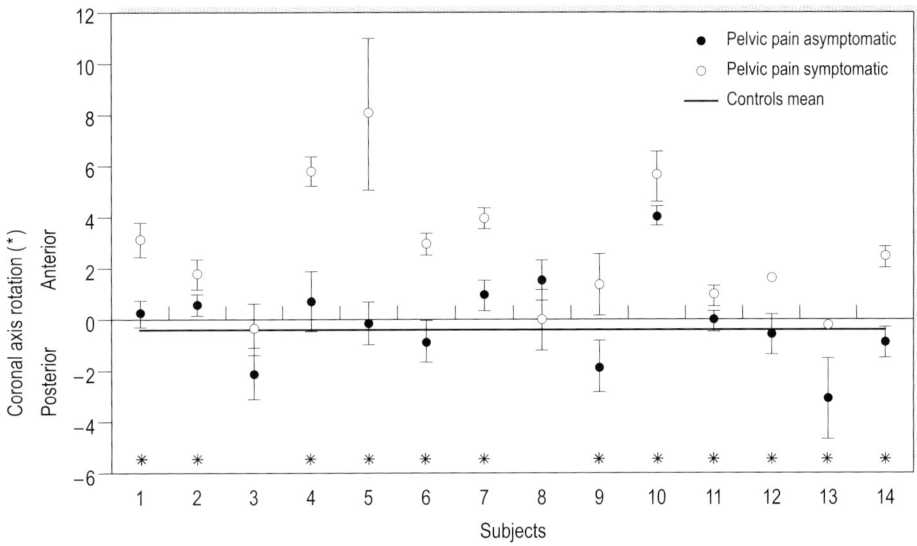

Fig. 25.3 A comparison of coronal axis angular motion at single-leg support in each subject with PPGP. Mean coronal axis motion for control subjects is depicted as a solid line. Error bars denote 2× standard error for each subject. * Significant at $P < 0.05$.

Table 25.1 Comparison of angular and translational motion of the left and right innominates on the side of hip flexion in control subjects and subjects with posterior pelvic girdle pain

		A: control subjects					B: posterior pelvic pain subjects				
		Left hip flexion		Right hip flexion			Asymptomatic hip flexion		Symptomatic hip flexion		
Motion segment	Axis of motion	Mean	SD	Mean	SD	*P* value	Mean	SD	Mean	SD	*P* value
Femur	Coronal	70.00	5.25	73.00	5.50	0.08	73.25	7.00	74.50	4.50	0.28
Innominate angular (°)	Coronal	–8.50	3.50	–10.00	3.50	0.05	–7.50	3.00	–10.00	3.25	0.04*
	Sagittal	–6.00	3.50	–7.75	5.00	0.18	–5.00	5.50	–6.25	4.00	0.44
	Vertical	4.50	4.50	3.50	3.00	0.39	3.75	2.50	4.75	1.75	0.27
Innominate translation (mm)	Antero-posterior	3.50	2.50	4.00	3.00	0.49	2.00	4.00	2.00	3.75	0.70
	Medio-lateral	–5.50	3.00	–5.50	2.50	0.74	–5.50	2.00	–6.50	3.00	0.36
	Vertical	–6.50	3.00	–7.50	3.50	0.46	–4.00	3.50	–5.00	2.00	0.76

Negative coronal value, posterior; negative sagittal value, toward flexed hip; negative vertical value, toward flexed hip; negative anteroposterior value, posterior; negative mediolateral translation, toward flexed hip; negative vertical translation, superior.
** significant at $P < 0.05$*

coronal axis angular motion of the innominate occurred at a mean (range) 73.0° (10.0) femoral flexion. The innominate concurrently side flexed toward the side of hip flexion, and rotated about the vertical axis away from the side of hip flexion.

On the side of hip flexion for the PPGP group, posterior rotation of the innominate also occurred with femoral flexion (Table 25.1B). A pattern of side flexion of the innominate, and rotation about the vertical axis away from the side of hip

Table 25.2 Comparison of angular and translational motion of the innominates on the side of single leg support in control subjects and subjects with posterior pelvic girdle pain

		A: control subjects					B: posterior pelvic pain subjects				
		Left single leg support		Right single leg support			Asymptomatic single leg support		Symptomatic single leg support		
Motion segment	Axis of motion	Mean	SD	Mean	SD	*P* value	Mean	SD	Mean	SD	*P* value
Femur	Coronal	1.50	3.00	1.50	2.50	0.79	1.75	3.50	1.75	3.25	0.86
Innominate angular (°)	Coronal	0.00	2.00	–0.50	3.00	0.88	0.50	1.50	2.00	2.00	0.02*
	Sagittal	–6.00	2.50	–5.75	2.50	0.46	–4.75	3.25	–3.75	3.00	0.42
	Vertical	3.50	2.75	4.50	4.50	0.17	5.00	2.50	3.75	2.75	0.09
Innominate translation (mm)	Antero-posterior	–4.50	6.00	–2.50	4.00	0.13	–4.00	2.50	–6.00	2.75	0.02*
	Medio-lateral	–6.50	3.25	–6.50	3.00	0.96	–7.00	3.25	–5.00	2.50	0.03*
	Vertical	–4.50	2.50	–3.50	2.50	0.19	3.50	2.25	2.00	3.00	0.04*

Negative coronal value, posterior; negative sagittal value, toward flexed hip; negative vertical value, toward flexed hip; negative anteroposterior value, posterior; negative mediolateral translation, toward flexed hip; negative vertical translation, superior.
** significant at P < 0.05*

Table 25.3 Comparison of angular and translational motion of the innominates between control subjects and subjects with posterior pelvic girdle pain

		A: hip flexion					B: single-leg support				
		Controls Right		Pelvic pain group Symptomatic			Controls Right		Pelvic pain group Symptomatic		
Motion segment	Axis of motion	Mean	SD	Mean	SD	*P* value	Mean	SD	Mean	SD	*P* value
Femur	Coronal	73.00	5.50	74.50	4.50	0.45	1.50	2.50	1.75	3.25	0.67
Innominate angular (°)	Coronal	–10.00	3.50	–10.00	3.25	0.16	–0.50	3.00	2.00	2.00	<0.01*
	Sagittal	–7.75	5.00	–6.25	4.00	0.94	–5.75	2.50	–3.75	3.00	0.12
	Vertical	3.50	3.00	4.75	1.75	0.46	4.50	4.50	3.75	2.75	0.90
Innominate translation (mm)	Antero-posterior	4.00	3.00	2.00	3.75	0.05	–2.50	4.00	–6.00	2.75	0.02*
	Medio-lateral	–5.50	2.50	–6.50	3.00	0.94	–6.50	3.00	–5.00	2.50	0.13
	Vertical	–7.50	3.50	–5.00	2.00	0.04*	–3.50	2.50	2.00	3.00	<0.001*

Negative coronal value, posterior; negative sagittal value, toward flexed hip; negative vertical value, toward flexed hip; negative anteroposterior value, posterior; negative mediolateral translation, toward flexed hip; negative vertical translation, superior.
** significant at P < 0.05*

flexion, occurred on both the asymptomatic and symptomatic sides during hip flexion.

Translation of the innominate relative to the sacral segment was associated with this angular motion during hip flexion. In both the control group and the PPGP group, the innominate translated anteriorly, superiorly, and laterally (gapping away from the sacrum) as the innominate posteriorly rotated (Table 25.1). No significant difference was found between sides in either the controls or the PPGP group.

Intrapelvic motion on the side of single-leg support

The contralateral limb maintained single-leg support during the standing hip flexion movement. Posterior rotation of the weight-bearing innominate occurred about the coronal axis in control subjects (Table 25.2A). A concurrent pattern of side flexion of the innominate toward, and rotation about, the vertical axis away from the side of hip flexion also occurred. The weight-bearing innominate translated posteriorly, superiorly and medially (toward the sacrum) (Table 25.2A). No significant difference was found in the pattern of either angular or translational motion of the weight-bearing innominate during single-leg support in control subjects.

The angular and translational motion of the weight-bearing innominate on the side of single-leg support, in subjects with PPGP, is depicted in Table 25.2B. The weight-bearing innominate anteriorly rotated significantly more (P = 0.02) about the coronal axis on the symptomatic in comparison to the asymptomatic side. Concurrently, the innominate side flexed toward, and rotated away from the side of hip flexion on both the symptomatic and asymptomatic sides. The innominate translated inferiorly, posteriorly, and medially (toward the sacrum) relative to the sacral segment (Table 25.2B). Posterior translation of the innominate relative to the sacral segment was significantly greater (P = 0.02) on the symptomatic side than the asymptomatic side, whereas inferior translation of the innominate was significantly less (P = 0.04) on the symptomatic side. Medial translation, or compression, of the innominate was also significantly less (P = 0.03) on the symptomatic side in comparison with the asymptomatic side (Table 25.2B).

Further comparison of coronal axis motion on the symptomatic side and asymptomatic side of single-leg support was performed for each subject with posterior pelvic pain (see Fig. 25.3). The mean range of posterior rotation on the side of single-leg support in control subjects was depicted as a solid line for comparison to the symptomatic group. A significant change toward anterior rotation of the innominate occurred in twelve of the fourteen posterior pelvic pain subjects on the symptomatic side; that is in subjects 1, 2, 4–7, 9–14 (see Fig. 25.3).

Comparison of control subjects and subjects with posterior pelvic girdle pain

During the hip flexion component of the standing hip flexion movement there was no significant difference in patterning of angular or translational motion between groups on the side of hip flexion (Table 25.3A).

On the side of single-leg support, a significant difference in the pattern of angular and translational motion of the innominate between controls and symptomatic subjects was determined (Table 25.3B). In the control group, posterior rotation of the weight-bearing innominate occurred on the side of single-leg support; however, in the PPGP group, anterior rotation occurred on the symptomatic side ($P < 0.01$). A pattern of posterior, superior and medial translation occurred concurrently with posterior rotation of the innominate in control subjects; however, inferior, posterior, and medial translation occurred with anterior rotation of the innominate in the symptomatic subjects.

Temporal relationship of muscle recruitment

Control subjects

When subjects with no history of lumbopelvic pain flexed their hip in standing, the onset of OI and multifidus EMG activity on the side of standing on one leg occurred prior to initiation of the task (Fig. 25.4A). In contrast, the onset of biceps femoris, adductor longus, gluteus maximus, gluteus medius, and TFL EMG occurred after initiation of motion. There was no significant difference in onset of EMG activity between sides in control subjects for all seven muscles (Fig. 25.4A). The epoch data verified that OI and multifidus activated first, followed by adductors (Fig. 25.5A). There was little change in EMG amplitude of gluteus maximus, gluteus medius, and TFL until four to five epochs (200–250 ms) after initiation of motion, and bicep femoris EMG decreased (Fig. 25.5A).

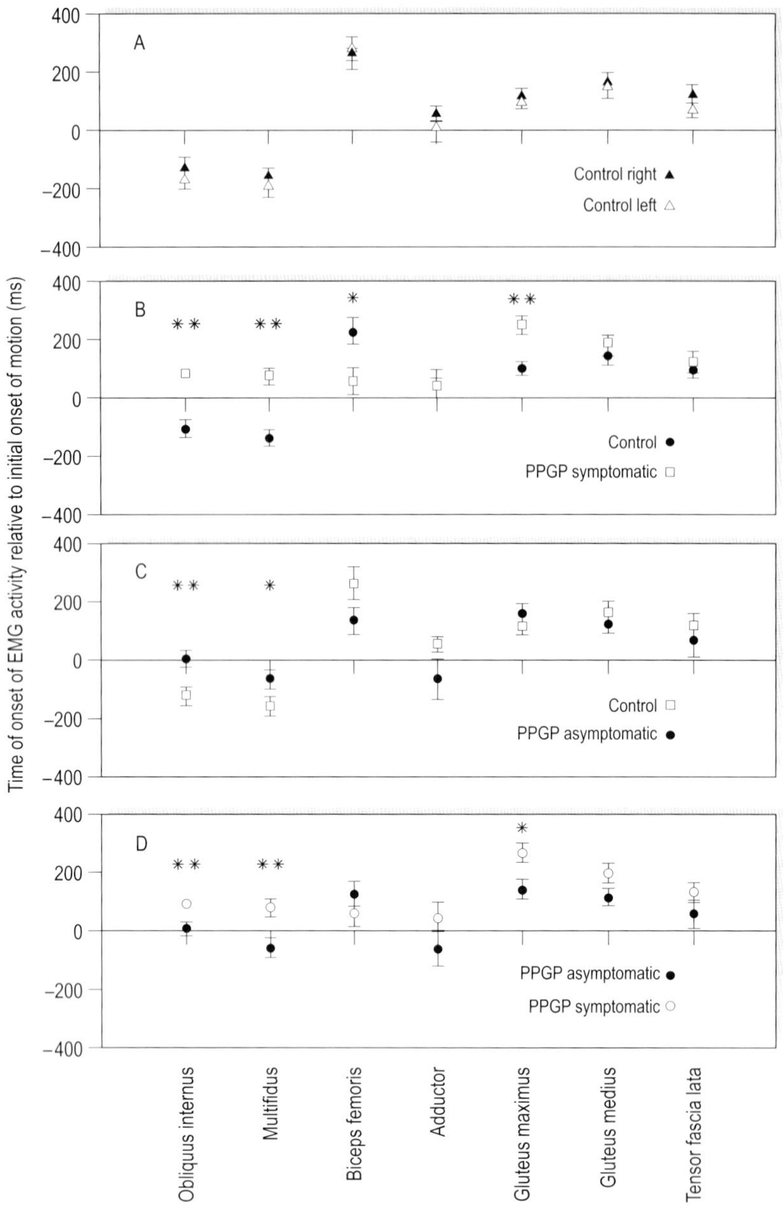

Fig. 25.4 Mean time of EMG onset for the supporting leg during hip flexion in standing in (A) control subjects; (B) control subjects versus PPGP subjects on the symptomatic side; (C) control subjects versus PPGP subjects on the asymptomatic side; (D) asymptomatic versus symptomatic side in PPGP subjects. $^*P \leq 0.05$; $^{**}P \leq 0.01$. (Reproduced with permission from © AMTA P/L.)

Comparison of muscle recruitment between controls and subjects with posterior pelvic girdle pain

In comparison to the control subjects, the EMG onsets of OI, multifidus, and gluteus maximus were significantly delayed ($P \leq 0.01$) on the symptomatic side in subjects with PPGP (see Fig. 25.4B). The onset of OI and multifidus EMG occurred more than 20 ms after onset of motion. In contrast, onset of bicep femoris EMG occurred significantly earlier ($P < 0.03$) on the symptomatic side, in comparison to controls (Fig. 25.4B). The general features of the temporal findings are consistent with epoch data (Fig. 25.5A). Comparison of EMG onsets for the asymptomatic side in the PPGP group and control subjects also showed a significant difference in temporal parameters for OI and multifidus activation (Figs 25.4C and 25.5B). Activation of OI was significantly delayed ($P \leq 0.01$) in comparison to control subjects, as was onset of activation of multifidus ($P = 0.05$). When onset of EMG activity on the symptomatic side was compared to the asymptomatic side in the PPGP group, there was a significant delay in the onset of activation in OI, multifidus, and gluteus maximus on the symptomatic side (Fig. 25.4D).

Discussion

The pattern of intrapelvic motion

Intrasubject comparisons: control group

Hip motion toward 90° of femoral flexion produced posterior rotation of the non-weight-bearing innominate (side of hip flexion) in the controls, consistent with previous research (Jacob & Kissling 1995, Sturesson et al 2000). A concurrent pattern of side flexion toward the side of hip flexion, and rotation about the vertical axis away from the side of hip flexion was found. In addition, a concurrent translational motion occurred (anterior, superior and lateral) during hip flexion. This pattern of translation is consistent with the model of arthrokinematic motion of the SIJ proposed by Lee (2004).

During this same movement, the weight-bearing innominate (side of single-leg support) posteriorly rotated; a finding consistent with previous research (Sturesson et al 2000). Posterior rotation of the innominate, or relative sacral nutation, is thought to occur as a consequence of the self-bracing mechanism of the pelvis and is essential for optimal load transfer during single-leg support (Snijders et al 1993, Vleeming et al 1995b). In addition, this study found a concurrent side flexion of the innominate toward, and axial rotation away from the side of hip flexion. This pattern of side flexion and contralateral axial rotation was identical to the pattern of sagittal and axial angular motion determined at the contralateral innominate. The

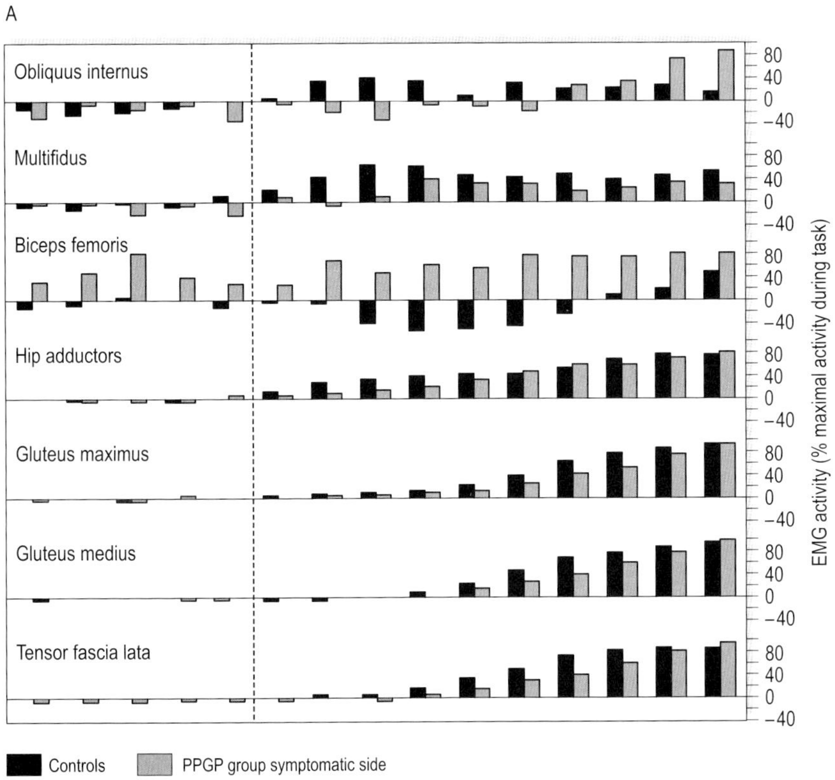

Fig. 25.5 Electromyographic (EMG) amplitude during 50 ms epochs before and after initiation of motion. (A) Comparison of control subjects and subjects with PPGP on the symptomatic side. *Continued*

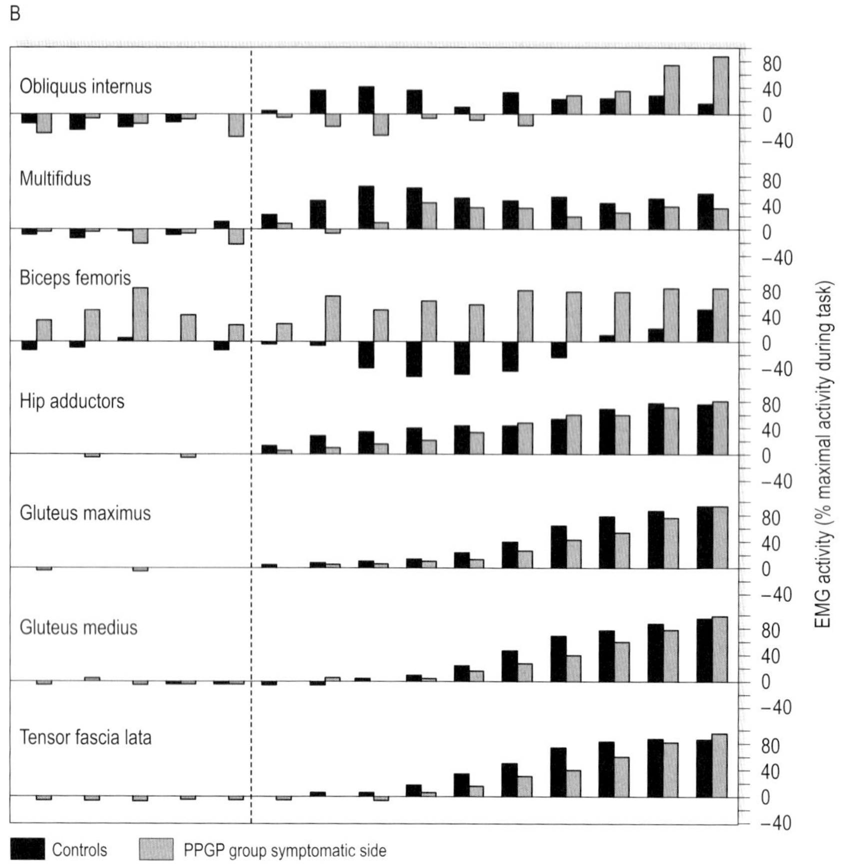

Fig. 25.5 *cont'd* Electromyographic (EMG) amplitude during 50 ms epochs before and after initiation of motion. (B) Comparison of control subjects and subjects with PPGP on the asymptomatic side. Activity above zero indicates an increase in EMG activity. Note the onset of OI and multifidus occurred within 1–2 epochs of the initiation of motion (dotted line) in control subjects, and onset of OI and multifidus was delayed more than three epochs after initiation of motion in subjects with PPGP on the symptomatic side. (Reproduced with permission from © AMTA P/L).

biomechanical analysis of the data assumed that movement of the innominates occurred relative to a stable sacrum, however further investigation is required to investigate whether the results reflect movement of the sacrum between the innominates.

Translational motion in a superior, posterior, and medial direction occurred during single-leg support. Although both the non-weight-bearing and weight-bearing innominates posteriorly rotated during standing hip flexion, the pattern of the concurrent translation between the innominate and sacral segments on the non-weight-bearing and weight-bearing sides differed. This variation of translational motion might reflect variations in muscle activation and the different compressive forces acting on the innominate to maintain stability for single-leg support. DonTigny (1995) proposed that posterior translation of the innominate relative to the sacrum during weight bearing might occur due to the activation of posterior hip musculature such as gluteus maximus. During hip flexion gluteus maximus would not be activated and therefore the forces affecting translation would alter. In regard to the medial translation, or compression that occurred during single-leg support, Richardson et al (2002) noted that a co-contraction of multifidus and transversus abdominis increased SIJ stiffness. The recruitment of these muscles by controls prior to single-leg support may therefore have augmented SIJ compression as a component of an optimal lumbopelvic stabilization strategy.

Intrasubject comparisons: posterior pelvic pain group

Femoral flexion produced posterior rotation of the non-weight-bearing innominate on both the symptomatic and asymptomatic side. The pattern of side flexion, rotation, and translation of the non-weight-bearing innominate did not differ between the asymptomatic and symptomatic sides.

On the side of single-leg support, anterior rotation of the weight-bearing innominate occurred in subjects with PPGP, similar to the findings of Mens et al (1999). In addition, the present study found that the concurrent translational motion of the weight-bearing innominate differed in PPGP patients. As the innominate rotated anteriorly it translated inferiorly and posteriorly; a pattern hypothesized to be consistent with less intrapelvic compression (Lee 2004). As medial translation, or compression was significantly decreased on the symptomatic side, the results suggest that compression onto the SIJ *was* decreased with the altered pattern of bone motion found on the side of pelvic dysfunction. It is also interesting to note that all of the subjects in the PPGP group reported increased symptoms with vertical loading through the pelvis. This might suggest they were unable to adequately compress the weight-bearing SIJ and maintain self-bracing of the pelvis (Snijders et al 1998) in order to control vertical shear loads.

The two groups: intersubject comparisons

A comparison of both the angular and translational motion of the non-weight-bearing innominate on the side of hip flexion between control subjects and matched subjects with posterior pelvic pain showed no significant difference. Interestingly, clinical assessment of posterior rotation of the innominate on the side of hip flexion (the Stork test) as a method of distinguishing normal joint motion from SIJ dysfunction (Mitchell 1995) has been found to be unreliable and unspecific (Vincent-Smith & Gibbons 1999). This study further validates such conclusions.

A significant difference was noted in the pattern of angular motion of the weight-bearing innominate during single-leg support when the control group (posterior rotation) was compared to the posterior pelvic pain group (anterior rotation). Vleeming et al (1995b) suggest that anterior rotation of the innominate (sacral counternutation) disengages the self-bracing mechanism of the pelvis and consequently diminishes the ability to transfer loads between the spine and legs. The positive clinical tests noted in the PPGP group might reflect their inability to posteriorly rotate the weight-bearing innominate on the symptomatic side. It is also possible that subjects lacked the ability to create sufficient compression due to altered motor control of the musculature known to stabilize the pelvis, such as transversus abdominis, lumbosacral multifidus, and gluteus maximus.

The pattern of lumbopelvic muscle recruitment prior to single-leg support

The present results indicate that EMG onsets of OI and multifidus occurred prior to initiation of motion in control subjects. This is consistent with previous research that has identified feedforward activation of TrA, OI and multifidus in association with limb movements that challenge the stability of the spine (Hodges & Richardson 1997b, Moseley et al 2002). Previous studies have suggested that TrA and the lower, horizontally oriented fibers of OI, might contribute to compression of the SIJ (Richardson et al 2002). Similarly, lumbar multifidus activation might increase tension on posterior SI ligaments and the posterior layer of the thoracolumbar fascia, and induce a nutation force on the sacrum (Willard 1997). Preactivation of OI and multifidus, as determined in this study, may therefore contribute to compression of the SIJ prior to initiation of single-leg stance, while influencing the motion pattern between the innominate and sacrum that is required during activation of the self-bracing mechanism for optimal pelvic stabilization and load transference (Vleeming et al 1995b).

In the PPGP group the onset of OI, multifidus, gluteus maximus, and bicep femoris EMG was significantly different on the symptomatic side compared to the asymptomatic side, and control subjects. OI and multifidus activation occurred more than 80 ms after initiation of motion and cannot be considered to be feedforward. This would suggest a change in the motor control strategy on the symptomatic side in subjects with PPGP. The delayed onset of OI and multifidus activation might have diminished the effectiveness of stabilizing mechanisms at the SIJ prior to increased vertical loading through the pelvis. Delayed activation of gluteus maximus might also have altered compression of the SIJ, with a subsequent failure of the mechanisms required for optimal load transference through the pelvis (Vleeming et al 1995b). The early onset of bicep femoris activation on the symptomatic side might have occurred to augment force closure across the SIJ via connections to the sacrotuberous ligament and the posterior layer of the thoracolumbar fascia (Vleeming et al 1989b). It is interesting to note that the altered pattern of OI and multifidus EMG activity also occurred on the asymptomatic side. Altered recruitment of OI and multifidus was not specific to the side of PPGP and positive clinical assessment testing, however onset of gluteus maximus was only delayed on the symptomatic side.

Clinical implications

The significant difference in the pattern of innominate rotation that occurred between the controls (posterior rotation) and the PPGP group on their symptomatic side (anterior rotation) might provide a means of evaluating or distinguishing patients with pelvic girdle dysfunction from other sources of low back or posterior hip pain. The ability to maintain the self-braced alignment of the pelvic bones during a weight-bearing activity that increased vertical loading through the pelvis was distinguishable using motion analysis technology, and yet is this possible in the clinic? Recent research has shown that physical therapists are able to reliably detect as little as 2° change of sagittal plane rotation of simulated pelvic bone motion (Goff et al 2004). It is therefore possible that palpation of relative bone motion between the innominate and sacrum, as single-leg support is induced during a hip flexion task (the Stork test on the support side; see Fig. 25.1B), might provide a means of clinically evaluating the ability to maintain the self-braced alignment of the pelvic bones. Therapists have been shown to have 91% agreement and good reliability in determining the pattern of pelvic bone motion during the Stork test on the support side (Hungerford et al 2006). Further investigation is required to determine the validity and specificity of this test in distinguishing pelvic girdle dysfunction.

Identification of an altered pattern of muscle recruitment in subjects with PPGP is significant for the conservative management of lumbopelvic pain. Previous research has shown specific exercise treatments are effective in altering pain and functional disability in patients with segmental lumbar instability and altered motor recruitment patterns (O'Sullivan et al 1997, 2000). Further research is required to determine if the altered pattern of muscle recruitment identified in subjects with PPGP might be similarly improved with specific exercise intervention, and whether a return to normal muscle recruitment pattern also improves patterning of intrapelvic motion.

Summary

This study has shown for the first time that subjects with a clinical diagnosis of PPGP show both an altered pattern of intrapelvic motion and delayed onset of EMG activity of OI, multifidus, and gluteus maximus on the side of single-leg support, compared to control subjects. A pattern of anterior rotation of the innominate occurred only on the symptomatic side, whereas posterior rotation occurred in controls and on the asymptomatic side in subjects with PPGP. The delay in onset of OI and multifidus EMG as subjects stood onto one leg occurred on both the symptomatic and asymptomatic side in the PPGP group, and gluteus maximus was delayed only on the symptomatic side. In comparison, bicep femoris activation occurred earlier in subjects with PPGP. Changes to SIJ compression, altered alignment of the sacrum and innominate during weight bearing, and a change to lumbopelvic muscle activation might indicate a failure of the self-bracing mechanism of the pelvis. The loss of lumbopelvic stability during increased loading through the pelvis may also be related to the pain reported during standing and walking. This research will hopefully provide impetus to further studies into pelvic girdle dysfunction and mechanisms by which we can be more specific in diagnosis and treatment of the lumbopelvic region.

References

Buyruk HM, Snijders CJ, Vleeming A et al 1999 Measurements of sacroiliac joint stiffness in peripartum pelvic patients with Doppler imaging of vibrations. European Journal of Radiology 83:159–163

Carmichael J 1987 Inter and intra-examiner reliability of palpation of the sacroiliac joint dysfunction. Journal of Manipulative and Physiological Therapeutics 10: 164–171

Damen L, Buyruk HM, Guler-Ulysal F et al 2001 Pelvic pain during pregnancy is associated with asymmetric laxity of the sacroiliac joints. Acta Obstetricia et Gynecologica Scandinavica 80:1019–1024

Damen L, Buyruk HM, Guler-Uysal F et al 2002 Prognostic value of asymmetric laxity of the sacroiliac joints in pregnancy-related pelvic pain. Spine 27:2820

Domholdt E 1993. Physical therapy research: principles and applications. WB Saunders, Philadelphia, PA

DonTigny RL 1995 Function of the lumbo-sacroiliac complex as a self-compensating force couple with a variable, force-dependent transverse axis. In: Vleeming A et al (eds) Second Interdisciplinary World Congress on Low Back Pain, San Diego, CA, p501–512

Fortin J, Dwyer A, West S et al 1994 Sacroiliac joint

referral patterns upon application of a new injection/ arthrography technique. I: Asymptomatic volunteers. Spine 19:1475–1482

Gilleard W 1999 Reliability of 3Dimensional motion analysis of sacroiliac joint motion in normal subjects during drop tests. Proceedings of the Fifth IOC World Congress of Sports Sciences, Sydney, Australia

Goff L, Gilleard W, Adams R 2004 Reliability and agreement of experienced manual physiotherapists in determining simulated sacroiliac joint motion. Eighth International Physiotherapy Congress, Adelaide, Australia, p123

Hodges P 2000 Dealing with the challenges to spinal stability: mechanisms of control of the trunk. Seventh International Federation of Orthopaedic Manipulative Therapists, Perth, Australia

Hodges P, Richardson C 1997a Feedforward contraction of transversus abdominis is not influenced by the direction of arm movement. Experimental Brain Research 114:362–370

Hodges P, Richardson C 1997b Contraction of the abdominal muscles associated with movement of the lower limb. Physical Therapy 77:1132–1144

Hungerford B, Gilleard W, Hodges P 2003 Evidence of altered lumbo-pelvic muscle recruitment in the presence of sacroiliac joint pain. Spine 28:1593–1600

Hungerford B, Gilleard W, Lee D 2004 Altered patterns of pelvic bone motion determined in subjects with posterior pelvic pain using skin markers. Clinical Biomechanics 19:456–464

Hungerford B, Gilleard W, Moran M, Emmerson C 2006 Evaluation of the reliability of therapists to palpate intra-pelvic motion using the Stork test on the support side. J Physical Therapy (submitted)

Jacob H, Kissling R 1995 The mobility of the sacroiliac joints in healthy volunteers between 20 and 50 years of age. Clinical Biomechanics 10:352–361

Lee D 2004 The pelvic girdle: an approach to examination and treatment of the lumbo-pelvic-hip region. Edinburgh: Churchill Livingstone

Lee D, Vleeming A 2000 Current concepts of pelvic impairment. Seventh International Federation of Orthopaedic Manipulative Therapists, Perth, Australia

Maslen B, Ackland T 1994 Radiographic study of skin displacement errors in the foot and ankle during standing. Clinical Biomechanics 9:291–296

Mens J, Vleeming A, Snijders C et al 2001 Reliability and validity of the active straight leg raise test in posterior pelvic pain since pregnancy. Spine 26:1167–1171

Mens JMA, Vleeming A, Snijders CJ et al 1999 The active straight leg raising test and mobility of the pelvic joints. European Spine Journal 8:468–473

Mitchell FJ 1995 The muscle energy manual, vol 1. MET Press, East Lansing

Mooney V, Pozos R, Vleeming A et al 1997 Coupled motion of contralateral latissimus dorsi and gluteus maximus: its role in sacroiliac stabilization. In: Vleeming A et al (eds) Movement, stability and low back pain. Churchill Livingstone, Edinburgh, p115–122

Moseley G, Hodges P, Gandevia S 2002 Deep and superficial fibres of multifidus are differentially active during arm movements. Spine 27:E29–E36

O'Sullivan P, Twomey L, Allison G 1997 Evaluation of specific stabilizing exercise in treatment of chronic low back pain with radiologic diagnosis of spondylosis or spondylolisthesis. Spine 22:2959–2967

O'Sullivan P, Chan R, Demuth N et al 2000 Efficacy of a lumbar stability program for persons with recurrent low back pain. Seventh International Federation of Orthopaedic Manipulative Therapists, Perth, Australia, p48

O'Sullivan PB, Beales DJ, Beetham JA et al 2002 Altered motor control strategies in subjects with sacroiliac joint pain during the active straight leg raise test. Spine 27: E1–E8

Panjabi MM 1992 The stabilising system of the spine. Part 2: neutral zone and stability hypothesis. Journal of Spinal Disorders 5:390–397

Richardson CA, Snijders CJ, Hides JA et al 2002 The relationship between transversus abdominis muscles, sacroiliac joint mechanics, and low back pain. Spine 27:399–405

Rogers M, Pai Y 1990 Dynamic transitions in stance support accompanying leg flexion movements in man. Experimental Brain Research 81:398–402

Schwarzer AC, Aprill CN, Bogduk N 1995 The sacroiliac joint in chronic low back pain. Spine 20(1):31–37

Sim J, Reid N 1999 Statistical inference by confidence intervals: issues of interpretation and utilization. Physical Therapy 79:186–195

Snijders C, Vleeming A, Stoeckart R 1993 Transfer of lumbosacral load to iliac bones & legs. Part 1: biomechanics of self bracing and its significance for treatment and exercise. Clinical Biomechanics 8:285–294

Snijders C, Ribbers M, de Bakker H et al 1998 EMG recordings of abdominal & back muscles in various standing postures: validation of a biomechanical model on sacroiliac joint stability. Journal of Electromyography and Kinesiology 8:205–214

Sturesson B, Udén A, Vleeming A 2000 A radiological analysis of movements of the sacroiliac joint during the standing hip flexion test. Spine 25:364–368

Tylkowski CM, Simon SR, Mansour JM 1982 Internal rotation gait in spastic cerebral palsy in the hip. Paper presented at the Proceedings of the Tenth Open Scientific Meeting of the Hip Society, St Louis, p89–125

Vincent-Smith B, Gibbons P 1999 Inter-examiner and intra-examiner reliability of the standing hip flexion test. Manual Therapy 4:87–93

Vleeming A, van Wingerden JP, Snijders CJ et al 1989a Load application to the sacrotuberous ligament: influences on sacroiliac joint mechanics. Clinical Biomechanics 4:204–209

Vleeming A, Stoeckart C, Snijders C 1989b The sacrotuberous ligament: a conceptual approach to its dynamic role in stabilising the sacroiliac joint. Clinical Biomechanics 4:201–203

Vleeming A, Volkers ACW, Snijders CJ, Stoeckart R 1990 Relation between form and function in the sacroiliac joint. 2: biomechanical aspects. Spine 15:133–136

Vleeming A, Buyruk J, Stoeckart R et al 1992 An integrated therapy for peripartum pelvic instability: a study of the biomechanical effects of pelvic belts. American Journal of Obstetrics and Gynaecology 166:1243–1247

Vleeming A, Pool-Goudzwaard A, Stoeckart R et al 1995a The posterior layer of the thoraco-lumbar fascia: its function in load transfer from spine to legs. Spine 20:753–758

Vleeming A, Snijders C, Stoeckart R et al 1995b A new light on low back pain. Second Interdisciplinary World Congress on Low Back Pain, San Diego, CA

Vleeming A, Pool-Goudzwaard AL, Hammudoghlu D et al 1996 The function of the long dorsal sacroiliac ligament: its implication for understanding low back pain. Spine 21:556–562

Vleeming A, de Vries HJ, Mens JM, van Wingerden JP 2002 Possible role of the long dorsal sacroiliac ligament in women with peripartum pelvic pain. Acta Obstetrics Gynecology Scandinavica 81:430

Walheim GG, Selvik G 1984 Mobility of the pubic symphysis. Clinical Orthopaedics and Related Research 191:129–135

Willard FH 1997 The muscular, ligamentous and neural structure of the low back and its relation to back pain. In: Vleeming A et al (eds) Movement, stability and low back pain. Churchill Livingstone, Edinburgh, p3–35

PART THREE

Section Three

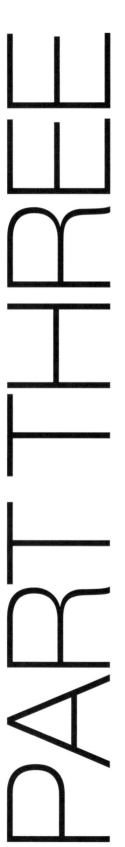

Diagnostic methods: Low back

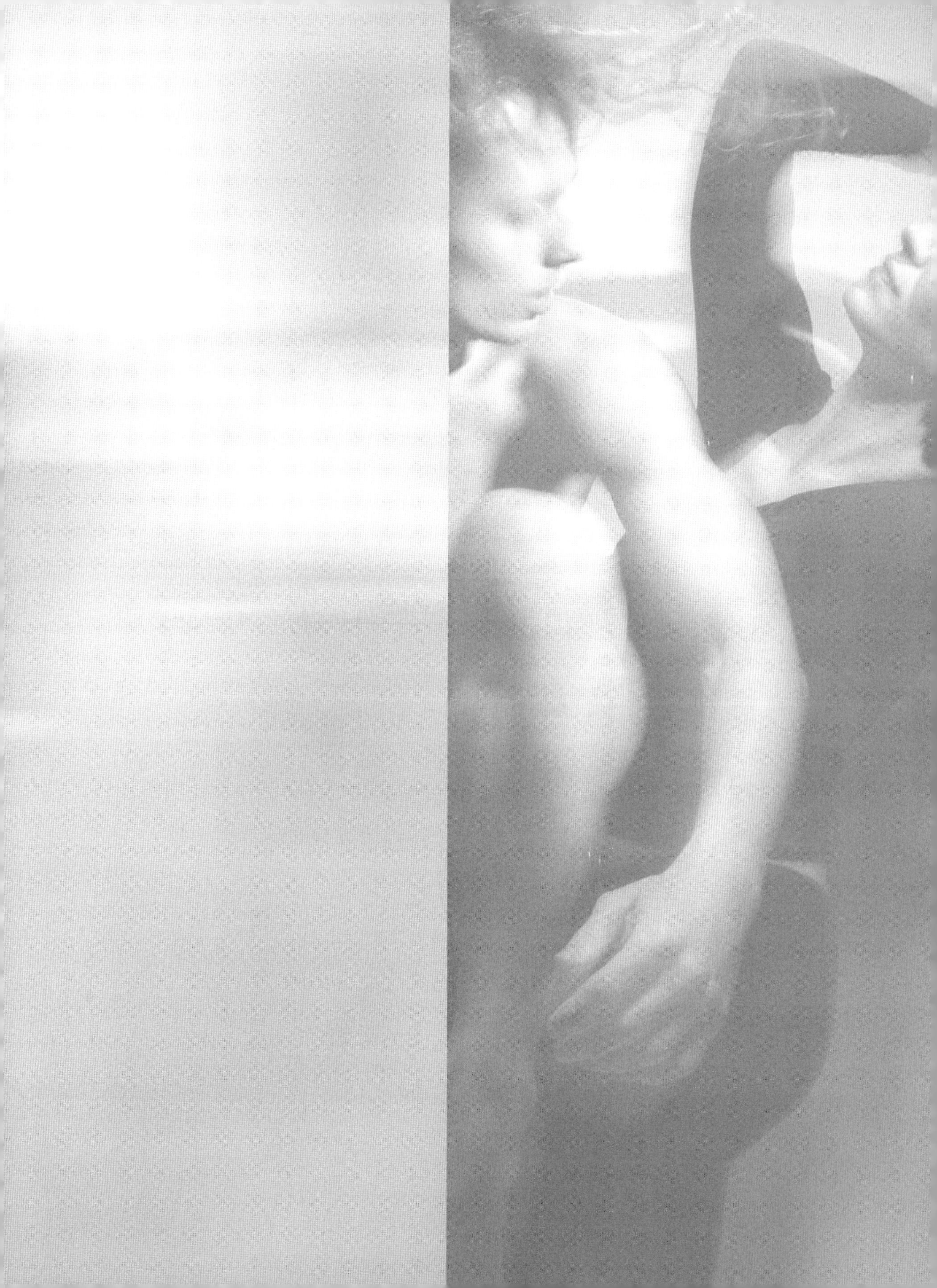

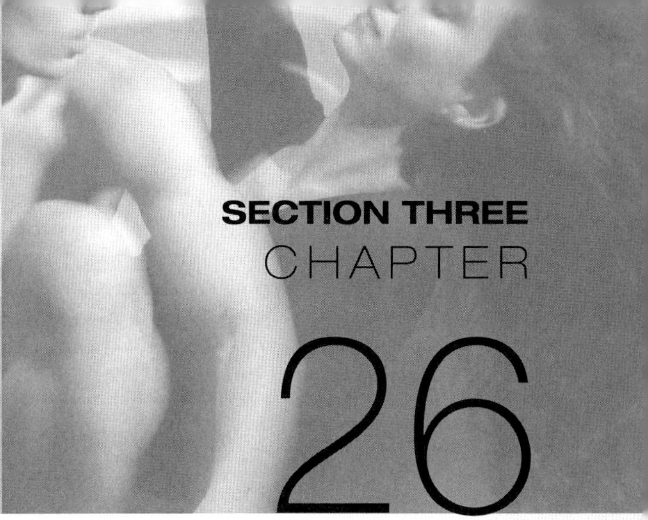

SECTION THREE
CHAPTER
26

Differential diagnosis of low back pain

Stanley V Paris and James Viti

The differential diagnosis of sacroiliac from low back pain is difficult.
(Stoddard 1959)

Introduction

There are two distinct ways of viewing low back pain. The first is the pathoanatomical model wherein the origin of the pain is determined and the stage of the condition is stated. The second is to accept that it is not possible to reach agreement on the pathoanatomical model and that it is therefore more practical simply to state where the pain is felt and what influences it in terms of its centralization and lessening in intensity.

This author has adopted the pathoanatomical model in the clinical belief that pain is the latent result of dysfunction/impairments in usually more than one tissue, and that to treat just the pain without paying attention to the underlying dysfunction will produce only a short-term result. When symptoms return they do so in an older patient and at a more chronic stage, making direct treatment of the pathoanatomical causes more difficult.

As stated, there is usually more than one dysfunction present before the level of noxious stimuli reaches the patient's awareness for pain. In this model the goal is to define the sources of dysfunction whether they are the source of pain (e.g. facet, disc, sacroiliac) or contribute to the source of pain (e.g. short leg, stiff hip). These authors also recognize that pain and the resulting complaints have a great deal to do with the individual's culture, personality, and activity status. However, these latter aspects will not be the focus of this chapter.

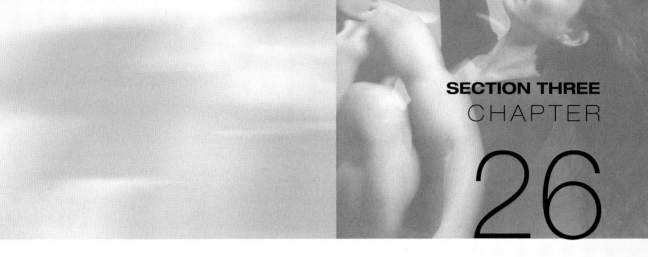

Most structures of the spine are innervated and are thus capable of giving rise to pain. For years it was thought that the disc was the largest aneuronal structure in the spine, if not the body, and that the disc only gave rise to pain when a protrusion came to rest on a nerve (Cyriax 1947, 1950). Now we know that the disc is exquisitely innervated (Roberts et al 1995) in its neurovascular capsule and that although the internal disc is not innervated, it becomes so when degeneration results in the invasion of blood vessels with accompanying nerve supply.

The sensation of pain occurs when the sum of nociception from one or more sources reaches the individual's threshold of awareness. The more actively engaged the individual, the higher their threshold for pain due in large part to the increased firing of mechanoreceptors (Wyke 1972) that will serve to operate the gate control mechanism to pain first described by Melzack & Wall (1965).

The accompanying list of common syndromes identifies structures that are innervated and thus might give rise to nociception. The first response to nociception is not pain but involuntary muscle splinting. Although this 'primitive reflex' will tend to hold the segment against further stress, it also increases the 'load' on the spine, which in turn adds further stress to the disc. The more stress on the disc, the more rapidly it will dehydrate, bulge outwards, and stress the nociceptive outer annulus. Thus these authors hold that regardless of the dysfunction the muscles will become involved and therefore increase the load on the disc which in turn may add to the sum of nociception which will eventually reach the threshold for pain.

Kirkaldy-Willis (1990) spoke of the 'degenerative cascade' and drew attention to the fact that if there were more than modest degenerative changes in the facet joints, the disc would become involved, and vice versa. In fact, he stated that it was impossible to have an operative disc lesion without there being additional changes such as instability and facet joint degeneration. Therefore to treat a single pathoanatomical structure without considering the totality of contributing factors is a rather short-sighted approach to spine care. The concept of 'summation,' wherein back pain is the 'sum' of dysfunctions rather than from a single source is much needed in back care. Surgery without manual therapy to muscles, facets, hip, and leg is just not going to have the results that could be obtained with a broader approach that integrates manual therapy, medicine, and surgery.

As a manual physical therapist who has specialized in manipulative therapy of the joints and myofascia, I (Paris) have been encouraged with the state of recent research that supports the fact that conservative care is equal to or better than surgical care even in the management of patients with paresis (DuBourg et al 2002). Furthermore, it has been shown that manual physical therapy working with medicine obtains results significantly better than surgery (Saal & Saal 1989). Thus conservative care should now become the focus of back pain management and it is hoped that this chapter contributes to that evolution.

Classification of syndromes and their treatment

The principal syndromes of the lumbar spine and pelvis that give rise to low back and leg pains are listed below. Within each syndrome there are several subsyndromes (Paris 2002). They are listed here not in order of their severity but in order of their frequency:

- myofascial states
- facet dysfunction
- ligamentous weakness and instability
- sacroiliac (SI) dysfunction
- disc dysfunction
- spondylolisthesis
- central canal and lateral foraminal stenosis
- kissing lumbar spines (Baastrup's disease)
- thoracolumbar syndrome
- lesion complex.

Myofascial states

As stated in the Introduction, changes in the myofascia will invariably accompany back pain, regardless of its origin. Not all myofascial changes, particularly those relating to changes in tone, require treatment, but they always require consideration. 'Tone' is here defined as the normal elasticity of a muscle to stretch or touch. When we palpate a muscle and speak of its 'tone', we are actually speaking of its response to our touch as it elastically (linear response) contracts against our deforming palpation in order to protect its muscle spindles from further deformation.

Hypertonic states

Spasm

There is no doubt that 'spasm' is one of the most misused terms in orthopedics because it is frequently used to describe any noted change in muscles.

True spasm is defined as a 'sudden involuntary contraction of one or more muscle groups' (*Stedman's Concise Medical Dictionary for the Health Professions* 1997). Thus patients who are rigidly splinting their back in flexion or any other posture are not demonstrating 'spasm' but rather what this author recognizes as 'muscle splinting.' There are several types of muscle splinting, some of which can benefit from treatment whereas others can be ignored while attention is directed at the cause. Thus the term 'spasm' should be reserved for sudden involuntary twitches of muscle denoting such possibilities as pain, instability, or apprehension.

Treatment: Treat the cause of spasm.

Hypertrophy

Hypertrophy commonly results from muscle training as in body building. Such muscles are at an increased tone even at rest and might unduly load the spine, impede nutrition at rest, and enable extreme weight to be lifted contributing to such fatigue fractures as spondylolisthesis.

Involuntary splinting

This is the most common of the hypertonic muscle states, usually involving the multifidus group, and will invariably coexist with most underlying dysfunctions. No doubt the muscle response is produced by nociception in an effort to splint the back from further stress and injury. It will be relieved immediately by lying down *with adequate support*. Unfortunately, muscle splinting increases the load on the spinal segments and should the nociception actually arise from the disc this would invariably aggravate the situation.

Treatment: Ignore the muscle behavior and treat the causes.

Chemical splinting

Should involuntary splinting continue it will result in the retention of waste products, which will give rise to back pain. The author considers that much of low back pain is due to persistent muscle splinting secondary to the underlying disc, facet, or sacroiliac problem. Another cause of chemical muscle splinting is from simple overuse, as can be experienced in, say, the quadriceps after an unaccustomed run or climb. The muscles retaining waste metabolites will appear to have an elevated resting tone and are tender and doughy to touch. Massage is of great help to relieve this discomfort and promote motion, and some patients learn that by 'cracking' their back they can relieve this discomfort. The mechanism here is believed to be the firing of type III articular mechanoreceptors, which, like Golgi tendon apparatuses (GTOs), are inhibitory of muscle tone (Wyke 1972).

Treatment: Heat, deep massage, stretching the muscle, and finding the causes. Discourage the self-cracking, as this usually takes place at a mobile or hypermobile joint with ligamentous weakness (see below).

Voluntary splinting

Should nociception reach the threshold for pain, the patient might voluntarily splint the affected parts, holding them against segmental motion much as a person with a painful shoulder might hold the arm to the side.

Treatment: Movement needs to be encouraged based on the same principles expounded by Codman (1934) for the shoulder, i.e. repetitive motion. Of course, if the condition involves acute significant trauma, support, rather than movement, should be given initially.

Psychosomatic stress

The possibility that psychosomatic stress might result in altered low back function must not be ignored. Tension can give rise to headaches, clenching jaw, and temporomandibular joint dysfunction, and so why not to low back pain?

Hypotonic states

Disuse atrophy

Disuse atrophy will occur in any back which for either pain or stiffness has resulted in a loss of normal mobility. The muscle will appear to have lost bulk, lack normal tone and be somewhat fibrous to palpation.

Treatment: Manipulation to restore motion, heat and deep tissue massage for circulation followed by specific exercise to the weakened muscles.

Wasting and fibrosis

Like disuse atrophy, this condition is more likely the result of neurological or surgical interference with normal nerve conduction. The muscles waste and appear fibrositic.

Treatment: Heat and massage for circulation, exercises to hypertrophy remaining muscles and stabilization routines to protect the possibly permanently weakened segments.

Normal tone/shortened

Adaptive shortening

Adaptive shortening, which is initially a loss of sarcomeres and later a shortening of the intramuscular connective tissues, results from muscle being held in a shortened position. A typical example is the overweight male with a pendulous abdomen. This posture results in an increased lumbar lordosis leading to posterior muscle shortening and limited hip extension secondary to shortening of psoas and associated muscles. This example of adaptive shortening can contribute to spinal stenosis.

Treatment: Muscle stretching by either fatigue stretching or connective tissue massage.

Compartmental syndrome

When muscles in the lumbar spine hypertrophy, owing either to muscle splinting, instability, a change in the work environment, or body-building activities, they can become restricted in their fascial compartments, resulting in a chronic uni- or bilateral paravertebral back pain. The muscles will feel tender to the touch.

Treatment: Deep massage (Rolfing, connective tissue techniques) to the paravertebral area, plus sustained squats or stretching over a bolster placed across the lap while seated. The goal is to stretch out the connective envelope in which the muscle resides to make space for the return of sarcomeres.

Fibrositis

The authors consider this a nonentity. The 'nodules' that can be palpated in muscle are not presented until palpated for. This apparent contradiction is explained by the fact that the palpating finger stretches the muscle spindle causing the fiber in which it resides to contract thus giving rise to a 'nodule'-like feeling. These nodules are therefore a physiological response to touch. However, around the iliac crest, just lateral to multifidus insertion, there are a number of fatty nodules that seem to be without pathology but – like all structures – will be tender when the back is experiencing sufficient dysfunction.

Facet dysfunction

The spinal facet joints, particularly their posterior medial aspect, are perhaps the most innervated structures in the spine (Paris 1984). Since the 1930s, they have been identified as a source of pain and have been the subject of a number of studies involving the reproduction of pain by injecting hypertonic saline (Mooney & Robinson 1976).

We can identify five separate clinical states in the spinal facets, which should not come as a surprise, as all five can exist in other synovial joints, such as the knee, which, in common with the spinal facets, have meniscal inclusions. These states are described below.

Facet synovitis/hemarthrosis (acute sprain)

Acute synovitis or hemarthrosis is perhaps the most common source of acute, usually transient, low back pain. Its cause appears to be a strain or nipping of the sensitive facet capsule and its synovial lining following an awkward or forceful movement. Depending on the degree of noxious stimulation, it is accompanied by involuntary or voluntary muscle guarding. It is widely accepted that 80% of back pain resolves within 2 weeks and in the view of these authors most of these cases are facet injuries.

Typically, the injury occurs when the spine is moved in a sudden motion or in recovering with a twist from a forward bent position. Although three structures are designed to prevent capsular nipping [the elastic anterior capsule (ligamentum flavum), the intracapsular fibrous meniscoid, and the attachment of the multifidus muscle posteriorly], these mechanisms can fail and a painful nipping can result. The joint swells and the nipping is relieved. The initial pain is sharp and often quite localized and, in the cervical spine, can be readily palpated.

The signs and symptoms are of localized low back pain and minimal radiation, perhaps to the iliac crest and buttock (further if there is a memory of sciatic pain from past problems).

Movement, if limited, is most likely from the accompanying involuntary muscle holding and is not particularly uncomfortable. Loading the facet, as in backward bending and bending to the same side, is not painful at this stage.

The effusion would be expected to resolve in 2–3 days and, as with other joints, will leave behind some restrictions to movement. This will be the case especially if the injury resulted in hemarthrosis and thus the deposition of fibrinogen into the joint leading to the formation of intra-articular adhesions (Paris 2002). These restrictions help to splint the sensitive joint, thus enabling the muscle splinting to abate and the patient to move more freely. Such restrictions do, however, leave the joint less able to tolerate future insults, making it even more prone to reinjury, and resulting again in synovitis and hemarthrosis. Restrictions of facets also serve to limit nutrition to the intervertebral disc.

Treatment: Manipulation to adjacent segments can facilitate early return to movement due to the manipulation's relaxing or inhibiting effect on muscles. Manipulation to the injured joint is not recommended for some 10 days because of the possibility of accompanying hemarthrosis. Medication for pain relief and assurance of a timely recovery are sufficient.

Facet stiffness (restrictions)

Spinal facet restriction is very common and is a painless condition, as is initial stiffness in joints of the extremities. However, stiffness leads to loss of nutrition and hence aids degeneration. This might be true – especially in the spine – where stiff facets combined with adaptive muscle shortening can lead to interference with disc nutrition and precipitate disc degeneration, herniation, and prolapse.

As stiff joints do not necessarily hurt, they are usually detected on examination for back pain from other causes. Segmental restrictions are detected with passive motion testing (motion palpation; Gonella et al 1982); adhesions have been demonstrated by the present author (Paris 1991).

Treatment: Manipulation directed specifically at the involved joint and in the direction of the restriction.

Facet painful entrapment

The patient reports with acute low back pain and postural deviation away from the painful side. The postural change came on immediately following the injury. Any effort to resume normal alignment is accompanied by a local and sharp pain on one side of the back. The pain does not radiate, but might – a day or so later – migrate up the spine owing to painful involuntary muscle guarding, leading to chemical muscle holding.

The pathology of this diagnosis has never been demonstrated but the logic of its presence is persuasive (Kraft & Levinthal 1951), especially given the effectiveness of the treatment. Pathological specimens have shown enlarged facet capsules and intra-articular fatty cysts, which are believed to be innervated (Kirkaldy-Willis, unpublished data).

Treatment: Manipulation is used, employing a lumbar rotary technique, which is, in effect, a distraction of the facet joint in order to release the entrapped facet capsule. On occasion, an isometric contraction of multifidus might pull the capsule from the joint space.

Facet mechanical block

In contrast to painful block, a mechanical block is relatively painless but again is immediate following an awkward motion. The patient quite simply becomes suddenly fixed in a laterally shifted position. Any attempt to straighten upward is met with difficulty, and the patient often reports being 'stuck' and in need of having it 'cracked.' The exact mechanism is speculative. However, as spinal facets contain menisci, and on occasion loose bodies, and such joints elsewhere in the body (the knee, craniomandibular joint, and wrist) are known to become stuck or locked, it is surely possible that the spinal facets might also lock.

Treatment: Distraction manipulation as for a painful block.

Chronic facet dysfunction

This condition results from repeated strains and sprains to the facet joints and is no different from degenerative arthrosis affecting synovial joints elsewhere in the body. Stiffness and pain is felt on rising, with stiffness easing and pain increasing towards the end of the day. A facet block can be diagnostic if both the traditional joint as well as its medial compartment is injected.

Ligamentous weakness and instability

The term 'instability' has received considerable attention since the 1990s. Instability will occur when the osseoligamentous and neuromuscular components of the segment are unable to hold the spine against slippage in neutral during sitting and standing and during movement against aberrant motions.

Ligamentous laxity can be a source of pain in peripheral joints such as the knee, glenohumeral, and acromioclavicular joints. It is now accepted that the same situation is commonly present in the spine (Kirkaldy-Willis 1990, Nachemson 1985). The structures responsible for passive spinal stability are initially the ligamentous structures, including the outer annulus of the intervertebral disc, which is likewise made up of type I stress-resistant collagen. The facet joints also play a variable role in passive spinal stabilization and their surgical removal will help to create instability. Additionally, the posterior muscles of the spine are important in achieving stabilization, especially the muscle multifidus. In some quarters, a great deal of attention has been given to the stabilizing role of the transverse abdominus, which no doubt is important but as a result it would seem that too little attention has been given to the remaining abdominal muscles especially the obliques.

In the authors' opinion, ligamentous weakness precedes segmental ligamentous instability, and instability is a precursor of the clinically apparent disc condition perhaps requiring surgery with or without fusion. A stable spine appears far less likely to present with a clinically obvious disc problem. As the outer annulus of the disc is type I collagen as are ligaments and tendons, the outer annulus must also be considered a ligament.

The pain of ligamentous weakness is characteristic. It begins with a dull ache in the back, which, as the day wears on, appears to spread to the muscles (the muscles are actually in chemical muscle holding). This ache can be relieved by a change in position, movement, and massage or by 'self-cracking' of the back. The 'self-cracking' is not to be recommended as it severely stresses the disc, leading to further instability, and although it might provide temporary relief, it does so at the expense of stability.

Given that ligamentous weakness also involves the annulus fibrosus, transient neurological signs might occur, as might a transient lateral shift, again toward the end of the day. Such a lateral shift can be considered to be a sign of instability, and is not unlike letting the air out of a car tire when parked on an incline: the car will shift sideways down the incline. Reinflation will set the car uphill once again, and a night's rest will straighten the spine – at least initially.

Causes of spinal instability are, no doubt, to be found in postural misuse and abuse, smoking and poor nutrition. The clinical signs and symptoms of instability (Paris 1985) include:

- A visible or palpable step or rotary deformity, which is present on standing but which reduces on lying.
- Hypertonicity of the muscles on standing that disappears on lying.
- Hypermobility on motion passive palpation: grade 5 or 6 (Gonnella et al 1982).
- Shaking or trembling of the lumbar spine on forward bending.
- More difficulty in coming upright than going into forward bending.
- A history of 'catches' and 'giving way'.

Treatment: The key to treatment is in understanding that while gymnasts have lost their osseoligamentous stability, they are quite stable (as long as they do not get fatigued) because of their superb neuromuscular training. That, then, is the way for all patients who have instability – neuromuscular training. Manipulation to any neighboring stiff joints might also assist.

Sacroiliac dysfunction

The sacroiliac joint is listed fourth in this presentation because, in the authors' opinion, it is the fourth most common cause of low back and pelvic pain, preceded only by muscular, facet joint syndromes, and ligamentous weakness.

The principal source of pain arising from the sacroiliac (SI) is, no doubt, the richly innervated, strong, deep posterior SI ligaments (Paris 1983), which are designed to resist principally vertical stresses and some element of rotation in the female. The iliolumbar ligament is also a key SI ligament and, when strained, will also give rise to lateral low back pain, which can be confused with sacroiliac pain.

It is the authors' opinion that stiff sacroiliac joints are not painful and that stiffness leading to osseous fusion is the natural condition, especially for the male SI (Paris 1983).

Acute strain

Acute strain is most commonly caused by a fall on one of the ischial tuberosities. If the ligaments are strong, they will resist a displacement but it might be quite painful for a few days. The pain is local as is the tenderness.

Treatment: Modalities or medication for pain relief. If severe and persisting beyond 1 week, the joint should be re-examined for hypermobility and, if present, treated as recommended below.

Hypermobility

Hypermobility is caused by repeated sprains and strains, such as in falls, poor postural habits, as in one-leg standing, and vigorous positions in sexual intercourse wherein the thighs are repeatedly forced toward the chest – this is especially the case in those with restricted hip motion. All of the above activities cause the ilium to rotate posteriorly. Once the joint is hypermobile it will ache on prolonged standing, especially one-legged standing and will be eased almost immediately by lying supine. Standing rotates the ilium posteriorly in the female whereas lying rotates it anteriorly. The pain is also increased, as with all ligamentous and discogenic pains, in the days just prior to the menstrual flow.

Treatment: Begin with an explanation of the stresses that are causing the problem and how to avoid most, if not all, of them. If the hip joints are restricted, they should be manipulated. If the SI pain is acute or severe, a Scultetus binder or sacroiliac belt is recommended. Relief by either the binder or belt is generally confirmatory of the diagnosis. Both must be placed uncomfortably low to support the sacrum between the ilium and should be placed while the subject is lying to correct the tendency of a hypermobile SI to go into backward rotation while standing.

Displacement (subluxation)

The hypermobile sacroiliac is most likely to result in a displacement and a resultant 'lock' of the irregular articular surfaces. The pain that was intermittent during the preceding period of hypermobility is now of a lower degree but is constant – even in lying.

Treatment: Manipulation. Once the manipulation has succeeded, the joint is usually found to be hypermobile and will benefit from support.

It should be noted that the previous three conditions are either aggravated or relieved by stress tests to the SI. Such tests are inconclusive if they are not specific to the supporting ligaments of the joint. Intra-articular injections have mixed results, as the anesthetic will fail to infiltrate the large posterior sacroiliac ligaments and of course the associated iliolumbar ligaments, and will, quite probably, burst through a synovial recess in the anterior capsule mistaken by some as an SI tear (Neville et al 1996). Injections given by numerous releases into the posterior ligaments, especially at the upper pole of the joint at the level of S1 and S2, would appear to be more effective.

Disc dysfunction

In virtually all patients with a clinically evident disc protrusion or rupture (presence of paresis) there is first a preceding history of ligamentous weakness and/or spinal instability. This raises the possibility that disc prolapses are the result of failure to intervene with conservative care, i.e. manual physical therapy.

For a clinical disc protrusion and/or prolapse to be diagnosed, there must be demonstrable neurological signs other than pain below the knee and limited straight leg raising. Straight leg raise can be limited by hip, sacroiliac, and muscular tenderness. Objective muscle weakness (paresis) and loss of skin sensation are indicative of nerve root involvement. Reduced or absent reflexes are less indicative.

An analysis of the literature now shows that even in the presence of paresis, conservative care is equal to or better than disc surgery and that aggressive conservative care is better than either (Saal & Saal 1989).

The nonoperative treatment will depend on the stage of the condition.

Immediate stage

This stage occurs when the patient, who has a history of ligamentous weakness and/or instability, performs an awkward or unguarded action and feels something 'give' or 'tear' in his or her back. In such circumstances, especially if there is a history of low back pain and instability, it is a real possibility that the disc has just torn.

The patient should immediately stand erect and maintain a lordosis to close down the tear and help promote healing. However, most people who injure their back are wont to sit down and rest. Unfortunately, sitting increases the load on the disc and might well place the patient in a kyphosis, which opens the tear and allows the nucleus to imbibe fluids and expand out through the tear. The lordotic posture should be maintained with the assistance of taping for 2 weeks, after which the back can rest flat; flexion should be avoided for at least 6 weeks.

Acute stage

Here we presume that the disc is protruded/extruded and the nerve root is compromised and that the opportunity to contain it by having gone immediately into backward bending (lordosis) is lost. Any attempt to go into backward bending at this stage may increase the size of the protrusion bringing it more firmly onto the nerve thus increasing symptoms (McCall 1980, Spohr & Paris 1992).

Treatment: Treatment is medications for pain and rest alternated with movement. The rest should be in a position of comfort and movement should be minimal. For ambulation, a walker or crutches can be of assistance, depending of the degree of the symptoms.

Subacute

The symptoms will begin to recede some 3 to 5 days after injury. Now the patient should be encouraged to ambulate and get moving. A walker or crutches can help. Periods of moving should be alternated with rest on a firm surface with the back flat to assist in disc nutrition and to avoid strain on the disc. The outer annulus appears to be more vascular than the medial ligament at the knee and so healing of the tear can be expected (Paris 1990). Sitting is to be discouraged, especially in a soft sofa or automobile seat.

Settled stage

This stage begins about 3 weeks after onset. The patient is ambulatory.

Treatment: Backward bending to regain the lordosis and the erect position is the first priority should the lordosis have been lost. Repeated backward bending can centralize the pain and lessen the discomfort.

If neurological signs are present, positional distraction, which seeks to open the foramen and gently pull the outer annulus flat, thus temporarily relieving the nerve root pressure can now be commenced. Positional distraction is side lying over a bolster with the painful side uppermost and the involved segment positioned in such a manner as to achieve maximum foraminal opening without unduly stressing the disc (Paris 2002). Treatments begin at 5 min and rapidly progress to 30 min several times a day. It can be done as a home program.

Chronic stage

This is at about 12 weeks, when all primary healing has taken place, and in a patient who still has symptoms.

Treatment: As for the settled stage, if it has not already been carried out. In addition, fitness training and work-hardening can be added. Emphasis should also be placed on behavioral modification techniques. Admittedly, treatment is not very effective at this stage and a multidisciplinary program might need to be engaged.

Spondylolisthesis

There are several types of spondylolisthesis. The most common is from a fatigue fracture of the pars interarticularis. Whatever the cause, a palpable 'step' and/or 'rotation' can be detected in the back when standing. If the step or rotation disappears with lying, the slip can be considered to be unstable. X-ray confirmation should be taken at the end of the day, with the patient standing to maximize displacement. Lying films might fail to show a degenerative spondylolisthesis if it is unstable and has self-reduced with lying.

The symptoms are ligamentous and local. Up to a grade I displacement (one-fifth slip) might not be the source of the patient's symptoms, as many such subjects can be found to be without back pain. Only if the slip is advanced will neurological signs and symptoms result.

Treatment: This depends on whether or not the condition is stable or unstable. If it is stable, no treatment is called for, as the condition is unlikely to be the cause of any complaints. If it is unstable, posture, education, stretching (carefully) of the iliopsoas, and stabilization exercises of the deep spinal musculature are called for and are usually successful. Stabilization treatment has been shown to be effective in the treatment of this condition (Hides et al 2001, O'Sullivan et al 1997).

Central canal and lateral foraminal stenosis

The typical patient is middle-aged to elderly, short, and heavy framed, with a history of a lifestyle that is physically stressful to the lumbar spine; the patient is perhaps obese, diabetic, and has a history of smoking.

The signs and symptoms are extremely variable but include transient neurological signs and symptoms brought on by exercising, particularly in the afternoon. Neurovascular claudication occurs during walking, similar to vascular claudication, but is distinguished by the fact that forward bending tends to relieve the pain. The bicycle test is confirmatory. Riding a stationary bicycle with the back in lordosis will soon bring on leg pain, but riding the bicycle with the low back in kyphosis will delay or even prevent the onset of pain.

Treatment: Treatment can often be effective if the patient will be compliant. The goal is to flatten the lordosis and increase the physical fitness. Muscle stretching especially of the paravertebral and psoas, and fitness training such as pool therapy and unweighted treadmill exercising all play a role.

Kissing lumbar spines

Baastrup described a condition in which the spinous processes of the lumbar spine impinge on one another and give rise to arthritis and sclerotic changes, which can become quite painful. The condition is most common in short, stocky males at middle life. It is in these individuals that the spinous processes tend to be large and the disc spaces small. With middle age and the natural shrinking of the intervertebral disc, the spinous processes impinge on one another, producing central low back pain relieved by forward bending or pulling the knees to the chest (Baastrup 1933).

Treatment: Conservative treatment is limited beyond providing an explanation, stretching out any tight lumbar myofascia to lessen a static lordosis, pelvic tilt, negative-heel shoes, and abdominal strengthening, with perhaps counseling for weight loss. Surgical intervention to remodel the spinous process was recommended by Baastrup; others have recommended sclerosing injections, and still others have had success with medial branch rhizolysis.

Thoracolumbar syndrome

Perhaps first described by Maigne, this instability condition at the thorocolumbar junction gives rise to irritation of the lateral cutaneous nerve to the thigh and a 'radicular' type of pain referral to the area of the hip joint and surrounding tissues. There is usually tenderness where the nerve crosses the posterior iliac crest.

The condition appears to originate from the T11–L1 levels, sometimes secondary to stiffness or surgical fusion of the lower levels.

Treatment: Manipulation of the lower levels when possible, and stabilization exercises for the thoracolumbar region, produces good results.

Lesion complex

The preceding sections have presented some of the more common dysfunctions that can cause pain in the spine. Although they have been presented as single entities and given names somewhat comparable with diagnostic terms, it is important to note that most of those who present with symptoms have signs and symptoms not simply of one syndrome but of several, and therein lies the difficulty of a differential diagnosis and the reason for the term 'lesion complex.' Furthermore as stated in the Introduction, patients rarely report with a single entity as the cause of their pain and disability but rather a number of entities that, in 'sum,' result in nociception crossing their threshold of awareness to pain.

Summary

The authors feel that the majority of back pain is the result of the following list of syndromes:

- Myofascial states
- Facet dysfunction
- Ligamentous weakness and instability
- Sacroiliac dysfunction
- Disc dysfunction
- Spondylolisthesis
- Central canal and lateral foraminal stenosis
- Kissing lumbar spines (Baastrup's disease)
- Thoracolumbar syndrome
- Lesion complex.

Since back pain can arise from one or a combination of the above listed sources, it is important for the practicing clinician to do a thorough examination in order to attempt to identify and treat the cause of the pain and its contributing factors, rather than treat the pain itself (Paris 1992). It is the authors' opinion that this will lead to a more permanent or lasting resolution of the symptoms and improvement in function.

References

Baastrup C 1933 On the spinous processes of the lumbar vertebrae and the soft tissues between them, and on pathological changes in that region. Acta Radiologica 14:52

Codman EA 1934 The shoulder. Thomas Todd Company, Boston, MA

Cyriax JH 1947 Textbook of orthopaedic medicine, vol. I. Diagnosis of soft tissue lesions. Cassell, London

Cyriax JH 1950 Textbook of orthopaedic medicine, vol. II. Treatment by manipulation and deep massage. Cassell, London

Dubourg G, Rozenberg S, Fautrel B et al 2002 A pilot study on the recovery from paresis after lumbar disc herniation. Spine 27(13):1426–1432

Gonella C, Paris SV, Kutner M 1982 Reliability in evaluating passive intervertebral motion. Physical Therapy 62(4):436–444

Hides JA, Jull GA, Richardson CA 2001 Long-term effects of specific stabilizing exercises for first-episode low back pain. Spine 26:E243–E248

Kirkaldy-Willis WH 1990 Segmental instability, the lumbar spine. WB Saunders, Philadelphia, PA

Kraft GL, Levinthal DH 1951 Facet synovial impingement; a new concept in the etiology of the lumbar vertebral derangement. Surgery, Gynecology and Obstetrics 93(4):439–444

McCall I 1980 In: The lumbar spine and low back pain, 2nd edn. Pitman, London

Melzack R, Wall PD 1965 Pain mechanisms: a new theory. Science 150(699):971–979

Mooney VT, Robinson J 1976 The facet syndrome. Clinical Orthopaedics 115:149–156

Nachemson A 1985 Lumbar spine instability: a critical update and symposium summary. Spine 10:254

Neville C, Graham-Smith A, Patla CE 1996 Sacroiliac joint instability, diagnostically confirmed: a case study poster presentation. American Physical Therapy Association, Atlanta, GA

O'Sullivan PB, Phyty GD, Twomey LT, Allison GT 1997 Evaluation of specific stabilizing exercise in the treatment of chronic low back pain with radiologic diagnosis of spondylolisis or spondylolisthesis. Spine 22(24):2959–2967

Paris SV 1983 Anatomy as related to function and pain. Orthopedic Clinics of North America 14(3):475–489

Paris SV 1984 Functional anatomy of the lumbar spine. University Microfilms International, Ann Arbor, MI

Paris SV 1985 Physical signs of instability. Spine 10(3): 277–279

Paris SV 1990 Healing of the lumbar intervertebral disc. Proceedings of the Canadian Manual Therapy Association, Canada

Paris SV 1991 Physical therapy approach to facet, disc and sacroiliac syndromes of the lumbar spine. In: White AH (ed) Conservative care of low back pain. Williams & Wilkins, Baltimore, MD

Paris SV 1992 Differential diagnosis of sacroiliac joint

from lumbar spine dysfunction. First Interdisciplinary World Congress on Low Back Pain and its Relation to the Sacroiliac Joint. University of California, San Diego, p313–326

Paris SV 2002 Introduction to spinal evaluation and manipulation. University of St Augustine for Health Sciences, St Augustine, USA

Roberts S, Eisenstein SM, Menage J et al 1995 Mechanoreceptors in intervertebral discs. Spine 20(24):2645–2651

Saal JA, Saal JS 1989 Nonoperative treatment of herniated lumbar intervertebral disc with radiculopathy: an outome study. Spine 14(4):431–437

Spohr C, Paris SV 1992 Discomyelogram, a fluoroscopic study of disc protrusion. Proceedings of the Fifth IFOMT Congress, Vail, CO

Stedman TL 1997 Stedman's concise medical dictionary for the health professions. Williams and Wilkins, Baltimore, MD, p810

Stoddard A 1959 Manual of osteopathic technique. Hutchinson, London

Wyke B 1972 Articular neurology. Physiotherapy 58(3): 94–99

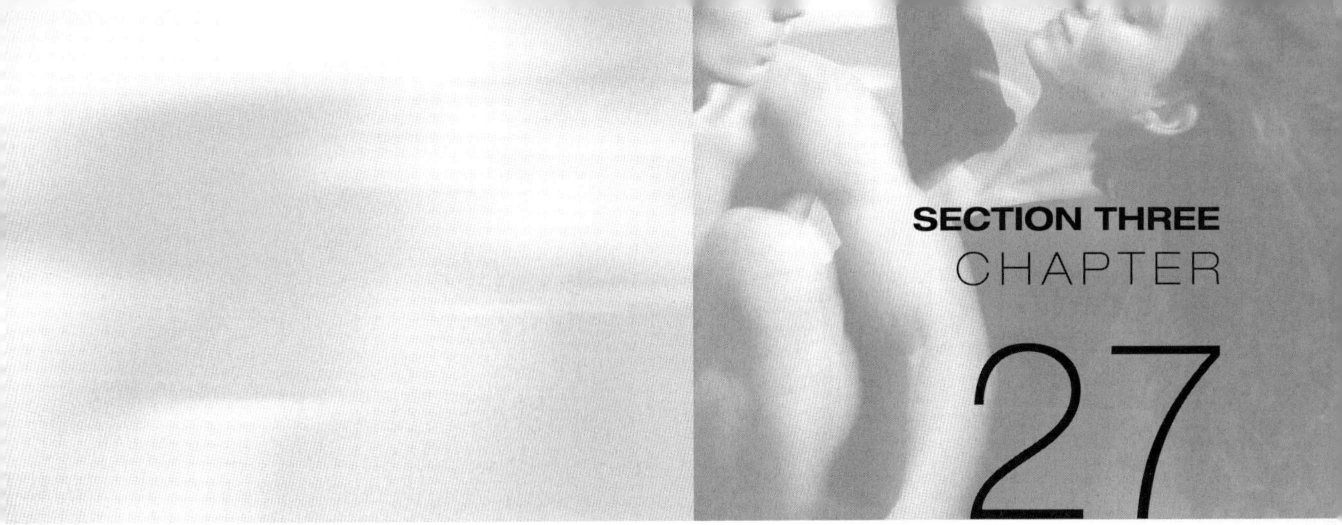

SECTION THREE CHAPTER 27

Conditions of weight bearing: asymmetrical overload syndrome (AOS)

James A Porterfield and Carl DeRosa

Introduction

Questions: 'Does the presence of a leg length difference predispose the person to premature low back and hip degeneration?' and 'Is there an exact science of measurement to determine this skeletal asymmetry?'

The answers to these questions remain mixed (Brady et al 2003, Burke 2004, Giles & Taylor 1981, Gofton 1985, Gurney 2002, Juhl et al 2004, Tallroth et al 2005, White et al 2004). This chapter presents an anatomical and biomechanical model for the evaluation and treatment of the conditions of weight bearing that will be referred to as AOS (asymmetrical overload syndrome). The chapter is divided as follows: introduction, aging and degeneration, body types, assessment (subdivided into standing examination, assessment of the foot and gait analysis) and treatment. Finally, before the summary statement, we briefly describe asymmetrical biomechanics of each malady listed in Box 27.1.

The body responds to consistent stresses placed on it. There are two physical principles and laws that form the foundation of physical medicine: (1) the SAID principle (specific adaptation to imposed demand); and (2) Wolff's law. These two principles are coupled with the dynamics and physics of the loads and forces (stress and strain) absorbed by and transferred through the body. These laws describe the buildup and breakdown of the tissues in the neuromusculoskeletal system. As our bodies age, adaptively change, and become injured, the load-bearing tolerance of our systems decreases and our postures change, restorative activities diminish, and the chances for increased pain and dysfunction increase.

Box 27.1

Common maladies with asymmetrical overload syndrome

1. Lumbar segment spondylosis
2. Sacroiliac joint sprain/strain/osteoarthritis
3. Hip joint osteoarthritis
4. Greater trochanter bursitis
5. Piriformis syndrome
6. Iliotibial band friction syndrome (lateral epicondylitis)
7. Knee pain:
   a. tibiofemoral osteoarthritis (medial)
   b. patellofemoral osteoarthritis/anterior knee pain

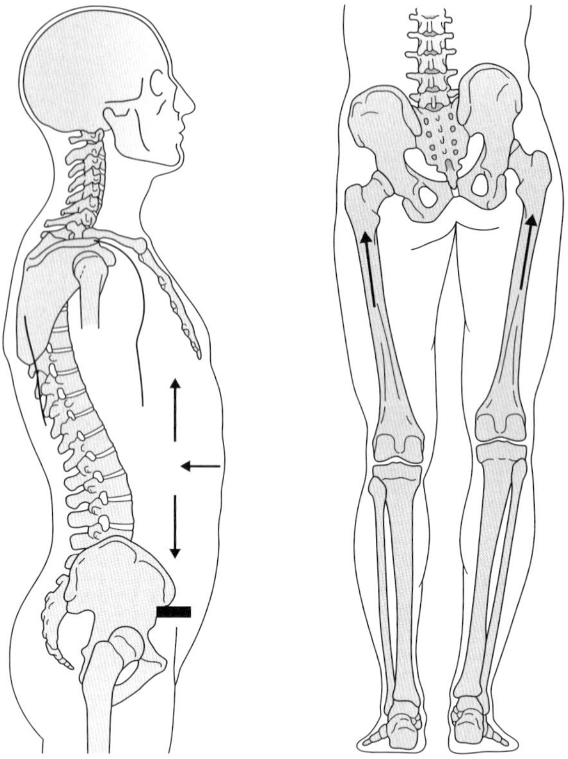

Fig. 27.1 Asymmetry created by changes in the antigravity posture in the frontal and sagittal planes predisposes the musculoskeletal tissues to injury and early degeneration.

Declining load-bearing tolerance enhances the potential for overload, and it is the overload that results in the painful condition. Skeletal asymmetry and changes in our posture both in the sagittal and frontal plane (Fig. 27.1) predispose the tissues to injury and early degeneration (Fann 2002). One of the primary goals of the examination process is to determine the 'overload.' In other words 'What are the abnormal often asymmetrical loads and forces from above down and below up that converge into and pass through the painful area, creating the overload?' Favorable clinical outcome depends on the ability to relate the knowledge of antigravity biomechanics to those loads and positions that reproduce the familiar pain.

The purpose of this chapter is to relate the degeneration of the neuromusculoskeletal system to asymmetrical loads, resulting in early system breakdown, and to analyze the biomechanics of common comparable maladies seen in the out-patient clinic.

Aging and degeneration

The skeletal system includes bone, articular cartilage, periosteum, intra- and extra-articular ligaments and tendons. These structures function as a unit: the muscles pull on the tendons, creating stresses and strain on the ligaments and periosteum, causing dynamics of the joint or segment in the spine, and eventually moving the bone. Most muscles are not attached to two fixed bones. For a body part to move, one attachment must be fixed or stabilized, creating a fixed point from which to pull. As we know, muscles function to stabilize and move, each generating loads to the skeleton. For example, it is easy to visualize the quadriceps moving the tibia forward on the femur when extending the knee in an open chain.

Similarly, loads are imparted to the vertebral segment (bone/disc/bone) as the weight line passes into and through it when one lifts an object from the floor and places it into another position. It is a chain of events that directs loads and forces through tissues. Excessive loads can cause injury, creating an injury cycle (Fig. 27.2). Injury causes swelling, swelling causes pain, pain causes increased pressure which decreases blood flow and increases fluid congestion. This congestion causes pH changes as a result of hypoxia and the introduction of healing chemicals. The area becomes acidic, decreasing the depolarization threshold of the pain-carrying nociceptive axon. This series of events inhibits and

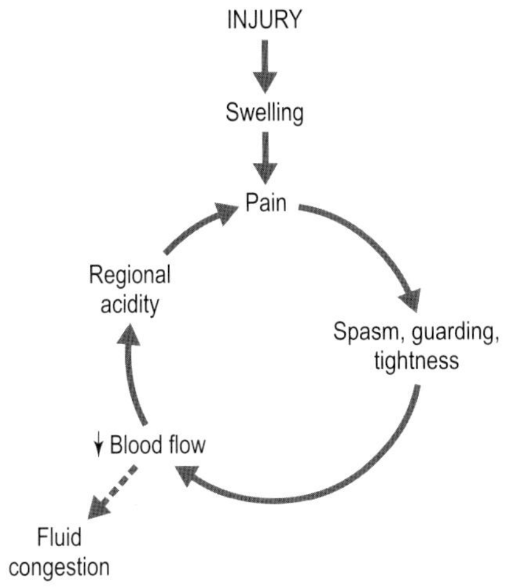

Fig. 27.2 The injury cycle is created as tissues become injured and swell.

decreases the load-bearing tolerance of the injured tissue. Injury weakens the musculoskeletal system. In essence, the load-bearing tolerances decrease with every exacerbation of pain (Buckwalter et al 2004, Hebdom & Hauselmann 2002, Kerin et al 2002, Ordeberg 2004). Limping is an example of this concept. The unconscious internal information system determines the contractile state and movement pattern that best minimizes pain. To complete the biomechanical and neurophysiological construct, overload causes injury, injury causes swelling, and swelling results in morning stiffness or stiffens after prolonged postures. The perception of morning stiffness is the best measure of overload the previous day. One primary clinical goal is to assist the patient in maintaining a high level of activity with decreased morning stiffness.

Body types

We are all a combination of three body types: ectomorph, endomorph, and mesomorph. The characteristics of each are as follows: the ectomorph is generally long and lean; the endomorph has excessive body fat and generally less overall body strength; the mesomorph is muscular and strong. The physiologic load-bearing tolerance is body-type dependent. The two extremes are those who have excess elastin in their structure, causing greater motion such as that seen in Ehlers–Danlos syndrome (Mao & Bristow 2001, Whitelaw 2004) and those individuals, primarily mesomorphic, who possess a very tight connective tissue structure, permitting less accommodation to the imposed demands of activity.

Because these two body types are commonly seen in the clinic, it appears logical to conclude that people who are of those two body types tend to have a greater potential for experiencing early skeletal break down, causing pain and disability.

Assessment

Two primary principles are inherent to the successful assessment and treatment of AOS. The first premise is that excessive and asymmetrical loads predispose the skeleton to early degeneration. Asymmetrical loads can be a result of muscular weakness and skeletal irregularities, such as leg length inequality and asymmetries in the structural balance of the feet. The second premise, as previously mentioned, is the reduced need to precisely identify the tissue of painful origin; instead, the focus should be to determine the biomechanics and dynamics of overload, i.e. determining those abnormal, or excessive, and often asymmetrical loads that converge into and pass through the injured area from above down and from below up, causing familiar pain (Fig. 27.3A–C). An example is a patient with low back pain whose pain is reproduced with backward bending, and in whom side bending to the right increases the familiar pain on the right. Once these biomechanics are determined, the treatment process is directed towards minimizing the fluid congestion, protecting the injured area from abrupt loads, while increasing strength and health. Integral to the successful management of the maladies detailed below is to teach the patient how to move and be active without reinjury, and to continue to strive to maximize their health. The key part of the total management with patients with mechanical musculoskeletal conditions is to improve their knowledge regarding the biomechanics, understand the importance of nutrition and exercise in improving their overall health and the discipline necessary to make that an ongoing activity.

Standing exam (Fig. 27.4)

Palpating bony landmarks during standing examination is common practice in the evaluation of the patient with low back pain. Four bony landmarks are the iliac crest, the anterior superior iliac spine, the posterior superior iliac spine and the greater trochanters (Porterfield & DeRosa 1998). A frontal plane asymmetry (FPA) is defined as these palpation

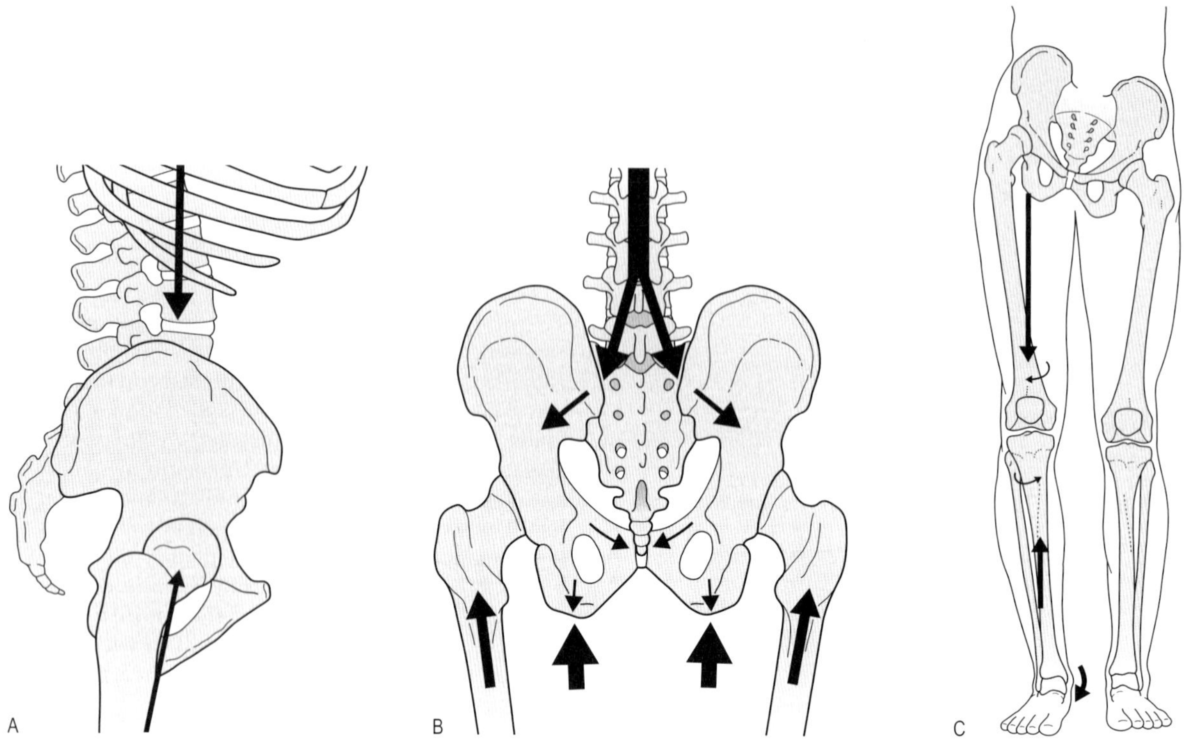

Fig. 27.3 Assessing loads and forces that converge into and pass through the injured body part from above down and below up. (A) Sagittal plane; (B and C) frontal plane views.

points being lower on one side as compared to the other. For the purpose of this chapter, we will use the example of a left FPA (Fig. 27.5) in which all points are low on the left. In addition to examining the posture in the frontal plane, the sagittal plane should also be assessed. Patients are commonly seen to have less stability of their trunk, resulting in a round-shouldered, forward head posture. This change in weight-bearing posture is often the result of fatigue and the gradual progressive loss of lean body mass as one ages. This posture adds to the overload, particularly at the base of the neck, lower aspect of the lumbar spine, and the anterior aspect of the shoulder. The key to successful management of both postural problems is to control the stresses that reach the region, increase strength to the neuromuscular system, and minimize fatigue.

The standing examination reveals information as to how the skeleton accepts loads from above. In addition to the above-mentioned frontal and sagittal plane asymmetries, the examiner might also palpate a difference in the resting position of one side of the pelvis as compared to the other (Beaudoin et al 1999). An example of this clinical finding is that the right iliac crest appears high, the posterior superior iliac spine (PSIS) on the right is lower than the left and the anterior superior iliac spine (ASIS) is high on the right. This is commonly interpreted as a positional fault whereby the right ilium is rotated backwards as compared to the left side of the pelvis, implying that one or both are in need of correction by manipulation. The painful side most often receives the primary attention. However, an alternative explanation of this antigravity finding is that this postural asymmetry is protective guarding, rather than a bone 'out of position.'

Often, the most painful side in this finding is on the side that appears to be rotated backwards, and backward bending and side bending over that side is painful. Therefore, it is reasonable to assume that the sagittal plane musculature is directed to increase contractile state to rotate the pelvis backwards, minimizing the compressive and shear loads to the lumbosacral segments.

If an FPA is seen in the standing examination, calibrated blocks are placed under one foot to determine the extent of the asymmetry. We use 10 cm (4 in) × 35.5 cm (14 in) × 0.3 cm ($^1/_8$ in) plastic

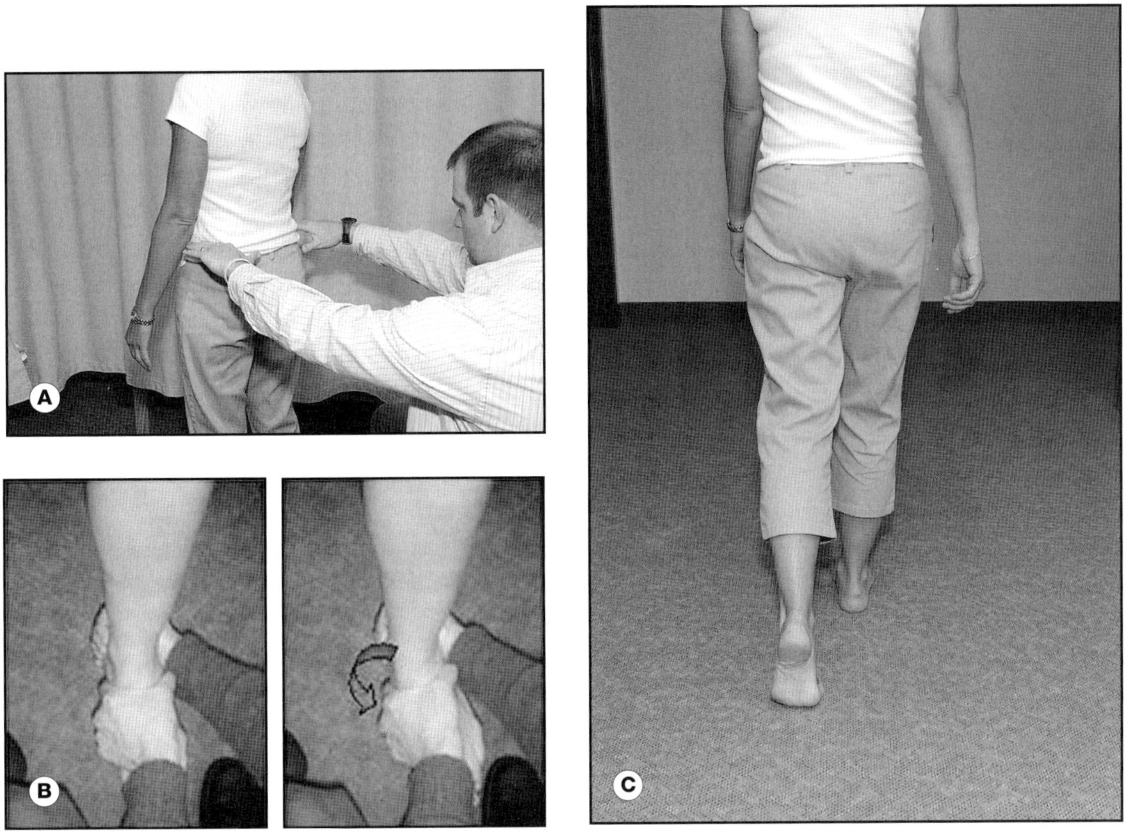

Fig. 27.4 Assessing skeletal asymmetry. (A) Standing examination: palpating four bony landmarks [iliac crest, posterior superior iliac spine (PSIS), anterior superior iliac spine (ASIS), greater trochanter] to determine positional symmetry. (B) Passive end range testing of the deltoid ligament complex of the foot. (C) Gait analysis.

blocks placed on top of each other to level the sacral base. The technique is gradually to add one block at a time, asking the patient to equalize the weight bearing on each foot at each level change. Pause for a few seconds to let the patient analyze the difference. Gradually decrease the sequence until the foot is on the floor. We suggest going through that sequence two or three times, because the response of the patient is critical. Most use words like 'It makes me feel more level,' 'I feel more balanced,' 'It takes the pressure off…' Responses like these highlight the need to change the antigravity weight-bearing posture. Orthotics can be fabricated to incorporate the frontal plane correction and longitudinal arch supports.

Analysis of the foot

The next aspect of the assessment of AOS is analyzing the symmetry of the feet. Analyzing the foot provides us with information about how the skeleton bears weight as a result of ground reaction forces.

This passive range of motion (ROM) testing determines the integrity of the deltoid ligament complex. The exam is very similar to valgus testing the medial collateral ligament of the knee. The deltoid ligament group stabilizes the movements of pronation of the foot during gait (see Fig. 27.4B).

Pronation is a combination of calcaneal eversion and midfoot rotation, and is essential for normal weight bearing while walking. It can be assessed by using both hands to direct a lateral and rotary force, taking the calcaneus and navicular down and away from the medial malleolus (see Fig. 27.4B). Often, asymmetrical laxity in the support tissues of the medial aspect of the ankle is prevalent on the short side. At heel strike, there is an increased movement between the rear foot and the ground creating increased loads to the medial tissues. This increase

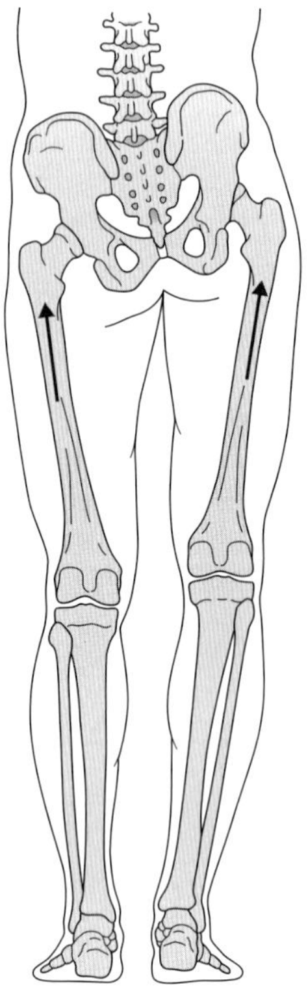

Fig. 27.5 Left frontal plane asymmetry (FPA). All four or a majority of bony landmarks are low on the left.

in movement translates to tibial internal rotation and genu valgus. This clinical finding is also seen in anterior knee pain which will be discussed below. This simple ROM test looking for asymmetry adds valuable information in the determination of overload. The last aspect in assessing AOS is to analyze walking.

Gait analysis

Gait analysis is a very important part of the assessment process (Kakushima et al 1999). Normal findings include a smooth transition of weight with equal movement from one side to another as the weight is transferred from one leg to the other during gait. An abnormal and very common finding in patients with AOS is an abrupt or excessive motion of the pelvis during stance phase, for example, the abrupt drop in the frontal plane of the left side of the pelvis during stance phase on the right. This translates to asymmetrical loading (overloading) in the frontal plane and the abruptness of the motion creates increased load and greater chances for injury. It is very difficult to successfully treat patients (i.e. unload the affected area) who cannot tolerate backward bending and side bending to the right in the low lumbar spine when they walk, as previously described. The loads directed to the spine in backward bending and side bending to the right are similar to those converging into the lumbosacral region as the pelvis drops down on the left during right stance. Backward bending and side bending replicate the converging loads from above down; the frontal plane drop seen during gait is from below up.

The pelvis dropping down to the left during right stance creates backward bending and side bending to the right from below up at the low lumbar spine. This is the key: to develop a three-dimensional appreciation of the anatomy and to be able to assess the overload from above down and from below up.

Excessive pronation of the rear and midfoot is also viewed while watching a patient walking briskly. The examiner is looking for asymmetry while evaluating the extent of genu valgus and tibial rotation during stance. Genu valgus alters the weight bearing of the hip and low back and can play a role in causing overload.

Analyzing gait with and without the correction also often reveals differences. The difference with adding a heel lift is a smoother less abrupt movement during the transition of weight from side to side, especially in those patients who, during the evaluation, describe a greater comfort while standing on a calibrated block.

Treatment

The treatment of AOS is based on centralizing the weight line through the skeleton by using heel lifts, increasing strength (health) of the neuromuscular system, and teaching the patient how to move and be active while protecting the injured area. In the most simplistic terms it is like hitting your thumb with a hammer. If one taps the thumb ten times and hits it once during the day, the pain in the thumb will increase in intensity and the sensitivity will increase significantly. Eventually, the pain and sensitivity will spread throughout the upper quarter; all from that afferent generator in the thumb. AOS is a repetitive overload condition, like hitting your thumb with a hammer. If the impact loads created by the hammer are not removed, the painful condition persists. The same exists in the conditions listed in Box 27.1. There is a relationship between abnormal biomechanics and early-onset degenerative changes of the musculoskeletal system, specifically the low back (Giles & Taylor 1981, Masset et al 1998, ten Brinke et al 1999), hip (Friberg 1983, Goel 1999, Johnson et al 1974, Krause et al 1976, Tapper & Hoover 1969), and the foot and ankle (Root et al 1977).

Common maladies of asymmetrical overload

With this general background, we can now review some common musculoskeletal conditions that might result from the presence of an FPA. Box 27.1 lists common conditions referred to as conditions of weight bearing: the asymmetrical overload syndrome (AOS). The example we will use for this explanation is a patient with a left FPA, all points low on the left, with increased laxity of the medial rear foot, most often accompanied by increased pronation on the left during the stance phase of gait. The following is a brief explanation of each malady listed in Box 27.1.

Lumbar segment spondylosis

In a left FPA, the pelvis drops down on the left and the lumbar spine side bends to the right, which increases the compressive loads on the right side of the lumbar spine and increases the tensile loads to the tissues on the left (Fig. 27.6). Figs 27.7 and 27.8 show how asymmetrical overload to the segment can cause structural breakdown of the posterior elements (facet joint) and at the bone/disc/bone interface (Latridis et al 2005). Changes are seen in the segment where the disc space narrows, the articular cartilage softens and fibrillates, and the subchondral bone becomes overloaded, stimulating bone growth and the formation of bone spurs.

It is easy to see how such structural changes alter the architecture of the intervertebral foramen and the lateral recess of the spinal canal. The lateral bending motion of the spine results in shear stress between the adjacent vertebral segments (Adams & Dolan 1995), which subjects the segment to significant increases in compression loads (MA Adams, personal communication).

Frontal plane correction levels the sacral base and 'decompresses' the region between the lower lumbar facets, decreases tension at one side of the annulus, and decreases compressive loading to the contralateral side of the intervertebral disc. This correction helps centralize the weight bearing at the base of the spine.

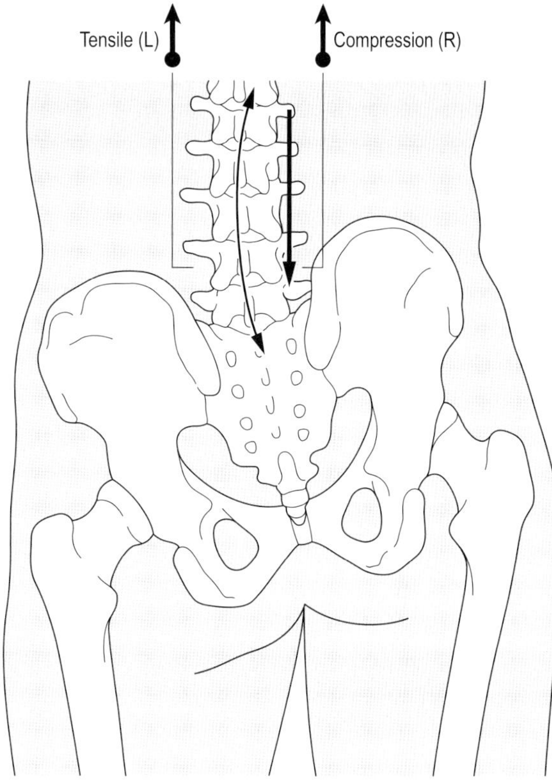

Fig. 27.6 Asymmetrical loads and forces imparted to the lumbar spine with a left frontal plane asymmetry. The spine is side bent to the right. There is increased tension on the left and increased compression and shear on the right.

Sacroiliac joint sprain/strain/osteoarthritis

The sacroiliac joints (SIJs) attenuate the stresses of compression and shear during weight bearing and movement (Puhakka et al 2004). As the pelvis drops on one side with a left FPA, the right SIJ orientation becomes more vertical and the contralateral side is more horizontal (Fig. 27.9). As a result, there is increased shear loading to the more vertically oriented right joint, and increased compression loading to the horizontally oriented left SIJ.

In our clinical experience, SIJ pain associated with frontal plane asymmetry is primarily associated with the 'long leg' side, suggesting that the shear loads are potentially more destructive. Pain in this area can be due to overload to any of the associated structures in this region.

The treatment process includes shifting the weight-bearing process to remove the nociceptive loads and forces, teaching the patient to move

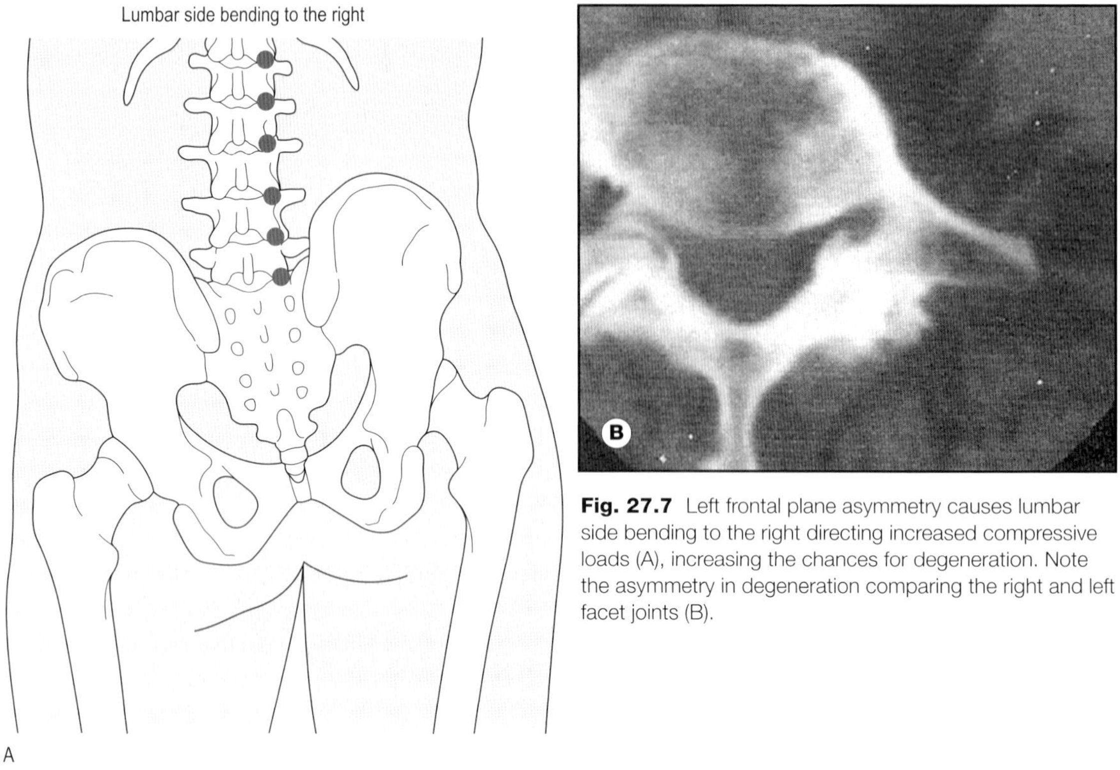

Fig. 27.7 Left frontal plane asymmetry causes lumbar side bending to the right directing increased compressive loads (A), increasing the chances for degeneration. Note the asymmetry in degeneration comparing the right and left facet joints (B).

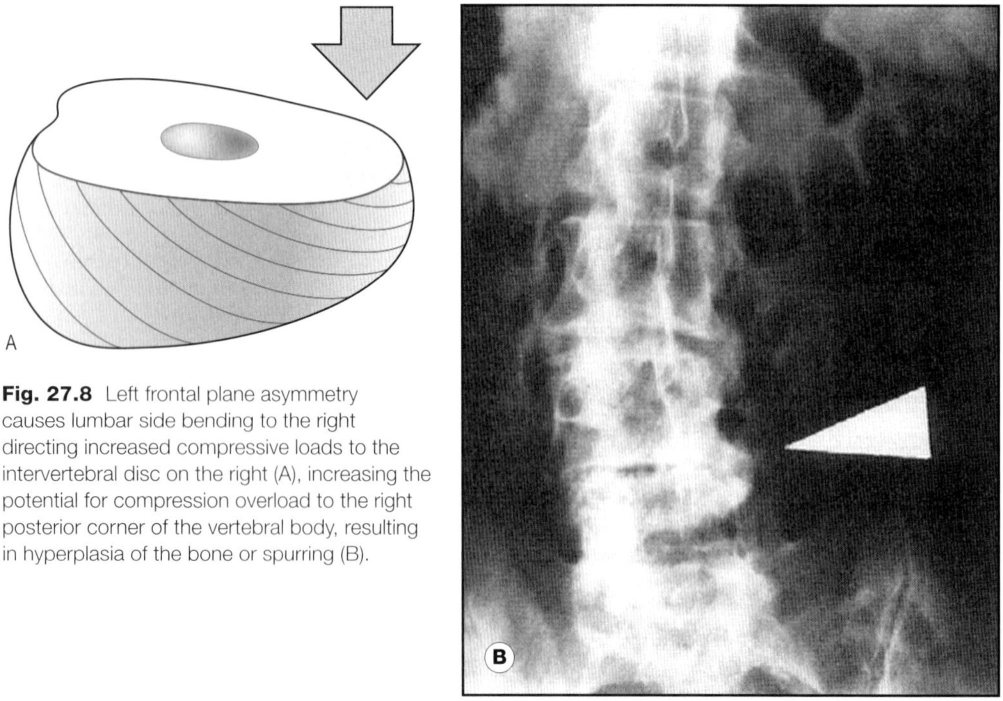

Fig. 27.8 Left frontal plane asymmetry causes lumbar side bending to the right directing increased compressive loads to the intervertebral disc on the right (A), increasing the potential for compression overload to the right posterior corner of the vertebral body, resulting in hyperplasia of the bone or spurring (B).

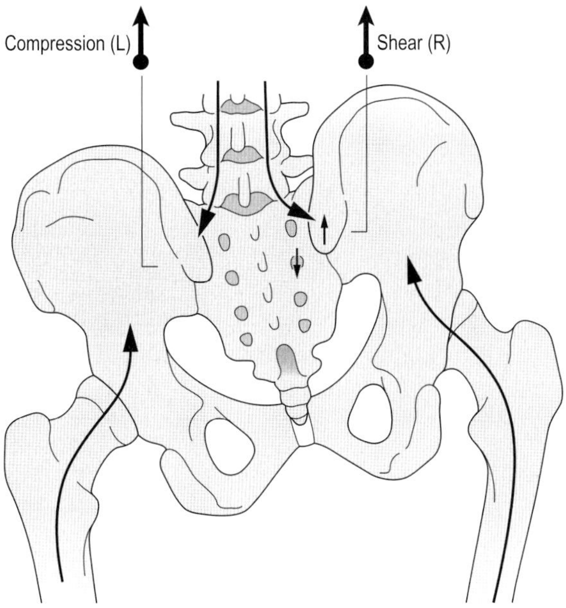

Fig. 27.9 Changes in loads and forces imparted to the sacroiliac joint with a left frontal plane asymmetry. The right joint is more vertical creating greater shear.

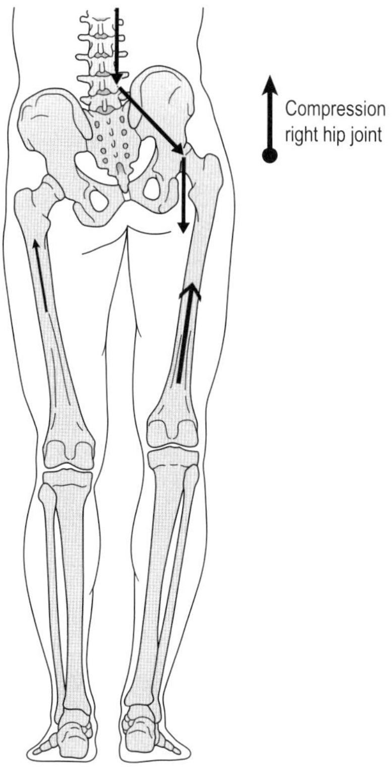

Fig. 27.10 Changes in the weight-bearing properties of the hip joints with a frontal plane asymmetry. Relative femoral adduction on the right directs the loads and forces more medially on the femoral head causing increased vertical loads and forces imparted to the right hip joint.

without reinjury, and developing increased strength and coordination of the muscles that work together to stabilize the sacroiliac joint (Vleeming et al 1996).

Hip joint osteoarthritis

The angle of inclination of the femoral neck and the position of the head of the femur in the acetabulum results in a complex series of forces including a bending moment to the femoral neck, and compressive loading to the femoral head. With a left FPA (Fig. 7.10), the right femur is adducted and the left femur is relatively abducted. This results in an increased bending moment at the femoral neck over the abducted left hip, and increased compressive loading to the adducted femoral head on the right. This adducted right hip is close pack. Friberg (1983) noted that the hip on the longer side in a limb length discrepancy translates to early-onset degeneration, and the literature is replete with discussions regarding limb length discrepancies associated with total hip arthroplasty (Brand & Yack 1996, Ranawat & Rodriguez 1997).

The question remains: 'Why, in the absence of trauma, would one hip show significantly earlier degeneration compared with the contralateral hip?' The answer is most likely related to the increased loads of skeletal asymmetry. Furthermore, the limb length discrepancy often seen after total hip joint arthroplasty might in fact be a pre-existing condition, rather than the result of the surgical procedure or weakness.

Greater trochanter bursitis (Fig. 27.11)

Functional and/or structural asymmetry also subjects the soft tissues at the hip to overload. A common diagnosis at the hip is greater trochanteric bursitis. The greater trochanteric bursa lies just under the aponeurosis of the gluteus maximus as the muscle courses inferior and lateral to attach to the fascia latae complex and the linea aspera.

The research remains focused on naming tissues at fault and devising treatment techniques that decrease the inflammatory process (Sayegh et al 2004, Shbeeb & Matteson 1996, Tortolani et al 2002). However, it stands to reason that this overload concept, especially in those who have no history of

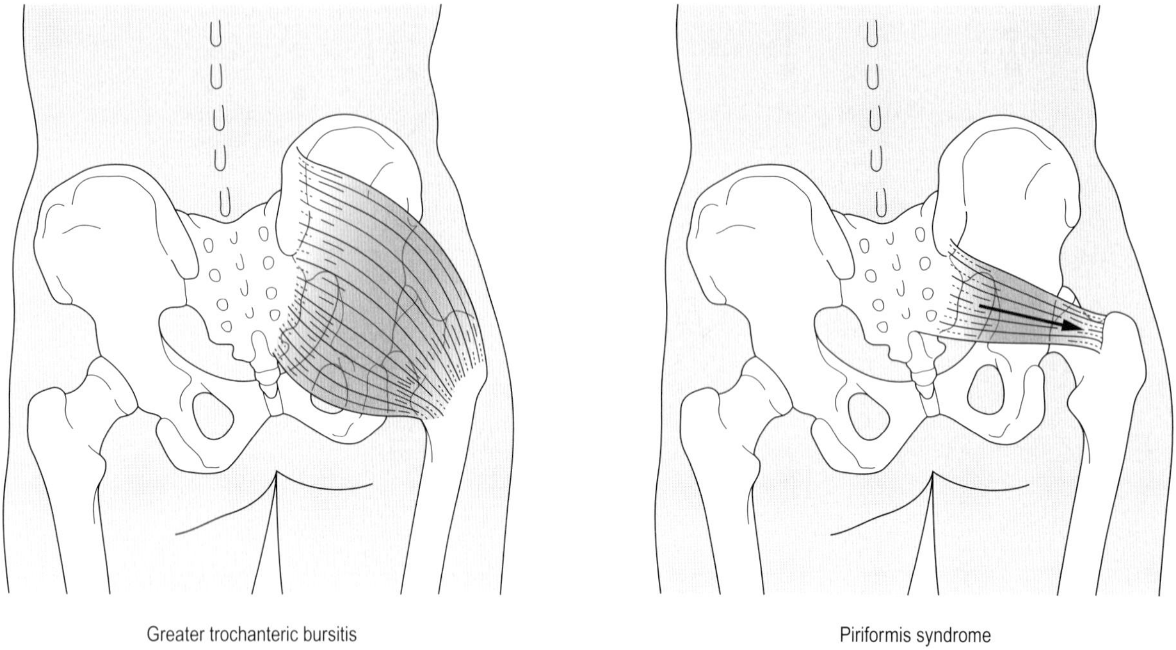

Fig. 27.11 As the pelvis drops down to the left there is an increased compression between the skin and aponeurosis of the gluteus maximus and the greater trochanter on the right, and an increased tensile stress to the tissues that travel from the sacrum to the superior aspect of the femur.

trauma, can injure any tissue involved, calling for further investigation.

An increased compressive stress to the bursal tissue occurs on the long leg (right) side as the pelvis tilts down to the left during stance phase on the right, creating a relative adduction of the femur (see Fig. 27.5). As the pelvis tilts down to the left, the right femur becomes adducted, resulting in increased compression between the aponeurosis of the gluteus maximus and the greater trochanter. As the gait continues, the femur creates shear to the bursae as it passes under the aponeurosis of the gluteus maximus during stance phase of gait. Compression and shear are most often responsible for tissue breakdown (overload) and in this scenario the greater trochanteric bursae are vulnerable to overload. These biomechanics are most often the explanation for the diagnosis of greater trochanteric bursitis in the patient with a gradual onset of symptoms and no history of blunt trauma.

It is difficult to predict exactly what tissue between the skin and the greater trochanter is causing the symptoms but the forces that reproduce the pain are clear. Indeed, if the forces that cause the injury are not addressed, long-term pain relief is unlikely.

An important component of the treatment process is centralizing (balancing) loads and forces by a frontal plane correction, and increased strength, power, and endurance of the frontal plane and sagittal plane muscles of the trunk.

Piriformis syndrome

Another common diagnosis at the region of the hip joint is piriformis syndrome, a condition described by persistent tenderness and irritation at the mid buttock (Broadhurst et al 2004, Papadopoulos & Khan 2004). For example, in a left FPA, the sacrum tilts down to the left in standing, or during right stance phase of gait, and the right femur relatively adducts (see Fig. 27.11). There is an increased tensile load imparted to the piriformis and related tissues as the origin at the pelvis moves away from the insertion located at the superior aspect of the right femur. Piriformis syndrome might be a misnomer as to naming the exact tissue involved in the painful syndrome, rather it is used as a term to depict tensile overuse syndromes of the deep rotators and abductors of the hip. Structural examination in standing and gait analysis reveals this finding.

Iliotibial band friction syndrome: lateral epicondylitis (Fig. 27.12)

Pain located at the outside of the knee is a very common condition with athletes, particularly runners and cyclists, who subject their skeletons to repetitive and excessive loads (Gunter & Schwellnus 2004, Kirk et al 2000). This malady is also seen in people who have frontal plane moments and movement in their lower extremities during stance phase in gait. The condition is easily identified because of the specific point tenderness at the lateral distal femur, which often radiates proximally and distally from that point.

This can be seen during the gait analysis, when the sacrum (pelvis) drops down and away from the weight-bearing limb during heel strike at a greater rate and amount than the other side (see Fig. 27.12). The relative hip adduction creates a varus (bowing-out) moment to the lower extremity from above. As a result, the femoral epicondyle located at the distal lateral femur increases compression and shear at the undersurface of the iliotibial band, causing tissue damage, swelling and pain at the lateral femoral epicondyle.

It is most often the combination of the compression and shear force that causes the connective tissue to break down, become inflamed, and cause pain. In the absence of a structural asymmetry, runners who frequently run on a crested road towards traffic, or run on a circular track in a direction where the painful limb is to the outside run an increased risk of injury. As with other conditions of weight bearing, fatigue plays a major role in the ability to stay active and under control (Gribble & Hertel 2004a, 2004b). Health maintenance and increases in strength throughout the trunk (Porterfield & DeRosa 1998) are the keys to successful management of any malady of AOS. One must take away and control the offending forces of injury before any long-term recovery can take place.

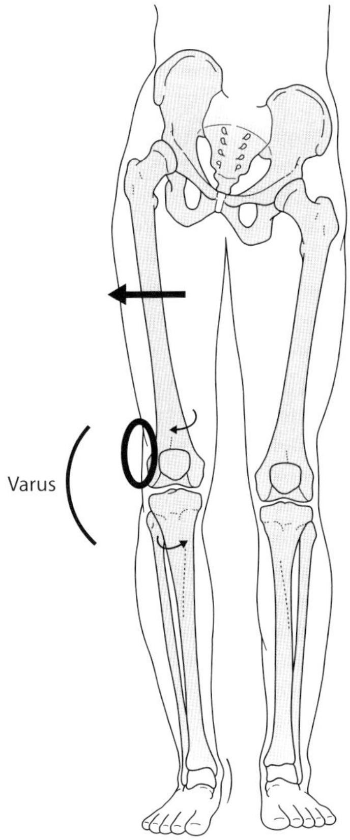

Fig. 27.12 A front view of a left frontal plane asymmetry showing the varus moment imparted to the right leg as the pelvis drops down on the left. As the right femur moves into adduction, the most lateral aspect of the distal femur (lateral epicondyle) moves out into the thick and fibrous undersurface of the distal aspect of the iliotibial band, potentially creating overload, tissue breakdown, swelling, and pain.

Knee pain: tibiofemoral osteoarthritis/patellofemoral osteoarthritis/anterior knee pain

Knee pain can be a result of many conditions (Brenner et al 2004, Dye et al 1985, Johnson et al 1998) (Fig. 27.13). The analysis of the forces as they migrate upward from the ground takes on more importance when discussing maladies of the knee.

Asymmetry in the feet can certainly accumulate and be a part of the asymmetrical biomechanics when discussing pelvis and low back pain, but it is the knee where most of the asymmetry from the foot is attenuated. High arched, rigid, cavus foot types pronate less, decreasing the shock absorption of the foot causing varus forces up from the floor, while pronated (lax) feet result in excessive internal rotation of the tibia, causing genu valgus and increased torque at the knee. As previously mentioned, a left fontal plane asymmetry causes varus from above and the foot can cause either varus or valgus and rotation at the knee. It is the analysis of the convergence of these forces from above and below that forms the foundation on which successful treatment can be rendered and descriptive functional outcomes can be derived. This practical

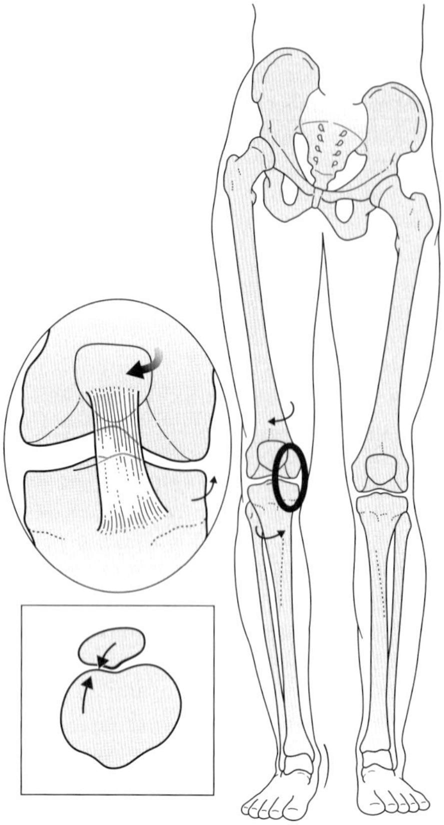

Fig. 27.13 Knee pain is often the result of excessive and repetitive compression, bending and twisting forces and loads from above and below. Medial tibiofemoral compression, lateral connective tissue tension, asymmetrical loads to the patellofemoral joint, and anterior knee pain are most common.

application of lower extremity biomechanics is the basis for explaining many mechanical knee problems, particularly those without a history of trauma and those with asymmetrical degenerative findings on X-ray.

Summary

There are numerous etiologies for the many musculoskeletal syndromes of the spine and the lower quarter and, unfortunately, naming the precise anatomic tissue that is the nociceptive source remains in question. With most clinical problems, it is likely that several tissues rather than one tissue contribute to the pain pattern. This chapter reviewed conditions of weight bearing with the primary emphasis on the potential clinical problems that accompany FPA. To successfully treat the conditions outlined in this chapter it is necessary to determine how the trunk and ground forces are converging into and passing through the region stimulating the nociceptive system.

The primary principle of this chapter is that painful conditions can be the result of tissue overload. And, overload conditions can be determined by analyzing the level of the pelvis in a frontal plane, observing the sagittal posture, passively assessing the symmetry of the foot, and observing the frontal and rotary plane motion of the pelvis and lower extremity during gait.

References

Adams MA, Dolan P 1995 Recent advances in lumbar spinal mechanics and their clinical significance. Clinical Biomechanics 10:3–19

Beaudoin L, Zabjek KF, Leroux MA et al 1999 Acute systematic and variable postural adaptations induced by an orthopaedic shoe lift in control subjects. Archives of Physical Medicine and Rehabilitation 80(3):348–349

Brady RJ, Dean JB, Skinner TM et al 2003 Limb length inequality: clinical implications for assessment and intervention. Journal of Orthopedic and Sports in Physical Therapy 33(5):221–234

Brand RA, Yack HJ 1996 Effects of leg length discrepancies on the forces at the hip joint. Clinical Orthopaedics 333:172–180

Brenner SS, Klotz U, Alscher DM et al 2004 Osteoarthritis of the knee – clinical assessments and inflammatory markers. Osteoarthritis Cartilage 12(6):469–475

Broadhurst NA, Simmons DN, Bond MJ 2004 Piriformis syndrome: correlation of muscle morphology with symptoms and signs. Archives in Physical Medicine and Rehabilitation 85(12):2036–2039

Buckwalter JA, Saltzman C, Brown T et al 2004 The impact of osteoarthritis: implications for research. Clinical Orthopedics 427:6–15

Burke W 2004 Leg length inequality in humans: a new neurophysiological approach. Neuroscience Letters 361:29–31

Dye SF, Boll DH, Dunigan PE et al 1985 An analysis of objective measurements including radionuclide imaging in young patients with patellofemoral pain. American Journal of Sports Medicine 13:432–436

Fann AV 2002 The prevalence of postural asymmetry in people with and without chronic low back pain. Archives in Physical Medicine and Rehabilitation 83(12):1736–1738

Friberg O 1983 Clinical symptoms and biomechanics of lumbar spine and hip joint in leg length inequality. Spine 8(6):643–651

Giles LG, Taylor JR 1981 Low-back pain associated with leg length inequality. Spine 6(5):510–521

Goel A 1999 Meralgia paresthetica secondary to limb length discrepancy: case report. Archives in Physical Medicine and Rehabilitation 80(3):348–349

Gofton JP 1985 Persistent low back pain and leg length disparity. Journal of Rheumatology 12(4):747–750
Gribble PA, Hertel J 2004a Effect of hip and ankle muscle fatigue on unipedal postural control. Journal of Electromyography and Kinesiology 14(6):641–646
Gribble PA, Hertel J 2004b Effect of lower-extremity muscle fatigue on postural control. Archives in Physical Medicine and Rehabilitation 85(4):589
Gunter P, Schwellnus MP 2004 Local corticosteroid injection in iliotibial band friction syndrome in runners: a randomized controlled trial. British Journal of Sports Medicine 38(3):269–272
Gurney B 2002 Leg length discrepancy. Gait Posture 15(2):195–206
Hebdom E, Hauselmann HJ 2002 Molecular aspects of pathogenesis in osteoarthritis: the role of inflammation. Cellular and Molecular Life Sciences 45–53
Johnson L, van Dyke GE, Green JR et al 1998 Clinical assessment of asymptomatic knees: comparison of men and women. Arthroscopy 4:347–359
Johnson RJ, Kettelcamp DB, Clark W et al 1974 Factors affecting late meniscectomy results. Journal of Bone and Joint Surgery 56(A):719–729
Juhl JH, Cremin TM, Russell JG et al 2004 Prevalence of frontal plane pelvic postural asymmetry – part 1. American Osteopathic Association 104(10):411–421
Kakushima M, Miyamoto K, Shimizu K 1999 The effect of leg length discrepancy on spinal motion during gait: three-dimensional analysis in healthy volunteers. European Spine Journal 8(1):40–45
Kerin A, Patwari P, Kuettner K et al 2002 Molecular basis of osteoarthritis: biomechanical aspect. Cellular & Molecular Life Sciences 27–35
Kirk KL, Kuklo T, Klemme W 2000 Iliotibial band friction syndrome. Orthopedics 23(11):1209–1214
Krause WR, Pope MH, Johnson RJ et al 1976 Mechanical changes in the knee after meniscectomy. Journal of Bone and Joint Surgery 58(A):599–604
Latridis JC, Maclean JJ, Ryan DD 2005 Mechanical damage to the intervertebral disc annulus fibrosus subjected to tensile loading. Journal of Biomechanics 38(3):557–565
Mao JR, Bristow J 2001 The Ehler–Danlos syndrome: on beyond collagen. Journal of Clincal Investigation 107(9):1063–1067
Masset DF, Piette A, Malchaire JB 1998 Relation between functional characteristics of the trunk and the occurrence of low back pain. Spine 23:359–365
Ordeberg G 2004 Characterization of joint pain in human OA. Novartis Foundation Symposium 260:105–115, discussion 115–121, 277–279
Papadopoulos EC, Khan SN 2004 Piriformis syndrome and low back pain: a new classification and review of the literature. Orthopedics Clinics of North America 35(1):65–71
Porterfield JA, DeRosa C 1998 Mechanical low back pain: perspectives in functional anatomy, 2nd edn. WB Saunders, Philadelphia, PA, p179–192
Puhakka KB, Jurik AG, Schiottz-Christensen B et al 2004 MRI abnormalities of sacroiliac joints in early spondylarthropathy: a 1-year follow-up study. Scandinavian Journal of Rheumatology 33(5):332–338
Ranawat CS, Rodriguez JA 1997 Functional leg-length inequality following total hip arthroplasty. Journal of Arthroplasty 12(4):359–364
Root M, Weed J, Orien W (eds) 1977 Abnormal and normal function of the foot. Clinical Biomechanics Corp., Los Angeles, CA, p134
Sayegh F, Potoupnis M, Kapetanos G 2004 Greater trochanter bursitis pain syndrome in females with chronic low back pain and sciatica. Acta Orthopaedica Belgica 70(5):423–428
Shbeeb MI, Matteson EL 1996 Trochanteric bursitis (greater trochanter pain syndrome). Mayo Clinic Proceedings 71(6):565–569
Tallroth K, Ylikoski M, Lamminen H et al 2005 Preoperative leg-length inequality and hip osteoarthrosis: a radiographic study of 100 consecutive arthroplasty patients. Skeletal Radiology 34:136–139
Tapper EM, Hoover NW 1969 Late results after meniscectomy. Journal of Bone and Joint Surgery 51(A):517–526
ten Brinke A, van der Aa HE, vander Palen J et al 1999 Is leg length discrepancy associated with the side of radiating pain in patients with a lumbar herniated disc? Spine 24:684–686
Tortolani PJ, Carbone JJ, Quartararo LG 2002 Greater trochanteric pain syndrome in patients referred to orthopedic spine specialists. Spine Journal 2(4):251–254
Vleeming A, Pool-Goudzwaard A, Hammudoghlu D et al 1996 The function of the long dorsal sacroiliac ligament: its implication for understanding low back pain. Spine Journal 21(5):556–562
White SC, Gilchrist LA, Wilk BE 2004 Asymmetric limb loading with true or simulated leg-length differences. Clinical Orthopedics 421:287–294
Whitelaw SE 2004 Ehlers–Danlos syndrome, classical type: case management. Dermatology in Nursing 16(5): 433–436

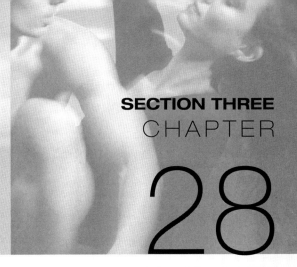

SECTION THREE

CHAPTER

28

Evidence-based clinical testing of the lumbar spine and pelvis

Mark Laslett

Introduction

Low back, buttock, groin, and referred lower extremity pain is common. The tissue origin of pain is typically a deep structure resulting in somatic referred pain distinguishable from radicular pain. It is commonly stated that 85% or more of patients have a 'nonspecific' source of pain (Nachemson & Jonsson 2000, van Tulder et al 1996, 1999, Waddell 1998), with the implication that diagnosis of the tissue origin of pain is not possible. Prior to the 1990s, this attitude had a real basis in fact. The Quebec Task Force on Activity-Related Spinal Disorders found that current methods of diagnosis were unreliable (Spitzer 1987). At that time, the clarity of diagnostic definitions and clinical criteria were confusing, contradictory and unsubstantiated. This problem persists, but in the last 15 years many of these difficulties have been examined using increasingly rigorous methods resulting in a greater understanding of the need for a diagnosis, and the means by which this may be achieved. This chapter outlines the current status of clinical diagnostics in the lumbar spine and pelvis and the reference standard methods of diagnosis of the source and causes of persistent lumbopelvic and referred lower extremity pain. Details are provided for the diagnostic accuracy of demographic, history, clinical finding, and test variables that have been evaluated in appropriate diagnostic studies.

The sources of chronic lumbopelvic and lower extremity pain

With the exception of painful hip joint pathologies, lower extremity pathologies are characterized by a small area of pain distribution, local signs, and pain provocation with specific movements. The hip joint can refer pain into the thigh and lower leg, but dominant pain is usually in the groin or hip region. Lower extremity pain referred from a disc, zygapophyseal joint (ZJ) or sacroiliac joint (SIJ), is characterized by dominant pain above the hip with dull aching pain of somatic referral diminishing in intensity the further it radiates into the limb. Nerve root/radicular pain produces dominant pain in the limb, with a sharp, twingeing, lancinating character in the distribution of a spinal segment. With the exception of the nerve root, the deep lumbar structures all produce similar pain and in similar distributions.

The most common structural sources of chronic low back pain (LBP) are the intervertebral disc, the ZJs and the SIJ (Bogduk 1995). These structures refer pain into the pelvis, groin, and lower extremity. When lower extremity pain is dominant, lower extremity pathology must be excluded but might be referred from a lumbosacral nerve root and associated dura mater.

The frequency of disc, ZJ, SIJ, and nerve root pain varies considerably depending on the patient population. However, approximate proportions may be estimated, based on available evidence (Table 28.1).

Sources of chronic low back and somatic referred pain

Lumbar intervertebral disc

The outer laminae of the annulus fibrosis and the vertebral endplates that form the inferior and superior boundaries of the intervertebral disc space are innervated by the sinuvertebral nerves, branches of the lumbar ventral rami and the gray rami communicantes (Bogduk & Twomey 1987, Bogduk et al 1981, Fagan et al 2003). Consequently, these structures are capable of producing back pain and somatic referred pain into the lower extremity (Brismar et al 1996, O'Neill et al 2002, Ohnmeiss 2002, Ohnmeiss et al 1997, Sehgal & Fortin 2000, Weinstein et al 1988). The original concept of internal disc disruption (IDD) (Crock 1986) was proposed to account for cases of disc pain with biochemical factors as the basis of painful pathology, rather than the mechanical aspects of disc herniation or protrusion. Evidence of biochemical substrates for pain within the disc have been found (Brown et al 1997, Weinstein et al 1988) and it is known that the nucleus is a potential irritant of the nerve roots (Olmarker et al 1993). Based on a consecutive series of chronic LBP patients receiving provocation discography, 39% (95%CI 29, 49) of patients will have IDD (Schwarzer et al 1995b).

Lindblom introduced discography in 1948. The technique involves penetration of the intervertebral disc under fluoroscopic guidance and introduction of contrast material into the disc core, to provide a nucleogram (Fig. 28.1). The key diagnostic factor is hydraulic distension of the disc to ascertain if it is mechanically sensitive, i.e. if the patient reports reproduction of the usual or familiar pain. Postdiscography axial CT images are acquired within one hour so that the pattern of annular fissuring is described (Aprill 1997). A high incidence of false positive responses to discography in an asymptomatic population was reported in 1968 (Holt 1968). The results of that study were re-evaluated and criticized on the basis that the subjects were prison inmates offered incentives to participate and other methodological flaws (Simmons et al 1988). The clinical and academic community remains polarized regarding the value of discography with proponents and detractors

Table 28.1 Sources of low back, pelvis or referred lower extremity pain

Structure/pathology	Prevalence	References
Disc pain (internal disc disruption)	39%	Schwarzer et al 1995b
Zygapophyseal joint	15–40% (increases with age)	Schwarzer et al 1995c, Schwarzer et al 1994a, Manchikanti et al 1999
Sacroiliac joint	6–13%	Schwarzer et al 1995a, Bogduk 1995
Nerve root (radicular pain)	2–10%	Deyo et al 1994, Govind 2004

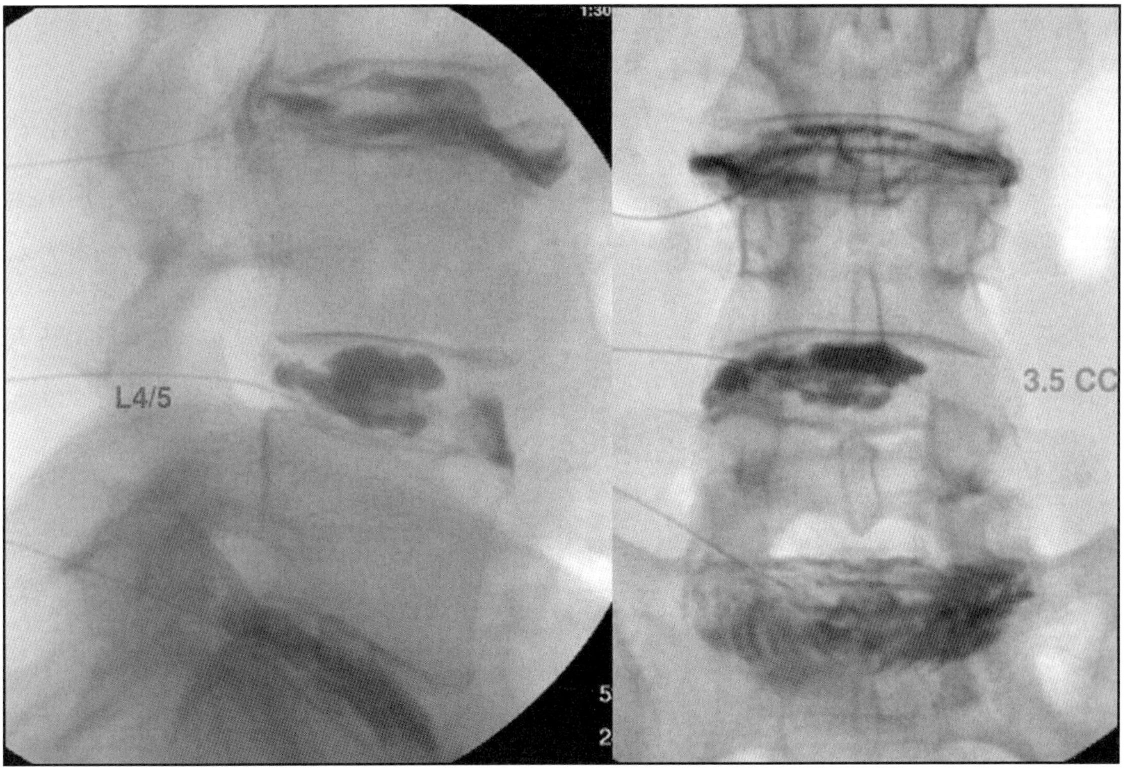

Fig. 28.1 Lateral and anteroposterior radiographs taken during lumbar discography at L3–L4, L4–L5, L5–S1. Only L4–L5 provoked pain at low pressures. (Courtesy of Charles N Aprill MD.)

seemingly equally convinced of their positions (Bogduk & Modic 1996). Although discography does appear to be painless in asymptomatic individuals (Walsh et al 1990), psychologic distress does confound interpretation of the pain response during hydraulic distension (Block et al 1996). Further evidence has been published concerning the problem of false-positive discography in normal subjects (Carragee et al 2000), but this too has been criticized because of methodological limitations, such as lack of adherence to the International Association for the Study of Pain (IASP) criteria for discography and reaching inappropriate conclusions from insufficient case numbers (Bogduk 2001). It appears that IDD is inherently associated with psychosocial distress. In Crock's original proposition, IDD could lead to depression and other signs of systemic illness through auto-immune reactions (Crock 1986). Subsequent research has shown that back pain patients with positive discograms are more distressed than patients with other serious causes of back pain such as symptomatic isthmic spondylolisthesis coming to surgery, and chronic vertebral osteomyelitis before diagnosis and treatment (Carragee 2001).

Regardless of the difficulties with, and controversy surrounding diagnostic discography, it remains the only means of directly challenging the intervertebral disc to detect if it is a source of LBP (Anderson 2004, Bogduk & McGuirk 2002, Executive Committee of the North American Spine Society 2004, Merskey & Bogduk 1994).

Lumbar zygapophyseal (facet) joints

The lumbar zygapophyseal joint (ZJ) is innervated by the medial branches of the dorsal rami emerging at the same segmental level, and the level above (Bogduk 1983). Identification of the ZJ as a source of LBP rests on the introduction of local anesthetic into the joint space (Fig. 28.2), or by performing nerve blocks to the medial branches of the dorsal rami at the two segmental levels supplying each joint.

Based on intra-articular injection of contrast and local anesthetic under radiographic guidance, an initial prevalence for ZJ-mediated back pain was 62% (Mooney & Robertson 1976). It was later realized that the capacity of the joint was less than the volume of injectate used in the 1976 study, and

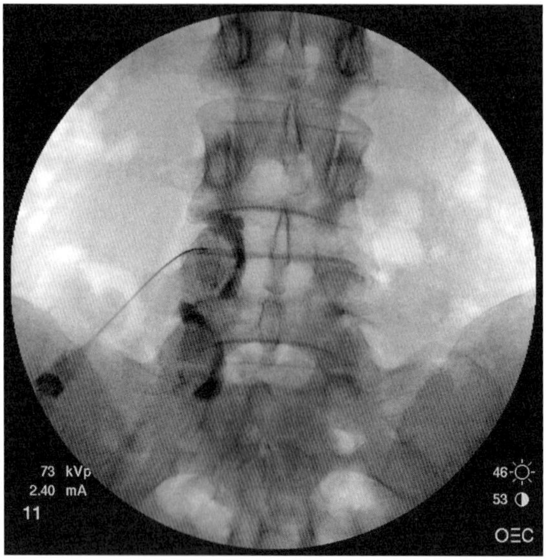

Fig. 28.2 Anteroposterior radiograph of intra-articular injection of contrast into the left L4–L5 zygapophyseal joint. (Courtesy of Charles N Aprill MD.)

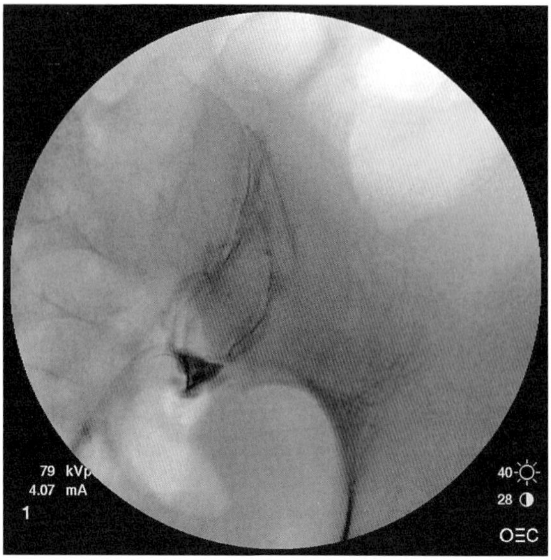

Fig. 28.3 Anteroposterior radiograph of injection of contrast into the left sacroiliac joint. (Courtesy of Charles N Aprill MD.)

decompression into the epidural space might have caused many false-positive responses (Moran et al 1988). Using fluoroscopic control and minimal volumes of injectate, the incidence of ZJ-mediated back pain was revised to about 17% of back pain patients (Moran et al 1988) or even less than 10% (Jackson et al 1988). More recent studies have shown that false-positive responses are about 30% (Manchikanti et al 2000b, Schwarzer et al 1994b) and the use of placebo-controlled or comparative double blocks is now considered best practice (Bogduk 1997b, Dreyfuss et al 2003). There is also evidence that whatever the cause of false-positive responses, somatization, depression, and generalized anxiety disorders are not responsible (Manchikanti et al 2001). Using these guidelines, the prevalence of ZJ-mediated pain in a general chronic back pain population is approximately 15% (Schwarzer et al 1995c), although in older populations the prevalence can be as high as 40% (Manchikanti et al 1999, Schwarzer et al 1994a). However, it is clear that the prevalence of pain of purely ZJ origin is low: about 4% (Schwarzer et al 1994a).

Sacroiliac joints

The SIJ is capable of small ranges of motion; this range of motion is not related to the presence or absence of pain (Sturesson 1999, Sturesson et al 1989). It receives innervation from the L5–S4 segments (Grob et al 1995, Willard 1997) and is capable of producing pain (Fortin et al 1994a, 1994b, Vilensky et al 2002). Identification of the SIJ as a source of LBP is dependent on substantial pain relief following intra-articular injection of local anesthetic into the joint space (Dreyfuss et al 1996, Fortin et al 1994a, Merskey & Bogduk 1994, Schwarzer et al 1995a) (Fig. 28.3).

Although it can be presumed that false-positive responses to an initial injection occur in the same way as for ZJ blocks, standards are not as well established in the case of the SIJ. Single blocks (Dreyfuss et al 1996, Schwarzer et al 1995a, Slipman et al 1998) and double comparative blocks (Laslett et al 2003, Maigne et al 1996) have been used in recent studies but the false-positive rate for single blocks is not established. Estimates of the prevalence of SIJ-mediated pain vary widely from < 1% (Cyriax 1975 p 546) to a range from 3.5% (Laslett 1997) to 30% (Bernard & Cassidy 1991, Schwarzer et al 1995a). In a review of the current literature, Bogduk estimated the prevalence to be in the vicinity of 13% (Bogduk 1995), which is consistent with the estimated prevalence of 12% in a pregnant population (Albert et al 2002). The relationship between the concepts of pelvic girdle pain and SIJ-mediated pain is unclear. In studies of pelvic girdle pain, symphysis pubis disorders are commonly associated with peripartum musculoskeletal problems. Albert et al (2000) make this distinction, but in a study of one pain provocation test, Östgaard et al (1994a, 1994b) referred only to 'posterior pelvic pain.' The latter authors considered symphysis pubis pain as irrelevant, arguing that there was no definable SIJ syndrome and considering posterior pelvic pain to be a more reasonable description of this subgroup of peripartum patients. The symptoms, signs, and clinical tests used to identify posterior pelvic pain syndrome are essentially the same as those used to clinically identify SIJ-mediated pain. In my opinion, it is likely that after exclusion of pain in the symphysis pubis, posterior pelvic pain and SIJ pain are the same clinical entity.

Nerve root (radicular) and dura mater

The nerve root and dura mater are capable of producing pain (Edgar & Nundy 1966, Garfin et al 1995, Groen et al 1988, 1990, Hunt et al 2001, Kallakuri et al 1998, Olmarker et al 1993, Rydevik 2002, Rydevik et al 1984). The reference standard of diagnosis is essentially based on clinical findings (Vroomen et al 1999) but clear distinctions between the concepts of somatic referred pain, nerve root irritation (radicular pain) and radiculopathy are essential (Bogduk & McGuirk 2002 p 28–30). Radicular pain is identified by its character (sharp/lancinating), myotomal location (a narrow band in the distribution of a spinal nerve), dominant location (the pain is dominant in the area of distribution, not in the back or buttock), and response to nerve tension tests [the radiating pain is provoked by straight leg raise (SLR) or femoral nerve tension tests] (Waddell 1998 p 17–19). Radiculopathy is not inherently painful but is evidence of interrupted nerve conduction. It is identified clinically by examining key muscles for weakness, the tendon reflexes for areflexia, and light touch sensitivity for anesthetic skin in a dermatomal distribution. Electrodiagnostic tests of nerve function can be used to augment these findings. Although the dura mater is stressed during tension testing of the neural structures (Hall & Elvey 1999), it will provoke somatic referred pain, not radicular pain. Thus, it is likely that local back or buttock pain provoked during tension tests is of dural origin, whereas peripheral pain in the nerve root distribution is likely to be mediated by nerve root irritation. A variation of the SLR test, the slump test (Maitland 1985, Philip et al 1989) adds cephalad movement of the cord with spinal flexion (Lew et al 1994) to the SLR and might be more informative than Lasegue's original description (Deville et al 2000). Selective epidural injection (Lieberman 2000, Stitz & Sommer 1999) is nonspecific as a diagnostic test (Cannon & Aprill 2000, Govind 2004, Narozny et al 2001, Saal 2002) but absence of temporary pain relief following fluoroscopically guided epidural anesthesia suggests that pain of nerve root and dura mater origin is unlikely.

Pathoanatomic causes of low back and referred lower extremity pain

Herniated lumbar disc causing radiculopathy

The most common cause of radicular pain and radiculopathy is a herniation of intervertebral disc material. Typically, the reference standard for diagnosis used in most past studies of diagnostic accuracy for clinical tests has been surgical demonstration of herniated disc material compressing a nerve root. Since the advent of advanced imaging techniques (CT and MRI), clinical evidence of radicular pain and radiculopathy with confirmatory imaging is now considered the reference standard diagnosis for herniated lumbar disc causing radiculopathy (Waddell 1998). A negative MRI study effectively rules out a herniated disc as a cause of radiculopathy. Although the prevalence of disc bulges, protrusions, and herniations in age- and sex-matched symptomatic and asymptomatic patients is similar, evidence of disc extrusion is strongly correlated with radiculopathy and radicular pain (specificity 87%) (Boos et al 1995). Consequently, imaging results must not be taken out of context of the history and clinical findings (Nachemson & Vingård 2000 p 234). The images confirm the diagnosis only if the imaging results clearly match the clinical findings.

Lumbar spinal stenosis

There is no gold standard method of diagnosis (Katz et al 1995). Spinal stenosis is a collective term that relates to evidence of narrowing of the central spinal canal or the exit foramina for the exiting lumbar nerve roots (Nachemson & Vingård 2000 p 214–216). Contrast myelography has largely been replaced by CT and MRI for diagnosis because they can provide quality visualization of the spinal canal and foraminae with less risk. Age-related structural changes are the most common causes of spinal stenosis (Katz et al 1995) but some patients have a constitutionally narrowed foramen and are more susceptible to the development of symptoms (Spivak 1998). Spinal stenosis is not a heterogeneous condition but can be subdivided into three categories: (1) central spinal stenosis; (2) lateral stenosis; and (3) foraminal stenosis (Postacchini 1999, Spivak 1998).

The finding of spinal stenosis on images is not diagnostic of a patient's complaint of back and referred lower extremity symptoms. At least 20% of individuals over the age of 60 have anatomical stenosis but are asymptomatic (Bozzao et al 2004). It has been emphasized that the diagnosis of *symptomatic* spinal stenosis rests on the history and clinical examination findings with appropriate imaging findings used for confirmation (Fritz et al 1998, Katz et al 1995, Kent et al 1992, Porter 1996, Radu & Menkes 1998, Spivak 1998).

The diagnostic accuracy of imaging, history, demographic, and physical examination variables in relation to reference standards

There are two important aspects to estimating the diagnostic value of clinical tests:

1. Reliability: interexaminer reliability is the degree to which different examiners agree on the result from a test when applied to the same patient.
2. Validity: the degree to which a test is able to identify the target disease, when the disease is known to be present (sensitivity), and the degree to which the test is able to identify cases known to be free of the disease (specificity).

This section considers interexaminer reliability and validity separately for each of the most common causes and sources of pain: disc, ZJ, SIJ, nerve root, and spinal stenosis. Data are scattered throughout the literature of the last 30 years and the quality of many studies is questionable in the light of current reporting standards for diagnostic studies (Bossuyt et al 2003, Irwig et al 2002). Generally, 95% confidence intervals are not reported in older studies, many of which do not provide the raw data or summaries of data that allow for postpublication reanalysis. Estimates of sensitivity and specificity are provided in the following tables with 95% confidence intervals where available, or when sufficient raw data have permitted calculation. In some instances an estimate of interexaminer reliability is available. The appropriate statistic for most assessments of interexaminer reliability is Cohen's kappa, because it accounts for chance agreements. It ranges in value from −1.0 to +1.0, where 0.0 reflects chance agreement, −1.0 reflects perfect disagreement between observers and +1.0 reflects perfect agreement (Fleiss 1981). Kappa scores in excess of 0.0 reflect agreement better than chance. Kappa scores between +0.21 to +0.40 reflect 'slight agreement'; +0.41 to +0.60 reflect 'moderate agreement'; +0.61 to +0.80 'good agreement'; and +0.81 to + 1.00 'excellent agreement' (Landis & Koch 1977).

Clinical features suggesting discogenic pain

Validity and reliability data are available for some clinical tests. Centralization, peripheralization, or the identification of a directional preference during a standardized repeated movements examination (Donelson et al 1991, McKenzie & May 2003, Werneke et al 1999), have a relationship to pain provocation during discography. The repeated movement examination utilizes, but is not limited to, assessment of pain intensity and distribution before, during, and after, single and sets of standardized movements. The movements are: standing flexion, standing extension, supine flexion (knees-to-chest), prone extension (the half push-up), rotation in flexion and lateral flexion in standing (side-gliding) (Fig. 28.4). Table 28.2 presents the data available from the literature on the diagnostic accuracy of the clinical findings in relation to pain provocation during discography. Figure 28.5 graphically illustrates the centralization phenomenon and its opposite behavior: peripheralization.

Clinical features suggesting facetogenic pain

Although pain arising from the ZJs was once thought to be common (Mooney & Robertson 1976), subsequent research has shown otherwise. There is evidence that no clinical 'facet syndrome' exists (Jackson 1992, Schwarzer et al 1994a). However, a cluster of clinical variables ('Revel's criteria') were found to have sensitivity of 92% and specificity of 80% in relation to a 75% reduction in pain following a single ZJ block (Revel et al 1998), although this has not been confirmed (Laslett et al 2004). Furthermore, evaluation against double ZJ blocks

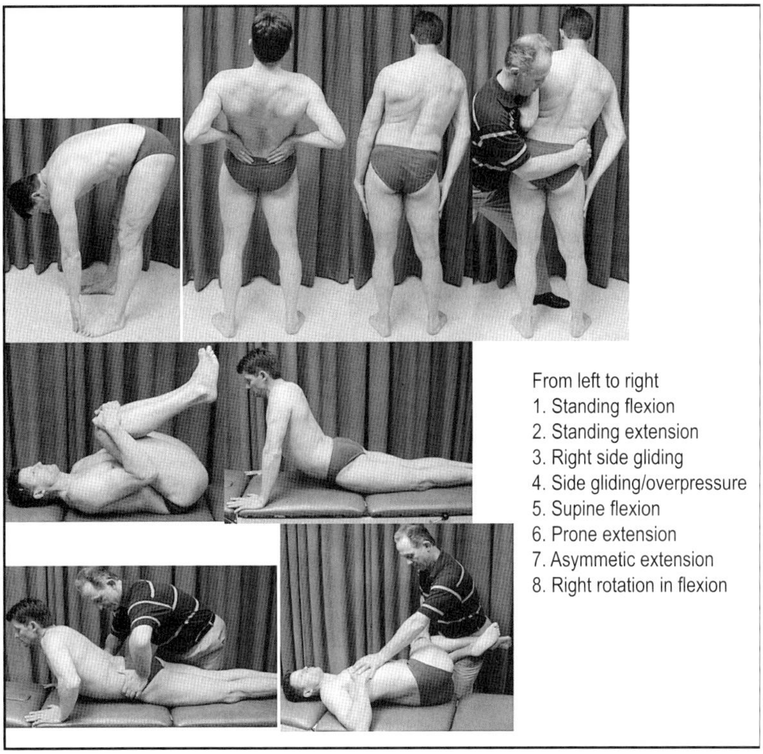

Fig. 28.4 Standardized test movements used in the repeated movements assessment for centralization, peripheralization or directional preference. (© University of Linköping, Sweden.)

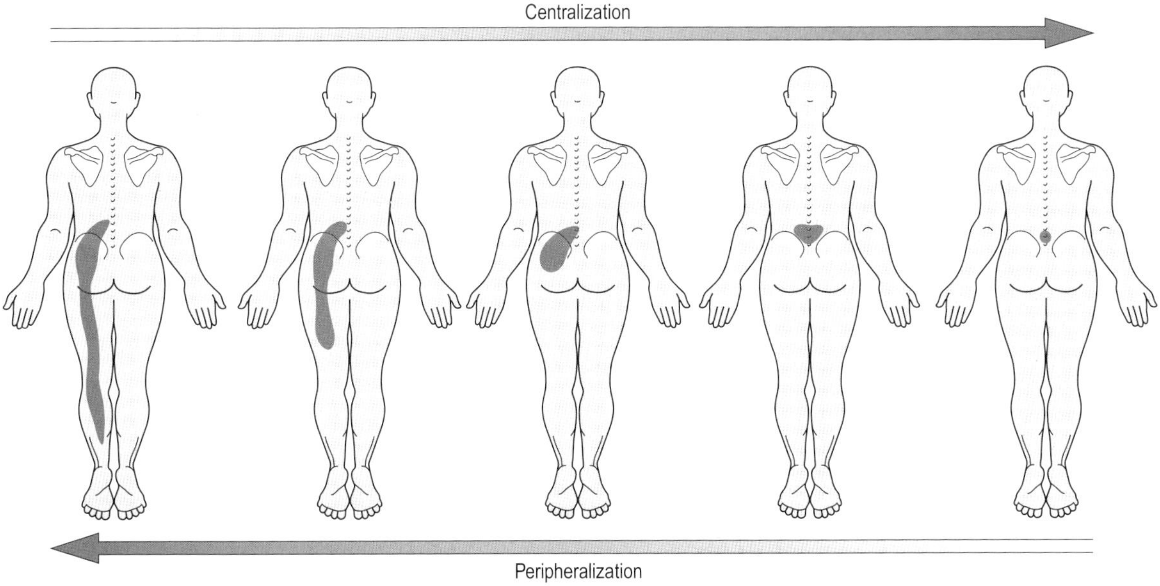

Fig. 28.5 Graphic representation of centralization and peripheralization of pain during repeated movements assessment.

Table 28.2 Diagnostic accuracy data of the clinical findings in relation to pain provocation during discography

	Validity		Reliability	
Variables	**% Sens (95% CI)**	**%Spec (95% CI)**	**Kappa (95% CI)**	**References**
Centralization or peripheralization	94* (82, 98)	52* (34, 69)		Donelson et al 1997, Bogduk 1997a*
Centralization (CP)	92 (75, 98) 25 (15, 37)	64 (43, 80) 96 (81, 99)	0.72 (0.35, 1.1) 0.79 (0.78, 0.81)	Donelson et al 1997*, Laslett et al 2005b, Kilpikoski et al 2002, Fritz et al 2000
Peripheralization	69* (44, 86) 11 (5, 22)	64* (43, 80) 79 (60, 91)		Donelson et al 1997 Laslett 2005
Directional preference	49 (37, 62)	91 (73, 98)	0.54 (0.12, 0.97)	Laslett 2005, Kilpikoski et al 2002
High intensity zone (MRI T2 weighted) vs exact or similar pain production discography	63 (51, 74)	97 (88, 99)	0.96 (0.89, 1.00) 0.57 (0.44, 0.70)	Aprill & Bogduk1992, Smith et al 1998
High intensity zone (MRI) vs exact or similar pain production	81	79		Lam et al 2000
Vibration vs discography	71 (55, 83)	63 (41, 81)	0.89 (0.82, 0.96)	Yrjämä & Vanharanta 1994
Moderate or major loss of lumbar extension	27 (18, 38)	88 (73, 95)		Laslett et al 2006b, Laslett 2005
History of PPE	32 (22, 44)	92 (75, 98)		Laslett et al 2006b, Laslett 2005
Patient report of VABLE	41 (30, 53)	83 (64, 93)		Laslett et al 2006b, Laslett 2005
Any one of Eloss, PEP or VABLE is present	69 (58, 79)	66 (47, 82)		Laslett et al 2006b, Laslett 2005
Any one of Eloss, PEP, VABLE or CP, is present	80 (70, 88)	50 (31, 69)		Laslett et al 2006b, Laslett 2005

**calculated from data in original report.*
%Sens, % sensitivity; %Spec, % specificity; CP, centralization; MRI, magnetic resonance imaging; PPE, persistent pain between episodes; VABLE, vulnerability in the neutral zone.

has shown that Revel's criteria are not predictive of a positive response (Manchikanti et al 2000a). Table 28.3 presents available data for diagnostic accuracy of clinical findings in relation to a double anesthetic block reference standard.

In essence, ZJ pain is more frequent in patients over 55 years. The high sensitivities for absence of pain with coughing, absence of pain in the spinal midline (Schwarzer et al 1994a), and no pain with the extension rotation test permit a statistical 'SnNout' (Sackett et al 2000), i.e. ZJ pain can be ruled out in the presence of coughing pain, midline pain, or pain-free extension rotation.

Clinical features suggesting sacroiliac joint pain

Clinical tests for SIJ 'dysfunction' are based on observation of observed abnormalities or asymmetries of position or motion (Magee 1992 p 309–328, van der Wurff et al 2000a). Typically, these tests require training in palpation skills. Clinical tests for SIJ pain are based on maneuvers intended to stress the SI joints and thus provoke familiar pain (Cyriax 1975 p 549–554, Magee 1992 p 309–328). Reliability of motion and mobility palpation tests are characterized by poor interexaminer reliability (Carmichael 1987, Freburger & Riddle 1999, Herzog et al 1989, Meijne et al 1999, O'Haire & Gibbons 2000, Potter & Rothstein 1985, Strender et al 1997, van der Wurff et al 2000a). Pain provocation tests generally perform better in reliability studies (Kokmeyer et al 2002, Laslett & Williams 1994, Potter & Rothstein 1985, van der Wurff et al 2000a). Multitest regimes do appear to be more reliable (Cibulka & Koldehoff 1999, Kokmeyer et al 2002), although the thigh thrust test [also called the PPPP test (Östgaard et al 1994a)] and Gaenslen's test appear to satisfy stringent evaluations for reliability (van der Wurff et al 2000a).

The validity of clinical tests for SIJ pain has been studied in a number of studies using a variety of designs. With the exception of one study (Östgaard et al 1994a), methodological quality was inadequate (van der Wurff et al 2000b). This one high-quality study used 'a history of posterior pelvic pain in pregnant women' as a reference standard, which has limited value in my opinion. A satisfactory reference standard for SIJ pain is a problem. Controlled intra-articular anesthetic blocks are the accepted reference standard for intra-articular sources of pain (Fortin

Table 28.3 Diagnostic accuracy of clinical findings in relation to an anesthetic block reference standard

	Validity		Reliability	
Variables	**%Sens (95% CI)**	**%Spec (95% CI)**	**Kappa**	**References**
5/7 Revel's criteria	13	84	66 (4–100)	Manchikanti et al 2000a, Petersen et al 2004
Absence of pain coughing	90	13		Manchikanti et al 2000a
Age over 65	21 39 (18, 64)	85 85 (77, 90)		Manchikanti et al 2000a, Laslett 2005
Ext/rotation test pain[a]	100 (87, 100) 90 (60, 98)	12 (7, 18) 35 (26, 46)		Schwarzer et al 1994c, Laslett et al 2006a
Walking is best	31 (13, 58)	92 (85, 96)		Laslett et al 2006a
Sitting is best	33 (14, 61)	90 (82, 94)		Laslett et al 2006a

% Sens, % sensitivity; %Spec, % specificity.
[a]The extension rotation test was also evaluated by Manchikanti et al (2000a) with results quite different to Schwarzer et al (1994) and my own results.

et al 1994a, Merskey & Bogduk 1994) but cannot be expected to identify or rule out extra-articular SIJ sources of pain (Laslett 1998, Maigne et al 1996). Since the van der Wurff et al review, results from a study comparing provocation SIJ tests with intra-articular blocks have been published (Laslett et al 2003, 2005a). Table 28.4 presents relevant data from that study and selected results from other studies on diagnostic accuracy of clinical findings.

Whereas Maigne et al (1996) state that the distraction, compression, sacral thrust, Gaenslen, Patrick, resisted hip external rotation, and symphysis pubis pressure tests were not useful predictors of double blocks, these authors did not provide data and did not report on composites of tests. Also, Slipman et al (1998) report that the Patrick, shear, standing extension, Gaenslen, Yeoman, sacral sulcus pressure tests or any combination were not predictive of a response to a single SIJ block; however, they did not provide data either. Figures 28.6 to 28.10 depict the five pain provocation tests: distraction, thigh thrust, Gaenslen's test, compression, and sacral thrust used in my studies.

Clinical features suggesting radicular pain/radiculopathy secondary to a herniated lumbar disc

Tests used to make this diagnosis have been evaluated in a number of studies. Table 28.5 presents

Table 28.4 Diagnostic accuracy data for clinical findings in relation to anesthetic blocks to the SIJ

	Validity		Reliability	
Variables	**% Sens (95% CI)**	**%Spec (95% CI)**	**Kappa (95% CI)**	**References**
≥ 3 positive provocation SIJ tests in non-centralizers	91 (62, 98)	83 (68, 96)	0.65 (0.41, 0.89)	Laslett et al 2003, Petersen et al 2004
At least 1 positive SIJ test	100 (81, 100)	44 (28, 61)	0.52–0.89 (0.26, 1.01)	Laslett et al 2005a, Laslett & Williams 1994
At least 2 positive SIJ tests	93 (72, 99)	66 (48, 80)	0.52–0.89 (0.26, 1.01)	Laslett et al 2005a, Laslett & Williams 1994
At least 3 positive SIJ tests	94 (72, 99)	78 (61, 89)	0.52–0.89 (0.26, 1.01)	Laslett et al 2005a, Laslett & Williams 1994
At least 4 positive SIJ tests	60 (36, 80)	81 (65, 91)	0.52–0.89 (0.26, 1.01)	Laslett et al 2005a, Laslett & Williams 1994
At least 5 positive SIJ tests	27 (11, 52)	88 (72, 95)	0.52–0.89 (0.26, 1.01)	Laslett et al 2005a, Laslett & Williams 1994
Any two provocation SIJ tests of D, C, TT, Sc	88 (64, 97)	78 (61, 89)	0.52–0.89 (0.26, 1.01)	Laslett et al 2005a, Laslett & Williams 1994
Sacral sulcus tenderness	95	9		Dreyfuss et al 1996
Better with manipulation	54 (36, 70)	78 (55, 91)		Dreyfuss et al 1996
Quantitative radionuclide bone scanning	46	89		Maigne et al 1998

% Sens, % sensitivity; %Spec, % specificity; C, compression test; cD, distraction test; S, sacral thrust test; SIJ, sacroiliac joint; TT, thigh thrust test.

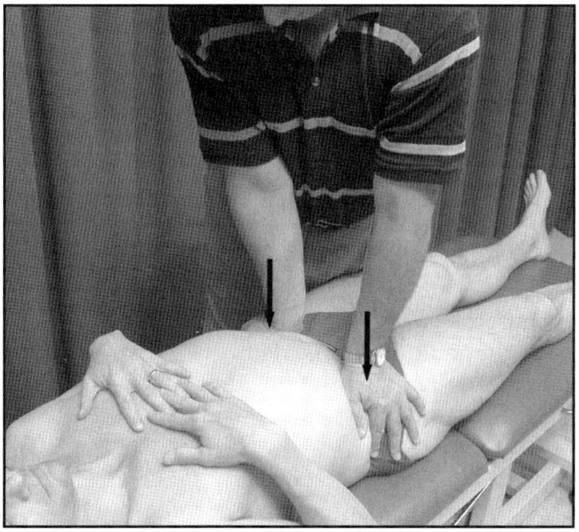

Fig. 28.6 Distraction sacroiliac joint provocation test. (Reproduced with permission from Laslett et al 2003.)

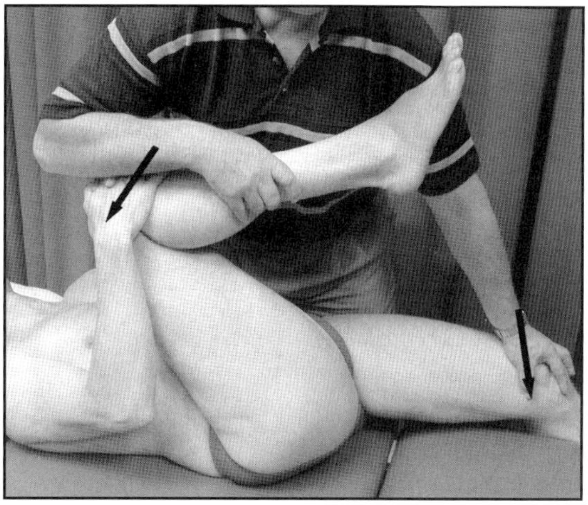

Fig. 28.8 Gaenslen's sacroiliac joint provocation test. (Reproduced with permission from Laslett et al 2003.)

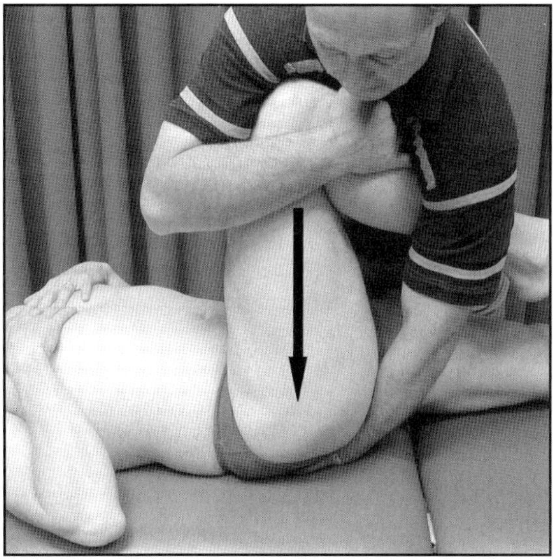

Fig. 28.7 Thigh thrust sacroiliac joint provocation test. (Reproduced with permission from Laslett et al 2003.)

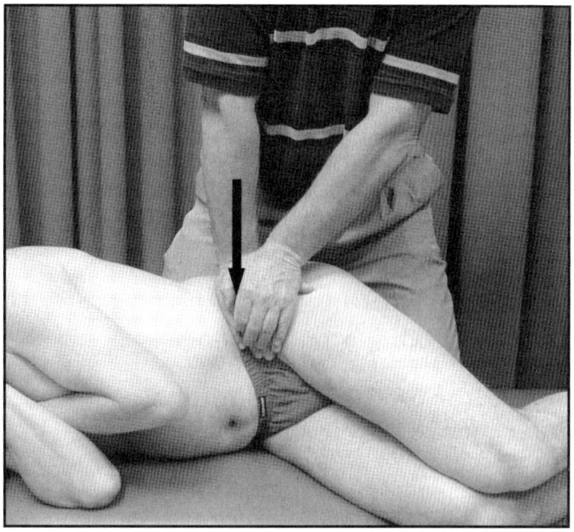

Fig. 28.9 Compression sacroiliac joint provocation test. (Reproduced with permission from Laslett et al 2003.)

the data available from the literature on diagnostic accuracy of clinical findings in relation to the reference standard of surgical findings.

It can be seen that, with the exception of an MRI showing neural compromise, all tests have either higher sensitivity or high specificity. Most of the tests for neurologic deficit have high specificity but low sensitivity because of several factors. A lumbar disc herniation can compress any one of the lumbar nerve roots depending on its particular pathoanatomy. Consequently, weak dorsiflexion, for example, is sensitive and specific to L4 root compression but will be 'negative', i.e. insensitive, to S1 root compression. As a single sign, it is therefore insensitive to herniated discs compressing any one of several nerve roots, but

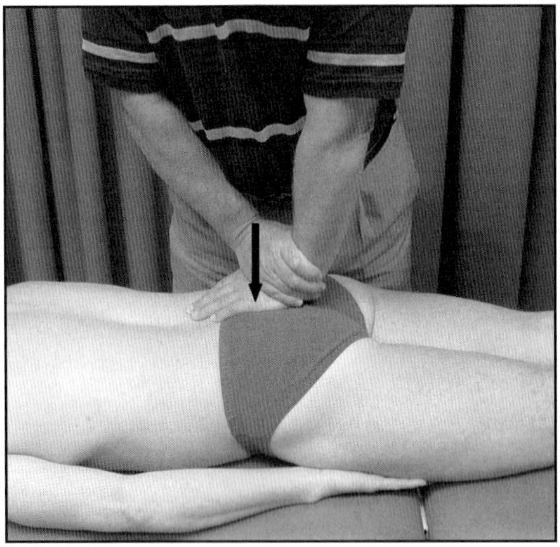

Fig. 28.10 Sacral thrust sacroiliac joint provocation test. (Reproduced with permission from Laslett et al 2003.)

as the great majority of radiculopathies are caused by herniations, it is highly specific to that disorder. The SLR test is sensitive but not specific because the majority of herniated discs produce a positive test, but specificity is low because there are many other different causes for a positive SLR. For example, a hamstring strain will produce a positive SLR.

Clinical features suggesting symptomatic spinal stenosis

While a pattern of neurogenic (pseudo) claudication is regarded as a key feature of symptomatic spinal stenosis, nearly 30% of patients with the diagnosis are not worse with walking. In addition, pain below the knee is also commonly associated with the diagnosis, but 30–60% do not have this symptom (Katz et al 1995). Table 28.6 provides data available from the literature for the diagnostic accuracy of clinical findings mostly in relation to findings during surgical decompression and surgical outcomes.

In one study (Katz et al 1995), multivariate analysis using age, no pain when seated, wide-based gait and thigh pain with 30 seconds of lumbar extension, predicted 49% of the variance in experts' confidence that spinal stenosis was the cause of pain. All patients where these experts were more that 80% confident that stenosis was the cause of pain had MRI or CT confirmation of the diagnosis.

What should be included in the clinical evaluation of back pain patients?

All patients should receive a comprehensive evaluation that includes basic diagnostic triage (Waddell 1998 p 9–25). This includes consideration of possible serious causes of lumbopelvic pain (Bogduk 2002 p 128).

Different clinicians use different methods and have different objectives. However, to fully utilize those data items with an evidential base for their diagnostic accuracy, the following variables should be included:

Demographic variables

- Age, occupation, social history.

Questions in the history

Medical and social history

- Some measure of disability and/or distress (questionnaires).
- Other diseases/medical conditions.

Pain onset

- Trauma?
- Original pain location.

Pain distribution

- Widespread pain/anatomic location.
- Is pain dominant in the spinal midline?
- Pain below the buttocks.
- Pain below the knees.
- Is pain dominant below the gluteal fold?

Pain quality

- Diffuse/aching.
- Lancinating/twingeing.

Pain response to activity

- Pain with walking/claudication.
- Positions and activities that are best and worst for symptoms.
- Positions and activities that influence pain intensity and distribution.
- Consistent?
- Does pain change location?

Table 28.5 Diagnostic accuracy data of clinical findings in relation to the reference standard of surgical findings of herniated disc causing radiculopathy

	Validity		Reliability	
Variable	**% Sens**	**%Spec**	**Kappa (95% CI)**	**References**
Ipsilateral SLR	91 (82, 94)	26 (16, 38)	0.36–0.81	Deville et al 2000, McCombe et al 1989
Contralateral SLR (cross SLR)	29 (24, 34)	88 (86, 90)	–0.02–0.74	Deville et al 2000, McCombe et al 1989
Weakness ankle DF	20–49	54–82	0.35–1.00	Hakelius 1970, McCombe et al 1989
Weakness ankle PF	60	95	0.02–0.65	Hakelius 1970, McCombe et al 1989
Weakness EHL	37	71	0.29–0.65	Hakelius 1970, McCombe et al 1989
Quads weakness	10	99	0.04–0.85	Hakelius 1970, McCombe et al 1989
Ankle reflex weak	50–52	62–63	0.20–0.39	Hakelius 1970, Spangfort 1972, McCombe et al 1989
Patellar reflex weak	40–70	93–97	0.13–0.23	Hakelius 1970, Spangfort 1972, McCombe et al 1989
Sensory loss	66	51	0.53–0.68	Kosteljanetz et al 1988, McCombe et al 1989
MRI shows disc herniation	96	24	0.74	Boos et al 1995
MRI shows neural compromise	83	87	0.90	Boos et al 1995
MRI shows disc degeneration	96	15	0.90	Boos et al 1995
MRI shows extrusion	41	87	0.90	Boos et al 1995
Depression	54	85		Boos et al 1995

% Sens, % sensitivity; %Spec, % specificity; EHL, extensor hallucis longus; MRI, magnetic resonance imaging; PF, plantar flexion; SLR, straight leg raise.

Physical examination

Observation

- Idiopathic scoliosis.
- Use of walking aids/wheelchairs.
- Vulnerability in neutral zone/supporting weight in flexion.
- Avoidance of neutral zone, jerky, uncontrolled motion.

Repeated movements testing (see Fig. 28.4)

- Centralization (see Fig. 28.5).
- Directional preference (see Fig. 28.5).

Neurological screening examination

- Motor/tendon reflex deficit.
- Sensory loss.

Specific tests

- SLR test:
  - provokes back or leg pain?
  - cross leg sign
  - at least four SIJ provocation tests (see Figs 28.6–28.10): preferred are distraction, thigh thrust, compression, sacral thrust. Gaenslen's and Faber have value.
- Active SLR test.

Table 28.6 Diagnostic accuracy data of clinical findings mostly in relation to findings during surgical decompression and surgical outcomes

	Validity		Reliability	
Variable	**% Sens (95% CI)**	**%Spec (95% CI)**	**Kappa (95% CI)**	**References**
Age > 65 years	77 (64, 90)	69 (53, 85)		Katz et al 1995
Pain below buttocks	88 (78, 98)	34 (18, 50)		Katz et al 1995
Pain below knees	56 (41, 71)	63 (46, 80)		Katz et al 1995
No pain when seated	46 (30, 62)	93 (84, 100)		Katz et al 1995
Symptoms improved when seated	52 (37, 67)	83 (70, 96)		Katz et al 1995
Symptoms worse with walking	71 (57, 85)	30 (14, 46)		Katz et al 1995
Wide based gait	43 (28, 58)	97 (91, 100)		Katz et al 1995
Abnormal Romberg result	39 (24, 54)	91 (81, 100)		Katz et al 1995
Vibration deficit	53 (38, 68)	81 (67, 95)		Katz et al 1995
Walking better holding onto shopping cart	63	67		Fritz et al 1997a
Leg symptoms worse walking, better sitting	81	16		Fritz et al 1997a
Best posture for symptoms is sitting	89	39		Fritz et al 1997a
Worst posture for symptoms is walking or standing	89	33		Fritz et al 1997a
No pain with lumbar flexion	79 (67, 91)	44 (27, 61)		Katz et al 1995
Thigh pain with 30 seconds lumbar extension	51 (36, 66)	69 (53, 85)		Katz et al 1995
Improved tolerance with lumbar flexion	50	92		Dong & Porter 1989
Earlier symptom onset on level vs inclined treadmill walking	68	83		Fritz et al 1997b
Longer recovery time after level vs inclined treadmill walking	82	68		Fritz et al 1997b

% Sens, % sensitivity; %Spec, % specificity.

Imaging

Radiographs

- Recent trauma.
- Screen for possible red flag condition.

MRI or CT

- Suspected herniated disc.
- Suspected spinal stenosis.
- Suspected red flag condition.

Clinical application

Many items from the history and clinical examination can be used in a clinical reasoning process leading to improved certainty about the source and cause of back and referred pain. Fig. 28.11 presents a proposed algorithm that utilizes those data items for which evidence exists regarding their predictive value. It begins with questions that rule out serious pathologies (Bogduk & McGuirk 2002 p 35–39), and nerve root pain (see above). Pain associated with hip joint pathology is revealed when hip joint movements provoke pain rather than lumbar spine movement and some SIJ tests (distraction, compression, and sacral thrust). The next step is to utilize information from the repeated movements evaluation (McKenzie & May 2003). If the symptoms can be made to centralize, or if there is a clear directional preference to one movement direction, discogenic pain is highly likely. In this event, further diagnostic procedures are unnecessary because an effective treatment strategy is available (Long et al 2004, Werneke & Hart 2001, 2003). The next step is to use information from SIJ provocation tests. If three or more provoke the pain, SIJ pain is highly likely. If there is a need to establish the SIJ as the source of pain, SIJ blocks are required. The next step is to consider the location of the dominant pain complaint. If midline pain is dominant, SIJ and ZJ pain are highly unlikely, leaving the disc as the probable source of pain. If this needs to be confirmed, provocation discography is indicated. If the dominant pain is other than in the spinal midline, evaluation of other data is helpful. Even though Revel's criteria have poor sensitivity, they are highly specific. In this eventuality, ZJ pain is likely and the patient should undergo ZJ blocks.

The next question is intended to identify radicular pain without radiculopathy. Typically, these disorders produce dominant lancinating pain in the lower limb in a narrow myotomally distributed band, plus nerve root tension signs. If there is dominant lower extremity pain without evidence of radicular pain, the patient should be investigated for lower extremity pathology such as undetected fractures, neoplasm, infection, peripheral vascular disease, etc. Psychosocial distress factors can also be a factor and must be considered here. If at this point in the algorithm it is clear that the dominant pain is above the gluteal fold, the intervertebral disc is the most likely source of pain based simply on epidemiological grounds. At this point some of the less powerful predictors of painful discography may be used to suggest which investigation is most appropriate and justifiable. Persistent pain between episodes (PPE) of acute back pain, a major loss of lumbar extension (ExtLoss), and 'vulnerability' in the 'neutral zone' (VABLE) are findings with modest specificity and are associated with positive discography. Further investigation with discography may establish or rule out the disc as the source of pain. If none of these clinical findings are present, the report that 'walking is the best activity for pain' is considered. In this eventuality, spinal stenosis and hip joint pain are unlikely, and a positive response to a screening ZJ block is likely. This patient should proceed directly to ZJ blocks and not undergo discography or screening SIJ blocks. If the patient is not 'best walking', exploration of the effect of walking and standing is valuable. Careful questioning regarding the pattern of claudication and the means by which relief is obtained (e.g. needing to sit or if standing still is sufficient), can suggest whether peripheral vascular disease is the likely cause or if spinal stenosis is more likely. Investigation can proceed depending on which mechanism is suggested.

The use of invasive and expensive technologies to establish the source and cause of chronic LBP needs to be justifiable. Bogduk & McGuirk (2002) have proposed an evidence-based clinical reasoning process in the form of three algorithms with the purpose of minimizing potential overuse of the procedures and maximizing utility of the information gained. The algorithm provided here integrates the most recent information, allows the clinician to skip certain steps, and may serve as a useful beginning point to Bogduk & McGuirk's tightly reasoned procedure. The current algorithm allows a simplification of Bogduk & McGuirk's (2002 p 181) second algorithm, 'an algorithm for the investigations of the synovial joints of the lumbar spine' and Fig. 28.12 is offered as an update.

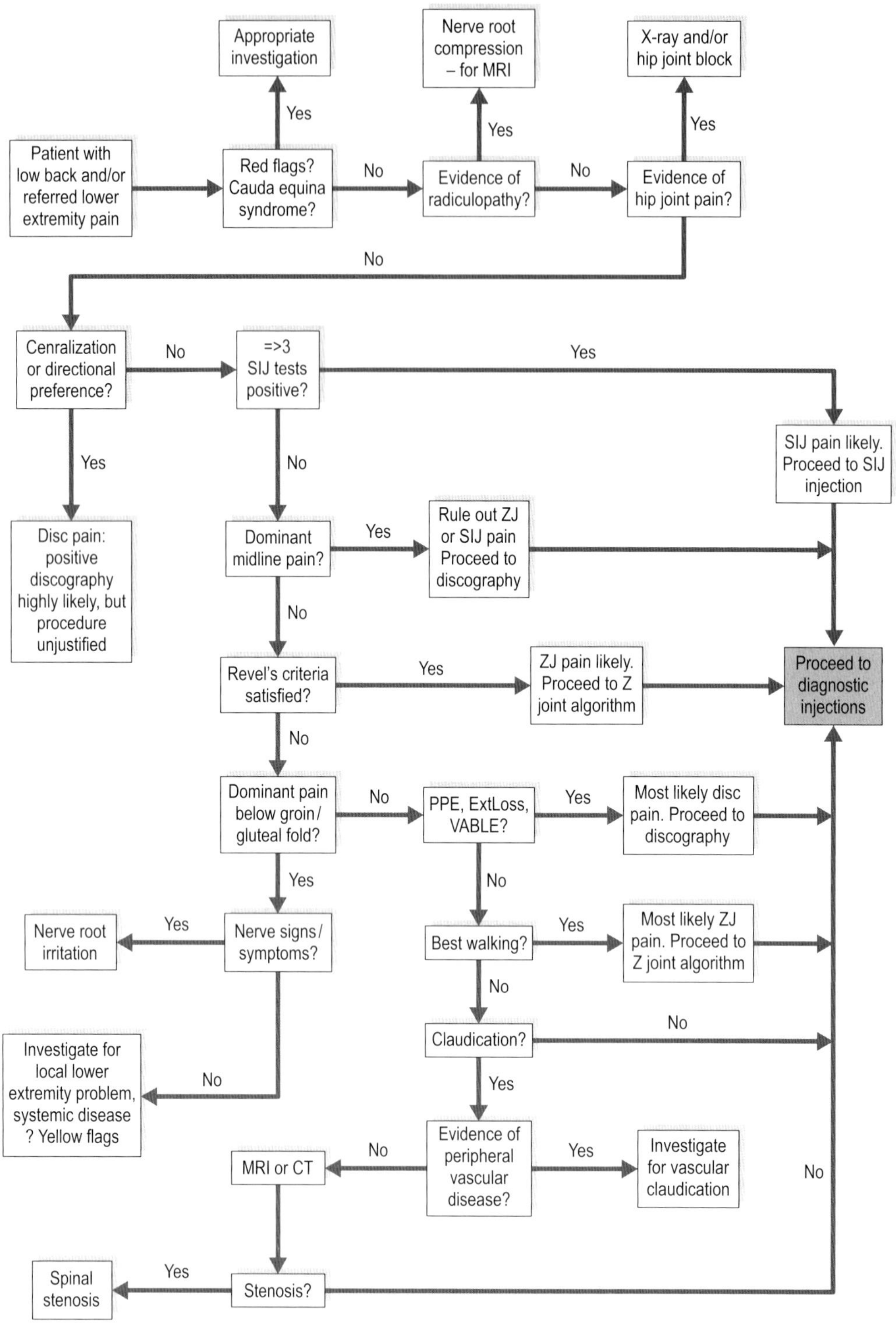

Fig. 28.11 Proposed algorithm for use of demographic, history and clinical examination findings in clinical assessment of chronic LBP patients. (With permission of the University of Linköping, Sweden.)

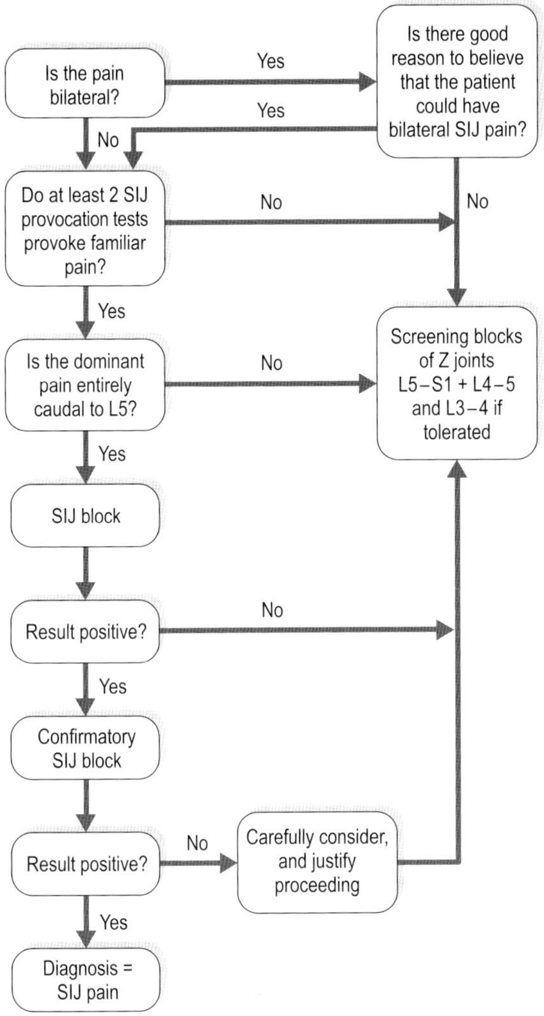

Fig. 28.12 Initial algorithm for investigation of synovial joints of the lumbar spine and pelvis. (With permission of the University of Linköping, Sweden.)

Summary

Diagnosis of the sources and causes of chronic LBP is possible in over 50% of cases using advanced imaging techniques and fluoroscopically guided diagnostic injection techniques. The clinical examination can provide information that enables the clinician to make a diagnosis in a significant proportion of cases while improving the quality of selection of patients for more sophisticated diagnostic interventions.

References

Albert H, Godskesen M, Westergaard J 2000 Evaluation of clinical tests used in classification procedures in pregnancy-related pelvic joint pain. European Spine Journal 9:161–166

Albert HB, Godskesen M, Westergaard JG 2002 Incidence of four syndromes of pregnancy-related pelvic joint pain. Spine 27(24):2831–2834

Anderson MW 2004 Lumbar discography: an update. Seminars in Roentgenology 39(1):52–67

Aprill CN 1997 Diagnostic disc injection. II Diagnostic lumbar disc injection. In: Frymoyer JW, et al (eds) The adult spine: principles and practice. Lippincott–Raven Publishers, Philadelphia, PA

Aprill C, Bogduk N 1992 High-intensity zone: a diagnostic sign of painful disc on magnetic resonance imaging. British Journal of Radiology 65(773):361–369

Bernard TN Jr, Cassidy JD 1991 The sacroiliac joint syndrome: pathophysiology, diagnosis, and management. In: Frymoyer JW (ed) The adult spine: principles and practice. Raven Press Ltd, New York

Block AR, Vanharanta H, Ohnmeiss DD et al 1996 Discographic pain report. Influence of psychological factors. Spine 21(3):334–338

Bogduk N 1983 The innervation of the lumbar spine. Spine 8(3):286–293

Bogduk N 1995 The anatomical basis for spinal pain syndromes. Journal of Manipulative and Physiological Therapeutics 18(9):603–605

Bogduk N 1997a Commentary on 'A prospective study of centralization and lumbar and referred pain: A predictor of symptomatic discs and annular competence'. The Pain Medicine Journal Club Journal 3(5):246–248

Bogduk N 1997b International Spinal Injection Society guidelines for the performance of spinal injection procedures. Part 1: Zygapophysial joint blocks. Clinical Journal of Pain 13(4):285–302

Bogduk N 2001 An analysis of the Carragee data on false-positive discography. International Spinal Injection Society Scientific Newsletter 4(2):3–10

Bogduk N 2002 Checklist for red flag clinical indicators prepared for Australian National Musculoskeletal Association. In: Bogduk N, McGuirk B (eds) Medical management of acute and chronic low back pain: an evidence based approach. Elsevier Science BV, Amsterdam

Bogduk N, McGuirk B 2002 Medical management of acute and chronic low back pain. Elsevier Science BV, Amsterdam

Bogduk N, Modic MT 1996 Controversy. Lumbar discography. Spine 21(3):402–404

Bogduk N, Twomey L 1987 Clinical anatomy of the lumbar spine. Churchill Livingstone, London

Bogduk N, Tynan W, Wilson AS 1981 The nerve supply to the human lumbar intervertebral discs. Journal of Anatomy 132(1):39–56

Boos N, Rieder R, Schade V et al 1995 Volvo Award in clinical sciences. The diagnostic accuracy of magnetic resonance imaging, work perception, and psychosocial factors in identifying symptomatic disc herniations. Spine 20(24):2613–2625

Bossuyt PM, Reitsma JB, Bruns DE 2003 Towards complete and accurate reporting of studies of diagnostic accuracy: the STARD initiative. British Medical Journal 326(7379):41–44

Bozzao A, Gallucci M, Masciocchi C et al 2004 Lumbar disk herniation: MR imaging assessment of natural history in patients treated without surgery. Radiology 185(1):135–141

Brismar H, Vucetic N, Svensson O 1996 Pain patterns in lumbar disc hernia: Drawings compared to surgical findings in 159 patients. Acta Orthopaedica Scandinavica 67(5):470–472

Brown MF, Hukkanen MV, McCarthy ID et al 1997 Sensory and sympathetic innervation of the vertebral endplate in patients with degenerative disc disease. Journal of Bone & Joint Surgery (UK) 79(1):147–153

Cannon DT, Aprill CN 2000 Lumbosacral epidural injections. Archives of Physical Medicine & Rehabilitation 81(March):S87–S98

Carmichael JP 1987 Inter- and intra-examiner reliability of palpation for sacroiliac joint dysfunction. Journal of Manipulative & Physiological Therapeutics 10(4): 164–171

Carragee EJ 2001 Psychological and functional profiles in select subjects with low back pain. The Spine Journal 1:198–204

Carragee EJ, Tanner CM, Khurana S et al 2000 The rates of false-positive lumbar discography in select patients without low back symptoms. Spine 25(11):1373–1381

Cibulka MT, Koldehoff R 1999 Clinical usefulness of a cluster of sacroiliac joint tests in patients with and without low back pain. Journal of Orthopedic and Sports Physical Therapy 29(2):83–99

Crock HV 1986 Internal disc disruption: a challenge to disc prolapse fifty years on. Presidential address: ISSLS. Spine 11(6):650–653

Cyriax J 1975 Textbook of orthopaedic medicine. Vol. 1: Diagnosis of soft tissue lesions, 6th edn. Ballière Tindall, London

Deville WLJM, van der Windt DAWM, Dzaferagic A et al 2000 The test of Lasegue: systematic review of the accuracy in diagnosing herniated discs. Spine 25(9):1140–1147

Deyo RA, Haselkorn J, Hoffman R et al 1994 Designing studies of diagnostic tests for low back pain or radiculopathy. Spine 19(suppl):2057S–2065S

Donelson R, Grant W, Kamps C et al 1991 Pain response to sagittal end range spinal motion: A multi-centered, prospective, randomized trial. Spine 16(suppl): S206–S212

Donelson R, Aprill C, Medcalf R, Grant WA 1997 Prospective study of centralization of lumbar and referred pain. A predictor of symptomatic discs and anular competence. Spine 22(10):1115–1122

Dong GX, Porter RW 1989 Walking and cycling tests in neurogenic and intermittent claudication. Spine 14(9):965–969

Dreyfuss PH, Michaelsen M, Pauza K et al 1996 The value of history and physical examination in diagnosing sacroiliac joint pain. Spine 21:2594–2602

Dreyfuss PH, Dreyer SJ, Vaccaro A 2003 Lumbar zygapophysial (facet) joint injections. The Spine Journal 3(Supplement):50–59

Edgar MA, Nundy S 1966 Innervation of the spinal dura mater. Journal of Neurology and Neurosurgery Psychiatry 29:530–534

Executive Committee of the North American Spine Society 2004 Position statement on discography. Spine 13(12):1343

Fagan A, Moore R, Vernon-Roberts B et al 2003 ISSLS prize winner. The innervation of the intervertebral disc: a quantitative analysis. Spine 28(23):2570–2576

Fleiss JL 1981 Statistical methods for rates and proportions. John Wiley and Sons, New York

Fortin JD, Aprill C, Pontieux RT et al 1994a Sacroiliac joint: pain referral maps upon applying a new injection/ arthrography technique. Part II: Clinical evaluation. Spine 19(13):1483–1489

Fortin JD, Dwyer AP, West S et al 1994b Sacroiliac joint: pain referral maps upon applying a new injection/ arthrography technique. Part 1: Asymptomatic volunteers. Spine 19:1475–1482

Freburger JK, Riddle DL 1999 Measurement of sacroiliac joint dysfunction: a multicenter intertester reliability study. Physical Therapy 79(12):1134–1141

Fritz JM, Erhard RE, Delitto A et al 1997a Preliminary results of the use of a two-stage treadmill test as a clinical diagnostic tool in the differential diagnosis of lumbar spinal stenosis. Journal of Spinal Disorders 10(5):410–416

Fritz JM, Erhard RE, Vignovic M 1997b A nonsurgical treatment approach for patients with lumbar spinal stenosis. Physical Therapy 77(9):962–973

Fritz JM, Delitto A, Welch WC, Erhard RE 1998 Lumbar spinal stenosis: a review of current concepts in evaluation, management, and outcome measurements. Archives of Physical Medicine & Rehabilitation 79:700–708

Fritz JM, Delitto A, Vignovic M, Busse RG 2000 Interrater reliability of judgments of the centralization phenomenon and status change during movement testing in patients with low back pain. Archives of Physical Medicine & Rehabilitation 81(1):57–61

Garfin SR, Rydevik B, Lind B, Massie J 1995 Spinal nerve root compression. Spine 20(16):1810–1820

Govind J 2004 Lumbar radicular pain. Australian Family Physician 33(6):409–412

Grob KR, Neuhuber WL, Kissling RO 1995 Innervation of the sacroiliac joint of the human. Rheumatology 54(2): 117–122

Groen GJ, Baljet B, Drukker J 1988 The innervation of the spinal dura mater: anatomy and clinical implications. Acta Neurochirgurie (Wien) 92(1–4):39–46

Groen GJ, Baljet B, Drukker J 1990 Nerves and nerve plexuses of the human vertebral column. American Journal of Anatomy 188(3):282–296

Hakelius A 1970 Prognosis in sciatica. Acta Orthopaedica Scandinavica 129 (suppl):1–70

Hall TM, Elvey RL 1999 Nerve trunk pain: physical diagnosis and treatment. Manual Therapy 4(2):63–73
Herzog W, Read LJ, Conway PJ et al 1989 Reliability of motion palpation procedures to detect sacroiliac joint fixations. Journal of Manipulative & Physiological Therapeutics 12(2):86–92
Holt EP 1968 The question of lumbar discography. Journal of Bone & Joint Surgery (US) 50:720
Hunt JL, Winkelstein BA, Rutkowski MD et al 2001 Repeated injury to the lumbar nerve roots produces enhanced mechanical allodynia and persistent spinal neuroinflammation. Spine 26(19):2073–2079
Irwig L, Bossuyt PM, Glasziou P 2002 Evidence base of clinical diagnosis: Designing studies to ensure that estimates of test accuracy are transferable. British Medical Journal 324(7338):669–671
Jackson RP 1992 The facet syndrome: myth or reality? Clinical Orthopedics & Related Research 279(June): 110–121
Jackson RP, Jacobs RR, Montesano PX 1988 Volvo award in clinical sciences.Facet joint injection in low-back pain. A prospective statistical study. Spine 13:966–971
Kallakuri S, Cavanaugh JM, Blagoev DC 1998 An immunohistochemical study of innervation of lumbar spinal dura and longitudinal ligaments. Spine 23(4): 403–411
Katz JN, Dalgas M, Stucki G, Lipson SG 1995 Degenerative lumbar spinal stenosis. Diagnostic value of the history and physical examination. Arthritis & Rheumatism 38(9):1236–1241
Kent DL, Haynor DR, Larson EB et al 1992 Diagnosis of lumbar spinal stenosis in adults: a meta-analysis of the accuracy of CT, MR and myelography. Americal Journal of Roentgenology 158(5):1135–1144
Kilpikoski S, Airaksinen O, Kankaanpaa M et al 2002 Interexaminer reliability of low back pain assessment using the McKenzie method. Spine 27(8):E207–E214
Kokmeyer DJ, van der Wurff P, Aufdemkampe G et al 2002 The reliability of multitest regimens with sacroiliac pain provocation tests. Journal of Manipulative & Physiological Therapeutics 25(1):42–48
Kosteljanetz M, Bang F, Schmidt-Olsen S 1988 The clinical significance of straight-leg-raising (Lasègue sign) in the diagnosis of prolapsed intervertebral disc. Spine 13:393–395
Lam KS, Carlin D, Mulholland RC 2000 Lumbar disc high-intensity zone: the value and significance of provocative discography in the determination of the discogenic pain source. European Spine Journal 9(1):36–41
Landis RJ, Koch GG 1977 The measurement of observer agreement for categorical data. Biometrics 33:159–174
Laslett M 1997 Pain provocation sacroiliac joint tests: Reliability and prevalence. In: Vleeming A, Mooney V (eds) Movement, stability and low back pain: the essential role of the pelvis. Churchill Livingstone, Edinburgh
Laslett M 1998 The value of the physical examination in diagnosis of painful sacroiliac joint pathologies (letter; comment). Spine 23(8):962–964
Laslett M 2005 The diagnostic accuracy of the clinical examination compared to available reference standards in chronic low back pain patients. Faculty of Health Sciences, Linköpings Universitet, 2005
Laslett M, Williams M 1994 The reliability of selected pain provocation tests for sacroiliac joint pathology. Spine 19(11):1243–1249
Laslett M, Young SB, Aprill CN et al 2003 Diagnosing painful sacroiliac joints: a validity study of a McKenzie evaluation and sacroiliac joint provocation tests. Australian Journal of Physiotherapy 49:89–97
Laslett M, Oberg B, Aprill CN et al 2004 Zygapophysial joint blocks in chronic low back pain: A test of Revel's model as a screening test. BMC Musculoskeletal Disorders 5(1):43
Laslett M, Aprill CN, McDonald B et al 2005a Diagnosis of sacroiliac joint pain: validity of individual provocation tests and composites of tests. Manual Therapy 10(30): 207–218
Laslett M, Oberg B, Aprill CN et al 2005b Centralization as a predictor of provocation discography results in chronic low back pain, and the influence of disability and distress on diagnostic power. The Spine Journal 5:370–380
Laslett M, Aprill CN, Tropp H et al 2006a Clinical predictors of screening lumbar zygapophyseal joint blocks: Development of clinical prediction rules. The Spine Journal 6(4):370–379
Laslett M, Oberg B, Aprill CN et al 2006b A study of clinical predictors of lumbar discogenic pain as determined by provocation discography. European Spine Journal (submitted)
Lew PC, Morrow CJ, Lew AM 1994 The effect of neck and leg flexion and their sequence on the lumbar spinal cord. Implications in low back pain and sciatica. Spine 19(21):2421–2424
Lieberman RM 2000 Letter to the editor: accuracy of blind versus fluoroscopically guided caudal epidural injection. Spine 25(6):760
Lindblom K 1948 Diagnostic puncture of intervertebral discs in sciatica. Acta Orthopaedica Scandinavica 17: 231–239
Long A, Donelson R, Fung T 2004 Does it matter which exercise?: A randomized control trial of exercise for low back pain. Spine 29(3):2593–2602
Magee DJ 1992 Orthopedic physical assessment, 2nd edn. WB Saunders, Philadelphia, PA
Maigne JY, Aivaliklis A, Pfefer F 1996 Results of sacroiliac joint double block and value of sacroiliac pain provocation tests in 54 patients with low back pain. Spine 21(16):1889–1892
Maigne JY, Boulahdour H, Chatellier G 1998 Value of quantitative radionuclide bone scanning in the diagnosis of sacroiliac joint syndrome in 32 patients with low back pain. European Spine Journal 7(4):328–331
Maitland GD 1985 The slump test: Examination and treatment. Australian Journal of Physiotherapy 31(6):215–219
Manchikanti L, Pampati VS, Pakanati RR et al 1999 Prevalence of patients facet joint pain in chronic low back pain. Pain Physician 2:59–64

Manchikanti L, Pampati V, Fellows B et al 2000a The inability of the clinical picture to characterize pain from facet joints. Pain Physician 3(2):158–166

Manchikanti L, Pampati V, Fellows B et al 2000b The diagnostic validity and therapeutic value of lumbar facet joint nerve blocks with or without adjuvent agents. Current Reviews in Pain 4(5):337–344

Manchikanti L, Pampati V, Fellows B et al 2001 Influence of psychological factors on the ability to diagnose chronic low back pain of facet joint origin. Pain Physician 4(4):349–357

McCombe PF, Fairbank JCT, Cockersole BC et al 1989 Reproducibility of physical signs in low back pain. Spine 14(9):908–918

McKenzie RA, May S 2003 Mechanical diagnosis and therapy: the lumbar spine, 2nd edn. Spinal Publication New Zealand Ltd, Waikanae, New Zealand

Meijne W, van Neerbos K, Aufdemkampe G, van der Wurff P 1999 Intraexaminer and interexaminer reliability of the Gillet test. Journal of Manipulative & Physiological Therapeutics 22(1):4–9

Merskey H, Bogduk N 1994 Classification of chronic pain: descriptions of chronic pain syndromes and definitions of pain terms, 2nd edn. IASP Press, Seattle

Mooney V, Robertson J 1976 The facet syndrome. Clinical Orthopedics & Related Research 115:149–156

Moran R, O'Connell D, Walsh MG 1988 The diagnostic value of facet joint injections. Spine 13(12):1407–1410

Nachemson AL, Jonsson E 2000 Neck and back pain – the scientific evidence of causes, diagnosis, and treatment. Lippincott Williams & Wilkins, Philadelphia, PA

Nachemson A, Vingård E 2000 Assessment of patients with neck and back pain: A best-evidence synthesis. In: Nachemson A, Jonsson E (eds) Neck and back pain: scientific evidence of causes, diagnosis and treatment. Lippincott Williams & Wilkins, Philadelphia, PA

Narozny M, Zanetti M, Boos N 2001 Therapeutic efficacy of selective nerve root blocks in the treatment of lumbar radicular leg pain. Swiss Medical Weekly 131(5–6): 75–80

O'Haire C, Gibbons P 2000 Inter-examiner and intra-examiner agreement for assessing sacroiliac anatomical landmarks using palpation and observation: pilot study. Manual Therapy 5(1):13–20

O'Neill CW, Kurgansky ME, Derby R, Ryan DP 2002 Disc stimulation and patterns of referred pain. Spine 27(24):2776–2781

Ohnmeiss DD 2002 Pain drawings in the evaluation of lumbar disc-related pain. Karolinska Institute, Sweden

Ohnmeiss DD, Vanharanta H, Ekholm J 1997 Degree of disc disruption and lower extremity pain. Spine 15(22):1600–1605

Olmarker K, Rydevik B, Nordborg C 1993 Autologous nucleus pulposus induces neurophysiologic and histologic changes in porcine cauda equina nerve roots. Spine 18(11):1425–1432

Östgaard HC, Zetherstrom G, Roos-Hansson E 1994a The posterior pelvic pain provocation test in pregnant women. European Spine Journal 153:1–3

Östgaard HC, Zetherstrom G, Roos-Hansson E et al 1994b Reduction of back and posterior pelvic pain in pregnancy. Spine 19(8):894–900

Petersen T, Olsen S, Laslett M et al 2004 Inter-tester reliability of a new diagnostic classification system for patients with non-specific low back pain. Australian Journal of Physiotherapy 50:85–91

Philip K, Lew P, Matyas TA 1989 The inter-therapist reliability of the slump test. Australian Journal of Physiotherapy 35(2):89–94

Porter RW 1996 Spinal stenosis and neurogenic claudication. Spine 21(17):2046–2052

Postacchini F 1999 Surgical management of lumbar spinal stenosis. Spine 24(10):1043–1047

Potter NA, Rothstein JM 1985 Intertester reliability for selected clinical tests of the sacroiliac joint. Physical Therapy 65(11):1671–1675

Radu AS, Menkes CJ 1998 Update on lumbar spinal stenosis. Retrospective study of 62 patients and review of the literature. Reviews in Rheumatology (English edn) 65(5):337–345

Revel M, Poiraudeau S, Auleley GR et al 1998 Capacity of the clinical picture to characterize low back pain relieved by facet joint anesthesia. Proposed criteria to identify patients with painful facet joints. Spine 23(18):1972–1977

Rydevik BL 2002 The effects of compression on the physiology of nerve roots. Journal of Manipulative & Physiological Therapeutics 15(1):62–66

Rydevik B, Brown MD, Lundborg G 1984 Pathoanatomy and pathophysiology of nerve root compression. Spine 9(1):7–15

Saal JS 2002 General principles of diagnostic testing as related to painful lumbar spine disorders: a critical appraisal of current diagnostic techniques. Spine 27(22):2538–2545

Sackett DL, Straus SE, Richardson WS et al 2000 Evidence-based medicine: how to practice and teach EBM. Churchill Livingstone, Edinburgh

Schwarzer AC, Aprill C, Derby R et al 1994a Clinical features of patients with pain stemming from the lumbar zygapophysial joints. Is the lumbar facet syndrome a clinical entity? Spine 19(10):1132–1137

Schwarzer AC, Aprill CN, Derby R 1994b The false-positive rate of uncontrolled diagnostic blocks of the lumbar zygapophysial joints. Pain 58(2):195–200

Schwarzer AC, Derby R, Aprill CN 1994c Pain from the lumbar zygapophysial joints: a test of two models. Journal of Spinal Disorders 7(4):331–336

Schwarzer AC, Aprill C, Bogduk N 1995a The sacroiliac joint in chronic low back pain. Spine 20(1):31–37

Schwarzer AC, Aprill C, Derby R et al 1995b The prevalence and clinical features of internal disc disruption in patients with chronic low back pain. Spine 20(17): 1878–1883

Schwarzer AC, Wang SC, Bogduk N et al 1995c Prevalence and clinical features of lumbar zygapophyseal joint pain: a study in an Australian population with chronic low back pain. Annals of Rheumatic Diseases 54(2):100–106

Sehgal N, Fortin JD 2000 Internal disc disruption and low back pain. Pain Physician 3(2):143–157

Simmons JW, Aprill CN, Dwyer AP et al 1988 A re-assessment of Holt's data on: 'The question of lumbar discography'. Clinical Orthopedics & Related Research 237(December):120–124

Slipman CW, Sterenfeld EB, Chou LH et al 1998 The predictive value of provocative sacroiliac joint stress maneuvers in the diagnosis of sacroiliac joint syndrome. Archives of Physical Medicine & Rehabilitation 79(3):288–292

Smith BM, Hurwitz EL, Solsberg D et al 1998 Interobserver reliability of detecting lumbar intervertebral disc high-intensity zone on magnetic resonance imaging and association of high-intensity zone with pain and anular disruption. Spine 23(19):2074–2080

Spangfort EV 1972 The lumbar disc herniation. A computer-aided analysis of 2,504 operations. Acta Orthopedica Scandinavica 142(suppl):1–95

Spitzer WO 1987 Scientific approach to the assessment and management of activity-related spinal disorders. A monograph for clinicians. Report of the Quebec Task Force on Spinal Disorders. Spine 12(7S)

Spivak JM 1998 Current concepts review: Degenerative lumbar spinal stenosis. Journal of Bone & Joint Surgery 80-A(7):1053–1066

Stitz MY, Sommer HM 1999 Accuracy of blind versus fluoroscopically guided caudal epidural injection. Spine 24(13):1371–1376

Strender L-E, Sjoblom A, Sundell K et al 1997 Interexaminer reliability in physical examination of patients with low back pain. Spine 22(7):814–820

Sturesson B 1999 Load and movement of the sacoiliac joint. Department of Orthopaedics, Lund University, Sweden

Sturesson B, Selvik G, Uden A 1989 Movements of the sacroiliac joints – a roentgen stereophotogrammetric analysis. Spine 14(2):162–165

van der Wurff P, Hagmeijer RH, Meyne W 2000a Clinical tests of the sacroiliac joint. A systemic methodological review. Part 1: reliability. Manual Therapy 5(1):30–36

van der Wurff P, Meyne W, Hagmeijer RHM 2000b Clinical tests of the sacroiliac joint: a systematic methodological review. Part 2: validity. Manual Therapy 5(2):89–96

van Tulder MW, Koes B, Bouter LM 1996 Low back pain in primary care: Effectiveness of diagnostic and therapeutic interventions. CIP-Gegevans Koninklijke Bibliotheek, Den Haag, the Netherlands

van Tulder MW, Koes BW, Assendelft WJJ, Bouter LM 1999 The effectiveness of conservative treatment of acute and chronic low back pain. CIP Gegevens Konoklijke Bibliotheek, Den Haag, the Netherlands

Vilensky JA, O'Connor BL, Fortin JD et al 2002 Histologic analysis of neural elements in the human sacroiliac joint. Spine 27(11):1202–1207

Vroomen PC, de Krom MC, Knottnerus JA 1999 Diagnostic value of history and physical examination in patients suspected of sciatica due to disc herniation: a systematic review. Journal of Neurology 246(10):899–906

Waddell G 1998 The back pain revolution. Churchill Livingstone, Edinburgh

Walsh TR, Weinstein JN, Spratt KF et al 1990 Lumbar discography in normal subjects. Journal of Bone & Joint Surgery (US) 72:1081–1088

Weinstein J, Claverie W, Gibson S 1988 The pain of discography. Spine 13(12):1344–1348

Werneke M, Hart DL 2001 Centralization phenomenon as a prognostic factor for chronic low back pain and disability. Spine 26(7):758–765

Werneke M, Hart DL 2003 Discriminant validity and relative precision for classifying patients with non-specific neck and low back pain by anatomic pain patterns. Spine 28(2):161–166

Werneke M, Hart DL, Cook D 1999 A descriptive study of the centralization phenomenon: A prospective analysis. Spine 24(7):676–683

Willard FH 1997 The muscular, ligamentous and neural structure of the low back and its relation to back pain. In: Vleeming A et al (eds) Movement, stability and low back pain: the essential role of the pelvis. Churchill Livingstone, Edinburgh

Yrjämä M, Vanharanta H 1994 Bony vibration stimulation: a new, non-invasive method for examining intradiscal pain. European Spine Journal 3:233–235

PART FOUR

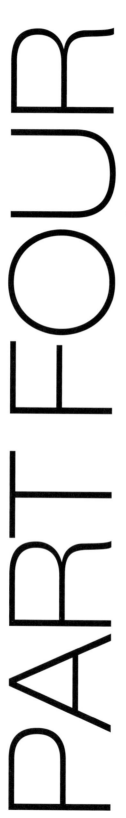

Guidelines

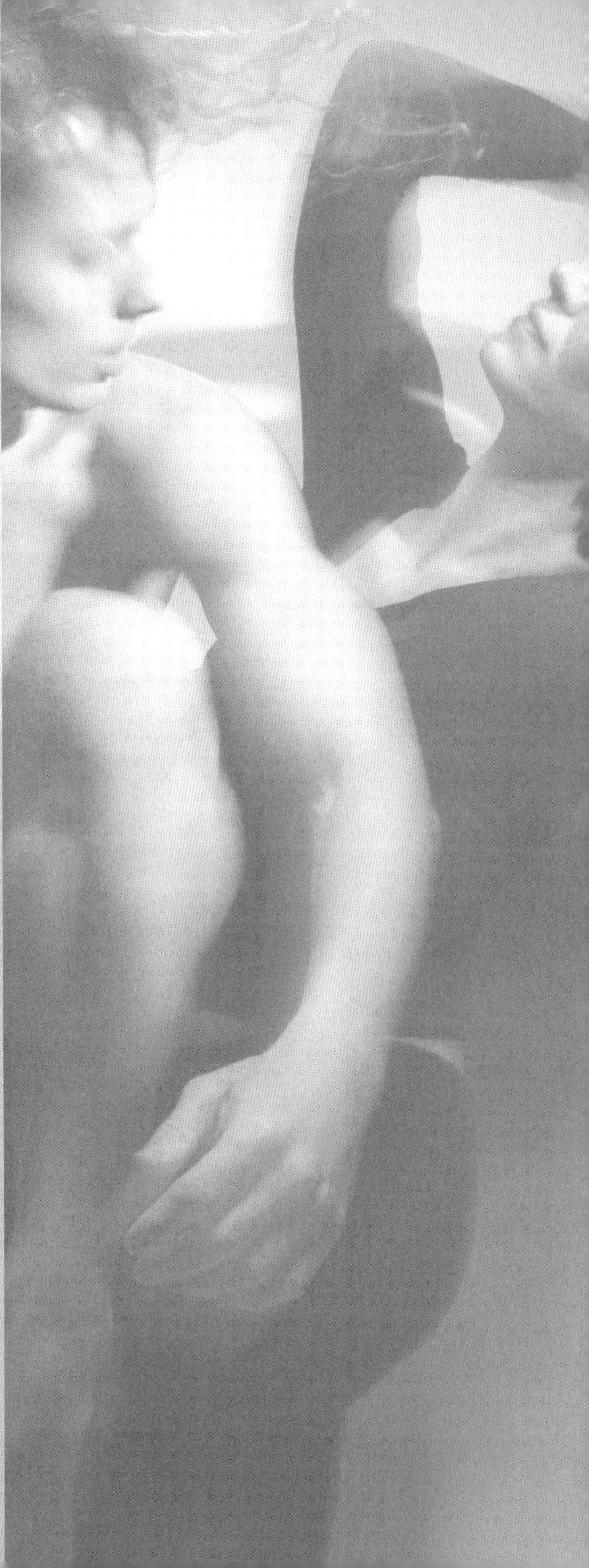

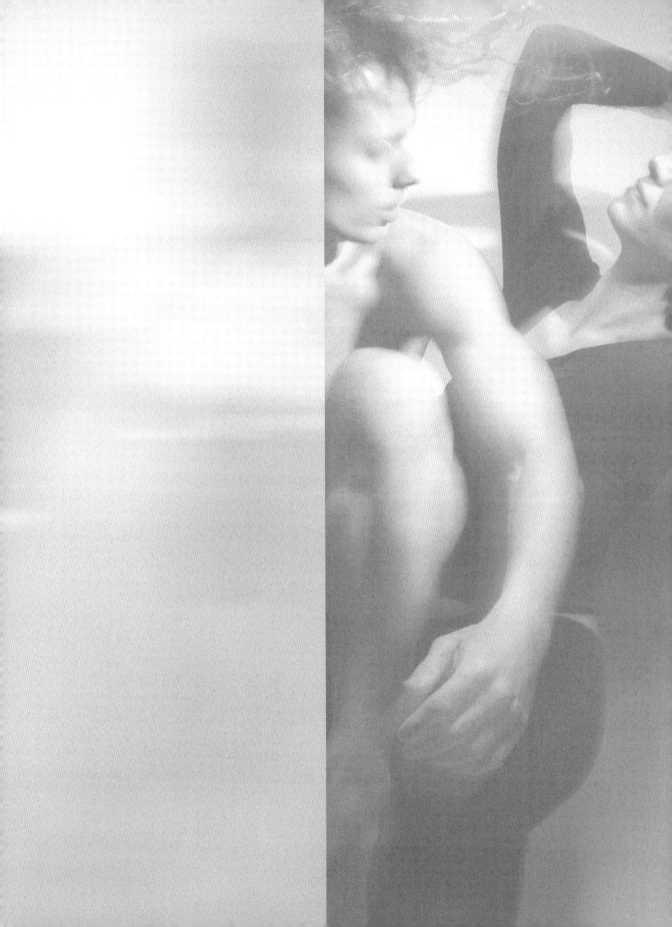

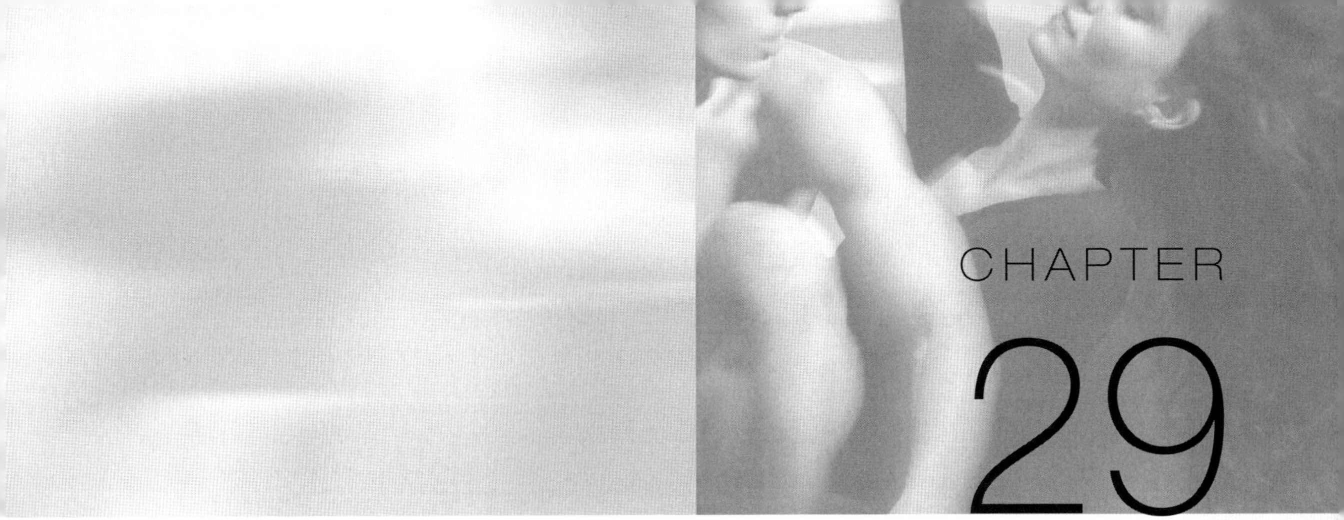

CHAPTER 29

European guidelines for prevention in low back pain

Gerd Müller on behalf of the COST B13 Working Group on European Guidelines for Prevention in Low Back Pain

Summary of the concepts of prevention in low back pain

- The general nature and course of commonly experienced low back pain (LBP) means that there is limited scope for preventing its incidence (first-time onset). Prevention, in the context of this guideline, is focused primarily on reduction of the impact and consequences of LBP.
- Primary causative mechanisms remain largely undetermined: risk factor modification will not necessarily achieve prevention.
- There is considerable scope, in principle, for prevention of the *consequences* of LBP, e.g. episodes (recurrence), care seeking, disability, and work loss.
- Different interventions and outcomes will be appropriate for different target populations (general population, workers, and children) yet inevitably there is overlap.
- Interventions that are essentially treatments in the clinical environment, focused on management of current symptoms, are not considered as 'prevention' for the purposes of this guideline: they are covered in the accompanying clinical guidelines.

Overarching comments

- Overall, there is limited robust evidence for numerous aspects of prevention in LBP.
- Nevertheless, there is evidence suggesting that prevention of various consequences of LBP is feasible.

- However, for those interventions where there is acceptable evidence, the effect sizes are rather modest.
- The most promising approaches seem to involve physical activity/exercise and appropriate (biopsychosocial) education, at least for adults.
- But no single intervention is likely to be effective to prevent the overall problem of LBP, owing to its multidimensional nature.
- Prevention in LBP is a societal as well as an individual concern.
- So, optimal progress on prevention in LBP will likely require a cultural shift in the way LBP is viewed, its relationship with activity and work, how it might best be tackled, and just what is reasonable to expect from preventive strategies.
- It is important to get all the players onside, but innovative studies are required to understand better the mechanisms and delivery of prevention in LBP.
- Anecdotally, individuals might report that various strategies work for them but in the absence of scientific evidence that does not mean they can be generally recommended for prevention; it is not known whether some of these strategies have disadvantageous long-term effects.
- Recommendations are based on systematic reviews, and scientific studies. The studies on which these recommendations are based were often variable and imprecise in specifying the interventions and outcomes investigated. Hence, it is not always possible to state exactly which outcomes will be influenced by a given intervention.

Summary of recommendations for the general population

- Physical exercise is recommended for prevention of sick leave due to LBP and for the occurrence or duration of further episodes (Level A). There is insufficient consistent evidence to recommend for or against any specific type or intensity of exercise (Level C).
- Information and education about back problems, if based on biopsychosocial principles, should be considered (Level C), but information and education focused principally on a biomedical or biomechanical model cannot be recommended (Level C).
- Back schools based on traditional biomedical/biomechanical information, advice and instruction are not recommended for prevention in LBP (Level A). High-intensity programs, which comprise both an educational/skills program and exercises, can be recommended for patients with recurrent and persistent back pain (Level B).
- Lumbar supports or back belts are not recommended (Level A).
- There is no robust evidence for or against recommending any specific chair or mattress for prevention in LBP (Level C), although persisting symptoms can be reduced with a medium-firm rather than a hard mattress (Level C).
- There is no evidence to support recommending manipulative treatment for prevention in LBP (Level D).
- Shoe insoles are not recommended in the prevention of back problems (Level A). There is insufficient evidence to recommend for or against correction of leg length (Level D).

Summary of recommendations for workers

- Physical exercise is recommended in the prevention of LBP (Level A), for prevention of recurrence of LBP (Level A) and for prevention of recurrence of sick leave due to LBP (Level C). There is insufficient evidence to recommend for or against any specific type or intensity of exercise (Level C).
- Back schools based on traditional biomedical/biomechanical information, advice and instruction are not recommended for prevention in LBP (Level A). There is insufficient evidence to recommend for or against psychosocial information delivered at the worksite (Level C), but information oriented toward promoting activity and improving coping may promote a positive shift in beliefs (Level C).
- Lumbar supports or back belts are not recommended (Level A).
- Shoe inserts/orthoses are not recommended (Level A). There is insufficient evidence to recommend for or against insoles, soft shoes, soft flooring or antifatigue mats (Level D).
- Temporary modified work and ergonomic workplace adaptations can be recommended to facilitate earlier return to work for workers sick listed due to LBP (Level B).
- There is insufficient consistent evidence to recommend physical ergonomics interventions alone for prevention in LBP (Level C). There is some evidence that, to be successful, a

physical ergonomics program would need an organizational dimension and involvement of the workers (Level B); there is insufficient evidence to specify precisely the useful content of such interventions (Level C).

- There is insufficient consistent evidence to recommend standalone work organizational interventions (Level C), yet such interventions could, in principle, enhance the effectiveness of physical ergonomics programs.
- Whereas multidimensional interventions at the workplace can be recommended (Level A), it is not possible to recommend which dimensions and in what balance.

Summary of recommendations for school age

- There is insufficient evidence to recommend for or against a generalized educational intervention for the prevention of LBP or its consequences in schoolchildren (Level C).
- Despite the intuitive appeal of the idea, there is no evidence that attempts to prevent LBP in schoolchildren will have any impact on LBP in adults (Level D).

Introduction

The high prevalence of LBP and the related costs to society have fostered many approaches to prevent this problem. Prevention in LBP is a societal as well as an individual concern. Prevention by the healthcare system would use some of the resources available at an early stage to reduce further consequences, e.g. loss of work or disability. For the individual, preventive measures might help to reduce the intensity or duration of pain episodes or its consequences.

In this guideline, recommendations concern common LBP, defined as pain and discomfort below the costal margin and above the inferior gluteal folds, with or without leg pain, and not attributed to recognizable, known specific pathology (e.g. infection, tumor, osteoporosis, ankylosing spondylitis). It covers both episodic and persistent symptoms: recurrent LBP is defined as a new episode after a symptom-free period, not an exacerbation of persistent LBP.

The distinction between acute LBP, usually defined as the duration of an episode persisting for less than 6 weeks, subacute LBP (between 6 and 12 weeks) and chronic LBP (12 weeks or more) is convenient for clinical purposes. It is less helpful when considering the matter of prevention, where back pain and its consequences tend to occur in an episodic manner (de Vet et al 2002).

The lifetime prevalence of LBP is reported as over 70% in industrialized countries (1-year prevalence 15% to 45%, adult incidence 5% per year). The prevalence rate during school age approaches that seen in adults (Taimela et al 1997, Watson et al 2002), increasing from childhood to adolescence (Balague et al 1999) and peaking between ages 35 and 55 (Andersson 1997). A role of genetic influence on liability to back pain is suggested from recent research (Hestbaek et al 2004, MacGregor et al 2004).

Acute LBP is usually considered to be self-limiting (recovery rate 90% within 6 weeks) but 2–7% of people develop chronic pain. Recurrent and chronic back pain is widely acknowledged to account for a substantial proportion of total workers' absenteeism. About half the days lost from work are accounted for by the 85% of people away from work for short periods (< 7 days), whereas the other half is accounted for by the 15% who are off work for > 1 month; this is reflected in the social costs of back pain, where some 80% of the healthcare and social costs are for the 10% with chronic pain and disability (Nachemson et al 2000).

These statistics, however, tend to be based on the clinically convenient classification of acute and chronic, which does not fully reflect the pattern of back pain among the population. Recent evidence shows that back pain manifests as an untidy pattern of symptomatic periods interspersed with less troublesome periods (Croft et al 1998, de Vet et al 2002, Hestbaek et al 2003a), although for some the symptoms (and associated disability) can become persistent. Around two-thirds of people are likely to experience relapses of pain over 12 months and around one-third are likely to have relapses of work absence (Hestbaek et al 2003b). These issues present interpretive difficulties when considering prevention, but are considered – so far as is practical – in the formulation of this guideline.

Importantly, for the scope of this guideline, back pain should be seen as an issue for all ages and all sectors of society: the prevalence in adolescents is similar to adults (Watson et al 2002), and the prevalence in workers generally does not dramatically differ from non-workers (Nachemson et al 2000). It is important to distinguish between the presence of symptoms, care seeking, work loss, and disability; these have different prevalence rates and are influenced by a varying balance of biological, psychological, and social factors (Burton 1997, Nachemson et al 2000). For instance, an episode of back pain can occur for no apparent reason or might result from some strenuous event (whether during work or leisure), whereas disability and sick leave are influenced largely by psychosocial factors (Waddell & Burton 2000).

The general nature and course of commonly experienced LBP means that there is limited scope for preventing its incidence (first-time onset). Therefore prevention, in the context of this guideline, is focused primarily on reduction of the impact and consequences of LBP. There is considerable scope, in principle, for prevention of the consequences of LBP, e.g. episodes (recurrence), care seeking, disability, and work loss. Different interventions and outcomes will be appropriate for different target populations (general population, workers, and children) yet inevitably there is overlap. Interventions that are essentially treatments in the clinical environment, focused on management of current symptoms, are not considered as 'prevention' for the purposes of this guideline: they are covered in the accompanying clinical guidelines.

The issue of risk factors for LBP is clearly highly relevant to the concept of prevention but the subject is poorly understood and inconsistently documented. The most powerful risk factor for a new episode of back pain is a previous history, where the 12-month risk is approximately doubled (Hestbaek et al 2003b). Beyond that, the most frequently reported risk factors are heavy physical work; frequent bending, twisting, lifting, pulling, and pushing; repetitive work; static postures; and vibrations (Andersson 1997). Psychosocial risk factors include stress, distress, anxiety, depression, cognitive functioning, pain behavior, job dissatisfaction, and mental stress at work (Andersson 1997, Hoogendoorn et al 2000, Linton 2000). However, there is limited evidence for these (purported) risk factors and those that are well documented frequently have small effect sizes, which – logically – will compromise the magnitude of preventive interventions. Alternatively, in some occupational groups more substantial effect sizes might be apparent in highly exposed groups. Some purported risk factors (e.g. smoking and obesity) can be more a matter of general health, yet might influence certain back pain outcomes. This guideline considers as wide a range of potential risk factors as is permitted by the available evidence on prevention. However, the risk for long-term incapacity, which is influenced by complex social factors (Waddell et al 2003), is generally beyond the scope of this guideline.

Objectives

The primary objective of the European Evidence-Based Guidelines is to provide a set of recommendations that can support existing and future national and international guidelines or future updates of existing back pain guidelines. This particular guideline intends to foster a realistic approach to improving prevention in respect of common (nonspecific) LBP in Europe by:

1. Providing recommendations on strategies to prevent LBP and/or its consequences in the general population, workers, and during school age.
2. Ensuring an evidence-based approach through the use of systematic reviews and existing evidence-based guidelines, supplemented (where necessary) by individual scientific studies.
3. Providing recommendations that are generally acceptable to a wide range of professions and agencies in all participating countries.
4. Enabling a multidisciplinary approach, stimulating collaboration between the various players potentially involved in prevention, thus promoting consistency across countries in Europe.
5. Identifying ineffective interventions to limit their use.
6. Pointing to areas where more research is needed.

The target population for this guideline on the prevention of LBP is individuals or groups that are going to develop new guidelines (national or local) or update existing guidelines, and the professional associations that will disseminate and implement these guidelines. Indirectly, these guidelines also aim to inform the general public, people with LBP, healthcare providers, health promotion agencies, industry/employers, educationalists, and policy makers in Europe.

When using this guideline as a basis, it is recommended that guideline development and implementation groups should undertake certain actions and procedures, not all of which could be accommodated under COST B13. These will include: taking patients' preferences into account; performing a pilot test among target users; undertaking external review, providing tools for application; consideration of organizational obstacles and cost implications; provision of criteria for monitoring and audit; provision of recommendations for implementation strategies (van Tulder et al 2004). In addition, in the absence of a review date for this guideline, it will be necessary to consider new scientific evidence as it becomes available.

Material and methods

The guideline on prevention in LBP was developed within the framework of the COST ACTION B13

'Low back pain: guidelines for its management', issued by the European Commission, Research Directorate-General, Department of Policy, Coordination and Strategy. The guidelines Working Group consisted of experts in the field of LBP research, four women and eight men with various professional backgrounds, representing nine countries. None of the 12 members believed they had any conflict of interest.

The working group for the prevention worked from May 2001 until December 2004, three subgroups were formed to accommodate the interventions and outcomes appropriate for prevention across the general population, workers, and during school age (the latter defined as < 18 years of age). The penultimate draft was sent for peer review to external experts, with the final draft being reviewed by the members of the Management Committee of COST B13. The full guidelines are available at: http://www.backpaineurope.org

Recommendations are based on systematic reviews, existing evidence-based guidelines, and scientific studies. The studies on which these recommendations are based were often variable and imprecise in specifying the interventions and outcomes investigated. Hence, it is not always possible to state exactly which outcomes will be influenced by a given intervention.

Evidence

The evidence underpinning the guideline recommendations was retrieved through systematic searches of the scientific literature up to the end of 2003; more recent studies were included until summer 2004, if available. Because of the nature of the subject matter, each subgroup (population, workers, and school age) formulated its own search criteria according to what was deemed appropriate, searching the major electronic databases (including the Cochrane Library), and then supplemented by citation tracking, personal databases, and expert knowledge. No language restrictions were imposed, but non-English articles were considered only if their language was covered by a member of the working group.

The working group determined that it was impossible to carry out a complete *de novo* systematic review of every aspect of prevention to an acceptable standard within an acceptable period of time. A strategy broadly conducive with the other guidelines in COST ACTION B13 was adopted: in the first instance, systematic reviews (and existing guidelines) were sought, supplemented by individual scientific studies where systematic reviews and evidence-based guidelines were not available. It was decided that evidence from narrative reviews should be excluded, unless they were a synthesis of multiple reviews. It was anticipated that the field of 'prevention' in LBP would have limited robust scientific evidence from randomized controlled trials (RCTs), which are not always appropriate or practicable in this area. Therefore the group decided that studies employing scientifically weaker designs (e.g. controlled trials, controlled before–after trials, and interrupted time series designs) should be included in the absence of RCTs. Longitudinal epidemiological studies were also included where the group felt these added useful information.

To reduce both individual and subgroup bias, the evidence was reviewed and discussed by the entire working group, as were the resultant recommendations. Sections were added to each subsection of the guidelines to reflect the discussion themes. The recommendations were considered separately for 'general population', 'workers', and 'school age'.

The strength of recommendations was based on the four-level rating system used for the other guidelines in the COST B13 program, but was slightly modified to take account of the nature of the available evidence:

- Level A: generally consistent findings provided by (a systematic review of) multiple RCTs.
- Level B: generally consistent findings provided by (a systematic review of) multiple weaker scientific studies.*
- Level C: one RCT/weaker scientific study, or inconsistent findings provided by (a systematic review of) multiple weaker scientific studies.*
- Level D: no RCTs or no weaker scientific studies.*

*The term 'weaker scientific studies' is taken to include non-randomized controlled trials, controlled before/after studies, interrupted time series designs, and longitudinal epidemiological studies. The 'level' is a grading of the strength of the evidence; it is an indicator of confidence in the recommendation, rather than its strength or effect size.

For this guideline, the review of the literature may best be summarized as systematic searching of the published scientific literature with mixed quantitative/qualitative evaluation of the evidence to produce best-synthesis recommendations.

Outcomes and interventions

The working group spent considerable time debating the focus of this guideline, and attempting to produce a working definition of 'prevention.'

The conceptual focus of the guideline was determined to be prevention of *future* aspects of LBP, as opposed to manifestations of the current spell. Taking account of the epidemiology of back pain, the working group concluded that prevention of the first onset of common LBP (especially in adults) is, to all intents and purposes, likely to be impracticable. Nevertheless, interventions directed at such were not excluded. The working group, in principle, recognized the distinction between 'primary' and 'secondary' prevention, but concluded [as have others (Jellema et al 2001)] that the distinction is difficult to determine in practice, and preferred not to use the terms.

Certain aspects of the back pain phenomenon are generally excluded from this guideline. Severe spinal injury and serious pathology are excluded by definition. In addition, prevention of structural changes such as 'degeneration,' along with risk factor modification, modification of psychosocial variables, and screening procedures (unless there is concomitant specific influence on back pain outcomes) are also excluded for adults. In recognition of widespread interest in back pain among schoolchildren, and the possibility of prevention of consequences later in life, the working group decided not to exclude general consideration of potentially modifiable risk factors for back pain in this population.

It is accepted that there is a vast number of 'interventions' that purportedly will 'prevent' (some aspect of) common LBP, but scientific evidence may be absolutely lacking. Not all possible interventions will be included in this guideline, largely because they are idiosyncratic, non-generalizable, or untested. That is not to say they cannot be shown effective at some future date.

Interventions directed at social change or altering the (sickness certification) behavior of clinicians were excluded. Provision of occupational health services was not considered to be a preventive intervention for the purposes of this guideline, and is the subject of other national guidelines (Staal et al 2003). However, the working group recognizes that occupational health has an important role in supporting and enhancing other interventions.

A broad categorization of included interventions would be: information/advice, activity/exercise, ergonomics, organizational change, furniture, clothing, and orthoses. Clearly, some interventions involve an active element, and some will concern avoidance, whereas others might involve less direct approaches, such as addressing inappropriate beliefs (Ihlebæk & Eriksen 2003) or interfacing with social reorganization (Scheel et al 2002). Specific interventions might not be universally applicable; rather they will be variously suited to the general population, workers, and school age. The working group recognized the potential for overlap with the accompanying clinical guidelines addressing acute and chronic back pain, and pelvic pain, and that these 'clinical' interventions might have a preventive effect on some outcomes. Furthermore, it was recognized that preventive interventions could not (and should not) exclude people with existing back symptoms. To accommodate these issues, it was decided that interventions that are essentially treatments focused on management of current symptoms in the clinical environment would not be considered as 'prevention' for the purposes of this guideline, unless the intervention has an explicit intent to prevent future consequences.

Judgment is necessary when using evidence statements to guide decision making, and it needs to be recognized that weak evidence statements on a particular relationship or effect do not necessarily mean that it is untrue or unimportant; it might simply reflect either insufficient evidence or the limitations of current scientific endeavor.

Of necessity, there will be some measure of overlap between interventions directed at the general population and workers. The same basic interventions might apply equally to both, but their nature and location of delivery will differ. It is possible that the evidence will overlap, and may not necessarily come to identical conclusions.

The working group recognizes that access to interventions, the ability to act on health advice, and the capacity to influence one's own health can be significantly influenced by socioeconomic variables, and it has been shown that clinical guidelines generally do not take the effects of socioeconomic position into account (Aldrich et al 2003); this is likely to be true also for other types of guideline. It is not the purpose of this guideline to address the socioeconomic position and its influences in respect of the recommendations given here. Yet the working group would urge target groups to take social inequalities into account when considering implementation and take steps to reach populations that are relatively disadvantaged, so as to avoid the risk of increasing health inequalities. Finally, the working group offers recommendations for future research that could improve our capacity for prevention in LBP.

Populations

The general population as a focus for prevention in back problems is the largest and most heterogeneous group. It includes different age groups, people with or without back pain, with or without specific spinal disorders, working and nonworking people and many other possible subgroups that might or might not be mutually exclusive. Information on preventing back pain in pregnancy was included.

In the workers' subgroup, employees with or without existing low back symptoms were targeted but interventions targeting workers consulting healthcare providers were excluded. Interventions to simply reduce return-to-work time were included only if there was follow-up focusing on the recurrence of LBP and/or consequences of LBP. The only exception to this rule was the intervention 'modified work', because this is not covered by the accompanying clinical guidelines.

Interventions aimed at preventing LBP in the workforce can be categorized into: (1) individual focus; (2) physical ergonomics; and (3) organizational ergonomics. All three categories were eligible, as long as they aimed to reduce LBP or its consequences among workers in the occupational setting. Numerous interventions include several additive dimensions, particularly for interventions described as 'physical ergonomics' – the following grouping was used: (1) physical ergonomic interventions (main component is a change focusing on biomechanical exposure at work); (2) organizational ergonomic interventions aiming at the work organization (alone or as the main dimension of the intervention); and (3) multidimensional interventions (interventions in which 'changing the physical and/or work organization' is present, but is not the main dimension). The included interventions are directed predominantly towards workers and their immediate environment.

Occupational health interventions concerning return to work were included when the intervention was the provision of 'modified work' for workers sick-listed due to LBP, and the intention was return to regular work. Non-healthcare interventions aiming at early return to work were also included if there was follow-up focusing on recurrence of (sick leave due to) LBP.

Workplace surveillance can be useful to identify factors associated with the risk of disability due to LBP (Ferguson & Marras 1997) but, because surveillance is not a preventive measure in itself, it was excluded. Similarly, medical assessment of 'fitness to work' was also excluded, although it is recognized that it could have a significant impact on lost work time.

Four types of factor are commonly found in the literature covering occupational epidemiology and ergonomics: (1) exposure to (purported) risk factors for LBP; (2) perceived exertion, discomfort or fatigue; (3) occurrence and/or recurrence of LBP; and (4) sick leave due to LBP. The evaluation of ergonomic interventions is often based on exposure to risk factors and on perceived exertion, discomfort, or fatigue – studies having these outcomes alone were excluded, but studies reporting on the occurrence and/or recurrence of (sick leave due to) LBP were included. Occasionally, the incidence rate of back injuries is used as an outcome measure, but it needs to be acknowledged that use of the concept of 'injury' is imprecise – the reporting of an injury can be driven more by legal and compensation requirements than objectively demonstrable injury. In view of the wide variety of outcome measures found in the literature (e.g. self-reported symptoms, sick leave, occupational back pain, low back injuries, compensable LBP), it was necessary to apply a 'consensus interpretation' when formulating recommendations.

Results

For the purpose of this chapter, the results of the two subgroups 'general population' and 'workers' are combined whenever possible. This section starts with the general results and recommendations applicable to both working and general populations, followed by the results that are specific to the workplace setting and finally the children's section.

Prevention in general population and workers

Physical exercise

There is evidence for positive effects of physical exercise to prevent (recurrent) episodes, the severity of episodes and sick leave due to LBP. In seven different reviews, RCTs on different types of physical exercise interventions have been evaluated (Gebhardt 1994, Lahad et al 1994, Linton & van Tulder 2001, Lühmann et al 2003, Tveito et al 2004, van Poppel et al 1997, Waddell & Burton 2001). All the authors' main conclusions were that physical exercise has a positive effect in the prevention of back pain, further episodes and work absence. Effect sizes were reported to be small to moderate. A recent meta-analysis (Kool et al 2004) demonstrated that the overall effect for studies with a follow-up period of 2 years or longer was positive. This indicates that recurrence of sick leave due to LBP can be reduced by physical exercise. There is no evidence that any particular type of exercise is superior to another.

Physical exercise is recommended to prevent work absenteeism due to back pain and the occurrence or duration of further back pain episodes (Level A). The effect size is moderate. There is insufficient evidence to recommend for or against any specific kind of exercise, or the frequency/ intensity of training (Level B). For pregnant women one systematic review (Young & Jewell 2003) concluded that water gymnastics has a preventive effect on future back pain.

Information and education

One systematic review (van Poppel et al 1997) found inconsistent results on the effect of information for prevention in back pain. More recently, a controlled trial of a public health multimedia campaign found improved beliefs about back pain, a reduction in days off work and reduced use of the healthcare system (Buchbinder et al 2001). One educational program (Versloot et al 1992), which has been included in several reviews, was not focused primarily on body mechanics, but on stress and coping strategies. This study showed a reduction in the duration of absenteeism among workers with prolonged absence compared to a control group. This is similar to the finding of Symonds et al (1995), who compared a traditional 'good posture' pamphlet to a psychosocial pamphlet focused on fear avoidance beliefs among workers. The latter pamphlet reduced the number of days of future work loss and the number of spells with extended absence (Symonds et al 1995). Linton & Ryberg (2001) investigated the effect of six-session cognitive behavioral group intervention in acute or subacute back patients, comparing it with usual care. The risk for long-term sick leave was significantly reduced in the intervention group.

The preventive effect of information alone might be weak. The effect size is likely to vary in combination with other interventions, such as physical exercise or treatment (the combination of physical exercise and information is discussed below in the back school section). Information might have a higher impact in a treatment setting, when people/patients are actually affected by a specific problem; they might be more susceptible to this information compared to a preventive setting, when the information is less relevant at the given time. This aspect is supported by the fact that information and education is an inherent and possibly important aspect of multidisciplinary programs.

A narrative review by Burton & Waddell (2002) made an attempt to distinguish studies by the content of the information being transmitted. They concluded that traditional approaches based on a biomedical model can convey negative messages about back pain with damaging effects on patients' beliefs and behaviors. By contrast, carefully selected and presented information based on a biopsychosocial model can have a positive effect. They estimated the power of written information to be relatively weak, nevertheless it might be cost-effective due to its low per-person costs. Recent studies (Buchbinder et al 2001, Burton et al 1999) variously reported positive results for beliefs, future disability, future work loss, and use of health care, but older studies reported inconsistent results. Those recent studies are strongly based on the fear avoidance concept, which fits the biopsychosocial model, whereas many of the older studies contain a mixture of biomechanical and psychosocial information. A problem occurs in pooling or judging these studies because the 'active ingredients' and the mixture of the messages vary considerably between the different studies. In conclusion, there is evidence from the more recent studies that information based on the biopsychosocial model, focusing particularly on beliefs, is potentially beneficial for reducing work loss, further spells of LBP and the utilization of health care. However, it is appreciated that this evidence is somewhat limited. By contrast, providing information based on a biomedical model or biomechanics principles has not been shown to have a positive effect for prevention in back pain.

As a conclusion, traditional information/advice/ instruction on biomechanics, lifting techniques, optimal postures, etc. is not recommended for prevention in LBP (Level A). Information and education about back pain, if based on biopsycho-social principles, should be considered for the general population; it improves back beliefs, and can have a positive influence on health and vocational outcomes, though the effect size may be relatively small (Level C).

Back schools and training

Two systematic reviews (Heymans et al 2004, Linton & van Tulder 2001) and one review that included systematic reviews and RCTs (Lühmann et al 1999) came to different conclusions on the effect of back schools. Linton et al and Lühmann focused on interventions based on the Swedish back school with emphasis on proper lifting techniques. Both reviews concluded that there is no positive effect on back pain or further work loss.

The recent Cochrane review (Heymans et al 2004) included 19 RCTs. Back school in this review was defined as a group intervention, conducted or supervised by a paramedical therapist or a medical specialist, which consisted of both an education/skills program and exercises. The review did not distinguish between preventive and therapeutic interventions; most studies were designed as therapeutic studies. The authors concluded that there was: (1) conflicting evidence on the effectiveness of back schools, compared with other treatments for acute or subacute pain, on further work loss; and (2) limited evidence that back schools show no differences in long-term recurrence rates of LBP episodes. The same evidence level was found when back schools were compared to placebo treatment or waiting list controls. The authors concluded that back schools might be effective for patients with recurrent and chronic pain, with the most promising interventions being those with a high intensity (3–5-week stay in specialized centers). The effect sizes of these interventions were judged small.

The conclusion that there is no positive effect of back schools (Linton & van Tulder 2001, Lühmann et al 2003) is different from the most recent review (Heymans et al 2004), reflecting different approaches and search strategies (more studies were included in the latter). The systematic review by Linton & van Tulder (2001) covers two RCTs (Daltroy et al 1997, Donchin et al 1990). The comprehensive study by Daltroy et al (1997) on 2543 postal workers investigated the effect of proper lifting techniques. The study group that was educated in the 'proper' lifting techniques according to the Swedish back school had no reduction in further episodes of back pain or days off work.

The most recent systematic review included 19 RCTs (Heymans et al 2004). Back school in this review was defined as a group intervention, conducted or supervised by a paramedical therapist or a medical specialist, and comprising an education and skills program including exercises. There was considerable variation between the RCTs with respect to several criteria: duration and content of program (minimum 3 × 45 minutes, maximum 3-week inpatient setting), duration of symptoms (acute, subacute, chronic patients), pain distribution (with or without pain radiation, or not described), control intervention (waiting list, placebo treatment, exercises, advice, spinal manipulation), demographics (age, gender).

The authors rated the methodological quality high in four studies and low in 15 studies. One aspect of the low quality of the studies was the poor description of the exact content of the interventions. In addition to the intensity of the program, this refers to the ratio between passive, educational elements and the active 'training' parts, as well as to the exact content and wording during the educational sessions. The latter is more difficult to describe and control compared to written information. However, the outcome might be highly influenced by the specific content of the education, in particular whether a biopsychosocial or a biomedical/biomechanical approach was emphasized. Seemingly, most studies used a combination of both, which makes it difficult to study subgroups with respect to the approach being used. A cost-effectiveness analysis was not possible.

In addition to the limitations of heterogeneity of the study populations, the low methodological quality of most of the studies and the inclusion of acute and chronic patients in all studies, it is uncertain if the findings from patients can be transferred to a general population setting. The conclusion of the authors (Heymans et al 2004) with respect to the effectiveness of very intensive (3–5 weeks) programs brings up a problem of definitions for 'back school' and 'multidisciplinary programs'.

In conclusion, back schools based on a biomechanical approach with emphasis on teaching lifting techniques are not recommended (Level A). High-intensity back schools, which comprise both an educational/skills program and exercises, can be recommended for patients with recurrent and persistent pain (Level B). The effect sizes of these interventions might be relatively small.

Mattresses and chairs

Several studies on the use of mattresses were found, but no systematic reviews. The design of the studies, their methodological quality and the results do not allow any conclusions with respect to prevention in back pain, though one good-quality RCT suggests that people with back problems might experience less pain with a medium-firm rather than a hard mattress (Kovacs et al 2003a). There is insufficient robust evidence to recommend for or against any specific mattresses for prevention in back pain (Level C), though existing persistent symptoms might reduce with a medium-firm rather than a hard mattress (Level C).

No acceptable evidence for any preventive aspects of chairs was found. The few studies retrieved had inappropriate methodology. There is insufficient evidence to recommend for or against any specific chairs for prevention in LBP (Level D).

Shoe insoles and correction of leg length discrepancies

No systematic reviews on the use of shoe insoles, shock-absorbing heel inserts, or orthoses for the prevention of back pain were found. Seven clinical trials with an intervention aiming at reducing back pain used different insoles: only two of those, the smallest studies with numerous methodological weaknesses, reported a beneficial effect from orthoses (Fauno et al 1993, Tooms et al 1987). A good-quality RCT among military conscripts, in which custom-made, semi-rigid biomechanical shoe orthoses were provided (no intervention in the control group) showed a statistically significant difference between the intervention and control group for 3-month prevalence of 'back or lower extremity problems' (Larsen et al 2002). However, a further look into the results of this RCT revealed that this was due to differences in the prevalence of shin splints and, to a lesser extent, Achilles tendonitis. For 'back problems' there was no difference at all between groups.

Two narrative reviews reported on correction of leg length inequality as a possible preventive measured for back pain (Brady et al 2003, Gurney & Pye 2002). They found 12 articles that investigated the link between limb length inequality and LBP, but any association was not supported unequivocally; the only association found was when the discrepancy was over 10 mm. All the intervention studies (none of which were RCTs or CTs) included in one of the reviews concerned patients with persistent LBP; the authors concluded that there are 'limited data to support lift therapy for *treatment* of LBP' (Brady et al 2003). Based on the above data there is no acceptable evidence for interventions aimed at correction of leg length discrepancy for prevention in LBP.

Back belts and lumbar supports

There is evidence of no effect from the use of back belts/lumbar supports in the prevention of LBP. In seven reviews, RCTs on the use of back belts have been evaluated. The reviews are essentially based on many of the same studies. The most recent reviews report the strongest evidence that lumbar supports are not effective for prevention in LBP. Most of the reviews concluded that there was strong evidence of no effect of back belts for prevention in LBP (Linton & van Tulder 2001, Maher 2000, Waddell & Burton 2001).

Back belts, supports and braces cover a variety of devices used by workers. They are often used in combination with other interventions, and it is then difficult to determine if a possible benefit may be due to back support or an educational component of an intervention. Additionally, compliance with wearing lumbar support varies substantially.

Back belts/lumbar supports are not recommended for prevention in LBP (Level A).

Workplace-specific interventions

Physical ergonomics

There is evidence from two systematic reviews. Westgaard & Winkel (1997) found a general lack of success from mechanical exposure interventions, whereas Linton & van Tulder (2001) offered a negative conclusion about the role of ergonomic interventions. Three subsequent good-quality studies (Brisson et al 1999, Evanoff et al 1999, Yassi et al 2001) reported that physical ergonomics interventions might reduce the prevalence and severity of LBP. The only RCT (Yassi et al 2001) did not find lower injury rates in the intervention groups. Two other recent good-quality studies did not report an improvement following changes intended to reduce exposure to physical risk factors (Fredriksson et al 2001, Smedley et al 2003). Physical ergonomic interventions that include an organizational dimension, actively involving the workers and leading to substantial changes in exposure to the risk factors, might (in principle) be the most effective. However, there is limited supportive evidence from one systematic review (Westgaard & Winkel 1997). In respect of reducing (reported) back injuries – occupational or compensable LBP in particular – there are several studies reporting physical ergonomics interventions to be successful, although only one (Evanoff et al 1999) was of high quality.

Two conditions for a successful intervention (organizational dimension and involvement of the workers) are stressed in the conclusion of the review by Westgaard & Winkel (1997), which deals with 'musculoskeletal health' in general. These two conditions are also explicitly present in two successful interventions (Brisson et al 1999, Evanoff et al 1999). The third condition, i.e. the need to substantially change the exposure to the purported risk factors, is discussed in two good-quality negative studies (Fredriksson et al 2001, Smedley et al 2003). Smedley et al (2003) considered that the improvement in exposure to physical risk factors measured in the study was too small for any reduction in back pain to be expected. In the other negative study (Fredriksson et al 2001), the workers stated that their level of physical exertion was higher after the implementation of the ergonomic changes. The opportunity to influence the work had also decreased. The authors concluded that it is important to pay attention to the psychological dimension of the intervention (Fredriksson et al 2001). One study found that the positive effects of the interventions occurred only for workers less than 40 years of age (Brisson et al 1999). Thus, it might be that ergonomic preventive interventions are less relevant for some subgroups of workers (e.g. the older ones or those with severe back disorders).

The magnitude of the effect differed between studies. It should be noted that the magnitude of a change is sensitive to the measure (relative or absolute decrease). Furthermore, work places exist where a majority of workers will develop LBP regardless of whether physical ergonomic interventions are implemented or not, hence the success of such interventions may depend on the mechanical exposure at work (Westgaard & Winkel 1997). For frequently occurring conditions such as LBP it is unrealistic to expect to reduce the prevalence to zero. For example, in one study the prevalence decreased from 73% to 56% in the intervention group, which appears substantial. However, the prevalence remained high at 15 months follow-up (Evanoff et al 1999).

Several additional remarks can be made about these outcomes: the rate of events such as compensable LBP is often low, leading to a lack of statistical power in the studies. The report of such events is strongly sensitive to organizational and administrative factors. One consequence of an intervention might be to actually increase the awareness of low back problems, including administrative notifications. This might be a problem for studies on LBP in general (Smedley et al 2003). Finally, LBP has not been the only (or necessarily the major) condition evaluated in numerous studies of physical ergonomics; whether LBP and other musculoskeletal disorders are equivalent in this respect remains to be determined.

There is insufficient consistent evidence to recommend physical ergonomics interventions alone for reduction of the prevalence and severity of LBP (Level C). There is insufficient consistent evidence to recommend physical ergonomics interventions alone for reduction of (reported) back injuries, occupational or compensable LBP (Level C). There is some evidence that, to be successful, a physical ergonomics program would need an organizational dimension and involvement of the workers (Level B). There is insufficient evidence to specify precisely the useful content of such interventions (Level C), and the size of any effect may be modest.

Organizational ergonomics

There is inconsistent evidence that work organization interventions are successful for reduction of LBP. This type of intervention is not studied separately in systematic reviews. One study (Charney 1997), reports positive results of an intervention dealing with work organization: the implementation of lift teams in ten hospitals in order to reduce lifts by nurses. However, the methodological quality of the Charney study is low (group size unknown). The effect of a reduction of daily working hours was studied in one intervention. The prevalence of LBP did not change significantly between the intervention and reference groups (Wergeland et al 2003).

However, previous comments dealing with physical ergonomics interventions stress that not taking into account the organizational aspects may have negative effects, and epidemiological studies indicate that work organizational factors (especially psychosocial factors) are associated with various dimensions of LBP. There is insufficient consistent evidence to recommend standalone work organizational interventions alone for prevention in LBP (Level C), yet such interventions could, in principle, enhance the effectiveness of physical ergonomics programs.

Multidimensional interventions

There is evidence from two systematic reviews (Gatty et al 2003, Tveito et al 2004) that multidimensional interventions (some of which included an ergonomics component) have a positive effect for prevention in LBP. Tveito et al concluded that comprehensive multidisciplinary and multimodal treatment interventions can have a positive effect for some, but not all, LBP outcomes (Tveito et al 2004).

One high-quality systematic review (Gatty et al 2003) included five studies classified as 'education and task modification.' Despite the mixed results of the studies, the authors of the review suggested that programs including education and task modification, addressing the specific problems identified in the workplace, involving the staff and the workers, can have positive results.

The review by Tveito et al (2004) described four multidisciplinary and multimodal treatment programs, and found moderate to limited evidence that these programs can have an effect on some outcomes (e.g. sick leave, recurrence, pain, costs), yet each program might influence only some of the outcomes.

Although multidimensional interventions at the workplace might be recommended to reduce some aspects of LBP, it is not possible to recommend which dimensions and in what balance (Level A). The size of any effect might be modest.

Modified work for return to work after sick leave

There is moderate evidence of positive effects of modified work to promote return to work after sick leave from regular work due to LBP. Studies on the effects on return to work of modified work have been evaluated in three reviews (Krause et al 1998, van der Beek et al 2000, van der Beek 2004). However, they included studies covering all workers with disabling injuries and workers with musculoskeletal disorders (not only LBP). Positive results (shorter return-to-work time) were found in one RCT (Loisel et al 1997), one controlled before–after study (Yassi et al 1995), and one prospective cohort study using interrupted time series (Anema et al 2004).

Modified work is often part of a multidimensional intervention, so that the separate effects of modified work and the other parts of the intervention cannot be disentangled (Yassi et al 1995). Also, quite a few interventions can be regarded as 'modified work', but there is substantial variation as to the content of these interventions. The three predominant categories are: (1) light duty or work restriction or adapted job tasks; (2) reduction in the working hours per day and/or working days per week; and (3) ergonomic changes to the workplace. Depending on the social system in different countries, modified work can also involve 'therapeutic return to work' or 'work trial.' It is difficult to separate what could be effective in these different scenarios. Hence, there is no evidence that any type of modified work is superior to another but, based on the studies of Loisel et al (1997) and Anema et al (2004), it can be concluded that there is evidence to support ergonomic workplace adaptations in respect of facilitating return to work. Moreover, there is an indication that this is not just an 'attention effect'; it has been reported that a physiotherapist worksite visit, including information and advice but without actual workplace adaptation, did not add any further value to the effects of a back-to-school-type of mini-intervention during which exercises and advice on work activities were given (Karjalainen et al 2004). There is general agreement among occupational health guidelines that modified work should be a temporary measure, and that there is no need for the worker to be pain free before returning to work (Staal et al 2003); modified work can be seen as a component of a wider range of rehabilitation strategies (Waddell & Burton 2004). It must be acknowledged that there are a number of problems with implementing modified work concerning knowledge, understanding, availability of alternative duties, and resistance from coworkers (van Duijn et al 2004), and procedures are needed to ensure restricted duties are appropriately lifted rather than being allowed to become permanent (Hiebert et al 2003).

Irrespective of the evidence on physical and organizational ergonomics to specifically influence outcomes, the working group endorses the pragmatic view that 'Work should be comfortable when we are well, and accommodating when we are ill' (Hadler 1997), and recognizes that ergonomics has a role in formulating modified work to facilitate early return to work (Waddell & Burton 2004). Temporary modified work (which might include ergonomic workplace adaptations) can be recommended, when needed, to facilitate earlier return to work for workers sick-listed due to LBP (Level B).

Prevention in school age

Several recent studies demonstrated that non-specific LBP in schoolchildren is much more frequent than previously thought. In addition, there is some evidence that back pain at young age has a predictive value on LBP as an adult (Harreby et al 1995). Despite the number of epidemiological studies of back pain at young age, studies evaluating the effects of interventions to prevent LBP or the consequences of LBP in schoolchildren are still sparse. As a result, the aim to formulate evidence-based guidelines for prevention in LBP among schoolchildren could not be accomplished. Yet evaluating modifiable (purported) risk factors for back pain and its consequences in schoolchildren is relevant to the development of preventive interventions, so these are incorporated below.

Intervention studies

In schoolchildren, only five school-based intervention studies that included the evaluation of back pain or the consequences of back pain could be located. All five studies evaluated intervention programs comprising a variable number of hours of education in back care principles (Balagué et al 1996, Cardon et al 2002, Feingold & Jacobs 2002, Mendez & Gomez-Conesa 2001, Storr-Paulsen

2002). The results of these intervention studies are promising but differences between the interventions and the limitations of the studies do not permit recommendation of backcare education for prevention of LBP in schoolchildren. There is insufficient evidence to recommend for or against a generalized educational intervention for the prevention of LBP or its consequences in schoolchildren (Level C).

Modifiable risk factors

The following, potentially modifiable, risk factors were located in the literature search: lifestyle factors (overweight/obesity, smoking, alcohol intake, eating habits, working, sports participation, physical inactivity and sedentary activities), physical factors (physical fitness, mobility and flexibility, muscular strength), school-related factors (school bags and school furniture) and psychosocial factors.

The carefully designed, prospective, population-based cohort study by Jones et al (2003) on the association between LBP and body mass index (BMI) reports that neither BMI nor its change over the follow-up year was associated with an increase in the risk of future LBP. There is no evidence for or against recommending weight control as a preventive action for LBP in schoolchildren. There is insufficient evidence to recommend for or against modification of eating habits or the modification of alcohol intake as a preventive measure for LBP in schoolchildren.

The 'association' between back pain and smoking among schoolchildren has been shown in four studies (Feldman et al 1999, Harreby et al 1999, Kristjansdottir & Rhee 2002, Lebkowski 1997). In contrast to these findings, Kovacs et al (2003b) found no association between LBP and cigarette smoking. According to Harreby et al (1999), smoking habits in schoolchildren might indirectly reflect psychosocial and social problems as the main causes in developing LBP. It can be concluded that there is no evidence that antismoking campaigns will have a preventive effect in LBP in schoolchildren.

In addition to three studies pointing out the risk for LBP in young athletes (Hutchinson 1999, McMeeken et al 2001, Ogon et al 2001), several studies evaluated the risk of physical activity and sports in nonathlete populations and found a gender-specific positive link between sports participation and back pain (Burton et al 1996, Harreby et al 1999, Korovessis et al 2004, Kovacs et al 2003b). According to the findings from five studies, the total amount of physical activity was not associated with back pain reports in schoolchildren (Cardon et al 2004, Feldman 2001, Iyer 2001, Watson et al 2003, Widhe 2001). In children and adolescents there are indications that high performance training in certain sports can increase the risk for back pain, whereas the relationship between leisure time physical activity and back pain suffers from inconsistencies. There is no evidence that performing sports or being physically active has a preventive effect on LBP in schoolchildren. There is also insufficient evidence to recommend a general limitation of involvement in competitive sports participation as a preventive measure for LBP in schoolchildren.

According to a recent study there is no correlation between back pain and fitness parameters in 9- to 11-year-old children (Cardon et al 2004). However, two earlier studies reported that poor self-reported physical fitness increased the risk for back pain in schoolchildren (Kristjansdottir & Rhee 2002, Sjolie 2002). Findings in the literature on the relationship between LBP and mobility and flexibility in schoolchildren are conflicting. In line with the review of Balagué et al it can be concluded that LBP in schoolchildren cannot simply be attributed to muscle weakness (Balagué et al 1999).

Sheir-Neiss et al (2003) reported that adolescents with back pain reported significantly more hours watching TV than those without back pain, and Grimmer and Williams (2000) found gender- and age-specific associations between the amount of time spent sitting and recent LBP. However, in two other studies the association between LBP and hours of leisure sitting was not significant (Kovacs et al 2003b, Watson et al 2003). From the present review it can be concluded that the association between LBP and sitting in schoolchildren remains unclear. Furthermore, a study evaluating whether the loading on young growing body structures, associated with poor prolonged sitting postures or sedentary behavior, has an impact later in life could not be located. There is insufficient evidence to recommend for or against modified sitting postures as a preventive action for LBP in schoolchildren.

Working increased the risk of suffering LBP in school-aged children (Feldman et al 2002). Similarly, Harreby et al (1999) found a positive association between LBP and jobs involving a heavy load on the lower back. Also, in the cross-sectional survey-based study of Watson et al (2003), children with a part-time job had a 60% increase in odds of reporting LBP, although among those with a part-time job there was no association with reporting lifting heavy items. Also, in the recent prospective study by Jones et al (2003), having a part-time job significantly increased the risk for LBP. It can be concluded that working is associated with reported LBP in European schoolchildren. However, there is no evidence that modification of working has a preventive effect on LBP in schoolchildren. Furthermore, study findings were not controlled for social class. There is insufficient evidence to recommend modification of working as a preventive measure for LBP in schoolchildren.

Various studies (Goodgold et al 2002, Grimmer & Williams 2000, Watson et al 2003) have reported no associations between backpack-related factors and back pain at a young age. Other studies, though, have described an association between backpack load and LBP (Negrini & Carabalona 2002, Siambanes et al 2004, Szpalski et al 2002). According to Negrini & Carabolona, other factors, such as fatigue and time spent carrying, might be directly related to back pain, in addition to the weight of the backpack. In line with the recent review by Mackenzie et al (2003), conflicting study results are found for the association between backpack-related factors and LBP in schoolchildren. A major problem is that, at best, many studies looked only once at the actual weight of back packs, yet large variations between the days of the week within the same class of the same school have been found (Negrini & Carabalona 2002). There is no consistent scientific evidence for or against recommending a clear limit to the weight of school bags (or for avoiding use of schoolbags), changing the type of school bag or the method of carrying the school bag as primary measures for reducing LBP in schoolchildren.

Studying school furniture, Milanese & Grimmer (2004), in a cross-sectional study, reported on 1269 schoolchildren aged 8–12 years from Australia. The smallest students showed the best fit with school furniture, whereas the tallest ones (fourth quartile) showed higher odds of reporting LBP. There have been attempts to prevent LBP by modifications of school furniture (Hopf et al 1996, Knusel & Jelk 1994, Linton 1994), and from a physiological point of view the need for adjustable and dynamic furniture seems reasonable to prevent present and future LBP. Whereas three studies (Denis et al 2003, Panagiotopoulou et al 2004, Parcells et al 1999) indicated a mismatch between students' bodily dimensions and classroom furniture, a possible association with LBP was not evaluated. The possible protective role of adjusted school furniture remains unclear. The association reported by Milanese & Grimmer (2004) is not confirmation that an intervention on school furniture would be appropriate to prevent LBP, as age cannot be excluded as a confounding variable.

According to a study by Balagué et al (1995), psychological factors that were labeled 'positive' were associated with a reduction of lumbar pain whereas those factors considered 'negative' were accompanied by an increase of this sort of pain. Moreover, in a recent study (Watson et al 2003) it was suggested that psychosocial factors are more important than mechanical factors for LBP occurring in young populations. In line with these findings, numerous recent studies in schoolchildren reported an association between back pain and psychological factors, such as morning tiredness and parental support (Kristjansdottir & Rhee 2002), poor well-being and, in particular, poor self-perceived fitness (Sjolie 2002), a higher degree of somatizing, diminished self-esteem, and augmented negative affect (Staes et al 2003), disliking going to school (Storr-Paulsen 2002), psychosomatic factors (van Gent et al 2003), life quality (Harreby et al 1999), and poor mental health (Feldman 2001). Furthermore, according to the prospective study of Jones et al (2003), high levels of adverse psychosocial exposure; the presence of conduct problems, such as anger, disobedience and violence; and high levels of hyperactivity were associated with an increased risk of developing LBP in adolescents.

Because back pain reports in schoolchildren are mainly associated with psychosocial factors, and because it is shown in the literature that LBP in the young is mostly benign and self-limiting (Burton et al 1996, Salminen et al 1999), it can be argued that there is limited scope for generalized prevention of LBP in schoolchildren and that medicalizing the symptoms in schoolchildren needs to be avoided (Balagué et al 2003, Burton 1996, Burton et al 1996). Furthermore, an aggregation of symptoms retrieved by questioning children can be misleading, and the definition of boundaries between pain as an experience, as opposed to pain as a sign of 'a medically significant' disease, is sometimes difficult. Children are in a general learning process, including expression of pain in an adequate and acceptable fashion, both socially and culturally. Therefore, it might be time to look at what pain, aches, disability and 'disease' mean to schoolchildren themselves, and not to simply apply adult definitions to assess children and LBP (Balagué et al 2003).

Summary

It is recommended that the following approaches are considered for further research into prevention in LBP. Future studies need to be of high quality; where possible they should be in the form of randomized controlled trials. It is also recommended that standards of evidence criteria for efficacy, effectiveness and dissemination should be taken into account (Society for Prevention Research 2004).

As a general recommendation, it is considered important that future studies include cost–benefit and risk–benefit analyses.

- Good-quality RCTs are needed to study the effectiveness of daily physical activity for prevention of LBP and for prevention of recurrence of LBP. In addition, the effectiveness of physical exercise as well as daily physical activity should be studied for prevention of (recurrence of) sick leave due to LBP.
- It is recommended that good-quality RCTs are performed on the role of information oriented toward reducing fear avoidance beliefs and improving coping strategies in the prevention of LBP.
- Good-quality RCTs are needed to determine the effectiveness of specific interventions aimed at specific risk/target groups and how and by whom these interventions are best delivered.
- Misconceptions about back pain are shown to be widespread in adults, and they play a role in the development of long-term disability (Goubert et al 2004). Further study is necessary to explore whether these misconceptions may be prevented by carefully selected and presented health promotion programs, with the merit of demedicalizing LBP.
- Good-quality RCTs are urgently needed to study the effectiveness of physical, psychosocial, and organizational ergonomic interventions on a large variety of outcomes, ranging from prevention of (recurrence of) LBP and prevention of (recurrence of) sick leave due to LBP up to compensable LBP.
- RCTs evaluating the possible positive effects of preventive programs and risk factor modifications at young age on adult LBP are advocated.
- From a physiological point of view, poor lifestyle habits and prolonged static sitting during school age on unadjusted furniture may play a role in the origin of LBP. Further study is appropriate to determine any effectiveness of school-based interventions (exercise/sport, desks/seating, backpacks/bags).
- Further study with a follow-up into adulthood is needed to evaluate whether or not the physical cumulative load experience on the lumbar spine (e.g. from heavy book-bag carrying or sitting on unadjusted furniture) during childhood and adolescence contributes to adult LBP.

References

Aldrich R, Kemp L, Williams JS et al 2003 Using socio-economic evidence in clinical practice guidelines. BMJ 327:1283–1285

Andersson GBJ 1997 The epidemiology of spinal disorders. In: (Frymoyer JW ed) The adult spine: principles and practice, p 93–141. Lippincott-Raven, Philadelphia

Anema JR, Cuelenaere B, van der Beek AJ et al 2004 The effectiveness of ergonomic interventions on return-to-work after low back pain: a prospective two year cohort study in six countries on low back pain patients sicklisted for 3–4 months. Occup Environ Med 61:289–294

Balagué F, Skovron ML, Nordin M, Dutoit G, Waldburger M 1995 Low back pain in schoolchildren: a study of familial and psychological factors. Spine 20:1265–1270

Balagué F, Nordin M, Dutoit G, Waldburger M 1996 Primary prevention, education, and low back pain among school children. Bulletin Hospital for Joint Diseases 55:130–134

Balagué F, Troussier B, Salminen JJ 1999 Non-specific low back pain in children and adolescents: risk factors. European Spine Journal 8:429–438

Balagué F, Dudler J, Nordin M 2003 Low back pain in children. Lancet 361:1403–1404

Brady RJ, Dean JB, Skinner TM, Gross MT 2003 Limb length inequality: clinical implications for assessment and intervention. J Orthop Sports Phys Ther 33: 221–234

Brisson C, Montreuil S, Punnett L 1999 Effects of ergonomics training program on workers with video display units. Scand J Work Environ Health 25:255–263

Buchbinder R, Jolley D, Wyatt M 2001 Population based intervention to change back pain beliefs and disability: three part evaluation. BMJ 322:1516–1520

Burton AK 1996 Low back pain in children and adolescents: to treat or not? Bulletin Hospital for Joint Diseases 55:127–129

Burton AK 1997 Back injury and work loss: Biomechanical and psychosocial influences. Spine 22:2575–2580

Burton AK, Waddell G 2002 Educational and informational approaches. In: (Linton SJ ed), New avenues for the prevention of chronic musculoskeletal pain and disability, p 245–258. Elsevier Science, Amsterdam

Burton AK, Clarke RD, McClune TD, Tillotson KM 1996 The natural history of low-back pain in adolescents. Spine 21:2323–2328

Burton AK, Waddell G, Tillotson KM, Summerton N 1999 Information and advice to patients with back pain can have a positive effect: a randomized controlled trial of a novel educational booklet in primary care. Spine 24:2484–2491

Cardon GM, De Clercq DLR, De Bourdeaudhuij IMM 2002 Back education efficacy in elementary schoolchildren: A 1-year follow-up study. Spine 27:299–305

Cardon G, De Bourdeaudhuij I, De Clercq D et al 2004 The significance of physical fitness and physical activity for self-reported back and neck pain in elementary schoolchildren. Pediatr Exerc Sci 16:1–11

Charney W 1997 The lift team method for reducing back injuries: a 10 hospital study. AAOHN 45:300–304

Croft PR, Macfarlane GJ, Papageorgiou AC, Thomas E, Silman AJ 1998 Outcome of low back pain in general practice: a prospective study. BMJ 316:1356–1359

Daltroy LH, Iversen MD, Larson MG et al 1997 A controlled trial of an educational program to prevent low back injuries. N Engl J Med 337:322–328

de Vet HCW, Heymans MW, Dunn KM et al 2002 Episodes of low back pain: A proposal for uniform definitions to be used in research. Spine 27:2409–2416

Denis J, Darko M, Tomislav G, Viera G 2003 Research on ergonomic characteristics of high school furniture. Wood Research 48:53–62

Donchin M, Woolf O, Kaplan L, Floman Y 1990 Secondary prevention of low-back pain: A clinical trial. Spine 15:1317–1320

Evanoff BA, Bohr PC, Wolf LD 1999 Effects of a participatory ergonomics team among hospital orderlies. American Journal of Industrial Medicine 35:358–365

Fauno P, Kalund S, Andreasen I, Jorgensen U 1993 Soreness in lower extremities and back is reduced by use of shock absorbing heel inserts. Int J Sports Med 14:288–290

Feingold AJ, Jacobs K 2002 The effect of education on backpack wearing and posture in a middle school population. Work 18:287–294

Feldman DE 2001 Risk factors for the development of low back pain in adolescence. American Journal of Epidemiology 154:30–36

Feldman DE, Rossignol M, Shrier L, Abenhaim L 1999 Smoking – A risk factor for development of low back pain in adolescents. Spine 24:2492–2496

Feldman DE, Shrier I, Rossignol M, Abenhaim L 2002 Work is a risk factor for adolescent musculoskeletal pain. J Occup Environm Med 44:956–961

Ferguson SS, Marras WS 1997 A literature review of low back disorder surveillance measures and risk factors. Clin Biomech 12:211–226

Fredriksson K, Bildtc C, Hägga G, Kilboma Å 2001 The impact on musculoskeletal disorders of changing physical and psychosocial work environment conditions in the automobile industry. International Journal of Industrial Ergonomics 28:31–45

Gatty CM, Turner M, Buitendorp DJ, Batman H 2003 The effectiveness of back pain and injury prevention programs in the workplace. Work 20:257–266

Gebhardt WA 1994 Effectiveness of training to prevent job-related back pain: a meta-analysis. Br J Clin Psych 33:574

Goodgold S, Corcoran M, Gamache D et al 2002 Backpack use in children. Pediatr Phys Ther 14:122–131

Goubert L, Crombez G, De Bourdeaudhuij I 2004 Low back pain, disability and back pain myths in a community sample: prevalence and interrelationships. Eur J Pain 8:385–394

Grimmer K, Williams M 2000 Gender-age environmental associates of adolescent low back pain. Appl Ergon 31:343–360

Gurney SR, Pye SA 2002 Leg length discrepancy. G & P 15:195–206

Hadler NM 1997 Back pain in the workplace. What you lift or how you lift matters far less than whether you lift or when. Spine 22:935–940

Harreby M, Neergaard K, Hesselsoe G, Kjer J 1995 Are radiologic changes in the thoracic and lumbar spine of adolescents risk factors for low back pain in adults? A 25-year prospective cohort study of 640 school children. Spine 20:2298–2302

Harreby M, Nygaard B, Jessen T et al 1999 Risk factors for low back pain in a cohort of 1389 Danish school children: an epidemiologic study. European Spine Journal 8:444–450

Hestbaek L, Leboeuf-Yde C, Engberg M et al 2003a The course of low back pain in a general population. Results from a 5-year prospective study. J Manipulative Physiol Ther 26:213–219

Hestbaek L, Leboeuf-Yde C, Manniche C 2003b Low back pain: what is the long-term course? A review of studies of general patient populations. European Spine Journal 12:149–165

Hestbaek L, Iachine IA, Leboeuf-Yde C, Kyvik KO, Manniche C 2004 Heredity of low back pain in a young population: A classical twin study. Twin Research 7:16–26

Heymans MW, van Tulder MW, Esmail R, Bombardier C, Koes BW 2004 Back schools for non-specific low back pain (Cochrane Review). In The Cochrane Library John Wiley & Sons, Ltd, Chichester

Hiebert R, Skovron ML, Nordin M, Crane M 2003 Work restrictions and outcome of non-specific low back pain. Spine 28:722–728

Hoogendoorn WE, van Poppel MNM, Bongers PM, Koes BW, Bouter LM 2000 Systematic review of psychosocial factors at work and in private life as risk factors for back pain. Spine 25:2114–2125

Hopf C, Schrot C, Rompe JD, Bodem F 1996 No upright sitting position due to alternative school furniture. Z Orthop Ihre Grenzgeb 134:22–25

Hutchinson MR 1999 Low back pain in elite rhythmic gymnasts. Med Sci Sports Exerc 31:1686–1688

Ihlebæk C, Eriksen HR 2003 Are the "myths" of low back pain alive in the general Norwegian population? Scand J Public Health 31:395–398

Iyer SR 2001 Schoolchildren and backpacks. J Sch Health 71:88

Jellema P, van Tulder MW, van Poppel MNM, Nachemson AL, Bouter LM 2001 Lumbar supports for prevention and treatment of low back pain. Spine 26:377–386

Jones GT Watson KD, Silman AJ, Symmons DPM, Macfarlane GJ 2003 Predictors of low back pain in

British schoolchildren: A population-based prospective cohort study. Pediatrics 111:822–828

Karjalainen K, Malmivaara A, Mutanen P et al 2004 Mini-intervention for subacute low back pain: two-year follow-up and modifiers of effectiveness. Spine 29:1069–1076

Knusel O, Jelk W 1994 Pezzi-balls and ergonomic furniture in the classroom. Results of a prospective longitudinal study. Schweiz Rundsch Med Prax 83:407–413

Kool J, de Bie R, Oesch P et al 2004 Exercise reduces sick leave in patients with non-acute non-specific low back pain: a meta-analysis. J Rehabil Med 36:49–62

Korovessis P, Koureas G, Papazisis Z 2004 Correlation between backpack weight and way of carrying, sagittal and frontal spinal curvatures, athletic activity, and dorsal and low back pain in schoolchildren and adolescents. J Spinal Disord Tech 17:33–40

Kovacs FM, Abraira V, Pena A et al 2003a Effect of firmness of mattress on chronic non-specific low-back pain: randomised, double-blind, controlled, multicentre trial. Lancet 362:1599–1604

Kovacs FM, Gestoso M, Gil del Real MT et al 2003b Risk factors for non-specific low back pain in schoolchildren and their parents: a population based study. Pain 103:259–268

Krause N, Dasinger LK, Neuhauser F 1998 Modified work and return to work: a review of the literature. J Occup Rehabil 8:113–139

Kristjansdottir G, Rhee H 2002 Risk factors of back pain frequency in schoolchildren: a search for explanations to a public health problem. Acta Paediatr 91:849–854

Lahad A, Malter A, Berg AO, Deyo R 1994 The effectiveness of four interventions for the prevention of low back pain. JAMA 272:1286–1291

Larsen K, Weidich F, Leboeuf-Yde C 2002 Can custom-made biomechanic shoe orthoses prevent problems in the back and lower extremities? A randomized, controlled intervention trial of 146 military conscripts. J Manipulative Physiol Ther 25:326–331

Lebkowski WJ 1997 Back pain in teenagers and young adults. Pol Merkuriusz Lek 2:111–112

Linton SJ 1994 The role of psychological factors in back pain and its remediation. Pain Reviews 1:231–243

Linton SJ 2000 A review of psychological risk factors in back and neck pain. Spine 25:1148–1156

Linton SJ, Ryberg M 2001 A cognitive-behavioral group intervention as prevention for persistent neck and back pain in a non-patient population: a randomized controlled trial. Pain 90:83–90

Linton SJ, van Tulder MW 2001 Preventive interventions for back and neck pain problems: What is the evidence? Spine 26:778–787

Loisel P, Abenhaim L, Durand P et al 1997 A population-based, randomized clinical trial on back pain management. Spine 22:2911–2918

Lühmann D, Kohlmann T, Raspe H 1999 Die wirksamkeit von rückenschulprogrammen in kontrollierten studien. Eine literaturübersicht. Zeitschrift für Ärztliche Fortbildung und Qualitätssicherung 93:341–348

Lühmann D, Müller VE, Raspe H 2003 Prävention von rückenschmerzen. Bertelsmann Foundation, Gütersloh, Germany

MacGregor AJ, Andrew T, Sambrook PN, Spector TD 2004 Structural, psychological, and genetic influences on low back and neck pain: A study of adult female twins. Arthr Rheumatism 51:160–167

Mackenzie WG, Sampath JS, Kruse RW, Sheir-Neiss GJ 2003 Backpacks in children. Clin Orthop 409:78–84

Maher CG 2000 A systematic review of workplace interventions to prevent low back pain. Australian Journal of Physiotherapy 46:259–269

McMeeken J, Tully E, Stillman B 2001 The experience of back pain in young Australians. Man Ther 6:213–220

Mendez FJ, Gomez-Conesa A 2001 Postural hygiene program to prevent low back pain. Spine 26:1280–1286

Milanese S, Grimmer K 2004 School furniture and the user population: an anthropometric perspective. Ergoomics 47:416–426

Nachemson AL, Waddell G, Norlund AI 2000 Epidemiology of neck and low back pain. In: Nachemson AL, Jonsson E (eds) Neck and back pain: The scientific evidence of causes, diagnosis and treatment. p 165–188. Lippincott Williams & Wilkins, Philadelphia

Negrini S, Carabalona R 2002 Backpacks on! Schoolchildren's perceptions of load, associations with back pain and factors determining the load. Spine 27: 187–195

Ogon M, Riedl-Huter C, Sterzinger W et al 2001 Radiologic abnormalities and low back pain in elite skiers. Clin Orthop 390:151–162

Panagiotopoulou G, Christoulas K, Papanckolaou A, Mandroukas K 2004 Classroom furniture dimensions and anthropometric measures in primary school. Appl Erg 35:121–128

Parcells C, Stommel M, Hubbard R 1999 Mismatch of classroom furniture and student body dimensions. J Adolescent Health 24:265–273

Salminen JJ, Erkintalo MO, Pentti J, Oksanen A, Kormano MJ 1999 Recurrent low back pain and early disc degeneration in the young. Spine 24:1316–1321

Scheel IB, Hagen KB, Herrin J, Carling C, Oxman AD 2002 Blind faith? The effects of promoting active sick leave for back pain patients: A cluster-randomized controlled trial. Spine 27:2734–2740

Sheir-Neiss GI, Kruse RW, Rahman T, Jacobson LP, Pelli JA 2003 The association of backpack use and back pain in adolescents. Spine 28:922–930

Siambanes D, Martinez JW, Butler EW, Haider TH 2004 Influence of school backpacks on adolescent back pain. J Pediatr Orthop 24:211–217

Sjolie AN 2002 Psychosocial correlates of low-back pain in adolescents. Eur Spine J 11:582–588

Smedley J, Trevelyan F, Inskip H et al 2003 Impact of ergonomic intervention on back pain among nurses. Scandinavian Journal of Work, Environment & Health 29:117–123

Staal JB, Hlobil H, van Tulder MW et al 2003 Occupational health guidelines for the management of low back pain:

an international comparison. Occup Environ Med 60: 618–626
Staes F, Stappaerts K, Lesaffre E, Vertommen H 2003 Low back pain in Flemish adolescents and the role of perceived social support and effect on the perception of back pain. Acta Paediatr 92:444–451
Storr-Paulsen A 2002 The body-consciousness in school – a back pain school. Ugeskr Laeger 165:37–41
Symonds TL, Burton AK, Tillotson KM, Main CJ 1995 Absence resulting from low back trouble can be reduced by psychosocial intervention at the work place. Spine 20:2738–2745
Szpalski M, Gunzburg R, Balagué F, Nordin M, Mélot C 2002 A 2-year prospective longitudinal study on low back pain in primary school children. European Spine Journal 11:459–464
Taimela S, Kujala UM, Salminen JJ, Viljanen T 1997 The prevalence of low back pain among children and adolescents: A nationwide, cohort-based questionnaire survey in Finland. Spine 22:1132–1136
Tooms RE, Griffin JW, Green S, Cagle K 1987 Effect of viscoelastic insoles on pain. Orthopedics 10:1143–1147
Tveito TH, Hysing M, Eriksen HR 2004 Low back pain interventions at the workplace: a systematic literature review. Occup Med 54:3–13
van der Beek AJ 2004 Werkaanpassingen vanwege klachten aan het bewegingsapparaat. (van Mechelen W, Twisk JWR eds) p 14–22 Elsevier Gezondheidszorg, Maarsen
van der Beek AJ, Frings-Dresen MHW, Elders LAM 2000 Effectiviteit van werkaanpassingen bij werhervatting na klachten aan het bewegingsapparaat. Tijdschrift voor Bedrijfs- en Verzekeringsgeneeskunde 8:137–143
van Duijn M, Miedema H, Elders L, Burdorf A 2004 Barriers for early return-to-work of workers with musculoskeletal disorders according to occupational health physicians and human resource managers. J Occup Rehabil 14:31–41
van Gent C, Dols JJCM, de Rover CM, Sing RAH, de Vet HCW 2003 The weight of schoolbags and the occurrence of neck, shoulder, and back pain in young adolescents. Spine 28:916–921
van Poppel MN, Koes BW, Smid T, Bouter LM 1997 A systematic review of controlled clinical trials on the prevention of back pain in industry. Occup Environ Med 54:841–847
van Tulder MW, Tuut M, Pennick V, Bombardier C, Assendelft WJJ 2004 Quality of primary care guidelines for acute low back pain. Spine 29:E357–E362
Versloot JM, Rozeman A, van Son AM, Van Akkerveeken PF 1992 The cost-effectiveness of a back school program in industry: a longitudinal controlled field study. Spine 17:22–27
Waddell G, Burton AK 2000 Occupational health guidelines for the management of low back pain at work - Evidence review. Faculty of Occupational Medicine, London
Waddell G, Burton AK 2001 Occupational health guidelines for the management of low back pain at work: evidence review. Occup Med 51:124–135
Waddell G, Burton AK 2004 Concepts of rehabilitation for the management of common health problems. The Stationery Office, Norwich
Waddell G, Burton AK, Main CJ 2003 Screening to identify people at risk of long-term incapacity for work. Royal Society of Medicine Press, London
Watson KD, Papageorgiou AC, Jones GT et al 2002 Low back pain in schoolchildren: occurrence and characteristics. Pain 97:87–92
Watson KD, Papageorgiou AC, Jones GT et al 2003 Low back pain in schoolchildren: the role of mechanical and psychosocial factors. Arch Dis Child 88:12–17
Wergeland EL, Veiersted B, Ingre M et al 2003 A shorter workday as a means of reducing the occurrence of musculoskeletal disorders. Scand J Work Environ Health 29:27–34
Westgaard RH, Winkel J 1997 Ergonomic intervention research for improved musculoskeletal health: A critical review. International Journal of Industrial Ergonomics 20:463–500
Widhe T 2001 Spine: posture, mobility and pain. A longitudinal study from childhood to adolescence. European Spine Journal 10:118–123
Yassi A, Tate R, Cooper JE et al 1995 Early intervention for back injuries in nurses at a large Canadian tertiary care hospital: an evaluation of the effectiveness and cost benefits of a two-year pilot project. Occup Med 45: 209–214
Yassi A, Cooper JE, Tate RB et al 2001 A randomized controlled trial to prevent patient lift and transfer injuries of health care workers. Spine 26:1739–1746
Young G, Jewell D 2003 Interventions for preventing and treating pelvic and back pain in pregnancy (Cochrane Review). In The Cochrane Library, Issue 4 John Wiley & Sons, Ltd, Chichester

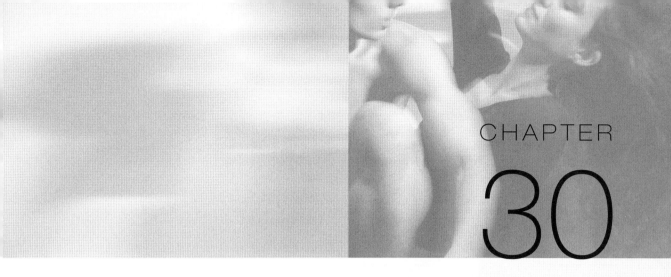

CHAPTER 30

Evidence-based medicine for acute and chronic low back pain: guidelines

Maurits van Tulder and Bart Koes

Low back pain (LBP) is a tremendous medical and socioeconomic problem. Many individual, psychosocial, and occupational risk factors for the onset of LBP have been identified, but their independent prognostic value is usually low. A number of factors have been identified that might increase the risk of chronic disability but no one single factor seems to have a strong impact. Exercises seem to be the only intervention that has proved to be effective for the prevention of LBP. Numerous randomized controlled trials and systematic reviews have been published on the effectiveness of treatment for LBP. These show strong evidence that advice to stay active and to treat the pain with nonsteroidal anti-inflammatory drugs (NSAIDs) and muscle relaxants are effective treatments for acute LBP. There is also strong evidence that exercise therapy, behavioral therapy and multidisciplinary pain treatment programs are effective for chronic LBP. However, treatment effects are usually small. Little is known about cost-effectiveness of interventions because there are hardly any high-quality, full economic evaluations. Future trials should include an economic evaluation. International guidelines on the management of acute LBP in primary care are consistent. Guidelines on chronic LBP are urgently needed. Implementation of guidelines is a major challenge for the future.

Introduction

Many people will experience one or more episodes of LBP in their life (Andersson 1997). Pain and disability – physical as well as psychosocial dysfunction – are the most important symptoms of nonspecific LBP. LBP can also have a major impact on the quality of life of patients. It is an important socioeconomic problem in Western countries because it is associated with high costs of healthcare utilization, work absenteeism, and disablement (Frymoyer & Cats-Baril 1991, van Tulder et al 1995, Webster & Snook 1990). In particular, the subgroup of patients with chronic back pain, which constitutes about 5–10% of patients with LBP, is responsible for most of the costs (Frymoyer & Cats-Baril 1991, Watson et al 1998).

LBP is usually defined as pain, muscle tension, or stiffness localized below the costal margin and above the inferior gluteal folds, with or without leg pain (sciatica). LBP is typically classified as being 'specific' or 'nonspecific.' Specific LBP refers to symptoms caused by a specific pathophysiologic mechanism, such as hernia nucleus pulposus (HNP), infection, inflammation, osteoporosis, rheumatoid arthritis, fracture, or tumor. In only about 10% of the patients specific underlying diseases can be identified (Deyo et al 1992). The vast majority of patients (up to 90%) are labeled as having nonspecific LBP, which is defined as symptoms without clear specific cause, i.e. LBP of unknown origin. Spinal abnormalities on X-rays and MRI are not strongly associated with nonspecific LBP because many people without any symptoms also show these abnormalities (Jensen et al 1994, van Tulder et al 1997a).

Nonspecific LBP is usually classified according to duration as acute (less than 6 weeks), subacute (between 6 weeks and 3 months), or chronic (longer than 3 months) (Frymoyer 1988). However, this traditional clinical view of acute and chronic LBP is inadequate, because population studies show that LBP typically has a persistent or recurrent course with fluctuating symptoms (von Korff & Saunders 1996). In general, most patients with an episode of nonspecific LBP will recover within a couple of weeks and have a good prognosis. But patients presenting with LBP might have had one or more previous episodes and acute attacks often occur as exacerbations of longstanding symptoms. Despite the epidemiological evidence that the course of LBP is more complex, most studies published up to now have used the traditional classification of acute, subacute, and chronic LBP. The management of acute, subacute, and chronic LBP differs.

During the last decades, many randomized controlled trials have been conducted and published on preventive interventions and conservative and alternative treatments for nonspecific LBP. The results of these trials have been summarized in a large number of systematic reviews (van Tulder & Koes 2003a, 2003b). Recently, the evidence from trials and reviews has formed the basis for clinical practice guidelines on the management of LBP that have been developed in various countries around the world (Koes et al 2001). This chapter provides an overview of the literature on diagnosis and treatment of nonspecific LBP and discusses the content of international clinical guidelines and their implementation.

Diagnosis

For most patients with acute LBP, a thorough history-taking and brief clinical examination is sufficient. It is well accepted that in most cases of acute LBP it is not possible to arrive at a diagnosis based on detectable pathological changes. Because of that several systems of diagnosis have been suggested, in which LBP is categorized based on pain distribution, pain behavior, functional disability, clinical signs, etc. However, none of these systems of classification has been critically validated. A simple and practical classification, which has gained international acceptance, is to divide acute LBP into three categories – the so-called 'diagnostic triage':

- serious spinal pathology
- nerve root pain/radicular pain
- nonspecific LBP.

The priority in the examination procedure follows this line of clinical reasoning. The first priority is to make sure that the problem is of musculoskeletal origin and to rule out nonspinal pathology. The next step is to exclude the presence of serious spinal pathology. Suspicion therefore is awakened by the history and/or the clinical examination and can be confirmed by further investigations. The next priority is to decide whether the patient has nerve root pain. The patient's pain distribution and pattern will indicate that, and the clinical examination will often support it. If that is not the case, the pain is classified as nonspecific LBP.

The initial clinical history taking should aim at identifying 'red flags' of possible serious spinal pathology [Royal College of General Practitioners (RCGP) 1999]. 'Red flags' are risk factors detected in an LBP patient's past medical history and symptomatology; they are associated with a higher risk of serious disorders causing LBP than in patients without these characteristics. If any red flags are present, further investigation (according to the suspected underlying pathology) will be required to exclude a serious underlying condition, e.g. infection, inflammatory rheumatic disease, or cancer. Individual red flags do not necessarily link to specific pathology but indicate a higher probability of a serious underlying condition, which might require further investigation. Multiple red flags certainly need further investigation. Red flags are signs in addition to LBP. These include (RCGP 1999):

- age of onset less than 20 years or more than 55 years
- recent history of violent trauma
- constant progressive, nonmechanical pain (no relief with bed rest)
- thoracic pain
- past medical history of malignant tumor
- prolonged use of corticosteroids
- drug abuse, immunosuppression, HIV
- systemically unwell
- unexplained weight loss
- widespread neurological symptoms (including cauda equina syndrome)
- structural deformity
- fever.

Cauda equina syndrome is likely to be present when patients describe bladder dysfunction (usually urinary retention, occasionally overflow incontinence), sphincter disturbance, saddle anesthesia, global or progressive weakness in the lower limbs, or gait disturbance. This requires urgent referral.

The initial examination serves other important purposes besides reaching a 'diagnosis.' A thorough history taking and physical examination enables an evaluation of the degree of pain and functional disability. This enables the healthcare professional to outline a management strategy that matches the magnitude of the problem. A careful initial examination also serves as a basis for credible information to the patient regarding diagnosis, management, and prognosis, and might help to reassure the patient.

There should be awareness of psychosocial factors from the first visit in primary care to identify patients with an increased risk of developing chronic disability. If there is no improvement in symptoms and with recurrent LBP, there is a need for assessment of psychosocial factors. Psychosocial 'yellow flags' should be reviewed in detail. These are factors that increase the risk of developing, or perpetuating, chronic pain and long-term disability including work loss associated with LBP (Kendall et al 1997). The identification of yellow flags should lead to appropriate cognitive and behavioral management. However, there is no evidence of the effectiveness of psychosocial assessment or intervention in acute LBP. Examples of yellow flags are (Kendall et al 1997):

- Inappropriate attitudes and beliefs about back pain (e.g. that back pain is harmful or potentially severely disabling, or high expectation of passive treatments rather than a belief that active participation will help).
- Inappropriate pain behavior (e.g. fear-avoidance behavior and reduced activity levels).
- Work-related problems or compensation issues (e.g. poor work satisfaction).
- Emotional problems (e.g. depression, anxiety, stress, tendency to low mood and withdrawal from social interaction).

Additional investigations are needed when specific spinal disorders are suspected on the basis of history and physical examination. In cases of sciatica, additional investigations are required only when other causes besides disc herniation are suspected or when disc surgery is seriously considered.

Radiological investigations are the primary additional investigation. Diagnostic imaging tests (including X-rays, CT, and MRI) are not routinely indicated for acute nonspecific LBP. Imaging tests should not be used in chronic LBP if there are no clear indications of possible serious pathology or radicular syndrome. A number of anatomical derangements can be revealed with X-rays that have a poor association with complaints and findings. Sometimes these findings will require further management (e.g. with fractures, which are symptomatic in only 10% of patients) but, more often, further management of these findings is unclear or unnecessary (e.g. with disc degeneration).

Magnetic resonance imaging (MRI) is the investigation of first choice when nerve root involvement needs to be demonstrated. It should be underlined that this expensive investigation is indicated only when the clinical picture of sciatica is sufficiently severe and longstanding to consider surgery. MRI is also the first choice option for demonstrating spinal malignancy. A radioisotope scan has sensitivity similar to MRI for showing malignant disease of the spine but it is much less specific. If neither is available, computed tomography (CT) scans are a good second choice.

In general, CT scans have a higher cost effectiveness when it comes to the demonstration of osseous abnormalities such as fractures. For demonstration of metastatic disease, however, CT scans are inferior to MRI scans (although they provide a reasonable alternative when MRI and radioisotope imaging are not available).

Laboratory investigations might point to cancer, inflammatory or infectious diseases, and diabetes or other metabolic disturbances. Increased calcium and alkaline phophatase levels might hint at malignant disease. Unfortunately, a normal erythrocyte sedimentation rate does not exclude malignancy because approximately 24% of patients with vertebral cancer have a normal sedimentation rate (van den Hoogen et al 1995).

The evidence from systematic reviews on diagnosis of back pain is now summarized.

History taking

One systematic review of nine studies evaluated the accuracy of history in diagnosing LBP in general practice (van den Hoogen et al 1995). The review found that history taking does not have a high sensitivity and high specificity for radiculopathy and ankylosing spondylitis. The combination of history and erythrocyte sedimentation rate had a relatively high diagnostic accuracy in vertebral cancer.

Physical examination

One systematic review of 17 studies found that the pooled diagnostic odds ratio for straight leg raising (SLR) for nerve root pain was 3.74 (95% CI 1.2–11.4); sensitivity for nerve root pain was high (1.0–0.88) but specificity was low (0.44–0.11) (Deville et al 2000). All included studies were surgical case series at nonprimary care level. Most studies evaluated the diagnostic value of SLR for disc prolapse. The pooled diagnostic odds ratio for the crossed SLR test was 4.39 (95% CI 0.74–25.9); with low sensitivity (0.44–0.23) and high specificity (0.95–0.86). The authors concluded that the studies do not enable a valid evaluation of diagnostic accuracy of the SLR test (Deville et al 2000).

Psychosocial risk factors

One systematic review was found of 11 cohort and 2 case-control studies evaluating psychosocial risk factors for the occurrence of LBP (Hoogendoorn et al 2000). Strong evidence was found for low social support in the workplace and low job satisfaction as risk factors for LBP. There was moderate evidence that psychosocial factors in private life are risk factors for LBP. There was also strong evidence that low job content had no effect on the occurrence of LBP. Conflicting evidence was found for a high work pace, high qualitative demands, and low job content.

Another systematic review found that there is strong evidence that psychosocial factors play an important role in chronic LBP and disability, and moderate evidence that they are important at a much earlier stage than previously believed (Linton 2000).

Diagnostic imaging

One systematic review was found that included 31 studies on the association between X-ray findings of the lumbar spine and nonspecific LBP (van Tulder et al 1997a). The results showed that degeneration, defined by the presence of disc space narrowing, osteophytes, and sclerosis, is consistently and positively associated with nonspecific LBP, with odds ratios ranging from 1.2 (95% CI 0.7–2.2) to 3.3 (95% CI 1.8–6.0). Spondylolysis/listhesis, spina bifida, transitional vertebrae, spondylosis, and Scheuermann's disease did not appear to be associated with LBP. There is no evidence on the association between degenerative signs at the acute stage and the transition to chronic symptoms.

A recent review of the diagnostic imaging literature (MRI, radionuclide scanning, CT, radiography) concluded that advanced imaging should be reserved for patients who are considering surgery or those in whom systemic disease is strongly suspected (Jarvik & Deyo 2002).

Treatment

Systematic reviews of randomized controlled trials on therapeutic interventions for back pain are promoted, conducted, and disseminated within the framework of the Cochrane Back Review Group (Bombardier et al 1997, Bouter et al 2003). In 1997, the Cochrane Back Review Group developed and published method guidelines for systematic reviews in this field. These method guidelines have recently been updated (van Tulder et al 2003a). The aim of these guidelines is to improve the quality of reviews, to facilitate comparison across reviews, and to enhance consistency among reviewers. The evidence on treatment of acute and chronic LBP is summarized below. Cochrane and other systematic reviews are used, with a recent edition of *Clinical Evidence*, in which these reviews have been updated with additional trials (van Tulder & Koes 2003a, 2003b). The evidence from systematic reviews on acute and subacute LBP is summarized in Table 30.1 and on chronic LBP in Table 30.2. Due to the heterogeneity of trials with regard to population, intervention, comparison, and outcomes included, most Cochrane reviews did not perform a meta-analysis. Consequently, overall estimates of the effect of each treatment modality are not provided. In general, effects are small.

Acute and subacute low back pain

(Table 30.1)

- **Acupuncture**: A Cochrane review did not find any randomized controlled trials (RCTs) of acupuncture specifically in people with acute LBP (van Tulder et al 1999).
- **Advice to stay active**: Two systematic reviews (one Cochrane review) and two subsequent RCTs (a total of eight RCTs) found that advice to stay active versus advice to rest in bed significantly increased the rate of recovery, reduced pain, reduced disability, and reduced time spent off work (Hagen et al 2000, Hilde et al 2003, Rozenberg et al 2002, Waddell et al 1997).
- **Analgesics (paracetamol, opioids)**: We found no placebo-controlled RCTs. Systematic reviews of three RCTs have found no consistent difference with analgesics versus NSAIDs in reducing pain (van Tulder et al 1997b).
- **Back exercises**: A Cochrane review and two additional RCTs (total of 14 RCTs) have found either no significant difference with back exercises versus other conservative treatments (e.g. manual therapy and analgesics) or inactive treatments (e.g. detuned ultrasound) in pain or disability, or have found that back exercises increase pain or disability (Chok et al 1999, Hides et al 1996, van Tulder et al 2000a).
- **Back schools**: Back school techniques vary widely, but essentially consist of repeated sessions of instruction about anatomy and function of the back and isometric exercises to strengthen the back. A Cochrane review of four RCTs found limited evidence that back schools versus placebo increased rates of recovery and reduced sick leave in the short term. The review found no significant difference in outcomes with back school versus physiotherapy, and found that a mini-back-school of one 45-minute session versus McKenzie exercises increased pain and sick leave (van Tulder et al 2000b). McKenzie exercises use self-generated stresses and forces to centralize pain from the legs and buttocks to the lower back. This method emphasizes self-care.
- **Bed rest**: A Cochrane review of eight RCTs have found that bed rest could be worse than no treatment, advice to stay active, back exercises, physiotherapy, spinal manipulation, or NSAIDs (Hagen et al 2003). Adverse effects of bed rest include joint stiffness, muscle wasting, loss of bone mineral density, pressure sores, and venous thromboembolism.
- **Behavioral therapy**: A Cochrane review including one RCT on acute LBP found that cognitive behavioral therapy (CBT) versus analgesics and exercises reduces acute LBP and disability (van Tulder et al 2000b). One additional RCT showed better pain relief compared with electromyographic biofeedback for patients with acute sciatica and a high risk for chronicity (Hasenbring et al 1999).
- **Epidural steroid injections**: A systematic review included two RCTs on acute LBP (Koes et al 1999). One RCT found that epidural steroids versus subcutaneous lidocaine injections increased the proportion of people who were pain free after 3 months. A second RCT found no significant difference in the proportion of people cured or improved with epidural steroids versus epidural saline, epidural bupivacaine, or dry needling.
- **Massage**: A Cochrane review found insufficient evidence from one RCT about the effects of massage compared with spinal manipulation or electrical stimulation (Furlan et al 2002).
- **Multidisciplinary treatment programs**: A Cochrane review in people with subacute LBP found limited evidence that multidisciplinary treatment, including a workplace visit, versus usual care by the attending physician reduced sick leave (Karjalainen et al 2001).
- **Muscle relaxants**: A Cochrane review of nine RCTs found that muscle relaxants versus placebo improve symptoms (including pain and function), but found no significant difference in outcomes among muscle relaxants. Adverse effects in people using muscle relaxants were common and included dependency, drowsiness, and dizziness (van Tulder et al 2003a).
- **NSAIDs**: A Cochrane review of 25 RCTs and two additional RCTs have found that NSAIDs versus placebo significantly increase the proportion of people with overall improvement after 1 week and significantly reduce the proportion of people requiring additional analgesics. No significant difference was found in pain relief with NSAIDs versus each other or

Table 30.1 Effectiveness of systematic reviews on conservative treatment for acute and subacute low back pain

Systematic review*	No. trials	Comparison	Results
Advise to stay active			
Waddell et al 1997	2	Bed rest	Faster recovery
	7	Usual care	Faster recovery, less chronic disability, less health care use, faster return to work
Hilde et al 2003	4	Bed rest	Inconsistent findings; small beneficial effects on functional status, sick leave
Analgesics			
van Tulder et al 1997	0	Placebo	
	3	NSAIDs	No difference in pain intensity
Back exercises			
van Tulder et al 2000c	8	Other treatment	No differences in pain intensity, functional status, overall improvement
	4	Inactive or no treatment	No differences in pain intensity, functional status
Back schools			
van Tulder et al 2000a	2	'Placebo'/no treatment	Faster recovery, no difference in pain relief, better physical outcomes
	2	Other treatments	Not more effective
Bed rest			
Hagen et al 2003	4	Advise to stay active	Inconsistent findings
	2	Short vs. long bed rest	No differences
	2	Exercises	No differences in pain intensity, functional status
Behavioral therapy			
van Tulder et al 1997	1	Usual care	Better on pain drawings, claimed impairment
Epidural steroid injections			
Koes et al 1999	2	Lidocaine, bupivacaine	Inconsistent findings
	1	Saline	No difference in proportion of people improved
Massage			
Furlan et al 2002	1	Spinal manipulation	No difference in pain
Multidisciplinary treatment			
Karjalainen et al 2001	2	Usual care	Faster return to work, fewer sick leaves, alleviates disability
Muscle relaxants			
van Tulder et al 2003b	1	Benzodiazepines vs. placebo	Better short-term pain relief and overall improvement Note: more CNS side effects
	8	Non-benzodiazepines vs. placebo	Better short-term pain relief and overall improvement Note: more CNS side effects
	2	Antispasticity drugs vs. placebo	Better short-term pain relief

Continued

Table 30.1 Effectiveness of systematic reviews on conservative treatment for acute and subacute low back pain—*cont'd*

Systematic review*	No. trials	Comparison	Results
NSAIDs			
van Tulder et al 2000d	9	Placebo	Inconsistent findings on pain relief; better global improvement; less analgesic use
	6	Other drugs	No differences
	3	Acetaminophen (paracetamol)	Inconsistent findings on pain relief
Spinal manipulation			
Assendelft et al 2003	1	Sham	Better short-term pain relief; no difference in function
	3	General practitioner care	No differences in pain, function
	5	Physical therapy or exercise	No differences in pain, function
	7	Ineffective therapies	Better short-term pain relief
	2	Back school	No differences in pain, function
Traction			
van der Heijden et al 1995	2	Placebo	No difference in global improvement
	2	Other treatment	Inconsistent findings

** Cochrane review if available, otherwise most recent systematic review; two reviews are included on advice to stay active, because the Cochrane review had defined advice to stay active as single treatment and Waddell et al (1997) used a broader definition and consequently included more trials.*

versus other treatments (paracetamol, opioids, muscle relaxants, and nondrug treatments) (Laws 1994, Pohjalainen et al 2000, van Tulder et al 2000d).

- **Spinal manipulation**: A systematic review of 16 RCTs on acute and subacute LBP found that spinal manipulation versus sham therapy significantly decreases pain but not function. Spinal manipulation was not more or less effective than general practitioner care, analgesics, physical therapy, exercises, or back school (Assendelft et al 2003).
- **Traction**: A systematic review of two RCTs found conflicting evidence on the effects of traction (van der Heijden et al 1995).
- **Electromyographic biofeedback; lumbar supports; temperature treatments (short wave diathermy, ultrasound, ice, heat); transcutaneous electrical nerve stimulation**: We found neither systematic reviews nor randomized controlled trials on the effects of these interventions for acute LBP.

Chronic low back pain (Table 30.2)

- **Acupuncture**: We found conflicting evidence from two systematic reviews (one Cochrane review) and two subsequent RCTs about effects of acupuncture compared with placebo or no treatment (Carlsson & Sjölund 2001, Cherkin et al 2001, Ernst & White 1998, van Tulder et al 1999).
- **Analgesics**: One RCT found that tramadol versus placebo decreased pain and increased functional status. A second RCT found that paracetamol versus diflunisal increased the proportion of people who rated the treatment as good or excellent (van Tulder et al 1997b).
- **Antidepressants**: One systematic review and six additional RCTs have found that antidepressants versus placebo provided significantly better pain relief, but have found no consistent difference in functioning or depression. Additional RCTs have found conflicting results on pain relief with

Table 30.2 Effectiveness of systematic reviews on conservative treatment for chronic low back pain

Systematic review*	No. trials	Comparison	Results
Acupuncture			
van Tulder et al 1999	3	No treatment	Conflicting evidence on pain relief and global improvement
	8	Placebo/sham treatment	Conflicting evidence on pain relief and global improvement
	2	Conventional treatment	Not more effective on pain relief and global improvement
Analgesics			
van Tulder et al 1997	1	NSAID	No difference on pain intensity; fewer patients improved
Antidepressants			
Salerno et al 2002	9	Placebo	Better pain relief; no difference in activities of daily living; more adverse effects
Back schools			
van Tulder et al 2000a	5	Other treatments	Better short-term effects on pain and functional disability; no long-term effects
	6	Waiting list controls	Conflicting evidence on short-term effects; no long-term effects
Behavioral therapy			
van Tulder et al 2000b	11	No treatment, waiting list controls	Moderate positive effect on pain intensity and small positive effects on generic functional status and behavioral outcomes
	2	Other treatments	Graded activity better return to work than usual care; no difference between behavioral treatment and exercise therapy
EMG biofeedback			
Note: very small sample size			
van Tulder et al 1997	3	Placebo, waiting list controls	No difference in pain intensity and functional status
Epidural steroid injections			
Nelemans et al 2000	4	Placebo	No difference in pain relief
	6	Pragmatic trials	No difference in pain relief compared with saline injections
Exercise			
van Tulder et al 2000c	6	Inactive treatment/ placebo	Conflicting evidence on pain, functional status and overall improvement
	3	Conventional physiotherapy	No differences on pain intensity, functional status, overall improvement or return to work
	3	Usual care by GP	Better pain relief, functional status and return to work
Facet joint injections			
Nelemans et al 2000	2	Placebo	No difference in pain relief
	1	Pragmatic trial	No difference in pain relief between facet joint injections and facet blocks

Continued

Table 30.2 Effectiveness of systematic reviews on conservative treatment for chronic low back pain—*cont'd*

Systematic review*	No. trials	Comparison	Results
Functional restoration			
Schonstein et al 2003	6	Usual care	Reduction in duration of sick leave; no difference in proportion of patients off work at 12 months
	5	Other interventions	Reduction in duration of sick leave; no difference in function
Local injections			
Nelemans et al 2000	5	Placebo	No difference in pain relief
	2	Pragmatic trials	No difference in pain relief
Lumbar supports			
van Tulder et al 2000c	1	Lumbar support plus corset vs. corset alone	Note: very small sample size and poor methodological quality Better subjective but not objective index after 4 and 8 weeks
Massage			
Furlan et al 2002	1	Inert treatment	Better short-term pain; better short- and long-term function
	7	Other active treatment	Worse immediate improvement in function and pain relief compared with spinal manipulation; better short-term function than acupuncture, self-care education and exercise; no differences in pain and no long-term differences
Multidisciplinary treatment			
Guzman et al 2001	10	Non-multidisciplinary treatment or usual care	Better improvement of pain and function; conflicting evidence on vocational outcomes
Muscle relaxants			
van Tulder et al 2003b	3	Benzodiazepines vs. placebo	Better short-term pain relief and overall improvement
	3	Non-benzodiazepines vs. placebo	Better short-term overall improvement; conflicting evidence on pain relief
NSAIDs			
Note: small sample sizes			
van Tulder et al 2000d	1	Placebo	Better short-term pain relief (data only in graphs)
	1	Acetaminophen (paracetamol)	No difference in short-term pain relief; better overall improvement
Spinal manipulation			
Assendelft et al 2003	3	Sham	No differences in pain, function
	4	General practitioner care	No differences in pain, function
	2	Physical therapy or exercise	No differences in pain, function
	4	Ineffective therapies	No differences in pain, function
	3	Back school	No differences in pain, function

Continued

Table 30.2 Effectiveness of systematic reviews on conservative treatment for chronic low back pain—*cont'd*

Systematic review*	No. trials	Comparison	Results
TENS			
Milne et al 2001	5	Placebo	No differences in pain, function
Traction			
			Note: most studies had small sample sizes and methodological flaws in design and conduct, which do not allow clear conclusions
van der Heijden et al 1995	1	Placebo	No difference in global improvement
	2	Conservative treatment	Better global improvement after 3–4 weeks

** Cochrane review if available, otherwise most recent systematic review.*

antidepressants versus each other or versus analgesics (Atkinson et al 1998, 1999, Dickens et al 2000, Hameroff et al 1982, 1984, Salerno et al 2002, Treves et al 1991).

- **Back schools**: A Cochrane review and one subsequent RCT have found that, in occupational settings, back schools versus no treatment improve short-term pain and reduce disability (Dalichau et al 1999, van Tulder et al 2000a); there were no long-term differences. There is conflicting evidence on the effects of back schools in primary or secondary care compared with waiting list controls.
- **Behavioral therapy**: A Cochrane review has found that behavioral therapy reduces pain and improves functional status and behavioral outcomes compared with no treatment, placebo, or waiting list control. The review found no significant difference in functional status, pain, or behavioral outcomes between different types of behavioral therapy, and found conflicting results with behavioral therapy versus other treatments (van Tulder et al 2000b).
- **Electromyographic biofeedback** One systematic review has found no difference in pain relief or functional status between electromyographic biofeedback and placebo or waiting list control, but found conflicting results on the effects of electromyographic biofeedback compared with other treatments (van Tulder et al 1997b).
- **Epidural steroid injections**: A Cochrane review has found no significant difference between epidural steroid injections and placebo, nor between epidural steroid injections and saline injections in pain relief after 6 weeks or 6 months (Nelemans et al 2000). Most of these trials included patients with sciatica.
- **Exercise**: A Cochrane review and nine additional RCTs have found that exercise improves pain and functional status compared with usual care by the general practitioner. RCTs have found conflicting evidence on the effects of different types of exercise, or exercise compared with inactive treatments (Bendix et al 1995, 1998, Friedrich et al 1998, Hildebrandt et al 2000, Kankaanpaa et al 1999, Kuukkanen & Malkia 2000, Mannion et al 1999, 2001a, 2001b, 2001c, O'Sullivan et al 1997, Soukup et al 1999, 2001, van Tulder et al 2000c).
- **Facet joint injections**: A Cochrane review found no significant difference in pain relief between facet joint injections and placebo or facet joint nerve blocks (Nelemans et al 2000). Most of these trials included patients with sciatica.
- **Functional restoration**: A Cochrane review has found that functional restoration programs with a cognitive behavioral approach plus physical training for workers with back pain reduced sick days but not the risk of being off work at 12 months compared with usual general practitioner care or with other interventions (Schonstein et al 2003).
- **Local injections**: A Cochrane review found that four out of five trials indicated that injection therapy was more effective than placebo injection, irrespective of the medication used. However, the meta-analysis showed that there

was no significant difference in pain relief. Two trials did not show any differences between local injection with bupivacaine and lidocaine or bupivacaine and methylprednisolone (Nelemans et al 2000). Most of these trials included patients with sciatica.

- **Lumbar supports**: We found insufficient evidence on the effects of lumbar supports (van Tulder et al 2000e).
- **Massage**: A Cochrane review found that massage combined with exercises and education is more effective than soft tissue massage only, remedial exercises and education only, and sham laser therapy. The review found conflicting evidence about the effects of massage compared with other treatments (Furlan et al 2002).
- **Multidisciplinary treatment programs**: A Cochrane review has found that intensive multidisciplinary biopsychosocial rehabilitation with functional restoration reduces pain and improves function compared with inpatient or outpatient non-multidisciplinary treatments or usual care. The review found no significant difference between less intensive multidisciplinary treatments and non-multidisciplinary treatment or usual care in pain or function (Guzman et al 2001).
- **Muscle relaxants**: A Cochrane review found better short-term pain relief and overall improvement with muscle relaxants compared to placebo. One RCT found that adverse effects in people using muscle relaxants are common and include dependency, drowsiness, and dizziness (van Tulder et al 2003a).
- **NSAIDs**: A Cochrane review and two additional RCTs have found no significant difference with NSAIDs versus each other for symptom outcomes. One RCT found that naproxen versus placebo increased pain relief. Two RCTs found conflicting evidence on the effects of NSAIDs versus other analgesics (Famaey et al 1998, van Tulder et al 2000d, Veenema et al 2000).
- **Spinal manipulation**: One systematic review identified 16 comparisons in 13 RCTs. The review found that spinal manipulation versus placebo did not improve pain and function (Assendelft et al 2003).
- **Traction**: One systematic review and two additional RCTs found no significant difference between traction and placebo or between traction plus massage and interferential treatment in pain relief or functional status (Beurskens et al 1995, van der Heijden et al 1995, Werners et al 1999).
- **Transcutaneous electrical nerve stimulation**: A Cochrane review found no significant difference in pain relief and function between transcutaneous electrical nerve stimulation and sham stimulation (Khadilkar et al 2005).

Guidelines

Since 1994 a number of clinical guidelines for the management of LBP in primary care have been developed in various countries worldwide in which the evidence from trials and reviews has been translated into clinically relevant recommendations. As the available evidence is international, one would expect that each country's guidelines would give more or less similar recommendations regarding diagnosis and treatment and, indeed, comparison of clinical guidelines for the management of LBP in primary care from 11 different countries showed that the content of the guidelines regarding the diagnostic classification (diagnostic triage) and the use of diagnostic and therapeutic interventions is quite similar. However, there were also some discrepancies in recommendations across guidelines (Koes et al 2001). Such differences might be due to incompleteness of the evidence, different levels of evidence, magnitude of effects, side effects and costs, differences in healthcare systems (organizational/financial), or differences in membership of guidelines committees. More recent guidelines might have included more recently published trials and, therefore, might end up with slightly different recommendations. Also, guidelines might have been based on systematic reviews that included trials in different languages; the majority of existing reviews have considered only studies published in a few languages, and several, only those published in English.

Recommendations in guidelines are based not only on scientific evidence but also on consensus. Guideline committees might consider various arguments differently, such as the magnitude of the effects, potential side effects, cost-effectiveness, and current routine practice and available resources in their country. In particular, as we know that effects in the field of LBP, if any, are usually small and short-term effects only, interpretation of effects might vary among guideline committees. Also, guideline committees might give different weight to other aspects, such as side effects and costs. The constitution of the guideline committees and the professional bodies the members they represent might introduce bias – either for or against a particular treatment. This does not necessarily mean that one guideline is better than another or that one is right and another is wrong. It merely shows that when translating the evidence into clinically relevant recommendations many aspects play a role, and that these aspects will vary locally or nationally.

European guidelines

To increase consistency in the management of nonspecific LBP across countries in Europe, the European Commission approved a program for the development of European guidelines for the management of LBP, called 'COST B13.' The main objectives of this COST action were:

- Developing European guidelines for the prevention, diagnosis, and treatment of nonspecific LBP.
- Ensuring an evidence-based approach through the use of systematic reviews and existing clinical guidelines.
- Enabling a multidisciplinary approach, stimulating collaboration between primary healthcare providers, and promoting consistency between providers and countries in Europe.
- Promoting implementation of these guidelines across Europe.

This project started in 1999 and the guidelines were finalized in 2004. To ensure an evidence-based approach, recommendations were based on Cochrane and other systematic reviews and on existing national guidelines. The European guidelines could be used as the basis for future national guidelines or future updates of existing national guidelines. The European guidelines could also help healthcare providers to make evidence-based decisions, improve the quality and outcome of health care, lead to a more rational and efficient use of resources, and identify gaps in the existing scientific evidence in order to prioritize future research.

The target population of the guidelines consists of healthcare providers, who are reached through individuals or groups that are going to develop new guidelines or update existing guidelines, and their professional associations that will disseminate and implement these guidelines. Indirectly, these guidelines also aim to inform the general public, LBP patients, and policy makers in Europe.

Four working groups have been initiated within this COST B13 action and it was these that produced the final guidelines on prevention, management of acute LBP, management of chronic LBP, and management of pelvic girdle pain. The experts in the working groups represented all countries that had issued guidelines for LBP or were developing guidelines and all relevant health professions. The recommendations for the management of acute and chronic LBP are summarized below and a full draft of the European guidelines can be seen at: http://www.backpaineurope.org

European guidelines on the management of acute low back pain

Summary of recommendations for diagnosis of acute nonspecific low back pain

- Case history and brief examination should be carried out.
- If history taking indicates possible serious spinal pathology or nerve root syndrome, carry out more extensive physical examination including neurological screening when appropriate.
- Undertake diagnostic triage at the first assessment as a basis for management decisions.
- Be aware of psychosocial factors and review them in detail if there is no improvement.
- Diagnostic imaging tests (including X-rays, CT, and MRI) are not routinely indicated for nonspecific LBP.
- Reassess those patients who do not resolve within a few weeks after the first visit, and those who are following a worsening course.

Summary of recommendations for treatment of acute nonspecific low back pain

- Give adequate information and reassure the patient.
- Do not prescribe bed rest as a treatment.
- Advise patients to stay active and continue normal daily activities including work if possible.
- Prescribe medication, if necessary, for pain relief. Preferably, this is to be taken at regular intervals. First choice is paracetamol; second choice NSAIDs.
- Consider adding a short course of muscle relaxant, on its own or added to NSAIDs, if

paracetamol or NSAIDs have failed to reduce pain.

- Consider (referral for) spinal manipulation for patients who are failing to return to normal activities.
- Multidisciplinary treatment programs in occupational settings might be an option for workers with subacute LBP and sick leave for more than 4–8 weeks.

European guidelines on the management of chronic low back pain

Summary of diagnosis in chronic low back pain

Patient assessment

- **Physical examination and case history**: The use of diagnostic triage, to exclude specific spinal pathology and nerve root pain, and the assessment of prognostic factors ('yellow flags') are recommended. We cannot recommend spinal palpatory tests, soft-tissue tests, and segmental range of motion or straight leg raising tests (Laseque) in the diagnosis of nonspecific chronic LBP.
- **Imaging**: We do not recommend imaging (plain radiography, CT, or MRI), bone scanning, SPECT, discography or facet nerve blocks for the diagnosis of nonspecific chronic LBP unless a specific cause is strongly suspected. MRI is the best imaging procedure for use in diagnosing patients with radicular symptoms, or for those in whom discitis or neoplasm is suspected.
- **Electromyography**: We cannot recommend electromyography for the diagnosis of nonspecific chronic LBP.

Prognostic factors

Assessment of work-related factors, psychosocial distress, depressive mood, severity of pain and functional impact, prior episodes of LBP, extreme symptom reporting, and patient expectations should be included in the diagnosis of patients with nonspecific chronic LBP.

Summary of treatment of chronic low back pain

Conservative treatments

Cognitive behavioral therapy, exercise therapy, brief educational interventions, and multidisciplinary (biopsychosocial) treatment can all be recommended for nonspecific chronic LBP. Back schools, and short courses of manipulation can also be considered. The use of physical therapy (TENS, heat/cold, traction, laser, ultrasound, short wave, interferential, massage, corsets) cannot be recommended.

Pharmacological treatments

Noradrenergic or noradrenergic–serotoninergic antidepressants, weak opioids and short-term uses of NSAIDs, muscle relaxants and capsicum plasters can be recommended for pain relief; strong opioids can be considered in patients who do not respond to all other treatment modalities.

Invasive treatments

Acupuncture, epidural corticosteroids, intra-articular (facet) steroid injections, local facet nerve blocks, intradiscal injections, trigger-point injections, botulinum toxin, prolotherapy, radiofrequency facet denervation, intradiscal radiofrequency lesioning, intradiscal electrothermal therapy, radiofrequency lesioning of the dorsal root ganglion, and spinal cord stimulation cannot be recommended for CLBP. Percutaneous electrical nerve stimulation (PENS) and neuroreflextherapy can be considered where available.

Surgery for nonspecific CLBP cannot be recommended unless 2 years of all other recommended conservative treatment (inclusive multidisciplinary approaches with combined programs of cognitive intervention and exercises) have failed, or such combined programs are not available, and then only in carefully selected patients.

Implementation of guidelines

Development and dissemination of guidelines does not automatically mean that healthcare providers will read, understand, and use the guidelines. Passive dissemination of information is generally ineffective and specific implementation strategies are necessary to establish changes in practice. Systematic reviews have shown that a clear and strong evidence base, clear messages, consistent messages across professions, clear sense of ownership, communication with all relevant stakeholders, charismatic leadership, continuity of care, continuous education, and continuous evaluation are successful ingredients for implementation of guidelines (Bero et al 1998, Grimshaw et al 2001, Grol 1997).

Recommendations for guideline development have been published (AGREE collaboration).

Guidelines should have a clear and strong evidence base and be based on systematic reviews. Guidelines that are not based on sound scientific evidence might effectively implement the wrong evidence. Also, there should be an explicit link between recommendations and evidence. Messages should be clear, specific, and unambiguous. Inconsistent recommendations across health professions can be confusing. Therefore, messages of the various healthcare providers involved in the management of LBP should be consistent. Communication with all relevant stakeholders (patients, professional organizations, and policy makers) is also important for successful implementation. Guideline committees should include representatives of all relevant stakeholders. Additionally, stakeholders should all have the opportunity to comment on the guidelines before publication. In that way, stakeholders will have a clear sense of ownership of the guidelines. It is also important to realize that development, publication, dissemination, implementation, and evaluation of guidelines is a continuous process. Continuous evaluation of the evidence, the guidelines and their implementation may result in improved implementation.

Several barriers to the implementation of guidelines have been identified. The practice behavior of health professionals can be influenced by a lack of knowledge, a shortage of time, disagreement with the guideline content, or reluctance from colleagues to adhere to the guideline. Furthermore, health professionals might 'get lost' in the large number of different guidelines received. Priority in getting evidence into practice is identifying barriers to change behavior of health professionals. However, patients also have specific views or beliefs and these may not correspond to the care proposed in the guidelines. Public health education might be important to overcome this barrier.

Summary

- LBP is a tremendous medical and socioeconomic problem.
- Many individual, psychosocial and occupational risk factors for the onset of LBP have been identified, but their independent prognostic value is usually low.
- A number of factors that might increase the risk of chronic disability have been identified, but no one single factor seems to have a strong impact.
- Exercise seems to be the only intervention that has proven to be effective for the prevention of LBP.
- There is strong evidence that advice to stay active and to take NSAIDs and muscle relaxants is effective for acute LBP.
- There is also strong evidence that exercise therapy, behavioral therapy, and multidisciplinary pain treatment programs are effective for chronic LBP.
- Little is known about cost-effectiveness of interventions because there are hardly any high-quality full economic evaluations.
- International guidelines on the management of acute LBP in primary care are consistent.
- Implementation of guidelines is a major challenge for the future.

References

Andersson GBJ 1997 The epidemiology of spinal disorders. In Frymoyer JW (ed) The adult spine: principles and practice. Lippincott-Raven, Philadelphia, PA, pp 93–141

Assendelft WJJ, Morton SC, Yu EI et al 2003 Spinal manipulative therapy for low back pain. A meta-analysis of effectiveness relative to other therapies. Ann Intern Med 138:871–881

Atkinson JH, Slater MA, Williams RA et al 1998 A placebo-controlled randomized clinical trial of nortriptyline for chronic low back pain. Pain 76:287–296

Atkinson JH, Slater MA, Wahlgren DR et al 1999 Effects of noradrenergic and serotonergic antidepressants on chronic low back pain intensity. Pain 83:137–145

Bendix AF, Bendix T, Ostenfeld S et al 1995 Active treatment programs for patients with chronic low back pain: a prospective, randomized, observer-blinded study. Eur Spine J 4:148–52

Bendix AF, Bendix T, Labriola M et al 1998 Functional restoration for chronic low back pain: two-year follow-up of two randomized clinical trials. Spine 23:717–725

Bero LA, Grilli R, Grimshaw JM et al 1998 Closing the gap between research and practice: an overview of systematic reviews of interventions to promote the implementation of research findings. The Cochrane Effective Practice and Organization of Care Review Group. Br Med J 317:465–468

Beurskens AJ, de Vet HCW, Köke AJ et al 1995 Efficacy of traction for non-specific low back pain: a randomised clinical trial. Lancet 346:1596–1600

Bombardier C, Esmail R, Nachemson AL and the Back Review Group Editorial Board 1997 The Cochrane Collaboration Back Review Group for Spinal Disorders. Spine 22:837–840

Bouter LM, Pennick V, Bombardier C and the Editorial Board of the Back Review Group 2003 Cochrane Back Review Group. Spine 28:1215–1218

Carlsson CPO, Sjölund BH 2001 Acupuncture for chronic low back pain: a randomized placebo-controlled study with long-term follow-up. Clin J Pain 17:296–305

Cherkin DC, Eisenberg D, Sherman KJ et al 2001 Randomized trial comparing traditional Chinese medical acupuncture, therapeutic massage, and self-care education for chronic low back pain. Arch Intern Med 161: 1081–1088

Chok B, Lee R, Latimer J et al 1999 Endurance training of the trunk extensor muscles in people with subacute low back pain. Phys Ther 79:1032–1042

Dalichau S, Scheele K, Perrey RM, Elliehausen H-J, Huebner J 1999 Ultraschallgestützte Haltungs-und Bewegungsanalyse der Lendenwirbelsäule zum Nachweis der Wirksamkeit einer Rückenschule. Zbl. Arbeitsmedizin 49:148–156

Deville WL, van der Windt DA, Dzaferagic A et al 2000 The test of Lasegue: systematic review of the accuracy in diagnosing herniated discs. Spine 25:1140–1147

Deyo RA, Rainville J, Kent DL 1992 What can the history and physical examination tell us about low back pain? JAMA 268:760–765

Dickens C, Jayson M, Sutton C et al 2000 The relationship between pain and depression in a trial using paroxetine in sufferers of chronic low back pain. Psychosomatics 41:490–499

Ernst E, White AR 1998 Acupuncture for back pain. A meta-analysis of randomized controlled trials. Arch Intern Med 158:2235–2241

Famaey JP, Bruhwyler J, Vandekerckhove K et al 1998 Open controlled randomised multicenter comparison of nimesulide and diclofenac in the treatment of subacute and chronic low back pain. J Drug Assess 1:349–368

Friedrich M, Gittler G, Halberstadt Y et al 1998 Combined exercise and motivation program: effect on the compliance and level of disability of patients with chronic low back pain: a randomized controlled trial. Arch Phys Med Rehabil 79:475–487

Frymoyer JW 1988 Back pain and sciatica. N Eng J Med 318:291–300

Frymoyer JW, Cats-Baril W 1991 An overview of the incidences and costs of low back pain. Orthop Clin N Am 22:263–271

Furlan AD, Brosseau L, Imamura M, Irvin E 2002 Massage for low-back pain: a systematic review within the framework of the Cochrane Collaboration Back Review Group. Spine 27:1896–1910

Grimshaw J, Shirran L, Thomas R 2001 Changing provider behavior: an overview of systematic reviews of interventions. Medical Care 29:II2–II45

Grol R 1997 Beliefs and evidence in changing clinical practice. Br Med J 315:418–421

Guzman J, Esmail R, Karjalainen K et al 2001 Multidisciplinary rehabilitation for chronic low back pain: systematic review. BMJ 322:1511–1516

Hagen EM, Eriksen HR, Ursin H 2000 Does early intervention with a light mobilization program reduce long-term sick leave for low back pain? Spine 25: 1973–1976

Hagen KB, Hilde G, Jamtvedt G et al 2003 Bed rest for acute low back pain and sciatica (Cochrane Review). In: The Cochrane Library, Issue 1. Update Software, Oxford

Hameroff SR, Cork RC, Scherer K et al 1982 Doxepin effects on chronic pain, depression and plasma opioids. J Clin Psychiatry 43:22–27

Hameroff SR, Weiss JL, Lerman JC et al 1984 Doxepin's effects on chronic pain and depression: a controlled study. J Clin Psychiatry 45:47–52

Hasenbring M, Ulrich HW, Hartmann M et al 1999 The efficacy of a risk factor-based cognitive behavioral intervention and electromyographic biofeedback in patients with acute sciatic pain: an attempt to prevent chronicity. Spine 24:2525–2535

Hides JA, Richardson CA, Jull GA 1996 Multifidus muscle recovery is not automatic after resolution of acute first episode low back pain. Spine 21:2763–2769

Hilde G, Hagen KB, Jamtvedt G et al 2003 Advice to stay active as a single treatment for low back pain and sciatica (Cochrane Review). In: The Cochrane Library, Issue 1. Update Software, Oxford

Hildebrandt VH, Proper KI, van den Berg R et al 2000 Cesar therapy is temporarily more effective in patients with chronic low back pain than the standard treatment by family practitioner: randomized, controlled and blinded clinical trial with 1 year follow-up [in Dutch]. Ned Tijdschr Geneesk 144:2258–2264

Hoogendoorn WE, van Poppel MNM, Bongers PM et al 2000 Systemic review of psychosocial factors at work and private life as risk factors for back pain. Spine 25:2114–2125

Jarvik JG, Deyo RA 2002 Diagnostic evaluation of low back pain with emphasis on imaging. Ann Intern Med 137:586–597

Jensen MC, Brant-Zawadzki MN, Obuchowski N 1994 Magnetic resonance imaging of the lumbar spine in people without back pain. N Engl J Med 331:69–73

Kankaanpaa M, Taimela S, Airaksinen O et al 1999 The efficacy of active rehabilitation in chronic low back pain. Effect on pain intensity, self-experienced disability, and lumbar fatigability. Spine 24:1034–1042

Karjalainen K, Malmivaara A, van Tulder M et al 2001 Multidisciplinary biopsychosocial rehabilitation for subacute low back pain in working-age adults. Spine 26:262–269

Kendall NAS, Linton SJ, Main CJ 1997 Guide to assessing psychosocial yellow flags in acute low back pain: risk factors for long-term disability and work loss. Accident Rehabilitation & Compensation Insurance Corporation of New Zealand and the National Health Committee, Wellington, New Zealand

Khadilkar A, Milne S, Brosseau L et al 2005 Transcutaneous electrical nerve stimulation for the treatment of chronic low back pain: a systematic review. Spine 30(23): 2657–2666

Koes BW, Scholten RJPM, Mens JMA et al 1999 Epidural

steroid injections for low back pain and sciatica: an updated systematic review of randomized clinical trials. Pain Digest 9:241–247

Koes BW, van Tulder MW, Ostelo R et al 2001 Clinical guidelines for the management of low back pain in primary care: an international comparison. Spine 26:2504–2513

Kuukkanen T, Malkia E 2000 Effects of a three-month therapeutic exercise programme on flexibility in subjects with low back pain. Physiother Res Int 5:46–61

Laws D 1994 Double blind parallel group investigation in general practice of the efficacy and tolerability of acemetacin, in comparison with diclofenac, in patients suffering with acute low back pain. Br J Clin Res 5: 55–64

Linton SJ 2000 A review of psychological risk factors in back and neck pain. Spine 25:1148–1156

Mannion AF, Muntener M, Taimela S et al 1999 A randomized clinical trial of three active therapies for chronic low back pain. Spine 24:2435–2448

Mannion AF, Junge A, Taimela S et al 2001a Active therapy for chronic low back pain: part 3. Factors influencing self-rated disability and its change following therapy. Spine 26:9209

Mannion AF, Muntener M, Taimela S et al 2001b Comparison of three active therapies for chronic low back pain: results of a randomized clinical trial with one-year follow-up. Rheumatology 40:7728

Mannion AF, Taimela S, Muntener M et al 2001c Active therapy for chronic low back pain part 1. Effects on back muscle activation, fatigability, and strength. Spine 26:897–908

Milne S, Welch V, Brosseau L et al 2001 Transcutaneous electrical nerve stimulation (TENS) for chronic low back pain. Cochrane Database Syst Rev (2)

Nelemans PJ, de Bie RA, de Vet HCW et al 2000 Injection therapy for subacute and chronic benign low back pain. In: The Cochrane Library, Issue 3. Oxford, Update Software

O'Sullivan PB, Twomey LT, Allison GT 1997 Evaluation of specific stabilizing exercise in the treatment of chronic low back pain with radiologic diagnosis of spondylolysis or spondylolisthesis. Spine 24:2959–2967

Pohjalainen T, Jekunen A, Autio L et al 2000 Treatment of acute low back pain with the COX-2 selective anti-inflammatory drug nimesulide: results of a randomised, double-blind comparative trial versus ibuprofen. Spine 25:1579–1585

Royal College of General Practitioners (RCGP) 1999 Clinical guidelines for the management of acute low back pain. RCGP, London

Rozenberg S, Delval C, Rezvani Y et al 2002 Bed rest or normal activity for patients with acute low back pain: a randomized controlled trial. Spine 27:1487–1493

Salerno SM, Browning R, Jackson JL 2002 The effect of antidepressant treatment in chronic back pain: a meta-analysis. Arch Intern Med 162:19–24

Schonstein E, Kenny DT, Keating J, Koes BW 2003 Work conditioning, work hardening and functional restoration for workers with back and neck pain (Cochrane Review). In: The Cochrane Library, Issue 1. Update Software, Oxford

Soukup MG, Glomsrod B, Lonn JH et al 1999 The effect of a Mensendieck exercise program as secondary prophylaxis for recurrent low back pain. A randomized, controlled trial with 12-month follow-up. Spine 24: 1585–1591

Soukup MG, Lonn J, Glomsrod B et al 2001 Exercises and education as secondary prevention for recurrent low back pain. Physiother Res Int 6:27–39

Treves R, Montane de la Roque P, Dumond JJ et al 1991 Prospective study of the analgesic action of clomipramine versus placebo in refractory low back pain and sciatica (68 cases) [in French]. Rev Rhum Mal Osteoartic 58:549–552

van den Hoogen HMM, Koes BW, van Eijk JThM, Bouter LM 1995 On the accuracy of history, physical examination and erythrocyte sedimentation rate in diagnosing low back pain in general practice. A criteria-based review of the literature. Spine 20:318–327

van der Heijden GJMG, Beurskens AJHM, Koes BW et al 1995 The efficacy of traction for back and neck pain: a systematic, blinded review of randomized clinical trial methods. Phys Ther 75:93–104

van Tulder MW, Koes BW 2003a Acute low back pain and sciatica. Clin Evid 9:1245–1259

van Tulder MW, Koes BW 2003b Chronic low back pain and sciatica. Clin Evid 9:1260–1276

van Tulder MW, Koes BW, Bouter LM 1995 A cost-of-illness study of back pain in the Netherlands. Pain 62: 233–240

van Tulder MW, Assendelft WJ, Koes BW, Bouter LM 1997a Spinal radiographic findings and nonspecific low back pain. A systematic review of observational studies. Spine 22:427–434

van Tulder MW, Koes BW, Bouter LM 1997b Conservative treatment of acute and chronic non-specific low back pain: a systematic review of randomized controlled trials of the most common interventions. Spine 22: 2128–2156

van Tulder MW, Cherkin DC, Berman B et al 1999 The effectiveness of acupuncture in the treatment of acute and chronic low back pain: a systematic review within the framework of the Cochrane Collaboration Back Review Group. Spine 24:1113–1123

van Tulder MW, Esmail R, Bombardier C, Koes BW 2000a Back schools for non-specific low back pain (Cochrane Review). In: The Cochrane Library, Issue 3. Update Software, Oxford

van Tulder MW, Ostelo RWJG, Vlaeyen JWS et al 2000b Behavioral treatment for chronic low back pain: a systematic review within the framework of the Cochrane Collaboration. Spine 25:2688–2699

van Tulder MW, Malmivaara M, Esmail R, Koes BW 2000c Exercise therapy for low back pain: a systematic review within the framework of the Cochrane Collaboration. Spine 25:2784–2796

van Tulder MW, Scholten RJPM, Koes BW, Deyo RA 2000d

Non-steroidal anti-inflammatory drugs for low back pain: a systematic review within the framework of the Cochrane Collaboration. Spine 25:2501–2513
van Tulder MW, Jellema P, Nachemson AL et al 2000e Lumbar supports for prevention and treatment of low back pain (Cochrane Review). In: The Cochrane Library, Issue 3. Update Software, Oxford
van Tulder MW, Furlan A, Bombardier C, Bouter L and the Editorial Board of the Cochrane Collaboration Back Review Group 2003a Updated method guidelines for systematic reviews in the Cochrane Collaboration Back Review Group. Spine 28:1290–1299
van Tulder MW, Touray T, Furlan AD et al 2003b Muscle relaxants for nonspecific low back pain: a systematic review within the framework of the Cochrane Collaboration. Spine 28:1978–1992
Veenema KR, Leahey N, Schneider S 2000 Ketorolac versus meperidine: ED treatment of severe musculoskeletal low back pain. Am J Emerg Med 18:404–407
von Korff M, Saunders K 1996 The course of back pain in primary care. Spine 21:2833–2837
Waddell G, Feder G, Lewis M 1997 Systematic reviews of bed rest and advice to stay active for acute low back pain. Br J Gen Pract 47:647–652
Watson PJ, Main CJ, Waddell G et al 1998 Medically certified work loss, recurrence and costs of wage compensation for back pain: a follow-up study of the working population of Jersey. Br J Rheumatol 37:82–86
Webster BS, Snook SH 1990 The cost of compensable low back pain. J Occup Med 32:13–15
Werners R, Pynsent PB, Bulstrode CJK 1999 Randomized trial comparing interferential therapy with motorized lumbar traction and massage in the management of low back pain in a primary care setting. Spine 24: 1579–1584

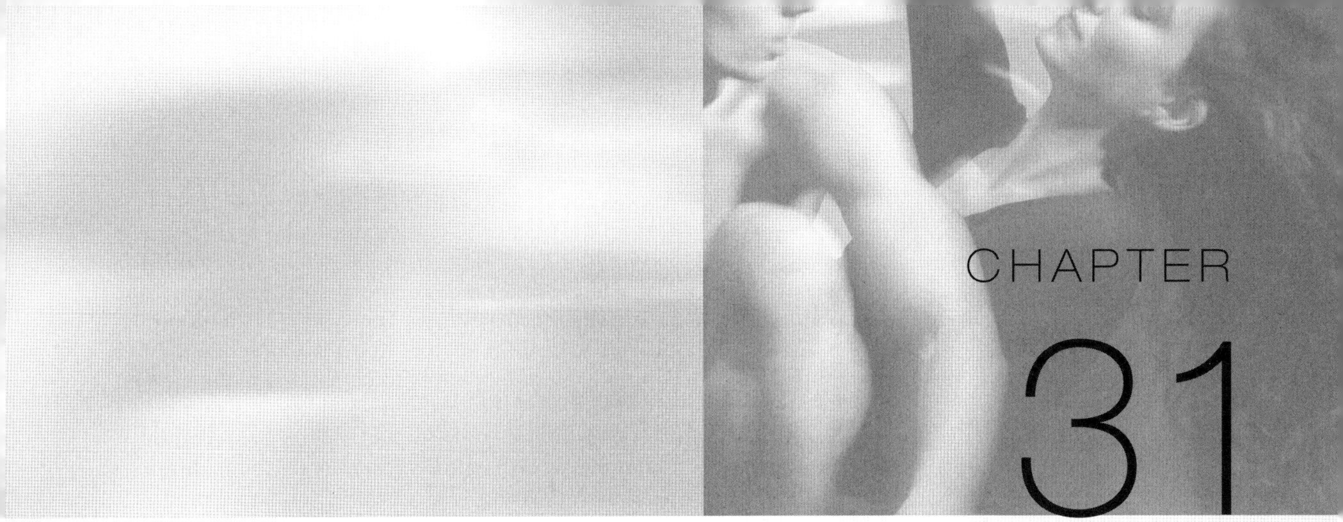

CHAPTER 31

European guidelines on the diagnosis and treatment of pelvic girdle pain

Andry Vleeming, HB Albert, HC Östgaard, B Stuge, and B Sturesson on behalf of the COST B13 Working Group on Pelvic Girdle Pain

Low back pain: guidelines for its management

The guidelines are developed within the framework of the COST ACTION B13 'Low back pain: guidelines for its management,' issued by the European Commission, Research Directorate-General, Department of Policy, Coordination and Strategy:

- Andry Vleeming (chairman): Clinical anatomist (the Netherlands)
- Hanne B Albert: Physical therapist (Denmark)
- Hans Christian Östgaard: Orthopedic surgeon (Sweden)
- Britt Stuge: Physical therapist (Norway)
- Bengt Sturesson: Orthopedic surgeon (Sweden).

Objectives

The focus of Working Group 4 (WG4) is to produce a guideline on pelvic girdle pain (PGP). The working group will formulate a rationale to support the proposition that PGP is a specific form of back pain. The guideline will provide recommendations on the diagnosis and treatment of pelvic girdle pain.

The guideline seeks to improve the clinical management of PGP by making recommendations that are acceptable to healthcare professionals and their respective organizations. Other objectives are to initiate new research and to promote consistency in definitions, diagnosis and treatment between the various healthcare providers.

Target population

The guideline is directed to professional national healthcare organizations that will disseminate and implement these guidelines among their members. The guideline is intended to inform policymakers, healthcare providers, the general public, and patients suffering from PGP.

Guideline pelvic girdle pain

This guideline was developed within the framework of the COST ACTION B13 'Low back pain: guidelines for its management,' issued by the European Commission, Research Directorate-General, Department of Policy, Coordination and Strategy. The guideline working group consisted of experts in the field of PGP who have been involved in primary, secondary, and tertiary healthcare as well as in research projects related to PGP patients. Working group 4 has five members, two orthopedic surgeons from Sweden, two physiotherapists from Denmark and Norway, and one clinical anatomist from the Netherlands. The over-representation of members from the Nordic countries is primarily the result of extensive clinical research on PGP conducted by these countries.

Evidence

To ensure an evidence-based approach, a strategy broadly conducive with the other guidelines in COST ACTION B13 was adopted. In the first instance, systematic reviews were sought, supplemented by individual scientific studies where systematic reviews were not available. Three subgroups were formed to explore: (1) basic information; (2) diagnostics and epidemiology; and (3) therapeutic interventions.

Because it became apparent that limited evidence-based knowledge was available in the form of randomized controlled trials (RCTs), a wider search of the literature was made, including basic studies. The literature search covered the period from the beginning of the 1890s to August 2004. The major databases were searched (without language restrictions), using Medline, the Cochrane library, the internet and any available dissertations on this subject. No national guidelines for PGP were identified. The progress of the subgroups was discussed at each meeting and the final report is based on group consensus.

A grading system was used to denote the strength of the evidence (see Chapter 29). This grading system is simple and easy to apply, and shows a large degree of consistency between the grading of therapeutic and preventive, prognostic and diagnostic studies. The system is based on the original ratings of the AHCPR Guidelines (1994) and levels of evidence recommended in the method guidelines of the Cochrane Back Review group.

Grading of evidence and strength of recommendations according to the guidelines of the acute group (Working Group 1) for therapy and prevention:

- **Level A**: Generally consistent findings provided by (a systematic review of) multiple high-quality randomized controlled trials (RCTs).
- **Level B**: Generally consistent findings provided by (a systematic review of) multiple low-quality RCTs or non-randomized controlled trials (CCTs).
- **Level C**: One RCT (either high or low quality) or inconsistent findings from (a systematic review of) multiple RCTs or CCTs.
- **Level D**: No RCTs or CCTs.

A checklist for the methodological quality of therapy/prevention studies was used to assess internal validity (Hagen et al 2000). The studies were ranked as high methodological quality studies (low risk of bias) and moderate to low methodological quality (high risk of bias). The studies were considered to be of high methodological quality when there was: adequate method of randomization, concealment of treatment allocation, drop-out rate described and acceptable, intention-to-treat analysis, blinding of observer/outcome assessor, and no co-interventions (Clarke & Oxman 1999).

Summary of basic studies, epidemiology and risk factors for pelvic girdle pain (PGP)

- Pelvic girdle pain (PGP) is a specific form of low back pain (LBP) that can occur separately or in conjunction with LBP.
- The 1990s saw increasing efforts among clinicians and researchers to study pain and the etiology of pelvic girdle pain. The working group proposes a definition for pelvic musculoskeletal pain under the title pelvic girdle pain (PGP), to exclude gynecological and/or urological disorders:

Pelvic girdle pain (PGP) generally arises in relation to pregnancy, trauma, osteoarthrosis and arthritis. Pain is experienced between the posterior iliac crest and the gluteal fold, particularly in the vicinity of the sacroiliac joints (SIJ). The pain may radiate in the posterior thigh and can also occur in conjunction with/or separately in the symphysis. The endurance capacity for standing, walking, and sitting is diminished. The diagnosis of PGP can be reached after exclusion of lumbar causes. The pain or functional disturbances in relation to PGP must be reproducible by specific clinical tests.

- Although it is possible to focus on and specify PGP, functionally the pelvis cannot be studied in isolation. PGP is related to nonoptimal stability of the pelvic girdle joints.
- The typical anatomy of the sacroiliac joint (SIJ) (which is characterized by a coarse cartilage texture, cartilage-covered grooves and ridges, a wedge-like shape of the sacrum, and a propeller-like shape of the joint surface) leads to the highest coefficient of friction of diarthrodial human joints. This friction can be altered according to the loading situation and serves to stabilize the pelvic girdle.
- Nutation of the sacrum (flexion of the sacrum relative to the iliac bones), is generally the result of load bearing and a functional adaptation to stabilize the pelvic girdle.
- More research is needed in patients with PGP to verify whether counternutation of the SIJ (anterior rotation of the iliac bones relative to the sacrum) in load-bearing situations is a typical sign of nonoptimal stability of the pelvic girdle.
- Optimal and nonoptimal stability is defined by the working group as follows:

Functional definition of general joint stability: The effective accommodation of the joints to each specific load demand through an adequately tailored joint compression, as a function of gravity, coordinated muscle and ligament forces, to produce effective joint reaction forces under changing conditions.

Optimal stability is achieved when the balance between performance (the level of stability) and effort is optimized to economize the use of energy.

Non-optimal joint stability implicates altered laxity/stiffness values leading to increased joint translations resulting in a new joint position and/or exaggerated/reduced joint compression, with a disturbed performance/effort ratio (Vleeming et al 2004).

- The incidence/point/prevalence of pregnant women suffering from PGP is about 20%. The evidence for this result is strong.
- Risk factors for developing PGP during pregnancy are most probably a history of previous LBP, and/or previous trauma to the pelvis. There is slight conflicting evidence (one study) against the following risk factors; pluripara and high work load. There is agreement that non risk factors are: contraceptive pills, time interval since last pregnancy, height, weight, smoking and most probably age (one study reports that young age is a risk factor).
- No studies have been published on the risk factors for the non-pregnant population to develop PGP, or which women or men are at risk of developing chronic PGP.

Summary of recommendations for diagnosis and imaging of PGP

- To make the diagnosis of PGP, the following tests are recommended for use during the clinical examination (see Appendix 1):
  - SIJ pain: posterior pelvic pain provocation test (P4), Patrick's faber test, palpation of the long dorsal SIJ ligament, and Gaenslen's test.
  - Symphysis: palpation of the symphysis and modified Trendelenburg's test of the pelvic girdle.
  - Functional pelvic test: active straight leg raise test (ASLR).
- It is recommended that a pain history be taken with specific attention paid to pain arising during prolonged standing and/or sitting. To ensure that the pain is in the pelvic girdle area, it is important that the precise area of pain be indicated: the patient should either point out the exact location on his/her body, or preferably shade in the painful area on a pain location diagram.
- There are limited indications for the use of conventional radiography due to its poor sensitivity in detecting the early stages of degeneration and arthritis of the SIJ.
- In most cases of nonankylosing spondylitis (non-AS) PGP, there is limited value for imaging.
- Magnetic resonance imaging (MRI) discriminates changes most effectively in and

around the SIJ. Early AS and tumors can be easily detected. To establish the diagnosis of PGP imaging techniques are generally only needed in AS, for patients showing 'red flag' signs, and when surgical intervention procedures are considered.
- Do not use scintigraphy for PGP.
- Use pain referral maps for PGP.
- Do not use local SIJ injections as a diagnostic tool for PGP. A combination of simple manual diagnostic tests, with high sensitivity and specificity, will analyze a broader spectrum of PGP complaints.

Recommendations for treatment of pelvic girdle pain

- Consider using physical therapy during pregnancy.
- We recommend an individualized treatment program, including specific stabilizing exercises, as part of a multifactorial treatment.
- Consider using water gymnastics (exercises) during pregnancy.
- Consider using acupuncture during pregnancy.
- Consider using therapeutic intra-articular SIJ injections for ankylosing spondylitis (under imaging guidance).
- Do not surgically fuse sacroiliac joints.

Recommendations for future research

Basic studies

- Verify whether counternutation of the SIJ (anterior rotation of the iliac bones relative to the sacrum) in load-bearing situations is a typical sign of nonoptimal stability of the pelvic girdle in PGP patients.

Diagnosis

- More studies are needed on diagnostic procedures for PGP. The diagnostic tests currently proposed need re-evaluation and trials for falsifications have to be set up.
- More research is needed to verify whether patients with PGP based on AS react to the same diagnostic procedures as do non-AS PGP patients.
- Studies are needed with fluoroscopic-guided intra-articular anesthetic SIJ blocks, together with local superficial injections of extra-articular SIJ ligaments and compared to manual diagnostic tests.
- Randomized trials are needed, as well as a universal protocol for diagnostic/follow-up procedures after fusion surgery.
- Further evaluate disease-specific outcome measures for PGP.

Treatment

- Different treatment modalities and applications should be investigated to establish evidence for specific recommendations. Future studies should include PGP patients in different cohorts, such as patients with AS. The methodological quality of a study is as important as the quality of the intervention studied. High methodological quality does not necessarily guarantee that a study offers a high quality of intervention. Relevant treatment modalities to be studied include comparison of:
  - exercise programs with and without the use of a pelvic belt
  - individualized physical therapy with group treatment
  - cognitive interventions with exercise programs. Study the effect of manipulation, mobilization, massage, and relaxation in PGP patients.
- Randomized trials are needed to establish the effect of fusion surgery in PGP patients not responding to nonoperative treatment.

A more extended version of this summary and overview of basic studies can be found at: http://www.europeanbackpain.org and in an article in *European Spine Journal* that will be published in 2006–7.

Summary

- It is concluded that pelvic girdle pain (PGP) is a specific form of low back pain (LBP) that can occur separately or in conjunction with LBP; a new definition of PGP is recommended.
- The incidence/point/prevalence of pregnant women suffering from PGP is about 20%. The evidence for this result is strong.
- Risk factors for developing PGP during pregnancy are most probably a history of

previous LBP and/or previous trauma to the pelvis. There is slight conflicting evidence against the following risk factors; pluripara and high work load. There is agreement that nonrisk factors are: contraceptive pills, time interval since last pregnancy, height, weight, smoking and – probably – age. No studies have been published on the risk factors for the *non-pregnant* population to develop PGP, or which women or men are at risk of developing chronic PGP.

- Several specific tests are recommended for the diagnosis of PGP. Those for sacroiliac pain are: the posterior pelvic pain provocation test (P4), Patrick's faber test, palpation of the long dorsal sacrolilac ligament, and Gaenslen's test. Those for symphyseal pain are: the palpation of the symphysis and modified Trendelenburg's test of the pelvic girdle. For functional testing of the pelvis, the active straight leg raise test (ASLR) is used.
- It is recommended that a pain history be taken with specific attention paid to pain arising during prolonged standing and/or sitting.
- There are limited indications for the use of conventional radiography in diagnosis because of its poor sensitivity in detecting the early stages of degeneration and arthritis of the sacroliac joints. Magnetic resonance imaging (MRI) discriminates changes most effectively in and around the sacroiliac joints. Early ankylosing spondylitis and tumors can be easily detected.
- To establish the diagnosis of PGP, imaging techniques are generally only needed in ankylosing spondylitis, for patients showing 'red flag' signs, and when surgical intervention procedures are considered.
- An individualized treatment program is recommended, including specific stabilizing exercises, as part of a multifactorial treatment. Physical therapy should be considered during pregnancy.
- Surgical fusion of the sacroiliac joints is not recommended. Severe traumatic cases of PGP can be an exception to this recommendation, but only when other nonoperative treatment modalities have failed by professionals with expert knowledge of the condition.
- Recommendations are made for future research on PGP.

Acknowledgement

The authors are grateful for the important contribution made by Diane Lee (PT) and Prof Dr FCT van der Helm to the basic part of this manuscript; especially in relation to the definition of joint stability.

References

Clarke M, Oxman AD 1999 Cochrane reviewers' handbook 4.0 [in Review Manager (RevMan) computer program, version 4]. The Cochrane Collaboration, Oxford

Hagen KB, Hilde G, Jamtvedt G, Winnem MF 2000 The Cochrane review of bed rest for acute low back pain and sciatica. Spine 25:2932–2939

Vleeming A, Albert HB, van der Helm FCT et al 2004 A definition of joint stability. In: European guidelines on the diagnosis and treatment of pelvic girdle pain. Cost action B13: low back pain: guidelines for its management, working group 4

Appendix 1

Definitions of pelvic girdle pain tests

Active straight leg raise test (ASLR)

The test is performed with patients in a supine position with straight leg and feet 20 cm apart. The test is performed after the instruction 'Try to raise your legs, one after the other, above the couch for 20 cm without bending the knee.' The patient is asked to score impairment on a six-point scale: 0 = not difficult at all; 1 = minimally difficult; 2 = somewhat difficult/difficult; 3 = fairly difficult; 4 = very difficult; 5 = unable to do. The scores on both sides are added, so that the sum score ranges from 0 to 10 (Mens 2001).

Gaenslen's test

The patient, lying supine, flexes the knee and hip of the same side, the thigh being crowded against the abdomen with the aid of both the patient's hands clasped about the flexed knee. The patient is then brought well to the side of the table, and the opposite thigh is slowly hyperextended by the examiner with gradually increasing force by pressure of the examiner's hand on the top of the knee. With the opposite hand, the examiner assists the patient in fixing the lumbar spine and pelvis by pressure over the patient's clasped hands. The test is positive if the patient experiences pain, either local or referred on the provoked side.

Long dorsal sacroiliac ligament test (LDL test)

The patient is lying prone and tested on tenderness on bilateral palpation of the LDL, directly under the caudal part of the posterior superior iliac spine. A skilled examiner scores the pain as positive or negative. The LDL test is scored on a scale from: 0 = no pain; 1 = mild pain; 2 = moderate pain; 3 = unbearable pain. Both sides are added so that the sum score ranges from 0 to 6. Studied on postpartum women (Vleeming et al 2002).

Instruction for the LDL test on a pregnant woman: The subject lies on her side with slight flexion in both hip and knee joints. If the palpation causes pain, that persists more than 5 seconds, after removal of the examiner's hand, it is recorded as pain. If the pain disappears within 5 seconds it is recorded as tenderness. Studied on pregnant women (Albert et al 2000).

Pain provocation of the symphysis by modified Trendelenburg's test

The patient stands on one leg, flexes the other at 90° in hip and knee. If pain is experienced in the symphysis the test is positive (Albert et al 2000).

Patrick's faber test

The subject lies supine. One leg is flexed, abducted, and externally rotated (faber is an abbreviation of flexion, abduction, and external rotation) so that the heel rests on the opposite knee. If pain is felt in the SI joints or in the symphysis the test is considered positive (test described by Albert et al 2000, Broadhurst & Bond 1998, Wormslev 1994).

Posterior pelvic pain provocation test

The test is performed with the woman supine and the hip flexed to an angle of 90° on the side to be examined: a light manual pressure is applied to the patient's flexed knee along the longitudinal axis of the femur while the pelvis is stabilized by the examiner's other hand resting on the patient's contralateral superior anterior iliac spine. The test is positive when the patient feels a familiar, well-localized pain deep in the gluteal area on the provoked side (Östgaard et al 1994); a similar test is described as posterior shear or 'thigh thrust' (Laslett & Williams 1994).

Symphysis pain palpation test

The subject lies supine. The entire front side of the pubic symphysis is palpated gently. If the palpation causes pain that persists more than 5 seconds after removal of the examiner's hand, it is recorded as pain. If the pain disappears within 5 seconds it is recorded as tenderness (Albert et al 2000).

References

Albert H, Godskesen M, Westergaard J 2000 Evaluation of clinical tests used in classification procedures in pregnancy-related pelvic joint pain. Eur Spine J 9: 161–166

Broadhurst NA, Bond MJ 1998 Pain provocation tests for the assessment of sacroiliac joint dysfunction. J Spinal Disord 11:341–345

Laslett M, Williams M 1994 The reliability of selected pain provocation tests for sacroiliac joint pathology. Spine 19:1243–1249

Mens JMA, Vleeming A, Snijders CJ et al 2001 Reliability and validity of the active straight leg raise test in posterior pelvic pain since pregnancy. Spine 26: 1167–1171

Östgaard HC, Zetherström G, Roos-Hansen E, Svanberg G (1994) The posterior pelvic pain provocation test in pregnant women. Eur Spine J 3:258–260

Vleeming A, de Vries HJ, Mens JMA, van Wingerden JP 2002 Possible role of the long dorsal sacroiliac ligament in women with peripartum pelvic pain. Acta Obstet Gynecol Scand 81:430–436

Wormslev M, Juul AM, Marques B et al 1994 Clinical examination of pelvic insufficiency during pregnancy. Scand J Rheumatol 23:96–102

PART FIVE

Section One

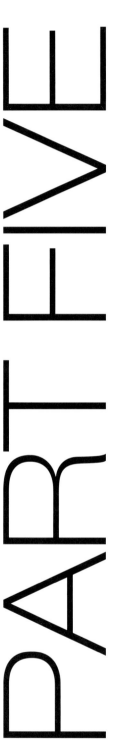

Effective training and treatment: Psychological, social and motivational aspects

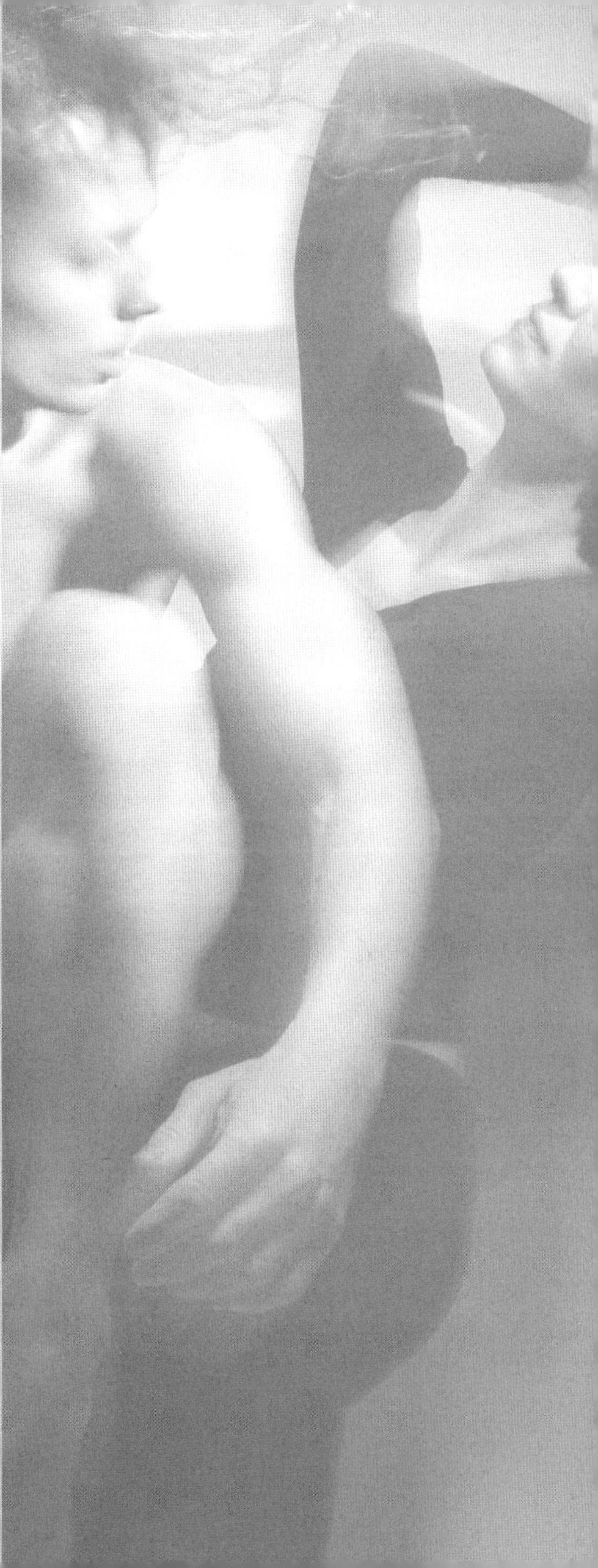

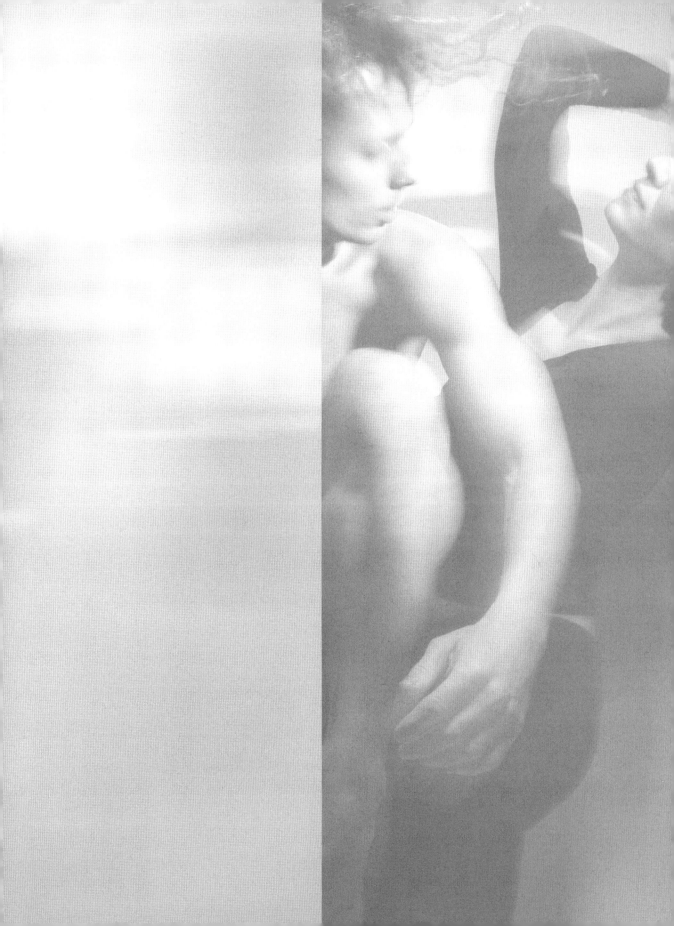

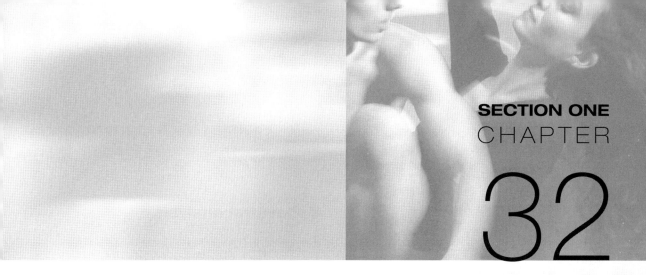

SECTION ONE
CHAPTER

32

Behavioral analysis, fear of movement/(re)injury, and cognitive–behavioral management of chronic low back pain

Johan WS Vlaeyen and Linda MG Vancleef

Introduction

Chronic musculoskeletal pain syndromes such as chronic low back pain (CLBP) are responsible for enormous costs for health care and society (Picavet & Schouten 2003, Verhaak et al 1998, Waddell 1987). The biomedical approach often proves insufficient to explain these pain conditions and, nowadays, the biopsychosocial view on pain offers the foundation for a better insight into how pain can become a persistent problem (Fordyce 1976, Turk & Flor 1999). The main assumption of the model is that pain and pain disability are not only influenced by organic pathology, if present, but also by biological, psychological, and social factors. As such, the distinction between somatogenic (real) and psychogenic (imaginary) pain is no longer considered relevant. In this chapter, the behavioral analysis of chronic pain will be discussed, with special attention to the role of pain-related fear in the development and maintenance of chronic pain, and the cognitive–behavioral management of chronic back pain.

Chronic back pain as a societal problem

Many people (60–90% of the population) suffer from low back pain (LBP) in the course of their lives, not all of whom seek health care (von Korff 1994). In the majority of patients who seek care and refrain from work, the problem of pain resolves within a few weeks. These patients return to work and resume their daily activities within 4–6 weeks of the onset of the complaints. However, in a small subgroup of patients (5–10% of the total population), back pain complaints persist for a period > 3 months and develop into a chronic pain problem. This relatively small group of back-pain patients is responsible for the largest amount of healthcare and societal costs of back problems (Goossens et al 1999, Nachemson 1992, Waddell 2004). What are the reasons for this group becoming chronic pain sufferers? One possibility could be that these patients have more serious impairments than those who resume daily activities earlier. However, no research supports this assumption. On the contrary, numerous studies have shown that there is no perfect relationship between impairment, pain, and disability (Peters et al 2005). Patients with back problems often show no physical injury and, conversely, not everyone who does show physical injury reports pain or disability (e.g. Jensen et al 1994). A biopsychosocial approach offers the foundations for a better insight into how pain can become a persistent problem (Turk & Flor 1999). The main assumption of this approach is that pain and pain disability are not only influenced by organic pathology, if present, but also by psychological and social factors. The interrelationship between the biological, psychological, and social factors, as well as their influence on the pain experience, is complex. For example, from a biomedical view, a return to work should be encouraged only when the underlying pathology has healed. Otherwise, the risk of (re)injury and repeated failure would increase, leading to the enhancement of chronicity. From this biomedical perspective, staying off work too long would be much safer than resuming work activities too early. The literature, however, supports the conjecture that an early return to work contributes to a decrease in long-term work disability in patients with musculoskeletal pain (Vowles et al 2004, Watson et al 2004). Their arguments include the recognition that musculoskeletal incidents are increased by the immediate consequences – such as diminished pain, increased attention from others, avoidance of unpleasant and fearful situations, and the stability of the sick role. In other words, the pain disability is subject to a graded shift from structural/mechanical to cognitive/environmental control. A number of studies suggested that this shift occurs quite rapidly, probably within 4–8 weeks of the onset of acute pain (Deyo et al 1986, Klenerman et al 1995, Philips & Grant 1991).

Behavioral analysis

Pain is now defined as not only a sensory experience, but also as an emotional one. The International Association for the Study of Pain (IASP) has proposed the following definition of pain:

> *An unpleasant sensory and emotional experience associated with actual or potential tissue damage, or described in terms of such damage.*

Emotional experiences can only be inferred by their effects at some observable level (Öhman 1987). Likewise, chronic pain can best be approached as a hypothetical construct that can be inferred by at least three partially independent response systems: overt pain behaviors, psychophysiological reactivity, and cognitive processes about pain and pain control (Vlaeyen et al 1989) (Fig. 32.1).

Overt pain behaviors

In the 1960s, the American psychologist Wilbert Fordyce pointed to the importance of behavioral dysfunction of the patient in analyzing the pain problem and treatment (Fordyce et al 1968). According to Fordyce, the pain behavior of the patient, rather than the pain complaint, needs to be the central issue. In making this statement, Fordyce acknowledged that the relationship between the pain experience and dysfunction is often far from perfect. Pain behavior was defined as behavior from which outsiders could infer that a

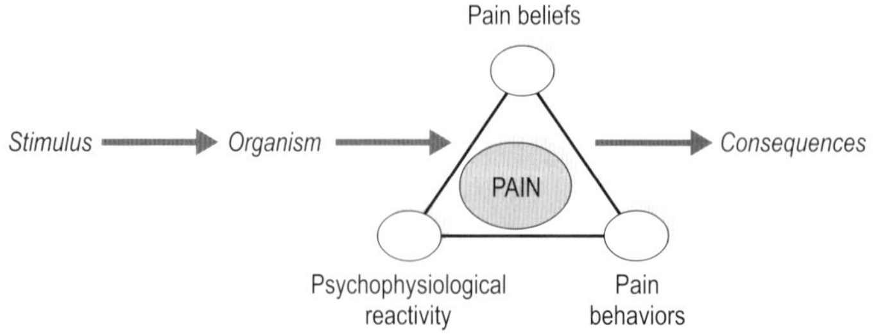

Fig. 32.1 Pain as a hypothetical construct, that can only be inferred by observable psychophysiological reactivity, pain cognitions, and pain behaviors. (Based on Öhman 1987 and Vlaeyen 1991.)

person suffers from pain. This behavior might vary considerably: painful grimace, moaning, taking pain medication, a disordered posture, bed rest, avoidance of and escape from activities, isolation, work leave, etc. It is highly likely that some of these have a communicative function. The origin of other behaviors is self-protective and recuperative (Williams 2002).

According to Fordyce, pain behaviors are likely to come under the control of short-term consequences through operant conditioning principles (Fordyce 1976). Acute pain elicits evolutionarily determined self-protective behaviors; when these are able to diminish pain, they are likely to increase in frequency. A patient who experiences that escaping activities reduces pain will stop doing those activities that produce pain and will avoid them on future occasions. Performing tasks during intense pain is a frustrating and difficult experience. Alternatively, others might criticize the patient because tasks are not performed as expected. By no longer performing these activities the patient might escape his or her own feelings of frustration and avoids criticism of others. The patient might also avoid some annoying tasks or responsibilities thanks to pain. In all the abovementioned situations, pain behavior is maintained through the avoidance of negative consequences, i.e. through negative reinforcement.

Pain behavior can also be maintained through positive reinforcement. Partners and family members might reinforce pain behavior by the way they give attention to the patient (Block 1981). Support and comprehension for the pain complaint by partners and family members should not, however, be banned. Pain behavior occurs less in patients who are adequately supported by family members. A possible explanation is that, in these families, not only are support and attention given in difficult situations, but also in situations without pain behavior or in situations in which the patient successfully copes with the pain. Indirect evidence for the role of positive reinforcement is provided by a study in which chronic pain patients were requested to perform physical tasks in the absence or presence of the spouse. In the presence of solicitous spouses, patients' pain behaviors increase, whereas the presence of punishing spouses tends to decrease pain behaviors compared to situations in which no spouses are present (Romano et al 1992).

A number of experimental studies have shown that verbal reports of pain intensity caused by repeated noxious stimuli of equal intensities can be modified through operant conditioning. Subjects who received verbal positive reinforcement from the experimenter after each trial if their report of pain intensity exceeded that of the previous trial reported significantly greater pain than the non-reinforced subjects (Jolliffe & Nicholas 2004). Of interest is that the effects of upward conditioning of pain reports appear to extinguish much more slowly in patients with chronic pain than in healthy controls (Flor et al 2002).

The general goal of the operant treatment approach is to increase healthy behaviors and activity levels, and to decrease pain behaviors and excess disability. For an extensive description we refer to Sanders (2002). In this treatment, (sometimes called graded activity), two important principles are followed: the establishment of baseline of the goal behaviors and the systematic and positive reinforcement of behaviors that are in line with those goals.

The treatment program always starts with a number of baseline trials in which the patient performs some exercises to the limit of tolerance ('until pain or discomfort make you stop'). The therapist then sets a quota of exercises to be performed each session. Initial quotas are below baseline levels but they are systematically increased towards a preset goal. During the treatment, a time-contingence between activity and rest is followed, rather than a pain-contingency. This means that the patient continues the activity until a certain amount of time has elapsed, and does not stop because of an increase in pain. In the preset exercise scheme, several moments of activity and rest are determined and, gradually, the activity levels are built up and the rest periods are reduced. Using such a time-contingency principle, the patient learns to work towards the preset agreements, despite the pain. When the patient reaches a preset goal, this is positively reinforced. The operant graded activity approach gives patients the opportunity to discover that they can perform much more than anticipated, despite the pain.

Because partners of patients can influence pain behavior to a considerable extent, they are involved as much as possible. They might be involved in a relatively intensive training in which they learn to identify pain behavior and healthy behavior and to pay more attention to the capabilities of their partner instead of pain behavior (Kole-Snijders et al 1999). They might also be involved in training the patient in communication skills to stimulate direct communication by the patient, at the expense of the indirect communicative function of pain behavior (Keefe et al 1999).

Psychophysiological reactivity

Emotional events, stress, and pain have an influence on physiological systems such as the heartbeat, respiration, and muscle tension. In many circumstances these psychophysiological reactions are adaptive and functional. In anxiety and fear, they are part of an energetic and motor preparation for fight and flight. When in pain, muscles become tightened to avoid further pain increases. Sustained muscle contraction is, however, accompanied by a reduction of oxygen in the muscles and a hypersensitivity of the receptors, which can paradoxically increase pain. A prolonged elevated muscle tension can cause pain, even long after the tension in the muscles is released. However, it is still unclear how important this mechanism is in the maintenance of pain problems.

Although the nature of the psychophysiological responses strongly depends on situational characteristics, strong and consistent individual differences exist in physiological reactions to stress. This phenomenon has been labeled response stereotypy. Response stereotypy has been extensively investigated in the chronic pain response. Indeed, a clinical hypothesis is that pain patients react to stressful situations with an automatic tensing of the muscles in the painful area. Although for a long time reliable data in favor of this hypothesis were lacking (Flor & Turk 1989), there are now several methodologically sound studies. Flor et al (1992) investigated the relationship between physiological parameters and both personally relevant and general stressors in several groups of chronic pain patients. Compared with nonpain patients, only patients with pain in the maxillary joint showed a stronger increase of the electromyographic (EMG) values of the maxillary joint muscles in the personal stress situation (talking about important life events). In particular, patients with CLBP responded by tensing the back muscles in the personal stress situation. This type of response stereotypy has also been shown to be associated with increased pain (Burns et al 1997).

The aim of relaxation exercises is to reduce muscle tension and psychophysiological reactivity. A commonly used technique is applied relaxation (Öst 1988), by which the patient learns to relax in an increasingly shorter span of time and, subsequently, to apply the relaxation response in diverse situations in which stress usually increases. Training can take place both individually and in groups, and consists of three phases: reconceptualization, skills training, and generalization. Skills training starts with progressive relaxation in which the patient learns to feel the difference between tensed and relaxed muscle groups, and progresses so that the patient can relax only the required muscle group. Thereafter, so-called cues are introduced. The goal of this phase is to bring about a conditioning between a cue (e.g. the word 'relax' or a visual stimulus) and the relaxed state. By means of these cues, the patient learns to execute the relaxation response during performance of daily activities, which facilitates generalization. Sometimes training is supported by EMG biofeedback (Donaldson et al 1994). To date, relatively little empirical support exists for the effectiveness of relaxation exercises with or without biofeedback, except for headache patients (Bogaards & ter Kuile 1994). One of the reasons for the limited effectiveness relates to the fact that most treatments pay too little attention to the implementation of the learnt relaxation response in personally relevant stressful situations. Therefore, it is necessary to determine the role of psychophysiologic stressors individually for all patients, so that specific treatment can be planned for each individual patient (Arena & Blanchard 2002).

Cognitive processes

The processes involved in making sense of pain are extensively elaborated in cognitive perspectives (Jensen et al 1999, Turk et al 1983). Cognitive processes have a substantial impact on pain. Attention is an important factor, but also the attributions and expectations about possibilities of control are of influence upon the pain experience.

Attention

It makes sense that pain interrupts ongoing activities and demands attention, even in situations when the current concern of the individual is not related to pain. Pain is an evolutionary signal of bodily threat that urges escape. Despite the fact that pain can be considered to be a 'false alarm' in many situations of chronic pain, pain continues to interrupt attention. Research has revealed that the interruptive quality of pain is amplified by its intensity, novelty, unpredictability, and threat value (Eccleston & Crombez 1999). Pain can also become the focus of attention because of its immediate relevance for the current goals of the individual. There are many examples in which the processing of pain-related information has priority and has immediate relevance for the goal of the individual. Patients might attempt to avoid the worsening of pain during physical activity. Patients might worry about the ineffectivity of previous medical interventions, and continue searching for other ways to manage their pain (Aldrich et al 2000). The feature these examples have in common is that the current goal of the individual is related to pain. In such situations, a hypervigilance to pain or pain-related information emerges (Crombez et al 2005). Attention is automatically shifted to pain or cues for pain (Peters et al 2002) and, once detected, attention dwells on pain and is difficult to disengage from (van Damme et al 2004). Hypervigilance to pain is largely automatic and emerges when pain has a high threat value. It is an unintentional and efficient process that occurs when the individual's current concern is to escape and avoid pain. Studies have revealed that attempts to suppress pain or fear can prove futile and might lead to a paradoxical increase of pain or anxious thoughts once the attempts at suppression are stopped (Koster et al 2003). Both the interruptive quality of pain and hypervigilance to pain are related to attributions about pain and expectations about the possibilities of having control of the situation.

Attributions and catastrophizing about pain

Attributions refer to the interpretation of events and the search for possible explanations of the complaints. For patients with chronic pain it is often difficult to make sense of the pain. Pain is of little diagnostic value for both the patient and the physician; pain is experienced as useless. Patients struggle with the 'mysterious' origin of their pain (Williams & Keefe 1991). Frequently, patients catastrophize about their pain. Although the criteria for catastrophizing about pain have never been explicitly stated, it has been broadly conceived of as an exaggerated negative orientation towards actual or anticipated pain experiences ('pain is the worst that can happen to me') (Sullivan et al 1995). Experimental studies have shown that a catastrophic style of thinking is related to higher pain intensity, worrying about pain, feelings of helplessness, and having difficulty directing attention away from the pain (Sullivan et al 2001). Catastrophizing about pain is also related to the personality characteristic negative affectivity, a general negative orientation towards oneself and the world. However, research has indicated that catastrophizing about pain is not always equated with this personality characteristic (Goubert et al 2004). Also, particular situations can facilitate catastrophizing about pain. Poor communication between patient and caregiver can, for example, give rise to catastrophizing about pain ('after many investigations the specialist still has not made a diagnosis; my condition will be so serious that he still has not dared to say something') (Houben et al 2005).

Expectations and perceived control

Self-efficacy is the confidence someone has in his or her own abilities to successfully perform specific tasks (Bandura 1977, Dolce et al 1986). This implies that the extent of self-efficacy varies according to the type of task. In this way, experienced self-efficacy for the performance of relaxation exercises might vary considerably from the self-efficacy for the performance of physical activities. Self-efficacy has been shown to be related to the extent to which patients suffer from their pain (Turner et al 2005).

Patients have expectations about which situations exacerbate pain and about the long-term consequences of pain. These expectations instigate avoidance behavior (Crombez et al 1998). A particular expectation in patients with chronic back pain is the fear of movement, which is (erroneously) assumed to be a possible cause of (re)injury (Vlaeyen et al 1995a). This is called 'kinesiophobia' (Kori et al 1990). The research findings on 'kinesiophobia' can be summarized as follows (see Vlaeyen & Linton 2000 for a review):

- In patients suffering from chronic musculoskeletal pain, pain-related fear is associated with impaired physical performance (Al-Obaidi et al 2000, Crombez et al 1999, Heuts et al 2004, Nederhand et al 2004, Vlaeyen et al 1995a) and increased self-reported disability (Asmundson et al 1997, Vlaeyen et al 1995b) (Fig. 32.2).
- In the open population, pain-related fear predicts future disability and health status (Buer & Linton 2002, Picavet et al 2002, Severeijns et al 2002).
- In patients with acute LBP, pain-related fear predicts future occupational disability (Fritz et al 2001).
- Educational interventions aimed at reducing negative attitudes and beliefs that mediate avoidance behavior reduce LBP-related absence from work (Buchbinder et al 2001, Moore et al 2000).

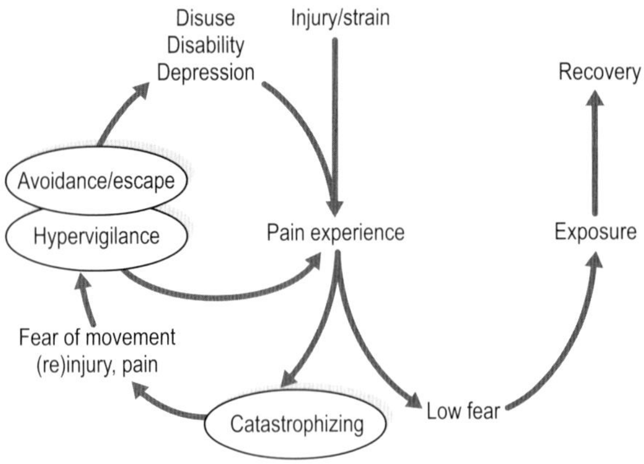

Fig 32.2 Cognitive–behavioral model of pain-related fear. If pain (e.g. caused by an injury or strain) is interpreted as threatening (pain catastrophizing), pain-related fear evolves. This leads to avoidance/escape, followed by disability, disuse and depression. The last will maintain the pain experiences, thereby fueling the vicious circle of increasing fear and avoidance. A more direct causal link between pain-related fear and pain is assumed to be mediated by hypervigilance. In patients who do not catastrophize, pain-related fear will probably not occur. These patients are likely to confront daily activities rapidly, leading to fast recovery. (Based on Vlaeyen et al 1995a, 1995b.)

Furthermore, Vowles & Gross (2003) found that work-specific fears were more important predictors of improved physical capability for work than changes in pain severity and fear of physical activity. Other studies found an association between fear-avoidance beliefs, work loss, and pain-related disability in both acute and chronic pain patients (e.g. Ciccone & Just 2001, Grotle et al 2004).

Reduction of pain-related fear in back pain

What treatment implications can be derived from the pain-related fear model? Peter Lang's (1979) bioinformational theory of fear predicts that two main conditions are needed to reduce fear: (1) the fear network needs to be activated; (2) new information needs to be available that disconfirms the fear expectations that are inherent to the fear memory. In clinical practice, several techniques are aimed at reducing fears in patients with chronic pain, with uneven success: verbal reassurance, education, physical exercise and/or graded activity, and exposure *in vivo* with behavioral experiments.

Verbal reassurance

Verbal reassurance generally consists of two classes of verbal cues: verbal statements intended to emotionally reassure patients directly, such as 'I wouldn't worry if I were you,' and verbal statements that indicate the absence of a medically relevant disease 'There is nothing wrong with your back' (Coia & Morley 1998). Doctors can tell their patients that they do not have the particular disease they fear, often supported by showing them negative test results, and sometimes by providing an alternative nondisease explanation such as stress, muscle pain, physical overuse. The major problem with verbal reassurance is its inherent ambiguity: 'How can it be that there is nothing wrong with my back and yet I still feel pain?' A surprisingly small number of studies have examined the effects of verbal reassurance and the overall conclusion is that it does not reduce fears and can even have paradoxical effects: in the long run, reassurance can increase fear in a number of patients (Donovan & Blake 2000, McDonald et al 1996). This is not surprising, as verbal reassurance does not activate the fear network (but rather attenuates it), and neither does it provide new information that disqualifies previous beliefs. What moderately fearful patients need is an explanation of their symptoms that is credible and that provides a better account for the current situation than the disease model. To achieve this in the area of chronic musculoskeletal pain, a number of researchers have developed education material aimed at modifying beliefs about hurting and harming.

Education

Another way of reducing levels of fear is providing new information about the irrationality of the feared consequences. Patients can be educated in such a way that they view their pain as a common condition that can be self-managed as a useful first step, rather than as a serious disease or a condition that needs careful protection. One of the major goals of the educational part is to increase the willingness of the patient to finally engage in activities they have been avoiding for a long time. The aim is to correct the misinterpretations and misconceptions that have occurred early on during the development of the pain-related fear. One study evaluated a booklet (the back book) especially designed for lay people in a group of patients consulting their family physician with a new pain episode (Burton et al 1999). Although there were no differences in pain, patients receiving the experimental booklet showed a statistically significant early improvement in beliefs; this was maintained at 1 year. A greater proportion of patients with an initially high pain-related fear who received the experimental booklet had clinically important reductions in pain-related fear at 2 weeks, followed by a clinically important improvement in their disability levels. Moore and colleagues examined the effects of a two-session group intervention for back pain patients in primary care that is based on education. Besides the group meeting, there was also one individual meeting and telephone conversation with the group leader, and with a psychologist experienced in chronic pain management (Moore et al 2000). The intervention was supplemented by educational materials (book and videos) supporting active management of back pain. A control group received usual care supplemented by a book on back pain care. Participants assigned to the self-care intervention showed significantly greater reductions in back-related worry and fear-avoidance beliefs than the control group. A population-based public health prevention program was carried out in Victoria, Australia (Buchbinder et al 2001). The program consisted of a large media campaign using television and radio commercials, printed advertisements, outdoor billboards, seminars, workplace visits and publicity articles using positive messages of back pain. Positive results for this unique project were found for back pain beliefs both among patients and among doctors, and a decline in number of claims for back pain, rates of days compensated and medical payments for claims for back pain. There is also evidence that sub-CLBP can be managed successfully with an approach that includes clinical examination combined with information for patients about the nature of the problem, provided in a manner designed to reduce fear and give them reason to resume light activity (Indahl et al 1998).

Physical exercise/operant-graded activity

Although most exercise and operant-graded activity programs were originally not designed to reduce pain-related fear, but rather to directly increase activity levels despite pain, these programs might have fear-reducing effects. A study by Mannion et al (1999) compared three sorts of active treatment: (1) modern active physiotherapy; (2) muscle reconditioning on training devices; and (3) low-impact aerobics. After therapy, significant reductions were observed in pain intensity, frequency, pain disability, pain catastrophizing, and pain-related fear. These effects were maintained over the subsequent 6 months, with the exception of the patients receiving physiotherapy, who increased their levels of pain-related fear and disability. A subsequent study suggested that the improvements are likely a result of the positive experience of completing the prescribed exercises without undue harm (Mannion et al 2001). Similar findings have been reported after an operant-graded activity program (Van Den Hout et al 2003).

Exposure *in vivo*

Philips (1987) was one of the first to argue for the systematic application of graded exposure to produce disconfirmations between expectations of pain and harm, the actual pain and the other consequences of the activity. She further suggested that:

> *These disconfirmations can be made more obvious to the sufferer by helping to clarify the expectations he/she is working with, and by delineating the conditions or stimuli which he feels are likely to fulfill his expectations. Repeated, graded, and controlled exposures to such situations under optimal conditions are likely to produce the largest and most powerful disconfirmations. (Philips 1987 p 279)*

Experimental support for this idea is provided by the match/mismatch model of pain, which states that people initially tend to overpredict how much pain they will experience but that after some exposures these predictions tend to be corrected to match with the actual experience (Rachman & Arntz 1991). A similar pattern was found in a sample of CLBP patients who were requested to perform four exercise bouts (two with each leg) at maximal force (Crombez et al 1996). During each exercise bout, the baseline pain, the expected pain, and experienced pain were recorded. As predicted, the CLBP patients initially overpredicted pain but, after repetition of the exercise bout, this overprediction was readily corrected. The expectancy did not seem to generalize to the exercise bout with the other leg as a small increase in pain expectancy re-emerged. Also, expectancies were immediately corrected after another performance. These findings have been replicated with two other physical activities: bending forward and straight leg raising (Goubert et al 2002).

In analogy with the treatment of phobias, graded exposure to back-stressing movements has been tested as a treatment approach for back pain patients reporting substantial fear of movement/(re)injury (for a detailed description of the exposure *in vivo* protocol, see Vlaeyen et al 2002b). In a first replicated single-case cross-over experiment, four CLBP patients who were referred for outpatient behavioral rehabilitation and who reported substantial fear of movement/(re)injury (TSK score > 40), were randomly assigned to one of two interventions (Vlaeyen et al 2001). In intervention A, patients received the exposure first, followed by operant-graded activity. In intervention B, the sequence of treatment modules was reversed. Daily measures of pain-related cognitions and fears were recorded with visual analog scales. Using time series analysis, we found that improvements only occurred during the exposure *in vivo*, and not during the graded activity, irrespective of the treatment order. Analysis of the pre–post-treatment differences also revealed that decreases in pain-related fear also concurred with decreases in pain catastrophizing and pain disability and in half of the cases also an increase in pain control. In a subsequent study, patients carried an ambulatory activity monitor at home for one week after each treatment module (Vlaeyen et al 2002b). Analyses revealed that decreases in pain-related fear again occurred at the introduction of the exposure module only. Additionally, these improvements concurred with decreases in pain disability, pain vigilance, and an increase in physical activity. In both studies, the exposure *in vivo* treatment was embedded in a multidisciplinary treatment program and this might have confounded the results. In two further studies, one of which was carried out in a different setting, the exposure *in vivo* was delivered as the sole treatment. Again, similar effects were found (Linton et al 2002, Vlaeyen et al 2002a). Because fear reductions occurred at the very beginning of the exposure treatment, during which education was also provided, a subsequent study was designed to disentangle the effects of education, graded activity, and graded exposure (de Jong et al 2005). After a 3-week no-treatment baseline measurement period, all patients received a psychoeducation session during which they were told that their pain was a common and benign condition that can be self-managed, rather than as a serious disease or a condition that needs careful protection, followed again by a 3-week no-treatment period. Then, random assignment to either 3-week exposure *in vivo* or 3-week graded activity occurred. Of interest was that psychoeducation reduced the reports of pain-related fear from all patients. However, fear was further reduced during exposure *in vivo*, but not during graded activity. Furthermore, perceived disability was not influenced by the educational session, and changed only during the exposure *in vivo* condition. These results suggest that education might reduce distress on a subjective level but that it does not change actual behaviors of the patients. Taken together, there is now preliminary evidence that graded exposure *in vivo* can be an effective treatment in patients with musculoskeletal pain who report substantial pain-related fear. Despite these promising results, interpretation should remain cautious because these studies had very small sample sizes. Randomized control trials with large samples and long-term follow-up measures are therefore warranted.

Summary

- As with other emotional experiences, pain is never directly observable in itself but can only be inferred through three observable systems: psychophysiological reactivity, overt pain behaviors, and cognitive processes about pain and pain control. A behavioral analysis specifies the causes and maintaining factors of overt behaviors, psychophysiological reactivity, and beliefs in terms of explicit environmental events that can be objectively identified and that are potentially manipulable.
- Pain disability occurs when individual goals are not met because of the pain, and can be subject to a graded shift from structural/mechanical to cognitive/environmental control. In back pain, this shift occurs quite rapidly, probably within 4–8 weeks. Similarly, the presence of demonstrable biomedical findings does not guarantee that psychological or social factors do not contribute to the level of pain disability.
- Avoidance behavior is postulated to be one of the core mechanisms in sustaining chronic pain disability. In the acute pain situation, avoidance of daily activities that increase pain is a spontaneous adaptive reaction of the individual; it usually allows the healing process to occur. In chronic pain patients, however, avoidance behavior appears to persist beyond

the expected healing time. Avoidance behavior can then be viewed as a dysfunctional response that promotes further disability, and a heightened awareness for somatic symptoms.

- Certain beliefs and expectations that patients hold about their pain influence the persistence of avoidance behavior. If the individual believes that further exposure to certain stimuli will increase pain, harm, and suffering, avoidance or escape will probably occur.
- Cognitive–behavioral approaches have been developed. These are not designed to remove pain, nor to teach patients how to be more stoic or let them believe that it is all in their mind. The aim is to decrease pain disability levels and to provide patients with the opportunity to learn and practice skills to cope better with pain. For this, behavioral and biomedical sciences are integrated in a transdisciplinary working model, characterized by active patient participation. These treatments appear effective and successful for a large number of patients.
- A specific group of patients is in need of a treatment for their pain that focuses on the irrational beliefs that pain is a signal of impending threat to the body. The associated fear of movement/(re)injury appears to play a pivotal role in the maintenance and exacerbation of chronic pain disability. Exposure-based treatments are developed to diminish the catastrophic cognitions and to gradually increase the activity levels of patients in line with their individual life goals. Such a treatment approach appears effective, although subsequent studies with larger samples and long-term follow-up data are needed.

References

Aldrich S, Eccleston C, Crombez G 2000 Worrying about chronic pain: vigilance to threat and misdirected problem solving. Behav Res Ther 38:457–470

Al-Obaidi SM, Nelson RM, Al-Awadhi S Al-Shuwaie N 2000 The role of anticipation and fear of pain in the persistence of avoidance behavior in patients with chronic low back pain, Spine 25:1126–1131

Arena JG, Blanchard EB 2002 Biofeedback for chronic pain disorders: a primer. In: Turk DC, Gatchel R (eds) Psychological approaches to chronic pain: a practitioner's handbook. The Guilford Press, New York, p159–186

Asmundson GJ, Norton GR, Allerdings MD 1997 Fear and avoidance in dysfunctional chronic back pain patients. Pain 69:231–236

Bandura A 1977 Self-efficacy: toward a unifying theory of behavioral change. Psychol Rev 84:191–215

Block AR 1981 Investigation of the response of the spouse to chronic pain behavior. Psychosom Med 43:415–422

Bogaards MC, ter Kuile MM 1994 Treatment of recurrent tension headache: a meta-analytic review. Clin J Pain 10:174–190

Buchbinder R, Jolley D, Wyatt M 2001 Population based intervention to change back pain beliefs and disability: three part evaluation. Br Med J 322:1516–1520

Buer N, Linton SJ 2002 Fear-avoidance beliefs and catastrophizing: occurrence and risk factor in back pain and ADL in the general population. Pain 99:485–491

Burns JW, Wiegner S, Derleth M et al 1997 Linking symptom-specific physiological reactivity to pain severity in chronic low back pain patients: a test of mediation and moderation models. Health Psychol 16:319–326

Burton AK, Waddell G, Tillotson KM, Summerton N 1999 Information and advice to patients with back pain can have a positive effect. A randomized controlled trial of a novel educational booklet in primary care. Spine 24:2484–2491

Ciccone DS, Just N 2001 Pain expectancy and work disability in patients with acute and chronic pain: a test of the fear avoidance hypothesis. The Journal of Pain 2:181–194

Coia P, Morley S 1998 Medical reassurance and patients' responses. J Psychosom Res 45:377–386

Crombez G, Vervaet L, Baeyens F et al 1996 Do pain expectancies cause pain in chronic low back patients? A clinical investigation. Behav Res Ther 34:919–925

Crombez G, Vervaet L, Lysens R et al 1998 Avoidance and confrontation of painful, back-straining movements in chronic back pain patients. Behav Modif 22:62–77

Crombez G, Vlaeyen JW, Heuts PH, Lysens R 1999 Pain-related fear is more disabling than pain itself: evidence on the role of pain-related fear in chronic back pain disability. Pain 80:329–339

Crombez G, Van Damme S, Eccleston C 2005 Hypervigilance to pain: an experimental and clinical analysis. Pain 116:4–7

de Jong JR, Vlaeyen JW, Onghena P et al 2005 Fear of movement/(re)injury in chronic low back pain: education or exposure in vivo as mediator to fear reduction? Clin J Pain 21:9–17

Deyo RA, Diehl AK, Rosenthal M 1986 How many days of bed rest for acute low back pain? A randomized clinical trial. N Engl J Med 315:1064–1070

Dolce JJ, Doleys DM, Raczynski JM et al The role of self-efficacy expectancies in the prediction of pain tolerance. Pain 27:261–272

Donaldson S, Romney D, Donaldson M, Skubick D 1994 Randomized study of the application of single motor unit biofeedback training to chronic low back pain. J Occ Rehab 4:23–37

Donovan JL, Blake DR 2000 Qualitative study of interpretation of reassurance among patients attending rheumatology clinics: 'just a touch of arthritis, doctor?' Br Med J 320:541–544

Eccleston C, Crombez G 1999 Pain demands attention: a cognitive-affective model of the interruptive function of pain. Psychol Bull 125:356–366

Flor H, Turk DC 1989 Psychophysiology of chronic pain: do chronic pain patients exhibit symptom-specific psychophysiological responses? Psychol Bull 105:215–259

Flor H, Schugens MM, Birbaumer N 1992 Discrimination of muscle tension in chronic pain patients and healthy controls. Biofeedback Self Reg 17:165–177

Flor H, Knost B, Birbaumer N 2002 The role of operant conditioning in chronic pain: an experimental investigation. Pain 95:111–118

Fordyce WE 1976 Behavioral methods for chronic pain and illness. Mosby, St Louis, MO

Fordyce WE, Fowler RS Jr, Lehmann JF, DeLateur BJ 1968 Some implications of learning in problems of chronic pain. J Chronic Dis 21:179–190

Fritz JM, George SZ, Delitto A 2001 The role of fear-avoidance beliefs in acute low back pain: relationships with current and future disability and work status. Pain 94:7–15

Goossens ME, Evers SM, Vlaeyen JW et al 1999 Principles of economic evaluation for interventions of chronic musculoskeletal pain. Eur J Pain 3:343–353

Goubert L, Francken G, Crombez G et al 2002 Exposure to physical movement in chronic back pain patients: no evidence for generalization across different movements. Behav Res Ther 40:415–429

Goubert L, Crombez G, Van Damme S 2004 The role of neuroticism, pain catastrophizing and pain-related fear in vigilance to pain: a structural equations approach. Pain 107:234–241

Grotle M, Vollestad NK, Veierod MB, Brox JI 2004 Fear-avoidance beliefs and distress in relation to disability in acute and chronic low back pain. Pain 112:343–352

Heuts PH, Vlaeyen JW, Roelofs J et al 2004 Pain-related fear and daily functioning in patients with osteoarthritis. Pain 110:228–235

Houben RM, Gijsen A, Peterson J et al 2005 Do health care providers' attitudes towards back pain predict their treatment recommendations? Differential predictive validity of implicit and explicit attitude measures. Pain 114:491–498

Indahl A, Haldorsen EH, Holm S, Reikeras O, Ursin H 1998 Five-year follow-up study of a controlled clinical trial using light mobilization and an informative approach to low back pain. Spine 23:2625–2630

Jensen MC, Brant-Zawadzki MN, Obuchowski N et al 1994 Magnetic resonance imaging of the lumbar spine in people without back pain [see comments]. N Engl J Med 331:69–73

Jensen MP, Romano JM, Turner JA et al 1999 Patient beliefs predict patient functioning: further support for a cognitive–behavioural model of chronic pain. Pain 81:95–104

Jolliffe CD, Nicholas MK 2004 Verbally reinforcing pain reports: an experimental test of the operant model of chronic pain. Pain 107:167–175

Keefe FJ, Caldwell DS, Baucom D et al 1999 Spouse-assisted coping skills training in the management of knee pain in osteoarthritis: long-term follow-up results. Arth Care Res 12:101–111

Klenerman L, Slade PD, Stanley IM et al 1995 The prediction of chronicity in patients with an acute attack of low back pain in a general practice setting. Spine 20:478–484

Kole-Snijders AM, Vlaeyen JW, Goossens ME et al 1999 Chronic low-back pain: what does cognitive coping skills training add to operant behavioral treatment? Results of a randomized clinical trial. J Consult Clin Psychol 67:931–944

Kori SH, Miller RP, Todd DD 1990 Kinesiophobia: a new view of chronic pain behavior. Pain Management Jan/Feb:35–43

Koster EH, Rassin E, Crombez G, Naring GW 2003 The paradoxical effects of suppressing anxious thoughts during imminent threat. Behav Res Ther 41:1113–1120

Lang PJ 1979 A bio-informational theory of emotional imagery. Psychophysiology 16:495–512

Linton SJ, Overmeer T, Janson M et al 2002 Graded in vivo exposure treatment for fear-avoidant pain patients with functional disability: a case study. Cog Behav Ther 31:49–58

Mannion AF, Muntener M, Taimela S, Dvorak J 1999 A randomized clinical trial of three active therapies for chronic low back pain. Spine 24:2435–2448

Mannion AF, Muntener M, Taimela S, Dvorak J 2001 Comparison of three active therapies for chronic low back pain: results of a randomized clinical trial with one-year follow-up. Rheumatology 40:772–778

McDonald IG, Daly J, Jelinek VM et al 1996 Opening Pandora's box: the unpredictability of reassurance by a normal test result [see comments]. Br Med J 313: 329–332

Moore JE, Von Korff M, Cherkin D et al 2000 A randomized trial of a cognitive–behavioral program for enhancing back pain self care in a primary care setting. Pain 88:145–153

Nachemson AL 1992 Newest knowledge of low back pain. A critical look. Clin Orthop 17:8–20

Nederhand MJ, Ijzerman MJ, Hermens HJ 2004 Predictive value of fear avoidance in developing chronic neck pain disability: consequences for clinical decision making. Arch Phys Med Rehabil 85:496–501

Öhman A 1987 The psychophysiology of emotion: an evolutionary–cognitive perspective. Adv Psychophysiol 2:79–127

Öst LG 1988 Applied relaxation: description of an effective coping technique. Scand J Behav Ther 17:83–96

Peters ML, Vlaeyen JW, Kunnen AM 2002 Is pain-related fear a predictor of somatosensory hypervigilance in chronic low back pain patients? Behav Res Ther 40: 85–103

Peters ML, Vlaeyen JW, Weber WE 2005 The joint contribution of physical pathology, pain-related fear and catastrophizing to chronic back pain disability. Pain 113:45–50

Philips HC 1987 Avoidance behaviour and its role in sustaining chronic pain. Behav Res Ther 25:273–279

Philips HC, Grant L 1991 The evolution of chronic back pain problems: a longitudinal study. Behav Res Ther 29:435–441

Picavet HS, Schouten JS 2003 Musculoskeletal pain in the Netherlands: prevalences, consequences and risk groups, the DMC(3) study. Pain 102:167–178

Picavet HS, Vlaeyen JW, Schouten JS 2002 Pain catastrophizing and kinesiophobia: predictors of chronic low back pain. Am J Epidemiol 156:1028–1034

Rachman S, Arntz AR 1991 The overprediction and underprediction of pain. Clin Psychol Rev 11:339–355

Romano JM, Turner JA, Friedman LS et al 1992 Sequential analysis of chronic pain behaviors and spouse responses. J Consult Clin Psychol 60:777–782

Sanders S 2002 Operant treatment. Back to basics. In: Turk DC, Gatchel R (eds) Psychological approaches to pain management. A practitioner's handbook. The Guilford Press, New York, p128–137

Severeijns R, van den Hout M, Vlaeyen J, Picavet H 2002 Pain catastrophizing and general health status in a large Dutch community sample. Pain 99:367

Sullivan MJ, Bishop SR, Pivik J 1995 The pain catastrophizing scale: development and validation. Psychol Assess 7:524–532

Sullivan MJ, Thorn B, Haythornthwaite JA et al 2001 Theoretical perspectives on the relation between catastrophizing and pain. Clin J Pain 17:52–64

Turk DC, Flor H 1999 Chronic pain: a biobehavioral perspective. In: Gatchel R, Turk DC (eds) Psychosocial factors in pain. Critical perspectives. Guilford Press, New York, p18–34

Turk DC, Meichenbaum D, Genest M 1983 Pain and behavioral medicine. A cognitive–behavioral perspective. Guilford Press, New York

Turner JA, Ersek M, Kemp C 2005 Self-efficacy for managing pain is associated with disability, depression, and pain coping among retirement community residents with chronic pain. J Pain 6:471–479

Van Damme S, Crombez G, Eccleston C 2004 Disengagement from pain: the role of catastrophic thinking about pain. Pain 107:70–76

Van Den Hout JH, Vlaeyen JW, Heuts PH et al 2003 Secondary prevention of work-related disability in nonspecific low back pain: does problem-solving therapy help? A randomized clinical trial. Clin J Pain 19:87–96

Verhaak PF, Kerssens JJ, Dekker J et al 1998 Prevalence of chronic benign pain disorder among adults: a review of the literature. Pain 77:231–23

Vlaeyen JW, Linton SJ 2000 Fear-avoidance and its consequences in chronic musculoskeletal pain: a state of the art. Pain 85:317–332

Vlaeyen JW, Snijders AM, Schuerman SA et al 1989 Chronic pain and the three-systems model of emotions: a critical examination. Tijdschrift voor Psychiatrie 31:100–113

Vlaeyen JW, Kole-Snijders AM, Boeren RG, van Eek H 1995a Fear of movement/(re)injury in chronic low back pain and its relation to behavioral performance. Pain 62:363–372

Vlaeyen JW, Kole-Snijders AMJ, Rotteveel AM et al 1995b The role of fear of movement/(re)injury in pain disability. Journal of Occupational Rehabilitation 5: 235–252

Vlaeyen JW, de Jong J, Geilen M et al 2001 Graded exposure in vivo in the treatment of pain-related fear: a replicated single-case experimental design in four patients with chronic low back pain. Behav Res Ther 39:151–166

Vlaeyen JW, de Jong J, Geilen M et al 2002a The treatment of fear of movement/(re)injury in chronic low back pain: further evidence on the effectiveness of exposure in vivo. Clin J Pain 18:251–261

Vlaeyen JWS, de Jong JR, Sieben JM, Crombez G 2002b Graded exposure in vivo for pain-related fear. In: Turk DC, Gatchel E (eds) Psychological approaches to pain management. A practitioner's handbook. Guilford Press, New York, p210–233

von Korff M 1994 Studying the natural history of back pain. Spine 19:2041S–2046S

Vowles KE, Gross RT 2003 Work-related beliefs about injury and physical capability for work in individuals with chronic pain. Pain 101:291–298

Vowles KE, Gross RT, Sorrell JT 2004 Predicting work status following interdisciplinary treatment for chronic pain. Eur J Pain 8:351–358

Waddell G 1987 Volvo award in clinical sciences. A new clinical model for the treatment of low-back pain. Spine 12:632–644

Waddell G 2004 The back pain revolution, 2nd edn. Churchill Livingstone, New York

Watson PJ, Booker CK, Moores L, Main CJ 2004 Returning the chronically unemployed with low back pain to employment. Eur J Pain 8:359–369

Williams AC 2002 Facial expression of pain: an evolutionary account. Behav Brain Sci 25:439–455, discussion 455–488

Williams DA, Keefe FJ 1991 Pain beliefs and the use of cognitive–behavioral coping strategies. Pain 46:185–90

PART FIVE

Section Two

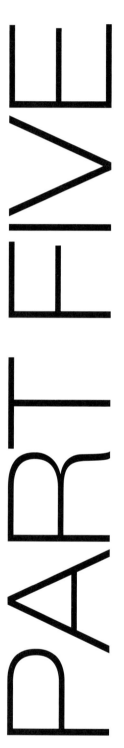

Effective training and treatment: Motor control

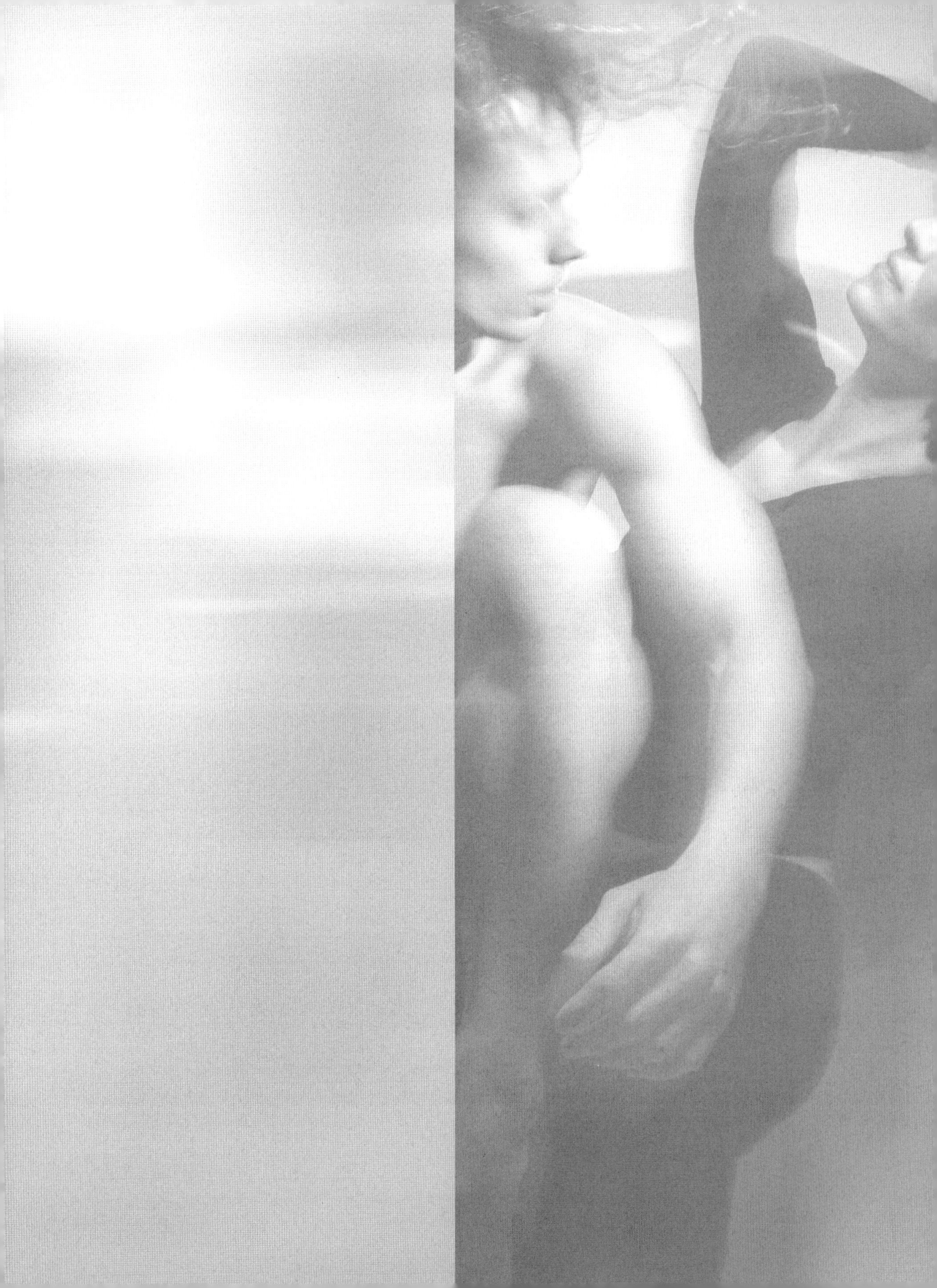

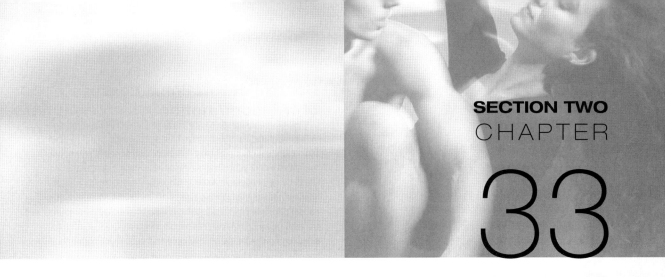

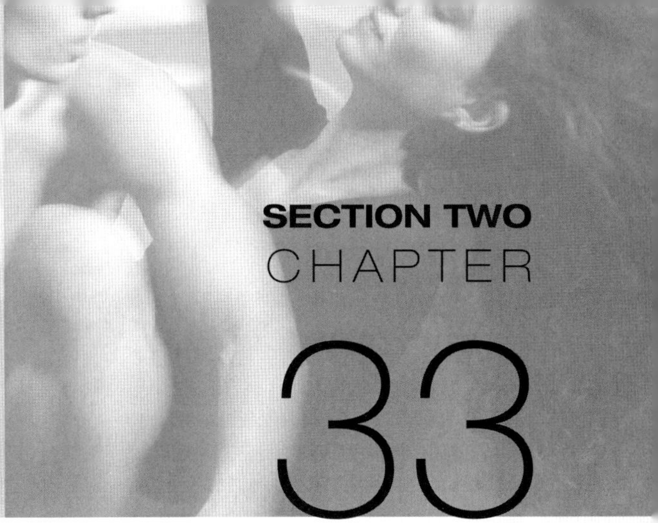

SECTION TWO
CHAPTER
33

Functional control of the spine

Paul W Hodges and Jacek Cholewicki

Introduction

Control of the function of the spine and pelvis is complex. It is well accepted that the spine is inherently unstable and depends on the contribution of muscles. In a static sense, stability is assured if the spine maintains or returns to an equilibrium position (i.e. point of minimum potential energy) if perturbed. In an unstable system, perturbation would induce movement away from an equilibrium position. To meet the demands placed on the spine, Panjabi (1992) recognized that lumbopelvic stability is dependent not only on the contribution of the passive elements (including the intervertebral discs, ligaments, joint capsules, and facet joints), but also on the active elements (muscles) and the controller (nervous system). In effect, stability is dependent on stiffness derived from passive structures and from active elements, and both are directly and indirectly dependent on activity controlled by the nervous system. Therefore, the concept of lumbopelvic stability should be discussed from the dynamical system point of view, which encompasses simultaneously both the spine and pelvis (plant) and the central nervous system (CNS) (controller).

The challenge for the controller is immense. The CNS must determine the requirements for stability and then plan appropriate strategies to meet those demands. In some circumstances the challenge is predictable and the CNS can plan or select strategies in advance, but when the challenge is unpredictable muscle activity must be initiated rapidly in response to the disturbance. Both situations are dependent on accurate proprioceptive information regarding the position and motion of the lumbar spine and pelvis and an accurate internal model(s) of the interaction between the body and forces. Our understanding of how the CNS meets these demands is based on data from empirical studies of response strategies and predictions from biomechanical models. Integration of the results from these somewhat divergent paradigms has led to confusion in the understanding of lumbopelvic control mechanisms. However, careful consideration of the available experimental data and their shortcomings as well as the limitations of the current modeling approaches could provide insight into the complexity of the system and help reconcile the field.

There are six degrees of freedom at each intervertebral segment (three rotations and three translations) and buckling of the spine can involve any combination of these. Conventional models of spine stability consider control of rotations, without consideration of the control of translations. Although the models have provided critical data to understand spinal stability, they do not provide a complete understanding of functional control of the spine. Thus differences in strategies of muscle activity to maintain stability predicted from modeling and muscle activity recorded in empirical studies may be at least partly explained on the basis of modeling limitations.

Further problems arise when considering the control of the spine during movement. Current models are static and cannot deal with the stability of the spine when it moves through an intended trajectory. For instance, if the spine is moving and is perturbed from the intended trajectory, the CNS must respond not only to control buckling of the spine but also to return the spine to the intended path, i.e. it must maintain the stability of the motion. To fully understand spine function as a dynamical system, the CNS must be modeled with equal diligence as the spine. Adding further complexity is the possibility that the CNS must also integrate the necessity for spinal movement associated with respiration and postural equilibrium, in conjunction with meeting the relatively simple demands for spinal stability. Each of these factors is important to consider when interpreting the coordination of trunk muscle activity to meet the demands of optimal function of the lumbar spine and pelvis.

The purpose of this chapter is to consider the requirements for functional control of the spine and to expand the concept of stability to encompass dynamic situations, beyond the limitations of the current models. From this perspective, it might be easier to consider how this control can be modified in low back and pelvic pain, and what the implications for rehabilitation of these disorders are.

Control of rotational degrees of freedom/motion

A key factor in the control of spinal stability is the prevention of buckling. When all of the muscles are removed, the spine buckles with compressive load of as little as 90 N (~9 kG) (Crisco et al 1992). This finding indicates that the spine is vulnerable to such loading and emphasizes the importance of the muscle and control systems. Numerous studies have modeled the control of buckling forces to estimate stability and muscular contributions to stability (Bergmark 1989, Cholewicki & McGill 1996, Crisco & Panjabi 1991, Gardner-Morse et al 1995, Granata et al 2001). In general, these models have considered control of buckling in terms of rotational degrees of freedom around three orthogonal axes (Fig. 33.1A). On the basis of these

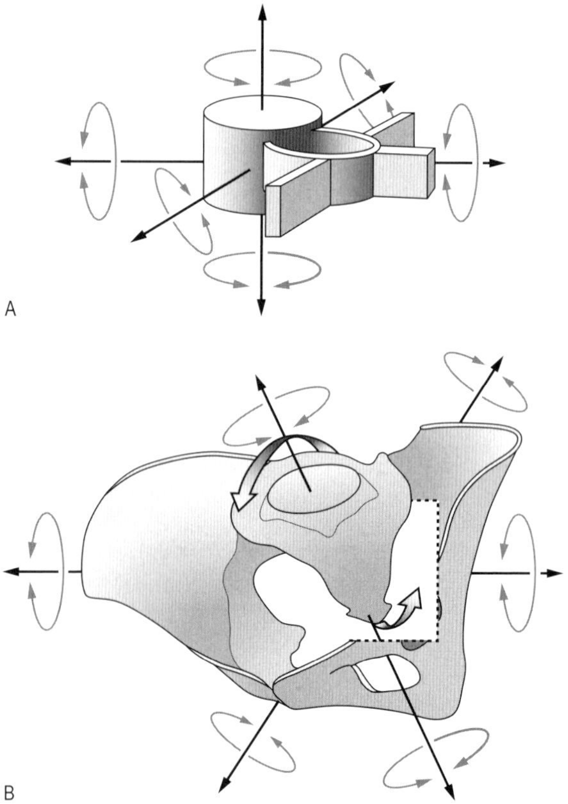

A

B

Fig. 33.1 (A) Optimal spinal control requires consideration of all six degrees of freedom (three rotations and three translations). (B) Control of the pelvis involves control of six degrees of freedom of pelvic motion as well as the control of the translations and rotations between the segments of the pelvis including the sacroiliac joints.

models it has been argued that stability depends on the contribution of muscles that act as 'guy ropes' (Crisco & Panjabi 1991). Activity of these muscles is clearly essential to maintain the stability of the spine and to prevent buckling behavior in response to loading (Fig. 33.2).

Simultaneous coactivation of many muscle groups increases spine stiffness (Cholewicki et al 1997, Gardner-Morse & Stokes 1998, Granata & Marras 2000). Several investigators have attempted to identify the relative contributions of different muscles to the control of stability as defined by such models. A range of approaches have been used: prediction of patterns of spine deformation due to changes in muscle activity (Gardner-Morse et al 1995), and comparison of relative contribution of muscles via a knockout procedure (Cholewicki & Van Vliet 2002), and comparison of stability between muscles that cross many versus few segments (Crisco & Panjabi 1991). Although these studies suggest that the antagonist co-contraction of large muscles that act as 'guy ropes' provide a critical contribution, the general outcome is that many muscles contribute to stability and the relative contribution varies with many factors, including the task, posture, and moment direction. Notably, sufficient stiffness can be achieved, at least in neutral posture, with minimal levels of co-contraction of abdominal and paraspinal muscles (Cholewicki et al 1997).

In terms of motor control, the nervous system is likely to coordinate muscle activity in a carefully planned sequence to match the internal and external forces placed on the spine. During high load tasks, such as lifting (Cholewicki et al 1991), and other strong trunk exertions (Zetterberg et al 1987), significant co-contraction of antagonist trunk muscles is expected and observed. Similar patterns of co-contraction have been identified in tasks in which the load is unpredictable (van Dieen & de Looze 1999) and when the potential risk (or perceived risk) to the spine is greater, such as when tasks are performed by people with low back pain (LBP) (Radebold et al 2000).

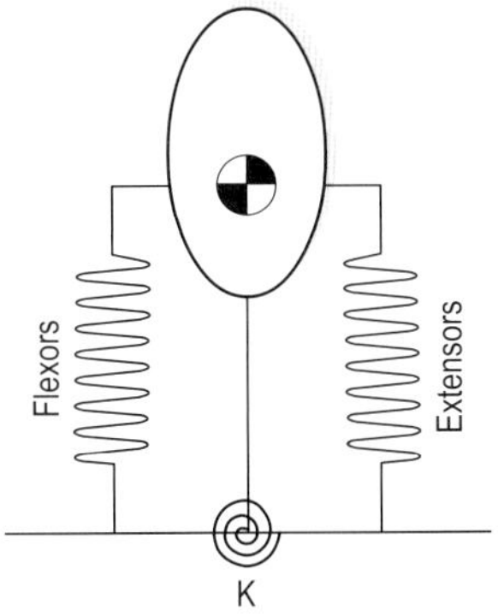

Fig. 33.2 Simple model of co-contraction of antagonist muscles and passive spine stiffness (K) to control stability of a motion segment.

Although antagonist co-contraction is sufficient to achieve static stability, more complex patterns of muscle activity have been observed in many situations, particularly in those involving movement. In these tasks the CNS must carefully balance the internal and external forces with an 'adaptive' strategy of muscle activity that allows a movement along the intended trajectory while resisting any perturbations. For instance, during walking, rather than maintaining tonic unchanging activity of the trunk muscles throughout the gait cycle, the activity of most muscles is modulated such that greatest activity occurs in conjunction with foot strike when reactive forces are greatest (Fig. 33.3). Other peaks of muscle activity occur at times of maximal trunk rotation (Saunders et al 2005). In another example, during shoulder flexion, which imposes a reactive moment on the trunk causing it to flex, the trunk muscles do not co-contract to increase stiffness of the spine, which would be a valid strategy for increasing stability in a static sense, but instead they respond in a triphasic manner with alternating flexor and extensor bursts of activity to match the moments imposed on the spine, which is an appropriate strategy to assure stability in a dynamic sense (Hodges & Richardson 1997, Hodges et al 1999) (Fig. 33.4). Clearly, controlled activation of a group of muscles is critical. However, as existing models consider control of stability in terms of rotations at an instant in time (quasi static), and omit other elements of stability such as the control of translations and control of motion, these models are unlikely to provide full explanation for all strategies utilized by the CNS to meet the various demands imposed on the spine.

One factor that is difficult to explain by existing models is the potential contribution of the deeply placed muscles such as transversus abdominis (Hodges & Richardson 1997) and multifidus (Hides et al 1996, Kaigle et al 1997). Activity of these muscles is consistently identified as a component of the strategies implemented by the CNS in association with perturbations to the spine and pelvis. Recent data suggest that when the potential contribution of these muscles to spinal control is modeled in terms of the control of rotation buckling of the spine, their contribution is limited, particularly when transversus abdominis is modeled as a trunk flexor

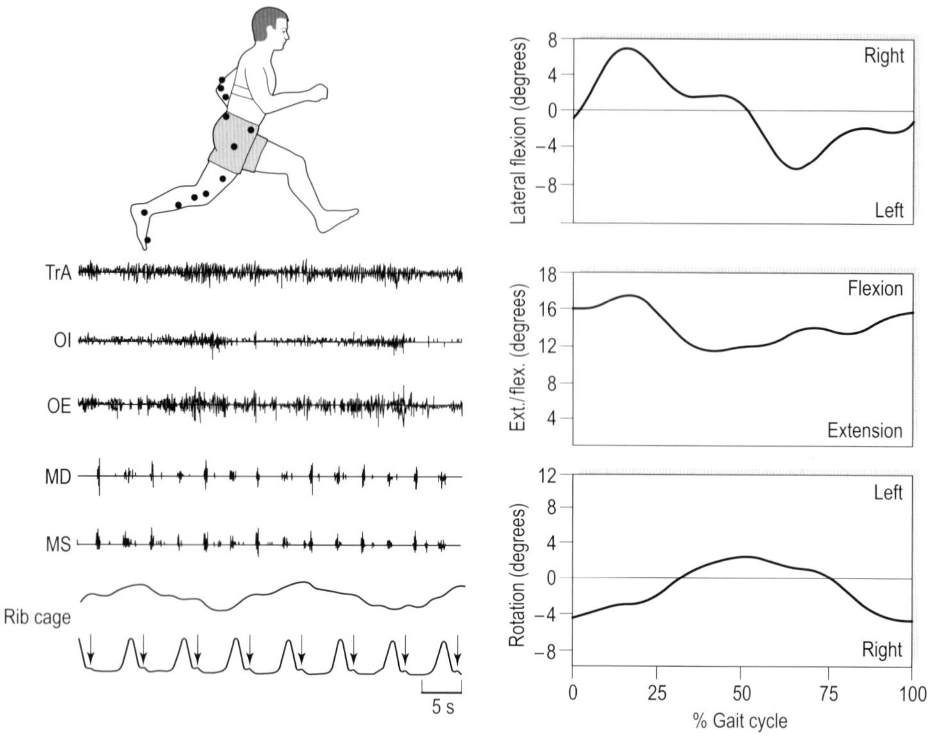

Fig. 33.3 During locomotor tasks, movement of the lumbar spine and pelvis is required to contribute to propulsion of the body, shock absorption, and control of energy expenditure. This motion is controlled not by simple co-contraction of large trunk muscles, but by a carefully timed sequence of muscle activity that is matched to the demands of the movement (direction and force). MD, multifidus deep fibers; MS, multifidus superficial fibers; OE, obliquus exernus abdominis; OI, obliquus internus abdominis; TrA, transversus abdominis. (Adapted from Saunders et al 2004b, 2005.)

or lateral flexor (Kavcic et al 2004). However, when control of rotation is studied *in vivo* in pigs when additional effects of increased tension in the middle layer of the thoracolumbar fascia (Barker et al 2006, Hodges et al 2003a) and increased intra-abdominal pressure (Hodges et al 2003a, 2003b), contraction of transversus abdominis has been found to have an effect on control of intervertebral motion (Fig. 33.5). However, it is important to point out that there are some limitations to these experimental studies as well. It is difficult to separate whether decreased spine motion resulted from the stiffer spine or from the changes in end conditions, such as the stiffer abdominal content. However, as stiffness of the abdominal content is modulated by contraction of these muscles, their action provides a direct or indirect control of spine stability.

As well as the smaller contribution of these muscles to spinal stability in terms of control of rotational buckling, there might be other advantages for the CNS to include activity of these muscles. For instance, most trunk muscles also generate variable amounts of torque around different spinal levels. If the configuration of the spine is to be maintained, then the torque resulting from contraction of a muscle must be counteracted by co-contraction with an antagonist muscle. For this reason the CNS might, at times, utilize activity of the deep muscles to provide a simplified means to influence stability at a single level without the control problem of coordinating activity of multiple muscles. Furthermore, numerous functions such as breathing and balance are potentially compromised by co-contraction of larger trunk muscles and provision of some control by the deeper muscle may be advantageous (see below). An additional consideration is that it is well recognized that muscle attachment to each segment is critical for control of intersegmental buckling (Bergmark 1989, Crisco & Panjabi 1991). If a single segment is left with no muscle attachment, despite strong contraction of the superficial muscles, the spine as a system is

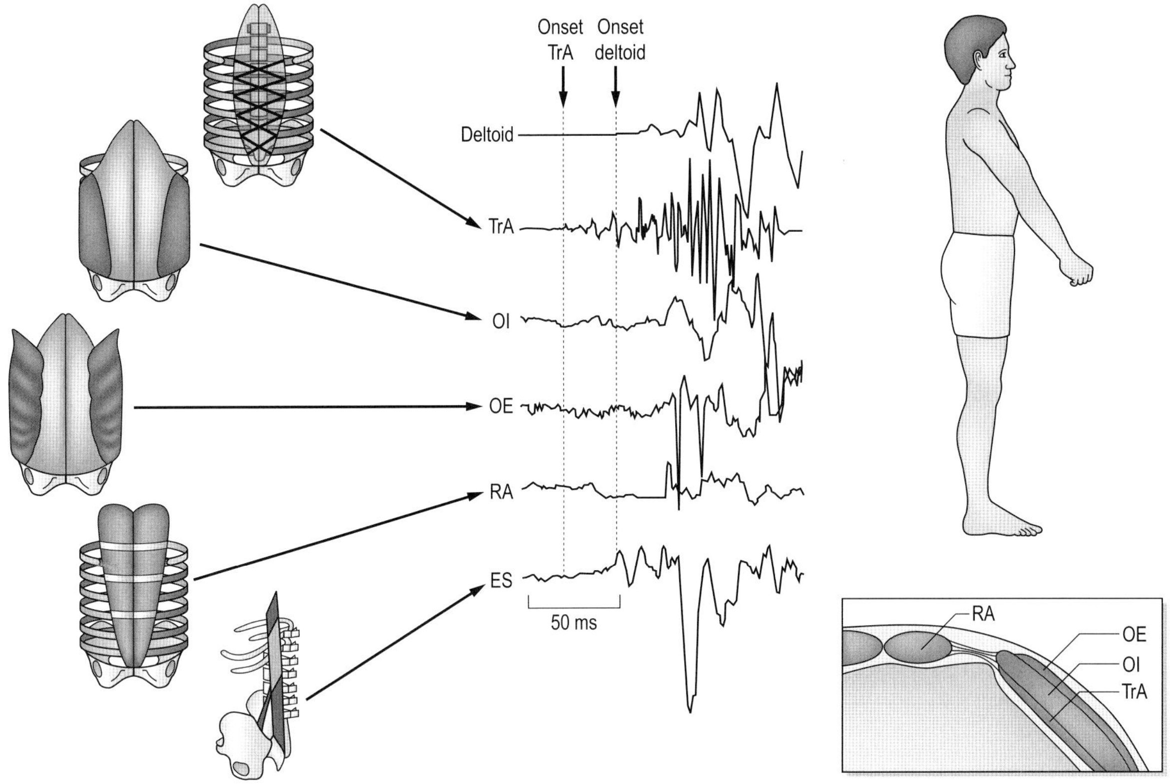

Fig. 33.4 In association with rapid movement of an arm, activity of the trunk muscles does not involve simple co-contraction, but instead muscle activity is carefully sequenced to balance the demands for dynamic stability of the spine. This strategy involves early activity of transversus abdominis (TrA) and early activity of the trunk extensors (erector spinae: ES) to control the flexion moment acting on the trunk. ES, erector spinae; OE, obliquus exernus abdominis; OI, obliquus internus abdominis; RA, rectus abdominis. (Adapted from Hodges & Richardson 1997.)

not controllable and cannot be stabilized (Crisco & Panjabi 1991). Finally, it is possible that stiffness, rather than motion of each intervertebral joint, is fine-tuned by the deep paraspinal muscles, so that when large trunk muscles exert different moments at different spinal levels, a uniform motion of the entire spine results.

Control of translations

Translations in the intervertebral joints, as components of possible buckling modes, must be also controlled (see Fig. 33.1A). For instance, radiological studies of motion of the centers of rotation of the lumbar segments have identified that people with clinical signs of instability exhibit abnormal translation relative to rotation as compared to healthy individuals (Schneider et al 2005). Control of translations is particularly important for the stability of the joints of the pelvis, chiefly the sacroiliac joints (SIJs), which are exposed to considerable shear forces due to their orientation and the requirement to transfer loads from the sacrum to the ilia (Snijders et al 1995) (see Fig. 33.1B). Passive mechanisms do contribute to control of translations. For instance, the direction of the facet joints in the lumbar spine resists posteroanterior translation in standing (except in individuals with spondylolisthesis). In the pelvis, the wedge shape of the SIJs, the undulated nature of the joint surfaces, and the high friction coefficient of the cartilage all play a part in the control of downward translation of the sacrum in upright postures (Snijders et al 1995). However, contribution of muscles is essential (Snijders et al 1995).

Due to the mathematical complexity of additional degrees of freedom, translational motions have not been included in the existing models of spine stability. It is well accepted that few muscles

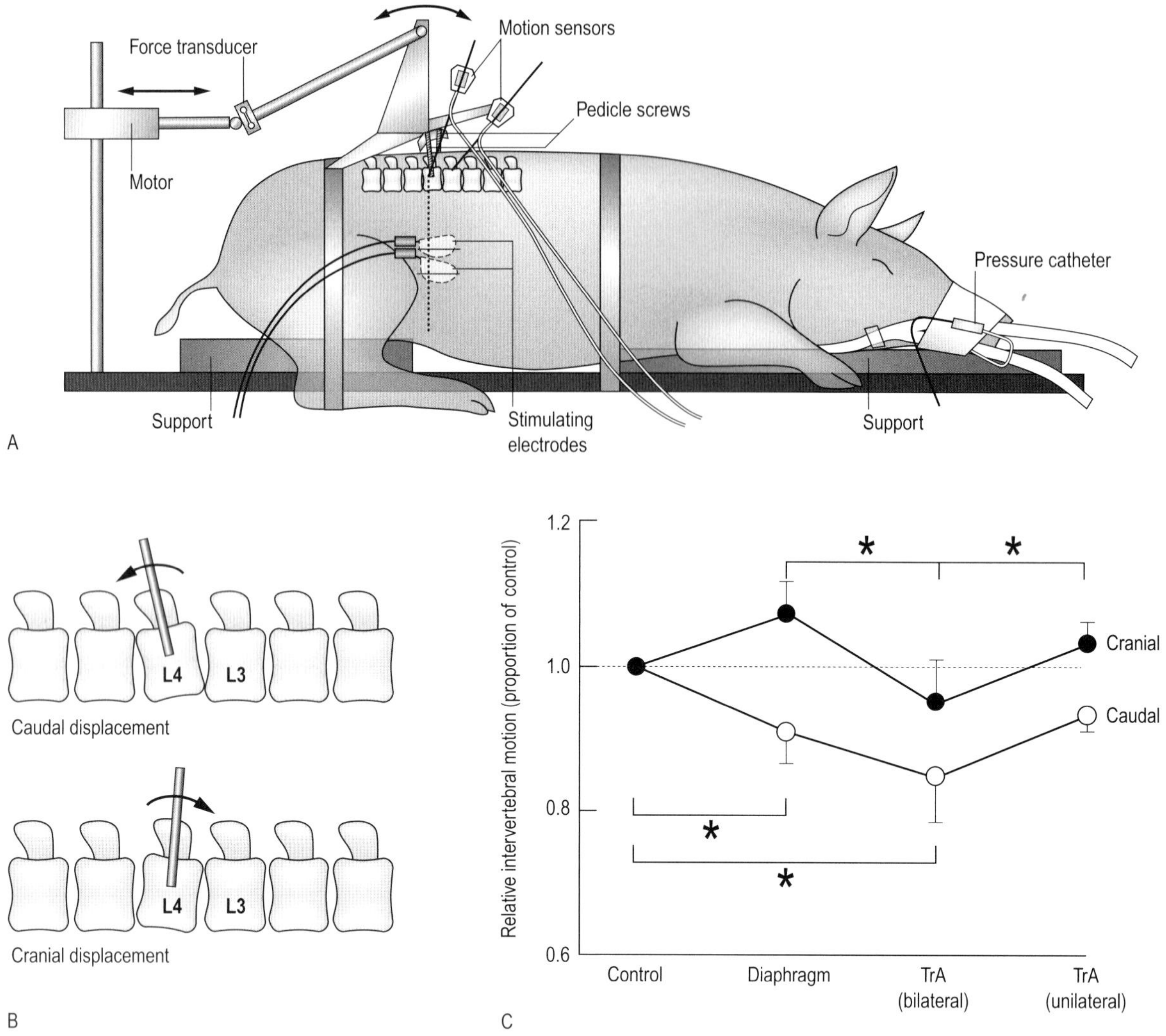

Fig. 33.5 Activity of transversus abdominis (TrA) and the diaphragm, when stimulated electrically in pigs, reduces the relative intervertebral motion of the spine. (A) The L4 vertebra was rotated with a motor attached to pedicle screws. Motion of L3 and L4 was recorded with movement sensors attached to the spinous processes. (B) Caudal and cranial displacement was applied. (C) Relative intervertebral motion was reduced during caudal displacements with diaphragm and bilateral TrA activity. With cranial displacement, diaphragm, but not TrA activity increased relative intervertebral motion. This difference in response is likely to be due to the effect of the attachment of TrA via the thoracolumbar fascia. (Reproduced with permission from Hodges et al 2003a.)

have an ideal moment arm to control translations (Bogduk 1997) due to their longitudinal orientation, perpendicular to the direction of translation. In general, it has been regarded that many trunk muscles possess a small force vector component in the translation direction and therefore have some potential to control shear motion (Potvin et al 1991). In addition, the activity of trunk muscles, aiming to control rotation, and body mass also exert compression force, which stiffens the spine and helps control translations (Gardner-Morse & Stokes 2001, Janevic et al 1991). Further consideration of these issues has been limited.

Although spine compression from co-contraction of large trunk muscles can provide an adequate solution in some circumstances, it might not be an ideal strategy in all situations. One issue to consider is that intervertebral translation at a single segment cannot be controlled by co-contraction of larger superficial muscles as these muscles cross several levels. In this case, if the CNS increases muscle activity to an extent sufficient to maintain control of translation at a specific segment, all other levels are compressed to a similar extent. This has possible consequences for spinal movement and other functions such as balance and respiration. Second, excessive or sustained compressive load on the spine for an extended period has been argued to lead to changes in passive elements of the spine (Adams et al 1996) and increased risk for LBP (Kumar 1990, Norman et al 1998). Third, if co-contraction is utilized to control translations, this is likely to stiffen the trunk and reduce movement, which might be required for other functions.

Although co-contraction of the large superficial muscles contributes to control of translations, contraction of muscles such as the diaphragm, transversus abdominis, and multifidus might provide an alternative or supplementary strategy. Recent data suggest that increased intra-abdominal pressure from contraction of the muscles of the abdominal wall (diaphragm, transversus abdominis, pelvic floor) increases the stiffness of the spine to a posteroanterior translation in humans (Hodges et al 2005c, Shirley et al 2003) and pigs (Hodges et al 2003b). Furthermore, tension of the middle layer of the thoracolumbar fascia in human cadaver spines reduces intervertebral translations due to flexion/extension loading of the spine (Guggenheim & Barker, unpublished observations). From another perspective, the deeper fibers of multifidus have the potential to provide compression over two intervertebral joints, which can provide a mechanism for more selective increases in control of intervertebral translation. Panjabi (1992) considered this to be a major advantage to the CNS. A key advantage of utilization of these muscles by the CNS to contribute to control of translation is that, as mentioned above, they produce minimal torque and thus can provide a simple solution to control translation without the complexities involved in control of unwanted torques. However, the above-outlined mechanisms still await detailed biomechanical calculations to verify their efficacy and to estimate the magnitude of their effects.

Dynamic control of the lumbar spine and pelvis

A key limitation to the current understanding of control of the spine function is that few tasks involve static control of the spine. Even during quiet standing the spine is continually moving. For instance numerous studies have identified small repetitive motions of spine and pelvis in association with breathing, which is thought to counteract the disturbance to postural equilibrium caused by breathing (Gurfinkel et al 1971, Hodges et al 2002). Thus in most spine functions, a dynamic control of stability must be considered, rather than static equilibrium. That is, the CNS must control the stability of the spine's trajectory through which it travels and prevent excessive deviations from this trajectory due to perturbations from internal and external forces.

Current models consider the stability of the spine in a static sense and not when the spine is moving through an intended trajectory. The demands and strategies for controlling stability of a static equilibrium versus stability of motion are rarely the same. For instance, at a moment in time during trunk flexion, static models might predict that antagonist co-contraction is required to optimize stability; however, such a strategy could limit the intended path of the trunk motion into flexion (Fig. 33.6). Thus ideal control of the spine will require control of the muscles of the spine and pelvis in a dynamic sense to match the demands for stable movement.

At this point it is important to expand the concept of stability to dynamic situations to provide a common base for further discussion. Unlike the stability of a static system, in which the maintenance of a static equilibrium configuration is concerned, the stability of a dynamic system deals with constancy of the intended trajectory through which the system is moving. In general terms, a trajectory is defined by a time series of variables that describe the state of the system. In kinematic terms, these variables will be position, velocity, and acceleration at each degree of freedom of each intervertebral joint, in a spine example. However, trajectory can also include other variables that describe dynamic systems, such as temperature or pressure. Thus, let us define stability of a dynamic system as the ability to maintain the desired trajectory despite kinetic, kinematic, or control disturbances. It is important to point out that this definition is inclusive of static situations, in which the desired trajectory is reduced to a fixed configuration. Thus, in a lumbopelvic example, a trajectory might be the desired or necessary motion (position, velocity, and acceleration) in all intervertebral joints to accomplish a certain task. Stability of such a system will determine how far the variables describing the motion will deviate

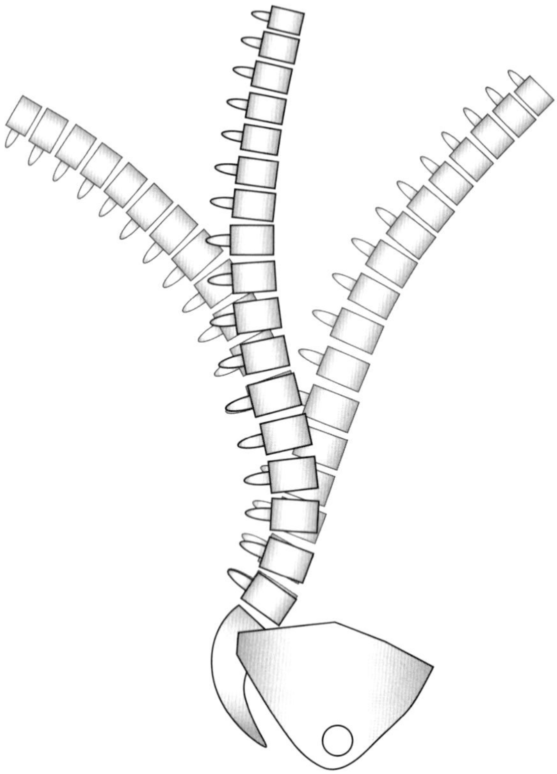

Fig. 33.6 Dynamic control of the spine involves control of the trajectory of spinal motion. Note that the concept of intervertebral buckling is encompassed by the concept of stability of motion, as the intervertebral kinematics describe (system's state variables) the intended trajectory.

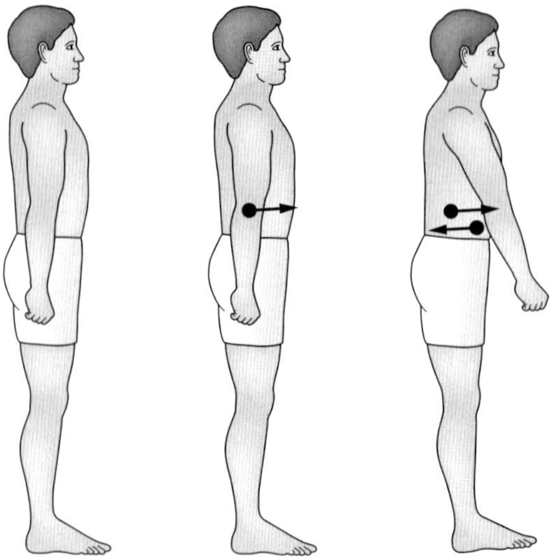

Fig. 33.7 In a dynamic system the nervous system can use the inertia of body segments to assist with the control of stability. Prior to movement of a limb, early activity of the paraspinal muscles initiates a trunk extension movement that may accelerate the trunk forwards such that the inertia of the body helps oppose the reactive moments from the arm movement.

from their intended values. An example is gait, which can be described very precisely by a series of angles, velocities, and accelerations at various joints. A perturbation, such as a slip or trip, will disturb this pattern. In a stable situation, the controller (the CNS) will quickly restore the movements to the original pattern. The stability might be lost when the perturbation is too large or the controller is inadequate and the intended kinematic trajectory will not be restored (e.g. fall).

Adjustment of stiffness via muscle activity (e.g. co-contraction of antagonist trunk muscles) is the only parameter available to control spine stability in a static sense. In dynamic situations, inertia and damping also contribute to the system's impedance to perturbations in addition to stiffness. As a result, many more control strategies are available to the CNS to assure stability of the desired spine motion or configuration. For example, the CNS might use inertia to control stability of the spine.

An illustration of this idea comes from studies of arm movement. When a limb is moved, reactive moments are imposed on the trunk that are equal in amplitude but opposite in direction to those of the moving limb (Belenkii et al 1967, Bouisset & Zattara 1981). Prior to such movements, the CNS initiates a pattern of muscle activity of the trunk and lower limbs to prepare the body for the perturbation from these moments. This strategy involves activity of trunk muscles. For instance, activity of the paraspinal muscles precedes that of the deltoid muscle of the arm to prepare the trunk for the reactive flexion moment from the arm movement (Aruin & Latash 1995, Belenkii et al 1967, Hodges & Richardson 1997). An important observation is that this activity does not just stiffen the spine, but also moves the spine into extension prior to the onset of the movement (Fig. 33.7). Momentum of the trunk in the opposite direction provides a logical strategy to utilize the inertia of the trunk to counteract the reactive forces and limit the motion of the trunk into flexion.

Furthermore, allowing the spine to have some 'give' to move rather than simple stiffening might reduce the reaction forces arising from displacement perturbations. If a displacement (or energy) perturbation is imposed on a stiff spine, the reaction force

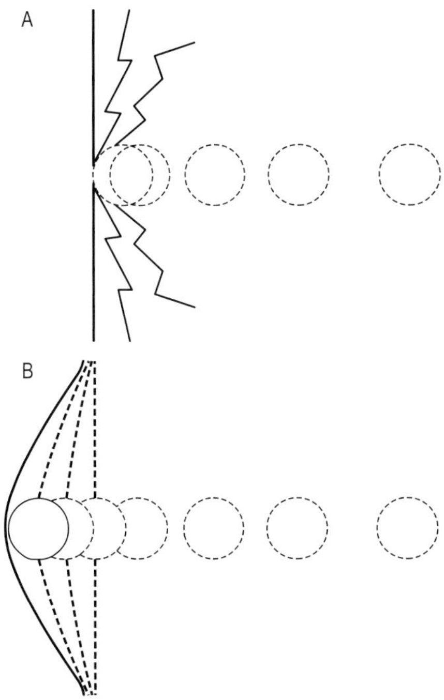

Fig. 33.8 'Give' in the spine is likely to help reduce the impact of imposed perturbations. When a ball hits a stiff surface, the resultant force is applied over a short period of time with high peak load. If instead the ball hits a flexible surface, the same energy is applied, but the resultant force is distributed over a longer time and the peak load is reduced. Via this mechanism, having 'give' in the spine rather than maximal stiffness, provides a different strategy to reduce the impact of perturbations on the spine.

will be high. However, if the same perturbation is applied to a flexible spine, the peak reaction force will be reduced (Fig. 33.8). Consider a skyscraper; if the building is stiff, when an earthquake strikes the building will topple. However, if the foundation is flexible, allowing the building to move, the building will remain standing. Function of the spine as a flexible column, rather than a stiff rod, is critical to absorb and dissipate energy imposed on the spine by external perturbations and to maintain optimal spinal function. Recent data suggest that when people with recurrent LBP perform arm movements they are less likely to use movement (or inertia strategy) to prepare for perturbations, and as a result have greater resultant displacement of the spine (Mok et al 2004a).

An additional consideration is that movement may also reduce the energy demands of a task. For instance, during walking vertical displacement of the center of mass is limited by motion of the pelvis and spine. Failure to allow movement to control displacement of the center of mass would increase the energy demands of the task (Perry 1992). Thus, stable movement rather than simple stiffening of the spine presents a number of benefits to the CNS, including improved energy absorption and energy efficiency. Many other movement strategies could be utilized by the CNS to contribute to the optimal dynamic control of the spine, which we are only beginning to understand.

Selection of response strategy

To meet the challenges of constantly changing demands in dynamic control of the spine and pelvis, the CNS must utilize varying strategies to move and control movement of the trunk. The relative contribution of muscles to spine stability changes constantly, based on the demands of the task. During walking, the constant modulation of EMG activity of the trunk muscles provides an illustration of this control. Alternating activity of the trunk muscles produces and controls movement in each plane in conjunction with satisfying the mechanical demands to progress the body forwards and to control internal and external forces on the trunk (Saunders et al 2005). It might also be desirable to tune the overall trunk stiffness to synchronize its natural frequency to the frequency of a repetitive task such as walking or running. Thus, a number of factors are likely to contribute to the selection of strategy for optimal control.

The selection of appropriate control strategies by the CNS is likely to be associated with the real or perceived risk to the spine. Spinal stiffening by co-contraction of antagonist trunk muscles, which represents one end of the spectrum of options for control of dynamic stability of the spine, provides a simple solution for the CNS to control the demands for spinal stability (Fig. 33.9). In contrast, dynamic control of movement requires much more careful precision of the timing and pattern (muscles and amplitude) of muscle activity. As a result, dynamic control of the spine has a greater potential for error. Thus in situations of high real or perceived risk to the spine, the CNS might opt to limit the possibility of error and utilize a strategy to stiffen the spine and increase the 'safety margin.' Although this might have consequences, such as the potential for greater resultant displacements, as described above, the potential for the error is reduced. In contrast, when the real or perceived risk to the spine is low the CNS could opt to use a more versatile strategy involving

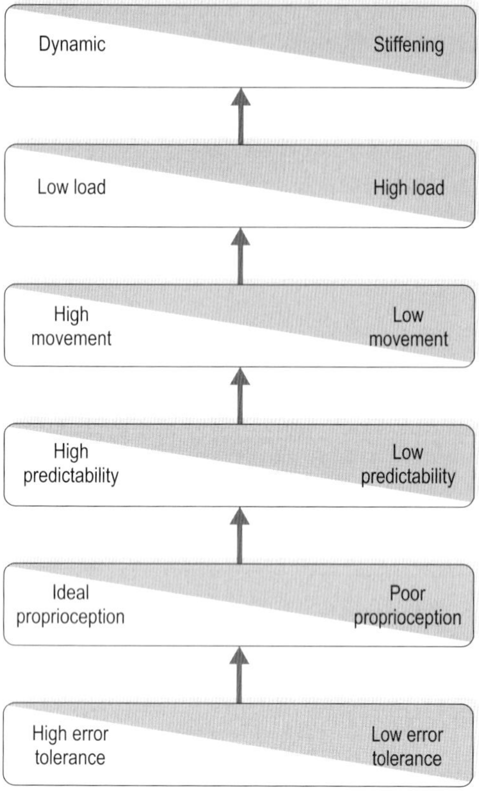

Fig. 33.9 Dynamic control of the spine involves a spectrum of control strategies that range from co-contraction stiffening to more dynamic control strategies that involve carefully timed muscle activity and movement. Multiple factors such as load, movement, predictability, proprioceptive function and error tolerance are likely to influence the selection of the appropriate dynamic control strategy.

carefully timed muscle activity and movement, which might be more efficient and more optimal in the long term, but with greater risk for error if the timing or magnitude of the perturbation is misjudged or not possible to accurately predict.

Issues that might influence the selection of strategy based on the real or perceived risk include, but are not limited to, load, predictability, availability of accurate proprioceptive information, and the real or perceived potential for injury and/or pain (Fig. 33.9). In this framework it would be predicted that the CNS would limit movement and use high levels of co-contraction in association with lifting large masses from the floor (Cholewicki et al 1991), but might use more flexible strategies involving movement and alternating contraction of trunk muscles when performing a low load task such as arm movement (Aruin & Latash 1995, Hodges & Richardson 1997). Similarly, when lifting an unknown mass, the CNS would be predicted to select a strategy that involves co-contraction in comparison to a more dynamic strategy when lifting a known mass. These predictions have been confirmed experimentally (van Dieen & de Looze 1999).

If the information from sensory receptors (e.g. proprioceptive information from the spine, visual information of the nature of an impending load based on its size and form) is accurate, the CNS is likely to be able to use more dynamic strategies (see Fig. 33.9). Whereas a static strategy might be required if the position of the spine cannot be accurately defined, which can occur in situations such as LBP in which reduced proprioception is a common finding. The CNS might also use a stiffening strategy if there is a greater risk (or perceived greater risk) to the spine, due to osseoligamentous insufficiency or anticipation of pain. In other words, the strategy might be selected on the basis of the perceived tolerance for errors in control (see below). Thus multiple factors or combinations of factors might be involved in the selection of strategies between the extremes in the spectrum from static to dynamic.

An important consideration is that the nature of the task will also impact on strategy selection. If the task requires movement such as a golf swing then the CNS has no choice but to control spine motion. However, if movement is not essential (such as during some lifting styles), it can be restricted with some reduction of movement efficiency (e.g. loss of counter-rotation of the shoulders and pelvis in gait resulting in en bloc movement of the trunk; Lamoth et al 2002), can be compensated at other joints (e.g. restriction of lumbar movement and increased hip movement in forward bending; Paquet et al 1994), or movement may be prevented and the task of spinal stability reduced to a situation approaching static control (see Fig. 33.9).

The selection of stability strategy will depend on many factors associated with the task (load, movement requirement, predictability) and the status of the system (real or perceived risk); and the threshold to adapt the strategy or switch between different strategies is likely to vary between individuals. A further consideration of the potential contribution of muscles such as transversus abdominis, diaphragm, pelvic floor, and multifidus to dynamic stability of the lumbar spine and pelvis is that during movement these muscles might provide a strategy to simplify the control of translations without compromising the intended movement trajectory. For instance, contraction of multifidus that is evoked electrically in pigs has been shown to improve the quality of control of intervertebral motion, without restricting the overall range of motion of the spine (Kaigle et al 1995). This goal to provide control during movement would be consistent with the sustained tonic activity of many of these muscles that has been reported during repetitive arm movements (Hodges & Gandevia 2000a) and walking (Saunders et al 2004a).

The concept of 'switching' between various control strategies is also well illustrated with studies of adaptation to novel perturbations (Franklin et al 2003, Milner & Franklin 2005). In the initial phases, subjects utilized muscle co-contraction and wrist joint stiffening during arm movement to resist unknown force perturbations. With practice, subjects learned to compensate very specifically in the direction of force perturbations by creating an internal dynamics model. It is clear from the above discussion that we are dealing with a complex dynamical control system. In engineering terms, such a control can be described as 'adaptive' and 'switching' between various internal models of the system. The adaptability involves updating and tuning of the parameters of the internal model as well as the controller to meet challenges of the changing environment. Thus proprioceptive feedback and other inputs are likely to lead to ongoing tuning of the trunk muscle response to accurately meet movement demands. This adaptation can also involve switching between various models and control strategies when task objectives change. For example, if the perceived risk to the spine is increased due to the threat of pain, the CNS might switch from a more dynamic strategy to a static stiffening to increase the 'safety margin.'

Thus, investigation of the dynamic control of lumbopelvic stability is the next major challenge facing our understanding of functional control of the spine and pelvis. Without consideration of this requirement, current models are unlikely to provide further insight into the strategies selected by the CNS to control the spine in most human functions. The challenge for the CNS in this context is immense. To determine or predict the requirements for control and then plan appropriate strategies to control a selected trajectory of motion requires the CNS to have a detailed internal model of the dynamics of the body and its interaction with the environment as well as a finely tuned proprioceptive apparatus to determine the status of the body at any instant in time. Although dynamic control of the spine is only beginning to be understood, it is important to recognize that this control is likely to be further complicated by the contribution of the trunk muscles and trunk movement to other functions such as respiration/continence and control of whole body equilibrium. In a dynamically stable system the stability of these functions must also be maintained.

Contribution of the spine and trunk muscles to respiration and continence

In addition to the control of movement and stability of the spine and pelvis, trunk muscles also have important respiratory and continence functions. In addition, breathing involves movement of the spine – inspiration is associated with extension and expiration with flexion. The diaphragm is the principal muscle of inspiration. It depresses the central tendon to increase the vertical dimensions of the thorax and elevates the lower ribs which, due to the bucket handle action of the ribs, increases the transverse diameter of the rib cage (Mead 1979) (Fig. 33.10). The relative displacement of the ribs and central tendon depend on the resistance of the abdominal contents to diaphragm descent (De Troyer 1997). Other muscles, such as the erector spinae and latissimus dorsi, extend the spine to assist inspiration and oppose deflationary forces transmitted to the vertebral column by rib cage articulations (Cala et al 1992). During strong expiratory efforts activity of the paraspinal muscles is also likely to be required to counteract the flexion moment from activity of the expiratory abdominal muscles.

The abdominal muscles deflate the rib cage and elevate the diaphragm to assist expiration (De Troyer 1997) (see Fig. 33.10). The contribution of abdominal muscles to expiration varies between anatomical regions of the muscle (Urquhart & Hodges 2005). The middle fibers of transversus abdominis, which attach to the thoracolumbar fascia, have the lowest threshold for respiratory activation (Urquhart & Hodges 2005). Although many authors argue that abdominal muscles are not active during quiet breathing and expiration is a passive process involving elastic recoil of the ribcage and lung, recent data suggest that some regions of the muscles are active during most respiratory cycles (Urquhart & Hodges 2005).

Activity of the pelvic floor muscles, although having limited potential to assist airflow, is likely

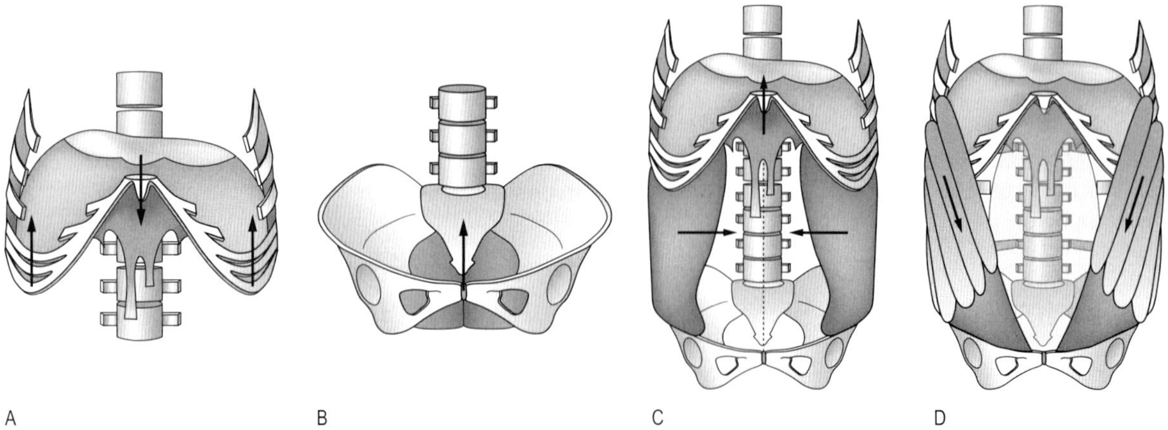

Fig. 33.10 Contribution of the muscles of the abdominal cavity to respiration. (A) Diaphragm contraction depresses the central tendon and elevates the lower ribs. (B) Pelvic floor muscle activity prevents depression of the floor when intra-abdominal pressure is increased. (C) Transversus abdominis activity narrows the waist and elevates the diaphragm via displacement of the abdominal contents. (D) The superficial abdominal muscles, including obliquus externus abdominis (shown) depress the rib cage and increase intra-abdominal pressure.

to be required during breathing to support the abdominal contents and control continence in association with variation in intra-abdominal pressure during respiration (Campbell & Green 1955) (see Fig. 33.10). In quiet breathing, intra-abdominal pressure is increased during inspiration by contraction of the diaphragm. Recent data indicate that pelvic floor muscle activity increases phasically during quiet breathing in standing, consistent with this proposal, although its activity is more closely linked to periods of increased abdominal muscle activity than intra-abdominal pressure (Hodges et al 2007). During loaded breathing when abdominal muscle activity increases to assist expiration, there are peaks in intra-abdominal pressure with both inspiration and expiration (Campbell & Green 1955). Recent data suggest that a larger peak in pelvic floor muscle activity accompanies the abdominal muscle activity (Hodges et al 2007).

The respiratory functions of the trunk muscles must be coordinated with the demands for these muscles to contribute to spinal control. It is well established that respiratory muscles contribute to the strategies used by the CNS to control the trunk. For instance, activity of the diaphragm and transversus abdominis is initiated prior to rapid limb movements (Hodges & Richardson 1997), and tonically during repetitive movements of the arm (Hodges & Gandevia 2000a, 2000b) and walking (Saunders et al 2004a). Furthermore, diaphragm activity is associated with trunk extension efforts in quadriplegic patients (Sinderby et al 1992), and intercostal muscles are active during trunk rotation (Rimmer et al 1995). The challenge for the CNS is to coordinate the postural and respiratory functions. Under normal conditions these functions can be coordinated. For instance, during repetitive arm movement the diaphragm is tonically active, consistent with the demand to control spinal stability, but this activity is phasically modulated in conjunction with breathing to maintain airflow (Fig. 33.11). Furthermore, the activity is also phasically modulated with arm movement, to provide additional support to the trunk at times of peak reactive force (Hodges & Gandevia 2000b). Similar responses of the abdominal muscles have been identified in walking (Saunders et al 2004a).

Under certain conditions the coordination of these two functions is compromised. For instance, breathing is restricted during lifting (Hagins et al 2004, Pietrek et al 2000). A potential conflict exists in the activity of abdominal muscles during simultaneous lifting and ventilatory challenge (McGill et al 1995). This conflict arises from the need to increase spine stiffness via muscle co-contraction and the need for the same muscles to assist in respiration. Breathing is also restricted when sprinting for short distances (Francis 1997). Sprint velocity cannot be maintained if a runner inspires during a race (Francis 1997). Conversely, activity of the trunk muscles in association with spinal stability may be compromised when respiratory demand is increased. For instance, when

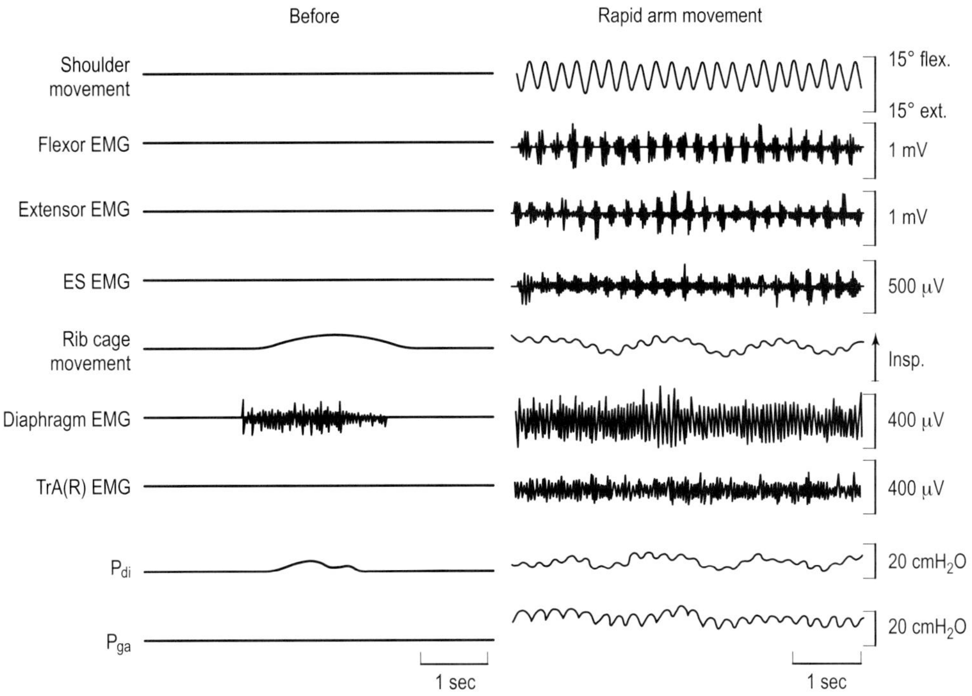

Fig. 33.11 During quiet breathing the diaphragm is active during inspiration. When an arm is moved repetitively while breathing, diaphragm activity is tonic with superimposed phasic modulation of amplitude in association with breathing and arm movements. Tonic activity results in a sustained increase in intra-abdominal (P_{ga}) and transdiaphragmatic (P_{di}) pressure, which is consistent with the requirement to control the spine. EMG, electromyography; ES, erector spinae; TrA, transversus abdominis. (Adapted from Hodges & Gandevia 2000b.)

breathing with an increased dead-space to induce hypercapnea, postural activity of the diaphragm is reduced during repetitive arm movement, which repetitively challenges spinal stability (Hodges et al 2001b). This also occurs when people with chronic airways disease move an arm rapidly and repetitively (Hodges et al 2000).

Reduced contribution of the trunk muscles to spinal stability during periods of increased respiratory demand may compromise control of spinal stability during exercise. However, it could be argued based on recent data that entrainment of breathing and locomotion may ensure that periods of peak impact on the spine (i.e. footstrike) do not occur when stability of the spine is likely to be impaired by reduced activity of the trunk muscles (Hodges & Saunders 2001). Alternatively, activity of other trunk muscles may increase to compensate for the decreased contribution of deeper trunk muscles. Consistent with this proposal recent data from a study of support surface translations suggest that postural activity of oblique abdominal muscles increases when respiration is increased (Hodges et al 2005b). Furthermore spinal loading is increased by muscle co-contraction when lifting while breathing with increased respiratory demand (McGill et al 1995).

In addition to the contribution of trunk muscles to airflow, trunk muscles also move the spine and pelvis in a manner that counteracts the body sway due to breathing. Movement of the spine and pelvis, and activity of lumbopelvic muscles, is time locked to the respiratory movement of the rib cage and abdomen (Gurfinkel et al 1971, Hodges et al 2002) and matches the displacement of the center of mass induced by breathing. The contribution of this movement to control of body sway is supported by the observation that sway with breathing is increased if the contribution of lower limb segments is eliminated, for instance by having the subject kneel on the force plate (Bouisset & Zattara 1990). Furthermore, motion of the center of pressure is increased with breathing in people with LBP (Gagey 1986, Grimstone & Hodges 2003), consistent with the finding that stiffness of the spine is increased in this population.

In terms of continence mechanisms, the demand to coordinate functions appears less complex. Activity of the pelvic floor muscles may contribute to lumbopelvic control in a number of ways. For instance pelvic floor muscles support the abdominal contents when intra-abdominal pressure is increased. This provides an indirect contribution to spinal control via pressure and tension in the thoracolumbar fascia (Hodges et al 2007). The effect of pelvic floor muscle activity on the thoracolumbar fascia is due to the dependency of tension in this structure on the pressure in the abdominal cavity (Tesh et al 1987). In addition, tension in the pelvic floor muscles increases the stiffness of the SIJs in women (Pool-Goudzwaard et al 2004).

The demand for pelvic floor muscle activity to contribute to continence is unlikely to compete with the demands for lumbopelvic control. That is, increased activity of the pelvic floor muscles would enhance both continence and lumbopelvic control. Consistent with this proposal, recent data indicate that activity of the pelvic floor muscles contributes to postural activity associated with perturbations to the spine from arm movement (Hodges et al 2007). However, if pelvic floor muscle activity is compromised, for example with stress urinary incontinence, the system may not be able to meet the demands of spinal control. Furthermore, recent data suggest that women with stress incontinence may have increased activity of the obliquus externus abdominis, which may overcome the activity of the pelvic floor muscles and lead to incontinence (Smith et al 2007). Together these changes may be associated with a combination of incontinence and poor dynamic control of the spine and pelvis.

It is important to consider that static models of spinal control do not take into account the interaction between spinal control, breathing and continence. This is important because although activation of a muscle such as obliquus externus abdominis might provide an optimal contribution to stability in a specific task when co-contracting with the paraspinal muscles, this could restrict the ability of the individual to expand the rib cage to inspire. Thus static strategies for spinal stability that stiffen the spine and prevent spinal and rib cage movement are likely to be unsustainable due to their effect on the essential demands of breathing. Without consideration of effects such as this, it is unlikely that static models will explain the strategies used by the CNS to control the spine. From another perspective it is important to consider that deficits in respiration and continence may lead to compromised spinal control.

Although it is difficult to confirm that increased respiratory demand and incontinence decrease the capability of the trunk muscles to maintain spinal stability, data from several cross-sectional (Finkelstein 2002, Smith et al 2006) and longitudinal (Smith et al 2005) studies suggest that the incidence of back pain is increased in populations with these disorders. Most notably, recent data suggest that breathing difficulties and incontinence are associated with increased odds for development of LBP (Smith et al 2005). Future studies are required to understand the physiological relationship between these disorders.

Contribution of the spine to balance control

Another critical issue is that trunk movement is required to maintain balance and postural equilibrium. For example, when the support surface is translated, the CNS must move the center of mass of the body over a new base of support. If the translation is slow or small, equilibrium can be maintained by contraction of ankle muscles to move the body as an inverted pendulum over the new base of support ('ankle strategy') (Horak & Nashner 1986). However, if the movement is fast or of large amplitude, torque at the ankle is not sufficient and hip muscle activity is required to move the center of mass quickly over the new base (Fig. 33.12). In this case, if the floor translates forwards, the hip is extended to move the center of mass forwards (Runge et al 1999). In a similar manner if balance is maintained on a short beam that is shorter than the length of the feet, sufficient ankle torque cannot be generated to maintain equilibrium and a hip strategy is required to displace the center of mass (Horak & Nashner 1986).

If spinal stability is controlled statically, and movement of the spine is restricted, the contribution of the spine to control of balance would be reduced. Recent data from studies with passive (Gruneberg et al 2004) and active (Van Dieen et al 2004) mechanisms to reduce trunk movement have shown decreased equilibrium control. Notably, recent data suggest that people with LBP have poor ability to maintain balance when standing on a short beam (Mole et al 2004). In this case the short base of support renders the ankle strategy ineffective as the lever arm is reduced and a hip strategy must be adopted. Reduced balance control in people with back pain when standing on this surface is likely to be explained by an inability to control balance with

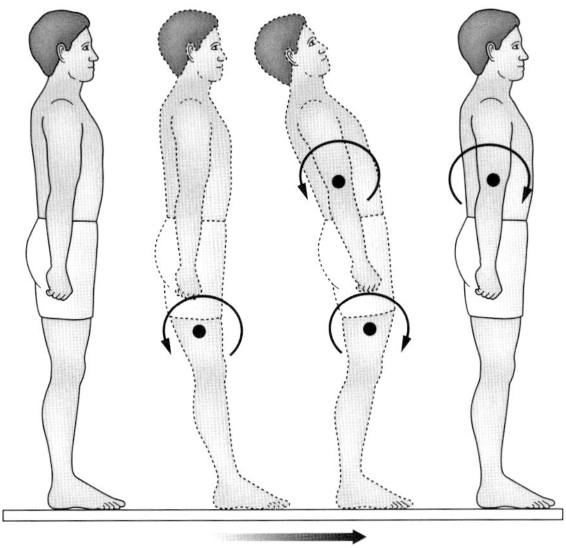

Fig. 33.12 If the support surface moves rapidly forwards, the center of mass falls behind the new base of support due to the inertia of the trunk. In order to regain balance the center of mass of the body must be moved forwards. This can be achieved by trunk and hip movement.

movement of the hip and trunk (Mok et al 2004b). Thus consideration of the contribution of the spine and pelvis to active strategies for control of equilibrium is required to understand the functional control of the spine.

Changes in functional control with lumbopelvic pain

Pain in the lumbopelvic region is associated with a variety of changes in movement and activity of the trunk muscles. Many of these changes are likely to affect the stability of the spine and pelvis, but the nature of these changes is complicated. A major issue is that some changes are consistent with reduced stability whereas others are associated with increased stability when it is considered in the static sense. For instance, studies of people with LBP have reported increased co-contraction of flexor and extensor muscles when a load is released from the trunk (Radebold et al 2000) (Fig. 33.13), increased activity of erector spinae muscles during gait (Arendt-Nielsen et al 1996), increased erector spinae activity during a sit-up (Soderberg & Barr 1983), increased bracing of the abdominal muscles during an active straight leg raise (O'Sullivan et al 2002), increased activity of obliquus externus abdominis with shoulder flexion in people with experimentally induced pain (Hodges et al 2003c) or when pain is anticipated (Moseley et al 2004). These findings suggest that static stability of the spine is increased. Consistent with this argument is the finding that motion of the spine is often compromised in people with back pain. For instance people with LBP less frequently prepare the spine with movement during rapid arm movements (leading to increased resultant motion of the spine) (Mok et al 2004a), intervertebral motion is decreased during trunk flexion (Kaigle et al 1998), and counter-rotation of the shoulders and pelvis is reduced during locomotion (Lamoth et al 2002).

However, other data suggest that activity of transversus abdominis (Hodges & Richardson 1996) (Fig. 33.14) and multifidus (MacDonald et al 2004) is delayed in association with arm movements, tonic activity of transversus abdominis is reduced during walking (Saunders et al 2004b), and with repetitive arm movements during experimentally induced LBP (Hodges et al 2003c). Furthermore, there is evidence for decreased cross-sectional area (Hides et al 1994), increased fatiguability (Roy et al 1989), and increased intramuscular fat in the paraspinal muscles (Alaranta et al 1993). Although these factors do not directly measure activity, they do suggest functional changes in the muscle. Findings of reduced activity of the deeper muscles could suggest decreased spine stability, particularly in view of recent data that provide evidence for a contribution of these muscles to spinal control (Barker et al 2006, Hodges et al 2001a, 2003a, 2005c). Kinematic data also suggest that intervertebral translation is abnormal in people with spondylolisthesis (Schneider et al 2005) and buckling has been observed with fluoroscopy in a single subject during a weight-lifting effort (Cholewicki & McGill 1996). How can these findings be reconciled?

Clearly there is variability in the adaptation of the trunk muscles in people with lumbopelvic pain. Findings such as these suggest that there is no consistent adaptation of muscle control during pain. But is there a common goal that underpins the adaptation to pain? An obvious first consideration is that not all patients with LBP will be the same, and there are likely to be subgroups with different clusters of movement and control changes. Numerous authors have aimed to identify subgroups in the LBP population (Dankaerts et al 2006, Moffroid et al 1994).

Despite the variability, it has been suggested that an underlying principle is that the CNS might adapt to pain or injury by increasing spinal stiffness to increase the safety margin. In this case the nervous

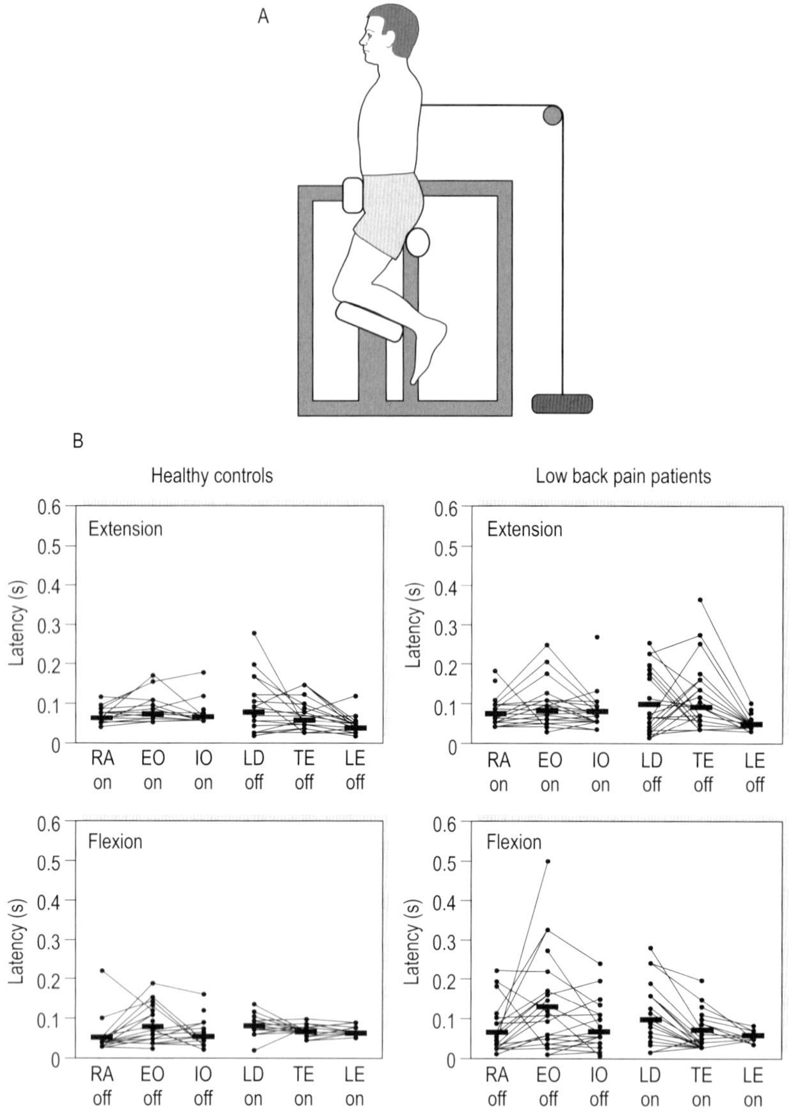

Fig. 33.13 When a mass is attached to the trunk posteriorly, activity of the trunk flexor muscles is required to maintain the body upright. If the mass is removed suddenly, activity of the trunk muscles must be reduced to prevent the body from moving forward. When this task is performed by people with back pain, the latency to turn off the trunk muscles is increased (although the muscle that is delayed varies between individuals) and there is a greater period of co-contraction between the flexors and extensors of the trunk. (Reproduced with permission from Radebold et al 2000.)

system may adopt a strategy to increase stiffness of the spine by increased co-contraction of trunk muscles. This may represent a 'switch' in strategy amongst the options available for dynamic control as mentioned above. Rather than using a variety of strategies to match stability demands, the CNS appears to stiffen the spine with reduced flexibility of movement choices (Fig. 33.15). With this strategy, the CNS would decrease the potential for error, limit the impact of an unanticipated perturbation to the spine, and limit the potential for further injury. In effect, the CNS, rather than selecting a strategy from a spectrum of dynamic possibilities that are perfectly matched to the demands of the task, may select a simple solution that provides reasonable quality of control over a number of situations. However, because many muscles can achieve the same goal (that is, a 'redundant' system), different individuals

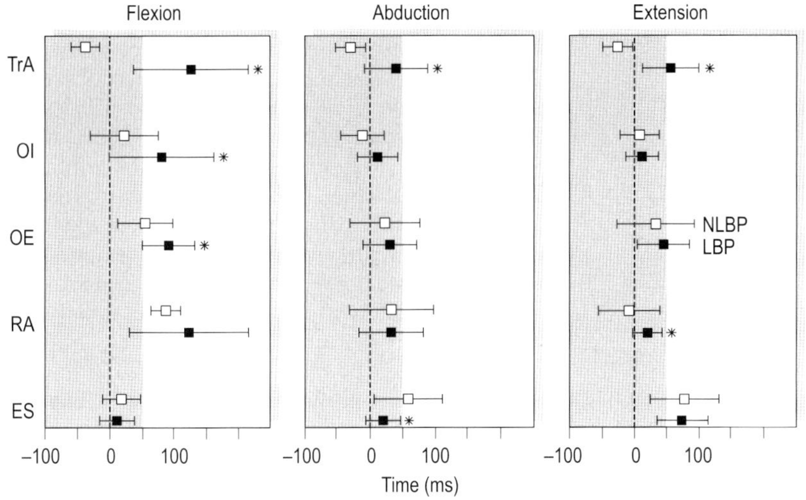

Fig. 33.14 Movement of an arm is normally associated with early activity of the trunk muscles, including transversus abdominis (TrA). However, people with LBP have a consistent delay in the onset of activity of this muscle with movement of the arm in multiple directions. Onset of activity of other muscles is variable between directions of movement. ES, erector spinae; LBP, low back pain; NLBP, non-low back pain; OE, obliquus exernus abdominis; OI, obliquus internus abdominis; RA, rectus abdominis. (Reproduced with permission from Hodges & Richardson 1996.)

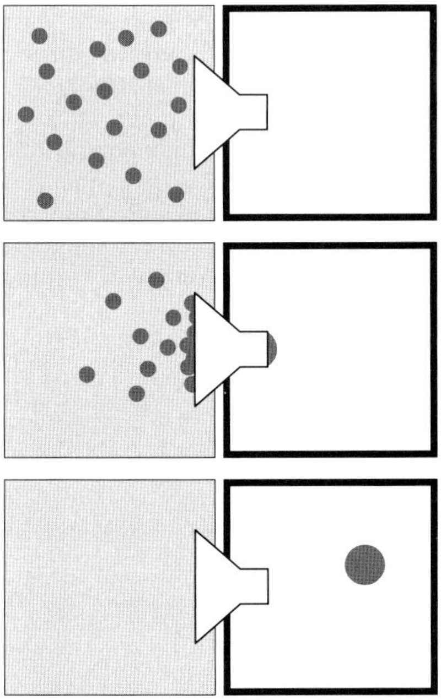

Fig. 33.15 Dynamic control of the spine involves a variety of strategies that can be used flexibly to meet the demands of the range of elements that must be controlled. In low back pain it appears that a common strategy is to reduce the multiple alternatives to a simplified solution to increase the stiffness of the trunk.

may select different combinations of muscle activity to achieve this goal and the strategy may differ between different tasks. Data from modeling studies indicate that simulation of a range of strategies adopted by people with LBP increases stability (van Dieen et al 2003a) (Fig. 33.16). Furthermore, the goal might be achieved to varying degrees by different individuals. For instance, some individuals may brace and stiffen the spine completely, whereas others may rely on co-contraction of superficial muscles, but also control intervertebral motion to some extent.

In general, it is argued that the CNS adopts a co-contraction strategy to compensate for reduced osseoligamentous stability of the spine (Panjabi 1992, van Dieen et al 2003a, 2003b). However, similar changes in motor control may be replicated when pain is induced experimentally by injection of hypertonic saline (Hodges et al 2003c) and the osseoligamentous instability is not changed. Furthermore, similar changes might occur even when pain is anticipated, but not present (Moseley et al 2004). For example, if painful electrical shocks to the back are provided every time an arm is moved, the response of the obliquus externus abdominis is augmented and occurs earlier in association with arm movement. However, this is maintained after the painful stimulation is no longer linked to the arm movement (Moseley & Hodges 2005). Thus, it

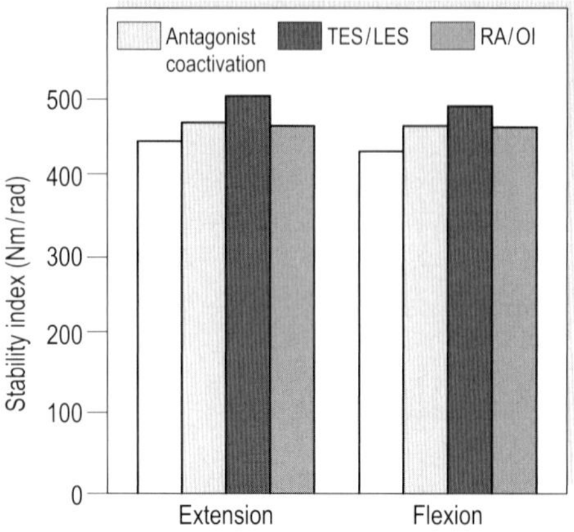

Fig. 33.16 A feature of low back pain is the large variability in changes in muscle activity between individuals. Using an electromyography driven model it is possible to calculate an index of the stability of the spine. When a variety of strategies that are adopted by people with low back pain are simulated in the model, the stability index is increased, suggesting that despite the variability, the adaptation to pain has a common goal. LES, lumbar erector spinae; OI, obliquus internus abdominis; RA, rectus abdominis; TES, thoracic erector spinae. (Reproduced with permission from van Dieen et al 2003a.)

appears that adaptation may occur in a number of situations when the real or perceived stability of the spine is decreased, when there is a real or perceived risk of further injury, or when there is a real or perceived risk of pain (Fig. 33.17). When considering dynamic control of the spine, it is important to perfectly match muscle activity to the movement demands to maintain stability of the trajectory and all other components of spinal control. However, as mentioned above this dynamic strategy has the potential for error. In a healthy system, where there is tolerance for errors, this is not problematic. However, if the real or perceived tolerance for errors is reduced (due to osseoligamentous insufficiency, pain, poor proprioception, etc.), the CNS might adopt a static strategy to increase spinal stiffness (see Fig. 33.17). Thus, rather than using a range of control alternatives, the CNS might choose a simple solution, but with variation between individuals and tasks due to the redundancy of the system.

The adaptation to pain to increase activity of superficial muscles and increase spinal stiffness that is exhibited by many people with LBP could have negative consequences for the spine. Although a strategy to increase stiffness and stability may provide an advantage in the short term, in the long term this may have consequences due to increased loading, restriction of movement and inadequate fine-tuning of trunk movement. One consequence of the increased spinal stiffness is that muscle co-contraction would increase the compressive load on the spine (Fig. 33.18). Although there is debate whether increased loading is detrimental to the spine, it is plausible that high cumulative load may lead to mechanical and physiological changes (Kumar 1990, Norman et al 1998). Recent data suggest that load on the spine is greater during lifting in people with LBP (Marras et al 2004).

In addition, if increased stability and stiffness decreases the potential for spine movement, this could also have a number of negative consequences. First, it would reduce the potential contribution of movement to control perturbations to the spine via the use of inertia and 'give' to limit impact on the spine. Recent data confirm that people with LBP who do not use preparatory trunk motion end up with greater displacements in the spine as a result

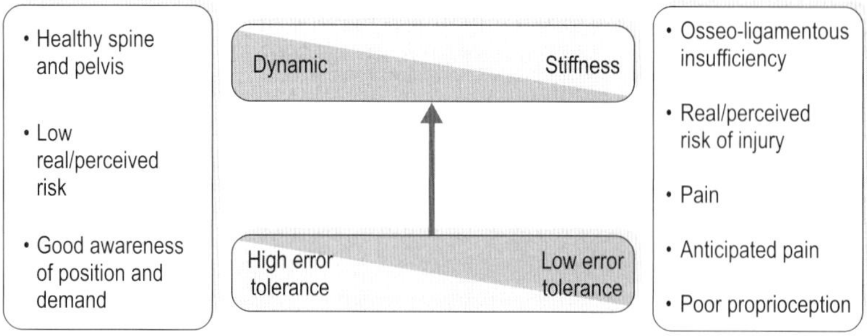

Fig. 33.17 The selection of dynamic control strategy between the extremes of dynamic and stiffening alternatives is likely to be influenced by the tolerance for errors. In a healthy situation the tolerance for errors is high and it is possible to use a dynamic strategy in many situations. However, if the tolerance for errors is reduced due to real or perceived risk of pain or injury or other factors, the nervous system may be forced to use a simple stiffening strategy with a lesser risk of errors and greater static stability.

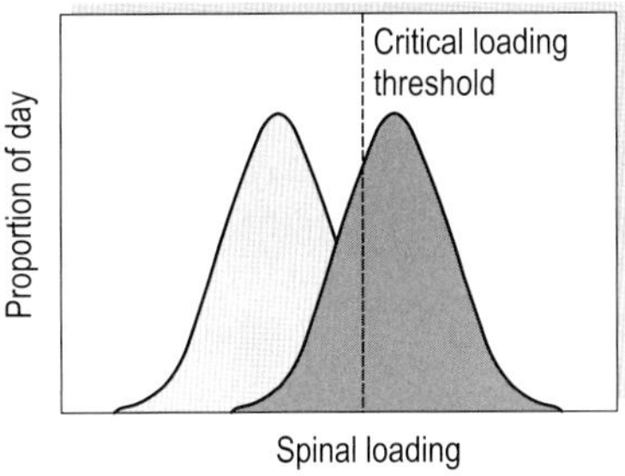

Fig. 33.18 Loading on the spine varies throughout the day depending on functional activities. However, for the majority of the day the loading is within a healthy range. However, if the nervous system adopts a strategy of increased spinal stiffness through co-contraction of antagonist trunk muscles, this will increase spinal loading. This would effectively shift the curve to the right and increase the average level of loading.

of the arm movement (Mok et al 2004a). Second, if spine movement is reduced, the contribution of spinal motion to respiration and the postural compensation for breathing would be reduced. Consistent with this proposal it has been shown that people with LBP sway more with breathing (Gagey 1986, Grimstone & Hodges 2003) and have increased vertical motion of the rib cage with breathing (Hodges et al 2005a). This latter finding may suggest restricted ability to use anteroposterior and lateral motion of the abdominal wall and rib cage due to increased activity of the superficial abdominal muscles. Third, increased spinal stiffness may limit the contribution of spinal movement to control of postural equilibrium. Again, recent data confirm that people with LBP are less able to use a hip strategy to maintain balance when standing on a short support base (Mok et al 2004b). A final consideration is that if the CNS adopts a control strategy that relies on spine stiffening rather than movement, this may limit the ability of the CNS to perform some tasks. Although the stiffening strategy may be suitable for tasks when movement can be restricted (i.e. movement is not required, can be compensated elsewhere, or can be reduced without preventing the task from being completed), when movement is obligatory, an appropriate strategy may not be available. For instance, when standing on one leg it is essential to shift the center of mass over the stance leg. Inappropriate control of the spine in this context through trunk stiffening, makes the above task difficult to execute (Hungerford et al 2003).

A final negative consequence of the increased spine stiffness strategy is that the CNS might then not perceive the need to incorporate activity of the deep muscles into spinal control of stability due to their redundancy. Based on the data indicating the activity of the deep muscles may contribute to spinal control, it is important to note that the activity of the deep muscles may not be completely replicated by activity of the larger more superficial muscles especially in the dynamic situations. This is likely to leave the entire spinal system and its control vulnerable.

For the reasons outlined above, it could be argued that the muscle co-contraction strategy with its short-term benefit, may lead to increased risk of back pain recurrence if it does not resolve. It is well accepted that previous back pain is a strong predictor of future back injury (Greene et al 2001). The failure of resolution of changes in trunk muscle control may be a mechanism underlying this finding. Data from numerous studies of individuals with a history of pain, but no pain at the time of testing, indicate that changes in motor control persist after the resolution of symptoms (Hodges & Richardson 1996). This implies that motor strategies don't resolve spontaneously after cessation of pain, at least in some individuals. The possibility that abnormal muscle activation leads to LBP is supported by recent data that suggest that delayed offset of activity of the abdominal muscles predicts LBP (Cholewicki et al 2005). However this was a predictor not only in those with a history of LBP. Furthermore, reduced cross-sectional area of multifidus that is not restored by specific training, is associated with increased risk of back pain recurrence compared to individuals who did receive such training (Hides et al 2001). A key issue to consider is why some individuals go on to have back pain recurrence while others do not? Further work is required to determine possible factors that may contribute to back pain recurrence, but recent data suggest that the failure of resolution of the motor adaptation may be linked to unhelpful attitudes and beliefs about pain (Moseley & Hodges, unpublished data). As persistence or recurrence of LBP (Burton et al 1995, Susan et al 2002) and pain-related attitudes are associated with changes in motor strategy (Watson & Booker 1997), this might provide a physiological link between psychological factors and back pain recurrence.

In summary, there could be a common behavioral goal that underpins the motor adaptation to pain. This goal appears to present an option to increase spinal stiffness. However, due to the redundancy in the motor system, the specific strategies are likely to vary between individuals and tasks, which can explain some of the variability identified in the literature. Although effective in the short-term, simple muscle co-contraction might have long-term consequences that contribute to the recurrence of pain.

Implications for exercise management

Consideration of control of the spine as a dynamic system has considerable implications for exercise management. The first consideration is that training patients to adopt a strategy associated with optimal static control of the spine is unlikely to be ideal as it is likely to limit the potential for the CNS to take advantage of the dynamic nature of spinal control, thus limiting the potential to use the spectrum of dynamic solutions to human movement. Furthermore, it has the potential to compromise the other functions that require spinal movement (e.g. balance, breathing and continence). The ideal solution would be to retrain the flexibility of the CNS to use all components of optimal dynamic control that includes co-contraction stiffening strategies as one of the range of solutions that can be matched to movement demands.

Optimal rehabilitation requires a comprehensive approach to restore dynamic control (Fig. 33.19). To retrain dynamic control it would be essential to reduce the reliance on a stiffening strategy, which might initially involve reduction of activity of superficial muscles, although the strategy adopted by each individual must be assessed. The next goal would be to train appropriate use of strategies that allow dynamic function including movement and breathing. This would involve training of deep muscle activation as a component of dynamic control of the spine, training of dynamic control of more superficial torque producers, rehabilitation of proprioceptive function, modification of real/perceived error tolerance, retraining of static control as one strategy to be used as required, and rehabilitation of dynamic strategies with balance and breathing training. A third goal is to manage the attitudes and beliefs about pain that might be associated with poor response recovery and non-resolution of symptoms.

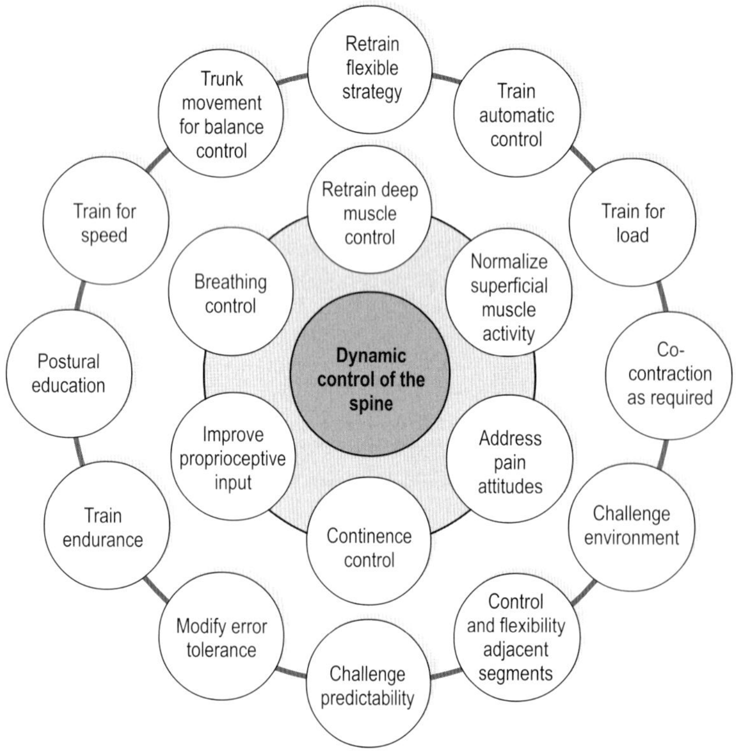

Fig. 33.19 Components that require consideration in order to reach optimal dynamic control of the spine in the management of patients with low back pain.

Adoption of approaches incorporating features of these recommendations have been shown to be effective in the management of chronic LBP associated with spondylolisthesis (O'Sullivan et al 1997), pregnancy-related pelvic pain (Stuge et al 2004), non-specific LBP (Ferreira 2005), and in conjunction with other strategies such as education about physiology of pain (Moseley 2002). Other data suggest that these strategies may also reduce the recurrence of back pain after an acute episode (Hides et al 2001).

Summary

Understanding the functional control of the spine requires consideration of spinal stability as a dynamical system with interaction between the spine and the nervous system. This model involves a spectrum of solutions to control the stability of all components including stability of the movement trajectory, rotational and translational buckling, breathing, balance, continence and many other factors. This dynamic control includes strategies ranging from static stiffening to fine-tuned feed-forward and feedback strategies that involve movement, deep muscle activity and carefully controlled patterns of muscle response to meet the dynamic movement demands. When people experience LBP, it appears common to adopt strategies near the static end of the control spectrum. Although these solutions may be ideal in the short term, they may have negative long-term consequences. In management of patients with LBP, the aim must be to restore normal dynamic control of the spine, which involves restoration of the multitude of control choices to match every movement alternative.

References

Adams MA, McMillan DW, Green TP et al 1996 Sustained loading generates stress concentrations in lumbar intervertebral discs. Spine 21:434–438

Alaranta H, Tallroth K, Soukka A, Heliaara M 1993 Fat content of lumbar extensor muscles in low back disability: a radiographic and clinical comparison. Journal of Spinal Disorders 6:137–140

Arendt-Nielsen L, Graven-Nielsen T, Svarrer H et al 1996 The influence of low back pain on muscle activity and coordination during gait: a clinical and experimental study. Pain 64:231–240

Aruin AS, Latash ML 1995 Directional specificity of postural muscles in feed-forward postural reactions during fast voluntary arm movements. Experimental Brain Research 103:323–332

Barker PJ, Guggenheimer K, Grkovic I et al 2006 Effects of tensioning the lumbar fasciae on segmental stiffness during flexion and extension. Spine 31:397–405

Belenkii V, Gurfinkel VS, Paltsev Y 1967 Elements of control of voluntary movements. Biofizika 12:135–141

Bergmark A 1989 Stability of the lumbar spine. A study in mechanical engineering. Acta Orthopedica Scandinavica 60:1–54

Bogduk N 1997 Clinical anatomy of the lumbar spine and sacrum, 3rd edn. Churchill Livingstone, London

Bouisset S, Zattara M 1981 A sequence of postural adjustments precedes voluntary movement. Neuroscience Letters 22:263–270

Bouisset S, Zattara M 1990 Segmental movement as a perturbation to balance? Facts and concepts. In: Winters JM, Woo SL-Y (eds) Multiple muscle systems: biomechanics and movement organisation. Springer-Verlag, New York, p498–506

Burton A, Tillotson K, Main C et al 1995 Psychosocial predictors of outcome in acute and subchronic low back trouble. Spine 20:722–728

Cala SJ, Edyvean J, Engel LA 1992 Chest wall and trunk muscle activity during inspiratory loading. Journal of Applied Physiology 73:2373–2381

Campbell EJM, Green JH 1955 The behaviour of the abdominal muscles and the intra-abdominal pressure during quiet breathing and increased pulmonary ventilation. Journal of Physiology (London) 127:423–426

Cholewicki J, McGill SM 1996 Mechanical stability of the in vivo lumbar spine: Implications for injury and chronic low back pain. Clinical Biomechanics 11:1–15

Cholewicki J, Van Vliet IJ 2002 Relative contribution of trunk muscles to the stability of the lumbar spine during isometric exertions. Clinical Biomechanics 17:99–105

Cholewicki J, McGill SM, Norman RW 1991 Lumbar spine loading during the lifting of extremely heavy weights. Medicine and Science in Sports and Exercise 23: 1179–1186

Cholewicki J, Panjabi MM, Khachatryan A 1997 Stabilizing function of trunk flexor-extensor muscles around a neutral spine posture. Spine 22:2207–2212

Cholewicki J, Silfies S, Shah R et al 2005 Delayed trunk muscle reflex responses increase the risk of low back pain injuries. Spine 30(23):2614–2620

Crisco JJ, Panjabi MM 1991 The intersegmental and multisegmental muscles of the lumbar spine: A biomechanical model comparing lateral stabilising potential. Spine 7:793–799

Crisco JJ, Panjabi MM, Yamamoto I et al 1992 Euler stability of the human ligamentous lumbar spine. Part II: Experiment. Clinical Biomechanics 7:27–32

Dankaerts W, O'Sullivan PB, Straker LM et al 2006 The inter-examiner reliability of a classification method for non-specific chronic low back pain patients with motor control impairment. Manual Therapy 11:28–39

De Troyer A 1997 Mechanics of the chest wall muscles. In: Miller A, Bianchi A, Bishop B (eds) Neural control of the respiratory muscles. CRC Press, Boca Raton, FL, p59–76

Ferreira PH 2005 Effectiveness of specific stabilisation exercises for chronic low back pain. School of Physiotherapy. The University of Sydney, Australia

Finkelstein MM 2002 Medical conditions, medications, and urinary incontinence. Analysis of a population-based survey. Canadian Family Physician 48:96–101

Francis C 1997 Training for speeded. Faccioni Speed and Conditioning Consultants, Canberra, Australia

Franklin DW, Osu R, Burdet E et al 2003 Adaptation to stable and unstable dynamics achieved by combined impedance control and inverse dynamics model. Journal of Neurophysiology 90:3270–3282

Gagey P 1986 Postural disorders among workers on building sites. In Bles W, Brandt T (eds) Disorders of posture and gait. Elsevier, Amsterdam, p253–268

Gardner-Morse MG, Stokes IA 1998 The effects of abdominal muscle coactivation on lumbar spine stability. Spine 23:86–91

Gardner-Morse MG, Stokes IA 2001 Trunk stiffness increases with steady-state effort. Journal of Biomechanics 34:457–463

Gardner-Morse M, Stokes IA, Laible JP 1995 Role of muscles in lumbar spine stability in maximum extension efforts. Journal of Orthopaedic Research 13:802–808

Granata KP, Marras WS 2000 Cost–benefit of muscle cocontraction in protecting against spinal instability. Spine 25:1398–1404

Granata KP, Orishimo KF, Sanford AH 2001 Trunk muscle coactivation in preparation for sudden load. Journal of Electromyography and Kinesiology 11:247–254

Greene HS, Cholewicki J, Galloway MT et al 2001 A history of low back injury is a risk factor for recurrent back injuries in varsity athletes. Am J Sports Med 29:795–800

Grimstone SK, Hodges PW 2003 Impaired postural compensation for respiration in people with recurrent low back pain. Exp Brain Res 151:218–224

Gruneberg C, Bloem BR, Honegger F et al 2004 The influence of artificially increased hip and trunk stiffness on balance control in man. Exp Brain Res 157: 472–485

Gurfinkel VS, Kots YM, Paltsev EI et al 1971 The compensation of respiratory disturbances of erect posture of man as an example of the organisation of interarticular interaction. In: Gelfard IM et al (eds) Models of the structural functional organisation of certain biological systems. MIT Press, Cambridge, MA, p382–395

Hagins M, Pietrek M, Sheikhzadeh A et al 2004 The effects of breath control on intra-abdominal pressure during lifting tasks. Spine 29:464–469

Hides JA, Stokes MJ, Saide M et al 1994 Evidence of lumbar multifidus muscle wasting ipsilateral to symptoms in patients with acute/subacute low back pain. Spine 19:165–177

Hides JA, Richardson CA, Jull GA 1996 Multifidus muscle recovery is not automatic after resolution of acute, first-episode low back pain. Spine 21:2763–2769

Hides JA, Jull GA, Richardson CA 2001 Long term effects of specific stabilizing exercises for first episode low back pain. Spine 26:243–248

Hodges PW, Gandevia S 2000a Activation of the human diaphragm during a repetitive postural task. Journal of Physiology 522:165–175

Hodges PW, Gandevia S 2000b Changes in intra-abdominal pressure during postural and respiratory activation of the human diaphragm. Journal of Applied Physiology 89:967–976

Hodges PW, Richardson CA 1996 Inefficient muscular stabilisation of the lumbar spine associated with low back pain: a motor control evaluation of transversus abdominis. Spine 21:2640–2650

Hodges PW, Richardson CA 1997 Feedforward contraction of transversus abdominis in not influenced by the direction of arm movement. Experimental Brain Research 114:362–370

Hodges PW, Saunders S 2001 Coordination of the respiratory and locomotor activities of the abdominal muscles during walking in humans. IUPS. Christchurch, New Zealand

Hodges PW, Cresswell AG, Thorstensson A 1999 Preparatory trunk motion accompanies rapid upper limb movement. Experimental Brain Research 124:69–79

Hodges PW, McKenzie DK, Heijnen I et al 2000 Reduced contribution of the diaphragm to postural control in patients with severe chronic airflow limitation. Proceedings of the Annual Sceintific Meeting of the Thoracic Society of Australia and New Zealand. Melbourne, Australia

Hodges PW, Cresswell AG, Daggfeldt K et al 2001a In vivo measurement of the effect of intra-abdominal pressure on the human spine. Journal of Biomechanics 34: 347–353

Hodges PW, Heijnen I, Gandevia SC 2001b Reduced postural activity of the diaphragm in humans when respiratory demand is increased. Journal of Physiology 537:999–1008

Hodges PW, Gurfinkel VS, Brumagne S et al 2002b Coexistence of stability and mobility in postural control: evidence from postural compensation for respiration. Experimental Brain Research 144:293–302

Hodges PW, Kaigle Holm A, Holm S et al 2003a Intervertebral stiffness of the spine is increased by evoked contraction of transversus abdominis and the diaphragm: in vivo porcine studies. Spine 28: 2594–2601

Hodges PW, Kaigle-Holm A, Holm S et al 2003b Postero-anterior stiffness of the lumbar spine is increased by contraction of transversus abdominis and the diaphragm: porcine studies. Fourteenth International Congress of the World Confederation for Physical Therapy. Barcelona, Spain

Hodges PW, Moseley GL, Gabrielsson AH et al 2003c Acute experimental pain changes postural recruitment of the trunk muscles in pain-free humans. Experimental Brain Research 151:262–271

Hodges PW, Smith D, Chang A et al 2005a Breathing pattern changes and low back pain. 3rd World Congress of International Society for Physical and Rehabilitation Medicine. Sao Paulo, Brazil

Hodges PW, Smith M, Grigorenko A et al 2005b Trunk muscle response to support surface translation in sitting: Normal control and effects of respiration. International Society for Posture and Gait Research. Marseille, France

Hodges PW, Eriksson AE, Shirley D et al 2005c Intra-abdominal pressure increases stiffness of the lumbar spine. Journal of Biomechanics 38:1873–1880

Hodges PW, Sapsford R, Pengel LHM (2007) Postural and respiratory functions of the pelvic floor muscles. Neurourology and Urodynamics (in press)

Horak F, Nashner LM 1986 Central programming of postural movements: Adaptation to altered support-surface configurations. Journal of Neurophysiology 55:1369–1381

Hungerford B, Hodges P, Gilleard W 2003 Evidence of altered lumbo-pelvic muscle recruitment in the presence of posterior pelvic pain and failed load transfer through the pelvis. Spine 28(14):1593–1600

Janevic J, Ashton-Miller JA, Schultz AB 1991 Large compressive preloads decrease lumbar motion segment flexibility. Journal of Orthopedic Research 9:228–236

Kaigle AM, Holm SH, Hansson TH 1997 Volvo Award winner in biomechanical studies. Kinematic behavior of the porcine lumbar spine: a chronic lesion model. Spine 22:2796–2806

Kaigle AM, Wessberg P, Hansson TH 1998 Muscular and kinematic behavior of the lumbar spine during flexion-extension. Journal of Spinal Disorders 11:163–174

Kavcic N, Grenier S, McGill SM 2004 Determining the stabilizing role of individual torso muscles during rehabilitation exercises. Spine 29:1254–1265

Kumar S 1990 Cumulative load as a risk factor for back pain. Spine 15:1311–1316

Lamoth CJ, Meijer OG, Wuisman PI et al 2002 Pelvis–thorax coordination in the transverse plane during walking in persons with nonspecific low back pain. Spine 27:E92–E99

MacDonald D, Moseley GL, Hodges PW 2004 The function of the lumbar multifidus in unilateral low back pain. World Congress of Low Back and Pelvic Pain. Melbourne, Australia

Marras WS, Ferguson SA, Burr D et al 2004 Spine loading in patients with low back pain during asymmetric lifting exertions. The Spine Journal 4:64–75

McGill SM, Sharratt MT, Seguin JP 1995 Loads on spinal tissues during simultaneous lifting and ventilatory challenge. Ergonomics 38:1772–1792

Mead J 1979 Functional significance of the area of apposition of diaphragm to rib cage. American Review of Respiratory Disease 119:31–32

Milner TE, Franklin DW 2005 Impedance control and internal model use during the initial stage of adaptation to novel dynamics in humans. Journal of Physiology 567:651–664

Moffroid MT, Haugh LD, Henry SM et al 1994 Distinguishable groups of musculoskeletal low back pain patients and asymptomatic control subjects based on physical measures of the NIOSH Low Back Atlas. Spine 19:1350–1358

Mok N, Brauer S, Hodges PW 2004a Different range and temporal pattern of lumbopelvic motion accompanies rapid upper limb flexion in people with low back pain. In: Vleeming A et al (eds) Fifteenth Interdisciplinary World Congress on Low Back and Pelvic Pain. Melbourne, Australia, p295

Mok N, Brauer S, Hodges PW 2004b Hip strategy for balance control in quiet standing is reduced in people with low back pain. Spine 29(6):E107–E112

Moseley GL 2002 Combined physiotherapy and education is efficacious for chronic low back pain. Australian Journal of Physiotherapy 48:297–302

Moseley GL, Hodges PW 2005 Are the changes in postural control associated with low back pain caused by pain interference? Clinical Journal of Pain 21:323–329

Moseley GL, Nicholas MK, Hodges PW 2004 Does anticipation of back pain predispose to back trouble? Brain 127:2339–2347

Norman R, Wells R, Neumann P et al 1998 A comparison of peak vs cumulative physical work exposure risk factors for the reporting of low back pain in the automotive industry. Clinical Biomechanics 13:561–573

O'Sullivan PB, Twomey LT, Allison GT 1997 Evaluation of specific stabilizing exercise in the treatment of chronic low back pain with radiologic diagnosis of spondylolysis or spondylolisthesis. Spine 22:2959–2967

O'Sullivan PB, Beales DJ, Beetham JA et al 2002 Altered motor control strategies in subjects with sacroiliac joint pain during the active straight-leg-raise test. Spine 27: E1–E8

Panjabi MM 1992 The stabilizing system of the spine. Part I. Function, dysfunction, adaptation, and enhancement. Journal of Spinal Disorders 5:383–389

Paquet N, Malouin F, Richards CL 1994 Hip–spine movement interaction and muscle activation patterns during sagittal trunk movements in low back pain patients. Spine 19:596–603

Perry J 1992 Gait analysis: normal and pathological functioned. Slack Inc, Thorofare, NJ

Pietrek M, Sheikhzadeh A, Nordin M et al 2000 Biomechanical modeling of intra-abdominal pressure generation should include the transversus abdominis. Journal of Biomechanics 33:787–790

Pool-Goudzwaard A, van Dijke GH, van Gurp M et al 2004 Contribution of pelvic floor muscles to stiffness of the pelvic ring. Clinical Biomechanics 19:564–571

Potvin JR, McGill SM, Norman RW 1991 Trunk muscle and lumbar ligament contributions to dynamic lifts with varying degrees of trunk flexion. Spine 16:1099–1107

Radebold A, Cholewicki J, Panjabi MM et al 2000 Muscle response pattern to sudden trunk loading in healthy individuals and in patients with chronic low back pain. Spine 25:947–954

Rimmer KP, Ford GT, Whitelaw WA 1995 Interaction between postural and respiratory control of human intercostal muscles. Journal of Applied Physiology 79:1556–1561

Roy SH, DeLuca CJ, Casavant DA 1989 Lumbar muscle fatigue and chronic low back pain. Spine 14:992–1001

Runge CF, Shupert CL, Horak FB et al 1999 Ankle and hip postural strategies defined by joint torques. Gait Posture 10:161–170

Saunders S, Coppieters M, Hodges PW 2004a Reduced tonic activity of the deep trunk muscle during locomotion in people with low back pain. World Congress of Low Back and Pelvic Pain. Melbourne, Australia

Saunders S, Rath D, Hodges PW 2004b Respiratory and postural activation of the trunk muscles changes with mode and speed of locomotion. Gait Posture 20(3): 280–290

Saunders SW, Schache A, Rath D et al 2005 Changes in three dimensional lumbo-pelvic kinematics and trunk muscle activity with speed and mode of locomotion. Clinical Biomechanics 20:784–793

Schneider G, Pearcy MJ, Bogduk N 2005 Abnormal motion in spondylolytic spondylolisthesis. Spine 30:1159–1164

Shirley D, Hodges PW, Eriksson AEM et al 2003 Spinal stiffness changes throughout the respiratory cycle. Journal of Applied Physiology 95(4):1467–1475

Sinderby C, Ingvarsson P, Sullivan L et al 1992 The role of the diaphragm in trunk extension in tetraplegia. Paraplegia 30:389–395

Smith M, Russell A, Hodges PW 2005 Incontinence and breathing disorders are associated with development of back pain. Eleventh World Congress on Pain. Sydney, Australia

Smith MD, Russell A, Hodges PW 2006 Disorders of breathing and continence have a stronger association with back pain than obesity and physical activity. Australian Journal of Physiotherapy 52:11–16

Smith MD, Coppieters M, Hodges PW 2007 Postural response of the pelvic floor and abdominal muscles in women with and without incontinence. Neurourology and Urodynamics (in press)

Snijders CJ, Vleeming A, Stoeckart R et al 1995 Biomechanical modelling of sacroiliac joint stability in different postures. Spine: State of the Art Reviews 9:419–432

Soderberg GL, Barr JO 1983 Muscular function in chronic low-back dysfunction. Spine 8:79–85

Stuge B, Laerum E, Kirkesola G et al 2004 The efficacy of a treatment program focusing on specific stabilizing exercises for pelvic girdle pain after pregnancy: a randomized controlled trial. Spine29:351–359

Susan H, Picavet J, Vlaeyen J et al 2002 Pain catastrophizing and kinesiophobia: Predictors of chronic low back pain. American Journal of Epidemiology 156:1028–1034

Tesh KM, ShawDunn J, Evans JH 1987 The abdominal muscles and vertebral stability. Spine 12:501–508

Urquhart DM, Hodges PW 2005 Postural activity of the abdominal muscle varies between regions body and between body positions. Gait and Posture 22(4):295–301

van Dieen JH, de Looze MP 1999 Directionality of anticipatory activation of trunk muscles in a lifting task depends on load knowledge. Experimental Brain Research 128:397–404

van Dieen JH, Cholewicki J, Radebold A 2003a Trunk muscle recruitment patterns in patients with low back pain enhance the stability of the lumbar spine. Spine 28:834–841

van Dieen JH, Selen LP, Cholewicki J 2003b Trunk muscle activation in low-back pain patients, an analysis of the literature. Journal of Electromyography and Kinesiology 13:333–351

van Dieen JH, Mok N, Coppieters MW et al 2004 Increased cocontraction of trunk muscles as a cause of impaired balance control. International Society for the Study of the Lumbar Spine. Porto, Portugal

Watson PJ, Booker CK 1997 Evidence for the role of psychological factors in abnormal paraspinal activity in patients with chronic low back pain. Journal of Musculoskeletal Pain 5:41–56

Zetterberg C, Andersson GB, Schultz AB 1987 The activity of individual trunk muscles during heavy physical loading. Spine 12:1035–1040

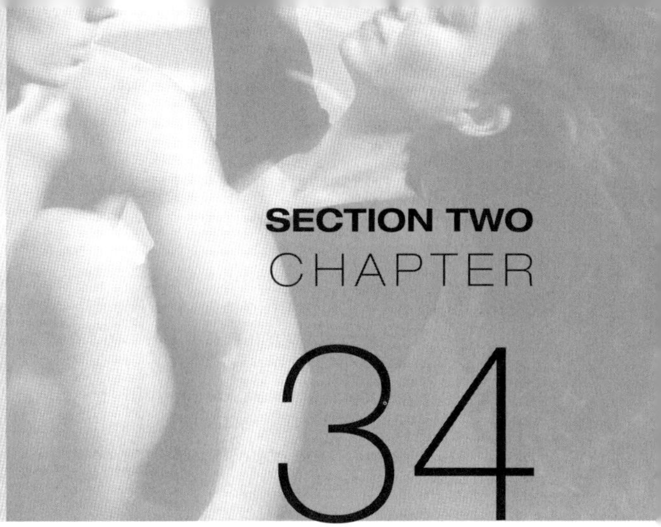

SECTION TWO
CHAPTER
34

Motor control in chronic pain: new ideas for effective intervention

G Lorimer Moseley

Introduction

Horse trainers know that when a racehorse breaks a leg it is best to send it off to greener pastures, not because the leg won't heal but because the horse won't again reach peak performance. Racing humans might be no different: one classic example is that of a world champion sprinter who 'pulled a hamstring' on the twenty-first stride of the 200 m at a big event. The following year, after successful rehabilitation and no signs or symptoms, that athlete still showed a visible limp at the twenty-first stride of the 200 m. Such phenomena suggest a complex relationship between pain and motor control, a relationship so intimate that pain and motor output may represent two dimensions of a common neural event (Melzack 1996). This possibility raises interesting issues for clinicians who target reduction in pain via alteration of motor control because it suggests that myriad factors may influence motor output and motor learning. Those factors probably become more important as pain becomes chronic because the central nervous system (CNS) undergoes profound changes which result in: (1) increased synaptic efficacy of central pain networks; and (2) changes in cortical representation of the painful and adjacent parts.

This chapter proposes new directions for management of chronic back and pelvic pain by first drawing on the wealth of data on neural changes associated with chronic pain and the impact of psychological factors on motor output and then integrating those data with established principles of motor control training for low back and pelvic pain.

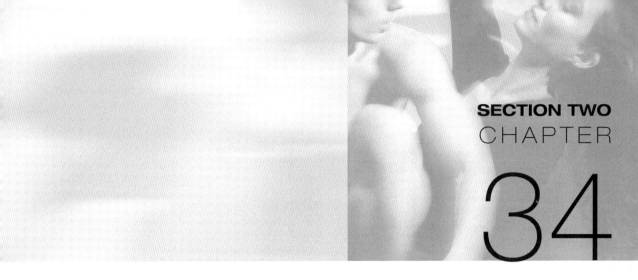

Cortical changes associated with chronic pain

The CNS is highly dynamic. Functional organization and neural stimulus–response profiles vary according to use and changes can be rapid but can also be long lasting. Broadly speaking, two types of change seem to occur: increased synaptic efficacy of nociceptive and pain networks and altered functional organization of cortical representation of the affected body part.

Enhanced synaptic efficacy of nociceptive and pain networks

Discussion of the neural mechanisms involved in enhanced synaptic efficacy associated with pain is beyond the scope of the current work. However, conceptualization of the phenomenon is critical. It is first useful to understand a popular working model of the brain outlined in Melzack's neuromatrix theory (Melzack 1990). This theory, which was proposed to explain pain in missing or paralyzed body parts, suggests that each output of the brain can be conceptualized as the result of activation of a particular neurosignature. The neuromatrix theory goes on to argue that each neurosignature trifurcates to effect an experience and a motor and endocrine output. Thus, according to the neuromatrix theory, pain and motor output are dimensions of one process. As is the case with any theory of the brain, empirical data are difficult to obtain. Notwithstanding, however, it is a useful theory with which to understand the cortical changes associated with chronic pain.

To further elucidate this issue, one can utilize the metaphor of the brain as an orchestra, with each tune analogous to a neurosignature (Butler & Moseley 2003). In this metaphor, the orchestra can normally play a wide range of tunes, can learn new tunes easily, can adapt old tunes, and can improvise quickly. Should the orchestra play one tune (e.g. the pain tune) repeatedly, it not only gets better at playing that tune, it is more easily initiated, adaptability reduces, and improvization suffers. In much the same way, the brain that continually activates the pain neurosignature becomes better at doing so such that fewer and less threatening inputs are required to activate it and it becomes the dominant brain output. In such situations, things that didn't hurt now do (allodynia) and things that used to hurt, now hurt more (hyperalgesia). Allodynia and hyperalgesia can also be mediated by spinal and peripheral changes, but the impact of cortically mediated changes are probably more profound and can involve inputs from across sensory, psychological, and environmental domains.

There are substantial data concerning short- and long-term changes at each stage of the nociceptive pathway: the superficial (Moore et al 2000, Zhuo 2000) and deep (Svendsen et al 2000) dorsal horn; the thalamus (Lenz et al 2000); the cortex (Flor 2000); and across these areas (Pertovaara 2000). Much of the research in this area has been paraphrased in a clinician and lay-friendly manner in Butler & Moseley (2003).

Altered cortical representation of the painful body part

The body is represented throughout the brain. We can consider these representations as virtual bodies. We can also consider entire systems as having a 'representation' (Janig & Baron 2003), called a 'neural correlate' by others (Jeannerod 1994), and herein conceptualized as virtual systems. The most commonly studied virtual bodies are those 'held' in the primary somatosensory (S1) and the primary motor (M1) cortex. Those cortices are most often studied probably because they are intuitively likely to be important and because they are accessible to a range of experimental techniques that are used to investigate brain function. With chronic pain, changes occur in both S1 and M1. Broadly speaking, the organization of S1 changes such that the virtual body part becomes larger. For example, when the S1 response to stimulation of the back and finger was compared between patients with chronic low back pain and matched controls, two findings were apparent (Flor et al 1997). First, the focus of the response, which is thought to reflect where in S1 the virtual body part is located, was more medial in patients than it was in controls. That can be interpreted as illustrative of an enlarged virtual back. The second notable response was that patients showed a bigger response to back stimulation, but not finger stimulation, than controls. That can be interpreted as being illustrative of the increased synaptic efficacy of the neurosignature for back pain, discussed earlier. Both findings correlated with the duration of back pain.

Changes in M1 associated with chronic pain involve changes in excitability (Valeriani et al 1999) and organization (Juottonen et al 2002). It is reasonable to propose that such changes in the motor system manifest in reduced motor control and may offer an explanation for the difficulty that patients with chronic spinal pain have in isolating certain muscles or learning and performing fine motor skills. Thus, the patient with chronic pain is faced with two issues that are likely to hamper rehabilitation: sensitivity of the pain neurosignature and incongruence between the virtual body and the actual body and between virtual movement and executed movement. In order to understand why these issues are important, it is helpful to first explore the relationship between pain and motor control.

Current paradigms of pain and motor control

Current explanatory models for the relationship between pain and motor control include the vicious cycle (Travell et al 1942, for all intents and purposes equivalent to the muscle tension model), the pain adaptation model (Lund et al 1991), and the neuromuscular activation model (Sterling et al 2001). The muscle tension model has been refuted fairly convincingly. For example, Matre et al (1998) found that while the stretch reflex was increased during experimentally induced pain, there was no change in the corresponding H-reflex, which indicates no change in the excitability of the α motorneuron pool. Other studies are corroborative of that work (Capra & Ro 2000, Svensson et al 1998, Zedka et al 1999).

Almost all data that support the pain adaptation model have been obtained from limb studies, in which muscles can be given clear agonist and antagonist roles. The main effect of pain on muscle activity appears to be reduced activity of the agonist and although the model stipulates that there is an opposite effect (i.e. augmentation) on the antagonist, data are less convincing. Nonetheless, the physiology of the pain adaptation model has conventionally been argued to involve spinal mechanisms, but it seems equally feasible that both tonic and supraspinal mechanisms could account for the stipulated effects. Indeed, more recent writings acknowledge that the mechanisms are probably more complex than short-loop spinal mechanisms. Although there are a great many studies that investigate the pain adaptation model [the interested reader is referred to Graven-Nielsen's group, which has done the majority of this work (Arendt-Nielsen et al 1996, Svensson et al 1998)], there are limited data relevant to spinal control. That is not altogether surprising because application of a model concerning agonist and antagonist muscle activity to the spine and pelvis can not account for the complex and variable relationship between muscles, even within tasks. Still, in so far as it proposes that changes in muscle activity are task-dependent and serve to limit movement, the pain adaptation model is supported by the majority of studies (Arendt-Nielsen et al 1996, Hodges & Richardson 1996, Lamoth et al 2006, Watson et al 1997).

Proponents of the pain adaptation model and of the neuromuscular activation model, at least in regards to spinal pain, commonly presume that the changes in motor control reflect only a response to pain. However, changes in motor output might also be part of the pain state itself. That view would be consistent with proposals put forward by pre-eminent thinkers in pain science, proposals that emphasize the intimacy between pain and motor control. Patrick Wall's reality–virtual reality theory (Fig. 34.1) implies that input to the brain is analyzed according to what should be done about it (Wall 1994) and Ronald Melzack's neuromatrix theory (Fig. 34.2) proposes that motor and experience 'commands' emanate from a single neural phenomenon called a neurosignature, and that the neurosignature can be modified by internal and external inputs.

Inherent to the reality–virtual reality theory is the assumption that the brain creates a reality based on the available sensory information and the internal perceptual state. According to that model, when the brain, or more accurately the central nervous system, is unable to select the appropriate motor response, it diverts to a virtual reality system and attempts to create a motor response that matches that virtual

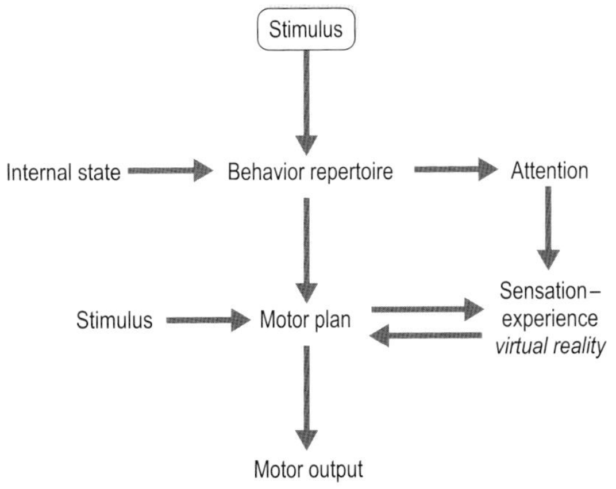

Fig. 34.1 The reality–virtual reality theory. (Adapted from Wall 1994.)

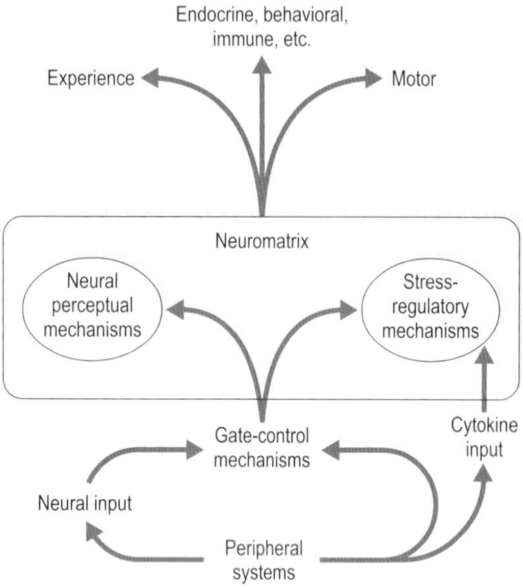

Fig. 34.2 The neuromatrix theory. (Adapted from Melzack 1990.)

reality. Wall proposed that this situation occurs during pain and thus, motor output is inherent to pain. In its application to chronic pain, the reality–virtual reality theory has some similarities with a model offered by Aldrich and colleagues (2000), in which chronic pain is conceptualized as chronic vigilance to threat. In that model, chronic vigilance to threat may lead to continued and unsuccessful attempts to escape. In either case the motor/behavioral component is responsive to threat and occurs in parallel rather than in response to pain.

The neuromatrix theory presents a conceptual framework about which the treatment approaches of our group have been built. As such, further discussion of this theory is appropriate here. The neuromatrix theory built on an earlier theory of pattern generators (Melzack & Casey 1968), which in turn was proposed because available models could not account for some common pain phenomena (e.g. phantom limb pain and post-stroke central pain). Three assumptions underlie the neuromatrix theory. First, that all the experiences that humans might have in response to input to the brain might also be possible without these inputs (dreaming is one example of such a situation). Second, that the same neural mechanisms are responsible for an experience regardless of whether they are evoked by peripheral input or not. According to this assumption, noxious stimuli do not cause the experience of pain but might trigger a neural mechanism within the brain that produces pain. Third, that experiential and motor output originate in a common neural mechanism. For example, factors that impact on pain will also impact on motor output.

Although methodological limitations mean that neither can be empirically evaluated, the basic tenet of both the neuromatrix theory and Wall's proposal is that pain is as motoric as it is experiential. The neuromatrix theory conceptualizes a complex network of neurons that incorporates the cortex, thalamus, and limbic system (although it may be more appropriate to incorporate spinal neurons, which also have extensive afferent and efferent connections). The theory proposes that the neuromatrix is essentially genetically determined but is modified by learning; the connections are both divergent, allowing parallel processing, and convergent, allowing interaction between components and modulation of processes. The neurosignature is a continuous outflow from the neuromatrix that trifurcates to project to: (1) a conceptual neural center that converts it to awareness, the so-called 'sentient neural hub'; (2) motor systems that effect the appropriate motor response; and (3) endocrine, immune, and homeostatic systems. Like the reality–virtual reality theory, motor output is no longer conceptualized as the result of afferent processes, responsive to pain, but the result of efferent processes, in parallel with pain.

The primary weakness of both the reality–virtual reality theory and the neuromatrix theory is the lack of biological substrate or neuroanatomical locations particular to the components or functions of each. Although important, the lack of empirical data does not reduce the relevance of either model because their strength lies in providing a framework with which to understand physiology and guide treatment.

Nonetheless, neuroimaging studies offer relevant information. For example, brain areas most consistently observed to be active during pain are conventionally understood to be motoric rather than sensory, for example the anterior cingulate cortex (ACC), premotor and motor cortices [see Ingvar & Hsieh (1999) for a review]. Specifically, the ACC is thought to play a complex and pivotal role in: (1) coordinating the perception of bodily threat with other areas involved in selection and planning of an appropriate behavioral/motor response strategy; and, intriguingly, (2) establishing an emotional valence of pain (Price 2000). These functions are evidenced by the fact that the ACC projects directly to motor and supplementary motor areas (Price 2000), and receives direct projections from reticular formation neurons, which in turn have demonstrated clear relevance to escape behavior and fear responses, but not to sensory-discriminative aspects of pain. Those formation neurons include nucleus gigantocellularis (Willis 1985) and periaqueductal gray nucleus (Mayer & Price 1976).

Overwhelmingly, the distal origins of these neural mechanisms are second-order wide dynamic range (WDR) spinal neurons that also project to limbic centers (Vogt et al 1993), the activity of which relates to affective/emotional–motivational functions (Bushnell 1995). Notably, it is the WDR second-order neuron that undergoes most rapid and substantial change in chronic pain (Svendsen et al 2000), which raises the possibility of a common affective–emoto-motor mechanism.

To summarize, in the same way that activation of S1 and S2 cortices are seen as subserving sensory–discriminative dimensions of pain, it appears likely that premotor and motor areas subserve motor dimensions of pain. In fact, although intuitive according to structural–pathological models of pain, it seems scientifically dubious to interpret motor cortical activity during pain as a response to pain, but sensory cortical activity as part of pain itself. According to modern models of pain such as the neuromatrix theory, and because WDR neurons project predominantly to affective and motor areas, it is reasonable to propose that pain has an affective–motor dimension.

Pain and postural adjustments of the trunk muscles

A series of studies undertaken in the 1990s by Hodges and colleagues demonstrated that when people who have a long history of recurrent back pain move a limb, they control their trunk muscles differently to people who have no back trouble [see Hodges (1999) for review]. This work sparked a revolution in the treatment of patients with low back pain. Subsequently, numerous research groups have undertaken physiological studies investigating the role of the trunk muscles in spinal control and clinical studies that investigate the efficacy of treatment aimed at regaining normal control. The experts have no doubt contributed heavily to the current book and their work is best discussed by them. However, Hodges' early work also raised a number of questions about why those people with recurrent low back pain, but who were pain-free at the time of testing, appeared to use a different strategy to control their spine even though they appeared to be moving their arm in the same way. Why do these people have altered control? Is it a cause or a consequence of their back pain? Or both? Does the change in control reflect disruption of the system, caused by distraction associated with pain? Or by stress? Or fear? Perhaps it is not a disruption so much as a functional adaptation. These questions formed the basis of a series of studies that underpin the clinical explorations discussed in the final section of this chapter.

1. Is altered postural control of the trunk muscles a cause of pain or a consequence of pain, or both?

Extensive data show that transversus abdominis (TrA) makes an important contribution to stiffness between vertebral segments [see Hodges (1999) for review] and that postural activity of this muscle during limb movements is consistent with such a contribution to spinal control (Hodges & Richardson 1999). It follows then that delayed or reduced activity of TrA may be associated with reduction of fine control or increased load of spinal structures, both of which may increase the likelihood of nociceptive stimulation and injury. Thus, it is reasonable to suggest that altered control of this muscle in people who suffer recurrent episodes of low back pain, may be causing the problem.

Although feasible, it is not the only possible explanation for that finding. In fact, the opposite relationship may be true; perhaps recurrent episodes of back pain cause altered control of TrA. That possibility was tested by inducing experimental back pain in asymptomatic subjects (Hodges et al 2003) and evaluating the effect on the timing and amplitude of postural adjustments of the abdominal muscles (including TrA) during arm movements.

Intramuscular injection of hypertonic saline elicits pain of moderate to strong intensity and with similar sensory characteristics to the pain reported by people with nonexperimental pain. That said, it should be noted that any investigation that involves experimentally induced pain is limited in its generalizability because experimentally induced pain is fundamentally different to nonexperimental pain; it is known by the subjects not to be damaging (presumably very few people would give consent to participate if this were not made very clear), it is of a known time course and is associated with a known nociceptive stimulus. Extensive research in our group attests to this. For example, on the

McGill Pain Questionnaire (Melzack 1975), on which patients select words that best describe their pain and those words are selected from affective–emotional, sensory–discriminate or evaluative domains, words in the affective–emotional category are seldom selected (Moseley et al 2005). This is in contrast to clinical populations who select words from across domains (Melzack 1975). Despite that limitation, when hypertonic saline was injected into the longissimus muscle of asymptomatic subjects, there was a change in control of the trunk muscles during arm movements. Specifically, subjects appeared to adopt a similar control strategy to that observed in the recurrent back pain patients – augmentation of at least one superficial trunk muscle and a systematic delay and reduction in the magnitude of the response in TrA (Fig. 34.3).

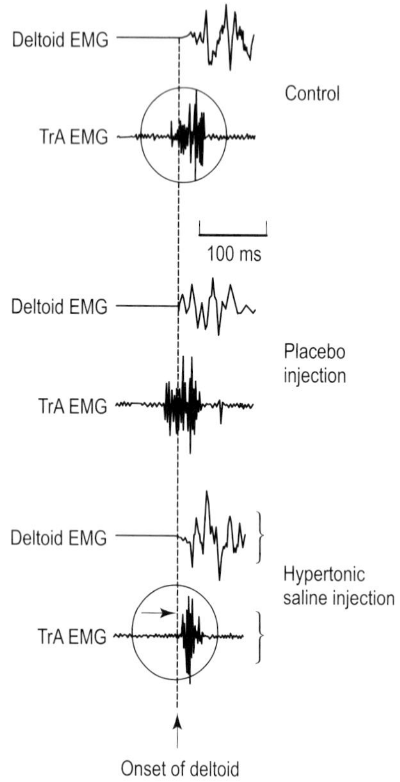

Fig. 34.3 Raw data from a representative subject showing electromyographic (EMG) activity in deltoid and transversus abdominus (TrA) during forward movement of the contralateral arm in standing. Note that the onset of TrA, relative to that of deltoid, occurs later during pain induced by injection of hypertonic saline into longissimus than it does during control or after placebo (isotonic saline, non-painful) injection. Vertical dashed line marks onset of deltoid EMG, horizontal arrow demonstrates delay in TrA EMG onset.

This finding demonstrated that low back pain can cause the motor control changes seen in patients. Importantly, however, it did not exclude the possibility that the opposite relationship also exists – that altered motor control can cause back trouble. That is, altered postural control appears to be a consequence of back pain, but may also be a cause of back pain.

2. Is the effect of pain simply due to reduced performance caused by the distracting effect of pain?

Pain demands central resources and it is well recognized that CNS performance is disrupted by pain. If the effect of pain on postural adjustments reflected such an effect, then that effect should also be elicited by a non-painful attention-demanding task. That proposal was tested in two separate studies with asymptomatic subjects. The first study involved a dual-task paradigm in which subjects performed arm movements while they also participated in a cognitive task (Moseley et al 2004c). That work demonstrated that a non-painful attention-demanding task did have an effect on postural control of the trunk muscles but that effect was different to that observed during pain. However, in the same way that experimentally induced pain is different to non-experimental pain, the attentional demand of a cognitive task may be fundamentally different, or utilize distinct CNS resources, to pain.

The second study attempted to overcome that issue by investigating the nature of motor control change imparted by experimentally induced pain (Moseley & Hodges 2004a). This study used painful cutaneous shock evoked via the initiation of deltoid muscle activity associated with arm movement (Fig. 34.4). This paradigm attempted to impart to the subjects a close association between arm movement and back pain (i.e. 'arm movement causes back pain'). If the alteration in postural adjustments imparted by experimentally induced back pain does reflect a specific demand on CNS performance, then the impact should follow a given pattern: changes in motor control should be greatest at the onset of pain or fear (Crombez et al 1994), the responses should habituate with repeated exposure as the threat value of the pain subsides, and the responses should be absent immediately when the threat of pain is removed (Crombez et al 1997, 1998). This pattern did not occur. Rather, the response gradually changed over

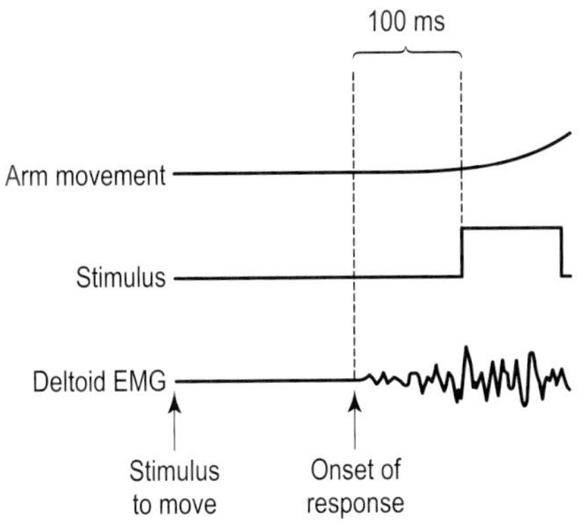

Fig. 34.4 Painful cutaneous stimulus was delivered 100 ms after the onset of electromyography in deltoid. The stimulus occurred at approximately the same time as the onset of arm movement. This paradigm aimed to provide the quasi-illusion that arm movement causes back pain.

a number of trials, and then gradually returned to control values once the painful stimuli were removed. In short, the findings corroborated those of the first study and suggested that the motor control changes associated with pain are not simply because pain demands attentional resources.

3. Is the effect of pain a general response to stress?

Stress changes motor control and pain is stressful. Can the effect of pain be replicated by nonpainful but stressful situations? This possibility was tested by performing the same cognitive task described earlier in a stressful environment, which was produced by arguments within the laboratory and by telling the subject that we thought they would find this (difficult) task easy (Moseley et al 2004c). There was an effect of stress on the trunk muscles, in particular on the deep trunk muscles, TrA and multifidus. Although the data showed that stress was sufficient to impact on deep trunk muscle control, the effect was again different to that observed during pain. That is, the effect of pain on motor control of the trunk muscles is probably not simply a response to stress.

4. Is the effect evoked by the expectation of back pain?

If the effect is evoked by the expectation of back pain, then it is reasonable to suggest that pain itself may not cause the effect, but that the effect might be part of a protective response of which pain is also a part. This possibility was tested by inducing an expectation of back pain elicited by painful cutaneous stimulation to the back (Moseley et al 2004b). This work showed that expecting back pain is sufficient to initiate a similar strategy to that observed during experimental pain and to that observed in patients with recurrent problems (Fig. 34.5). That is, the alteration in trunk muscle control might reflect a protective strategy associated with the expectation of pain or injury.

5. Why might some patients maintain such a strategic attempt to protect against pain or injury even if they are pain free?

The body of data raises the possibility that while alteration of motor control is a fairly consistent finding during back pain, resolution of motor control changes may not always occur. To test this possibility, individual subject data obtained using the arm movement–cutaneous stimulation paradigm were evaluated (Moseley & Hodges 2004b). In most subjects, motor control was normalized quickly once painful stimuli were removed. However, in ~15% of subjects, motor control of the trunk muscles did not normalize, even after 45 pain-free trials. Closer inspection of data from those subjects showed that nonresolution of motor control strategy was associated with a loss of normal variability in the response. Retrospective evaluation of the threat of back pain, a generic construct estimated via several self-report questionnaires, showed that the subjects in whom motor control strategy did not resolve were characterized by cognitions consistent with an extreme threat value of back pain. That is, the data suggest that nonresolution of motor control strategy after back pain is associated with an increased threat value of back pain. Notably, patients who have chronic back pain are characterized by such cognitions. Perhaps then, psychological aspects of low back pain, such as increased threat value of pain, are critical in determining recurrence and chronicity, via sustained alteration in motor control and consequent risk to spinal structures. This possibility is currently being tested in a prospective design.

A working model of threat, pain, and motor control

The threat–response model of chronic pain and motor control (Moseley & Hodges 2005) (Fig. 34.6)

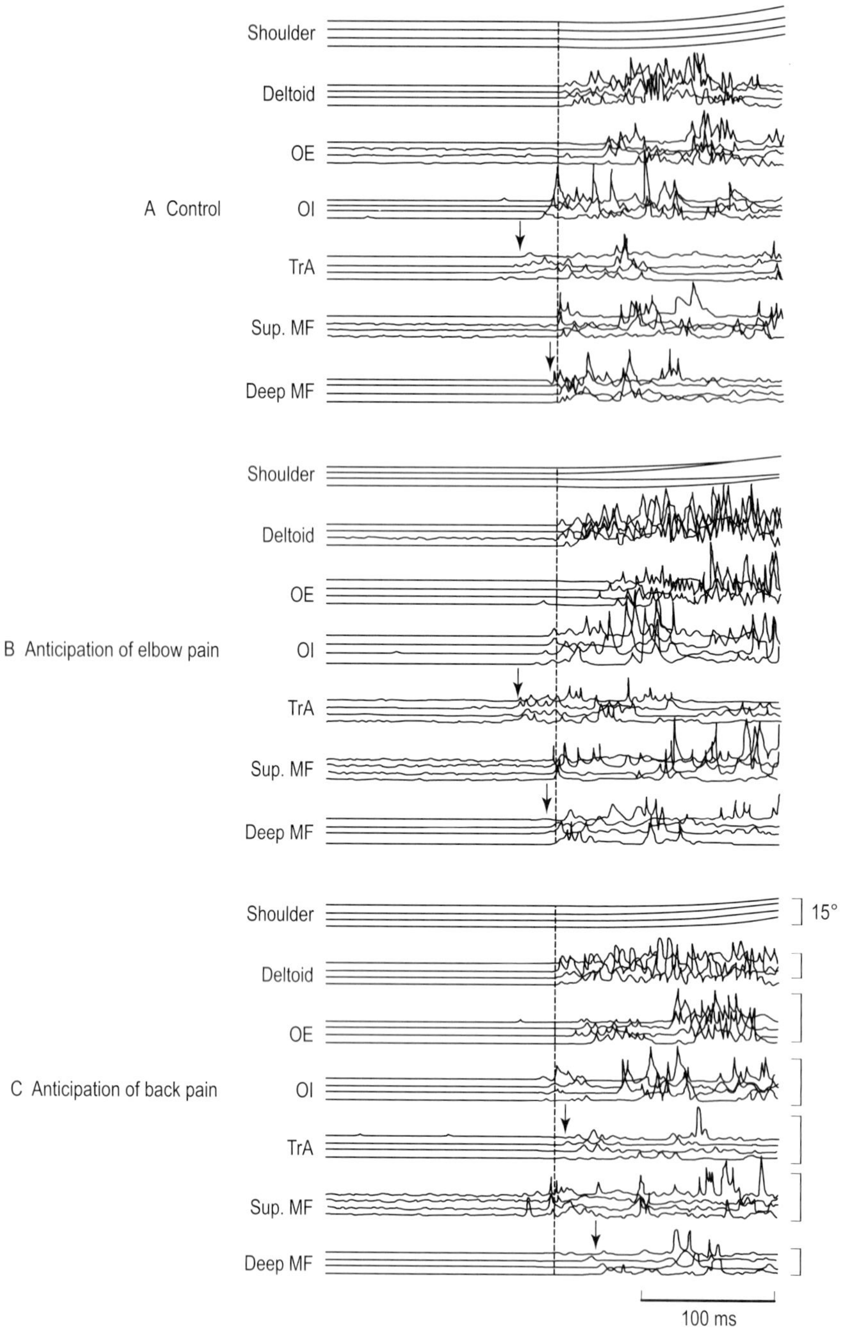

Fig. 34.5 Expectation of back pain alters postural adjustments of the deep trunk muscles. Rectified raw electromyographic (EMG) data for five trials from a representative subject performing forward arm movements in standing during (A) control; (B) expectation of elbow pain; and (C) expectation of back pain. Data are shown for obliquus externus (OE), internus (OI), transversus abdominus (TrA), superficial (Sup. MF), and deep (Deep MF) fibers of lumbar multifidus. Vertical downward arrows mark approximate onset of TrA and Deep MF. Vertical line marks onset of deltoid EMG. (Reproduced with permission from Moseley et al 2004c.)

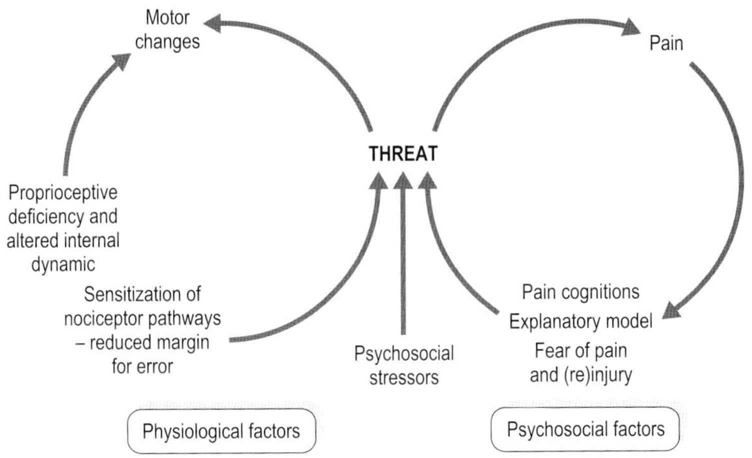

Fig. 34.6 Threat response model. (Reproduced with permission from Moseley & Hodges 2005.)

was proposed in an attempt to integrate the data discussed above. That model builds on both the neuromatrix theory and fear avoidance models of chronic pain and disability [see Vlaeyen & Crombez (1999) for a review]. The two basic principles of the threat-based model of chronic pain and motor control are that: (1) pain is produced by the brain when the brain perceives that threat to body tissue exists and that action is required; and (2) pain and motor control are intimately related, consistent with the conceptual bifurcation of a single pain neurosignature [see also Moseley (2003b)]. These principles imply that any input from across sensory, psychological, and environmental domains that increases the perceived threat to body tissue should also increase pain and have an impact on motor output. That is, it is the perception of threat to body tissue that underpins the relationship between pain and motor control. The threat–response model of pain and motor control implies two approaches to treatment – approaches that target motor control changes and approaches that reduce the perception of threat to body tissue.

Novel treatment approaches have been developed and evidence regarding the effects and utility of those approaches are slowly building. Several studies have investigated the effect on pain and motor control of educating patients about the biology of pain and chronic pain (Moseley 2002, 2003a, 2003c, 2004a, Moseley et al 2004a). That work has led to the development of a lay-friendly text that provides mechanisms by which modern understandings of the biology of pain can be explained to patients (Butler & Moseley 2003). The primary effects of explaining pain to patients appear to be a reduction in the perceived threat to body tissue, reduced disability and pain, and improved outcome of bimodal and multidisciplinary programs for people with chronic intractable pain. Notably, within the context of the current chapter, such changes imply that a substantial effect will also be imparted on motor control changes coexistent with pain. Current work is focusing on evaluating these changes more precisely.

The second avenue by which we have attempted to target the threat value of pain is by adopting a model of assessment and management that focuses on threat. That is, what threatening inputs are contributing to the pain state? In many respects, these new directions are analogous to common approaches to anxiety disorder, in which 'graduated exposure and response prevention' is the operational mantra. These new directions are also analogous to established principles of physical management, which inadvertently perhaps are driven according to the same mantra. That said, the physiological and psychosocial complexities of chronic back and pelvic pain have led to several novel approaches to application of these principles.

When no movement is too much movement

An earlier section of this chapter emphasized enhanced synaptic efficacy as a consequence and cause of chronic pain. It is appropriate to consider the impact of enhanced synaptic efficacy on rehabilitation via the threat–response model or via the neuromatrix theory, both of which are consistent with the metaphor of the orchestra in the brain. The primary manifestation of enhanced synaptic efficacy of nociceptive and pain networks is that less threatening input can cause pain. The biological complexity of the CNS means that threatening cues can emerge from across domains (e.g. sensory somatic, sensory nonsomatic, cognitive, emotional, environmental). In extreme, but anecdotally not overly rare cases, even benign and subtle movement-relevant motor tasks can activate the sensitized pain system. This type of phenomenon has been observed using functional magnetic resonance imaging during performance of a simple abdominal task in a patient with chronic low back pain (Moseley 2005b). Moreover, in some chronic pain states associated with marked sensitization of pain networks, even imagined movements can cause pain and swelling, even though no detectable muscle activity is present (Moseley 2004c).

So, when no movement appears to be too much movement, the threat–response model would suggest that one has to reduce the threat associated with that movement. Possible strategies by which this might be achieved are manipulating the environment, facilitating the patient to imagine performing the movement in a pain-free manner (imagined movements activate the same cortical and subcortical mechanisms as executed movements) (Lotze et al 1999), manipulating other sensory inputs by performing (or imagining) the movement in different postures, in different emotional states, etc. Extensive coverage of these principles has been presented elsewhere (Butler & Moseley 2003, Moseley 2003b, Moseley & Hodges 2005) and the interested reader is referred to those sources.

When the virtual body and the actual body don't match

An earlier section emphasized that chronic pain is associated with reorganization within the brain. One manifestation of this organization is that the virtual body becomes distorted and the delineation of body parts may become smudged. Aside from making skill aquisition difficult (think now of chronic low back pain patients who seem to not have any knowledge of where their pelvis is in space), such a situation will presumably produce a mismatch between motor output and sensory feedback. This type of sensorimotor mismatch is of great interest to clinicians interested in conditions characterized by marked distortions in the virtual body, for example phantom limb pain, focal dystonia and stroke, but are also pertinent in situations where changes are more subtle.

It has been proposed, consistent with Wall's reality–virtual reality theory mentioned earlier, that pain may be generated within the motor control system (McCabe et al 2005). Accordingly, it is proposed that assimilation of available information allows the motor control system to predict a certain response from the sensory system, and 'controllers' within the system compare the desired state with the motor command required to achieve it, thus permitting a precise motor output dependent on current and desired states. In effect, the consequence of this chain of actions is that sensory events are analyzed in terms of the appropriate motor response. It follows, therefore, that if error occurs within this system, for example because of a disrupted virtual body, then the above system is alerted and pain may result. Aspects of this have recently been reproduced experimentally in the limbs of asymptomatic volunteers by using a mirror to distort sensory feedback (McCabe et al 2005). This theory, put forward by McCabe and colleagues is similar in some aspects to theories of sensorimotor mismatch applied to different contexts by others, for example, distorted sensory feedback post-stroke preventing acquisition of appropriate motor outputs via a disruption within the control system. Although the proposal, that disruption within this system causes pain, remains to be verified, it raises the possibility that in such states: (1) the motor command will remain inaccurate, and therefore continue to contribute to a pain state regardless of training; and (2) it is first necessary to 'train the brain' before appropriate motor skills can be acquired. Training the brain in this sense will probably aim to normalize changes in both the sensory and motor cortices. Based on a distinct but related theoretical rationale, discussion of which is beyond the scope of this work, our group and others have explored several approaches to training the brain in limb studies (Acerra et al 2006, Moseley 2004b, 2005a). We are currently evaluating similar approaches in back pain patients.

Summary

Rapid advances in knowledge across the pain sciences raise new possibilities for management. The current chapter proposes that future directions should be driven by several key principles: (1) chronic pain is associated with physiological changes that mean that there is enhanced synaptic efficacy of nociceptive and pain networks; (2) that pain and motor control are intimately related; (3) that both pain and motor changes are produced by the brain when body tissue is perceived to be in danger; such that (4) any input that has an effect on perceived threat will also have an effect on motor control. Based on those principles, our group is exploring two broad areas of therapeutic possibility. First, reduction of threat via education about pain biology ('explaining pain') and graduated exposure to threatening cues (graded exposure and response prevention). Second, 'training the brain' prior to skill acquisition, in an attempt to normalize cortical changes and any sensorimotor mismatch that may prevent successful rehabilitation.

Acknowledgements

Research discussed in this chapter was supported by funding from the National Health & Medical Research Council of Australia; The Private Practice Trust Fund, Royal Brisbane & Women's Hospital; Division of Physiotherapy, The University of Queensland; The Pain Management Research Institute, The University of Sydney & Prince of Wales Medical Research Institute, Sydney. GLM is supported by a Nuffield Oxford Medical Fellowship and is currently on leave from the School of Physiotherapy, The University of Sydney.

References

Acerra N, Souvlis T, Moseley GL 2006 Common findings in stroke, complex regional pain syndrome and phantom limb pain. Implications and future directions. J Rehabil Med (in press)

Aldrich S, Eccleston C, Crombez G 2000 Worrying about chronic pain: vigilance to threat and misdirected problem solving. Behav Res Ther 38:457–470

Arendt-Nielsen L, Graven-Nielsen T, Svarrer H, Svensson P 1996 The influence of low back pain on muscle activity and coordination during gait: a clinical and experimental study. Pain 64:231–240

Bushnell MC 1995 Thalamic processing of sensory-discriminative and affective-motivational dimensions of pain. In: Besson JM, Guilbaud G, Ollat H (eds) Forebrain areas involved in pain processing. Eurotext, Paris, p63–77

Butler D, Moseley GL 2003 Explain pain. NOI Group Publishing, Adelaide, Australia, p114

Capra NF, Ro JY 2000 Experimental muscle pain produces central modulation of proprioceptive signals arising from jaw muscle spindles. Pain 86:151–162

Comerford M, Mottram S 2001 Movement stability dysfunction – contemporary developments. Man Ther 6:15–26

Crombez G, Baeyens F, Eelen P 1994 Sensory and temporal information about impending pain: the influence of predictability on pain. Behav Res Ther 32:611–622

Crombez G, Eccleston C, Baeyens F, Eelen P 1997 Habituation and the interference of pain with task performance. Pain 70:149–154

Crombez G, Eccleston C, Baeyens F, Eelen P 1998 Attentional disruption is enhanced by the threat of pain. Behav Res Ther 36:195–204

Flor H 2000 The functional organization of the brain in chronic pain. Prog Brain Res 129:313–322

Flor H, Braun C, Elbert T, Birbaumer N 1997 Extensive reorganization of primary somatosensory cortex in chronic back pain patients. Neurosci Lett 224:5–8

Hodges PW 1999 Is there a role for transversus abdominis in lumbo-pelvic stability? Man Ther 4:74–86

Hodges PW, Richardson CA 1996 Inefficient muscular stabilization of the lumbar spine associated with low back pain. A motor control evaluation of transversus abdominis. Spine 21:2640–2650

Hodges PW, Richardson CA 1999 Transversus abdominis and the superficial abdominal muscles are controlled independently in a postural task. Neurosci Lett 265: 91–94

Hodges PW, Cresswell AG, Daggfeldt K, Thorstensson A 2001 In vivo measurement of the effect of intra-abdominal pressure on the human spine. J Biomech 34:347–353

Hodges PW, Moseley GL, Gabrielsson A, Gandevia SC 2003 Experimental muscle pain changes feedforward postural responses of the trunk muscles. Exp Brain Res 151:262–271

Ingvar M, Hsieh J 1999 The image of pain. In: Wall P, Melzack R (eds) The textbook of pain. Churchill Livingstone, Edinburgh, p215–234

Janig W, Baron R 2003 Complex regional pain syndrome: mystery explained? Lancet (Neurology) 2:687–697

Jeannerod M 1994 The representing brain: neural correlates of motor intention and imagery. Brain Behav Sci 17: 187–245

Juottonen K, Gockel M, Silen T et al 2002 Altered central sensorimotor processing in patients with complex regional pain syndrome. Pain 98:315–323

Lamoth CUC, Meijer OG, Daffertshofer A et al 2006 Effects of chronic low back pain on trunk coordination and back muscle activity during walking: changes in motor control. European Spine Journal 15(1):23–40

Lenz FA, Lee J-I, Garonzik IM et al 2000 Plasticity of pain-related neuronal activity in the human thalamus. Prog Brain Res 2000:259–273

Lotze M, Montoya P, Erb M et al 1999 Activation of cortical and cerebellar motor areas during executed and imagined hand movements: an fMRI study. J Cogn Neurosci 11(5):491–501

Lund JP, Donga R, Widmer CG, Stohler CS 1991 The pain-adaptation model: A discussion of the relationship between chronic musculoskeletal pain and motor activity. Can J Physiol Pharmacol 69:683–694

Matre DA, Sinkjaer T, Svensson P, Arendt-Nielsen L 1998 Experimental muscle pain increases the human stretch reflex. Pain 75:331–339

Mayer DJ, Price DD 1976 Central nervous system mechanisms of analgesia. Pain 1:51–58

McCabe C, Haigh R, Halligan P, Blake D 2005 Simulating sensory-motor incongruence in healthy volunteers: implications for a cortical model of pain. Rheumatology 44(4):509–516

Melzack R 1975 The McGill Pain Questionnaire: major properties and scoring methods. Pain 1:277–299

Melzack R 1990 Phantom limbs and the concept of a neuromatrix. Trends Neurosci 13:88–92

Melzack R 1996 Gate control theory. On the evolution of pain concepts. Pain Forum 5:128–138

Melzack R, Casey KL 1968 Sensory, motivational, and central control determinants of pain: a new conceptual model. In: Kenshalo DR (ed) The skin senses. Thomas, Springfield, IL, p423–443

Moore KA, Baba H, Woolf CJ 2000 Synaptic transmission and plasticity in the superficial dorsal horn. Prog Brain Res 2000:63–80

Moseley GL 2002 Combined physiotherapy and education is effective for chronic low back pain. A randomised controlled trial. Aust J Physiother 48:297–302

Moseley GL 2003a Joining forces: combining cognition-targeted motor control training with group or individual pain physiology education: a successful treatment for chronic low back pain. J Man Manip Ther 11:88–94

Moseley GL 2003b A pain neuromatrix approach to patients with chronic pain. Man Ther 8:130–140

Moseley GL 2003c Unravelling the barriers to re-conceptualisation of the problem in chronic pain: the actual and perceived ability of patients and health professionals to understand the neurophysiology. J Pain 4:184–189

Moseley GL 2004a Evidence for a direct relationship between cognitive and physical change during an education intervention in people with chronic low back pain. Eur J Pain 8:39–45

Moseley GL 2004b Graded motor imagery is effective for long-standing complex regional pain syndrome. Pain 108:192–198

Moseley GL 2004c Imagined movements cause pain and swelling in a patient with complex regional pain syndrome. Neurology 62:1644

Moseley GL 2005a Is successful rehabilitation of complex regional pain syndrome simply sustained attention to the affected limb? A randomised clinical trial. Pain 114(1–2):54–61

Moseley GL 2005b Widespread brain activity during an abdominal task markedly reduced after pain physiology education – fMRI evaluation of a single patient with chronic low back pain. Aust J Physiother 51(1):49–52

Moseley GL, Hodges PW 2004a Are the changes in postural control associated with low back pain caused by pain interference? Clin J Pain 21(4):323–329

Moseley GL, Hodges PW 2004b Loss of normal variability in postural adjustments is associated with non-resolution of postural control after experimental back pain. Behav Neurosci 120(2):474–476

Moseley GL, Hodges PW 2005 Chronic pain and motor control. In: Jull G, Boyling J (eds) Grieves modern manual therapy of the vertebral column. Churchill Livingstone, Edinburgh

Moseley GL, Hodges PW, Nicholas MK 2004a A randomized controlled trial of intensive neurophysiology education in chronic low back pain. Clin J Pain 20:324–330

Moseley GL, Nicholas MK, Hodges PW 2004b Does anticipation of back pain predispose to back trouble? Brain 127:2339–2347

Moseley GL, Nicholas MK, Hodges PW 2004c Pain differs from non-painful attention-demanding or stressful tasks in its effect on postural control patterns of trunk muscles. Exp Brain Res 156:64–71

Moseley GL, Sim DF, Henry ML, Souvlis T 2005 Experimental hand pain delays recognition of the contralateral hand – evidence for a perceptual bias in acute pain. Cog Brain Res 25:188–194

Pertovaara A 2000 Plasticity in descending pain modulatory systems. Prog Brain Res 2000:231–242

Price DD 2000 Psychological mechanisms of pain and analgesia, vol. 15. IASP Press, Seattle, p223

Sterling M, Jull G, Wright A 2001 The effect of musculoskeletal pain on motor activity and control. J Pain 2:135–145

Svendsen F, Hole K, Tjolsen A 2000 Long-term potentiation in single wide dynamic range neurons induced by noxious stimulation in intact and spinalized rats. Prog Brain Res 2000:153–161

Svensson P, De Laat A, Graven-Nielsen T, Arendt-Nielsen L 1998 Experimental jaw-muscle pain does not change heteronymous H-reflexes in the human temporalis muscle. Exp Brain Res 121:311–318

Travell J, Rinzler S, Herman M 1942 Pain and disability of the shoulder and arm. Treatment by intramuscular infiltration with procaine hydrochloride. J Am Med Assoc 120:417–422

Valeriani M, Restuccia D, Di Lazzaro V et al 1999 Inhibition of the human primary motor area by painful heat stimulation of the skin. Clin Neurophysiol 110:1475–1480

Vlaeyen JW, Crombez G 1999 Fear of movement/(re)injury, avoidance and pain disability in chronic low back pain patients. Man Ther 4:187–195

Vogt BA, Sikes RW, Rogt LJ 1993 Anterior cingulate cortex and the medial pain system. In: Vogt BA, Gabriel M (eds) Neurobiology of cingulate cortex and limbic thalamus: a comprehensive handbook. Birkhauser, Boston, MA

Wall P 1994 Introduction to the edition after this one. Editorial. In: Wall P, Melzack R (eds) The textbook of pain. Churchill Livingstone, Edinburgh, p1–7

Watson PJ, Booker CK, Main CJ 1997 Evidence for the role of psychological factors in abnormal paraspinal activity in patients with chronic low back pain. J Musculoskel Pain 5:41–56

Willis WD 1985 The pain system. Karger, New York

Zedka M, Prochazka A, Knight B 1999 Voluntary and reflex control of human back muscles during induced pain. J Physiol (Lond) 520:591–604

Zhuo M 2000 Silent glutamatergic synapses and long-term facilitation in spinal dorsal horn neurons. Prog Brain Res 2000: 101–113

PART FIVE

Section Three

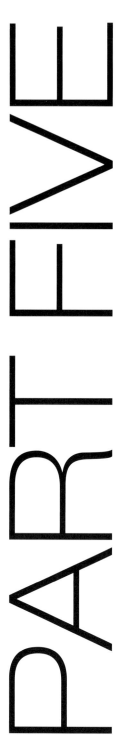

Effective training and treatment: Different views on effective training and treatment

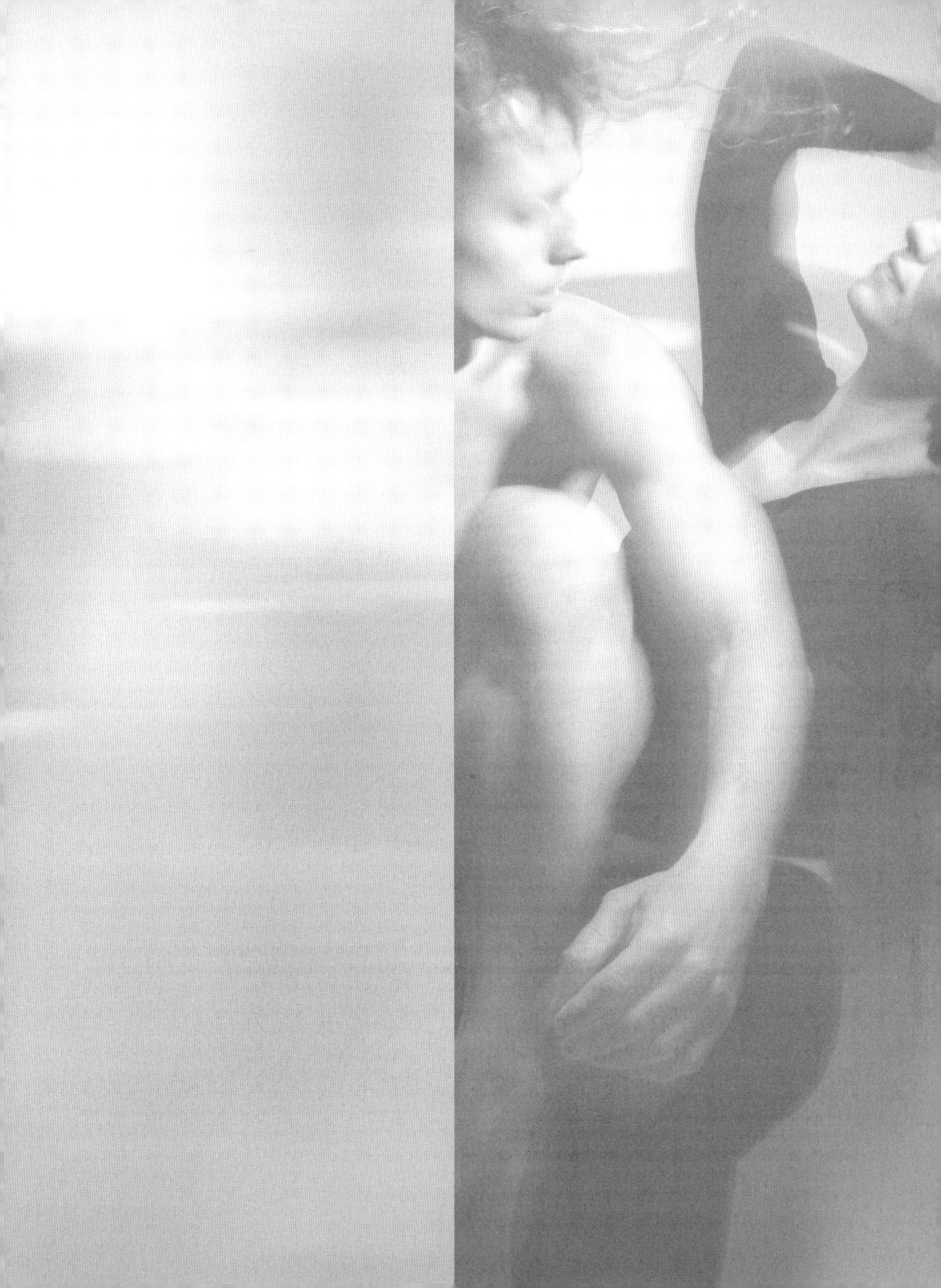

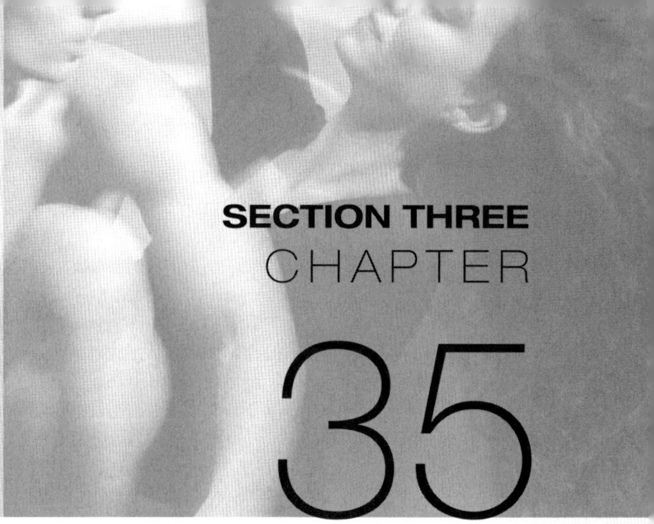

SECTION THREE
CHAPTER

35

The painful and unstable lumbar spine: a foundation and approach for restabilization

Stuart M McGill

Introduction

Much scientific and clinical effort has been directed towards developing exercise together with other protocols for treatment of the unstable spine. Although many have claimed that 'stabilization exercises' were used in their study, one must wonder 'How did they know the exercises were actually stabilizing?' 'How did they know the spine needed a stabilization approach at the outset?' This chapter attempts to introduce some of the notions necessary to understand stability and instability, and fosters discussion of appropriate progressive therapeutic exercise. A critical point must be made up front regarding clinical skill. Designing and prescribing therapeutic exercise is not about getting a patient to perform stabilization exercises. It is about finding the subtle techniques and precision in form, and motion and motor patterns that ensure that the exercise is building a patient's back rather than tearing it down. This requires not only knowledge of the science and basic forms of exercises but also the many details noticed by the better clinicians in the world. Determining the starting point for an exercise progression, sparing damaged joints, creating truly stabilizing muscle coactivation patterns, are all part of ensuring that the program helps an individual patient. Clinical trials in which a group of bad backs are given a standard dose of exercise will never reveal the true efficacy of the approach, nor will they reflect the importance of clinical skill. The best clinicians have many tools in their toolbox. The 'average' clinicians follow the teachings and cookbook guides of their gurus. This chapter is intended to enhance the foundation to enable better use of clinical tools and facilitate better clinical decisions. Some introductory notions are introduced here. For the interested reader, more extensive references together with tabulated data of specific muscle activation profiles, resultant spine loads, and algorithms for patient assessment, provocative testing, exercise design and prescription for the wide variety of unstable backs, can be found in the author's review chapters and original papers listed at: http://www.ahs.uwaterloo.ca/kin/people/StuMcGill.html or in the textbooks *Low back disorders: evidence-based prevention and rehabilitation* (McGill 2002) or *Ultimate back fitness and performance* (McGill 2006).

The clinical backdrop

In many traditional approaches to designing low back exercise, an emphasis has been placed on the immediate restoration, or enhancement, of spine range of motion and muscle strength. Generally, this approach has not been sufficiently efficacious in reducing back troubles; in fact, a review of the evidence suggests only a weak link with improving back symptoms while some studies suggest a link with negative outcome in significant numbers of people (McGill 1998). It appears that the emphasis on early restoration of spine range of motion continues to be driven by legislative definitions of low back disability – namely loss of range of motion. Thus, therapeutic success is often judged on motion restored. Not surprisingly recent work suggests little correlation between range of motion (ROM) and work disability ratings (Parks et al 2003). The developing philosophy based on mechanisms of injury and stability is developed here – that a spine must first be stable before moments and forces are produced to enhance performance but to do so in a way that spares the spine from potentially injurious load. Preliminary field evidence (although not yet definitive for all) suggests that the approach has promise.

Finally, no clinician will be successful without removing the cause. Provocative testing and detailed interviews help to identify the motions and loads that exacerbate symptoms. In my opinion, a large component of successful clinical outcome is due to the removal of the cause of the troubles from the patient's daily tasks. For this reason, the reader is briefly familiarized with injury mechanisms to ultimately minimize the risk of inadvertently prescribing routines that produce unnecessarily high loads on damaged tissues.

What causes instability? The links between mechanical overload, tissue damage, aberrant motor patterns and instability

Tissue damage results in a loss of stiffness in the supporting tissues allowing unstable joint behavior. Excellent progress has been made in the laboratory documenting specific instabilities from tissue damage in flexion–extension, lateral bend and axial rotation modes in animal preparations (Oxland et al 1991); however, understanding the injury process in humans (the cause of back troubles in real life) is not straightforward. For example, there is a tendency among those reporting or describing the back injury to identify a single specific event as the cause of the damage, such as lifting a box and twisting. This description of low back injury is common, particularly among the occupational/medical community, which is often required to identify a single event when filling out injury reporting forms. However, relatively few low back injuries occur from a single event. Rather, the culminating injury event was preceded by a history of excessive loading which gradually, but progressively, reduced the level of tolerance to tissue failure (McGill 1997). Thus other scenarios where subfailure loads (both repeated and prolonged) can result in injury are probably more important.

The links between injury mechanisms and instability have perhaps been hampered by the focus on exposure to a single variable – namely acute, or single maximum exposure to, lumbar compression. A few studies have suggested higher levels of compression exposure increased the risk of low back dysfunction (e.g. Ferguson et al 2005), although the correlation was low. Further some studies show that higher rates of low back dysfunction occur when levels of lumbar compression are reasonably low. Are there other mechanical variables that modulate the risk of low back dysfunctions? Joint shear has been shown to be very important as a metric for injury risk in the Norman et al (1998) study, particularly cumulative shear over a work day. In a series of work, the Waterloo group (McGill & Kippers 1994, McGill & Norman 1987, McGill et al 2000b) has shown that if the spine maintains a neutral curvature (the torso is flexed forward about the hips, neither flexing nor extending the spine itself) then the dominant low back extensors with their unique force vector direction (specifically longissimus thoracis and iliocostalis lumborum) support the shear reaction forces caused by the action of gravity on the flexed torso, resulting in a lowering of the shear load experienced by the joint. These forces would normally be borne by the disc and facet joints. However, if the individual elects to flex the spine itself when bending forward, sufficiently so to stretch the posterior ligaments with full spinal flexion, then the architecture of the interspinous ligaments causes anterior shear forces (Heylings 1978) to add to the shearing reaction from gravity (Fig. 35.1). Furthermore, ligamentous involvement disables the lumbar muscles (specifically noted above) from supporting the reaction shear as they reorientate to a line of action more parallel to the compressive axis (McGill et al 2000b). With full spine flexion and a modest amount of gravitational reaction shear it is not difficult to exceed shear failure loads of the spine, which have been found to be 2000–2800 Newtons in adult cadavers (Cripton et al 1995). This paragraph suggests that personal work technique, or more specifically, spine motion can affect the risk of spine damage. This is just one example of many.

Those reporting debilitating low back pain conclusively suffer simultaneous changes in their motor control systems. Recognizing these changes is important because they affect the stabilizing system and are therefore a focal point for optimal rehabilitation. Richardson et al (1999) have produced a comprehensive review of this literature and make a case for targeting specific muscle groups during rehabilitation. Specifically, their objective is to re-educate faulty motor control patterns postinjury. The challenge is to train the stabilizing system during steady-state activities together with stabilizing during rapid voluntary motions and to withstand sudden surprise loads. Our work documenting perturbed motor patterns focuses on biomechanical consequences. Paradoxically, many patients with back pain move in patterns to exacerbate pain! A major motor deficit appears to be 'gluteal amnesia' [erector spinae (ES) and hamstring dominance when lifting and rising from a chair] (McGill et al 2003). We believe from our stability analysis that this issue is much more important than other 'minor patterns', such as TrA, as evidenced from timing delays – greater delays exist in latissimus dorsi for example. Delays were observed in many muscles in those performing a more functional torso quick release study (Reeves et al 2005) and in fact were a powerful discriminator of those with a history of back troubles. This evidence coupled with our stability analyses suggest that the practice of 'drawing in' of the abdominal wall with intentional isolated activation of TrA compromises stability despite it being commonly taught to those who need stability. As will be shown, stability is enhanced with co-contraction of all muscles and that the muscles should be positioned away from the spine – not drawn towards it.

Preventing damaging tissue overload

Although there is not space to document the many mechanisms of back tissue damage in this brief chapter (see McGill 2002), a few guidelines are listed here:

1. First and foremost, design work tasks that facilitate variety:
   - Too much of any single activity leads to trouble. Relief of cumulative tissue strains are accomplished with posture changes, or better yet, other tasks that have different musculoskeletal demands.
2. During all demanding loading tasks, avoid fully flexed or bent spine postures (preserving a neutral curve in the spine). Of course the word 'demanding' needs to be interpreted within the context of the individual:
   - Disc herniation cannot occur.
   - Ligaments cannot be damaged as they are slack.
   - The anterior shearing effect from ligament involvement is minimized and the posterior supporting shear of the musculature is maximized.
   - Compressive testing of lumbar motion units has shown increases in tolerance with partial flexion but decreased ability to withstand compressive load at full flexion.
3. Choose a posture to minimize the reaction torque on the low back so long as 2 (above) is not compromised (keep the hand loads close):
   - Neutral spine is still maintained but sometimes the load can be brought closer to the spine with bent knees (squat lift) or relatively straight knees (stoop lift). The key is to reduce the torque which has been shown to be a dominant risk factor.
4. Consider the 'transmissible vector.' Attempt to direct external forces through the low back, minimizing the moment arm that causes high torques and crushing muscle forces:

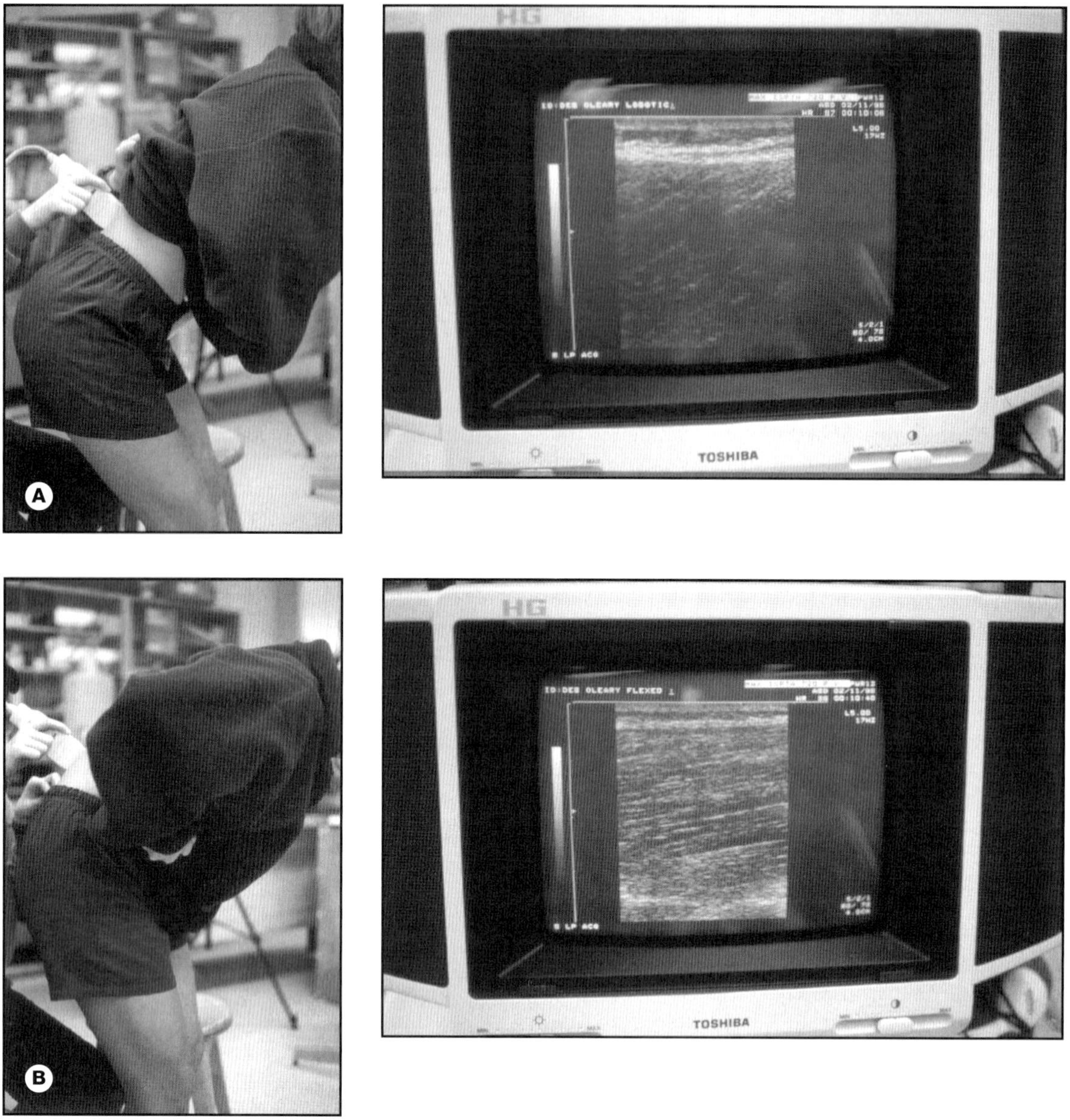

Fig. 35.1 The oblique angle of the lumbar portions of the iliocostalis lumborum and longissimus thoracis protects the spine against large anterior shear forces. However, this ability is a function of spine curvature. (A) A neutral spine and the oblique angle of these muscles as viewed with an ultrasound imager to be about 45°. (B) The loss of this angle to about 10° with spine flexion so that anterior shear forces cannot be counteracted. This is another reason to consider adopting a neutral spine during flexed weight-holding tasks with the muscles braced to ensure sufficient stability.

- This occurs when using pulling forces to open a door, vacuuming and other household chores, etc.

5. Use technique to minimize the actual weight of the load being handled:
   - A log-lifting example demonstrates how an entire log could be lifted into the back of a truck while only ever lifting half of its weight at any point in time (the log is lifted one end at a time).

6. Allow time for the disc nucleus to 'equilibrate' and ligaments to regain stiffness after prolonged flexion (e.g. sitting or stooping) and do not immediately perform strenuous exertions:

- After prolonged sitting or stooping, spend time standing to allow the nuclear material within the disc to equilibrate and equalize the stress on the annulus, and allow the ligaments to regain their rest length and provide protective stiffness to the lumbar spine. This can be expended to many special jobs, for example, for ambulance attendants it is important to be aware of the spine posture when traveling to the emergency scene. Don't sit in a slouched posture with the spine flexed, but rather sit upright. In this way the spine will be best prepared for strenuous work without a warm-up.

7. Avoid lifting or spine bending exercise shortly after rising from bed:
   - Forward bending stresses on the disc and ligaments are higher after rising from bed compared with later in the day (at least 1 hour after rising) causing discs to become injured at lower levels of load and degree of bending.
8. Prestress and stabilize the spine even during 'light' tasks:
   - Lightly co-contract the stabilizing musculature to stiffen the spine, even during 'light' tasks such as picking up a pencil.
9. Avoid twisting and the simultaneous generation of high twisting torques:
   - Twisting reduces the intrinsic strength of the disc annulus by disabling some of its supporting fibers while increasing the stress in the remaining fibers under load.
   - Generating twisting torque with the spine untwisted may not be as problematic nor is twisting lightly without substantial torque.
10. Use momentum when exerting force to reduce the spine load (rather than 'always lift slowly and smoothly' – this is an ill-founded recommendation for many skilled workers):
    - This is a skill that sometimes needs to be developed.
    - Dangerous for heavy loads and should not be attempted.
    - It is possible that a transfer of momentum from the upper trunk to the load can start moving an awkwardly placed load without undue low back.
11. Avoid prolonged sitting:
    - Prolonged sitting is associated with discogenic troubles.
    - When required to sit for long periods, adjust posture often, stand up, at least every 50 minutes, and extend the spine and/or, if possible, walk for a few minutes.
    - Organize work to break-up bouts of prolonged sitting into shorter periods that are better tolerated by the spine.
12. Consider the best rest-break strategies (customize this principle for different job classifications and demands):
    - Workers engaged in sedentary work would be best served by frequent, dynamic breaks to reduce tissue stress accumulation.
    - Workers engaged in dynamic work may be better served with longer and more 'restful' breaks.
13. Provide protective clothing to foster joint conserving postures:
    - Provide coveralls for dirty material handling, heavy aprons for sharp metals, knee pads for those who work at ground level, etc.
14. Practice joint-conserving kinematics movement patterns:
    - Some workers need to constantly re-groove motion patterns, for example locking the lumbar spine when lifting and rotating about the hips.
15. Maintain a reasonable level of fitness.
16. Think about interactions between several of these guidelines:
    - Some people have difficulty rolling over in bed, for example, when their backs are painful. Nearly all of them can be taught to manage their pain and still accomplish this task by combining muscle bracing with transmissible force vector steerage and a momentum transfer.

Instability as a cause of injury

Although biomechanists have been able to successfully explain how strenuous exertions cause specific low back tissue damage, explaining how injury occurs from tasks such as picking up a pencil from the floor has been more challenging. Evidence suggests that such injuries are real, and result from the spine 'buckling' or exhibiting unstable behavior. But this buckling mechanism can occur during far more challenging exertions as well.

A number of years ago, we were investigating the mechanics of powerlifter spines as they lifted extremely heavy loads – we were using video fluoroscopy to view their vertebrae in the sagittal plane. We happened to capture one injury on the fluoroscopic motion film – the first such observation that we know of. During the injury incident, just as the semi-squating lifter had lifted the load about 10 cm off the floor, the L2–L3 joint briefly rotated towards full flexion; all other lumbar joints maintained their static positions (not fully flexed) (Cholewicki & McGill 1992). The spine buckled! Sophisticated modeling analysis has revealed that buckling can occur from a motor control error where a short and temporary reduction in activation to one, or more, of the intersegmental muscles would cause rotation of just a single joint so that passive or other tissues become irritated or possibly injured (Cholewicki & McGill 1996). Conversely too much force in a single muscle could have led to the buckle (Brown & McGill 2005). So instability is both a cause and consequence of injury.

On stability: the foundation

This section briefly formalizes the notion of stability from a spine perspective. During the 1980s, Professor Anders Bergmark of Sweden very elegantly formalized stability in a spine model with joint stiffness and 40 muscles (Bergmark 1987). In this classic work, Bergmark formalized mathematically the concepts of 'energy wells', stiffness, stability, and instability. For the most part, this seminal work went unrecognized, largely because the engineers who understood the mechanics did not have the biological–clinical perspective, and the clinicians were hindered in the interpretation and implications of the engineering–mechanics. This pioneering effort, together with its continued evolution by several others has been synthesized in detail in McGill (2002).

The concept of stability begins with potential energy (PE), which for the purposes here, is of two basic forms. In the first form, objects have potential energy by virtue of their height above a datum:

$$PE = \text{mass} \times \text{gravity} \times \text{height}$$

Critical to measuring stability are the notions of energy 'wells' and minimum potential energy. If a ball is placed into a bowl it is stable, because if a force was applied to the ball (or a perturbation) the ball will rise up the side of the bowl but then come to rest again in the position of least potential energy at the bottom of the bowl – or the 'energy well.' As noted by Bergmark, 'stable equilibrium prevails when the potential energy of the system is minimum.' The system is made more stable by deepening the bowl and/or by increasing the steepness of the sides of the bowl.

Potential energy by virtue of height is only useful for illustrating the concept. Potential energy as a function of stiffness and storage of elastic energy is actually used for musculoskeletal application. Elastic potential energy is calculated from stiffness (k) and deformation (x) in the elastic element:

$$PE = 1/2 \times k \times x^2$$

In other words the greater the stiffness (k) the greater the steepness of the sides of the bowl (from the previous analogy), and the more stable the structure. Thus stiffness creates stability. Active muscle produces a stiff member and, in fact, the greater the activation of the muscle, the greater this stiffness; it has long been known that joint stiffness increases rapidly and nonlinearly with muscle activation such that only very modest levels of muscle activity create sufficiently stiff, and stable joints. The motor control system is able to control stability of the joints through coordinated muscle coactivation and to a lesser degree by placing joints in positions that modulate passive stiffness contribution. However, a faulty motor control system can lead to inappropriate magnitudes of muscle force, and stiffness, allowing a 'valley' for the 'ball to roll out' or clinically, for a joint to buckle or undergo shear translation [see Cholewicki & McGill (1996) for mathematical detail]. In clinical terms, the full complement of the stabilizing musculature must work harmoniously to both ensure stability together with generation of the required moment and desired joint movement. But only one muscle with inappropriate activation amplitude can produce instability, or at least unstable behavior could result at lower applied loads. Muscle stiffness is always stabilizing but muscle force, either too high or too low, can be destabilizing (Brown & McGill 2005).

In our series of papers, stabilization exercises were quantified and ranked for muscle activation magnitudes together with the resultant spine load (see Kavcic et al 2004a, 2004b). Furthermore, Cholewicki's work (Cholewicki & McGill 1996) has demonstrated that sufficient stability of the lumbar spine is achieved, in an undeviated spine, in most people with modest levels of coactivation of the paraspinal and abdominal wall muscles. This means that people, from patients to athletes, must be able to maintain sufficient stability in all activities – with low, but continuous, muscle activation. Thus, maintaining a stability 'margin of safety' when performing tasks, particularly the tasks of daily living, is not compromised by insufficient strength but rather by insufficient endurance. We are now beginning to understand the mechanistic pathway of those studies showing the efficacy of endurance training for the muscles that stabilize the spine (Biering-Sorensen 1984).

Finally, our understanding of shear stability has recently been enhanced. Shear stability is interesting for several reasons but the primary one is that many unstable spines are provoked with shear loading. Those muscles running parallel to the spine, and with direct attachment (e.g. psoas, quadratus, multifidus) become stiff when activated. When stiff, they resist transverse shearing. An analogy can be created by using a sock filled with fresh concrete. When wet, the sock cannot resist shear load but once the concrete sets, or as the muscle becomes active and stiff, it buttresses shear easily. In this way these muscles add stability via compression to the buckling mode together with direct buttressing of shear, hence added shear stability.

All muscles influence stability

Interestingly, muscle stiffness is always stabilizing, but muscle force might contribute to stability or it might reduce it if it is inappropriately large or small. There is no such thing as a muscle that is the best stabilizer of the back (Kavcic et al 2004b). There is a common notion that 'local' stabilizers are more important than 'global' ones. This notion is incorrect – generally, those muscles with the largest moment arms and capacity for stiffness (those furthest from the spine) are the more stabilizing on a relative basis. In addition, the most important stabilizers continually change as the task changes (Fig. 35.2). In addition, different stabilizing exercises produce different amount of spine stability (Kavcic et al 2004b).

In summary, the muscular and motor control system must satisfy the requirements to sustain postures, create movements, brace against sudden motion or unexpected forces, build pressure, and assist challenged breathing, all the while ensuring sufficient stability. Virtually all muscles play a role in ensuring stability but their importance at any point in time is determined by the unique combination of the demands just listed. Specific muscles by their architecture have different stabilizing abilities. The lumbar longissimus and iliocostalis have been mentioned (see Fig. 35.1); quadratus lumborum is a major stabilizer given its lateral attachments to every vertebral transverse process and the iliac creast and rib cage. The abdominal obliques, with their criss-crossing design buttress many modes of stability challenge. Rectus abdominis is critical as

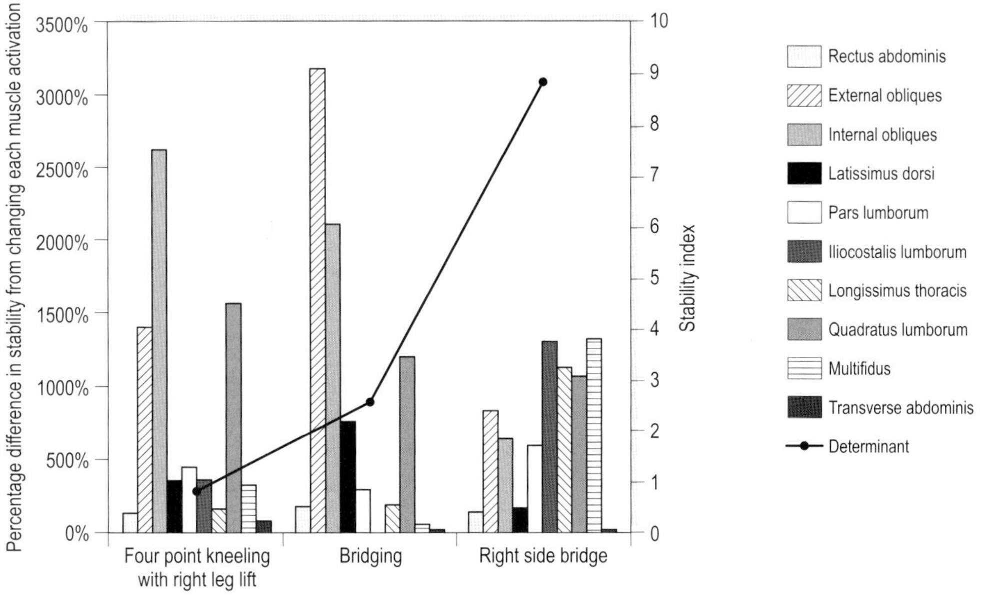

Fig. 35.2 The contribution of some torso muscles to spine stability is shown in three exercises performed by a single person. The most important contributors continually change. In this individual, the four point kneeling and back bridge show that the obliques of the abdominal wall together with quadratus are most important. Changing the task increases the role of quadratus lumborum, latissumus dorsi, iliocostalis, longissimus and multifidus as seen in the side bridge exercise. Subtle shifts in posture and technique would change these relative contributions.

the anterior anchor of the abdominal wall muscles. We are also starting to uncover evidence that there is a 'super binding' effect when all abdominal muscles are activated simultaneously such that the measured torso stiffness is larger than the sum of their individual stiffnesses – once again it would appear to be counterproductive to focus activation on just one muscle. These are simple examples of which there are many. Training a single muscle, or at least focusing on the activation of a single muscle appears to lead to dysfunction or at least compromised function!

Some thoughts on evaluating the potentially unstable patient – provocative testing

The issue here is not about identifying the tissues that cause pain – this is a dead-end pursuit unless one is a surgeon looking to 'cut the specific pain out.' Identifying the pain-causing tissue is also irrelevant for identifying and prescribing the best therapeutic exercise. Critical is the understanding of the motions/loads that exacerbate the pain so that these can be identified and removed from the patient's movements and postures that form their daily activities. It is also very important to ensure that the exercise prescription does not incorporate the pain exacerbator. All sorts of specific tests are designed to provoke with loads, postures, and motions. The best one for segmental instability that results in pain that we have found was described by Magee (1997) and trialed by our own group (Hicks et al 2005) (Fig. 35.3). The test was trialed in multiple centers and turned out to be the best predictor of which patients would do well with 'stability' exercises.

A program of staged progressions – the 'ultimate approach'

The evidence suggests that a systematic, staged, and very purposefully designed rehabilitation and performance-based program is best for the back. It must recognize the need to correct nonoptimal components of a patient's movement scheme, spare the joints, train muscle patterns, and performance qualities. For rehabilitation purposes, our program follows three general stages. Building the stable back for performance objectives follows a longer, five-stage process that ensures a foundation for eventual strength, speed, and power training (Box 35.1). The exercise components of each stage are carefully considered to reduce spine loading, and enhance muscular coactivation to ensure stability

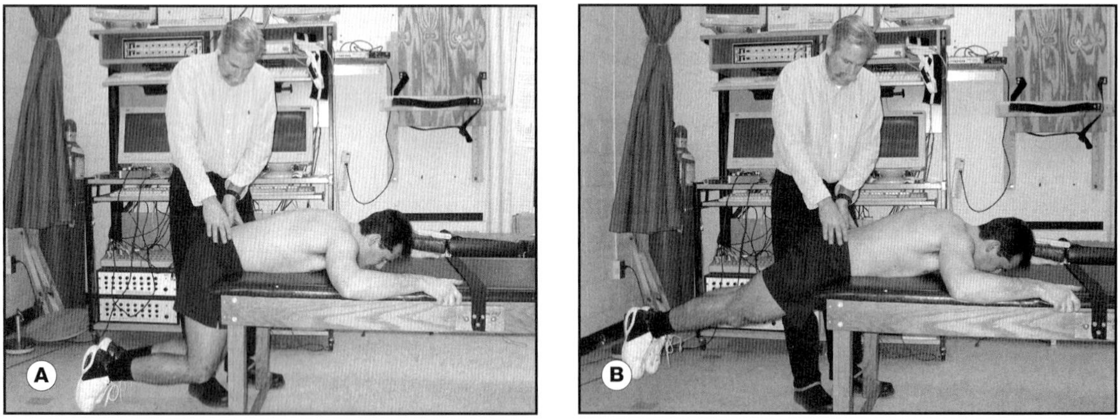

Fig. 35.3 The patient lies prone with the body on a table but with the legs over the edge and the feet on the floor (A), the torso musculature is relaxed. The clinician then applies direct force downward onto each spinous process in turn (starting at the sacrum, then L5, L4, L3, etc.). Unstable segments are identified when the patient reports pain. Then the patient raises the legs off the floor to contract the back extensors (B). The clinician once again applies force on each spinous process. By virtue of their lines of action, the lumbar extensors will reduce shearing instability if present. If pain is present in the resting position but then disappears or subsides with the active co-contraction, the test is positive. This test proves that activating the extensors stabilizes the shear instability and eliminates the pain. Now the challenge is to incorporate these extensor motor patterns into exercise prescriptions to carry over to daily activities.

Box 35.1

Rehabilitation and building a stable back for performance

For rehabilitation

- Stage 1: Groove motion patterns, motor patterns and corrective exercise:
  - basic movement patterns through to complex activity-specific patterns
  - basic balance-challenges through to complex balance-specific environments
- Stage 2: Build whole body and joint stability:
  - build stability while sparing the joints
  - ensure sufficient stability commensurate for the demands of the task
- Stage 3: Increase endurance:
  - basic endurance training to build the foundation for eventual strength
  - activity-specific endurance (duration, intensity)

For performance add

- Stage 4: Build strength:
  - spare the joints while maximizing neuromuscular compartment challenge
  - speed strength and multi-articular functional strength
  - optimal timing and 'steering' of strength
- Stage 5: Develop power, agility:
  - develop ultimate performance with the foundation laid in stages 1–4

Overlay for all stages

- The position of performance
- The balance environment

within the demand of the task. It is emphasized that these are only a few examples that might, or might not, be suitable for an individual.

Stage 1: Grooving motion/motor patterns and corrective exercise

In my consulting, I see the result of prescribed exercises that cause back troubles, or that are detrimental to performance in athletes/workers/patients. Where does one start in the process of finding the most appropriate and suitable exercise? Generally, we blend several perspectives, beginning with qualitative approaches and finishing with quantitative information. First, we assess the patient's current exercise status within our own knowledge of spine tissue loads that result from various activities. Then we blend our knowledge of injury mechanisms to qualify an individual for a specific exercise progression. We then make an 'educated' guess as to the best program and monitor patient progress to ensure a positive slope in the improvement in symptoms and function. In this way we act as 'medical detectives' where we try to view the person, and then the exercises, all within the context of the person's sporting and lifestyle environment. When I am teaching physicians, physical therapists, or conditioning experts to 'view' the client/patient, I suggest that they approach the task as if they are the student. What can they learn from the patient that will help them prescribe the optimal program? What do they see when they observe the client move, or sit, or stand? What do they hear when the client answers their questions? What do they feel when assessing co-contraction and muscle dominance in a particular test?

Many provocative tests are described that exacerbate pain – to identify movements and muscle activation patterns that are painful and must be avoided. Any exercise that causes pain is inhibiting and excellent form will not be achieved – working through the pain with the back is rarely successful. If the patient has pain he or she is doing the exercise incorrectly or – more likely – is doing the wrong exercise. Other provocative tests identify when an individual is ready for specific training objectives. For example, training torso torsion causes troubles for people who do not have the foundation.

Aberrant motion can indicate poor lumbar control, which needs addressing; this can be seen about several axes. For example, although many individuals are sufficiently strong in torso flexion and extension, they fail the following test (Fig. 35.4). Placing a person with poor torsional control in a cable pulling exercise to produce twisting torque could be problematic – corrective exercise would be required first. In this example, a rotational disconnect of the rib cage and pelvis during this test can indicate that more work is required for enhancing lumbar control.

Locking the rib cage onto the pelvis: the abdominal brace

For many unstable patients, learning to lock the rib cage on the pelvis is essential for pain control, injury prevention and for performance.

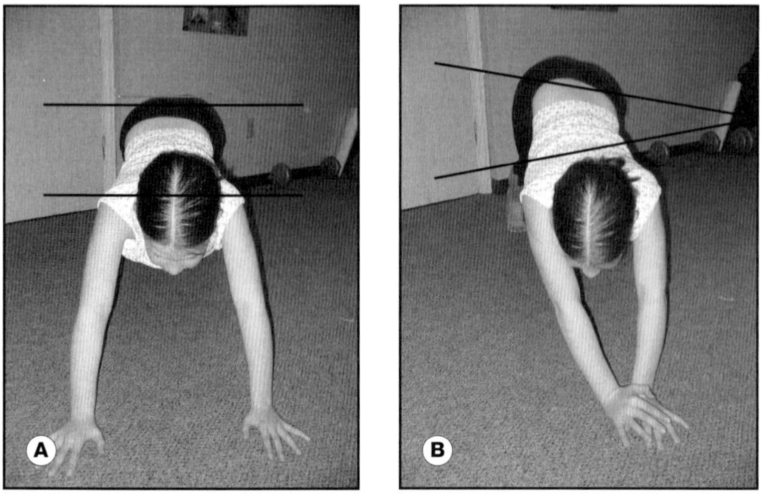

Fig. 35.4 Starting in the push-up position one hand is lifted over to the other. The pelvis and ribcage should remain locked. The elevated pelvis (shown in B) indicated poor lumbar torsional control.

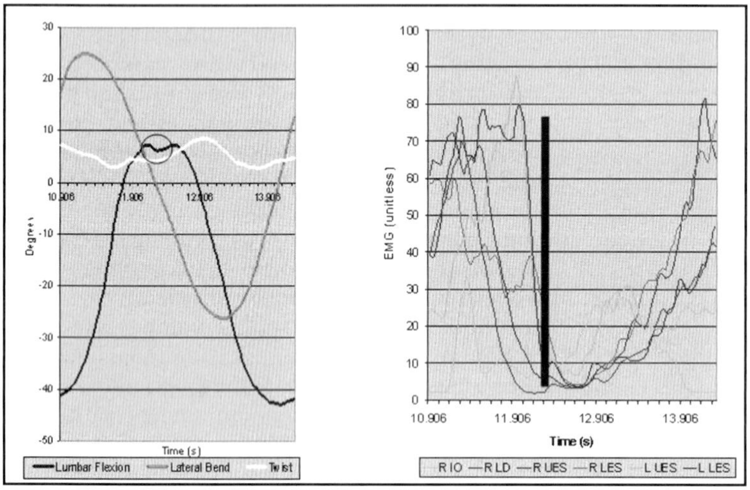

Fig. 35.5 The spine experiences instability (seen and heard as a clunk) during torso rotation in a standing position (circled in the left panel). The unstable event occurs as the torso passes through the upright posture at the instant that the muscle activity drops to a minimum and the instant of insufficient stability (indicated with the line in the right panel). RIO, right int. oblique; RLD, right latissimus dorsi; RUES, right upper erector spinea at T9; RLES, right lower erector spinea at L3; LUES and LLES are left side muscles.

In the following example a patient was exhibiting very graphic instability – the spine 'clunked' (this could also be heard) during circular motions of the trunk as he passed through the upright posture. Interestingly, and predictably, it was at this instant that all muscle activation levels dropped, resulting in insufficient stiffness (see Fig. 35.5). Teaching him the abdominal brace while moving buttressed the instability and removed the symptoms and accompanying sciatica – this was the beginning of his recovery to normal life. Many patients cannot stabilize with spine motion and need to be taught to lock the rib cage on the pelvis. An example of an exercise to establish the locking pattern between the rib cage and pelvis is the wall roll (Fig. 35.6). The motion pattern is accompanied by the abdominal brace motor pattern. The brace involves the co-contraction of the abdominal wall muscles without

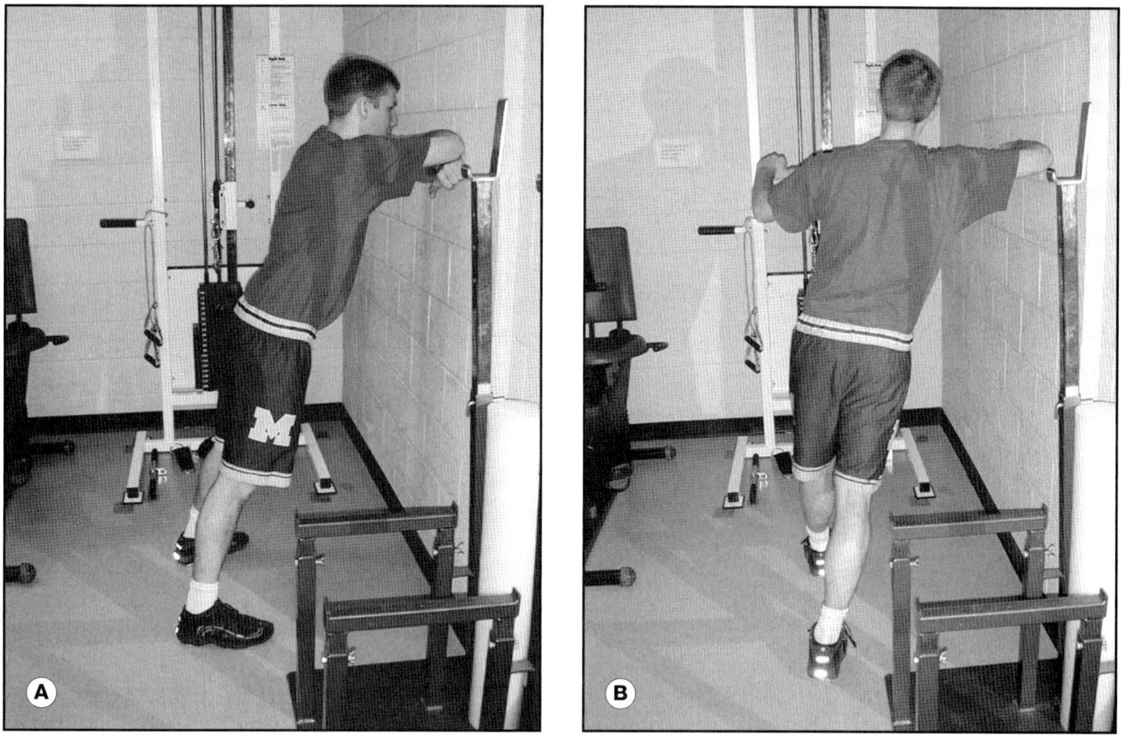

Fig. 35.6 The wall roll begins with the patient in the 'plank' with both elbows planted on the wall. The abdominals are braced and the ribcage is 'locked' on the pelvis. The individual pivots on the balls of the feet pulling one elbow off the wall. No spine motion is permitted. This is considered correct exercise and is suitable for many chronic backs.

pulling the navel in. This causes contraction of virtually all torso muscles enhancing stability (McGill 2006).

Building squat patterns

A good back needs healthy gluteal muscle function, because performance and safety demands balanced hip power about each axis. This section describes some hip motor patterns that inhibit performance and compromise back health, together with providing an example of corrective training progressions to address them.

The 'crossed-pelvis syndrome' (Janda 1996) occurs when the gluteal complex is inhibited during squatting patterns in those with a history of back troubles (together with some others as well). Interestingly, we still do not know if the crossed-pelvis syndrome exists prior to back troubles or is a consequence of having them. Nonetheless, the syndrome is noticeable in both athletes and normals referred to our research clinic (McGill 2006). This results in two concerns. First, those with aberrant gluteal patterns cannot spare their backs during squatting patterns because they use the hamstrings and erector spinae to drive the extension motion. Subsequently, the erector spinae forces load up the lumbar spine. Healthy gluteal patterns are needed to spare the back. Second, it is impossible to rebuild optimal squat performance, either for strength or hip extensor power, without well-integrated hip extensor patterns. In fact, the source of the failure for many athletes to properly rehabilitate is due to the emphasis on strengthening philosophies without first addressing the aberrant gluteal patterns. A strength and power athlete will continue to be compromised with chronic back troubles until these motor patterns are addressed.

Retraining the gluteals cannot be performed with traditional squat exercises that utilize a barbell on the back. Performing a traditional squat requires little hip abduction. Consequently, there is little gluteus medius activation and the gluteus maximus activation is delayed during the squat until lower squat angles are reached (McGill 2006). It is a quadriceps exercise! In contrast to the traditional squat, a one-legged squat activates the gluteus medius immediately to assist in the frontal plane hip drive necessary for leaping, running, etc., together with sooner integration of gluteus maximus higher in the squat motion.

For the chronic deconditioned patient we may begin with simply isolating gluteus medius with the clamshell exercise (Fig. 35.7). An example of a more progressive exercise – the one-legged squat matrix – is shown in Fig. 35.8.

Stage 2: Building whole body and joint stability

Spine stability is intended to control motion to minimize pain, and grooves in the motor patterns minimize the risk of unstable behavior during any sort of task or perturbation. Whole body stability is not spine stability and involves maintaining a dynamic balance, but in performance terms it includes honing the ability to 'steer' forces through the linkage in the optimal way. We have spent a number of years quantifying and exercise searching for those which enhance stabilizing patterns of muscle activation, yet spare the spine of large loads. From this collective work we developed the 'Big 3' – the curl-up, the side bridge, and the birddog (Figs 35.9, 35.10, 35.11, and 35.12). Briefly, a sample of the collection of work used in their development is as follows.

Given the architectural and electromyographic (EMG) evidence for quadratus lumborum as a spine stabilizer, the optimal technique to maximize activation but minimize the spine load appears to be the side bridge (see Fig. 35.10) – beginners bridge from the knees whereas advanced bridges are from the feet. When supported with the feet and elbow, the lumbar compression is a modest 2500 N but the quadratus closest to the floor appears to be active up to 50% of maximum voluntary contraction (the obliques experience similar challenge) (Juker et al 1998). Advanced technique to enhance the motor challenge is to roll from one elbow over to the other while abdominally bracing rather than repeated 'hiking' the hips off the floor into the bridge position

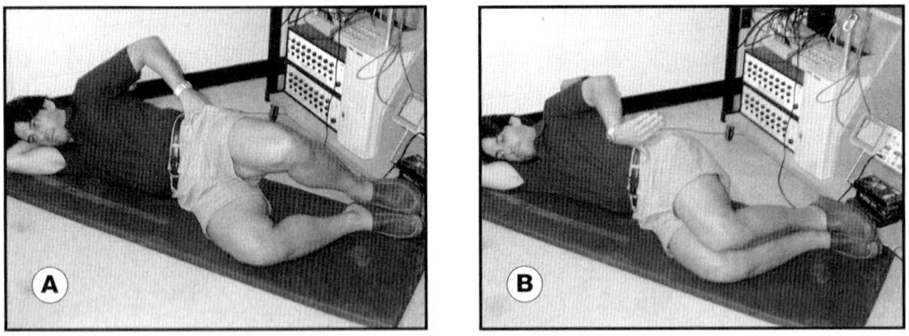

Fig. 35.7 Training gluteus medius into the motor pattern schema. Anchoring the thumb on the anterior superior iliac spine (ASIS) and reaching around with the finger tips should position them to land on gluteus medius. Opening the knees like a clam shell will allow the person to feel the gluteus medius activation.

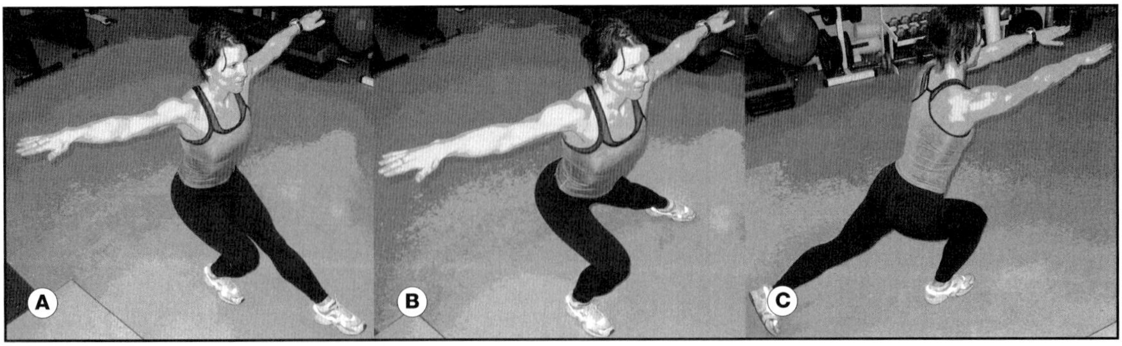

Fig. 35.8 Single-legged squat progressions with the leg to the front (A), side (B), and behind (C). The abdominals are braced, the lumbar spine neutral and the mental focus of the person is on hip extension torque. The hips are drifted posteriorly during the descent to place more emphasis on the gluteals for hip extension.

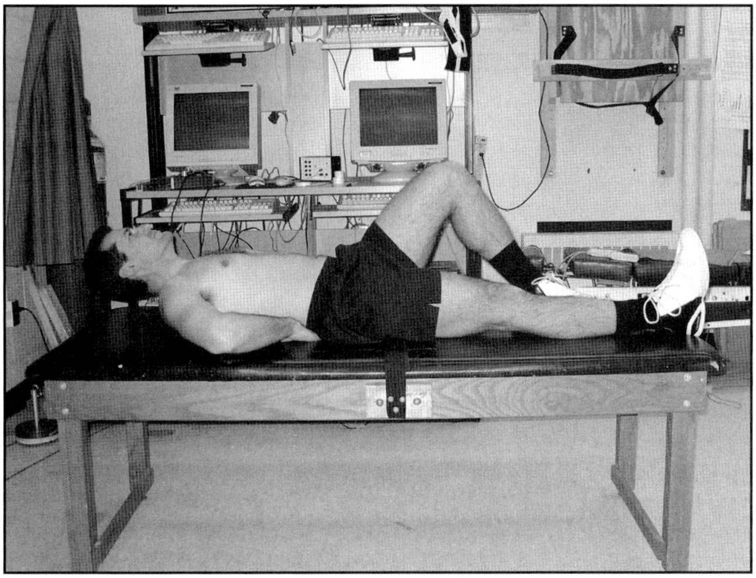

Fig. 35.9 The curl-up, where the head and shoulders are raised off the ground with the hands under the lumbar region to help stabilize the pelvis and support the neutral spine. Only one leg is bent to assist in pelvic stabilization and preservation of a 'neutral' lumbar curve. Additional progressive challenge can be created by raising the elbows from the floor and generating an abdominal brace or co-contraction.

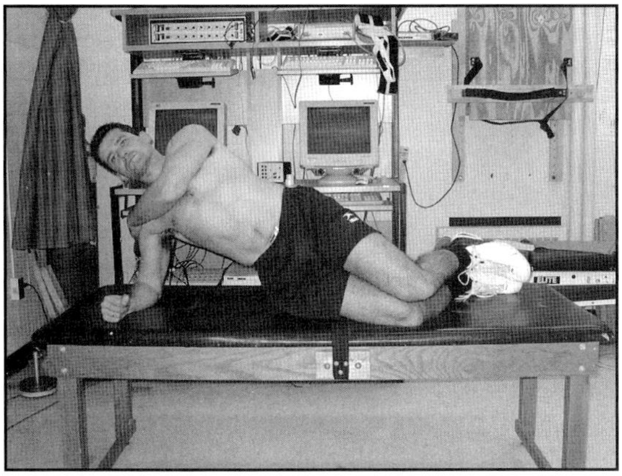

Fig. 35.10 The horizontal isometric side bridge. Supporting the lower body with the knees on the floor reduces the demand further for those who are more concerned with minimizing spine load to pain-free tolerable levels.

(see Fig. 35.11). Higher levels of activation would be reached with the feet on a labile surface (Vera Garcia et al 2000).

Calibrated intramuscular and surface EMG evidence suggests that the various types of curl-ups challenge mainly rectus abdominis, as psoas and abdominal wall (internal and external oblique, transverse abdominis) activity is relatively low. Sit-ups (both straight leg and bent knee) are characterized by higher psoas activation and higher low back compressive loads that approach and can exceed NIOSH occupational guidelines, whereas leg raises cause even higher activation and also spine compression [the interested reader is directed to Axler & McGill (1997) for actual data]. It is also interesting that myoelectric evidence suggests that there is little functional distinction between an 'upper' and 'lower' rectus abdominis in most people but, in contrast, the obliques are regionally activated with 'upper' and 'lower' motor point areas together with medial and lateral components. Transverse abdominis and internal oblique are selectively activated by dynamically 'hollowing' in the abdominal wall, whereas an isometric abdominal brace coactivates the entire abdominal wall and rectus abdominis, together with the extensors to ensure stability in virtually all modes of possible instability (McGill 2006). Several relevant observations were made regarding abdominal exercises in our investigations. It is interesting to note that the often-recommended 'press-heels' sit-up, which has been hypothesized to activate hamstrings and neurally inhibit psoas, was actually confirmed to increase psoas activation! [Original data can be found in Juker et al (1998); we note here that some clinicans and coaches who intentionally wish to train psoas will find this data informative.]

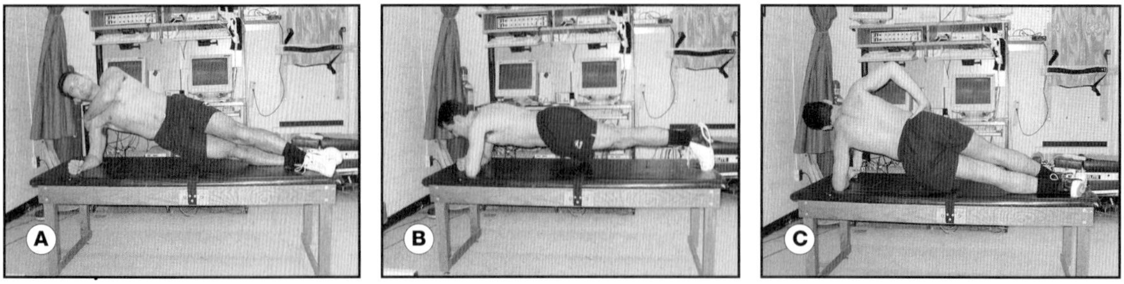

Fig. 35.11 Advanced side bridges are accomplished by supporting the body with the feet to enhance the muscle challenge, but also the spine load. Following each side bridge hold, one 'rolls' from one elbow to the other while abdominally bracing, locking the pelvis and the rib cage.

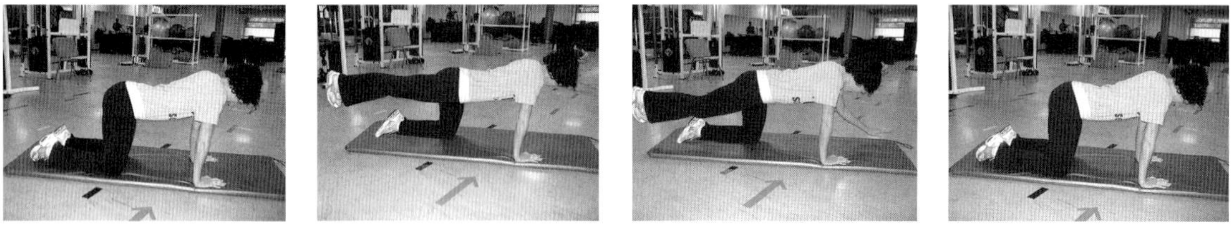

Fig. 35.12 The birddog is achieved with the individual raising the opposite arm and leg simultaneously. One should avoid raising either the arm or the leg past horizontal. The objective is to be able to hold the limbs parallel to the floor for about six to eight seconds. Good form includes a neutral spine and abdominal bracing. Some patients will start with simple raising of a hand or knee from the floor; more advanced patients will perform the 'sweep the floor' move with the arm and leg to develop stabilizing motion patterns. These are just examples within a much larger progression matched to the patient.

Once again, the horizontal side support appears to have merit as it challenges the lateral obliques and transverse abdominis without high lumbar compressive loading.

Most traditional extensor exercises are characterized by very high spine loads, which result from externally applied compressive and shear forces (either from free weights or resistance machines). From our search for methods to activate the extensors (including longissimus, iliocostalis and multifidii) with minimal spine loading, it appears that the single leg extension hold minimizes the spine load (< 2500 N) and activates one side of the lumbar extensors to approximately 18% of maximum voluntary contraction (MVC) (Callaghan et al 1998). Simultaneous leg extension with contralateral arm raise ('birddog') increases the unilateral extensor muscle challenge (approximately 27% MVC in one side of the lumbar extensors and 45% MVC in the other side of the thoracic extensors) but also increases lumbar compression to well over 3000 N (see Fig. 35.12). This exercise can be enhanced with abdominal bracing and deliberate 'mental imaging' of activation of each level of the local extensors. The often-performed exercise of lying prone on the floor and raising the upper body and legs off the floor is contraindicated for anyone at risk of low back injury, or reinjury. In this task, the lumbar region pays a high compression penalty to a hyperextended spine (usually much higher than 4000 N), which transfers load to the facets and crushes the interspinous ligament.

In general, we recommend that these isometric holds be held no longer than 7–8 seconds given recent evidence from near infrared spectroscopy indicating rapid loss of available oxygen in the torso muscles contracting at these levels – short relaxation of the muscle restores oxygen (McGill et al 2000a).

Challenges to the spine during daily activity include the maintenance of stability during stable, steady-state posture maintenance, and during unexpected loading events together with ballistic movement that is prehensively planned. This has motivated some clinicians to utilize labile surfaces such as gym balls. Certainly, these labile surfaces challenge the motor system to meet the dynamic tasks of daily living. But is this type of training of concern for some patients? Our recent quantification of elevated spine loads and muscle coactivation when performing a curl-up on labile surfaces (Vera Garcia et al 2000) suggests that the rehabilitation program should begin on stable surfaces. Labile surfaces should be introduced once the spine load-bearing capacity has been sufficiently restored. The point is that there is no ideal exercise for all unstable spines. Examine the patient and use the information to make wise choices in exercise design, choice of starting load, rate and type of progression. A few examples have been offered here.

Full progression of these with specific technique details is shown and described in *Ultimate back fitness and performance* (McGill 2006). More 'athletic' progressions can be developed. For example, performing the traditional push-up with a staggered hand placement, or with labile balls under the hands, facilitates the stabilizing torso mechanism (McGill 2004) (Fig. 35.13).

Stage 3: Endurance

Endurance is a pillar for training virtually every unstable individual with very few exceptions. There is a progression to building endurance. Typically, endurance is built first with repeated sets in patients, and then for some athletes the progression continues with longer holds.

Early endurance progressions usually begin with the isometric holds performed in the curl-ups, bridges, and birddog exercises. These should be held no longer than 7 or 8 seconds. The duration is based on recent evidence from near infrared spectroscopy indicating rapid loss of available oxygen in torso muscles contracting at these levels. Short relaxation of the muscle restores oxygen. The endurance objectives are achieved by building-up repetitions of the exertions rather than by increasing the duration of each hold.

Motivated by the evidence for the superiority of extensor endurance over strength as a benchmark for good back health, we documented normal ratios of endurance times for the torso flexors relative to the extensors and lateral musculature. These values may be used to identify endurance deficits – both absolute values and for one muscle group relative to another – and to establish reasonable endurance goals for patients (McGill et al 1999).

The reverse pyramid for endurance training

This approach to designing endurance sets is founded in the Russian tradition of maintaining excellent technique and form: 'Do as much as you can while you are as fresh as you can be.' For example, if one were to design sets for the side-bridge exercise using five repetitions then the workout would look like this. Five repetitions on the right side would be followed by five on the left. Rest. Then four on the right and four on the left. Finally, three on the right and then three on the left. Finished. Good technique is facilitated as the repetitions are reduced with each fatiguing set. This is generally used to build the endurance base; the objective of maintaining sufficient oxygen levels is met so that the failure mechanism is not oxygen starvation.

Training for endurance events

Some individuals will eventually need to train constant and prolonged contraction in the torso. An example of such a person would be a garbage collector or a long-distance swimmer. There are no specific guidelines here beyond seeking the optimal challenge for the back. Traditional endurance overload principles will be utilized within the activity-specific endurance demands. These types of

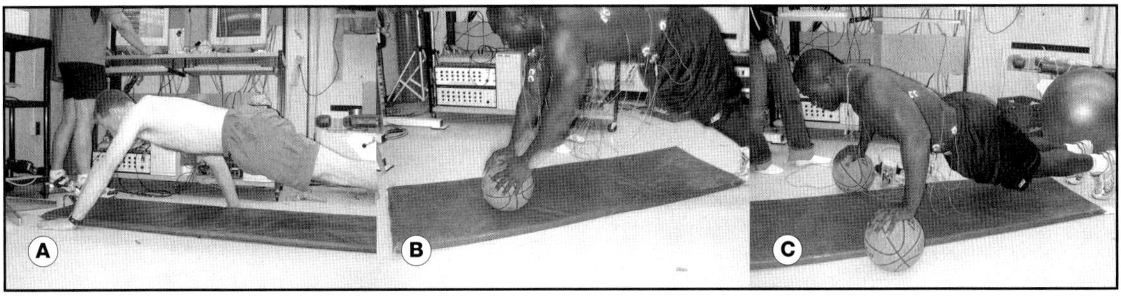

Fig. 35.13 Progressions of push-ups to facilitate abdominal activation for stability. In particular, moving the typical hand placement to a staggered position, with one forward and the other beside the lower ribs (A), and using a ball under the hands for lability are excellent techniques (B,C). Focus is on lumbar control with the rib cage locked to the pelvis.

individuals will obviously train with much longer durations for a repetition, up to several minutes, or even hours in some cases.

Stage 4: Strength training considerations

Training ultimate strength without injury is a difficult challenge. When searching for ways to obtain maximum myoelectric activity from the back extensor muscles, we discovered that isometric back extensor exercises do not recruit the full pool of motor units. Many more motor units fire with some extensor motion. For example, maximal-effort deadlifts appear to activate only a very limited number of the motor units possible with isometric contraction. There are many techniques to overcome this limitation presented in McGill (2006). An example of abdominal strengthening in a way that enhances overall strength and performance comprises of overhead cable pulls shown in Fig. 35.14. The spine is protected with a neutral posture and enhances performance for throwers, martial artists or any others needing abdominal strengthening and lumbar stability in upright postures to control objects or opponents.

Stage 5: Power

The emphasis is on developing power at the hips, as power development in the spine is very detrimental to the unstable spine. Developing spine power compromises both safety and performance. Note that power is the product of force × velocity and if either – force or velocity – is high then the other should generally be kept low. Finally, plyometric training of the torso muscles is very desirable for performance but again is only mentioned here as the final stages of exercise progression for the athletes with unstable spines and who have mastered stages 1–4. These examples are important to illustrate that an unstable spine can be properly conditioned to the level allowing world class performance.

Summary

A few examples of therapeutic exercise to address instability over a wide range of patient capabilities have been introduced here. It is part of an approach that should be considered as another tool for the toolbox of clinicians. The better clinicians have many tools and know when to try working with one tool, when to try different progressions of exercise, and when to try another tool.

Acknowledgments

The author wishes to acknowledge the contributions of many colleagues who have contributed to the collection of works reported here. Also the continual financial support from the Natural Science and Engineering Research Council, Canada has made this series of work possible.

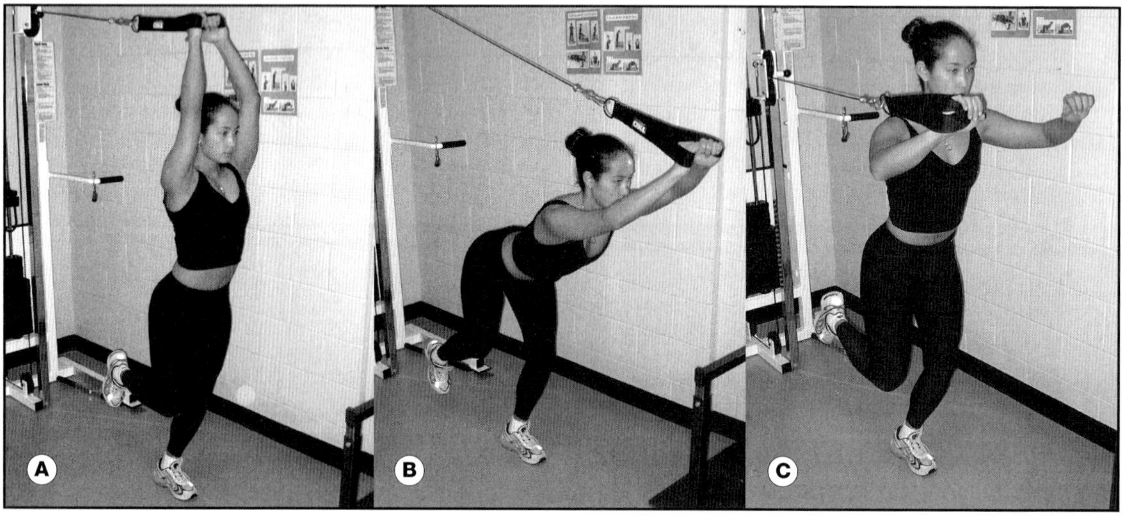

Fig. 35.14 Overhead cable pulls are a whole body exercise integrating the abdominals in a technique to enhance short-range stiffness, control and strength. Focus is on abdominal bracing, and a neutral spine. Labile surfaces under the feet can be incorporated.

References

Axler CT, McGill SM 1997 Low back loads over a variety of abdominal exercises: Searching for the safest abdominal challenge. Med Sci Sports Ex 29:804–811

Bergmark A 1987 Mechanical stability of the human lumbar spine. Doctoral dissertation, Department of Solid Mechanics, Lund University, Sweden

Biering-Sorensen F 1984 Physical measurements as risk indicators for low back trouble over a one year period. Spine 9:106–119

Brown SH, McGill SM 2005 Muscle force-stiffness characteristics influence joint stability. Clin Biomech 20(9):917–922

Callaghan JP, Gunning JL, McGill SM 1998 Relationship between lumbar spine load and muscle activity during extensor exercises. Physical Therapy 78:8–18

Cholewicki J, McGill SM 1992 Lumbar posterior ligament involvement during extremely heavy lifts estimated from fluoroscopic measurements. J Biomech 25(1): 17–28

Cholewicki J, McGill SM 1996 Mechanical stability of the in vivo lumbar spine: Implications for injury and chronic low back pain. Clin Biomech 11(1):1–15

Cripton P, Berleman U, Visarino H et al 1995 Response of the lumbar spine due to shear loading. In: Injury prevention through biomechanics. Symposium proceedings, 4–5 May, Wayne State University, TX

Ferguson SA, Marras WS, Burr D 2005 Workplace design guidelines for asymptomatic vs. low back injured workers. Appl Ergonom 36(1): 85–95

Heylings DJ 1978 Supraspinous and interspinous ligaments of the human lumbar spine. J Anat 123:127–131

Hicks GE, Fritz JM, Delitto A, McGill SM 2005 Preliminary development of a clinical prediction role for determining which patients with low back pain will respond to stabilization exercise program. Arch Phys Med Rehab 86(9):1753–1762

Janda V 1996 Evaluaton of muscle imbalance. In: Liebenson C (ed) Rehabilitation of the spine: a practioner's manual. Lippincott, Williams and Wilkins, Baltimore, MD

Juker D, McGill SM, Kropf P, Steffen T 1998 Quantitative intramuscular myoelectric activity of lumbar portions of psoas and the abdominal wall during a wide variety of tasks. Med Sci Sports Ex 30(2):301–310

Kavcic N, Grenier S, McGill S 2004a Determining the stabilizing role of individual torso muscles during rehabilitation exercises. Spine 29(11):1254–1265

Kavcic N, Grenier SG, McGill SM 2004b Quantifying tissue loads and spine stability while performing commonly prescribed stabilization exercises. Spine 29(20): 2319–2329

Magee D 1997 Orthopaedic physical assessment, 3rd edn. WB Saunders, Philadelphia, PA

McGill SM 1997 ISB keynote lecture – the biomechanics of low back injury: implications on current practice in industry and the clinic. J Biomech 30:465–476

McGill SM 1998 Low back exercises: Evidence for improving exercise programs. Physical Therapy 78:754–765

McGill SM 2002 Low back disorders: evidence based prevention and rehabilitation. Human Kinetics Publishers, Champaign, IL

McGill SM 2006 Ultimate back fitness and performance, 3rd edn. Wabuno Publishers, Waterloo, Canada. Online. Available: www.backfitpro.com

McGill SM, Kippers V 1994 Transfers of loads between lumbar tissues during the flexion–relaxation phenomenon. Spine 19:2190–2196

McGill SM, Norman RW 1987 Effects of an anatomically detailed erector spinae model on L4/L5 disc compression and shear. J Biomech 20:591–600

McGill SM, Childs A, Liebenson C 1999 Endurance times for stabilization exercises: Clinical targets for testing and training from a normal database. Arch Phys Med Rehab 80:941–944

McGill SM, Highson R, Parks K 2000a Erector spinae oxygenation during prolonged contractions: implications for prolonged work. Ergonomics 43:486–493

McGill SM, Parks K, Hughson R 2000b Changes in lumbar lordosis modify the role of the extensor muscles. Clin Biomech 15(10):777–780

McGill SM, Grenier S, Bluhm M et al 2003 Previous history of LBP with work loss is related to lingering effects in biomechanical, physiological, personal and psychosocial characteristics. Ergonomics 46(7):731–746

Norman RW, Wells R, Neumann P et al 1998 A comparison of peak vs. cumulative physical work exposure risk factors for the reporting of low back pain in the automotive industry. Clin Biomech 13:561–573

Oxland TR, Panjabi MM, Southern EP, Duranceau JJ 1991 An anatomic basis for spinal instability: a porcine trauma model. J Orthop Res 9:452–462

Parks KA, Crichton KS, Goldford RJ, McGill SM 2003 On the validity of ratings of impairment for low back disorders. Spine 28(4):380–384

Reeves NP, Cholewicki J, Milner TE 2005 Muscle reflex classification for low back pain. J Electromyogr Kinesiol 5(1):53–60

Richardson C, Jull G, Hodges P, Hides J 1999 Therapeutic exercise for spinal segmental stabilization in low back pain. Churchill Livingstone, Edinburgh

Vera Garcia FJ, Grenier SG, McGill SM 2000 Abdominal response during curl-ups on both stable and labile surfaces. Phys Ther 80(6):564–569

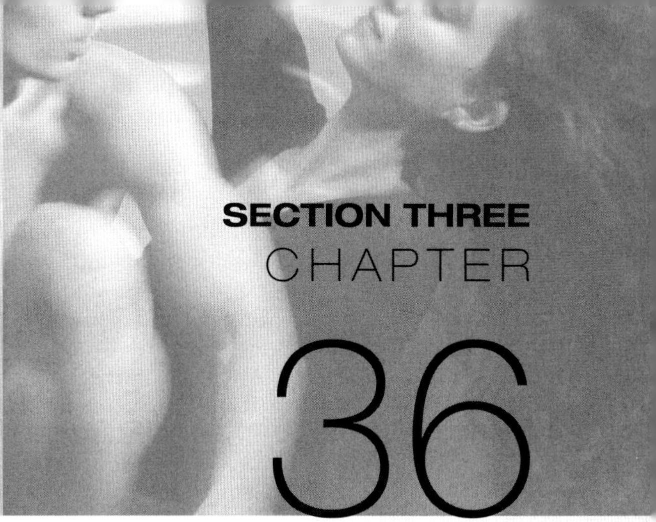

SECTION THREE

CHAPTER

36

Important aspects for efficacy of treatment with specific stabilizing exercises for postpartum pelvic girdle pain

B Stuge, NK Vøllestad

Introduction

In 1839, the Swedish obstetrician Cederschjöld wrote:

> *So long as the pelvic joints are very loose the woman cannot move herself in bed without pains and cannot get out of bed at all by herself. Even if she is helped up on her feet, she cannot walk, but feels as if her body wants, as it were, to drop down between her legs. If this affection is neglected, it may become a protracted one, with the risk of to some extent persisting forever, or else inflammation may arise, which through suppuration and hectic fever may lead to death (quoted in Genell 1949 p 9)*

More than one hundred years later, Genell (1949) described a case where the orthopedists advised a pregnant woman with pelvic girdle pain (PGP) to have an abortion. They believed the condition would cause her to become an invalid. Others have also stated that pain developed during pregnancy frequently continued after childbirth and might be exacerbated by an additional further pregnancy, and could thus constitute a direct cause of disability (Farbot 1952).

Today, low back pain (LBP) and pelvic girdle pain (PGP) account for the majority of sick leave among pregnant women in Scandinavian countries (Grunfeld & Qvigstad 1991, Sydsjo et al 1998). In several studies, pregnancy-related LBP and PGP are reported to have a negative effect on many daily activities such as walking, lifting, climbing stairs, lying flat on the back, turning in bed, housework, exercise, employment, leisure, sexual life, hobbies, and personal relationships (Hansen et al 1999, MacLennan

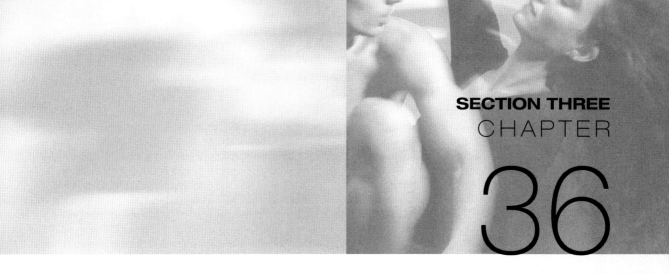

& MacLennan 1997, Mens et al 1996, Wormslev et al 1994). Women with postpartum LBP and PGP report a significantly lower health-related quality of life than that reported by healthy women (Hauken 1998), and lack of physical ability is found to be a major factor affecting quality of life (Olsson & Nilsson-Wikmar 2004, Stuge et al 2004a, Wågsæther 1998). It is a serious problem for the individual and for society that a number of young women develop chronic PGP after childbirth and are unable to earn a living. It has also been a problem that healthcare providers have only limited knowledge about effective treatment for this group of patients.

In a systematic review, nine controlled clinical trials of physical therapy with a total of 1350 pregnant and postpartum subjects were reviewed (Stuge et al 2003). Different exercise programs were examined. Except for three high-quality studies, the internal validity of the trials was moderate to low. The review did not reveal any strong evidence for treatment of PGP. Subsequently, we performed a randomized controlled trial demonstrating positive effect of a treatment program focusing on stabilizing exercises (Stuge et al 2004a). This chapter presents and discusses the prevalence of and diagnostic criteria for PGP, and the theoretical rationale for the treatment program we used. Hopefully, this will give a better understanding of clinical implementation of treatment for PGP.

Prevalence

Lumbopelvic pain has been stated to be culturally specific and more common in the Scandinavian countries than the rest of the world (Endresen 1995b, MacLennan 1991). However, studies show that lumbopelvic pain is a rather common problem in many countries. It has been reported in Africa (Bjorklund & Bergstrom 2000, Nwuga 1982), America (Dumas et al 1995, Fast et al 1987), Asia (Moon et al 2000, Suputtitada et al 2002, To & Wong 2003, Turgut et al 1998), Australia (Bullock et al 1987), and Europe (Albert et al 2000, Endresen 1995a, Kristiansson et al 1996, Mantle et al 1977, Mens et al 1996, Orvieto et al 1994, Östgaard & Andersson 1992, Östgaard et al 1991, Padua et al 2002, Sihvonen et al 1998), irrespective of the socioeconomics in these very disparate countries (van Dongen et al 1999). According to Wu et al (2004), nine studies using specific criteria for PGP demonstrated a mean PGP prevalence of 24% in pregnancy (range 4–42%). This is in agreement with Albert et al (2001), who found clinically examined pelvic joint pain in 20% of a sample of 2269 pregnant women. According to this finding, approximately 20% of all pregnant women suffer from PGP sufficiently serious to require medical help.

Lumbopelvic pain during pregnancy regresses spontaneously soon after delivery and disappears in most women within 6 months of delivery (Damen et al 2002, Kogstad 1988, Östgaard & Andersson 1992, Östgaard et al 1997). Few studies have examined the long-term prevalence of postpartum lumbopelvic pain. However, approximately 20% of those who suffered from lumbopelvic pain during pregnancy reported persisting pain 2 and 3 years postpartum (Noren et al 2002, To & Wong 2003). Albert et al (2001) found that 9% of women diagnosed with PGP during pregnancy were still suffering from daily pain from the pelvic joints 2 years after delivery.

Diagnosing pelvic girdle pain

Lumbopelvic pain in relation to pregnancy should be classified into LBP and PGP (Östgaard et al 1994a), and possibly further divided into subgroups of PGP (Albert et al 1997, 2001). To date, however, there has been no consensus on internationally accepted criteria on how to diagnose or categorize PGP. Objective diagnostic criteria are lacking (Östgaard 1997b). Pain cannot be related to any specific radiographic finding and no correlation has been found between the degree of symphyseal widening and pain in the pelvis (Abramson & Roberts 1934, Bjorklund et al 1997). Despite the development of imaging, including computerized tomography and magnetic resonance tomography, it is still necessary to rely on a thorough history and an examination including clinical tests when diagnosing PGP (Östgaard 1997a).

Characteristic symptoms and cardinal pain for PGP are located to the sacrum, the regions of the posterior superior iliac spine and/or the pubic symphysis (Mens et al 1996, Östgaard et al 1991). Other regions frequently indicated as painful are the groin and the coccyx. One of the characteristics Cederschjöld described in 1839 was the difficulty or almost inability to move the lower limbs (quoted in Genell 1949). Difficulty in walking has been confirmed by recent studies and proposed as a diagnostic sign for PGP (Dorman 1995, Sturesson et al 1997).

Because of low reliability and validity of most tests, a diagnosis should probably not be made on the basis of one test only. A multiple-test score is stated to be a more favorable method (Kristiansson

& Svardsudd 1996, van der Wurff et al 2000). Criteria based on history, pain drawings, and a combination of tests have been used in several studies on PGP (Fortin et al 1994, Noren et al 1997, Östgaard et al 1994b, Wedenberg et al 2000). The combination of the active straight leg raise (ASLR) test (Mens et al 2001), the posterior pelvic pain provocation (P4) test (Östgaard et al 1994a) and the long dorsal sacroiliac ligament (LDL) test (Vleeming et al 2002), combined with specific inclusion and exclusion criteria is proposed to differentiate between LBP and PGP (Vleeming et al 2002). Thus, the subjects in our intervention study were included based on history, pain location, positive P4 test and/or ASLR test, and additionally positive LDL test and/or pain provocation of the symphysis (Stuge et al 2004a).

Because similar and overlapping pathomechanisms might be involved between PGP and LBP it is important to exclude other possible diagnoses, such as lumbosacral vertebral disc ruptures (Ashkan et al 1998, LaBan et al 1983, Östgaard et al 1991), myofascial states, facet dysfunction, disc dysfunction, spondylolisthesis (Paris 1997), osteitis pubis (Andrews & Carek 1998), and gynecological disorders (Moen et al 1990).

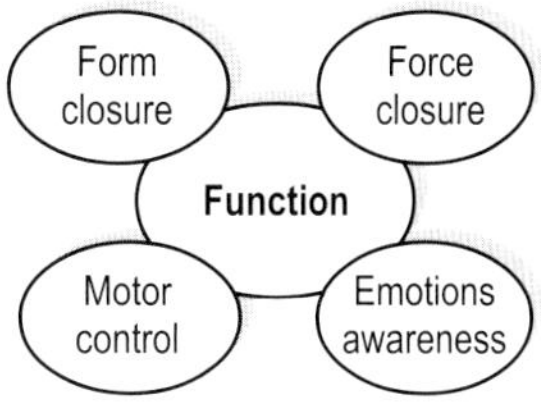

Fig. 36.1 An integrated model of function of the lumbopelvic region. [Adapted from Lee (2001) and Lee & Vleeming (2000).]

A treatment program focusing on specific stabilizing exercises

Theoretical rationale for stabilizing exercises

PGP has commonly been regarded as a problem of instability. However, despite the existence of different models that describe the stability of the lumbopelvic region, a generally accepted definition of stability has been lacking. In 1992, Panjabi presented a model of the spinal system consisting of three subsystems: the passive, the active and the neural subsystem. Lee (2001) and Lee & Vleeming (2000) further developed this model into a more integrated model of function of the lumbopelvic region (Fig. 36.1). They used the terms form closure (passive subsystem), force closure (active subsystem), motor control (neural subsystem) and added emotions/awareness as a fourth component. Any one or more of the subsystems might not function appropriately, thus affecting the overall stability of the lumbopelvic system.

Various muscles are assumed to contribute to force closure of the sacroiliac joints (SIJs) and there has been growing interest in how the neuromuscular system supports and controls the spinal segment. Bergmark (1989) described two functional muscle systems linked to spinal stabilization as the local and the global muscle systems. The muscles of the local muscle system are deep and anatomically closely related to the individual vertebrae, thus capable of increasing spinal segmental stiffness. Muscles of the global system are primarily the larger torque-producing muscles and are anatomically more distant from the joint but important for controlling spinal orientation and balancing external loads.

During recent years, there has been increased focus on the local muscle system, including musculus transversus abdominis (TrA), obliquus internus, multifidus, pelvic floor, and the diaphragm. It has been shown that the TrA is recruited prior to all other abdominal muscles and that its activation is directly linked to the development of intra-abdominal pressure (Hodges et al 2003, 2005, Richardson et al 1999). TrA is said to play an important role in stabilizing the lumbar column (Hodges & Richardson 1996, Richardson et al 1999) and the pelvis (Richardson et al 2002). Richardson et al (2002) found that contraction of the TrA significantly decreased the laxity of the SIJ. These findings support the use of TrA contractions for stabilization of the lumbopelvic region. However, also other muscles such as the pelvic floor muscles (PFM) could have contributed to the decreased SIJ laxity, but this was not assessed in the study. There is also some evidence for a coactivation of the abdominal muscles and the PFM in healthy subjects (Bø & Stien 1994, Critchley 2002, Neumann & Gill 2002, Sapsford et al 2001), although the importance of this is debated (Bø et al 2003). According to a biomechanical study in embalmed specimens, the PFM have the capability to increase stiffness of the pelvic ring and hence stabilize the pelvis in females (Pool-Goudzwaard et al 2004).

According to Vleeming et al (1997), an increase in tension in the thoracolumbar fascia can lead to compression on the SIJ, increasing force closure. A more recent study (Barker et al 2004) confirmed that low levels of tension are effectively transmitted between the TrA and the lumbar fascia, and may thereby influence intersegmental movement. It has further been shown that SIJ stiffness is significantly increased by activation of especially the erector spinae, the biceps femoris and the gluteus maximus muscles, even though some cocontraction of other muscles occurred (van Wingerden et al 2004). The finding that SIJ stiffness increased even with slight muscle activity supports the notion that load transfer from spine to legs improves when muscle activity compresses the SIJs and prevents shear forces.

Lumbopelvic stability and control in subjects with pelvic girdle pain

Several studies indicate altered lumbopelvic support and stability in subjects with PGP (Avery et al 2000, Commissaris et al 2002, Dorman 1995, Mens et al 2001, Mooney et al 2001, O'Sullivan et al 2002, Pool-Goudzwaard 2003, Sturesson et al 1997, Wu et al 2002). In contrast to healthy subjects, anterior rotation of the iliac bones is found in subjects with PGP (Hungerford et al 2004, Mens et al 1999). This might be indicative of failure of the self-bracing mechanism and load transfer through the pelvis, with a resultant decrease in the ability to oppose vertical shear loads during weight bearing. Furthermore, in subjects with pain over the SIJ compared to control subjects, a delayed onset of the oblique internus, multifidus, and gluteus maximus activity of the supporting leg during hip flexion was found on the symptomatic side (Hungerford et al 2003). The biceps femoris, however, showed an earlier onset of electromyographic activity on the symptomatic side in subjects with pain over the SIJ than in controls. These findings suggest an alteration in the strategy for lumbopelvic stabilization that may disrupt load transfer through the pelvis. Hence, treatment for PGP should probably aim to improve motor control and stability of the lumbopelvic region, and was thus the aim of the intervention in our study (Stuge et al 2004a).

The specific stabilizing exercise program

The main focus in our treatment program was exercise and training (Fig. 36.2). The treatment was based on specific training of the transversely oriented abdominal muscles with coactivation of the lumbar multifidus at the lumbosacral region (Richardson et al 1999), training of gluteus maximus, latissimus dorsi, the oblique abdominal muscles (Vleeming et al 1997), erector spinae, quadratus lumborum, and hip adductor and abductor muscles. The stabilization program consisted of three phases. During the first phase, the aim was to contract the local muscles without any movement of extremities and trunk. The second phase was aimed at using the local muscles to keep the lumbopelvic region stabilized during movements of the extremities and, in the third phase, during trunk movements. After the initial phase of stabilization of the lumbopelvic region, strength and coordination were trained (O'Sullivan 2000). Loading was progressively increased throughout the intervention period. However, attention was also paid to body awareness training and ergonomic advice in specific, real-life situations (e.g. lifting and carrying a child). When indicated, joint mobilization, massage, relaxation and stretching were performed.

The women were required to exercise for 30–60 minutes 3 days a week for 18–20 weeks, a training regimen in accordance with recommended guidelines (American College of Sports Medicine 1998). Individual guidance by the physical therapist and adjustments of the exercise program were performed once a week or every second week (on average 11 sessions). Individual records registered details such as resistance and number of repetitions. The sling exercise equipment TerapiMaster, as described by Ljunggren et al (1997), was used to facilitate the exercise progression for most of the exercises. The participants borrowed the equipment and had it installed at home during the intervention period, making it possible to perform most of the training at home. Compliance was measured by a training diary. The exercises were not to provoke pain and the subjects were encouraged to activate the transversely oriented abdominal muscles regularly during daily activities.

Women with PGP often experience pain during weight bearing, which is unavoidable when caring for a newborn. Using suspension by slings reduces the weight bearing and makes it possible to exercise without pain. By using the sling exercise apparatus, exercises could easily be down- and upgraded to obtain individual adjustment of load. A systematic increase of load level together with a training diary was reported to increase motivation and adherence to the exercise program. The ability to exercise at home with apparatus that is easy to use was important for this group of patients. The

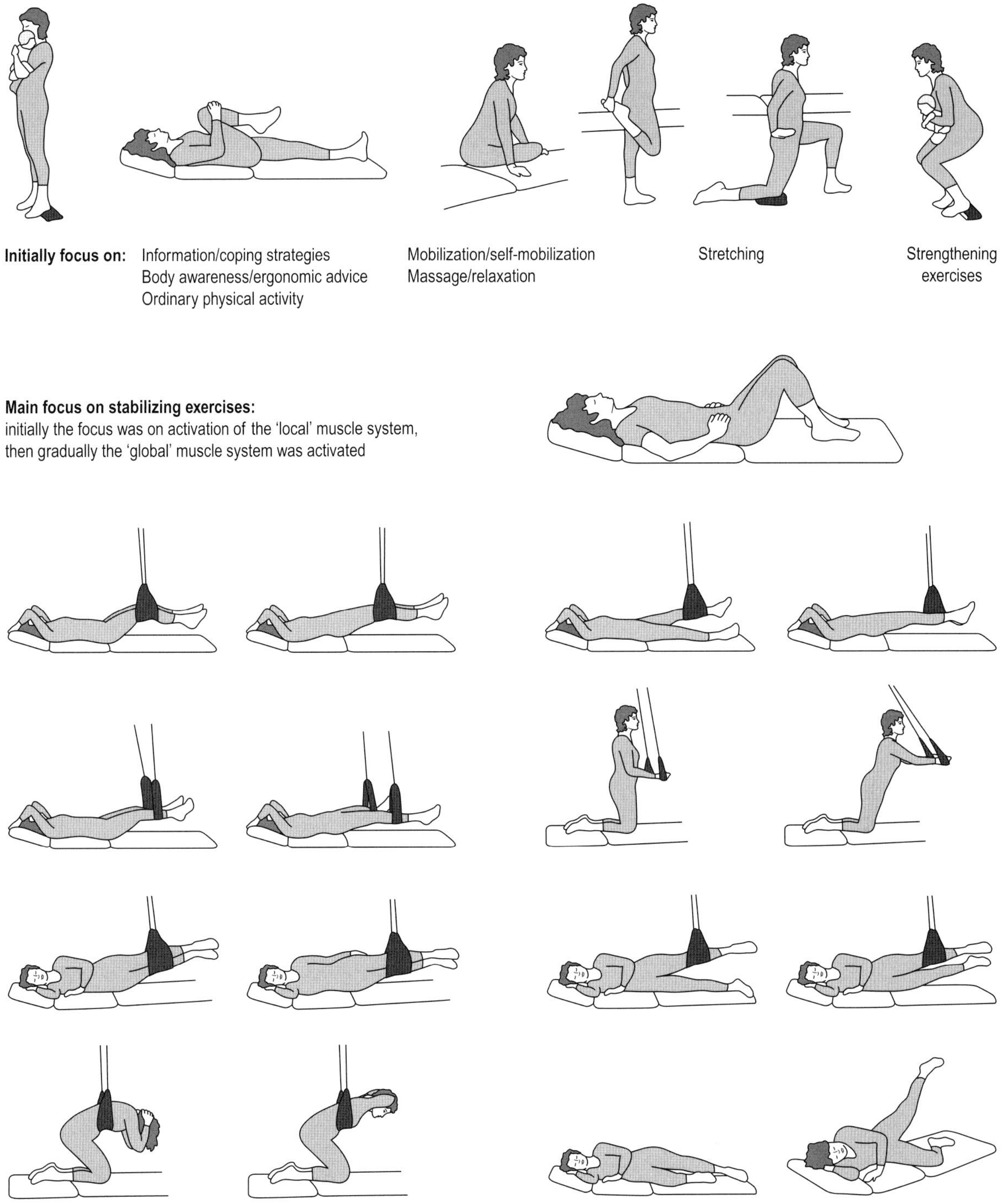
Initially focus on:
Information/coping strategies
Body awareness/ergonomic advice
Ordinary physical activity
Mobilization/self-mobilization
Massage/relaxation
Stretching
Strengthening exercises
Main focus on stabilizing exercises:
initially the focus was on activation of the 'local' muscle system, then gradually the 'global' muscle system was activated

Fig. 36.2 Key elements in the intervention program.

unstable environment of a sling also challenges the sensorimotor system to increase co-contraction of the muscles surrounding the joints (DeSerres & Milner 1991). Furthermore, the slings allow slow controlled closed kinetic chain exercises with focus on joint position, to increase co-contraction as well as to decrease the shear forces in the joint (Lutz et al 1993).

Individual adaptation of the exercises

The sequence of the exercises was individually chosen, in relation to the problems experienced. For a patient complaining of pain localized to the pubic symphysis and associated with tender adductors, a suspended and relaxed abduction/adduction exercise could be chosen as the first exercise (see Fig. 36.2). Graded progression was added when relaxation and the experience that exercising does not provoke pain were attained. For most patients with pain located over one or both SIJs, an appropriate exercise to start with could be a buttock-lift. An alternative to a buttock-lift with one or two legs on the ground is to suspend the legs in a sling, and then contracting the deep muscles, gluteus maximus, and the latissimus dorsi. The thoracolumbar fascia will thereby be facilitated and pain provocation from biceps femoris and the long dorsal sacroiliac ligament may be eliminated by avoiding weight bearing. If the patient's main problem was to transfer her baby into or out of bed, an initial exercise could be to lean forward while maintaining control of the pelvic girdle and the spine (see Fig. 36.2). In such a situation the focus would be on maintaining the neutral position of the lumbopelvic region while leaning forward as far as she could go without losing control or provoking pain. The position was held for 10 seconds while the patient was breathing normally.

The difference between stability and rigidity (inflexibility, stiffness) was emphasized to the patients. Rigidity was considered unfavorable. Specific exercises for each patient were taken out of a fixed menu of exercises (examples given in Fig. 36.2). The goal was to execute three sets of ten repetitions of each exercise 3 days a week. The number of exercises and repetitions was determined by the quality of the execution of the exercise. The exercises should not trigger a trembling of the lumbosacral region or provoke pain, either during the exercise program or at any time afterwards. However, the patients were encouraged to feel the difference between pain and muscle soreness; the latter was considered positive.

The results of a randomized controlled trial with a 2-year follow-up

Based on specific inclusion criteria, 81 women with PGP were included in a randomized controlled trial 6–16 weeks postpartum (Stuge et al 2004a). Forty women were assigned to the exercise group and 41 to the control group (receiving individualized physical therapy without specific exercises). The treatment groups were comparable at baseline (Tables 36.1 and 36.2) and there were no drop-outs. Consistent results were seen with positive effect on pain, disability and quality of life, in favor of the exercise group (Figs 36.3, 36.4, and 36.5). The treatment program focusing on specific stabilizing exercises (SSE) showed statistically and clinically significant better results compared to physical therapy modalities without SSE [$P = 0.001$ for all scales, except for the Short Form 36 (SF-36) mental health scores] (Stuge et al 2004a). After treatment, disability was reduced by more than 50% for the exercise group compared to negligible changes in the control group. Furthermore, 75% of the subjects in the exercise group scored lower than 25 on the Oswestry Low Back Pain Disability Questionnaire (OSW), compared to 25% in the control group ($P < 0.001$). The minimal clinically important difference for the OSW is reported to be 4–6 points for low back pain (Beurskens et al 1996, Fritz & Irrgang 2001, Grotle et al 2004). A mean change of 6 points was found within the control group versus 23 points within the exercise group from baseline to after treatment. One year postpartum the results were maintained. Thus, a large and clinically important change was found within the exercise group.

Even though both groups had improved after treatment with regard to evening pain (see Fig. 36.3), the improvement was significantly larger in the exercise group (Stuge et al 2004a). Hence, the difference in median evening pain after treatment was 30 mm on a visual analog scale (VAS). According to the results obtained in studies of low back pain the minimal clinically important difference for pain measured by VAS is 10–20 mm on a scale from 0 to 100 as used in our study (Beurskens et al 1996, Grotle et al 2004, Hagg et al 2003). The changes as well as the group differences exceed this range. Thus, it seems that individualized physical therapy with specific stabilizing exercises is effective in achieving clinically important improvements in women with PGP after pregnancy.

The long-term effect two years after delivery revealed that the significant differences between the

Table 36.1 Patient characteristics with demographic and other background variables at baseline. Data are given as mean (SD) or number (%)

	All (*N* = 81)	SSEG (*N* = 40)	CG (*N* = 41)
Age (years)	32 (4)	32 (4)	32 (4)
Height (cm)	168 (6)	169 (5)	167 (6)
Weight (kg)	68 (11)	69 (11)	67 (10)
Education (years at school)	16 (3)	16 (3)	16 (2)
Parity	2 (1)	2 (1)	2 (1)
Birth weight of baby (kg)	4 (1)	4 (1)	4 (1)
Time since last delivery (weeks)	10 (3)	10 (3)	9 (3)
Duration of present pain (months)	8 (4)	7 (3)	8 (5)
PGP started in pregnancy month	4 (2)	4 (2)	4 (2)
PGP experienced by mother or sister	27 (33%)	11 (28%)	16 (39%)
A 'catching' feeling of the leg when walking*	56 (70%)	28 (70%)	28 (68%)
LBP before pregnancy	39 (48%)	18 (45%)	21 (51%)
Previously 'damaged' pelvis	2 (3%)	1 (3%)	1 (2%)
PGP during last pregnancy	78 (96%)	37 (93%)	41 (100%)
LBP during last pregnancy	51 (64%)	26 (65%)	25 (61%)
Much pain during menstruation and ovariation	37 (46%)	18 (45%)	19 (46%)
Regular physical activity before pregnancy	58 (72%)	27 (68%)	31 (76%)
On sick leave during pregnancy because of PGP***	64 (82%)	32 (80%)	32 (70%)
Lying on back during delivery	44 (54%)	21 (53%)	23 (56%)
Cesarian section	7 (9%)	3 (8%)	4 (10%)
Incontinence	31 (38%)	14 (35%)	17 (42%)
Smoking	6 (7%)	3 (8%)	3 (7%)
Use of medication for PGP**	5 (6%)	3 (8%)	2 (5%)

** 1 missing, ** 2 missing, *** 3 missing*
CG, control group; LBP, low back pain; PGP, pelvic girdle pain; SSEG, specific stabilizing exercise group.

groups persisted with continued low levels of pain (Fig. 36.3) and disability (Fig. 36.4) in the exercise group (Stuge et al 2004b). All 81 women returned the questionnaires for the 2-year follow-up. Sixteen were excluded from the analysis (ten from the control group and six from the exercise group), mainly due to new pregnancies. The two groups (exercise group = 34, control group = 31) were still comparable at baseline. Statistically and clinically significant differences between the groups in functional status and pain ($P = 0.005$), and physical health (SF-36) ($P = 0.05$) were maintained 2 years after delivery. No or minimal disability was found in 85% of the exercise group as compared to 47% in the control group. No significant further changes were seen within the exercise group from 1-year to the 2-year follow-up. The control group showed statistically and clinically significant improvement in functional status (OSW) with a median change in score of 6.0 (interquartile ranges −12 to 0) ($P < 0.001$), but no statistically significant improvement of pain intensity ($P > 0.12$). No or minimal evening pain was reported by 68% in the exercise group versus 23% in the control group ($P = 0.001$). The scores of SF-36 2 years after delivery revealed that significant differences persisted between the groups in physical functioning ($P = 0.002$), role physical ($P = 0.05$), and bodily pain ($P = 0.001$), whereas no significant differences were seen for the other five subscales (see Fig. 36.5). Both groups demonstrated scores

Table 36.2 Outcome measures at baseline for all included subjects. Data given as mean (SD)

	All (*N* = 81)	SSEG (*N* = 40)	CG (*N* = 41)
Functional status			
Oswestry disability index (0–100)	42 (15)	53 (19)	54 (16)
Disability rating index (0–100)	54 (18)	53 (19)	54 (16)
Pain intensity			
Morning pain at worst (100 mm VAS)	40 (23)	36 (22)	44 (23)
Evening pain at worst (100 mm VAS)	61 (22)	57 (23)	65 (20)
Physical tests			
ASLR test (0–10)	4 (2)	4 (2)	4 (2)
ASLR test with compression	4 (2)	4 (2)	3 (2)
ASLR test with 'arm activation'	3 (2)	3 (2)	3 (2)
Hip adduction strength test (Newton)	146 (54)	141 (52)	149 (57)
Hip abduction strength test (Newton)	184 (64)	175 (67)	192 (61)
Sørensen test (seconds)	102 (61)	89 (60)	115 (59)
P4 test positive left and right (N, %)	61 (75%)	33 (83%)	28 (68%)

ASLR, active straight leg raise; CG, control group; P4, posterior pelvic pain provocation; SSEG, specific stabilizing exercise group.

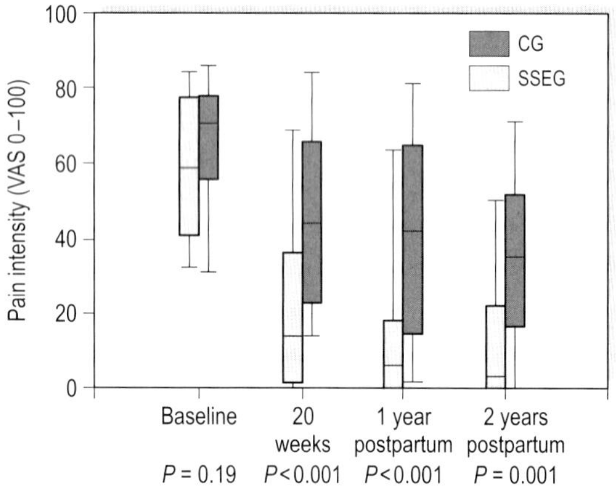

Fig. 36.3 Scores of evening pain intensity at worst (VAS 0–100) at baseline, after therapy (20 weeks), 1 and 2 years postpartum. The boxes show quartiles, medians (middle line), and 10th and 90th percentiles at the ends. CG, control group; SSEG, specific stabilizing exercise group; VAS, visual analog scale.

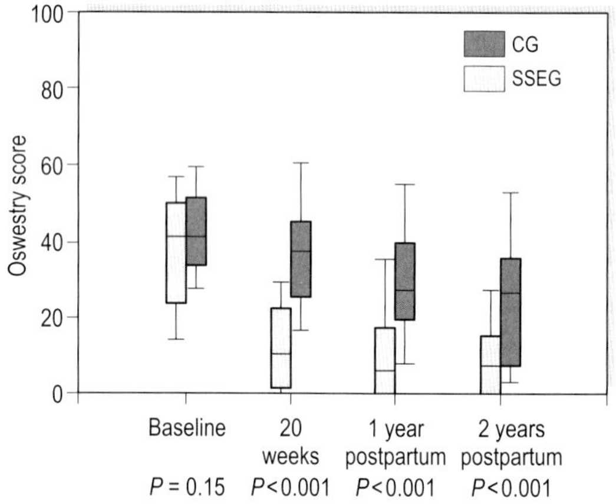

Fig. 36.4 Scores of functional status (Oswestry Low Back Pain Disability Questionnaire) at baseline, after therapy (20 weeks), 1 and 2 years postpartum. The boxes show quartiles, medians (middle line), and 10th and 90th percentiles at the ends. CG, control group; SSEG, specific stabilizing exercise group.

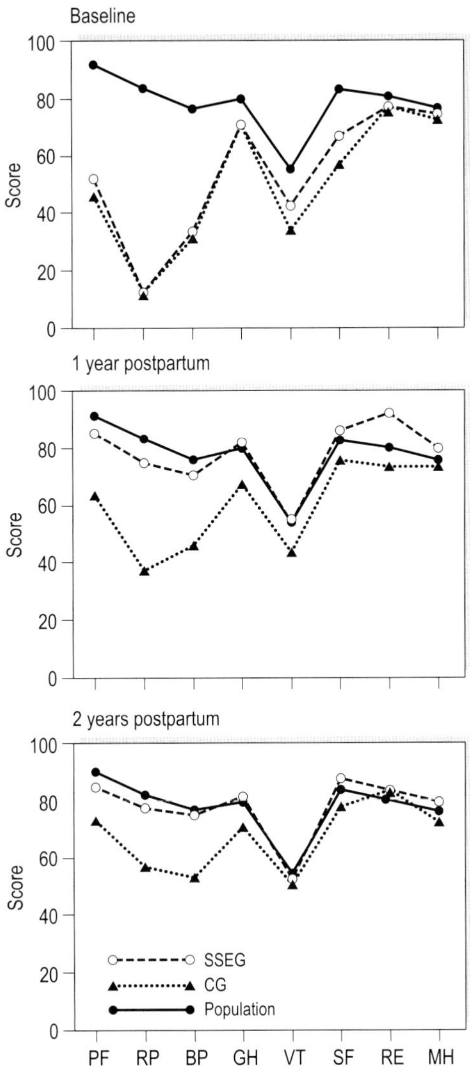

Fig. 36.5 Scores of health-related quality of life (SF-36) are presented as mean values at baseline, 1-year follow-up and 2-year follow-up. Standard deviations and confidence intervals of mean are given in Table 36.2. BP, bodily pain; CG, control group; GH, general health; MH, mental health; PF, physical functioning; Population, mean scores from a general Norwegian population (women 30–39 years old; Loge & Kaasa 1998); RE, role emotional; RP, role physical; SF, social functioning; SSEG, specific stabilizing exercise group; VT, vitality. (Reproduced with permission from Stuge et al 2004b.)

for the mental health scales similar to females of the same age in the Norwegian population (Loge & Kaasa 1998). Also, in another study of women with lumbopelvic pain, reduction in quality of life was mostly related to physical ability (Olsson & Nilsson-Wikmar 2004).

Possible reasons for the effect of the stabilizing exercise intervention

Only one study has previously investigated treatment for postpartum PGP (Mens et al 2000). The authors of that study concluded that exercises of the diagonal trunk muscle system were not superior to training of the longitudinal trunk muscle system or to no exercises. Their results thus led to quite different conclusions from ours. However, as discussed previously (Stuge et al 2006) there are several differences between the two studies regarding the interventions, including types of exercise, dosage, duration, individualization, and supervision. To understand possible reasons to explain the positive effects of an intervention with SSE, some principles of the intervention will now be discussed.

Stabilizing exercises

As described above, the treatment program in our study that included SSE was effective in relieving pain and improving functioning compared to treatment without SSE. The SSEs were defined as exercises for specific activation of the local and the global muscle system, specifically focusing on control of the lumbopelvic region and coordination of muscle recruitment. The intentions of the exercises were first to improve force closure and motor control, and subsequently to develop adequate strength and endurance to manage the physical demands as a mother of a newborn child.

Unlike the study by Mens et al (2000), the focus in the initial stage of our treatment program was to specifically train contraction of the deep muscle system, independently of the superficial muscles. Deep local muscles are thought to provide the fine-tuning of the intersegmental motion as a component of the complex interdependent activity of the trunk muscles to stabilize the lumbopelvic region (Hodges & Moseley 2003). The deep muscles are said to provide control of intersegmental motion that is not specific to the direction of force, whereas the superficial, global muscles control the orientation of the spine (Moseley et al 2002). Because probably all trunk muscles are required for lumbopelvic control and functional stability of the spine, activity of the global muscles was gradually added to the exercise program (Cholewicki et al 2003, Hodges & Moseley 2003, van Dieen et al 2003).

Exercise programs for patients with lumbopelvic pain have traditionally focused on strength and general fitness. However, research suggests that a key impairment in the muscle system is one of motor control rather than one of only strength (Richardson et al 1999). It is reasoned that such impairments need to be addressed specifically before, or at least in conjunction with, more general exercise programs (Jull & Richardson 2000).

Interventions similar to ours but applied to LBP patients and focusing on reorganization of the control of the deep and superficial trunk muscles through motor learning strategies have shown reduced pain and disability, and reduced recurrence of pain (Hides et al 2001, O'Sullivan et al 1997). Furthermore, a recent unpublished systematic review of 12 randomized controlled trials has been conducted to assess the efficacy of SSE in the treatment of pain of spinal and pelvic origin (Ferreira et al 2006). Single trials reported that SSE were effective in the treatment of cervicogenic headache and associated neck pain (Jull et al 2002), pelvic pain (Stuge et al 2004a), and in preventing recurrences after an acute episode of LBP (Hides et al 2001). SSEs were also effective in reducing pain and disability in chronic, but not in acute LBP (Hides et al 1996, O'Sullivan et al 1997, Rasmussen-Barr et al 2003). The review revealed, however, that the nature of the SSE programs varied and was not standardized.

Despite the importance of motor control, a certain muscular strength is a fundamental physical factor necessary for health, functional ability, and enhanced quality of life (Kraemer et al 2002). To date, few systematic reviews in this area have addressed the clinical relevance of type, quality, and approach of exercise (Hilde & Bo 1998, Liddle et al 2004). In addition to focusing on motor control, we followed accepted exercise principles for muscular strength and endurance (Kraemer et al 2002). Muscle strengthening, some aspects of flexibility and cardiovascular endurance training were included. Our program consisted of strengthening and muscular endurance exercises using progressive resistance exercise with the patients' body weight as resistance, stretching and to a lesser extent range of movement exercises. In addition, behavioral support and positive coping strategies and ergonomic advice were included in our exercise intervention. These aspects were highlighted in a recent systematic review identifying essential treatment characteristics to achieve and maintain successful results with exercise in LBP patients (Liddle et al 2004).

Individualization

Individualization of the treatment was another principle followed. The selection of and dosage of the exercises were individually chosen. However, the exercises were taken from a standardized exercise menu. Also, when indicated, joint mobilization was performed and might have contributed to the outcome changes. The inclusion of exercise co-interventions introduces a confounding influence when assessing the effectiveness of exercise programs. Unequal provision of care apart from treatment under evaluation is considered as performance bias and may reduce the internal validity of a randomized controlled trial (Juni et al 2001). In our study, mobilization was part of the treatment program in both treatment groups and thus was not regarded as a co-intervention. This type of design is particularly commonplace in pragmatic trials (Liddle et al 2004), and does not answer whether any specific element of an intervention is more important than another. Hence, we do not know if mobilization was a necessary part of the intervention.

However, heterogeneity of problems among PGP patients highlights the need for an individual problem-solving approach. It is unlikely that all women with PGP would profit from the same treatment. A 'one-size-fits-all' approach to the prescription of therapeutic exercise is not rationally based (Jull & Richardson 2000). On the other hand, in clinical practice, sometimes 'the more treatment modalities, the better' is the guiding practice to ensure positive results. Perhaps in some cases it would be wise to leave something out. Most probably there are subgroups of PGP that require different treatment modalities; this should be further investigated.

Partial supervision of the individual patient was emphasized in the exercise group. This involved initial instruction in exercises to be performed independently and with periodic follow-up from the therapist to adjust the program accordingly. Supervision of exercises is critically important in improving quality of exercise performance. A strong correlation between the quality of exercise performance and decrease in pain has been found (Friedrich et al 1996). Supervision and regular follow-up enable the therapist to adjust a program according to the patients' progress and might contribute to the maintenance of exercise benefits (Liddle et al 2004). Our supervised exercise program is in strong contrast to exercises guided by a videotape, as used in the study by Mens et al (2000). Results of a systematic review of studies in which exercise was the primary intervention for chronic LBP showed that when both experimental and control groups were given supervised exercise programs of variable content, both groups achieved a positive result (Liddle et al 2004). The control group in our study (Stuge et al 2004a) was advised to perform general exercises; however, they were not given a systematic exercise program. Even though they were supervised and met their therapist equally often, the exercise dosage was much lower in the control group.

Compliance

Compliance is essential for proper interpretation of the effect of an exercise intervention. Exercising three times a week, which is considered optimal (Kraemer et al 2002), can be hard to achieve for women with a newborn child. Clinical experience shows that for these patients it is a challenge to get continuity in an outpatient exercise program. In our study, the subjects reported to accomplish on average 80% of exercising three times a week for 15–20 weeks. This compliance was surprisingly high, also compared to other studies (Mens et al 2000, Östgaard et al 1997, Sluijs et al 1993).

The women reported that reasons for the high compliance were the possibility of exercising at home and the guidance by the therapist. In the study by Mens et al (2000) the subjects were supposed to exercise at home only. In their study, however, four subjects (25%) in the exercise group stopped exercising because of pain provoked by the exercises. The therapist's role in supporting and counseling, prolonged supervision and simple and convenient regimens tailored to the patient situation or daily routine play an essential role in compliance (Friedrich et al 1996, 1998, Sluijs et al 1993). It has been pointed out that patients need to understand *why*, not just *what* to do, to facilitate empowerment and commitment to change (Liddle et al 2004, Lively 2002). Another factor reported to be important for compliance was experience of continual improvement. In our study the women could follow their improvement through the use of an exercise diary. Schneiders et al (1998) found that patients receiving additional written and illustrated instruction had a significantly higher compliance to home-based exercises compared to patients who received verbal instruction alone. In accordance with what was emphasized by Liddle et al (2004), frequency and type of exercise was recorded in each exercise session in the present study, and probably has influenced both the compliance and the results of the SSE program.

The results of our study indicate beneficial long-term effects of a treatment program focusing on SSE as described above. These effects may be caused by the efficient motor control strategies obtained, and the ability to dynamically control and stabilize the lumbopelvic region during daily activities. In addition, the experiences achieved during exercising may also possibly contribute through reduced fear of pain and fear of physical activity. Thus, possible fear-avoidance behavior was avoided.

Summary

We recommend treating postpartum PGP with a treatment program focusing on stabilizing exercises. However, exercises for enhancing lumbopelvic control and stability should involve the entire spinal musculature. Focusing only on global muscles, and without individual guidance, seems insufficient. Thus, no fixed program can be recommended, rather the exercises must be chosen during close collaboration between therapist and patient. More studies are needed to enhance our knowledge of different aspects of stabilizing exercise interventions, such as individualization, choice, order and dosage of exercises, supervision and compliance, and how these interact with different subgroups of patients.

References

Abramson D, Roberts S 1934 Relaxation of the pelvic joints in pregnancy. Surgery Gynecology Obstetrics 58:595–613

Albert H, Godskesen M, Westergaard J et al 1997 Circulating levels of relaxin are normal in pregnant women with pelvic pain. European Journal of Obstetrics & Gynecology and Reproductive Biology 74(1):19–22

Albert H, Godskesen M, Westergaard J 2000 Evaluation of clinical tests used in classification procedures in pregnancy-related pelvic joint pain. European Spine Journal 9(2):161–166

Albert H, Godskesen M, Westergaard J 2001 Prognosis in four syndromes of pregnancy-related pelvic pain. Acta Obstetricia et Gynecologica Scandinavica 80(6): 505–510

American College of Sports Medicine 1998 The recommended quantity and quality of exercise for developing and maintaining cardiorespiratory and muscular fitnes, and flexibility in healthy adults. Medicine, Science in Sports, Exercise 30(6):975–991

Andrews SK, Carek PJ 1998 Osteitis pubis: a diagnosis for the family physician. Journal of American Board of Family Practice 11:291–295

Ashkan K, Casey AT, Powell M et al 1998 Back pain during pregnancy and after childbirth: an unusual cause not to miss. Journal of the Royal Society of Medicine 91(2): 88–90

Avery AF, O'Sullivan PB, McCallum M 2000 Evidence of pelvic floor muscle dysfunction in subjects with chronic sacro-iliac joint pain syndrome. IFOMT 2000 Conference Proceeding, IFOMT, Perth, Australia, p35–38

Barker PJ, Briggs CA, Bogeski G 2004 Tensile transmission across the lumbar fasciae in unembalmed cadavers – effects of tension to various muscular attachments. Spine 29(2):129–138

Bergmark A 1989 Stability of the lumbar spine – a study in mechanical engineering. Acta Orthopaedica Scandinavica 60:3–54

Beurskens AJHM, Devet HCW, Koke AJA 1996 Responsiveness of functional status in low back pain: a comparison of different instruments. Pain 65(1):71–76

Bjorklund K, Bergstrom S 2000 Is pelvic pain in pregnancy a welfare complaint? Acta Obstetricia et Gynecologica Scandinavica 79(1):24–30

Bjorklund K, Lindgren PG, Bergstrom S et al 1997 Sonographic assessment of symphyseal joint distention intra partum. Acta Obstetricia et Gynecologica Scandinavica 76(3):227–232

Bø K, Stien R 1994 Needle EMG registration of striated urethral wall and pelvic floor muscle-activity patterns during cough, Valsalva, abdominal, hip adductor, and gluteal muscle contractions in nulliparous healthy females. Neurourology and Urodynamics 13(1):35–41

Bø K, Sherburn M, Allen T 2003 Transabdominal ultrasound measurement of pelvic floor muscle activity when activated directly or via a transversus abdominis muscle contraction. Neurourology and Urodynamics 22(6):582–588

Bullock JE, Jull GA, Bullock MI 1987 The relationship of low back pain to postural changes during pregnancy. Australian Journal of Physiotherapy 33:10–17

Cholewicki J, van Dieen JH, Arsenault AB 2003 Muscle function and dysfunction in the spine. Journal of Electromyography and Kinesiology 13(4):303–304

Commissaris DA, Nilsson-Wikmar LB, van Dieen JH, Hirschfeld H 2002 Joint coordination during whole-body lifting in women with low back pain after pregnancy. Archives of Physical Medicine and Rehabilitation 83(9):1279–1289

Critchley D 2002 Instructing pelvic floor contraction facilitates transversus abdominis thickness increase during low-abdominal hollowing. Physiotherapy Research International 7(2):65–75

Damen L, Buyruk H M, Guler-Uysal F et al 2002 The prognostic value of asymmetric laxity of the sacroiliac joints in pregnancy-related pelvic pain. Spine 27(24): 2820–2824

DeSerres SJ, Milner TE 1991 Wrist muscle activation patterns and stiffness associated with stable and unstable mechanical loads. Experimental Brain Research 86(2):451–458

Dorman TA 1995 Failure of self bracing at the sacroiliac joints: the slipping clutch syndrome. In: Vleeming A et al (eds) Second Interdisciplinary World Congress on Low back Pain. San Diego, CA, p651–656

Dumas GA, Reid JG, Wolfe LA et al 1995 Exercise, posture, and back pain during pregnancy. Part 2: exercise and back pain. Clinical Biomechanics 10(2):104–109

Endresen EH 1995a Pelvic pain and low back pain in pregnant women – an epidemiological study. Scandinavian Journal of Rheumatology 24(3):135–141

Endresen EH 1995b Pelvic floor relaxation – a condition with many names and uncertain criteria. Tidsskrift Norske Laegeforening 115(26):3271–3273

Farbot E 1952 The relationship of the effect and pain of pregnancy to the anatomy of the pelvis. The Roentgen Departement, Elverum and Stavanger, Norway

Fast A, Shapiro D, Ducommun EJ et al 1987 Low back pain in pregnancy. Spine 12(4): 368–371

Ferreira PH, Ferreira ML, Maher CG et al 2006 Specific stabilisation exercise for spinal and pelvic pain: a systematic review. Australian Journal of Physiotherapy 52:79–88

Fortin JD, Aprill CN, Ponthieux B et al 1994 Sacroiliac joint: pain referral maps upon applying a new injection/arthrography technique. Part II: clinical evaluation. Spine 19(13):1483–1489

Friedrich M, Cermak T, Maderbacher P 1996 The effect of brochure use versus therapist teaching on patients performing therapeutic exercise and on changes in impairment status. Physical Therapy 76(10):1082–1088

Friedrich M, Gittler G, Halberstadt Y et al 1998 Combined exercise and motivation program: Effect on the compliance and level of disability of patients with chronic low back pain: a randomized controlled trial. Archives of Physical Medicine and Rehabilitation 79(5):475–487

Fritz JM, Irrgang JJ 2001 A comparison of a modified Oswestry Low Back Pain Disability Questionnaire and the Quebec Back Pain Disability Scale. Physical Therapy 81(2):776–788

Genell S 1949 Studies on insufficientia pelvis (gravidarum et puerperarum). The Women's Clinic, Malmö, Sweden

Grotle M, Brox JL, Vøllestad NK 2004 Concurrent comparison of responsiveness in pain and functional status measurements used for patients with low back pain. Spine 29(21):E492–E501

Grunfeld B, Qvigstad E 1991 Disease during pregnancy Sick-listing among pregnant women in Oslo. Tidsskrift Norske Laegeforening 111(10):1269–1272

Hagg O, Fritzell P, Nordwall A 2003 The clinical importance of changes in outcome scores after treatment for chronic low back pain. European Spine Journal 12(1):12–20

Hansen A, Jensen DV, Wormslev M et al 1999, Symptom-giving pelvic girdle relaxation in pregnancy II: symptoms and clinical signs. Acta Obstetricia et Gynecologica Scandinavica 78(2):111–115

Hauken MA 1998 En klinisk studie av livskvalitet hos kvinner med langvarige bekkenløsningsplager. Universitetet i Bergen, Det medisinske fakultet, Institutt for samfunnsmedisinske fag, seksjon for sykepleievitenskap

Hides JA, Richardson CA, Jull GA 1996 Multifidus muscle recovery is not automatic after resolution of acute, first-episode low back pain. Spine 21(23):2763–2769

Hides JA, Jull GA, Richardson CA 2001 Long-term effects of specific stabilizing exercises for first-episode low back pain. Spine 26(11):E243–E248

Hilde G, Bø K 1998 Effect of exercise in the treatment of chronic low back pain: a systematic review, emphasising type and dose of exercise. Physical Therapy Reviews 3:107–117

Hodges PW, Moseley GL 2003 Pain and motor control of the lumbopelvic region: effect and possible mechanisms Journal of Electromyography and Kinesiology 13: 361–370

Hodges PW, Richardson CA 1996 Inefficient muscular stabilization of the lumbar spine associated with low back pain. A motor control evaluation of transversus abdominis. Spine 21(22):2640–2650

Hodges P, Holm AK, Holm S et al 2003 Intervertebral stiffness of the spine is increased by evoked contraction of transversus abdominis and the diaphragm: in vivo porcine studies. Spine 28(23):2594–2601

Hodges PW, Eriksson AEM, Shirley D et al 2005 Intra-abdominal pressure increases stiffness of the lumbar spine. Journal of Biomechanics 38(9):1873–1880

Hungerford B, Gilleard W, Hodges P 2003 Evidence of altered lumbopelvic muscle recruitment in the presence of sacroiliac joint pain. Spine 28(14):1593–1600

Hungerford B, Gilleard W, Lee D 2004 Altered patterns of pelvic bone motion determined in subjects with posterior pelvic pain using skin markers. Clinical Biomechanics 19:456–464

Jull GA, Richardson CA 2000 Motor control problems in patients with spinal pain: a new direction for therapeutic exercise. Journal of Manipulative and Physiological Therapeutics 23(2):115–117

Jull G, Trott P, Potter H et al 2002 A randomized controlled trial of exercise and manipulative therapy for cervicogenic headache. Spine 27(17):1835–1843

Juni P, Altman DG, Egger M 2001 Systematic reviews in health care – assessing the quality of controlled clinical trials. British Medical Journal 323(7303):42–46

Kogstad O 1988 Backache after labor. Who will have it and what is the diagnosis? Tidsskrift Norske Laegeforening 108(14):1120–1122

Kraemer WJ, Adams K, Cafarelli E et al 2002 Progression models in resistance training for healthy adults. Medicine & Science in Sports & Exercise 34(2):364–380

Kristiansson P, Svardsudd K 1996 Discriminatory power of tests applied in back pain during pregnancy. Spine 21(20):2337–2343

Kristiansson P, Svardsudd K, von Schoultz B 1996 Back pain during pregnancy: a prospective study. Spine 21(6):702–709

LaBan MM, Perrin JC, Latimer FR 1983 Pregnancy and the herniated lumbar disc. Archives of Physical Medicine and Rehabilitation 64(7):319–321

Lee D 2001 An integrated model of joint function and its clinical application. In: Vleeming A et al (eds) Fourth Interdisciplinary World Congress on Low Back, Pelvic Pain Moving from Structure to Function. Montreal, Canada, p137–152

Lee D, Vleeming A 2000 Current concepts on pelvic pain. Conference Proceedings of the Seventh Scientific Conference of the International Federation of Orthopaedic Manipulative Therapists. Perth, Australia, p 118–123

Liddle SD, Baxter GD, Gracey JH 2004 Exercise and chronic low back pain: what works? Pain 107:176–190

Lively MW 2002 Sports medicine approach to low back pain. Southern Medical Journal 95(6):642–646

Ljunggren AE, Weber H, Kogstad O et al 1997 Effect of exercise on sick leave due to low back pain. A randomized, comparative, long-term study. Spine 22(14): 1610–1616

Loge JH, Kaasa S 1998 Short form 36 (SF-36) health survey: normative data from the general Norwegian population. Scandinavian Journal of Social Medicine 26(4):250–258

Lutz GE, Palmitier RA, An KN et al 1993 Comparison of tibiofemoral joint forces during open-kinetic-chain and closed-kinetic-chain exercises. Journal of Bone and Joint Surgery – American 75A(5):732–739

MacLennan AH 1991 The role of the hormone relaxin in human reproduction and pelvic girdle relaxation. Scandinavian Journal of Rheumatology Suppl 88:7–15

MacLennan AH, MacLennan SC 1997 Symptom-giving pelvic girdle relaxation of pregnancy, postnatal pelvic joint syndrome and developmental dysplasia of the hip. The Norwegian Association for Women with Pelvic Girdle Relaxation. Acta Obstetricia et Gynecologica Scandinavica 76(8):760–764

Mantle MJ, Greenwood RM, Currey HL 1977 Backache in pregnancy. Rheumatology and Rehabilitation 16(2): 95–101

Mens JM, Vleeming A, Stoeckart R et al 1996 Understanding peripartum pelvic pain. Implications of a patient survey. Spine 21(11):1363–1369

Mens JM, Vleeming A, Snijders CJ et al 1999 The active straight leg raising test and mobility of the pelvic joints. European Spine Journal 8(6):468–474

Mens JM, Snijders CJ, Stam HJ 2000 Diagonal trunk muscle exercises in peripartum pelvic pain: a randomized clinical trial. Physical Therapy 80(12):1164–1173

Mens JM, Vleeming A, Snijders CJ et al 2001 Reliability and validity of the active straight leg raise test in posterior pelvic pain since pregnancy. Spine 26(10):1167–1171

Moen MH, Kogstad O, Biornstad N et al 1990 Symptomatic pelvic girdle relaxation Clinical aspects. Tidsskrift Norske Laegeforening 110(17):2211–2212

Moon WN, Kim MY, Suh SW 2000 Incidence and risk factors of pelvic pain in pregnancy. Journal of Korean Spine Surgery 7(2):259–263

Mooney V, Pozos R, Vleeming A et al 2001 Exercise treatment for sacroiliac pain. Orthopedics 24(1):29–32

Moseley GL, Hodges PW, Gandevia SC 2002 Deep and superficial fibers of the lumbar multifidus muscle are differentially active during voluntary arm movements. Spine 27(2):E29–E36

Neumann P, Gill V 2002 Pelvic floor and abdominal muscle interaction: EMG activity and intra-abdominal pressure. International Urogynecology Journal 13(2): 125–132

Noren L, Östgaard S, Nielsen TF et al 1997 Reduction of sick leave for lumbar back and posterior pelvic pain in pregnancy. Spine 22(18):2157–2160

Noren L, Östgaard S, Johansson G et al 2002 Lumbar back and posterior pelvic pain during pregnancy: a 3-year follow- up. European Spine Journal 11(3):267–271

Nwuga VCB 1982 Pregnancy and back pain among upper-class Nigerian women. Australian Journal of Physiotherapy 28:8–11

O'Sullivan PB 2000 Lumbar segmental 'instability': clinical presentation and specific stabilizing exercise management. Manual Therapy 5(1):2–12

O'Sullivan PB, Phyty GD, Twomey LT et al 1997 Evaluation of specific stabilizing exercise in the treatment of chronic low back pain with radiologic diagnosis of spondylolysis or spondylolisthesis. Spine 22(24):2959–2967

O'Sullivan PB, Beales DJ, Beetham JA et al 2002 Altered motor control strategies in subjects with sacroiliac joint pain during the active straight-leg-raise test. Spine 27(1): E1–E8

Olsson C, Nilsson-Wikmar L 2004 Health-related quality of life and physical ability among pregnant women with and without back pain in late pregnancy. Acta Obstetricia et Gynecologica Scandinavica 83(4):351–357

Orvieto R, Achiron A, BenRafael Z et al 1994 Low-back pain of pregnancy. Acta Obstetricia et Gynecologica Scandinavica 73(3):209–214

Östgaard HC 1997 Lumbar back and posterior pelvic pain in pregnancy. In: Vleeming A et al (eds) Movement, stability and low back pain. The essential role of the pelvis. Churchill Livingstone, New York, p411–420

Östgaard HC, Andersson GB 1992 Postpartum low-back pain. Spine 17(1):53–55

Östgaard HC, Andersson GB, Karlsson K 1991 Prevalence of back pain in pregnancy. Spine 16(5):549–552

Östgaard HC, Zetherstrom G, Roos-Hansson E 1994a The posterior pelvic pain provocation test in pregnant women. European Spine Journal 3(5):258–260

Östgaard HC, Zetherstrom G, Roos-Hansson E et al 1994b Reduction of back and posterior pelvic pain in pregnancy. Spine 19(8):894–900

Östgaard HC, Zetherstrom G, Roos-Hansson E 1997 Back pain in relation to pregnancy: a 6-year follow-up. Spine 22(24):2945–2950

Padua L, Padua R, Bondi R et al 2002 Patient-oriented assessment of back pain in pregnancy. European Spine Journal 11(3):272–275

Panjabi MM 1992 The stabilizing system of the spine. 1. Function, dysfunction, adaptation, and enhancement. Journal of Spinal Disorders 5(4):383–389

Paris SV 1997 Differential diagnosis of lumbar back and pelvic pain. In: Vleeming A et al (eds) Movement, Stability and Low Back Pain. The essential role of the pelvis. Churchill Livingstone, New York p319–330

Pool-Goudzwaard A 2003 Biomechanics of the sacroiliac joints and the pelvic floor. Thesis. Erasmus University, Rotterdam

Pool-Goudzwaard A, van Dijke G H, van Gurp M et al 2004 Contribution of pelvic floor muscles to stiffness of the pelvic ring. Clinical Biomechanics 19(6):564–571

Rasmussen-Barr E, Nilsson-Wikmar L, Arvidsson I 2003 Stabilizing training compared with manual treatment in sub-acute and chronic low-back pain. Manual Therapy 8(4):233–241

Richardson CA, Jull GA, Hodges PW et al 1999 Therapeutic exercise for spinal segmental stabilization in low back pain. Churchill Livingstone, London

Richardson CA, Snijders CJ, Hides JA et al 2002 The relation between the transversus abdominis muscles, sacroiliac joint mechanics, and low back pain. Spine 27(4):399–405

Sapsford RR, Hodges PW, Richardson CA et al 2001 Co-activation of the abdominal and pelvic floor muscles during voluntary exercises. Neurourology and Urodynamics 20(1):31–42

Schneiders AG, Zusman M, Singer KP 1998 Exercise therapy compliance in acute low back pain patients. Manual Therapy 3(3):147–152

Sihvonen T, Huttunen M, Makkonen M et al 1998 Functional changes in back muscle activity correlate with pain intensity and prediction of low back pain during pregnancy. Archives of Physical Medicine and Rehabilitation 79(10):1210–1212

Sluijs EM, Kok GJ, Vanderzee J 1993 Correlates of exercise adherence in physical therapy – response. Physical Therapy 73(11):786

Stuge B, Hilde G, Vollestad N 2003 Physical therapy for pregnancy-related low back and pelvic pain: a systematic review. Acta Obstetricia et Gynecologica Scandinavica 82(11): 983–990

Stuge B, Lærum E, Kirkesola G et al 2004a The efficacy of a treatment program focusing on specific stabilizing exercises for pelvic girdle pain after pregnancy. A randomized controlled trial. Spine 29(10):351–359

Stuge B, Veierød M B, Lærum E et al 2004b The efficacy of a treatment program focusing on specific stabilizing exercises for pelvic girdle pain after pregnancy. A two-year follow-up of a randomized clinical trial. Spine 29(10):E197–E203

Stuge B, Holm I, Vøllestad N 2006 To treat or not to treat postpartum pelvic girdle pain with stabilizing exercises? Manual Therapy 11(4):337–343

Sturesson B, Uden G, Uden A 1997 Pain pattern in pregnancy and catching of the leg in pregnant women with posterior pelvic pain. Spine 22(16):1880–1883

Suputtitada A, Wacharapreechanont T, Chaisayan P 2002 Effect of the sitting pelvic tilt exercise during the third trimester in primigravidas on back pain. Journal of the Medical Association of Thailand 85(suppl 1): S170–S179

Sydsjo A, Sydsjo G, Wijma B 1998 Increase in sick leave rates caused by back pain among pregnant Swedish women after amelioration of social benefits. A paradox. Spine 23(18):1986–1990

To WWK, Wong MWN 2003 Factors associated with back pain symptoms in pregnancy and the persistence of pain 2 years after pregnancy. Acta Obstetricia et Gynecologica Scandinavica 82(12):1086–1091

Turgut F, Turgut M, Cetinsahin M 1998 A prospective study of persistent back pain after pregnancy. European Journal of Obstetrics & Gynecology and Reproductive Biology 80(1):45–48

van der Wurff P, Meyne W, Hagmeijer R H 2000 Clinical tests of the sacroiliac joint. A systematic methodological review. Part 2: validity. Manual Therapy 5(2):89–96

van Dieen JH, Selen LPJ, Cholewicki J 2003 Trunk muscle activation in low-back pain patients, an analysis of the literature. Journal of Electromyography and Kinesiology 13(4):333–351

van Dongen PW, de Boer M, Lemmens WA et al 1999 Hypermobility and peripartum pelvic pain syndrome in pregnant South African women. European Journal of Obstetrics & Gynecology and Reproductive Biology 84(1):77–82

van Wingerden JP, Vleeming A, Buyruk HM et al 2004 Stabilization of the sacroiliac joint in vivo: verification of muscular contribution to force closure of the pelvis. European Spine Journal 13:199–205

Vleeming A, Snijders CJ, Stoeckart R et al 1997 The role of the sacroiliac joints in coupling between spine, pelvis, legs and arms. In: Vleeming A et al (eds) Movement, stability and low back pain. The essential role of the pelvis. Churchill Livingstone, New York, p53–71

Vleeming A, Vries HJ, Mens JM et al 2002 Possible role of the long dorsal sacroiliac ligament in women with peripartum pelvic pain. Acta Obstetricia et Gynecologica Scandinavica 81(5):430–436

Wågsæther KB 1998 Livskvalitetsskjema WHOQOL-100: oversettelse, tilpasning og validering – en studie av friske kvinner og kvinner med bekkenleddsyndrom. Universitetet i Bergen, Det medisinske og Det psykologiske fakultet, Norway

Wedenberg K, Moen B, Norling A 2000 A prospective randomized study comparing acupuncture with physiotherapy for low–back and pelvic pain in pregnancy. Acta Obstetricia et Gynecologica Scandinavica 79(5):331–335

Wormslev M, Juul AM, Marques B et al 1994 Clinical examination of pelvic insufficiency during pregnancy. An evaluation of the interobserver variation, the relation between clinical signs and pain and the relation between clinical signs and physical disability. Scandinavian Journal of Rheumatology 23(2):96–102

Wu W, Meijer OG, Jutte PC et al 2002 Gait in patients with pregnancy-related pain in the pelvis: an emphasis on the coordination of transverse pelvic and thoracic rotations. Clinical Biomechanics 17:678–686

Wu WH, Meijer OG, Uegaki K et al 2004 Pregnancy-related pelvic girdle pain (PPP). I: Terminology, clinical presentation, and prevalence. European Spine Journal 13:575–589

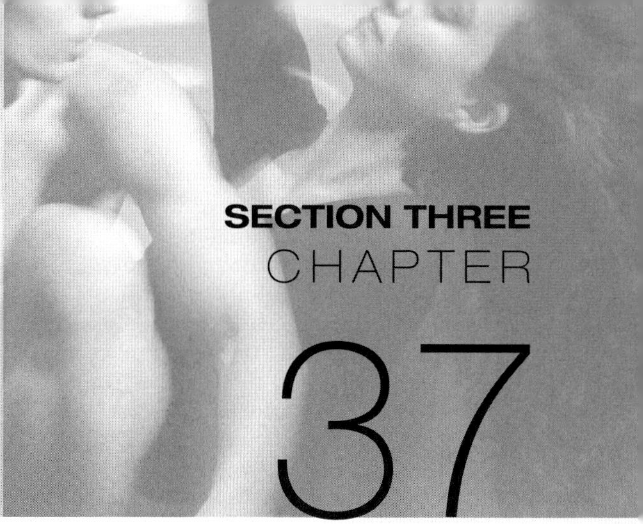

SECTION THREE

CHAPTER 37

Breathing pattern disorders and back pain

Leon Chaitow

Introduction

Hyperventilation (overbreathing) is a breathing pattern disorder (BPD) that produces a drop in arterial carbon dioxide ($PaCO_2$). It occurs when ventilation patterns exceed metabolic demands for oxygen (O_2; Schleifer et al 2002). When there is excessive loss of CO_2 due to an increase in the rate of flow of CO_2 from cells to lungs during hyperventilation, blood pH rises (normal is 7.4), creating respiratory alkalosis (Pryor & Prasad 2002). 'Hypocapnia' is the term used to describe deficiency of CO_2 in the blood resulting from hyperventilation and leading to respiratory alkalosis; 'hypoxia' describes one outcome of hypocapnia: a reduction of O_2 supply to the brain and to tissues, resulting in early fatigue (Nixon & Andrews 1996).

With the onset of respiratory alkalosis there is an immediate disruption in the acid–base equilibrium, triggering a chain of systemic physiological reactions, many of which have adverse implications for musculoskeletal health (Foster et al 2000). Some of the immediate effects of respiratory alkalosis include:

- Altered autonomic control together with a tendency for smooth muscles to constrict, leading to narrowing of blood vessels (as well as other tubular structures such as the intestines, urethra). This leads to reduced delivery of blood to tissues (Ford et al 1995).
- The Bohr effect, which states that an increase in alkalinity encourages the affinity of hemoglobin (Hb) for O_2. The Hb molecule is therefore less likely to release its O_2 in tissues that have become increasingly alkaline due to overbreathing (Levitsky 1995, Pryor & Prasad 2002).
- Reduced $PaCO_2$ increases O_2–Hb affinity, automatically leading to changes in serum calcium and red cell phosphate levels, with

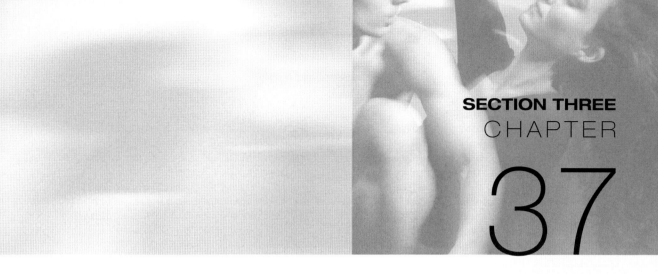

negative implications for neural function and muscle physiology (Enoka & Stuart 1992, George 1964), e.g. encouraging hyperirritability of motor and sensory neurons (Macefield & Burke 1991).
- Alkalosis increases feelings of anxiety and/or panic and associated balance control changes (Klein 1993).
- Hyperventilation is usually characterized by a shift from a diaphragmatic to a thoracic breathing pattern, which imposes biomechanical stress on the neck/shoulder region due to the excessive recruitment of sternocleidomastoid, scalene, and trapezius muscles in support of thoracic breathing (Schleifer et al 2002).

Epidemiology

Relative to men, women have a higher rate of respiration and a greater tendency to respiratory alkalosis, which is exaggerated during the luteal (progesterone) phase of the menstrual cycle. Hyperventilation syndrome (HVS) and breathing pattern disorders (BPD) are therefore female dominated, with a female:male ratio that ranges from 2:1 to 7:1 (Loeppky et al 2001).

Women may be more at risk of BPD because of hormonal influences, because progesterone stimulates respiration, and during the luteal (post ovulation/premenstrual) phase, CO_2 levels drop on average 25%. Additional stress can subsequently 'increase ventilation at a time when carbon dioxide levels are already low' (Damas-Mora et al 1980). There has been no definitive consensus as to the scale of hyperventilation and other functional breathing pattern disorders, although different researchers and clinicians have identified various medical/patient populations:

- Huey & West (1983) suggested that the range is anything from 3.5% to 28%.
- Timmons (1994) noted that 10% of patients attending cardiology clinics, diagnosed as having functional cardiovascular syndromes, are hyperventilators.
- Lum (1987) reported that in the United States as many as 10% of patients in a general internal medicine practice have hyperventilation syndrome as their primary diagnosis.
- Lum (1996) went further when highlighting the degree of what he saw as the widespread misdiagnosis of asthma:

  Thirty percent of cases of asthma are known to be induced by emotion or exercise, and many symptoms are common to hyperventilation and to asthma: intermittent, labored breathing; relief from bronchodilators (transient in hyperventilation); exercise; cough; fear, anxiety and panic. It is thus a matter of individual preference whether the clinician calls such cases asthma or hyperventilation. The distinction is important [because] treatment of hyperventilation cures the patient [while] the asthmatic is condemned to a life of medication.

- Tattersfield et al (2002) have confirmed that asthma can be relatively easily misdiagnosed, especially in patients with 'inappropriate hyperventilation, dysfunction of the vocal cords, or obstruction of the upper airway.' As to the size of this problem, Tattersfield et al (2002) report:

  Although asthma has no standard definition, a clinical diagnosis of asthma in young adults is a repeatable finding in populations with developed health services, and in such populations doctor-diagnosed asthma is typically reported by about 5% of those aged 20–44 years (Janson et al 1997) and in more than 10% of children. (The International Study of Asthma and Allergies in Childhood Steering Committee (ISAAC) 1999)

- Thomas et al (2005) agree with both Lum's and Tatterfield's assessments of the number of asthmatics who are in fact hyperventilators:

  Symptoms associated with functional breathing disorders have been reported as being common in secondary care settings, and can affect 29% of adults with current asthma in the community.

- To evaluate the levels of BPD in nonasthmatics, Thomas et al (2005) conducted a cross-sectional postal survey of adults without current asthma in a UK general practice. The instrument used was the Nijmegen questionnaire (see below). Positive screening scores were more common in women (14%, 7–20%) than men (2%, 0–5%, $P = 0.003$). Comparison with a previous survey showed that the prevalence of positive screening scores was higher in those with current asthma than those without (29% versus 8%, $P < 0.001$). This suggests that approximately one healthy adult in 12 has a dysfunctional breathing pattern.
- Numerous other subgroups and medical populations are also associated (not necessarily

causally) with hyperventilation tendencies, including people who are hypermobile (Bulbena et al 1993, Martin-Santos et al 1998, Muller et al 2003) as well as deconditioned individuals (Nixon & Andrews 1996), patients with fibromyalgia (Henriksson & Mense 1994) and/or patients with myofascial pain syndromes (Brucini et al 1981).

Although a disturbed breathing pattern can be the result of a variety of psychogenic and/or environmental triggers, it can at times coexist with organic disorders, making a comprehensive assessment essential to rule out any associated pathology. There are also conditions and situations in which overbreathing – and the resulting rise in pH – can be seen as normal responses to acidosis, for example in diabetic acidosis, renal or liver failure (Gardner 1994) and advanced pregnancy (Brownridge 1995). Hyperventilation is also normal in situations of hyperthermia (fever for example) where excessive ventilation has a heat-reducing function (Gardner 1994).

The likelihood is, however, that – as a rule – overbreathing results from something far less sinister and that it is due to pure habit. As Lum (1987) has stated:

> *Neurological considerations can leave little doubt that the habitually unstable breathing is the prime cause of symptoms. Why they breathe in this way must be a matter for speculation, but manifestly the salient characteristics are pure habit.*

This 'habit' will effectively set the individual's tolerance threshold for CO_2 at a low level, ensuring that the respiration rate remains rapid. Breathing retraining (see below) has as one of its aims the objective of raising the threshold of tolerance for CO_2, and so allowing a slower breathing rate to be well tolerated (Jennett 1994).

Does the widespread nature of BPD, whether mislabeled or not, have any significance for pain in general, and back pain in particular?

The relationship between BPD and musculoskeletal pain was evaluated in a pilot study, involving a convenience sample of approximately 110 individuals, by Perri & Halford (2003). The findings neatly summarize both the widespread nature of BPD and the question of linkage with other symptoms. This study showed that normal patterns of breathing are the exception rather than the rule. An overwhelming 75% of those studied exhibited faulty breathing mechanics. If the results of this study reflect the general population, as clinicians, your chances are three in four that the new patient you see today will have faulty breathing patterns. This really begs the question, 'Is there a direct correlation between faulty breathing mechanics and the experience of pain?' And an even more significant question of: 'Will correcting faulty breathing affect the experience of pain?'

A variety of percentages of different subgroups (including those who are well) can be shown to demonstrate disturbed breathing patterns. If as seems virtually certain, BPD frequently contributes to, and/or aggravates, back pain problems, the importance of evaluating all patients for BPD becomes clear (Chaitow 2004).

Biochemical and neurological influences of breathing pattern disorders

The biochemical effects of breathing pattern disorders (such as hyperventilation), leading as they do to systemic respiratory alkalosis (Foster et al 2001), as well as to modification of calcium, magnesium and potassium balance (Enoka & Stuart 1992) can be shown to alter motor function (Van Dieen et al 2003), to lower pain thresholds (Rhudy & Meagher 2000) and to increased sympathetic arousal (Dempsey et al 2002). Lum (1994b) has reported:

> *During moderate hyperventilation, loss of CO_2 ions from neurons stimulates neuronal activity, causing increased sensory and motor discharges, muscular tension and spasm, speeding of spinal reflexes, heightened perception (photophobia, hyperacusis) and other sensory disturbances.*

Hyperventilation decreases $PaCO_2$ (hypocapnia) and starts the acid–base changes that end as respiratory alkalosis. These changes in $PaCO_2$ produce secondary changes in plasma bicarbonate concentration. In chronic hypocapnia, changes in plasma bicarbonate occur as a result of adjustments in renal mechanisms that are attempting to restore homeostatic balance (Medias & Adrogue 2003). As Foster et al (2001) explain:

> *Respiratory alkalosis is an extremely common and complicated problem affecting virtually every organ system in the body [producing as it does] multiple metabolic abnormalities, from changes in potassium, phosphate, and calcium, to the development of a mild lactic acidosis. Hyperventilation syndrome is a common etiology of respiratory alkalosis.*

When the effects of respiratory alkalosis on human skeletal muscle metabolism have been examined (involving muscle biopsies), during submaximal exercise, a mismatch has been noted between pyruvate production and its oxidation, resulting in net lactate accumulation (LeBlanc et al 2002).

Mogyoros et al (1997) state:

> *The thresholds of human sensory and motor axons are altered during hyperventilation. Hyperventilation does not alter conduction velocity, refractoriness or super-normality, implying that the hyperventilation-induced increase in neuronal excitability is not the result of conventional depolarization, as seems to occur during ischaemia. These results suggest that hyperventilation has a rather selective action on the threshold channels… The greater expression of threshold channels in sensory [rather] than in motor fibres, can explain why hyperventilation induces paraesthesiae before fasciculation, and why only paraesthesiae occur during ischaemia.*

Seyal et al (1999) note that hyperventilation increases the excitability of both cutaneous and motor axons, and that in experimental animals, hyperventilation increases excitability of hippocampal neurons. Their research, involving healthy humans, demonstrates that hyperventilation increases the excitability of the human corticospinal system.

The evidence seems strong that the changes caused by hyperventilation are capable of interfering with motor control, normal muscular function, and pain perception (Chaitow 2004).

Effects of breathing pattern disorders on emotion and balance

Anxiety and apprehension are closely associated with altered breathing patterns, and breathing pattern disorders are in turn exaggerated by anxiety and apprehension (Balaban & Theyer 2001, Klein 1993). According to Balaban & Theyer (2001), links between balance control and anxiety are based on neural circuits that are shared by pathways that mediate autonomic control, vestibuloautonomic interactions, and anxiety. The core of this circuitry is a parabrachial nucleus network, which is a site of convergence of vestibular information processing and somatic and visceral sensory information processing, in pathways that appear to be involved in avoidance conditioning, anxiety, and conditioned fear. The amygdala appears to play a pivotal role in the transmission and interpretation of fear and anxiety. The neuronal interactions between the amygdala enable the individual to initiate adaptive behaviors to threat based on the nature of the threat and prior experience. There is mediation between the efferent pathways involving the amygdala, locus coeruleus, hypothalamus, and autonomic, neuro-endocrine, and skeletal–motor responses associated with fear and anxiety (Charney & Deutsch 1996).

The extremely complex relationship between balance and the nervous system (with its interoceptive, proprioceptive, and exteroceptive mechanisms) also involves a variety of somatic and visceral motor output pathways (Charney & Deutsch 1996). Maintaining body balance and equilibrium is a primary role of functionally coordinated muscles, acting in task-specific patterns, and this is dependent on normal motor control (Winters & Crago 2000).

Anxious, apprehensive thoughts have been shown to have an effect on the functioning of muscles. Lotze et al (1999) using functional MRI scans have demonstrated that the cortical activity involved in thinking about a movement is similar to the cortical activity associated with the movement itself. It appears that simply talking about painful experiences increases activity in associated muscles in chronic low back pain (LBP) patients (Flor et al 1992).

There is ample evidence that anxiety regarding movement, pain, and reinjury can all modify motor behavior, with implications for spinal stability (Chaitow 2004, Crombez et al 1999, Vlaeyen & Crombez 1999).

Abnormal breathing patterns such as hyperventilation lead to elevated reports of somatic symptoms, including disorientation. There is evidence that the central changes that accompany hyperventilation can influence balance system functioning. For example, healthy individuals exhibit a substantial increase in sway following voluntary hyperventilation, and this postural instability may be linked to peripheral and central changes in somatosensory function (Yardley & Redfern 2001).

LBP often involves altered muscle length relationships, postural changes, muscular imbalances, variations in location of the centers of mass and of pressure (Commerford & Motterm 2001a, 2001b) Unsurprisingly, in the presence of such changes, associated with chronic LBP, the speed and intensity of muscular contractions are commonly altered (Redebold et al 2000) with deep segmentally-related muscles losing both contraction speed and intensity; overactivity and tonic contraction occurs in the larger multisegmental muscles (Hodges & Richardson 1999, O'Sullivan et al 1997). All these changes lead to LBP patients moving differently when compared with healthy individuals (Selles et al 2001). Increased anxiety levels, caused or aggravated by disordered breathing patterns (such as hyperventilation) can amplify many of these changes. Put simply, the responses of the motor system alter under conditions of pain and anxiety, due to modified cerebral processing (Butler 2000).

There is good evidence that enhanced breathing function improves postural balance. Aust & Fischer (1997) investigated whether psychophysical breath work influences postural control. The method used involved optical patterns being projected onto a video screen, the test subjects having been instructed to shift their center of gravity according to the patterns projected. The patterns consisted of a line which had to be followed in the anterior–posterior and lateral plane, and a circle to be followed clockwise and counterclockwise. The results showed that those participants with some experience of breath training had significantly better results in the posturographic test with visual feedback. Additionally, the posturographic results immediately following 1 hour of breath work demonstrated clear improvements in body equilibrium, suggesting that breath work leads to a general improvement in maintaining equilibrium, which remains stable over time.

There is good evidence that breathing rehabilitation is a useful method for achieving reduced anxiety/panic levels and for improving postural control and somatic complaints, such as LBP (Aust & Fischer 1997, Han et al 1996, Lum 1994a).

Anxiety, breathing pattern disorders, and trigger points

Anxiety and other emotions have also been shown to encourage recruitment of a small number of motor units that display almost constant, or repeated, activity when influenced psychogenically. In one study, low-amplitude myoelectric activity (measured using surface electromyography) was evident even when muscles were not being employed in situations of mental stress (Waersted et al 1993):

> *A small pool of low-threshold motor units may be under considerable load for prolonged periods of time… motor units with Type 1 [postural] fibres are predominant among these. If the subject repeatedly recruits the same motor units, the overload may result in a metabolic crisis.*

This etiology parallels the proposed evolution of myofascial trigger points, as suggested by Simons et al (1999), with major implications for the development and exacerbation of myofascial pain conditions. Simons et al (1999) have also clearly demonstrated that an ischemic environment is a natural breeding ground for trigger points. This has recently been confirmed by remarkable techniques involving microanalytical assays of the milieu of living muscle in the region of active (i.e. pain-producing) trigger points (Shah et al 2005).

Biomechanical effects of breathing pattern disorders

Stability of the lumbar spine requires both passive stiffness, through the osseous and ligamentous structures, and active stiffness, through muscles. A spine, without muscles attached, would be unable to bear the compressive load it has to carry (Lucas & Bresler 1961, McGill 2002). Spinal instability occurs when either passive or active stiffness is disturbed. Muscle behavior alters in conditions of hypoxia and ischemia, and the effects of respiratory alkalosis and the Bohr effect ensure that both hypoxia and ischemia are more likely. Jammes et al (1997) have shown that:

- Prolonged and severe chronic hypoxemia markedly reduces muscle force generation by skeletal muscles and their endurance to fatigue.
- The diaphragm tolerates much more hypoxemia than do skeletal muscles, namely those that contain a large proportion of slow twitch oxidative fibers.
- Reduced oxygen supply to contracting muscles affects not only the metabolic paths but also modifies the gain of sensorimotor reflex loops.
- Chronic hypoxemia markedly reduces maximal force (F_{max}) and shortens the endurance time to fatigue.
- The consequences of chronic hypoxemia on force generation by skeletal muscles are much more accentuated than those exerted by acute hypoxia (Zattara-Hartmann et al 1995).
- Restoration of normal PaO_2 levels in these individuals improves maximal muscle performance immediately, perhaps through more efficient excitation–contraction coupling.

Jammes et al (1997) observed in relation to patients with chronic hypoxemia:

> *We noticed that reoxygenation paradoxically improved their muscle performances but reduced the motor unit recruitment. These facts lead one to suspect the existence of permanent skeletal muscle fatigue in chronic hypoxemic patients. Indeed, at constant strength of contraction, the occurrence of fatigue is signalled by an increase in ratio between integrated myoelectrical activity and muscle force. This is attributed to excitation-contraction uncoupling, which results partly from impaired calcium delivery and/or utilization in muscle fibers.*

This evidence strongly suggests that spinal stability is likely to be compromised by the effects of overbreathing.

The diaphragm, intra-abdominal pressure, and spinal stability

According to Schleifer et al (2002), hyperventilation can compromise spinal stability in a number of ways, including increasing any tendency to greater muscle tension, muscle spasm, amplified response to catecholamines, and muscle ischemia and hypoxia, as well as by interfering with the intra-abdominal pressure stabilization functions of the diaphragm.

There is evidence that increased intra-abdominal pressure (IAP), even with limited participation of the abdominal or back muscles, augments the stability of the spine (Hodges et al 2001, 2005).

Recent data confirm that the activity of the diaphragm occurs in association with tasks that challenge the stability of the spine (Hodges & Gandevia 2000a, 2000b, Hodges et al 1997). When, however, a challenge occurs that makes postural/stabilizing demands on the diaphragm at the same time that respiratory demands are occurring, it is the stability element that suffers.

Using a 10% CO_2 gas mixture to elevate breathing, McGill et al (1995) demonstrated that reduction in the support offered to the spine, by the muscles of the torso, can occur if there is both a load challenge to the low back and a breathing challenge (shovelling snow is given as an easily understood example in real-life rather than under research conditions):

> *Modulation of muscle activity needed to facilitate breathing may compromise the margin of safety of tissues that depend on constant muscle activity for support.*

Hodges et al (2001) demonstrated (using a long-tube breathing method) that after approximately 60 seconds of overbreathing the postural (tonic) and phasic functions of both the diaphragm and transversus abdominis are reduced or absent:

> *The present data suggest that increased central respiratory drive may attenuate the postural commands reaching motoneurons. This attenuation can affect the key inspiratory and expiratory muscles, and is likely to be co-ordinated at a premotoneuronal site.*

They further hypothesize:

> *Although investigation of spinal mechanics is required to confirm the extent to which spinal control is compromised by increases in respiratory demand, it is hypothesized that such a compromise may lead to increased potential for injury to spinal structures and reduced postural control. During strenuous exercise, when the physical stresses to the spine are greater, the physiological vulnerability of the spine to injury is likely to be increased.*

Studies by O'Sullivan et al (2002) have also indicated that people with sacroiliac pain have impaired recruitment of the diaphragm and pelvic floor. Leaving aside all other considerations outlined in this chapter, the influence of upper-chest (nondiaphragmatic) overbreathing alone can be seen to be capable of compromising spinal stability.

Breathing retraining

Reducing levels of apprehension, anxiety, and fear can be seen to have the potential for encouraging improvement in breathing patterns and all the negative symptoms that flow from these. There is good evidence that breathing rehabilitation is a useful method for achieving reduced anxiety/panic levels and for improving postural control and somatic complaints, such as LBP (Aust & Fischer 1997, Han et al 1996, Lum 1987, Nixon & Andrews 1996).

Breathing retraining has been used to successfully correct hyperventilation. In one study (Lum 1987) more than 1000 anxious and phobic patients were treated using a combination of breathing retraining, physical therapy, and relaxation. Symptoms were usually abolished in 1–6 months, with some younger patients requiring only a few weeks. At 12 months 75% were free of all symptoms, 20% had only mild symptoms and about one patient in 20 had intractable symptoms.

In another study (Han et al 1996), breathing therapy was evaluated in patients with hyperventilation syndrome (HVS) in which most of the patients met the criteria for an anxiety disorder. The diagnosis was based on the presence of several stress-related complaints, reproduced by voluntary hyperventilation, patients with organic diseases having been excluded. Therapy was conducted in the following sequence:

- brief, voluntary hyperventilation to reproduce the complaints in daily life
- reattribution of the cause of the symptoms to hyperventilation
- explaining the rationale of therapy-reduction of hyperventilation by acquiring an abdominal breathing pattern, with slowing down of expiration
- breathing retraining for 2–3 months by a physiotherapist.

After breathing therapy, the sum scores of the Nijmegen Questionnaire were markedly reduced. A canonical correlation analysis relating the changes of the various complaints to the modifications of breathing variables showed that the improvement of the complaints was correlated mainly with the slowing down of breathing frequency.

The Nijmegen Questionnaire provides a non-invasive test of high sensitivity (up to 91%) and specificity (up to 95%) (Vansteenkiste et al 1991). This easily administered, internationally validated diagnostic questionnaire is the simplest, kindest, and to date most accurate indicator of acute and chronic hyperventilation (Van Dixhoorn & Duivenvoorden 1985). The questionnaire enquires as to the following symptoms, and their intensity: constriction in the chest, shortness of breath, accelerated or deepened breathing, inability to breathe deeply, feeling tense, tightness around the mouth, stiffness in the fingers or arms, cold hands or feet, tingling fingers, bloated abdominal sensation, dizzy spells, blurred vision, feeling of confusion or losing touch with the environment.

Research evidence

Mehling & Hamel (2005) demonstrated that patients with moderate chronic low back pain, of average 1-year duration, improved significantly in pain and function from breathing rehabilitation methods, as much as from extensive physical therapy. The study involved 16 patients (mean age 49.7 years, 31.3% male) with chronic low back pain, who underwent breath therapy compared with 12 subjects with similar complaints (mean age 48.7 years, 41.7% male) who underwent physical therapy. It was found that:

- Patients improved in both groups regarding pain, with a visual analog scale of –2.7 with breath therapy, and –2.4 with physical therapy.
- There was a Short Form 36 (SF-36) score of +14.9 with breath therapy and +21.0 with physical therapy.
- Breath therapy recipients improved in function and in the physical and emotional role.
- Physical therapy patients improved in vitality.
- Average improvements were not different between the two groups.
- At 6–8 weeks, results showed a trend favoring breath therapy.
- At 6 months, a trend favoring physical therapy was seen.

Both the intervention and control groups received one introductory evaluation session of 60 minutes, and 12 individual therapy sessions of equal duration of 45 minutes over 6–8 weeks.

Summary

- It seems highly probable that chronic habitual breathing pattern disorders negatively influence motor control, neurological sensitization, muscle behavior, pain threshold, and balance.
- There is evidence that breathing rehabilitation can reverse these tendencies and restore more normal breathing patterns in many individuals. As with most features and functions not directly associated with the symptoms, unless BPDs are looked for and evaluated, they are unlikely to be recognized in a manual medicine setting (Chaitow et al 2002).
- Although seldom causative, BPD can be seen to potentially be a major factor in encouraging and maintaining musculoskeletal dysfunction in general, and back pain in particular.

References

Aust G, Fischer K 1997 Changes in body equilibrium response caused by breathing. A posturographic study with visual feedback. Laryngorhinootologie 76(10): 577–582

Balaban C, Thayer J 2001 Neurological bases for balance-anxiety links. Journal of Anxiety Disorders 15(1–2): 53–79

Brownridge P 1995 The nature and consequences of childbirth pain. European J Obstetrics & Gynaecology 59(Suppl):S9–S15

Brucini M, Duranti R, Galletti R 1981 Pain thresholds and electromyographic features of periarticular muscles in patients with osteoarthritis of the knee. Pain 10:57– 66

Bulbena A, Duro J, Porta M et al 1993 Anxiety disorders in the joint hypermobility syndrome. Psychiatry Research 46:59–68

Butler D 2000 The sensitive nervous system. Noigroup Publications, Adelaide, Australia, p89

Chaitow L 2004 Breathing pattern disorders, motor control, and LBP. Journal of Osteopathic Medicine 7(1):34–41

Chaitow L, Bradley D, Gilbert C 2002 Multidisciplinary approaches to breathing pattern disorders. Churchill Livingstone, Edinburgh

Charney D, Deutsch A 1996 A functional neuroanatomy of anxiety and fear: implications for the pathophysiology and treatment of anxiety disorders. Critical Reviews in Neurobiology 10:419–446

Commerford M, Mottram S 2001a Movement and stability dysfunction – contemporary developments. Manual Therapy 6:15–26

Commerford M, Mottram S 2001b Functional stability retraining. Principles and strategies for managing mechanical dysfunction. Manual Therapy 6:3–14

Crombez G, Vlaeyen J, Heurs P et al 1999 Fear of pain is more disabling than pain itself. Pain 80:329–340

Damas-Mora J, Davies L, Taylor W 1980 Menstrual respiratory changes and symptoms. British Journal of Psychiatry 136:492–497

Dempsey J, Sheel A, St Croix C 2002 Respiratory influences on sympathetic vasomotor outflow in humans. Respiratory Physiology & Neurobiology 130(1):3–20

Enoka R, Stuart D 1992 Neurobiology of muscle fatigue Journal of Applied Physiology 72:1631–1648

Flor H, Birmbaumer N, Schugens M et al 1992 Symptom specific psychophysiological responses in chronic pain patients. Psychophysiology 29:452–460

Ford M, Camilleri M, Hanson R 1995 Hyperventilation, central autonomic control, and colonic tone in humans. Gut 37:499–504

Foster G, Vaziri N, Sassoon C 2001 Respiratory alkalosis. Respiratory Care 46(4):384–91

Gardner W 1994 Diagnosis and organic causes of symptomatic hyperventilation. In: Timmons B, Ley R (eds) Behavioral and psychological approaches to breathing disorders. Plenum Press, New York, p99–113

George S 1964 Changes in serum calcium, serum phosphate and red cell phosphate during hyperventilation. New England Journal of Medicine 270:726–728

Han J, Stegen K, De Valck C et al 1996 Influence of breathing therapy on complaints, anxiety and breathing pattern in patients with hyperventilation syndrome and anxiety disorders. Journal of Psychosomatic Research 41(5):481–493

Henriksson K, Mense S 1994 Pain and nociception in FMS. Pain Reviews 1:245–260

Hodges P, Gandevia S 2000a Activation of the human diaphragm during a repetitive postural task. Journal of Physiology 522:165–175

Hodges P, Gandevia S 2000b Changes in intra–abdominal pressure during postural and respiratory activation of the human diaphragm. Journal of Applied Physiology 89:967

Hodges P, Richardson C 1999 Altered trunk muscle recruitment in people with LBP with upper limb movement at different speeds. Archives of Physical Medicine Rehabilitation 80:1005–1012

Hodges P, Butler J, McKenzie D 1997 Contraction of the human diaphragm during postural adjustments. Journal of Physiology 505:239–240

Hodges P, Heinjnen I, Gandevia S 2001 Postural activity of the diaphragm is reduced in humans when respiratory demand increases. Journal of Physiology 537(3): 999

Hodges P, Eriksson A, Shirley D 2005 Intra-abdominal pressure increases stiffness of the lumbar spine. Journal of Biomechanics 38(9):1873–1880

Huey S, West S 1983 Hyperventilation: its relation to symptom experience and anxiety. Journal of Abnormal Psychology 92:422–432

Jammes Y, Zattara-Hartmann M, Badier M 1997 Functional consequences of acute and chronic hypoxia on respiratory and skeletal muscles in mammals. Comparative Biochemistry and Physiology Part A: Physiology 118(1):15–22

Janson C, Chinn S, Jarvis D 1997 Physician-diagnosed asthma and drug utilization in the European Community Respiratory Health Survey. European Respiratory Journal 10:1795–1802

Jennett S 1994 Control of breathing and its disorders. In: Timmons B, Ley R (eds) Behavioral and psychological approaches to breathing disorders. Plenum Press, New York, p67–80

Klein D 1993 False suffocation alarms, spontaneous panics, and related conditions. Archives of General Psychiatry 50:306–317

LeBlanc P, Parolin M, Jones N 2002 Effects of respiratory alkalosis on human skeletal muscle metabolism at the onset of submaximal exercise. Journal of Physiology 544(Pt 1):303–313

Levitsky L 1995 Pulmonary physiology, 4th edn. McGraw Hill, New York

Loeppky J, Scotto P, Charlton G et al 2001 Ventilation is greater in women than men, but the increase during acute altitude hypoxia is the same. Respiration Physiology 125(3):225–237

Lotze M, Montoya P, Erb M et al. 1999 Activation of cortical and cerebellar motor areas during executed and imagined hand movements: an fMRI study. Journal of Cognitive Neuroscience 11:491–501

Lucas D, Bresler B 1961 Stability of the ligamentous spine. Biomechanics Laboratory, University of California, San Francisco, CA

Lum C 1996 Hyperventilation and asthma: the grey area. Biological Psychology 43(3):262
Lum L 1987 Hyperventilation syndromes in medicine and psychiatry. Journal of the Royal Society of Medicine 80(4):229–231
Lum L 1994a Editorial: hyperventilation and anxiety state. Journal Royal Society of Medicine Jan:1–4
Lum L 1994b Hyperventilation syndromes. In: Timmons B, Ley R (eds) Behavioral and psychological approaches to breathing disorders. Plenum Press, New York, p113–123
Macefield G, Burke D 1991 Parasthesia and tetany induced by voluntary hyperventilation. Brain 114:527–540
Martin-Santos R, Bulbena A, Porta M et al 1998 Association between joint hypermobility syndrome and panic disorder. American Journal of Psychiatry 55:1578–1583
McGill S 2002 Low back disorders: evidence-based prevention and rehabilitation. Human Kinetics, Champaign, IL
McGill S, Sharratt M, Seguin J 1995 Loads on spinal tissues during simultaneous lifting and ventilatory challenge. Ergonomics 38(9):1772–1792
Mehling W, Hamel K 2005 Randomized, controlled trial of breath therapy for patients with chronic low-back pain. Alternative Therapy and Health Medicine 11(4):44–52. Online. Available: http://www.breathexperience.com
Mogyoros I, Kiernan K, Burke D et al 1997 Excitability changes in human sensory and motor axons during hyperventilation and ischaemia. Brain 120(2):317–325
Muller K, Kreutzfeldt A, Schwesig R et al 2003 Hypermobility and chronic back pain. Manuelle Medizin 41:105–109
Nixon P, Andrews J 1996 A study of anaerobic threshold in chronic fatigue syndrome (CFS). Biological Psychology 43(3):264
O'Sullivan P, Twomey L, Allison G et al 1997 Altered patterns of abdominal muscle activation in patients with chronic LBP. Australian Physiotherapy 43:91–98
O'Sullivan P, Beales D, Beetham J et al 2002 Altered motor control strategies in subjects with sacroiliac joint pain during the active straight-leg-raise test. Spine 27:E1–E8
Perri M, Halford E 2003 Pain and faulty breathing: a pilot study. Journal of Bodywork and Movement Therapies 8(4):297–306
Pryor J, Prasad S 2002 Physiotherapy for respiratory and cardiac problems, 3rd edn. Churchill Livingstone, Edinburgh, p81
Rhudy J, Meagher M 2000 Fear and anxiety: divergent effects on human pain thresholds. Pain 84:65–75
Schleifer LM, Ley R, Spalding TW 2002 A hyperventilation theory of job stress and musculoskeletal disorders. American Journal of Independent Medicine 41(5): 420–432
Selles R, Wagenaar R, Smit T et al 2001 Disorders in trunk rotation during walking in patients with LBP: a dynamical systems approach. Clinical Biomechanics 16:175–181
Seyal M, Mull B, Gage B 1999 Increased excitability of the human corticospinal system with hyperventilation. Electroencephalography and Clinical Neurophysiology/ Electromyography and Motor Control 109(3):263–267
Shah J, Phillips T, Danoff J, Gerber L 2005 An in-vivo microanalytical technique for measuring the local biochemical milieu of human skeletal muscle. Journal of Applied Physiology 99(5):1977–1984
Simons D, Travell J, Simons L 1999 Myofascial pain and dysfunction: the trigger point manual. Vol 1, upper half of body, 2nd edn. Williams and Wilkins, Baltimore, MD
Tattersfield A et al 2002 Asthma. The Lancet 360(26): 1313–1322
The International Study of Asthma and Allergies in Childhood Steering Committee (ISAAC) 1999 Worldwide variations in the prevalence of asthma symptoms: the International Study of Asthma and Allergies in Childhood 1999. European Respiratory Journal 12: 315–335
Thomas M, McKinley R, Freeman E et al 2005 The prevalence of dysfunctional breathing in adults in the community with and without asthma. Primary Care Respiratory Journal 14(2):78–82
Timmons B 1994 Introduction In: Timmons B, Ley R (eds) Behavioral and psychological approaches to breathing disorders. Plenum Press, New York, p7
Van Dieen J, Selen L, Cholewicki J 2003 Trunk muscle activation in low-back pain patients, an analysis of the literature. Journal of Electromyography and Kinesiology 13:333–351
Van Dixhoorn J, Duivenvoorden H 1985 Efficacy of Nijmegen questionnaire in recognition of the hyperventilation syndrome. Journal of Psychosomatic Research 29:199–206
Vansteenkiste J, Rochette F, Demedts M 1991 Diagnostic tests of hyperventilation syndrome. European Respiratory Journal 4:393–399
Vlaeyen J, Crombez G 1999 Fear of movement.(re)injury, avoidance and pain disability in chronic LBP patients. Manual Therapy 4:187–195
Waersted M, Eken T, Westgaard R 1993 Psychogenic motor unit activity – a possible muscle injury mechanism studied in a healthy subject. Journal of Musculoskeletal Pain 1(3 and 4):185
Winters J, Crago P (eds) 2000 Biomechanics and neural control of posture and movement. Springer, New York
Yardley L, Redfern M 2001 Psychological factors influencing recovery from balance disorders. Journal of Anxiety Disorders 15(1–2):107–119
Zattara-Hartmann M, Badier M, Guillot C et al 1995 Maximal force and endurance to fatigue of respiratory and skeletal muscles in chronic hypoxemic patients: The effects of oxygen breathing. Muscle Nerve 18:495–502

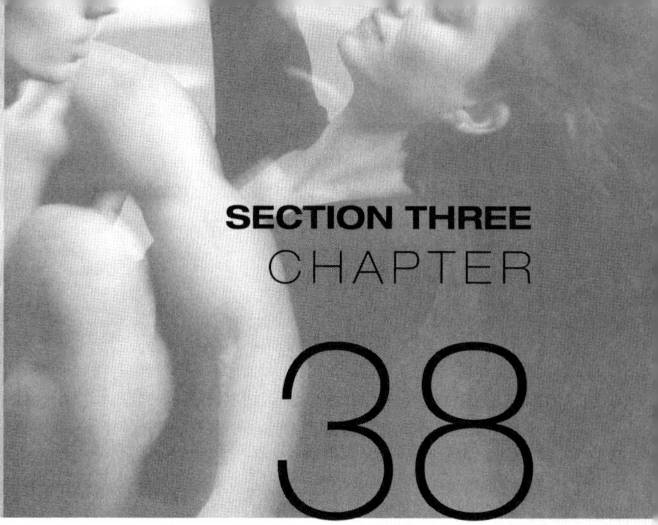

SECTION THREE
CHAPTER

38

Effective rehabilitation of lumbar and pelvic girdle pain

Vert Mooney

Introduction

It is the premise of this chapter that the effective rehabilitation of the lumbar and pelvic girdle pain can best be carried out in a rational manner by a progressive resistance exercise program. By appropriate evaluation, the selection of an exercise program that is most efficient and effective for the particular patient can be determined. Following that, a definable dose of therapeutic exercises is provided, and progressed in a stepwise manner until a plateau is reached. It is important that some objective measurement of treatment benefit be available and thus this chapter will discuss a method by which function can be tested.

It is the opinion of this author that an accurate insight into the role of exercises can best be achieved with the use of exercise equipment. This point of view apparently contrasts with other contributors to this text. Nonetheless, it is my hope to offer sufficient documentation in the text to justify that view. Because of the apparent discussion of exercise equipment only in this chapter, it is felt necessary that we start with a discussion of the historic development of the concepts of strength training.

Historic background

Surprisingly, the idea is not new. In 1865, Gustav Zander, a German physician who developed the idea, which he called 'medical mechanical therapy,' while at medical school opened a treatment center in Stockholm. He noted the importance of measured progress in exercise (Zander 1872) (Fig. 38.1). He developed 40 pieces of equipment, which were designed to isolate specific joint functions. By clever mechanical arrangement,

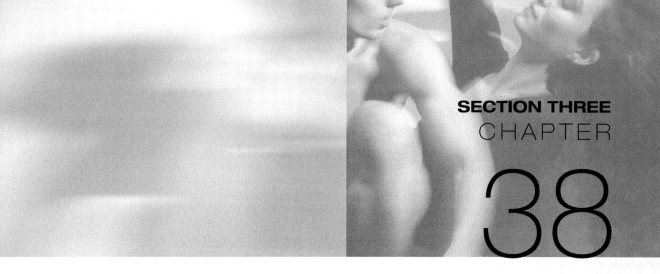

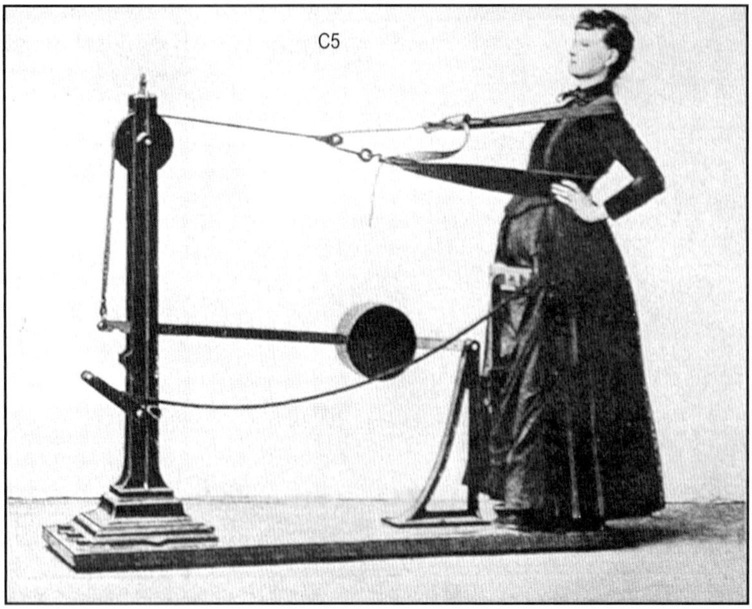

Fig. 38.1 Example of Zander Exercise Machine for strengthening low back extensors. This equipment was produced in the 1860s.

the amount of resistance could be varied. Thus, within the constraints of the particular machine, the number of repetitions at full range and the resistance was known and one could clearly identify the dose of therapeutic exercise. The response, in terms of symptoms and muscle size, was likewise notable.

By the turn of the twentieth century, there were over 200 facilities around the world with this equipment. The facilities were all quite similar in that the machines were laid out in a circuit; the patient was expected to move from one to the next to carry out a full exercise program. This, of course, was very much like the format in current health clubs.

Although Zander described his equipment as a therapeutic mechanical system of treatment, it did not attract the attention of the medical care community. Therapeutic exercise at that time was not considered an asset to the healing process. This was especially true in musculoskeletal abnormalities, where it was generally felt that prolonged rest and even immobilization was a more positive event in the healing process. Although general exercises were utilized in physical therapy at the time, these were largely focused at gaining range of motion and improved joint function. Neuromotor control was thought to be useful but strength was specifically not considered important.

The concept of progressive resistance exercises for strengthening as a medical treatment emerged from a former weight lifter who became an orthopedic surgeon – Thomas DeLorme. At the time of the Second World War, strength training was not considered important in the rehabilitation of joints. In the early 1940s, if military personnel injured their knees or had surgery, they were discharged from the service because they could not return to the high level of physical function demanded of active military. DeLorme, actually against instructions from his superior officer, took a group of Navy personnel with postoperative and injured knees and put them through the usual progressive strength training of a weight lifter. This had not been done before. Their muscles hypertrophied and they returned to normal function. It was thus accepted as a justifiable rehabilitation program. DeLorme first summarized the system of progressive exercises in 1945. However, he did not use any specific equipment and used weights tied to shoes as a mechanism of supplying progressive resistance.

Over the next several decades there was little interest in therapeutic exercise. Even for cardiac function, it was thought that rest was a more important factor. Eventually, however, with improved technology of monitoring, it became quite apparent that gradual progressive physical activity was not a deterrent to healing after a heart attack; actually, it was a positive event (Bruce 1973, Pilote et al 1992). Of course, with cardiac function, there are many mechanisms to monitor function, such as pulse rate, oxygen uptake, respiratory rate, and, of course, the electrical events of the heart itself as identified in the electrocardiogram. Using a combination of these various evaluation tools, standardized protocols as to appropriate physical activity could be created. Unfortunately, in the musculoskeletal system, there are far fewer tools to monitor function. In the case of the spine, it is even more difficult to test discrepancy from normal than with the extremities. At least, in evaluating the function of an injured extremity, one usually has the opportunity to test the other side for comparison to identify the expected level of normal for that individual.

A step forward in the monitoring of physical function was the reintroduction of exercise machines. The Zander equipment had faded from the scene. Expense was one factor but there was also a lack of endorsement of therapeutic benefit from the medical community. Active strength training exercises were usually done in high school gyms and basements of YMCAs. The exercise was in the form of medicine balls and free weights.

A true innovation in efficiency of exercise occurred to an entrepreneur, Arthur Jones. He had no medical background and, at that time, made a living by transporting exotic animals in his own airplanes from Africa to various zoos around the world. He was a relatively small man and looked toward bodybuilding to improve his image. His innovation was the use of a cam to spread the peak resistance throughout the entire arc of a joint range. If one is trying to strengthen the biceps with an elbow curl and a weight in the hand, the peak resistance is at the occasion where the elbow is fully extended, and the exercise becomes easier as the elbow is flexed. When an exercise machine is fit with a cam, which has a gradually increasing radius, one can arrange the mechanics so that the amount of resistance with the elbow fully extended is about the same as with it fully flexed. Jones named his innovation the 'nautilus exercise equipment.' The increasing size of the chambers of a nautilus shell is somewhat like the increasing radius of a cam (Jones 1970). The equipment was an immediate success and, along with numerous competitors, the entire health club business developed. The focus was exercise enthusiasts and the system remained under the radar of the medical community. Arthur Jones never published in medical journals. Most of his work is in *Iron Man Magazine*. Nonetheless, because of the machines, the modern health club has emerged, with all its chrome and mirrors, and is now attractive to men and women alike. Health clubs focus not only on bodybuilding but also on health maintenance and have a well-accepted place, at least under the heading of alternative medicine.

The Lumex Corporation, a competing exercise equipment manufacturer, purposely chose to market Cybex equipment to the medical community. This was an innovative design wherein the exercise to the joint had the speed of motion controlled by the machine. The transducers in the machine measured the torque or force the person was using to move the lever arm of the machine. The name coined for this unnatural type of exercise was 'isokinetic.' Unlike the nautilus, its introduction was in the medical literature (Thistle et al 1967). This was first thought to be a more precise system of exercise and was not conceived to be a test tool. Later on, the isokinetic equipment was used for testing as well as exercising. Thanks to computers and VCRs, a graphic display with specific patterns of joint function could be produced. It looked just mystical enough to be possibly scientific. Such measures as peak torque and average torque were computed. But it was difficult to recognize what these figures actually meant. In 1980, equipment for testing the lumbar spine was developed but it never became widely accepted as an exercise tool for the lumbar spine (Hasue et al 1980). Testing with this machine did document that, with back pain, the extensors, which are normally stronger than the torso flexors, become weaker whereas the torso flexors do not change at all. The equipment was later applied to clinical practice and became an adjunct to comprehensive, multimodality treatment for chronic back pain (Mayer et al 1985).

Another machine emerged for testing function in the lumbar spine. This was known as 'isodynamic' testing (Seeds et al 1987, 1988). This device could monitor not only lumbar function in the sagittal range but also simultaneous small range variation in lateral bend and rotation. It clearly demonstrated what was intuitively known already, that on the occasion of fatigue, substitution of alternative muscles varies the precise arc of motion in the biomechanical chain of integrated function. We move differently when we are fatigued. Widespread use of this testing system never proved to be helpful in a clinical sense.

In fact, after a decade of experience with the various machines described, their lack of effective clinical impact, lack of scientific credibility, and lack of protocol were described by Newton & Waddell (1993). Interestingly, although the equipment was in use, the authors did not discuss MedX™ exercise equipment.

MedX™, a specific type of equipment, had been developed by Arthur Jones after his sale of the Nautilus Company. This equipment was designed to have its use in the medical care system for chronic back problems, hence the name MedX™ (Fig. 38.2). It used isometric testing at various points in range to measure spinal strength. It also paid specific attention to isolation of lumbar extensor musculature with the purpose of forcing the multifidus and the erector spinae to be active. It was counterbalanced so all motion to the spine was caused by muscle activity without the assistance of gravity. Exercise was in both the eccentric and concentric mode (Graves et al 1990a, 1990b, Pollock et al 1991). This equipment is still widely used today and is the only one of the various machines designed for back strengthening still using computerized systems. Clinical experience with this equipment will be discussed later.

One of the problems always inherent in the use of specialized equipment is the expense. Many physical therapists had bought Cybex equipment, which was heavily marketed to them. In general, physical therapy is not a highly profitable business and it was considered an unnecessary overhead to purchase more expensive equipment. Most therapists prefer a hands-on mode of care. Thus, few physical therapy facilities have felt it necessary to utilize exercise equipment for the spine. Often, there will be rudimentary exercise equipment for the knee, and perhaps other joints. Strength training following knee surgery or shoulder surgery is now considered the standard of care. Such is not the case for the spine. There is seldom spinal strengthening equipment in the usual physical therapy centers.

However, a very simple training tool which has been used for years is a device known as a 'Roman chair.' In this system, individuals position themselves face down, supported by cushions at the pelvis. The torso, head, and upper extremities are unsupported. The feet and ankles are restrained on the posterior aspect to keep the body from tipping. The goal is to hold the body straight, either at 45° or parallel to the floor. For somebody with a painful or deconditioned back, this physical maneuver is extremely demanding.

For clinical application, a new device was designed to specifically treat people with painful backs. It was called the 'variable angle Roman chair.' With this device, the straightened body could be angulated in any position from neutral to 75° (15° from fully erect) (Fig. 38.3). In addition, by placing the hands and arms in various locations on the chest or on the head, varying amounts of greater weight were added to the torso, which produced varying amounts of resistance. Thus, both by changing the position of the treatment subject and the location of the arms, varying degrees of stress could be added to the erector spinae and multifidus muscles. Thus, a progressively greater amount of resistance could

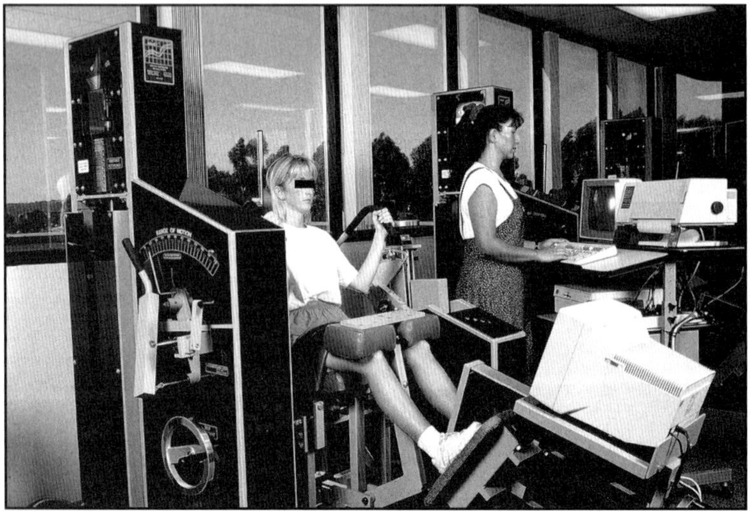

Fig. 38.2 The MedX™ Lumbar Strengthening Equipment. Notice the stabilization of the pelvis and the feedback of performance from the computer.

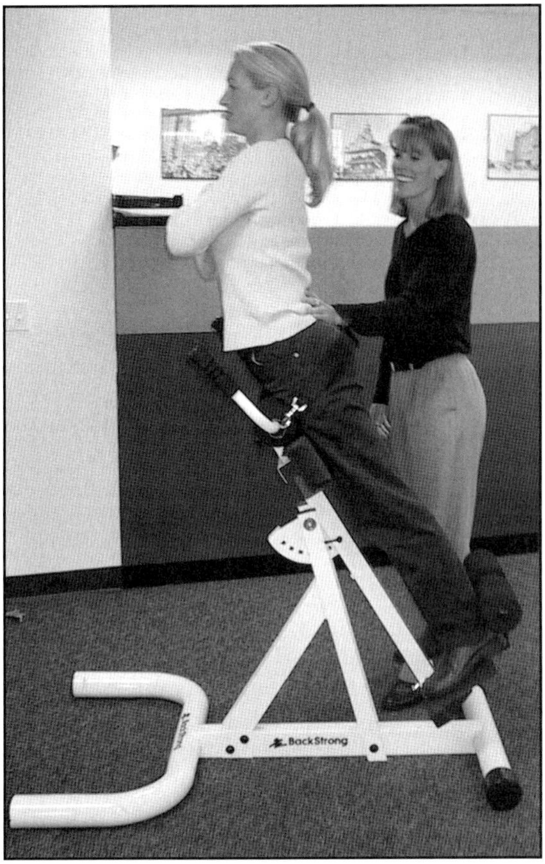

Fig. 38.3 A variable angle Roman chair. The angle from the horizontal can be adjusted so that the weight of the upper torso may increase resistance in extension of the spine.

be applied to the back. This was confirmed with EMG studies (Mayer et al 2002, Verna et al 2002) (Fig. 38.4).

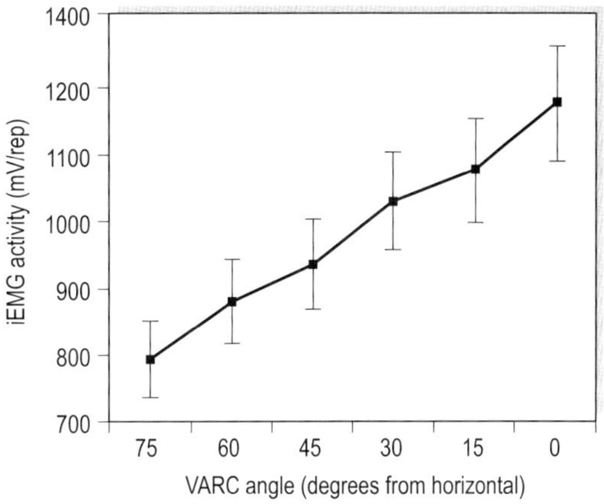

Fig. 38.4 A demonstration of increasing myoelectric (iEMG) activity of the lumbar extensors as one progresses from 75° to neutral or horizontal.

Justification for exercise treatment

It seems intuitively correct that exercise should be a positive event for any therapeutic maneuver to enhance tissue health. Prolonged inactivity is recognized to have a negative effect on physical as well as mental attributes. This was recognized by consensus of the recent Paris Task Force, which recommended that exercise programs should combine strength training, stretching and/or fitness (Abenhaim et al 2000). The American consensus report, the AHCPR Guidelines, likewise recommended an active exercise program, but offered no specifics (Bigos et al 1994).

However, is there evidence for a rationale for specific exercises? Certainly exercise treatment could be more generally effective if there is evidence for its use.

To answer this question, three different modes of exercise in back pain patients were used: active physiotherapy, muscle reconditioning on devices, or low-impact aerobics. The relative effectiveness of each was compared (Mannion et al 2001). By the test parameters used, all the patients seemed to improve roughly equally with increase in lumbar strength (Mannion et al 2001). As is typical of many articles concerning the comparison of one type of exercise versus the other, no specific rationale for the application of any of the exercises tested was presented. It was implied that all exercise is equally good in a therapeutic sense. That is the usual accepted attitude of the medical/physiotherapy community. However, that seems counterintuitive. If there is a rationale for training the injured knee, why not the injured back?

A specific mechanical diagnosis has been developed for sources of back pain that are thought to be discogenic. This is based on evaluation to determine specific direction of preference for exercises. Under this system of mechanical diagnosis, exercises are carried out in repeated extension of the lumbar spine or repeated flexion or slide–glide/rotation. The appropriate exercise is the one that achieves centralization of pain during repeated movements to end range (Donelson et al 1997, Fritz et al 2000, Kilby et al 1990, Kilpikoski et al 2002, McKenzie & May 2003, Razmjou et al 2000, Spratt et al 1993, Wernecke et al 1999, Wilson et al 1999).

In a study to clarify that the type of exercise *does* matter, a group of 312 acute, subacute, and chronic patients were evaluated for their direction of preference (Long et al 2004). In the unique research design, a third of the patients were assigned to an exercise program that corresponded to their direction of preference identified on initial evaluation. Another third of the group was assigned to an exercise program completely opposite to what was depicted as their direction of preference. The third group was assigned to an exercise program that was depicted as evidence based and used commonly taught multidirectional midrange lumbar exercises and stretches of the hip and thigh muscles.

In the results, 74% of the 312 people included in the study were shown to have a directional preference. For those who were assigned to the appropriately matched directional preference exercise, none got worse, 96% got better, and 40% resolved their symptoms. On the other hand, in the case of those who were assigned to mismatched exercises, the evidence-based group, about 18% got worse and most had no change. In the mismatched group, only 20% got any better at all. Thirty-four per cent of the mismatched group withdrew, while none in the matched group did. By far, most people had a directional preference to extension.

This was a clear demonstration by appropriate evaluation with the rationale that directional preference can be a guide to appropriate ranging exercises and lead to ultimate successful treatment. This was in a largely subacute group of patients. It was felt that directional preference was on account of the internal environment of the disc related to the exercise program and thus the source of the back pain was discogenic. The study certainly showed that all exercise is not the same. Appropriate testing could be a guide to more effective therapy.

As was noted earlier, when specific testing of flexor versus extensor strength was performed in patients with chronic back pain, the extensors were weaker than in normals (Mayer et al 1985, Smith et al 1985). At that time, it was not clear what caused this shift in strength. Although the equipment was more precise, even the idea that there was a loss of extensor strength was not easily accepted. Earlier work by Nachemson, with less precise equipment, had seemed to show that there was no difference (Nachemson & Lindh 1969).

With improving technology, however, progressive clarification of issues in muscle function in the spine became more apparent. Using specialized MRI techniques, it became clear that the most active musculature in spinal extension was the multifidus, which demonstrated greater fluid shifts than the long extensors or the psoas musculature (Flicker et al 1993). In patients with back pain, less effective metabolism was demonstrated.

The MRI has given us new insight as to changes occurring with chronic back pain. Parkkola et al (1993) demonstrated increased fatty infiltration and smaller size of the multifidus musculature in patients with chronic back pain than in normal subjects. The multifidus muscles were also smaller. The same findings were noted in a later study, which also compared myoelectric signals before and after extensor strengthening exercises (Mooney et al 1998) (Fig. 38.5). In addition to a significant increase in fatty infiltration with chronic back pain, the electromyographic (EMG) studies showed that, with exercise, neuromotor training could improve the efficiency of the lumbar extensors. This study demonstrated that, at the conclusion of an 8-week, 16-session training program, the amplitude of the multifidus musculature decreased by half for the same resistance, and the strength with training

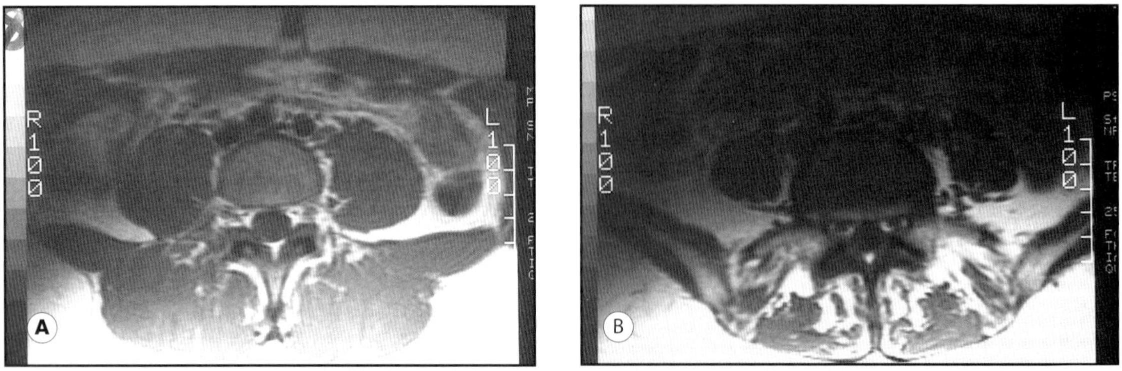

Fig. 38.5 A demonstration of extensive fatty infiltration in the multifidus musculature on an axial view of (A) a chronic back pain patient, compared to the musculature of (B) an individual without back pain.

increased an average of 65%. This was accompanied by resolution of the chronic pain.

The most definitive work concerning spinal musculature in normal and back pain patients came from the Physical Therapy Department of Queensland University of Australia. These studies used two tools, which gave a very accurate description of function. The first was ultrasound, which could assess muscle volume in real time; the second was wire electrodes to assess the function of the various muscles of the torso. The location of the electrodes was specifically identified with the help of the real time ultrasound.

Using the combined methodology of location by ultrasound and fine-wire electrode, it became apparent that the transversalis and multifidus worked in coordination to stabilize the torso several milliseconds before functional upper extremity activity was initiated. In the case of back pain, this pre-positioning stabilization was lost (Hodges & Richardson 1998). Actually, a more important observation from the standpoint of rationale for treatment was the observation that, shortly after first-time back pain, there was diminished size of the multifidus, apparently secondary to atrophy (Hides et al 1994). Taking this evidence into clinical practice, the group then demonstrated that, by pursuing a progressive resistance exercise program to strengthen the multifidus and transversalis muscles, at 1 year there was a 30% recurrence rate of back pain for exercised patients but an 80% recurrence rate for nonexercised patients (Hides et al 1996). Other studies had demonstrated that the multifidus was the first to fatigue in extensor exercise training and fatigued more rapidly in back pain patients (Ross et al 1993).

Given this information, it seems quite reasonable that another rationale in exercise treatment for back pain patients is a resistance exercise program to strengthen the lumbar extensors, especially the multifidus. In that the use of exercise equipment can allow measurement of baseline performance and monitor progression of training in terms of repetition and amount of resistance, there seems to be a reasonable rationale for such equipment to be used in rehabilitation. However, there has been an expression of some concern as to the peak loading of the disc if exercise is carried out on specialized equipment (McGill 1998).

There is good evidence that excessive flexion can cause disc damage (Adams & Dolan 1996). With repeated flexion and associated rotation, posterior disc herniations can be created (Wilder et al 1988). These authors also suggest that excess loading to the disc is a negative aspect of exercise. They present no documentation of adverse events, however. A very nice demonstration of a destabilized spine as a source of injury also came from this group.

To better understand spinal loads, they studied power lifters as they lifted extremely heavy loads (Cholewicki & McGill 1992). It was noted that, during the lifts, even though the subjects outwardly appeared to fully flex their spines, they kept their flexion 2–3° from full flexion at each joint. They even recorded an occasion where a lifter injured his joint and, in this in setting, using their specialized equipment, he had accidentally exceeded his full flexion angle by 0.5°. This demonstrates the spine is most prone to injury due to instability when the loading levels are high but there is a loss of motor control. They also can develop when the loads are low and muscles are not activated. The work of the Queensland group has demonstrated the loss of stability control by the transversalis and multifidus on the occasion of back pain presence. This phenomenon had actually been demonstrated earlier in Scandinavian studies (Cresswell & Thorstensson 1989). With loss of neuromotor control, as demonstrated in the injury of the power lifter in the study described above, back pain can also occur from injury. It seems justifiable that the best method to return neuromotor control to normal levels is a specific exercise program focused at the musculature that is most deficient. If the exercises are carried out with specialized equipment, the positions can be controlled and excessive displacement avoided, as had occurred in the case of the power lifter. These injuries also can occur with the use of free weights and calisthenics. Also, with the use of calisthenics, it is very difficult to progress the stress of exercises in a gradual manner because of the inability to measure the dose of exercise in the case of calisthenics. The dose–response phenomenon is the core to rational treatment throughout medicine.

Yet another phase of exercise should be justified. Certainly, strength and endurance do not exist alone in human performance. Aerobic capacity must make a significant contribution. Pure strength training cannot exist alone as a rehabilitation phenomenon. A study by Matheson et al (2002) analyzed the relative contributions of aerobic fitness and back strength and lift capacity. In this study, 45 healthy female participants were measured by three different maneuvers: they were strength tested isometrically on a dynamometer; aerobic capacity was tested on a treadmill with measurement of maximum oxygen uptake, and lift capacity was measured using a series of progressive weights by what is known as the epic lift capacity (Matheson et al 1995a, 1995b). It became apparent that the impact of aerobic capacity creates a predictive power of 43% of the variance in lifting capacity. This certainly justifies that any component of rehabilitation for back and pelvic pain should include aerobic capacity.

Thus, in contrast to the view that there is no justification for a specific exercise program, current evidence suggests that directional preference on repeated ranging, strength training for weakened or inhibited musculature, and aerobic capacity are important contributions to effective training. There, indeed, is a rationale.

We still haven't answered specifically the question asked of why isolation achieved by using the constraints of exercise equipment is important.

It is clear that our nervous system has the ability to substitute strong muscles for weakened muscles. Perhaps the best demonstration of that phenomenon was a study by Roy et al (1990), who, using power spectrum analysis, identified fatigability of musculature. Based on this analysis, when testing high-performance college rowers, Roy et al could identify with 93% accuracy those with back pain versus no back pain, even though their performance overall was equal (Roy et al 1990). In these rowers, the back pain caused early fatigability of the multifidus, yet they could still function at a high level of performance.

Perhaps a more dramatic demonstration of the phenomenon of substitution and its correction by isolation with equipment is in the case of adolescent scoliosis. Clinicians have long recognized that adolescent scoliosis can occur in very athletic young women. Often, they are expert swimmers. Apparently, muscle function is not a significant abnormality in scoliosis. On the other hand, when torso rotation is tested in all adolescent scoliotic subjects, it was found to be nonsymmetrical; it was weaker rotating one side versus the other (Mooney et al 2000). When subjects whose curvatures were less than a level appropriate for surgery were trained on a specific piece of equipment that could correct the strength imbalance of torso rotation, increase in curvature was stopped in all of the subjects and 80% improved by radiographic measurement (Mooney 2003). All of the subjects in this study had been very active physically, typical of their adolescent age group, yet only by isolating the torso-rotating musculature was any impact made on their spinal stabilization to resist the growth of scoliotic curvature.

Another dramatic demonstration of the value of focused, isolated resistance exercise is related to bone metabolism. In a remarkable study by Braith et al (1996), heart transplant recipients were randomized into treatment and control groups. The treatment group received lumbar extensor resistance exercises on specific equipment, to failure by fatigue, for one exercise session twice a week. Each exercise episode consisted of one set of 10–15 repetitions to volitional fatigue. The control group received no exercise but did receive medication, as did the exercise group.

As is typical for organ transplants, all of the patients received immunosuppressive drugs, which are well known to create osteoporosis. There was a 12–15% drop in bone mineral density because of these medications in all of the patients. Six months of resistance exercises, however, brought the bone mineral density to within 2.4% of baseline levels. Those who did not take part in an exercise program continued to lose bone mineral density. There were eight subjects in each group. This certainly is a demonstration of the specific therapeutic effect of isolated resistance exercises.

Clinical experience with strength training programs using exercise equipment

The pioneer program was that of Tom Mayer and Associates in Dallas. Following an extensive amount of preliminary work to establish functional testing, baselines of normal and protocols of treatment, an effective clinical program was packaged. The program was summarized with 2-year follow-up material in a classic article in the *Journal of the American Medical Association* (Mayer et al 1987). The results were remarkable. A treatment group of 116 patients with chronic back pain was compared to 72 patients who were not treated due to failure of their insurance companies to cover the cost; 87% of the treatment group were actively working in 2 years, compared with only 41% of the nontreated comparison group. About twice as many of the comparison group had additional spine surgery than the treatment group. The comparison group had approximately a five times higher rate of visits to health professionals than the treatment group. The reinjury rate in the treatment group was no higher than that of the general population, which was not the case for the nontreatment group. The study certainly demonstrated that, by testing the functional deficits and treating them with a combination of exercise, machine-based programs and general exercise and aerobic training associated with psychological support excellent results could be obtained. These studies were reproduced elsewhere with similar results (Hazard et al 1989). Certainly, activation according to protocols based on functional testing demonstrated effective treatment.

Other clinicians obtained similar results using different equipment (MedX™) but with the same philosophic basis. Nelson et al (1995) demonstrated that, at 1-year follow-up, 94% of 627 chronic back pain patients had good or excellent results. A control group was followed, who had been recommended for treatment but, for insurance-related reasons, could not pursue the program of progressive resistance exercises. It should be noted that, in the treatment group, on average the patients had tried and failed six different types of treatment program and that 89% had failed what was previously described as an exercise program. The results were similar for varied diagnoses such as mechanical strain, degenerative disc disease, lumbar disc syndrome, and spondylolisthesis. Thus, diagnosis made no specific difference as to the treatment protocol. Reutilization of the healthcare system within 1 year was 13% in the treated population but 42% in the controls who had not had active-exercise treatment. The specific point made in this study was the statement that a home exercise program or use of health clubs with insufficient supervision could not be an effective treatment. Almost all the patients had tried low-tech exercises and failed. A large number of these chronic low back patients had pain that was iatrogenically exacerbated. By encouraging passive modalities, patients were made dependent on healthcare systems for a limitless stream of 'feel-good' treatments. An active exercise program with measured progress can give appropriate feedback as to improvement.

A study from the same group focused specifically on the avoidance of surgery using a guided progressive specific exercise program using equipment (Nelson et al 1999). This study reviewed 651 cervical and lumbar surgical candidates. These were patients in whom a physician had recommended surgery or had a longstanding lesion that made them a surgical candidate. At follow-up, only 8.5% needed surgery. Of course, this demonstrated a considerable cost saving, which the authors, using the costs at that period of time, estimated to be $4.4 million, contrasted to $400,000 for the exercise program and for the patients who did ultimately require surgery. Here, again, the various clinical diagnoses did not change the outcomes.

Frequently, clinical studies are criticized for lacking a nontreatment control group to match the candidates for the test treatment. A study by Risch et al (1993) accomplished this difficult task. Subjects were randomized into an exercise program or a wait-list control group. In the treatment group, which was assigned to a 10-week, twice-a-week training program for the first 4 weeks and then once a week for the next 6 weeks, pain was measured by the West-Haven–Yale Multidimensional Pain Inventory. Following treatment, there was a significant improvement in pain, whereas in the control group receiving no treatment there was additional deterioration in degree of pain. The mental health inventory also demonstrated significant improvement in mental health in the treatment group with deterioration in the control group. The control group later received the exercise program and had similar results to the original exercise-treated group. The treatment group likewise had a significant increase in strength.

A theoretic advantage of exercise equipment is that treatment, to a significant extent, is not based on the charisma or analytical skills of the therapist. If a standardized protocol is used and appropriate precautions are taken, the personalities of the therapists should be rather irrelevant in the results. This hypothesis was challenged with yet another study (Leggett et al 1999). In this study, 412 patients were treated at two separate centers using the same treatment protocols. One was at San Diego as part of the UCSD Physical Therapy Treatment Program and the other was at the Physician's Neck and Back Clinic in Minneapolis, Minnesota. A total of 310 were treated in the San Diego clinic and 102 were in the Minneapolis clinic. In addition to strength testing, they had evaluation by SF-36 and had 1 year follow-up. All the patients had chronic low back pain and had usually failed several previous treatment programs. Sixty-two per cent of the San Diego group and 65% of the Minneapolis group had leg pain. Eleven per cent of the San Diego group had previous surgery, while 14% of the Minneapolis group had had surgery. Overall, 75% of the Minneapolis group and 82% of the San Diego group reported they were better as confirmed by SF-36 scores. There was significant improvement in range and strength in all of them. Probably most important was that the reuse of the healthcare system was 10% for the San Diego group and 12% for the Minneapolis group. A study about the same time of medical use with chronic back pain patients in North Carolina found that the annual rate of use of the healthcare system for that complaint was 73% (Daniels & Haughton 1987). This article, which had such similar results with a significant number of patients verified that these treatment protocols were probably more important than the personality of the therapist. The majority of the therapists in Minneapolis were physical therapists, while those in San Diego were exercise science graduates, such as exercise physiologists and athletic trainers. The assigned clinical diagnoses made no difference as to efficacy of care.

In this study, both groups used essentially the same protocol of twice-a-week strength training on MedX™ equipment with progress of resistance about 5% once the individual had achieved the capacity to do 20 repetitions. They also carried out aerobic exercises and general conditioning exercises on equipment for upper and lower extremities. No modalities were used, other than cold pack after exercises. Those who had achieved success with the treatment program did, indeed, have greater increase in strength based on isometric testing as well as dynamic testing than those who had failed. About 4% were made worse by the programs.

The above are not the only studies to demonstrate the benefit of exercise training for treatment of chronic back disorders. Each one, however, has a specific point to be made, which can be generalized into effective treatment. Based on our experience, there appears to be no justification to change.

Exercise treatment for pelvic pain

Pelvic pain is felt to have a different origin than lumbar pain. The facet joints, ligaments and soft tissue strains, and certainly the lumbar discs, are thought to be origins of lumbar pain. There often is referral of pain patterns into the lower extremity. However, pain emanating from the sacroiliac joint generally is more caudal and usually related to the buttocks. The incidence varies as to how much of the nonspecific back pain is from the sacroiliac joint. In one study, Fortin found the incidence to be about 13%, but 30% of those who had buttock pain (Fortin et al 1999). Incompetence of the sacroiliac joint is felt to be a cause of the pain and stabilization by a sacroiliac belt can often relieve the pain (Vleeming et al 1992).

An insight into the mechanism of achieving stability of the sacroiliac area was made by Vleeming et al, who noted the strong connection between the gluteus on one side and the latissimus dorsi on the other side by means of the thoracolumbar fascia (Vleeming et al 1995). We did a study on torso rotation equipment and found that, on the occasion of rotation, the gluteus on one side works in coordination with the latissimus dorsi on the other side. However, in patients with pelvic pain, the gluteal musculature was hyperactive compared to normals. Nonetheless, following training, the hyperactivity resolved and an EMG pattern similar to normals was achieved (Mooney et al 1997) (Fig. 38.6).

The myoelectric studies are of interest in that they attempt to show an attempt of the gluteus maximus to stabilize the sacroiliac joint although apparently unsuccessfully in the case of symptomatic pelvic pain. With training, however, the gluteus maximus reduces activity and the latissimus takes over a greater role, as is typical of normal function on torso rotation.

Back pain with pregnancy summarizes the complexity of identifying pain generators in the lumbopelvic area. Östgaard et al (1991) produced a study that tried to clarify the pain generators. In

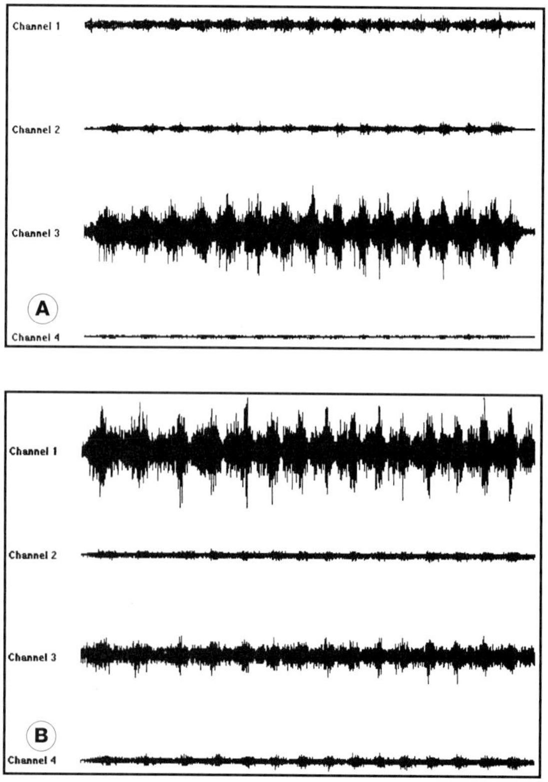

Fig. 38.6 Before (A) and after (B) torso-rotation training in an individual with a painful right sacroiliac joint. Hyperactive gluteal musculature is noted on channel 3 before but, after training, diminished activity is noted on the right gluteal with extensive activity on the contralateral latissimus dorsi.

a series of 855 pregnant women followed, starting in the twelfth week of pregnancy, 49% had back pain. The women were divided into three groups based on pain drawings demonstrating the localization of their pain; > 50% localized the pain to the sacroiliac area. In this group, the pain became worse during pregnancy. In the other groups, the pain got somewhat better. In the sacroiliac pain group, only 1% actually developed sciatica. This point emphasizes that the disc might not be a common cause of back pain during pregnancy. Another interesting study supporting this view is by Kristiansson (1995). In this study of 200 pregnant women, the back pain was correlated with their levels of relaxin. The incidence and severity were correlated to the relaxin levels.

Clinical tests for sacroiliac stability are difficult to achieve because nearly every test also challenges other joints and ligamentous structures. Östgaard has proposed separating the phenomenon of posterior pelvic pain from common back pain. To be assigned the label of 'posterior pelvic pain,' the pain should be in the buttock below the L5–S1 area and have a positive clinical test. Mens has developed a very simple test that does not apparently stress any other tissues than the sacroiliac joint (Mens et al 1995). In this test, the subject lies in a supine position and merely lifts the straight leg on the symptomatic side off the table several inches and holds it. When compared to the nonsymptomatic side, the leg on the symptomatic side feels much weaker. It can be corrected with manual pressure, pressing the iliac crests together, or with a pelvic belt. On the occasion of the use of the pelvic belt, the leg feels as strong as on the nonsymptomatic side.

This discussion is a short outline to explain our clinical experience with back pain in pregnancy. It started with several of our young therapists who had back pain on the occasion of their pregnancies. They were placed on the torso rotation machine (Fig. 38.7) and gradually increased their strength. This was highly successful in resolving back pain which was in the buttock area. For those who had pain in the lumbar area, strength training in a sagittal manner on the lumbar machines was more successful.

Another study, reinforcing the role of muscle stabilization of the sacroiliac joints, emerged once again from the Queensland group (Richardson et al 1999). This group has focused on specific exercises designed to stabilize segments of the spine and pelvis. Parallel to the concepts being displayed in this chapter, they felt it was important to carry out exercises with a specific rationale. They point out that conventional exercises generally work to increase the strength of the global muscles but it takes a specific exercise program to improve the dynamic stability of local muscles such as the transversalis and multifidus. Their studies have shown that the transversalis and multifidus function independently from the global abdominal muscles (Hodges & Richardson 1997). This has been

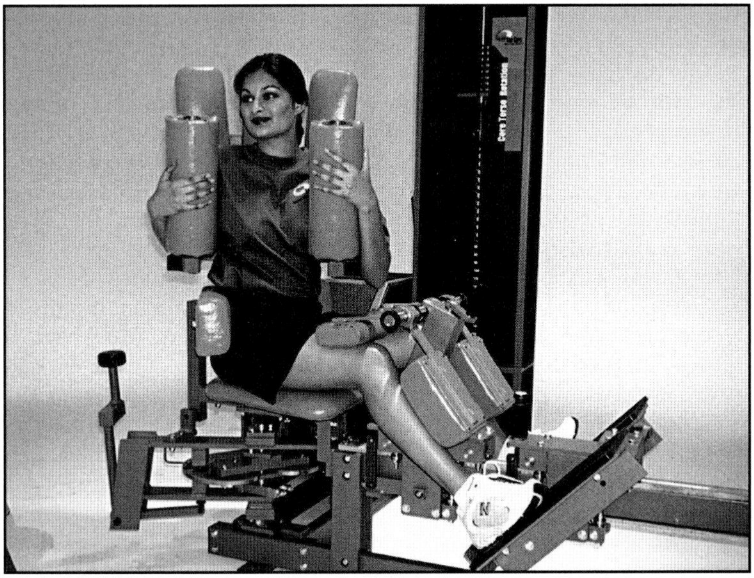

Fig. 38.7 Torso Rotation Machine. The pelvis is stabilized and the amount of resistance can be adjusted as well as the degree of rotation.

referred to as the self-bracing phenomenon (Snijders et al 1998). The specific study that documented this benefit used an exercise program in which retraction of the abdomen was the mechanism by which to achieve independent function of the transversalis. This could be documented by myoelectric studies as well as real-time ultrasound. With the advantage of those biofeedback systems, the efficacy of the retraction system was quantitated. The studies went on to demonstrate that, with effective retraction of the abdomen to create function of the transversus abdominis, the sacroiliac joint could be stabilized. Sacroiliac joint stabilization was demonstrated by transmission of a vibratory signal (Buyruk et al 1999). In a series of normal subjects, there was consistent demonstration of stabilization with documented function of the transversalis.

The achievement of the retraction exercises is somewhat difficult and is, of course, enhanced by the biofeedback of ultrasound and myoelectric signals. That type of feedback, however, is too complex for general clinical work.

Here again, the use of exercise equipment provides the ideal feedback to achieve strengthening of the transversalis. Using a torso-rotation exercise machine, one can gradually increase the resistance of the abdominal musculature, specifically the transversalis, due to the appropriate orientation of its fibers. That would be the reason why back pain of pregnancy and pelvic pain associated with sacroiliac dysfunction are effectively treated by torso rotation strengthening.

Measuring effective care

This chapter has discussed the rationale for using exercise equipment to enhance muscle strength. It is this author's opinion that it supplies a measurable, safe, and standardized system of strengthening. By isolating muscle function using equipment that has variable resistance attributes and effectively strengthens the 'weak links,' improvement in strength is easily demonstrated. But does that correlate with improvement? By itself, strength does not correlate with improvement but the subjective statement of the individual being treated is taken as a confirmation of efficacy. However, subjective comment is not really measurable. The lack of ability to truly measure improvement in the individual is one of the reasons that there are so many varied treatment programs for back and pelvic pain, both nonoperatively and surgically. In groups of patients, efficacy can be identified as percentage return to work, incidence of reuse of the medical care system, change in the use of medications and overall costs of care. Those measurements are not very reliable for the individual, however, due to numerous extraneous factors. Pain drawings can be of some benefit, as can the visual analog pain line. Again, these are subjective statements on the part of the treated person. Is it possible to have a more objective system to measure improvement following treatment?

Certainly, from society's standpoint, the amount of pain is somewhat irrelevant. From an economic standpoint, the question is, has treatment reduced disability? Disability implies the capacity to function independently and, for the economics of the problem, to be able to return to the workplace. The dilemma of how to measure disability is the great unanswered question in the industrialized world. Billions of dollars are spent to give support for disabled workers, but is the award justified? Certainly, in the US, a large amount of litigation revolves around that question. Each state tries to solve its problems by a separate set of rules to measure disability. California recently abolished its system, which had used description of pain as a significant factor in disability award, and has joined most other US states in measuring impairment, which then, by a 'consensus' formula, is converted to levels of disability. Only time will tell if this is fair.

What is really needed is an objective method to measure function. Matheson tried to simplify this problem by using a pictorial display of function rather than actually carrying out physical tests. However, relying on a few sets of standardized physical tests cannot fully summarize human function in the workplace. On the other hand, the more physical tests used, the more expensive, exhausting, and blurred the report will become. Thus, to try to simplify the system, the West Tool Sorts was devised. This slowly grew into Spinal Function Sorts, a set of 50 items, depicted in drawings, which had been selected from 230 items used in a rehabilitation clinic (Matheson & Matheson 1989). Later, Matheson devised similar tests for upper extremity function, known as the Hand Function Sort (Matheson & Matheson 1995). There are 62 pictures in the Hand Function Sort. Both of the Sorts allow classification of the individual into physical demand characteristics of sedentary, light, medium, and heavy, based on their statement of their capacity to carry out the functions depicted. Although effective in being able

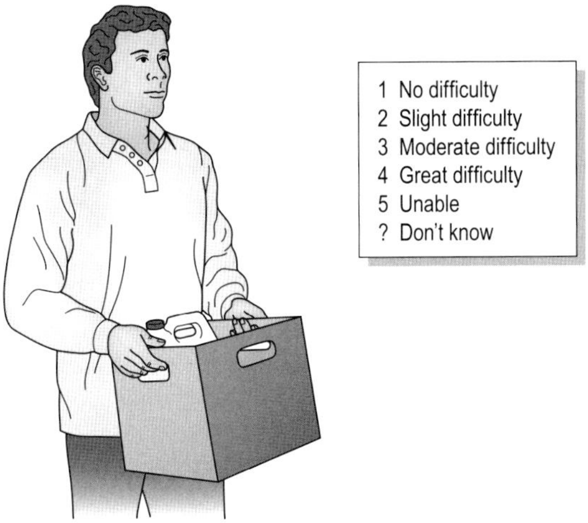
1 No difficulty
2 Slight difficulty
3 Moderate difficulty
4 Great difficulty
5 Unable
? Don't know

Fig. 38.8 An example of one of the 111 illustrations in the Multidimensional Task Ability Profile computerized function test. The individual selects the level of activity they perceive they can perform.

to label level of function, these tests were open to human error. The evaluee could skip items and the mathematics of summarizing the data was open to human error.

To supply a more efficient and error-proof system of pictorial functional analysis, the Multidimensional Task Ability Profile (eMTAP) was developed (Mooney et al 2003). This has 111 items depicted on a computer screen and individuals are asked on a five-level scale if they are able or unable to carry out the function depicted. They can also select a 'don't know' response (Fig. 38.8). The captions of the pictures are in various languages.

The obvious question is as to the validity of an individual's perception of his or her capacity compared to actual performance. We recently carried out a study to challenge that question (Mayer et al 2005). In this study, the eMTAP is compared to the Epic Lift Capacity Test (Matheson et al 1995a, 1995b). This is a standardized test using blinded weights where individuals are asked to go through six stages of progressive lifts. In so doing, their lift capacity is precisely identified. In the comparison study, 60 patients at two different treatment centers had both the eMTAP and the Epic Lift Capacity. The Spearman correlation between the Physical Demands Characteristics (PDC) measured from the eMTAP and lift capacity was 0.83. The Pearson correlation between the rating of perceived capacity from the eMTAP and the actual weight lifted during the Lift Capacity test was 0.89. These are excellent correlations and confirmed that perception of capacity is fairly close to actual achievement.

In another study to document the effectiveness of a restorative exercise program, 506 patients had baseline eMTAP and follow-up eMTAP testing. This was at the conclusion of treatment. There was a functional improvement averaging 30% and a pain reduction averaging 22%. Sixty-two per cent of the patients who were rated unemployable by PDC rating (below sedentary) became employable with ratings from sedentary to heavy. Reference assessing functional outcomes with new self-report instrument: Multidimensional Task Ability Profile (Mayer & Mooney unpublished data).

Summary

The purpose of this discussion has been to offer justification for a specific method of lumbar and pelvic girdle rehabilitation. The role of exercise equipment in rehabilitation has been explored. Its value in modern musculoskeletal care is emphasized by the reality that, in the case of professional athletes, musculoskeletal injuries are usually treated under the auspices of athletic trainers. They carry out a treatment program on exercise equipment, which every sports team has in their training room. They are not sent for home exercises. They certainly do not merely do calisthenics alone. If there were a more efficient or effective method of rehabilitation for these very expensive injured workers, it would be found.

Several clinical studies have been reviewed to document benefit. In most parts of the world, the ideal treatment program for lumbar and pelvic girdle pain has not been defined, as is demonstrated by the number of chapters in this text. A specific rationale has, however, been expressed in the discussion above.

Finally, a method of evaluating effective care has been demonstrated. It is this author's assumption that measuring function is more reliable than measuring pain. As the studies demonstrate, perception of function is about as reliable as actually testing function. In rehabilitation, a more reasonable goal than controlling pain is reducing disability.

The underlying goal of all aspects of medicine is, after the cause of the ailment is clarified, that treatment is best understood if there is a dose–response measurement system. The use of exercise equipment most easily accomplishes that goal.

References

Abenhaim L, Rossignol M, Valat B et al 2000 The role of activity in the therapeutic management of back pain. Report of the International Paris Task Force on Back Pain. Spine 25:1S–33S

Adams MA, Dolan P 1996 Recent advances in lumbar spine mechanics and their clinical significance. Clinical Biomechanics 10:3–19

Alaranta H, Tallroth K, Soukka A et al 1993 Fat content in lumbar extensor muscles and low back disability. Journal of Spinal Disorders 6:137–140

Bigos SJ, Bower R, Bocaln G et al 1994 Acute low back pain problems in adults, US Department of Health and Human Services. AHCPR, Rockville, MD, p137–141

Bruce RA 1973 Principles of exercise testing in exercise testing and exercise training in coronary heart disease. Academic Press, New York, p45–62

Buyruk HM, Stam HJ, Snidjers CJ et al 1999 Measurement of sacroiliac joint stiffness in peripartum pelvic pain patients with Doppler imaging of vibrations (DIV). European Journal of Obstetrics, Gynecology and Reproductive Biology 83:159–163

Cholewicki J, McGill SM 1992 Lumbar posterior ligament involvement during extremely heavy lifts estimated from fluoroscopic measurements. Journal of Biomechanics 25:17–28

Cresswell AG, Thorstensson A 1989 The role of the abdominal musculature in the elevation of the intra-abdominal pressure during specified tasks. Ergonomics 32:1237–1246

Daniels DL, Haughton VM 1987 Cranial and spinal magnetic resonance imaging: an atlas and guide. Raven Press, New York

Delorme TL 1945 Restoration of muscle power by heavy resistance exercises. Journal of Bone and Joint Surgery 27:645–667

Donelson R, Aprill C, Medcalf R et al 1997 A prospective study of centralization of lumbar and referred pain: a predictor of symptomatic discs and annular competence. Spine 22:1115–1122

Flicker PL, Fleckenstein JL, Ferry F et al 1993 Lumbar muscle usage in chronic low back pain: Magnetic resonance image evaluation. Spine 18(5):582–586

Fortin JD, Aprill CN, Ponthieux B et al 1999 Sacroiliac joint: pain referral maps applying a new injection/arthrography technique. Spine 19:1483–1489

Fritz J, Delitto A, Vignovic M et al 2000 Interrater reliability of judgments of the centralization phenomenon and status change during movement testing in patients with low back pain. Archives of Physical Medicine and Rehabilitation 81:57–61

Graves JE, Pollock ML, Carpenter D et al 1990a Quantitative assessment of full range of motion isometric lumbar extension strength. Spine 15:289–294

Graves JE, Pollock ML, Carpenter D et al 1990b Effect of training frequency and specificity on isometric lumbar extension strength. Spine 15:504–509

Hasue M, Fujiwara M, Kibuchi S et al 1980 A new method of quantitative measurement of abdominal and back muscle strength. Spine 5:143–148

Hazard RG, Fenwick JW, Kalish S et al 1989 Functional restoration with behavior support: a one-year prospective study of patients with chronic low back pain. Spine 14:157–161

Hides J, Stakes M, Saide M et al 1994 Evidence of multifidus wasting ipsilateral to symptoms in patients with acute/subacute low back pain. Spine 19(2):165–172

Hides J, Richardson C, Jull C et al 1996 Multifidus recovery is not automatic after resolution of acute, first episode low back pain. Spine 21(23):2763–2769

Hodges PW, Richardson CA 1997 Feed forward contraction of transversus abdominis is not influenced by the direction of arm movement. Experimental Brain Research 114:62–370

Hodges PW, Richardson CA 1998 Delayed postural contraction of transversus abdominis in low back pain associated with movement of the lower limbs. Journal of Spinal Disorders 11:46–56

Jones A 1970 A totally new concept in exercise and equipment. Iron Man Magazine November:32–34

Kilby J, Stigant M, Roberts A et al 1990 The reliability of back pain assessment by physiotherapists using a 'McKenzie algorithm'. Physiotherapy 76:579–583

Kilpikoski S, Airaksinen O, Kankaanpaa M et al 2002 Interexaminer reliability in low back pain assessment using the McKenzie method. Spine 27:E207–E214

Kristiansson P 1995 Relaxin – a marker for back pain during pregnancy. In: Vleeming A et al (eds) Second Interdisciplinary World Congress on Low Back Pain. San Diego, CA, p203–208

Leggett S, Mooney V, Matheson LN et al 1999 Restorative exercise for low back pain. Prospective two-center study with 1 year follow-up. Spine 24(9):889–898

Long A, Donelson R, Fung T et al 2004 Does it matter which exercise? A randomized control trial of exercise for low back pain. Spine 29(23):2593–2602

Mannion AF, Taimela S, Müntena M et al 2001 Active therapy or chronic low back pain. Spine 26(8):897–908

Matheson L, Matheson M 1989 Spinal function sort. Employment Potential Improvement Corporation. Wildwood, MO

Matheson L, Matheson M 1995 Hand function sort. Employment Potential Improvement Corporation. Wildwood, MO

Matheson L, Mooney V, Grant J et al 1995a A test to measure lift capacity of physically impaired adults. Part 1. Development and reliability testing. Spine 20(19):2119–2129

Matheson L, Mooney V, Holmes D et al 1995b A test to measure lift capacity of physically impaired adults: Part 2. Reactivity in a patient sample. Spine 20:2130–2134

Matheson L, Leggett S, Mooney V et al 2002 The contribution of aerobic fitness and back strength to lift capacity. Spine 27(11):1208–1212

Mayer T, Smith S, Keely J et al 1985 Quantification of lumbar function. Part 2: sagittal plane trunk strength in chronic low back pain patients. Spine 10:765–772

Mayer T, Gatchel R,Mayer H et al 1987 A prospective two-year study of functional restoration in industrial low back injury: an objective assessment procedure. Journal of the American Medical Association 258(13):1763–1767

Mayer J, Verna JL, Manini T et al 2002 Electromyographic activity of the trunk extensor muscles: effect of varying hip position and lumbar posture during roman chair exercise. Archives of Physical Medicine and Rehabilitation 83:1543–1546

Mayer J, Mooney V, Matheson L et al 2005 Reliability and validity of a new computer–administered pictorial activity and task sort. Journal of Occupational Rehabilitation 15(2):185–195

McGill S 1998 Low back exercises: evidence for improving exercise regimens. Physical Therapy 78(7):754–765

McKenzie R, May S 2003 Mechanical diagnosis and therapy, 2nd edn. Spinal Publications Ltd, New Zealand

Mens JMA, Vleeming A, Snidjers CJ et al 1995 Active straight leg raising. A clinical approach to the load transfer function of the pelvic girdle. In: Vleeming A et al (eds) Second Interdisciplinary World Congress on Low Back Pain. San Diego, CA, p205–208

Mooney V 2003 The role of measured resistance exercises in adolescent scoliosis. Orthopedics 26(2):167–171

Mooney V, Pozos R, Vleeming A et al 1997 Coupled motion of contralateral latissimus dorsi and gluteus maximus: its role in sacroiliac stabilization. In: Vleeming A et al (eds) Movement stability and low back pain – the essential role of the pelvis. Churchill Livingstone, Edinburgh, p115–122

Mooney V, Gulick J, Perlman M et al 1998 Relationships between myoelectric activity, strength and MRI of lumbar extensor muscles in back pain patients and normal subjects. Journal of Spinal Disorders 10:348–356

Mooney V, Gulick J, Perlman M et al 2000 A preliminary report on the effect of measured strength training in adolescent idiopathic scoliosis. Journal of Spinal Disorders 13(2):102–107

Mooney V, Matheson L, Leggett S et al 2003 Multi-dimensional task ability profile. Mind Trust. San Diego, CA

Nachemson A, Lindh M 1969 Measurement of abdominal and back muscle strength with and without low back pain. Canadian Journal of Rehabilitation Medicine 1:60–65

Nelson B, O'Reilly E, Miller M et al 1995 The clinical effects of intensive, specific exercise on chronic low back pain: a controlled study of 895 consecutive patients with 1-year follow-up. Orthopedics 18(10):971–981

Nelson B, Carpenter T, Priesinger T et al 1999 Can spine surgery be prevented by aggressive strengthening exercises? A prospective study of cervical and lumbar patients. Archives of Physical Medicine and Rehabilitation 80:20–25

Newton M, Waddell G 1993 Trunk strength testing with iso-machines. Part I: review of a decade of scientific evidence. Spine 18(7):801–811

Östgaard AC, Anderson GB, Karlson K et al 1991 Prevalence of back pain in pregnancy. Spine 16:549–552

Parkkola R, Rytokoski U, Kormans M et al 1993 Magnetic resonance imaging of the discs and trunk muscles in patients with chronic low back pain and healthy control subjects. Spine 18(7): 830–836

Pilote L, Thomas RJ, Dennis C et al 1992 Return to work after uncomplicated myocardial infarction: a trial of practice guidelines in the community. Annals of Internal Medicine 117:383–389

Pollock ML, Graves JE, Carpenter D et al 1991 Accuracy of counter-weighting to account for upper body mass in testing lumbar extension strength. Medicine and Science in Sports and Exercise 23(sup):66

Razmjou H, Kramer J, Yamada R et al 2000 Inter-tester reliability of the McKenzie evaluation of mechanical low back pain. Journal of Orthopaedic and Sports Physical Therapy 30:368–383

Richardson C, Jull G, Hodges PW et al 1999 Therapeutic exercise for spinal segmental stabilization in low back pain. Churchill Livingstone, London

Risch S, Norvell N, Pollock M et al 1993 Lumbar strengthning in chronic low back pain patients: Psychological and psychosocial benefits. Spine 18:232–238

Ross EC, Parnianpour M, Martin D et al 1993 The effect of resistance level on muscle coordination patterns and movement profiled during trunk extension. Spine 18:1829–1838

Roy SH, DeLuca CJ, Snidjer-Matheson L et al 1990 Fatigue recovery and low back pain in varsity rollers. Medicine and Science in Sports and Exercise 22:43–469

Seeds R, Levene J, Goldberg H et al 1987 Normative data for isolation B-100. Journal of Orthopaedic and Sports Physical Therapy 9:141–155

Seeds R, Levene J, Goldberg H et al 1988 Abnormal patient data for the isolation B-100. Journal of Orthopaedic and Sports Physical Therapy 10:121–133

Smith SS, Mayer TG, Gatchel R et al 1985 Quantification of lumbar function. Part 1: isometric and multispeed trunk strength measures in sagittal and axial planes in normal subjects. Spine 10:757–764

Snijders CJ, Slagter AHE, van Strik R et al 1995 Why leg-crossing? The influence of common postures on abdominal muscle activity. Spine 20(18):1989–1993

Spratt K, Weinstein J, Lehmann T et al 1993 Efficacy of flexion and extension treatment incorporating braces for low back pain patients with retrodisplacement, spondylolisthesis, or normal sagittal translation. Spine 18:1839–1849

Thistle H, Hyslop H, Moffroed M et al 1967 Isokinetic contraction: a new concept of resistive exercise. Archives of Physical Medicine and Rehabilitation 48:279–282

Verna JL, Mayer JM, Mooney V et al 2002 Back extension endurance and strength. Spine 27(16):1772–1777

Vleeming A, Buyruk M, Stoeckart RA 1992 A study of the biomechanical effects of pelvic belts. Am J Obstet Gynecol 162:535–543

Vleeming A, Pool-Goudzwaard AL, Stoeckart R 1995 The posterior layer of the thoracolumbar fascia: its function and local transfer for spine and legs. Spine 20:753–758

Werneke M, Hart DL et al 1999 A descriptive study of the

centralization phenomenon: a prospective analysis. Spine 24:676–683

Wilder DG, Pope MH et al 1988 The biomechanics of lumbar disc herniation and the effect of overload and instability. Journal of Spinal Disorders 1:16–32

Wilson L, Hall H et al 1999 Intertester reliability of a low back pain classification system. Spine 24:248–254

Zander G 1872 OM Medico-Mekaniska Instituteti Stockholm, J Nord Medical Archive. Band IV, 9, Stockholm

PART SIX

Integrating different views and opinions when dealing with a complex system

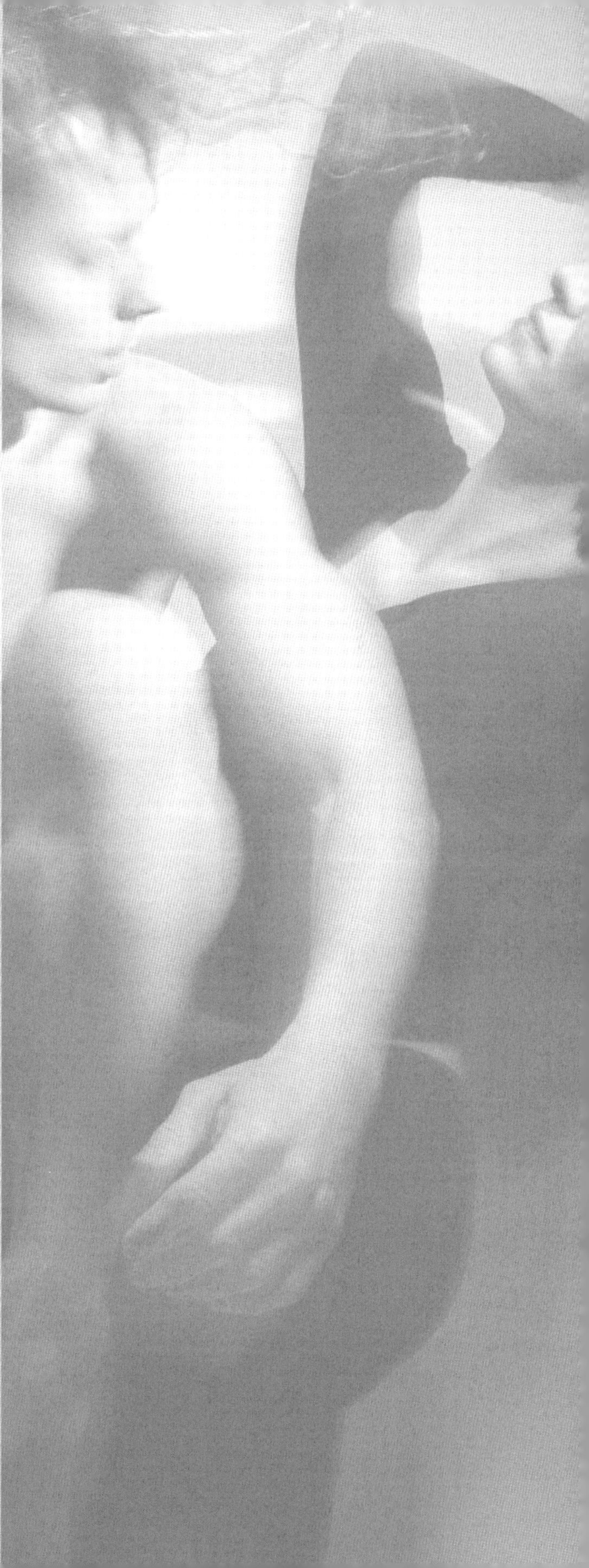

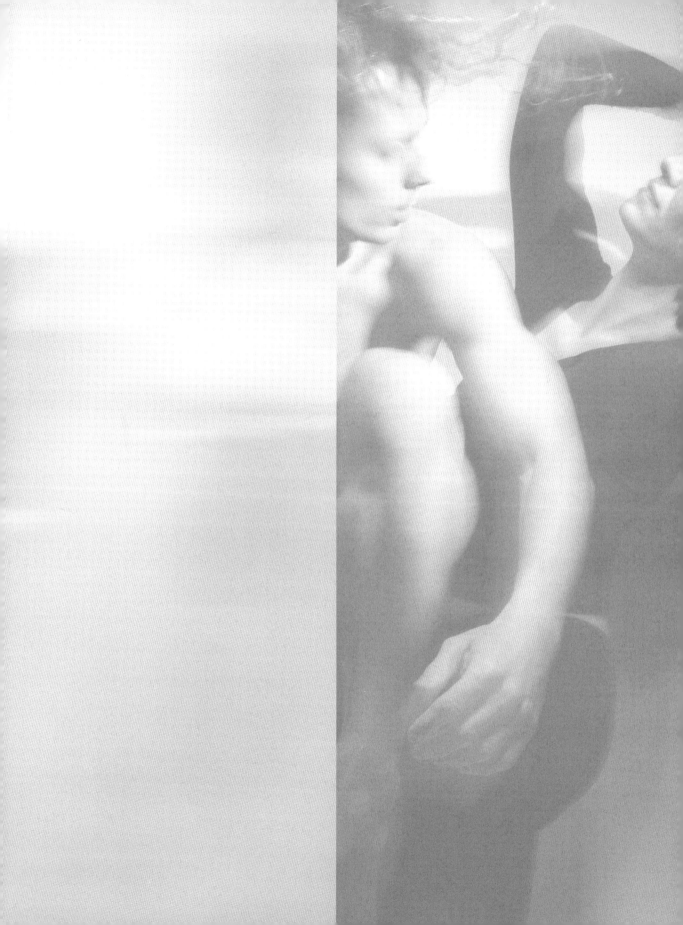

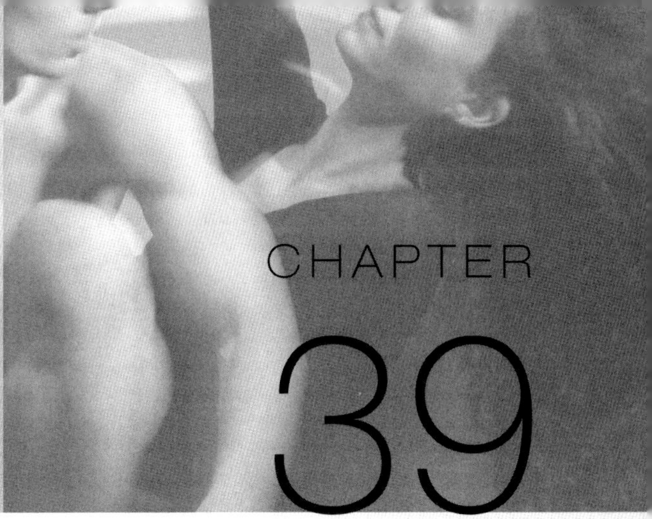

CHAPTER 39

An integrated approach for the management of low back and pelvic girdle pain: a case report

Diane Lee

Introduction

Low back pain (LBP) and pelvic girdle pain (PGP) have long been an endemic dilemma for most Western countries and significant funds and research have been dedicated to minimizing the economic impact of these conditions. In the past, researchers and clinicians had separate ideas regarding the best way to approach the problem. This separatist approach is slowly dissolving as interdisciplinary teams of researchers and clinicians evolve and begin to collaborate. The intent of this revision of *Movement, stability and lumbopelvic pain* was to bring together some of the current research and theoretical/clinical ideas related to the treatment of patients with LBP and PGP. This type of collaboration helps to identify what is known and what remains to be understood regarding the most effective way to assess and manage patients with LBP and/or PGP. As yet, there is not enough evidence to be totally *evidence-based* in clinical practice; however, collaborative efforts such as this help both the clinician and researcher to be *evidence-informed*.

The goal of this chapter is to present a case report to explain how the evidence can be clinically applied and to expose those areas which require further investigation. The case report will reveal one clinician's clinical reasoning process, which led to a treatment plan based on the science presented in this text. This is the clinical application of an integrated multimodal approach to the assessment and treatment of LBP and PGP.

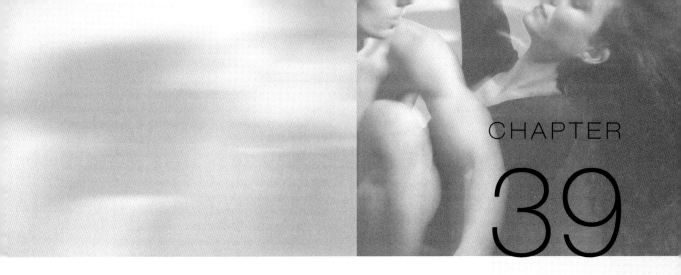

Julie's story

Julie is a 37-year-old lawyer with a 19-year history of LBP and PGP. From the age of 10 to 21 years she was involved in an intensive ballet program and had a brief professional dancing career. At the age of 18 years, Julie sustained a stress fracture of the pars interarticularis at L5 and subsequently wore a corset for several months. For 3 years she tried to continue dancing but frequent episodes of back pain forced her to retire at the age of 21. For the next 12 years she tried to maintain/improve her level of fitness through running/walking and a general gym program but this became increasingly difficult. In her words, her main problem during these early postinjury years was: 'A difficult to describe instability in my posture. I could feel good and strong in one moment and then I would turn a certain way or sit in a certain chair or lay down and it would all just let go.' She reported that she 'suddenly would feel like I couldn't breathe deeply and my legs were too turned out and my pelvis felt tucked under...' Being extremely in tune with her body as a dancer, Julie also felt that her breathing was impaired at times because her 'abs couldn't relax enough to allow it; it was as if all the wrong muscles were holding my body up.'

With these words she described the sensation of living with a maladaptive compensation strategy (O'Sullivan 2004 and see Chapter 33), which potentially involved overactivation of the global muscle system likely including the oblique abdominals, the erector spinae (ES) and the external rotators of the hip. Overactivation of these muscles can restrict or brace the lower rib cage as well as the hip joints and is clinically called 'chest-gripping' and/or 'butt-gripping' (Lee & Lee 2004b, 2004c). These strategies are commonly seen in patients who lack segmental spinal, intrapelvic and/or hip motion control.

One year ago, she lifted her niece and severely sprained both of her sacroiliac joints (SIJs). Fluroscopic arthrography after this incident revealed a posterior capsular tear of the left SIJ and a suspected ventral tear of the right. She tried many different treatment approaches (manual physiotherapy, chiropractic, osteopathy, craniosacral therapy, and various strengthening exercise programs) and found that her pain reduction, restored alignment, and improved function would last only a few days. Over time, the frequency of 'being out of alignment' progressed such that she now felt constantly 'out.' She felt her thorax was progressively shifting and rotating relative to her pelvis and noticed that her pelvis was posteriorly tilting as she tried to 'hold herself together' (Fig. 39.1).

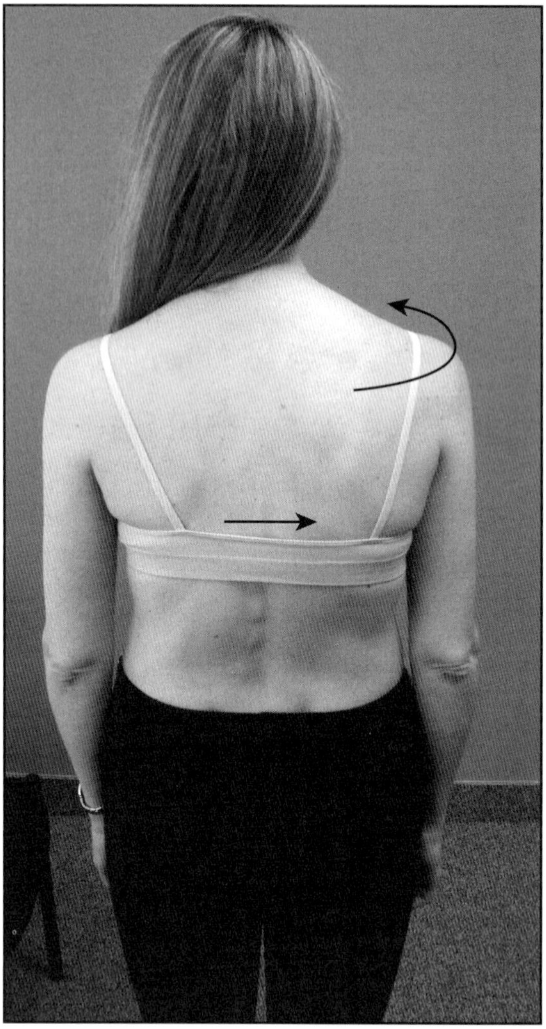

Fig. 39.1 Julie's posture in standing. Note the right lateral shift of the thorax (arrow) relative to the pelvis as well as the left sideflexion and left rotation (arrow). The lumbar lordosis is confined to one segment (L4–L5) and her pelvis is posteriorly tilted.

Her current pain was constant and located across her low back and upper posterior pelvic girdle [P4 score: 28/40 (Spadoni et al 2004)]. She reported episodic right anterior groin pain as well as midthoracic pain. Her pain was aggravated by bending, twisting, sitting, and walking [Patient Specific Functional Scale (PSFS; where 0 = unable to perform activity to 10 = able to perform at preinjury levels); Julie's PSFS bending score = 3/10, PSFS twisting score = 0/10, PSFS sitting score = 5/10]

(Stratford et al 1995, Westaway et al 1998). Her best sustained posture was standing and even this was limited in duration (20 minutes). She also described 'a feeling of swaying both in standing and sitting,' a feeling 'like walking on a ship at sea.' These symptoms are consistent with an impairment of postural equilibrium, a finding noted in subjects with LBP (Grimstone & Hodges 2003, Hodges 2003). Subjectively, Julie was describing a loss of segmental and intrapelvic motion control as well as a loss of regional control (thoracopelvic, pelvis/hip) in addition to difficulties with postural equilibrium.

Her X-rays revealed a mild scoliosis, a bone scan suggested signs of spondylosis at multiple levels of her lumbar spine and an MRI of the lumbar spine revealed mild disc bulges centrally at L2–L3 and L4–L5. Other than this, she was healthy and had no past history of surgery nor any trauma to her pelvic floor (pregnancies). There were no complaints of failed load transfer through the organs of her pelvic girdle such as stress urinary incontinence, organ prolapse or pelvic floor pain.

Objective examination

The findings from the initial objective examinations together with the suggested interventions are tabulated in Table 39.1.

Standing posture

Julie stood with her thorax shifted to the right and rotated to the left (relative to the pelvic girdle; see Fig. 39.1). Her pelvis was posteriorly tilted such that L5–S1 appeared flexed, L4–L5 extended and the rest of the thoracolumbar spine from T5 to L3 flexed. Collectively, this posture reflects a maladaptive stabilization strategy and suggests an asymmetric overactivation of the thoracopelvic stabilizers. In addition to what can be seen in Fig. 39.1, her right lower extremity was externally rotated in standing, a possible consequence of overactivation of the deep external rotators of the hip. These postural changes suggest that restoring a neutral spine, pelvic girdle and hip position would be an essential part of her treatment plan (O'Sullivan 2004; see also Chapter 36).

In addition to these postural findings, there was marked asymmetry in the resting position of both scapulae. Each scapula was downwardly rotated and anteriorly tilted as a consequence of the altered posture of the thorax and change in resting tone of the scapulothoracic stabilizers. Neither her shoulders nor her head/neck posture are being discussed as part of this case report.

Load transfer through the trunk in standing: movement tests

Forward bending

Julie bent forward with marked difficulty and her lumbopelvic pain increased. The strategy she used was primarily lumbar flexion with minimal anterior pelvic tilt, a strategy noted by van Wingerden et al (2004) in patients with PGP. Marked activation of the ES could be seen and felt on the right and the muscle failed to relax as it should at the limit of her available range (Fig. 39.2) (Shirado et al 1995). A consistent intrapelvic torsion occurred at the end of forward bending (Fig. 39.3) in that the right innominate anteriorly rotated further than the left and the sacrum rotated to the left; this is a physiological left intrapelvic torsion (see Chapter 18). It is not possible to determine the cause of the torsion at this point but it is important to note it.

Backward bending

In backward bending, the long thoracolumbar kyphosis (T5–L3) did not reverse and consequently Julie hinged into excessive extension at L4–L5. The L5–S1 segment remained flexed and her pelvic girdle did not posteriorly tilt relative to the femurs (extend at the hip joints). Once the hinging began at L4–L5 her LBP increased and she could not go through the pain.

Lateral bending/rotation

There was marked limitation of both right lateral bending, right rotation and left lateral translation of the thorax relative to the pelvic girdle, possibly due to an inability to eccentrically lengthen the vertical fibers of the left internal oblique (IO). Julie tended to 'collapse' easily into further left sideflexion, left rotation and right lateral translation.

Standing load transfer through the pelvic girdle to one leg: Stork test

Side of non-weight-bearing hip flexion

This test is useful for assessing the degree of compression within the SIJs (stiffness) and for detecting the presence of asymmetric force closure between the left and right sides of the pelvic girdle in standing (see Chapters 8 and 14). Optimally, the non-weight-bearing innominate should posteriorly rotate relative to the sacrum (Hungerford et al 2004; see also Chapter 25) and the amplitude of motion between sides should be symmetric (Buyruk et al 1995a, Damen et al 2001, 2002). In Julie's case, asymmetric motion was noted; the left innominate appeared to posteriorly rotate less (relative to the

Table 39.1 Summary of findings and treatment suggestions

Test	Finding	Suggested intervention
Standing posture	Thorax shifted right, rotated left, L5–S1 flexed, L4–L5 extended, T5–L3 flexed, right hip externally rotated (see Fig. 39.1)	Address posture in standing
Load transfer standing: movement tests		
Forward bending	Strategy: primary lumbar flexion with minimal anterior pelvic tilt. Left intrapelvic torsion present at end of forward bend. Failure of the right ES to relax at the end of range (see Fig. 39.2)	Release techniques for the right ES, retrain a better strategy for load transfer in forward bending (load sharing)
Backward bending	Strategy: inability to extend from T5–L3, excessive hinging at L4–L5, no active extension at L5–S1 or posterior pelvic tilt	Release techniques for the anterior abdomen (IO and EO if necessary) to allow the thorax to extend, retrain a better strategy for hip extension to decrease the stress on L4–L5
Lateral bending/rotation	Strategy: inability to right rotate and right lateral bend	Release techniques for the left lateral abdominal wall
Load transfer standing: one leg standing or Stork test		
Side of hip flexion	Asymmetric movement with the left innominate appearing to move less than the right (see Fig. 39.4A,B)	Motor control retraining to balance the forces within the pelvic girdle and to facilitate an optimal recruitment pattern during weight transfer to the left leg in single support
Side of single leg support	Unlocking of the left SIJ (see Fig. 39.5A) into internal and anterior rotation	
Load transfer supine: ASLR test		
ASLR: no compression	Unable to lift the left leg at all (see Fig. 39.6A). Score 5/5 left, 2/5 right	
ASLR: with compression of the pelvis	No improvement in the ability to lift the left leg (see Fig. 39.6C)	Suggests that further compression through stabilization training is not indicated at this time
ASLR: with decompression of the global system	Improved the ability to lift the left leg (see Fig. 39.6D)	Suggests that decompression of the global system is indicated at this time
Form closure analysis		
L5–S1	Excessive posterior translation in neutral and in flexion. The test provoked local pain when L5–S1 was translated posteriorly in both neutral and flexion No local system automatic control (see Fig. 39.7A,B,C)	Retraining of motor control for control of excessive neutral zone motion
Right SIJ	Decreased motion associated with muscular resistance in the elastic zone (see Fig. 39.8) No motion in the close-pack position	Release techniques for the muscles which are compressing the right SIJ
Left SIJ	Increased motion associated with pain when the passive restraints were stressed (+ve P4 test and +ve LDL test) No motion in the close-pack position	Retraining of motor control for control of neutral zone motion

Continued

Table 39.1 Summary of findings and treatment suggestions—*cont'd*

Test	Finding	Suggested intervention
Force closure/motor control analysis		
Response of the stabilizing muscles to a verbal cue: TrA	No differential activation of the left TrA from IO (RTUS) (see Fig. 39.9C)	Confirms that decompression of the left side of the trunk is necessary
Response of the stabilizing muscles to a verbal cue: dMF	Palpation: decreased tone and bulk on the left, difficult to palpate on the right due to excessive activity of the ES and resultant tension of the thoracolumbar fascia	Release techniques for the right ES Facilitation techniques for the dMF for isolation, then for endurance and strength training
Response of the stabilizing muscles to a verbal cue: pelvic floor	Inability to relax the right side of the pelvic floor seen via RTUS (see Fig. 39.12B) and associated with a tender trigger point in the right ischiococcygeus	Release techniques for the right ischiococcygeus
Response of the stabilizing muscles during ASLR	Left TrA fatigued before the left leg lowered, bladder shifted to the right as TrA relaxed (see Fig. 39.13). When decompression was applied to the left side of the trunk the bladder shift was minimized (see Fig. 39.14) and TrA remained contracted	Confirms that decompression of the left side of the trunk is necessary
The right hip	Overactivation of the right piriformis and obturator internus (right sided butt-gripping)	Release techniques for the external rotators of the hip combined with motor control retraining to facilitate centering of the hip joint during functional tasks

ASLR, active straight leg raise test; dMF, deep lumbosacral multifidus; EO, external oblique; ES, erector spinae; IO, internal oblique; LDL, long dorsal sacroiliac ligament test; P4, posterior pelvic pain provocation test; RTUS, real-time ultrasound; SIJ, sacroiliac joint; TrA, transversus abdominis.

sacrum) than the right (Fig. 39.4). This suggests that in standing, the left side of the pelvic girdle was under greater compression than the right.

Side of single leg support

During left single leg standing, the left innominate rotated internally and anteriorly relative to the sacrum (Fig. 39.5A). This is a sign of failed load transfer through this side of the pelvic girdle (Hungerford et al 2004; see also Chapter 25). Considering this in conjunction with the increased compression noted on the left side in the mobility portion of this test (side of hip flexion), it was likely that Julie was using a maladaptive compensatory strategy to try to stabilize the left SIJ. This is consistent with the findings of Sturesson et al (2000; see also Chapter 23), who found that women with clinically suspected instability of the SIJ had minimal (0.2°) motion of the innominate on the side of hip flexion during this test. Julie had less difficulty transferring her weight to the right lower extremity and was able to maintain a stable position of the right side of her pelvic girdle (Fig. 39.5B).

The findings from the one leg standing test suggest that Julie had a significant motor control problem in that she was unable to recruit the muscles of her lumbopelvic region so as to stabilize the joints of the pelvic girdle prior to any increase in loading (see Chapters 33 and 34). The specifics of her motor control deficit require further analysis before treatment can be planned; however, the findings from this test suggest that stability of the left SIJ during functional tasks and exercise will have to be monitored carefully.

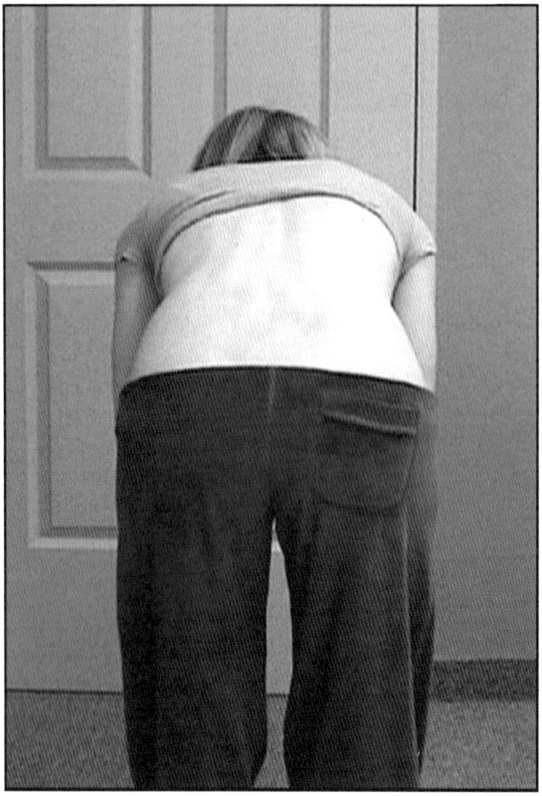

Fig. 39.2 Forward bending in standing. Note the asymmetry of her thorax in forward bending and the failure of the right ES to relax. The thorax remains shifted to the right and sideflexed to the left.

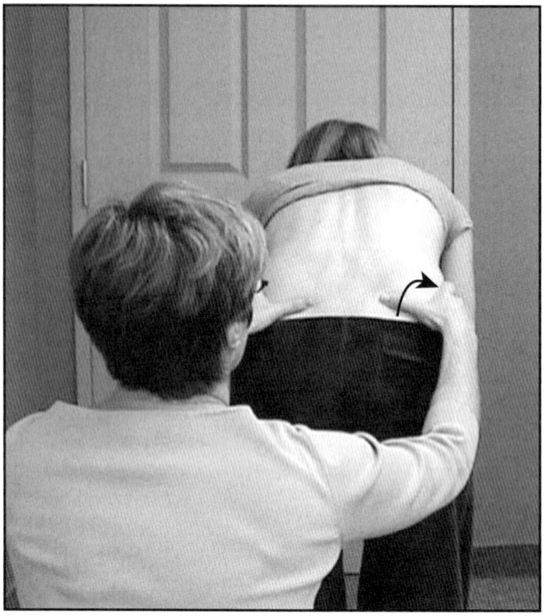

Fig. 39.3 A consistent intrapelvic torsion occurred each time Julie bent forward. The right innominate anteriorly rotated (arrow) relative to the left. This finding does not implicate a SIJ dysfunction, it merely suggests that something is causing the pelvis to twist as she forward bends.

Load transfer through the trunk and pelvic girdle in supine lying: active straight leg raise test

The ASLR is a load transfer test for the pelvic girdle in supine lying (Mens et al 1999, 2001, 2002) that has shown reliability, sensitivity, and specificity for patients with PGP after pregnancy. Julie could not lift her left leg off the table and scored 5/5 on this test (0 = no difficulty and 5 = inability to lift the leg) (Fig. 39.6A). She scored 2/5 on the right leg (fairly difficult) (Fig. 39.6B); her total score for the ASLR test was 7/10. She used a chest-gripping, bracing strategy for thoracopelvic stabilization with excessive activation of the oblique abdominals and the ES as a means to attempt this task. Compression of the pelvic girdle did not facilitate her ability to lift either leg regardless of where the compression was applied (anterior, posterior or oblique) (Fig. 39.6C). What did reduce the effort required to lift the left leg was *decompression* of the left side of the trunk (Fig. 39.6D), in other words lengthening of the left anterior and posterior thoracopelvic stabilizers (see Chapter 2). This is not part of the traditional ASLR test and is a clinical modification (Lee & Lee 2004a, 2004c) yet to be validated. Clinically, this finding suggests that her ability to effectively transfer load through the trunk and pelvic girdle to the left leg in supine would be facilitated if the thoracopelvic region was first decompressed by minimizing the ineffective compensatory strategy she was using to stabilize the trunk. Consequently, decompression techniques for the overactive global stabilizers should be introduced early in her treatment.

Form closure: neutral/elastic zone motion analysis

Analysis of the quantity and quality of motion in the neutral and elastic zones (form closure) requires tests for *articular* mobility and stability. Specifically, these tests examine the amplitude of motion of the neutral zone, the quality of the resistance provided by the active and passive elements in the elastic zone (muscles, capsule, and ligaments), as well as the provocation of any pain for each joint. The neutral

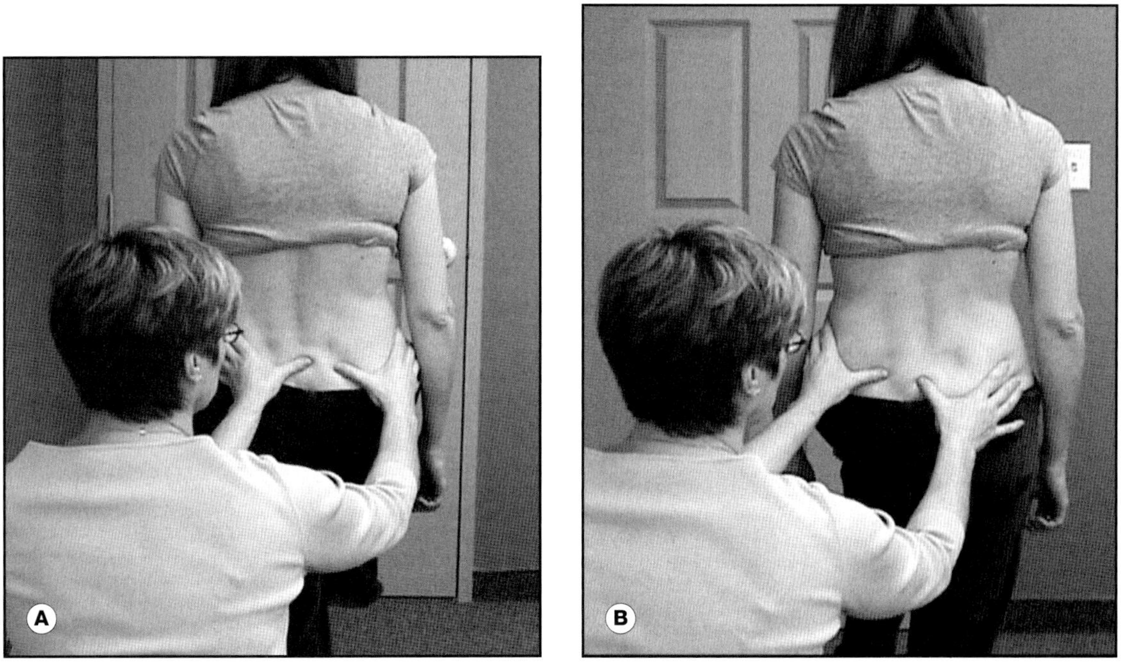

Fig. 39.4 One leg standing test – side of hip flexion. The test examines the ability of the innominate to posteriorly rotate relative to the sacrum during ipsilateral hip flexion. The motion should be symmetric between sides. (A) Note the small amount of posterior rotation of the right innominate during flexion of the right hip. (B) There is less posterior rotation of the left innominate during flexion of the left hip. This finding suggests that during this test the pelvic girdle is under more compression on the left side but does not indicate why.

and elastic zone analysis is first conducted with the joint in a neutral position (Lee & Lee 2004a). The amplitude of the neutral zone motion and the quality of the elastic zone resistance should be symmetric between sides [for the pelvic girdle (Buyruk et al 1995a, 1995b, Damen et al 2001)] or comparable to levels above and below (for the lumbar spine). The analysis is then done with the joint in a close-packed position. If the form closure mechanism is intact (the passive elements of the joint are healthy), the neutral zone of motion will be reduced to zero in this position (Lee & Lee 2004a).

With respect to the lumbar spine, excessive segmental translation (anterior or posterior) should not occur in neutral and should not provoke pain. All accessory motion should be eliminated when translation is tested in full segmental flexion or extension. In addition, when a load is applied to the trunk with the lumbar spine in a neutral sitting posture (e.g. resistance to arm elevation) no translation of the joint should be felt (O'Sullivan 2004). The muscles of the local system should contract to stabilize the neutral zone of motion prior to the load reaching the spinal segment (Richardson et al 1999; see also Chapter 33). The reliability, sensitivity, and specificity of these clinical tests remain unproven although extrapolation of the theoretical evidence supports this reasoning process (Hodges & Richardson 1996, 1997, Hungerford et al 2003).

In Julie's case, there was excessive posterior translation at L5–S1 in both neutral and in segmental flexion (Fig. 39.7) compared to L4–L5. Furthermore, the passive posterior translation tests in both neutral (Fig. 39.7A) and end range flexion (Fig. 39.7B) provoked her LBP. While in the neutral position at L5–S1, she was unable to control posterior translation at this segment when load was applied to her trunk by resisting elevation of her crossed arms, a test of automatic motor control (Fig. 39.7C). Thus, excessive posterior translation of L5–S1 during functional tasks and exercise would have to be monitored carefully in the treatment program.

With respect to her SIJs, there was asymmetry in the amplitude of motion in the neutral zone when anteroposterior translation between the innominate and sacrum was tested (Lee & Lee 2004a) (Fig. 39.8). The right SIJ was reduced compared

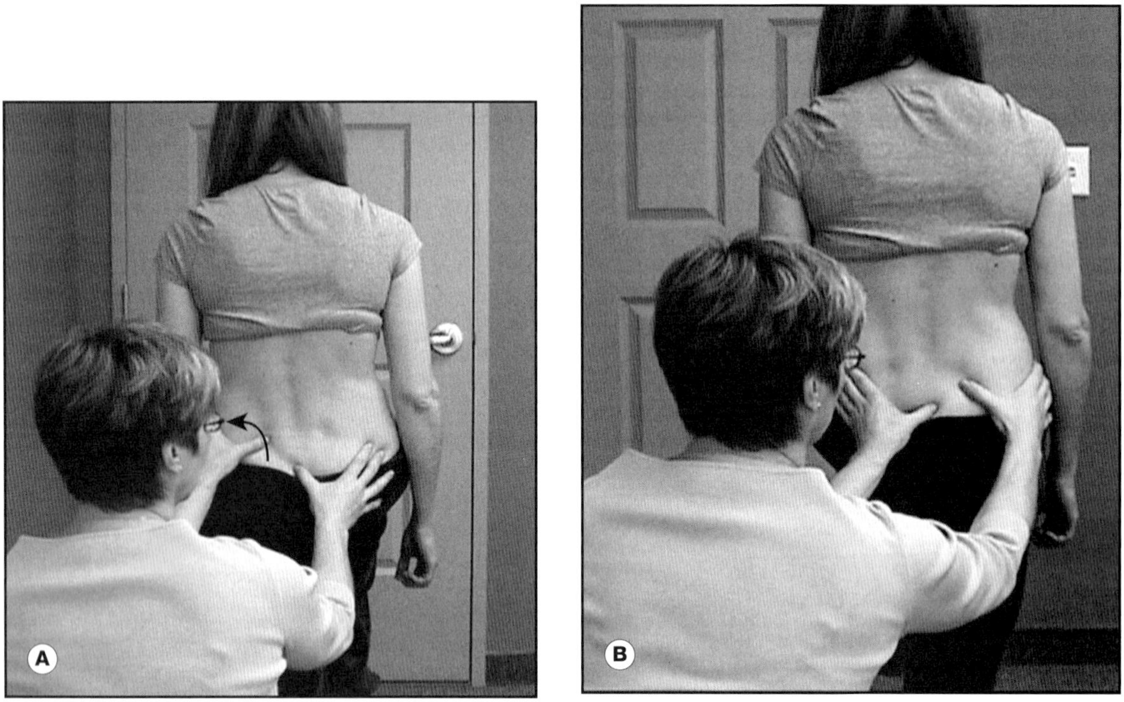

Fig. 39.5 One leg standing test – side of single leg support. (A) During left single leg standing Julie was unable to maintain stability of the left SIJ, the left innominate internally and anteriorly rotated relative to the sacrum (arrow). (B) During right single leg standing, Julie was able to maintain a stable SIJ (the right innominate remained posteriorly rotated) and transfer load effectively through the right lower extremity.

to the left and a muscular resistance was felt in the elastic zone. The amplitude of the left SIJ was increased and pain was provoked in the elastic zone. The posterior pelvic pain provocation (P4) test (see Chapter 24) was positive on the left and there was tenderness to palpation of the left long dorsal ligament (Vleeming et al 2002; see also Chapter 24).

The amplitude of motion of the SIJs was asymmetric in both standing and supine lying. In standing, the left SIJ moved less, in supine it moved more. This is characteristic of a motor control dysfunction (altered recruitment pattern of muscles) as opposed to a static joint dysfunction [fibrosis, ankylosis or ligamentous laxity (see Chapter 14)]. As the requirements for load transfer in standing are different than those for lying supine, different strategies for stabilization are often chosen and this suggests that the primary dysfunction is motor control. When the left and right SIJ were close-packed (sacrum nutated and the relevant innominate posteriorly rotated), the neutral zone of motion was reduced to zero. The passive elements of both joints were therefore healthy (although painful on the left) and this supports the clinical hypothesis that the asymmetry of motion was due to altered myofascial compression.

Force closure/motor control analysis

Response of the stabilizing muscle system to a verbal cue

Optimally, it is thought (though not yet known) that the transversus abdominis (TrA) and the deep multifidus (dMF) should co-contract bilaterally in response to a verbal cue to 'hollow or flatten' the lower abdomen (Richardson et al 1999) or to contract the pelvic floor (Sapsford et al 2001). This can be palpated clinically as well as observed via real-time ultrasound (RTUS) (Hides et al 1995, Lee & Lee 2004c, Richardson et al 1999, Whittaker 2004a, 2004b).

Transversus abdominis: Hypertonicity of the left superficial abdomen made palpation of Julie's left TrA difficult (see Chapter 4). There was a greater sense of superficial resting tone when trying to reach the left TrA, whereas the right side was relaxed

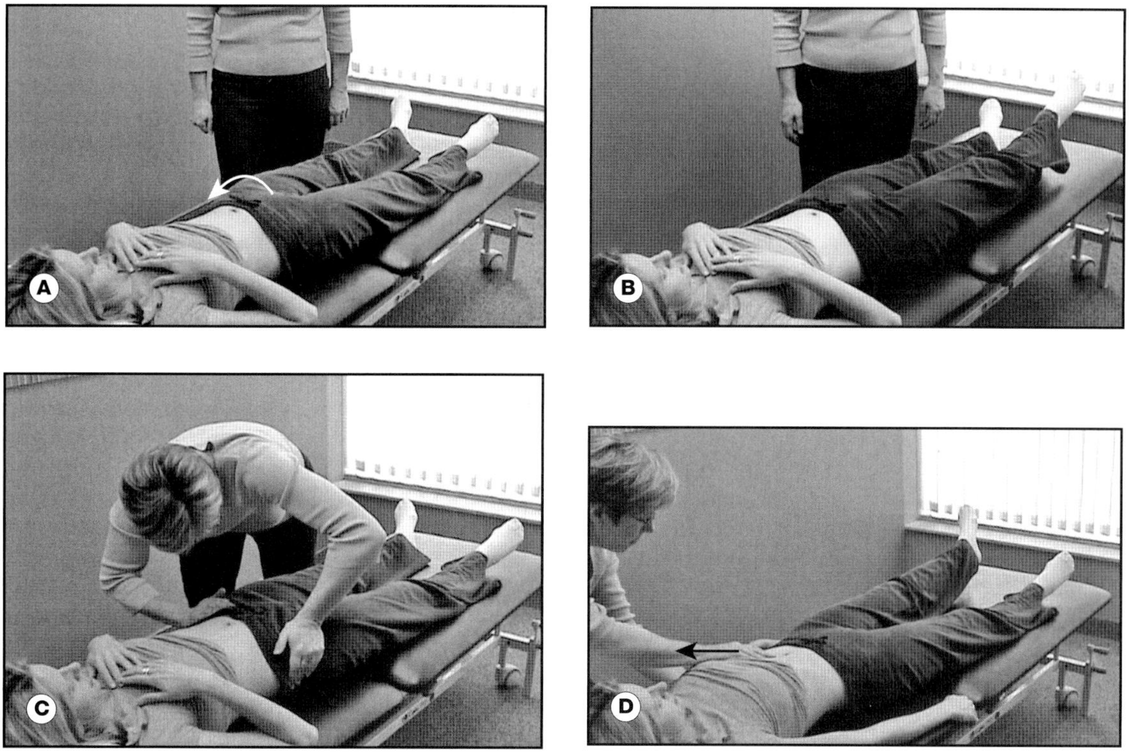

Fig. 39.6 Active straight leg raise (ASLR) test. (A) Julie could not lift the left leg off of the table and her pelvic girdle rotated to the left (arrow) when she tried. Excessive activation of the left oblique abdominals could be seen and felt during the left ASLR. (B) Julie had much less difficulty lifting the right leg off of the table. (C) Compression of the pelvic girdle did not facilitate her ability to lift the left leg. This suggests that stability training to increase force closure of her pelvic girdle would not improve her ability to perform this task *at this time*. (D) Using two hands to decompress the left side of the trunk (arrow) made it easier for Julie to lift the left leg. This decompression potentially reduces the impact of the maladaptive compensatory strategy and suggests that this should be the first focus of treatment.

and the deep abdomen could be palpated with ease. When given a command to recruit the lower abdominal wall, immediate bulging of the left lower abdomen and deep tensioning of the right lower abdomen was felt (Fig. 39.9A). This suggested early activation of the left IO, however without RTUS imaging (Fig. 39.9B,C,D) it is difficult to determine if TrA is contracting deep to the activation of the IO. Note in Fig. 39.9B the architectural change in girth of TrA, the lateral slide of the medial TrA fascia and the lateral corseting of this muscle with no change in the architecture of the IO. These changes should occur during an isolated contraction of TrA (Lee & Lee 2004c, Richardson et al 1999, Whittaker 2004a). Julie could not isolate the left TrA from the IO with any cue tried (Fig. 39.9C). The activation of the right side of her abdominal wall was normal (Fig. 39.9D). These findings confirmed that overactivation of the left oblique abdominals was present and that downtraining or relaxation of these muscles would be required early in the treatment program.

When Julie was asked to recruit the pelvic floor muscles ('Gently squeeze the muscles around your urethra as if to slowly stop your flow of urine.') no response was palpated on either side of the lower abdominal wall. Further assessment of the pelvic floor required either internal palpation or visualization via RTUS to confirm whether or not Julie was able to activate her pelvic floor in response to this command (see below).

Deep lumbosacral multifidus: Note the atrophy and possible fatty infiltration of the deep fibers of multifidus at both L5–S1 and the SIJs on her MRI in Fig. 39.10A,B (see Chapter 5). On palpation, the resting tone of the left dMF was markedly decreased and the atrophy was easily seen. The right lumbosacral dMF was difficult to palpate due to excessive tension in the fascia of the ES over the

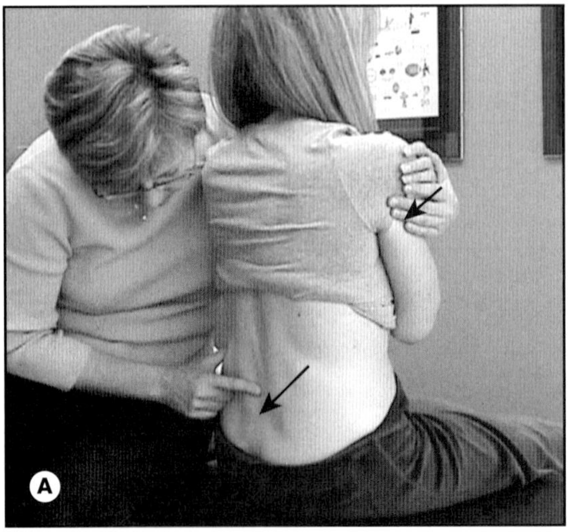

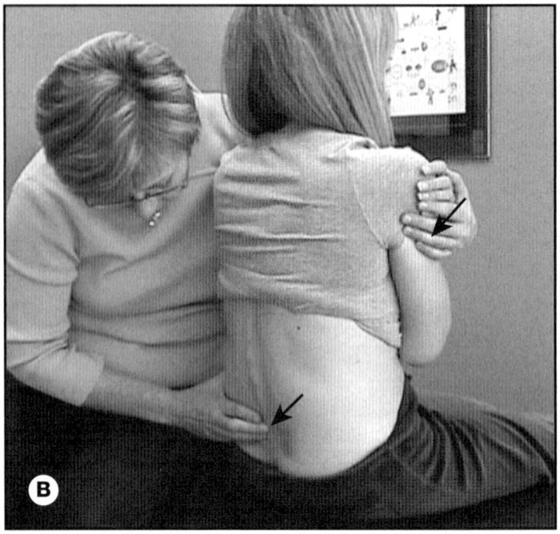

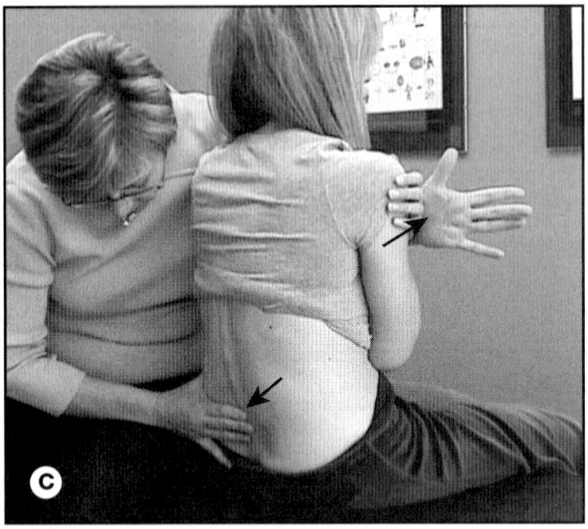

Fig. 39.7 There was an excessive amount of posterior translation (arrows) at L5–S1 both in (A) neutral and (B) flexion. (C) Julie could not control posterior translation at L5–S1 when an additional load was applied to her trunk through her upper extremities. This was tested by having her elevate her crossed arms against resistance (arrow). Optimally, there should be no posterior translation at L5–S1 (arrow) during this task.

dorsum of the sacrum and L5–S1 (see Chapter 3). This was likely due to overactivation of the right ES even at rest (note the response of this muscle in forward bending in Fig. 39.2). When asked to co-contract the deep stabilizing system with either an abdominal or pelvic floor cue, no response (swelling) was palpable in the left dMF and a further increase in tension of the fascia of the ES was felt on the right. Only a global phasic contraction could be seen on RTUS of either the left or right superficial multifidus at the lumbosacral junction. Initially, downtraining (relaxation) of the right ES would be required. Subsequently, both motor control retraining (timing of muscle activation and coactivation with the other muscles of the local

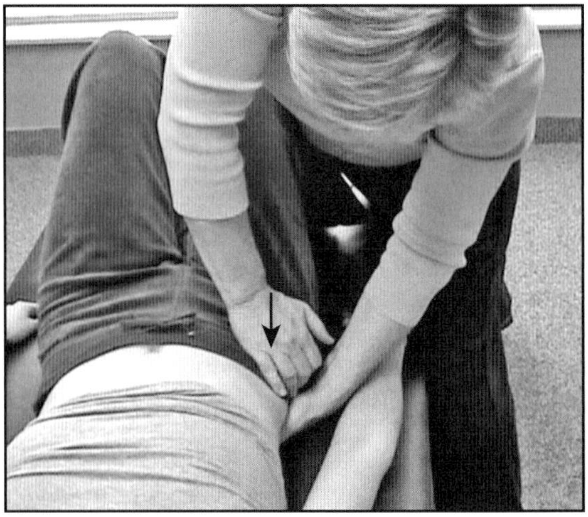

Fig. 39.8 Neutral and elastic zone analysis for the right sacrolilac joint (SIJ). Motion of the SIJs in the anteroposterior plane (arrow) should be symmetric with respect to both the amplitude and the quality of resistance. Julie's right SIJ had less motion and the elastic zone was more resistant (muscular). This suggests overactivation of at least one of the muscles that compresses the right SIJ (piriformis and/or ischiococcygeus).

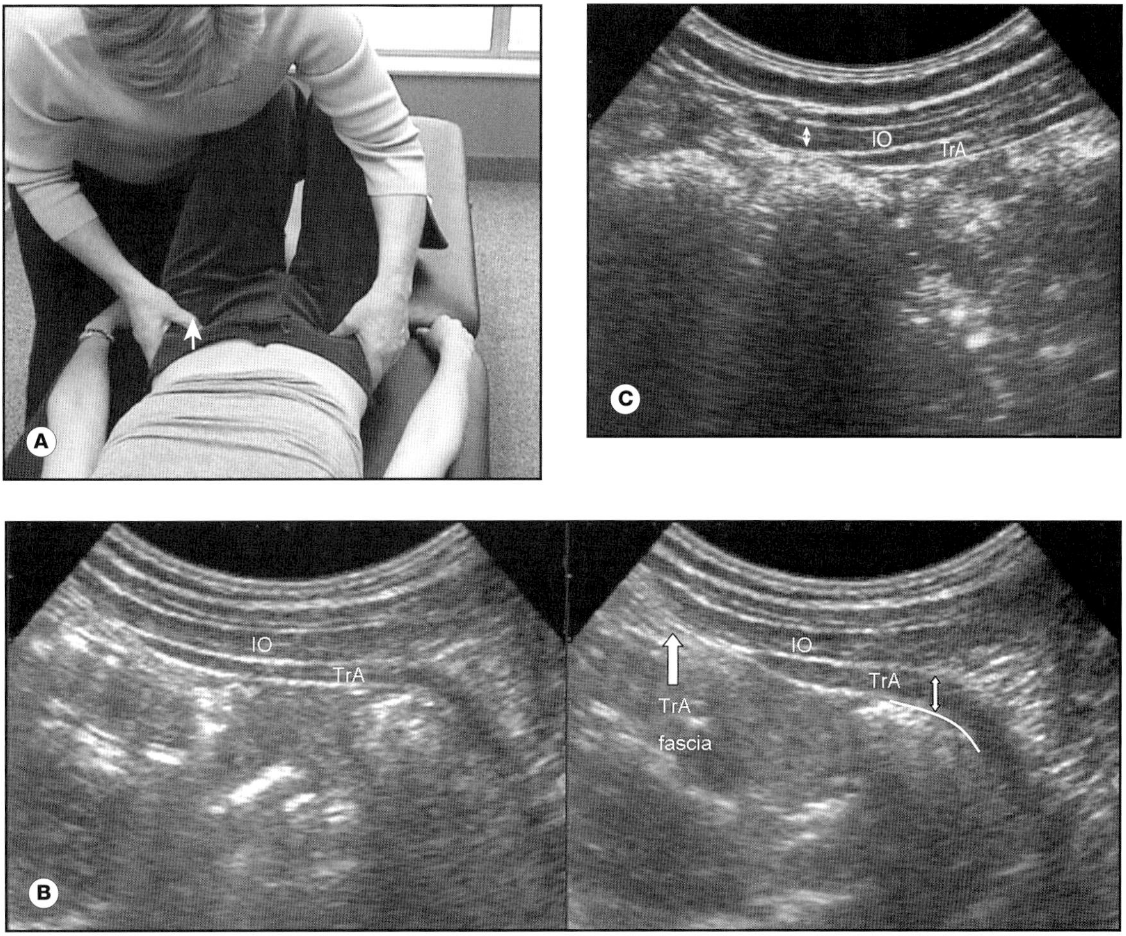

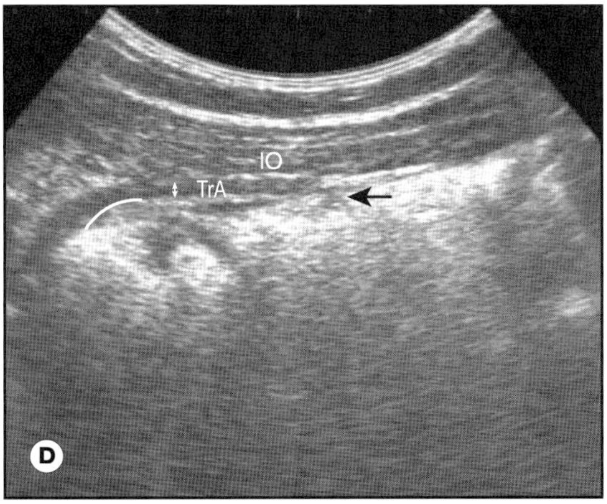

Fig. 39.9 Response of the local muscle system to a verbal cue. (A) When Julie was given a cue to contract the transversus abdominis (TrA; e.g. to think about connecting along a 'wire' between the two ASISs so as to hollow the lower abdomen) an immediate bulging of the left side of the abdomen and a deep tensioning of the right could be felt. Note how the left thumb has been pushed out of the abdomen by this bulging (small arrow on the therapist's right thumb). (B) The real-time ultrasound (RTUS) image on the left is a transverse view of the left lower lateral abdominal wall at rest (not Julie's). The RTUS image on the right is of an isolated contraction of TrA (not Julie's). Note the increase in girth of TrA (vertical double-headed arrow), the corseting of the muscle laterally (curved line) and the lateral slide of the medial TrA fascia. All of this occurs when an isolated contraction of TrA is produced. (C) RTUS image of Julie's left lower lateral abdominal wall during an attempt to isolate a contraction of TrA. Note the lack of activation of the TrA (no change in girth, no lateral corseting) compared to the increase in girth of the internal oblique (IO; vertical double-headed arrow). (D) RTUS image of Julie's right lower lateral abdominal wall during an attempt to isolate a contraction of TrA. Note the lateral slide of the medial TrA fascia (horizontal arrow) and the increase in girth (vertical double-headed arrow) as it corsets laterally (curved line) around the abdominal wall before any increase in girth is seen in the IO. This is an optimal isolated contraction of the right TrA.

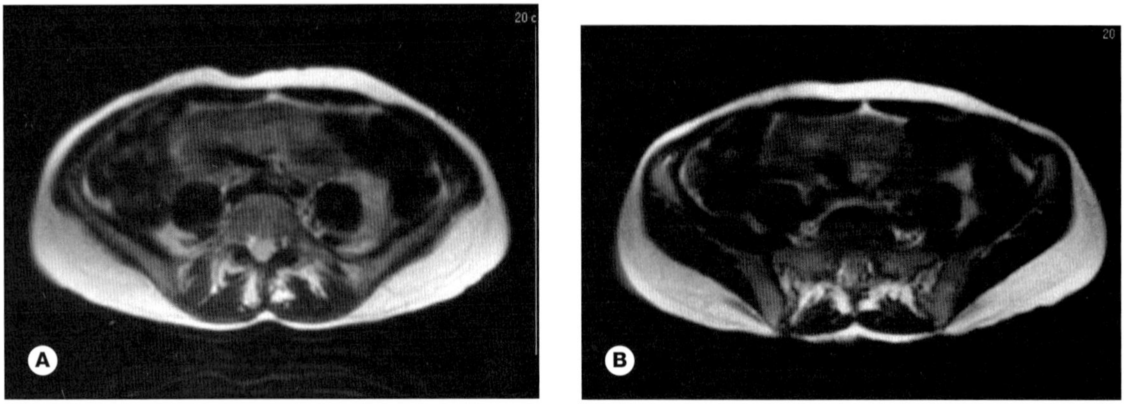

Fig. 39.10 (A) This is a MRI in the transverse plane at the level of L5. Note the fatty infiltration of the deep fibers of multifidus (bright white). (B) This MRI is at the level of the sacroiliac joints (SIJs). The fatty infiltration of the deep fibers of multifidus appears to extend caudally for three segments.

system) (O'Sullivan 2004, O'Sullivan et al 1997, Richardson & Jull 1995, Richardson et al 1999, Stuge et al 2004; see also Chapter 36) and muscle capacity training (strengthening, hypertrophy, and endurance) would be required to restore the role of this muscle for effective load transfer both for L5–S1 and the left side of the pelvic girdle. This would have to be restored before any exercises were given that challenged her lumbopelvic region in vertical loading through the left side of her pelvic girdle (single leg tasks on the left in either standing or four point kneeling) or in flexion loading through the lumbosacral junction (see Chapters 35 and 38). Training should therefore begin in positions that do not overly challenge her ability to stabilize vertically or in flexion (Lee & Lee 2004b, 2004c, O'Sullivan et al 1997, Richardson & Jull 1995, Richardson et al 1999, Stuge et al 2004).

The pelvic floor: Fig. 39.11A,B shows transverse suprapubic RTUS images of a normal bladder at rest (Fig. 39.11A) and in response to contraction of the pelvic floor (Fig. 39.11B). In comparison, note the image of Julie's bladder at rest (Fig. 39.11C), in particular the asymmetry of the bladder at the bottom of the image. This asymmetry suggests either that the endopelvic fascia on the left is lax (Ostrzenski & Osborne 1998) or that the pelvic floor muscles are hypertonic on the right. This can be confirmed via internal palpation or by observing what happens to the bladder shape when the pelvic floor contracts. When Julie was asked to gently contract her pelvic floor ('Squeeze the muscles around the urethra or gently lift the vagina') the asymmetry increased (Fig. 39.12A) and she was unable to completely relax the pelvic floor when cued to do so (Fig. 39.12B). The right side of the pelvic floor clearly could not let go (Fitzgerald & Kotarinos 2003a, 2003b) and was likely contributing to the muscular resistance felt in the elastic zone of the right SIJ. Subsequent external palpation of the right ischiococcygeus revealed an exquisitely tender trigger point in this muscle. These three findings suggest that decompression of the right SIJ and relaxation techniques for the right ischiococcygeus should be part of Julie's early treatment plan.

Response of the local and global stabilizing system during the ASLR test

The automatic recruitment pattern of both the local and global muscle systems during a functional task can also be assessed using real-time ultrasound (Ferreira et al 2004). When Julie attempted to lift her left leg, the left IO and TrA co-contracted initially and then the left TrA relaxed. As the left TrA relaxed and the thorax became more braced by the oblique abdominals, the bladder shifted to the right (Fig. 39.13) suggesting an alteration in the intra-abdominal pressure (this was not measured directly). When the left ALSR test was repeated and the trunk was simultaneously manually decompressed the bladder shift was less (Fig. 39.14). O'Sullivan et al (2002) noted a similar finding in PGP patients and that stabilization of the bladder occurred when compression was applied to the pelvic girdle. The subjects in O'Sullivan et al's study would likely require *more* compression of their pelvic girdle for the restoration of effective load transfer. For Julie, the ASLR test combined with RTUS imaging of the

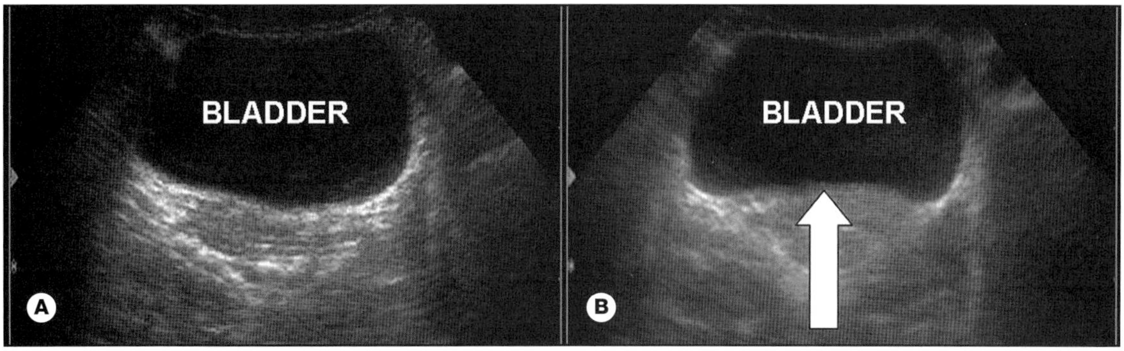

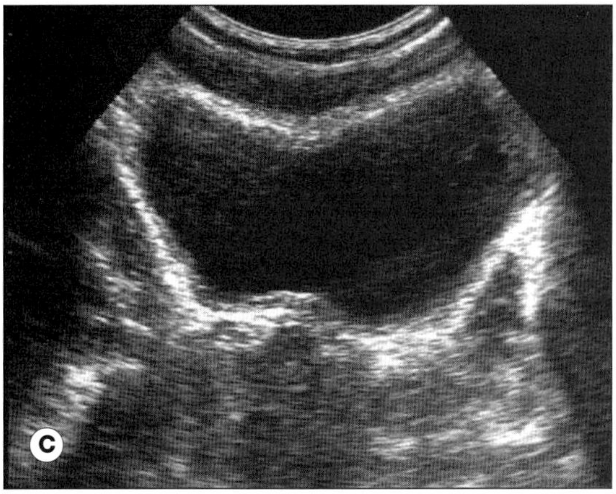

Fig. 39.11 (A) A transverse suprapubic RTUS image of a normal moderately full bladder at rest. (B) During a contraction of the pelvic floor the profile of the bladder changes and the inferior aspect of the image rises. (C) Transverse suprapubic real-time ultrasound (RTUS) image of Julie's bladder at rest. Note the asymmetry of the inferior border of this image compared to the normal bladder in (A). The profile of the bladder is by itself not diagnostic of any particular dysfunction. Either the endopelvic fascia on the left could be stretched or torn, or the pelvic floor muscles on the right could be hypertonic. Further tests are necessary to differentiate the cause of this asymmetry.

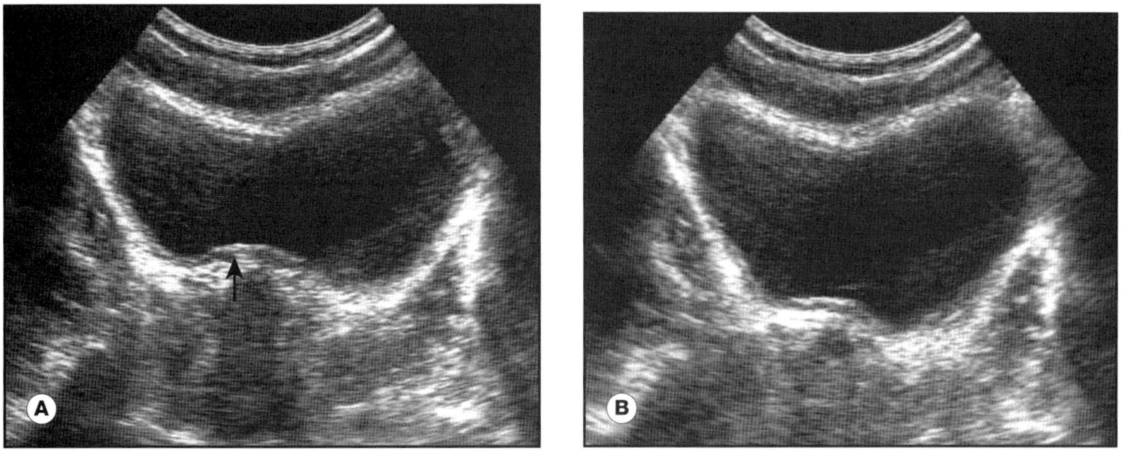

Fig. 39.12 (A) Response of the local system to a verbal cue. Note the change in the profile of Julie's bladder in response to a cue to squeeze the muscles around the urethra. In particular, note the increase in the asymmetry of the bladder on the right side (arrow); this is where the lift occurred. (B) Postcontraction image of Julie's bladder. Note the failure of the right side of the pelvic floor to relax completely after this contraction, the asymmetry persists and this finding suggests that there is hypertonicity of the levator ani muscle on the right.

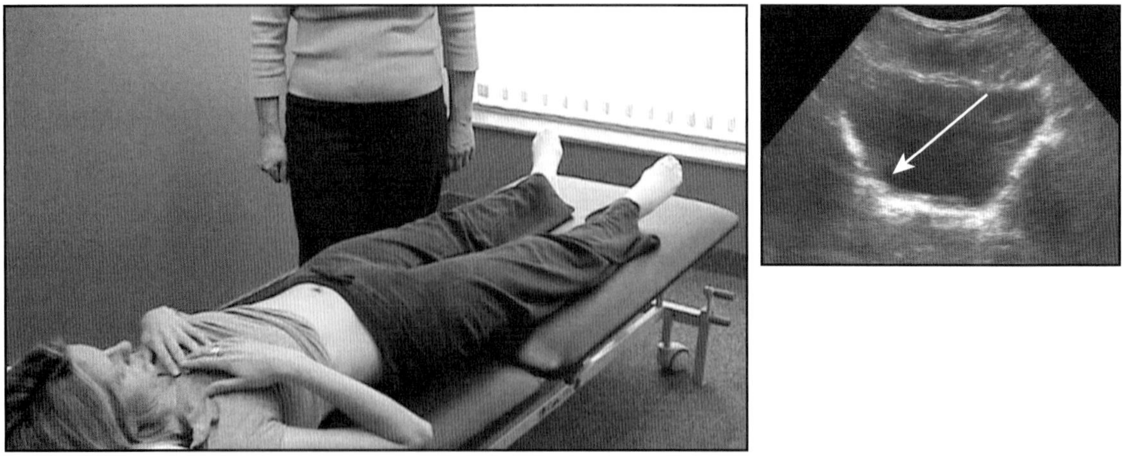

Fig. 39.13 The bladder shifted caudally and to the right during the left active straight leg raise (ASLR) test.

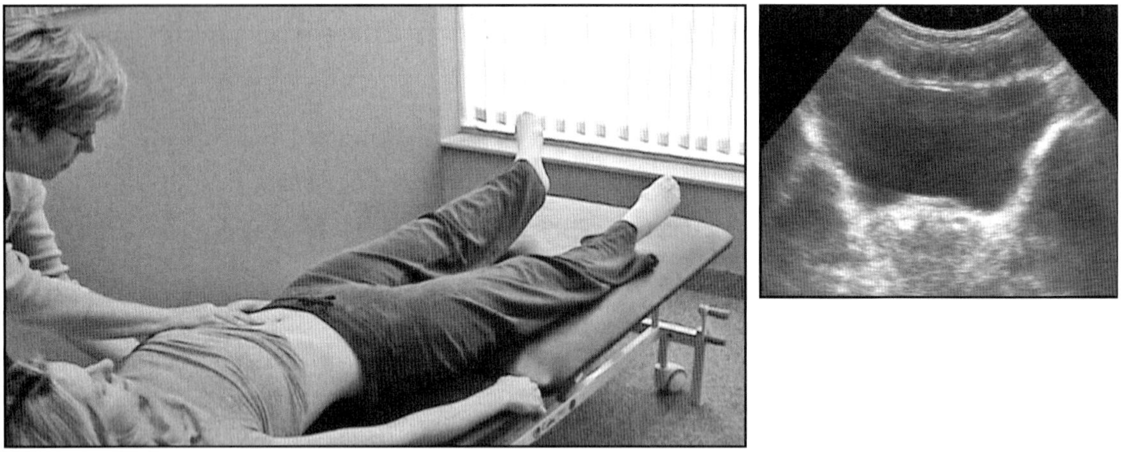

Fig. 39.14 The bladder shift was less when the trunk was manually decompressed on the left during the left active straight leg raise (ASLR) test.

bladder position suggests that her first treatment should be directed towards *reducing* compression in the lumbopelvic canister.

The right hip

A common compensatory strategy for failed load transfer through the pelvic girdle is to 'butt-grip.' This pattern usually involves overactivation of the deep external rotators of the hip joint including the piriformis and obturator internus. The overactivation and imbalance of these muscles can force the femoral head anteriorly (Fig. 39.15) and compress the structures of the anterior hip and subinguinal region. This can potentially be a source of groin pain and limit the range of motion at the hip, particularly combined flexion, adduction and internal rotation. Patients often complain of impingement and pain in their groin when crossing the affected leg. They tend to posture the affected extremity into external rotation both in standing and lying and the overactive muscles often have palpable trigger points. In Julie's case, she had overactivation of not only her right ischiococcygeus but also her piriformis and obturator internus. The piriformis and ischiococcygeus were likely compressing the right SIJ (thus reducing the neutral zone of motion and causing the muscular resistance in the elastic zone) and the piriformis and obturator internus were a potential source of the external rotation posturing of her right leg. Note the MRI of her pelvis and hip joints (Fig. 39.16). The anterior structures of the hip appear to be more compressed on the right

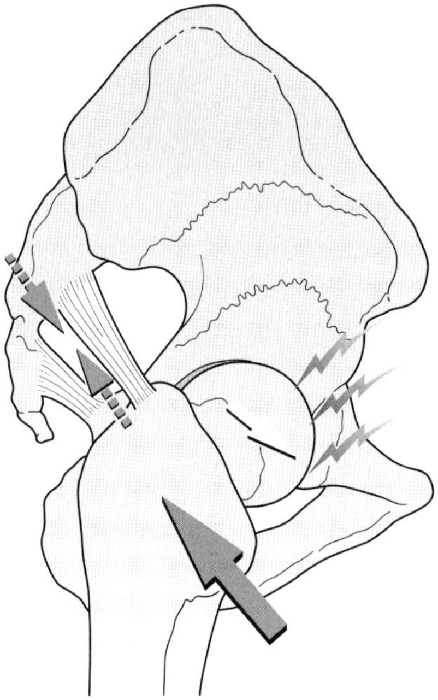

Fig. 39.15 Overactivation of the deep external rotators of the hip pulls the greater trochanter posterior (large arrow) and forces the femoral head anterior. This position compresses the structures of the anterior hip and the subinguinal region. (Reproduced with permission from Lee 2004.)

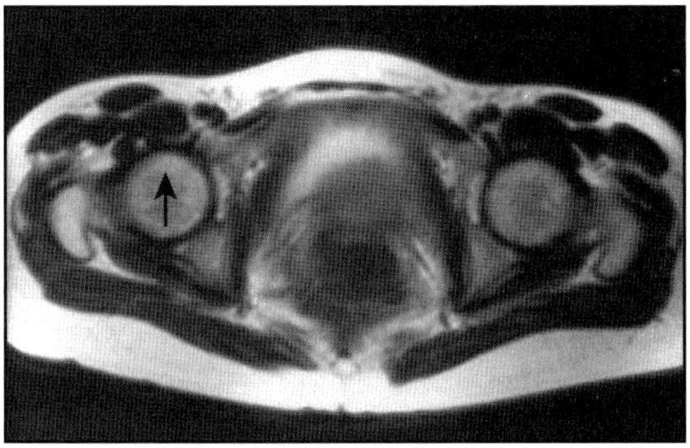

Fig. 39.16 This is an MRI through both hips and the pelvic floor. Note the anterior position of the right femoral head (arrow) and the resultant compression of the structures anterior to it.

and the right femur appears more externally rotated than the left. These findings support decompression or relaxation of these muscles as part of her early treatment plan along with techniques and exercises to center the femoral head during functional tasks in standing.

Intervention plan

An integrated approach to the management of LBP and PGP requires consideration and treatment of the multiple factors that led to the painful state. A careful review of the subjective examination will yield the history of events, the current location of symptoms and the activities that aggravate and/or relieve them. In addition, the patient's functional needs for work, sport and recreation require identification. All of this is important for building a patient-specific treatment plan (see Chapters 29, 30, and 31).

From the objective examination, the clinician will have an understanding of the patient's ability to transfer load in various postures and the strategies they use to do so. The clinician should also have identified the patient's current posture in standing, sitting and lying, their ability to move in and out of these postures (functional load transfer tests), the specific mobility and stability of each joint in the lumbopelvic–hip kinematic chain (form closure analysis), their ability to recruit the local muscle system on command as well as their ability to recruit both the local and global muscle system during specific tasks (force closure/motor control analysis). Through the examination process 'red and yellow flags' may or may not arise which lead the clinician to other tests (self-report questionnaires) regarding the emotional state and the role of fear-avoidance behavior in the clinical presentation (see Chapters 32 and 34).

Most patients will require a program which addresses their inability to functionally transfer loads secondary to:

- Maladaptive postures (standing, sitting, work/sport specific). Correction will require:
  - techniques to release tight/hypertonic muscles
  - techniques to restore mobility to stiff joints
  - techniques to align the skeleton (including both the trunk and extremities) optimally in standing, sitting and work-/sport-specific postures
  - techniques to stabilize the system and how to sustain the 'new' posture.
- Maladaptive movement strategies. Correction will require:
  - education regarding how to find the neutral spine/pelvis/lower extremity posture for sitting, standing, work- and sport-specific tasks and to move in and out of this posture without further aggravating the low back, pelvis or hip

- motor control training for optimal sequencing (timing) of local/global muscle activation in supported and unsupported postures (supine, sidelying , prone, sitting, four-point kneeling, standing, squats, lunges, etc.)
- muscle capacity training for strength and endurance of both the local and global muscle systems. Exercises should be specific to the individual's pattern of deficit and directed towards their functional needs
- proprioception and balance training (all of the above progressed to unstable surfaces such as rocker boards, foam rollers, and/or gym balls)
- movement pattern training for functional tasks of load transfer (getting in/out of chair/car, pushing, pulling, lifting, squats, work- and sport-specific needs); in other words the clinician needs to address how the patient should use their body more effectively to minimize loads and distribute forces throughout the kinematic chain for any task.

Julie's first treatment

Julie's treatment plan was developed using a clinical reasoning process that analyzed the assessment findings (see Table 39.1). The first goal was to use release techniques [neuromyofascial manual release techniques combined with dry needling (Gunn 1996)] to decompress the left side of the trunk (release the chest grip) and then to reassess the impact of this release on her ability to:

- perform an independent contraction of the lumbopelvic stabilizers, particularly TrA
- transfer load through the lumbar spine and pelvis.

These techniques were specifically directed to the vertical fibers of the left IO (Fig. 39.17A) and the right thoracic longissimus (part of the ES) (Fig. 39.17B).

Response to treatment

Once the vertical fibers of the left IO and the right thoracic longissimus (part of the ES) were relaxed, Julie could perform an isolated contraction of the left TrA. She could also co-contract the left and right TrA with an abdominal hollowing cue; however, there was no response in either the left or right dMF to this release. Consequently, during the same treatment session the dMF at L5–S1 was facilitated by first applying a 4-Hz alternating current through specifically placed acupuncture needles into the laminar fibers (Whittaker 2004c) (Fig. 39.18). While receiving this

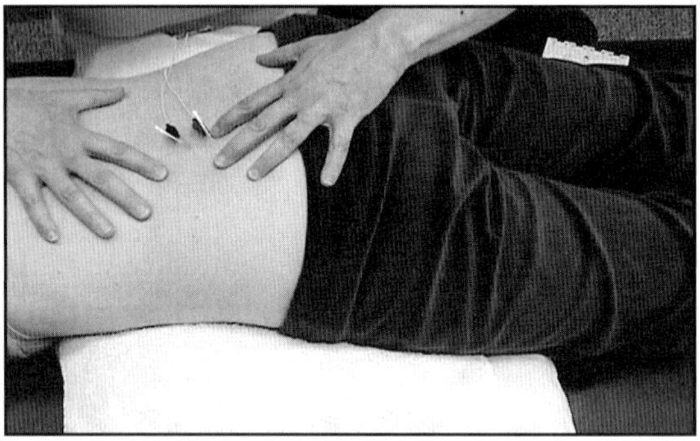

Fig. 39.18 Acustimulation of the deep fibers of multifidus helps the patient to 'remember' how to 'find the muscle.' The needles act as a conduit for the current to reach the deepest fibers of multifidus.

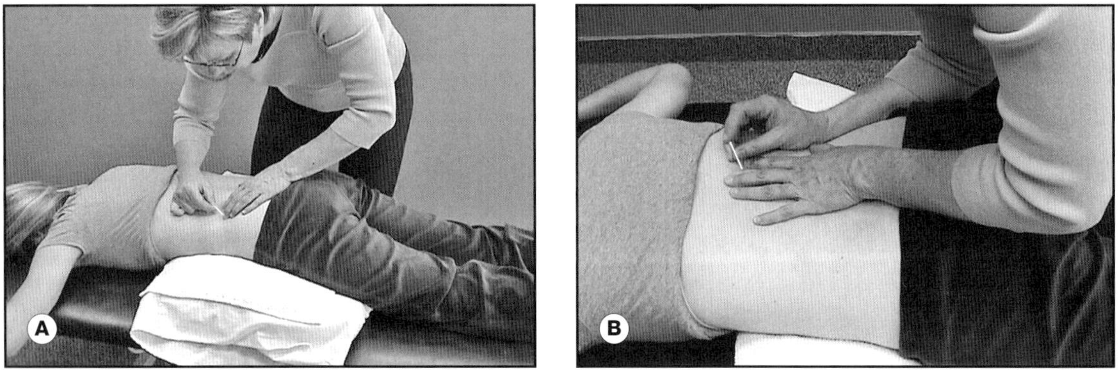

Fig. 39.17 (A) Dry needling release technique for the vertical fibers of the left IO. (B). Dry needling for the right thoracic longissimus. Alternatively, neuromyofascial release techniques could be used.

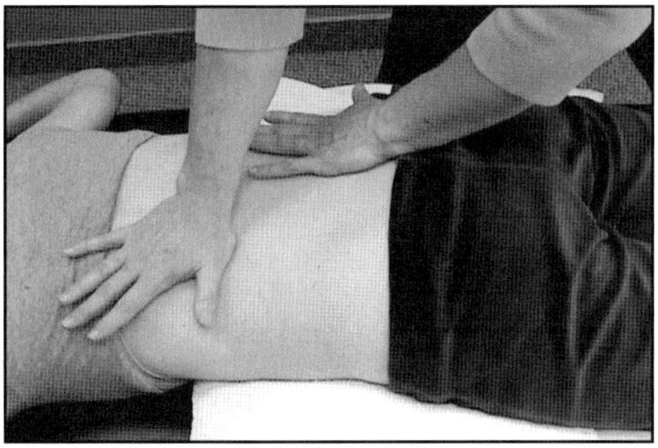

Fig. 39.19 One of Julie's home exercises was to use focused breathing (to open the areas beneath the therapist's hands) to relax the overactive global muscles. Verbal and tactile cues were used to facilitate the release of the global muscle system during this focused breath work.

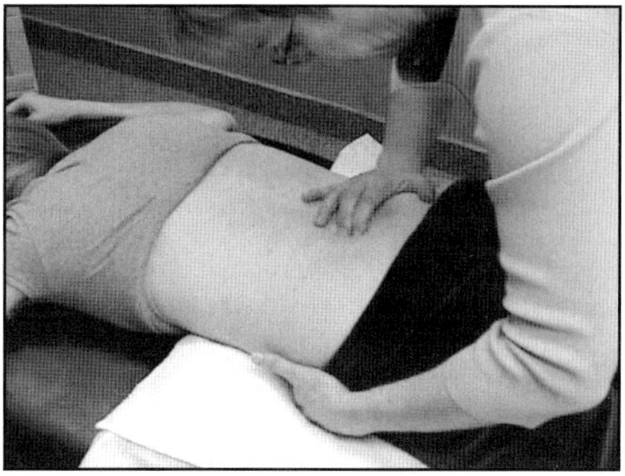

Fig. 39.20 Facilitation of the deep fibers of multifidus on the left at L5–S1. Julie's cue or image for facilitating a co-contraction of the left transversus abdominis (TrA) and the left deep multifidus (dMF) was to 'Imagine a guy wire from the inside of the ASIS through the pelvis to the lateral aspect of L5 and to connect along this line.' The therapist uses both verbal and tactile cues to create the image. When a proper co-contraction is produced, the therapist will feel a deep tension in the left anterior abdomen coupled with a slow swelling of the dMF. Ultimately, the goal is to produce a co-contraction of the left and right TrA and the left and right dMF, however cues often begin with a unilateral focus and progress to a bilateral cue once synergy occurs.

afferent input from the 4-Hz stimulation, Julie was advised to focus on the pulsing sensation in the area of her back where the current was being applied (no pain should occur with this technique) and to try to 'remember' the sensation of a deep muscle contraction at this level. The acustimulation was applied for 5 minutes following which Julie was given a specific cue for facilitating a connection to the dMF that resulted in a tonic swelling of the muscle (Lee & Lee 2004b, 2004c). The cue was combined with one for co-contraction with the TrA and the pelvic floor. She was able to achieve this easily after the release of the left IO and right ES. She was sent home with the following home exercises:

- To lie prone and breathe into the lateral and posterior aspects of her chest (Fig. 39.19). The aim was to relax the vertical fibers of the left IO and the right ES (Lee & Lee 2004b, 2004c).
- Following three or four focused breaths she was instructed to practice the cue (Fig. 39.20) for co-contraction of the dMF, TrA and pelvic floor and to maintain this co-contraction and breathe.

Julie's second treatment

Julie's second treatment began with a review of the breath work and the local system recruitment strategy taught in the first session. Subsequently, the emphasis of this session was to release the maladaptive compensatory strategy impacting the right hip joint and the right side of her pelvic girdle (release the butt-gripper). Neuromyofascial manual release techniques as well as dry needling were used for this (Fitzgerald & Kotarinos 2003b, Lee & Lee 2004b, 2004c) and directed towards the right ischiococcygeus, piriformis, and obturator internus.

Response to treatment

Once Julie could release/relax the muscles compressing her pelvis and hip (right pirformis, obturator internus, and the ischiococcygeus) the neutral zone of SIJ motion in the anteroposterior plane was more symmetric and the elastic zone had less muscular resistance on the right. She was now able to perform a left ASLR (score 2/5 on the left and 1/5 on the right for a total score of 3/10) (Fig. 39.21) if she consciously kept her:

- thorax relaxed (left IO and right ES)
- local system engaged with the combined cue taught in treatment session 1
- right hip/pelvic girdle relaxed.

The resting profile of her bladder (Fig. 39.22B) confirmed that she could now relax these muscles and during the ASLR test she was able to keep her bladder in a more central position. However if more compression was applied manually to her pelvic girdle, her ability to lift the left leg diminished

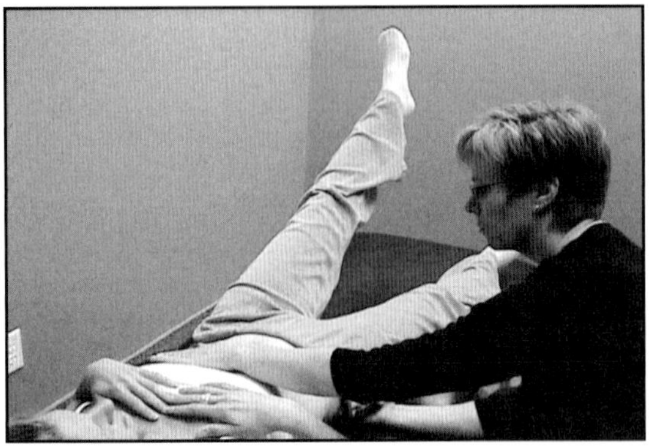

Fig. 39.21 The therapist is coaching Julie through the task of lifting her left leg by reminding her to keep the left side of her thorax relaxed and to breathe into this area, followed by gently activating the local system and simultaneously letting the right ischial tuberosity 'go wide,' i.e. relax the right lower buttock. After a few repetitions of this combined cue Julie could then lift her left leg with minimal effort and no pain. This is not about strength, but rather about motor control; strengthening and endurance of this pattern will follow.

(score 5/5). Therefore her pelvic girdle still could not tolerate too much compression and she was not given an SIJ belt.

Her home program now included the exercises from the first session (breath work and local system co-contraction training) as well as a release exercise for the trigger points in the posterior pelvis and buttock (Lee & Lee 2004b, 2004c).

Julie's third treatment

Julie was pleased with her progress in such a short period of time (3 days) and very committed to doing her part to facilitate her recovery. She understood that time, as well as strength and endurance training, was going to be required before she would see significant improvements in her ability to stand or sit for prolonged periods (see Chapter 36). She was encouraged, however, that a higher level of function was possible for her. Clinically, restoring hope and understanding through education of both the altered biomechanics as well as the neurophysiology of pain is critical in the early stages of rehabilitation (see Chapters 32 and 34) (Butler & Moseley 2003, Moseley 2003a, 2003b). Consequently, this treatment session focused on education, empowering her through knowledge. Her questions regarding the cascading events of the last 19 years, the impact of this on her pain neurophysiology and her biomechanics were discussed. Expectations from her, as well as from the treating practitioner, were considered, as well as the timelines and her future treatment options. She was advised to expect flare-ups of her symptoms during the recovery process until she learned how to pace her activities and was given tools to deal with these both physically and emotionally (Butler & Moseley 2003).

Exercise progressions for building timing, strength, and endurance of the dMF (ensuring synergy or coactivation with the other muscles of the local system) in a supported side-lying position

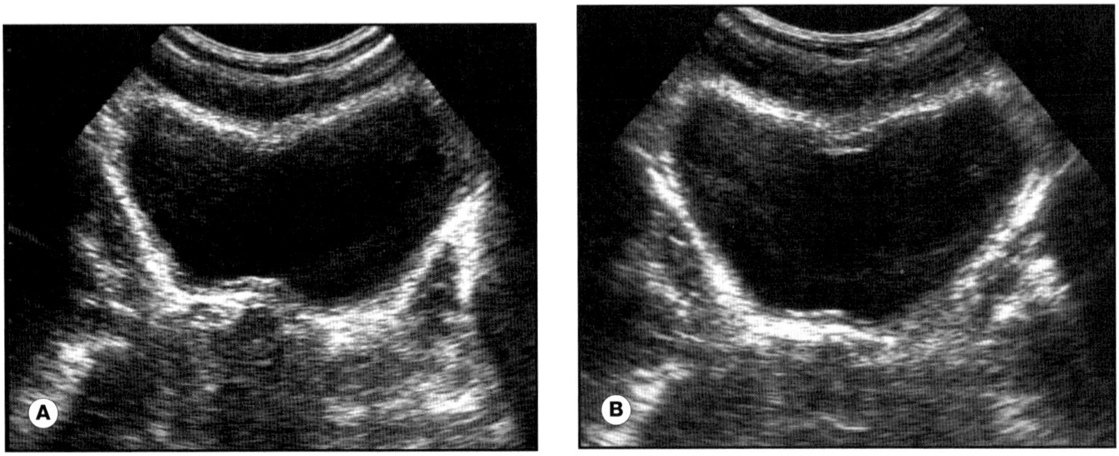

Fig. 39.22 (A) This is a transverse suprapubic RTUS image of Julie's resting bladder before she learned to relax the ischiococcygeus and the external rotators of the right hip. (B) RTUS image of Julie's resting bladder immediately after she stopped 'butt-gripping' for comparison. Note the change in shape of the right inferior aspect of the bladder.

were taught (Lee & Lee 2004b, 2004c, O'Sullivan et al 1997, Richardson & Jull 1995, Richardson et al 1999, Stuge et al 2004). She was given strategies to know whether or not she was performing the task optimally. She was reminded that it could take 4 to 6 weeks to build sufficient bulk in the dMF and that this would be required before functional progressions for vertical loading could be introduced. She was advised to avoid prolonged sitting if possible (take frequent breaks during the day) and to practice the local system recruitment strategies as frequently as possible.

Six weeks later

After 6 weeks of specific motor control training, Julie reported that her pain score (P4 scale) was now 20/40; down significantly from 28/40 (Spadoni et al 2004). With respect to her impairment status (ability to transfer loads in standing and supine lying, specific joint mobility/stability, etc.), Table 39.2 summarizes her findings 6 weeks into this program. Julie was now able to recruit a better motor plan for symmetric segmental stabilization of L5–S1 and both of her SIJs in forward bending (Fig. 39.23), one leg standing (Fig. 39.24) and during the ASLR test (ASLR score now 3/10) (Fig. 39.25). These changes were reflected in the PSFS score for forward bending, which had improved two points and was therefore significant (Westaway et al 1998). The rotation and sitting scores remain unchanged (both improved only 1 point). Further improvements in both rotation and sitting were anticipated as Julie continued to gain stability with mobility (ability to move in and out of neutral spine postures) and endurance for vertical loading tasks, the focus of this next stage of treatment.

As she was now able to independently and symmetrically recruit her local lumbopelvic muscle system (Fig. 39.26), Julie was ready to progress to exercises for restoring the neutral spine, pelvis and hip alignment and then to integrate these postures into functional tasks (sitting, forward bending, squats, etc.). Strategies for achieving a neutral spine and hip posture were first taught in standing (Fig. 39.27) and then in sitting (Fig. 39.28). She was shown how to move in and out of these postures using strategies which balanced the forces between her legs, pelvis and spine (Fig. 39.29). In addition to practicing these movement strategies, she was advised to continue with the breath work for releasing the left side of the thoracopelvic region [left external oblique (EO), IO], and to integrate

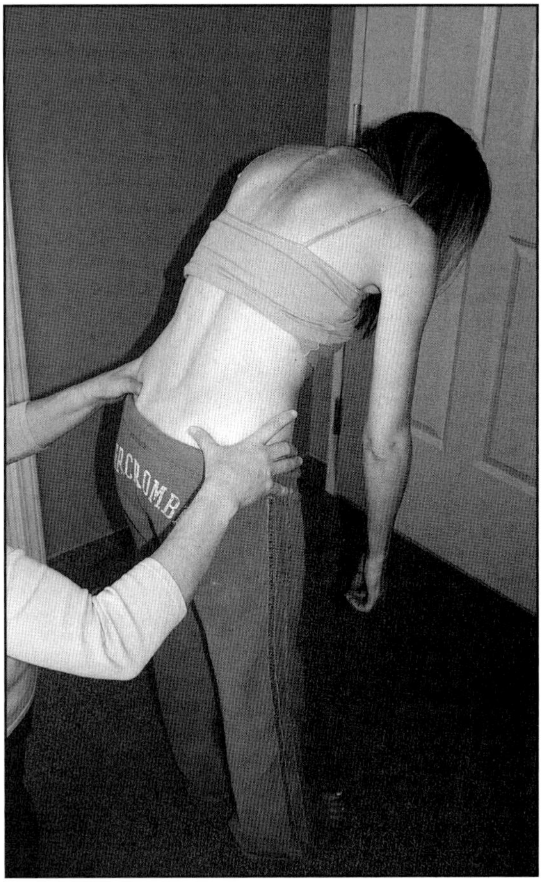

Fig. 39.23 Forward bending in standing: 6 weeks later. Note the intrapelvic symmetry compared to Figs 39.2 and 39.3. Julie still found it difficult to release her hips to allow her pelvis to anteriorly tilt.

the local system imagery during the functional integration exercises.

The key was to teach Julie how to remove the defensive posturing that she had embraced for so many years as a consequence of her pain and loss of motor control and replace it with postures and movement strategies that dispersed the forces throughout the entire kinematic chain ensuring that she had ways to control segmental spinal and intrapelvic loading and motion. Space precludes further discussion of the specifics of this functional retraining and the reader is referred to Lee & Lee (2004b, 2004c), Richardson et al (1999) and/or O'Sullivan (2004) for more clinical examples of how this approach is applied to patients with LBP and PGP.

Table 39.2 Summary of findings and treatment suggestions 6 weeks later

Test	Finding	Suggested intervention
Posture in standing/ sitting	No change as this had not been addressed in the first series of interventions	Address posture in standing and sitting (restore neutral spine/pelvis)
Load transfer standing: movement tests		
Forward bending	Strategy: better lumbopelvic strategy in that intrapelvic symmetry was maintained throughout forward bending. Increased activation of the right ES was still present at the end of flexion (see Fig. 39.23)	Continue to release the right ES and eventually progress to retrain symmetrical sequential thoracolumbar flexion. Restore neutral spine and then teach to move in/out of neutral symmetrically with a strategy that shares the load between the spine, pelvis and lower extremities
Backward bending	Strategy: able to extend the thoracolumbar spine with no hinging at L4–L5. Minimal posterior pelvic tilt	Continue to release the anterior abdominal wall to facilitate this motion. Restore neutral spine and then teach to move in/out of neutral symmetrically with a strategy that shares the load between the spine, pelvis and lower extremities
Lateral bending/ rotation	Strategy: still unable to freely rotate or lateral bend to the right	Continue to release the left lateral abdominal wall. Restore neutral spine and then teach to move in/out of neutral symmetrically with a strategy that shares the load between the spine, pelvis and lower extremities
Load transfer standing: one leg standing or Stork test		
Side of hip flexion	Symmetrical movement of the left and right SIJ	Continue to recruit the local muscle system and integrate into functional tasks for vertical loading
Side of single leg support	No unlocking of either SIJ (see Fig. 39.24) during single leg standing	
Load transfer supine: ASLR test		
ASLR: no compression	Could lift the left leg with minimal concentration Score 2/5 left, 1/5 right (see Fig. 39.25)	
ASLR: with compression of the pelvis	Manual compression decreased her ability to lift the left leg	
ASLR: with decompression of the global system	Manual decompression of the left thorax improved her ability to lift the left leg	Continue with release techniques (breathing and myofascial release, trigger point release when necessary)
Form closure analysis		
L5–S1	Much less posterior translation in neutral and in flexion. No palpable posterior translation occurred when resistance was applied to the trunk	Progress to vertical and loading in functional tasks (squats, forward bending)

Continued

Table 39.2 Summary of findings and treatment suggestions 6 weeks later–*cont'd*

Test	Finding	Suggested intervention
Right and left SIJ	Symmetric amplitude and resistance in both the neutral and elastic zones	Continue to recruit the local muscle system and integrate into functional tasks for vertical loading
Force closure/motor control analysis		
Response of the stabilizing muscles to a verbal cue: TrA	Isolation of the left TrA from the left IO now possible however the left TrA fatigued easily (see Fig. 39.26A)	Continue with release techniques for the left IO and right ES to decrease asymmetric global bracing and continue with cues to facilitate an independent contraction of the left TrA – build for endurance
Response of the stabilizing muscles to a verbal cue: dMF	Improved tone and bulk of both the left and right dMF, co-contraction with TrA noted bilaterally	Continue to use local system facilitation cues during functional tasks
Response of the stabilizing muscles to a verbal cue: pelvic floor	RTUS: bladder shape was symmetric at rest (see Fig. 39.26B) and a symmetric central lift was noted in response to a pelvic floor cue (see Fig. 39.26C). No palpable trigger point in the right ischiococcygeus	
Response of the stabilizing muscles during ASLR	No bladder shift with either ASLR left or right. Left TrA response was intermittent without manual decompression of the thorax	
The right hip	Right femoral head now centered in the acetabulum when supine but the right femur still shifts anterior in her habitual standing and sitting posture	Address posture in standing and sitting (restore neutral spine/pelvis) and then retrain vertical loading functional tasks with the femoral head centered (squats, sit to stand tasks)

ASLR, active straight leg raise test; dMF, deep lumbosacral multifidus; ES, erector spinae; IO, internal oblique; P4, posterior pelvic pain provocation test; RTUS, real-time ultrasound; SIJ, sacroiliac joint; TrA, transversus abdominis.

Summary

Julie's case is not uncommon in clinical practice. She has a combination of LBP and PGP from an injury sustained many years ago from which she never fully recovered. Consequently, she developed both an articular and a neuromuscular control problem in both her low back and pelvic girdle, as well as a sensitized nervous system. Increasingly, the evidence suggests that altered motor control that fails to optimally 'restore itself' plays a significant role in these challenging patients.

As always, more research is required to be truly evidence-based in the management of these patients; however, we first need to be able to identify subgroups of specific impairments. Following this, the specific tests for load transfer, form closure (mobility and stability) and force closure/motor control require investigation for their reliability, sensitivity and specificity for the subgroups of impairments. Only then will we have the ability to develop more sound studies (randomized and controlled) to test the efficacy of treatment programs that are specific to each subgroup. Until then, clinicians are encouraged to be evidence informed and to use a multimodal approach considering the biomechanical, neuromuscular, and emotional needs of the patient. Hopefully, collaboration between research teams and clinicians will continue so that the endemic dilemma of LBP and PGP eventually will be resolved.

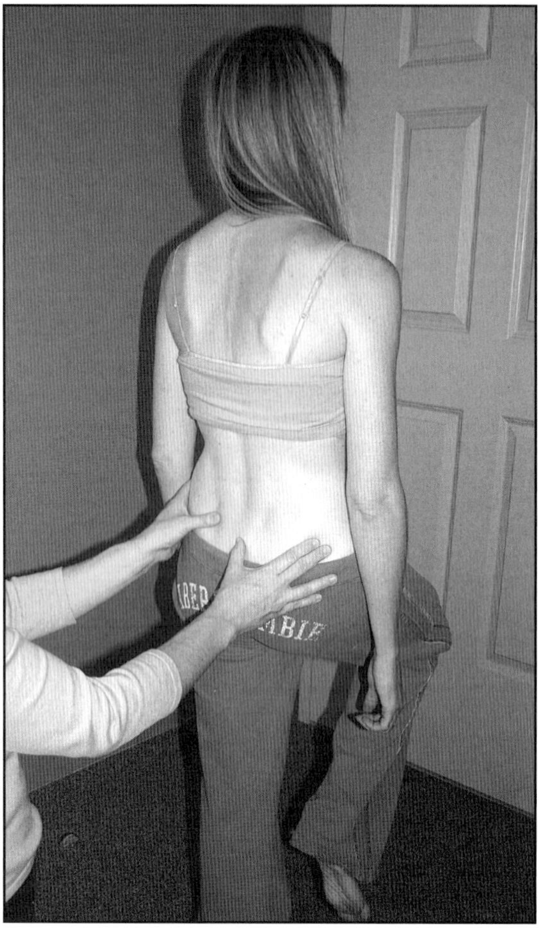

Fig. 39.24 One leg standing test: side of left single leg standing. Julie was now able to maintain stability of the left SIJ and hold this position for 10 seconds with ease.

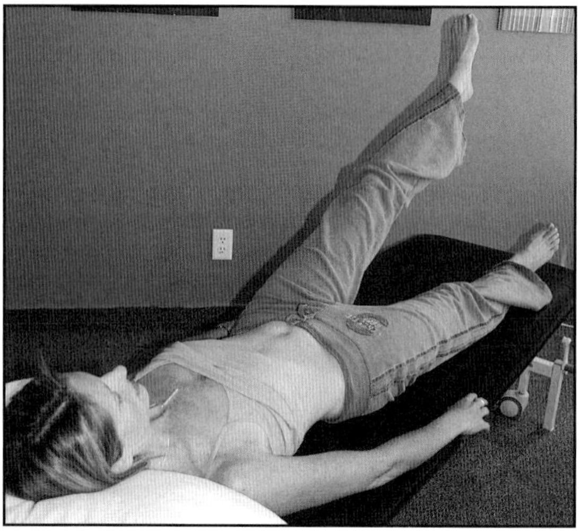

Fig. 39.25 Left active straight leg raise (ASLR) test. Julie could now lift her left leg off of the table with less effort and better alignment. When manual compression was applied to her pelvic girdle, the effort to lift the left leg increased whereas decompression of the thorax from the pelvis still reduced the required effort. This finding suggests that further decompression of the thorax from the pelvis is indicated while she simultaneously recruits the lumbopelvic local system.

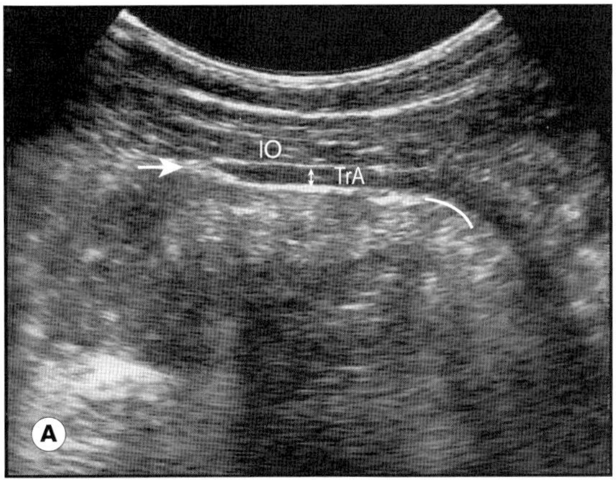

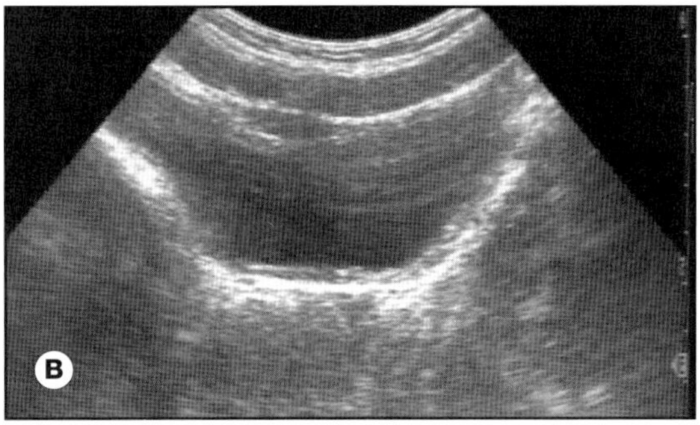

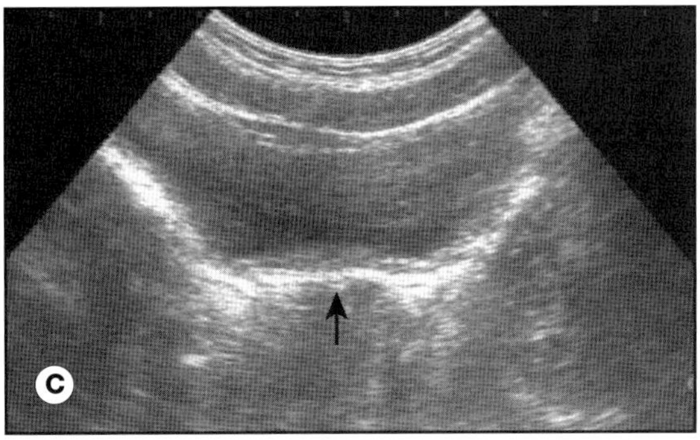

Fig. 39.26 Real-time ultrasound (RTUS) images of the lumbopelvic local muscle system. (A) Left lower lateral abdominal wall in response to a cue to gently hollow the lower abdomen. Compare this with Fig. 39.9(C). Note the relative increase in girth of the transversus abdominis (TrA; vertical double-headed arrow) and the corseting laterally (curved line). She could not yet maintain this isolated contraction for more than a few seconds. (B) This is a transverse suprapubic image of Julie's bladder at rest. Compare the profile of the inferior border of this bladder image to the ones in Figs 39.11C and 39.12B (6 weeks prior). This finding (coupled with the lack of a trigger point in the right ischiococcygeus and the symmetry of neutral zone motion of the sacroiliac joints) suggests that she was now able to relax the right ischiococcygeus. (C) Note the change in the profile of the bladder in response to a cue to squeeze the muscles around the urethra. The lift of the bladder is symmetric and central and suggests equal activation of the left and right levator ani muscles.

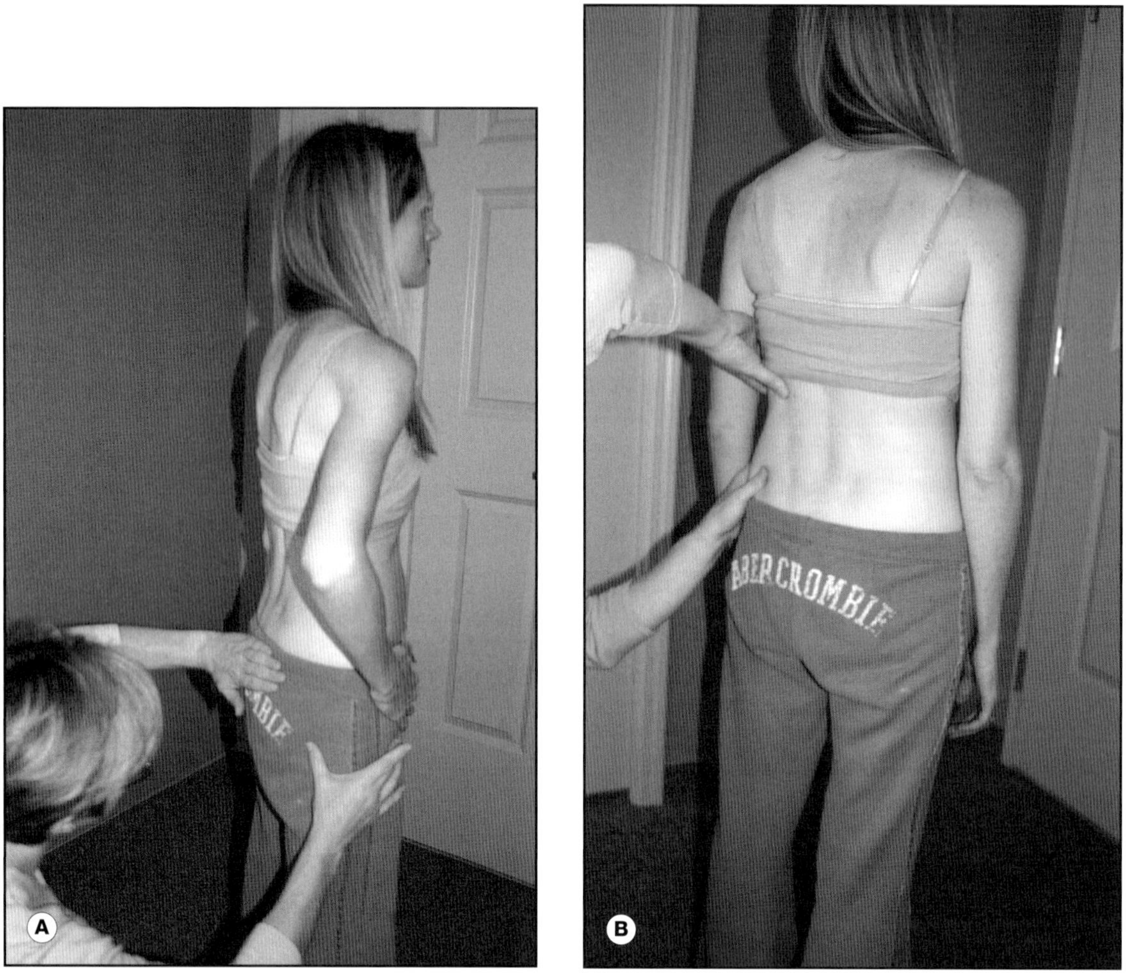

Fig. 39.27 Restoring neutral spine and hip in standing. (A) Julie was given cues to release the 'butt gripping' strategy that was forcing the right femur anterior when she stood. She was cued to think about opening a space in the posterior aspect of her right buttock and to allow the right femoral head to come posterior in the acetabulum. As she let go of the tendency to 'butt grip' on this side, the pelvic girdle released into a neutral position such that the anterior superior iliac spines (ASISs) and the pubic symphysis were in the same coronal plane (the pelvis was neither anteriorly nor posteriorly tilted). This helped to restore a gentle, even lumbar lordosis. (B) Julie was then taught how to correct the alignment of the thorax by opening the space between the rib cage and the pelvic girdle on the left and 'softening' the erector spinae (ES) on the right. Tactile and verbal cues are key elements for restoring a neutral spine position. Once achieved, this posture is usually associated with a sense of lightness (less tension/compression) and an improved ability to breathe. Several repetitions with less tactile and verbal feedback from the therapist are needed to ensure that the patient can find this posture on their own.

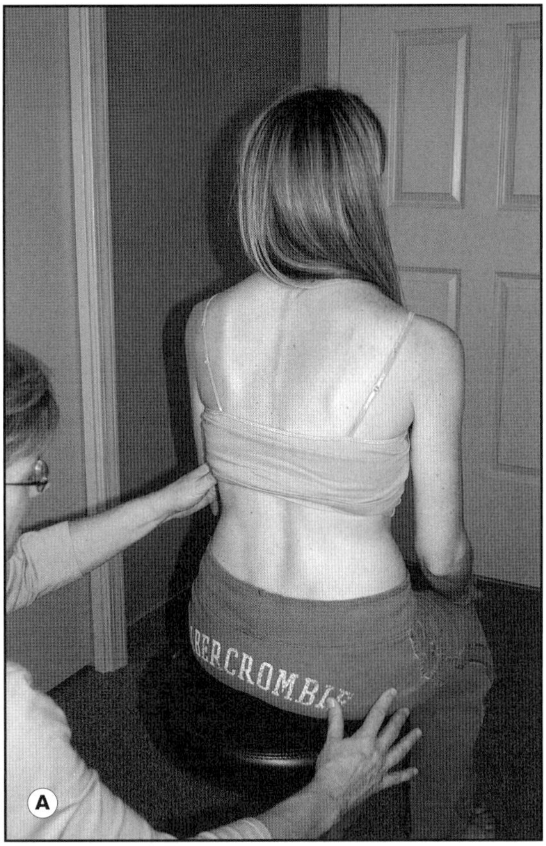

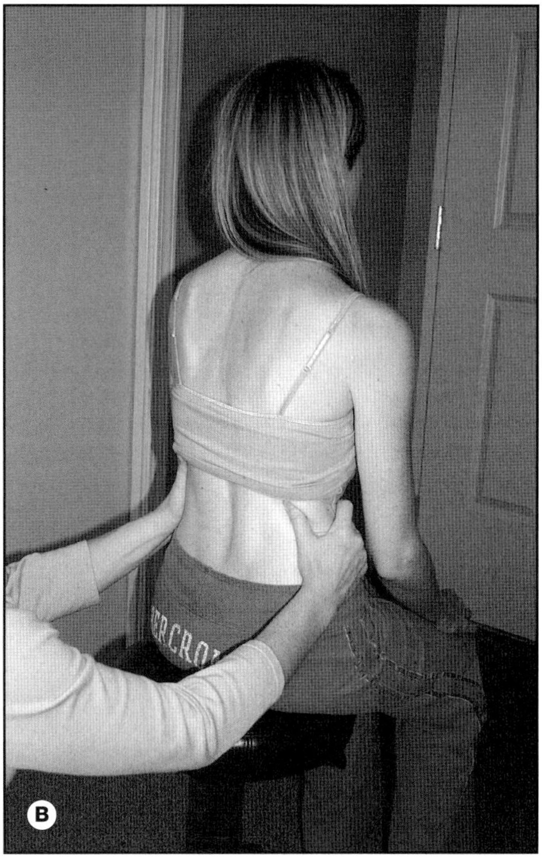

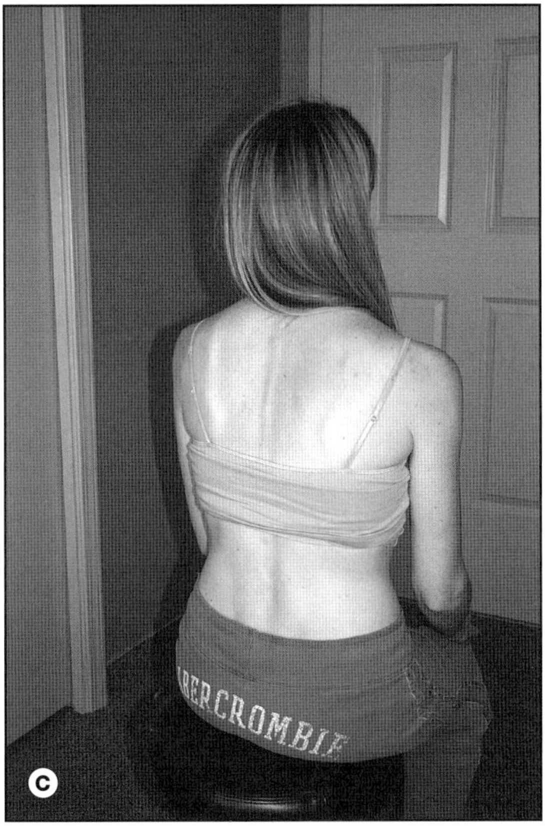

Fig. 39.28 Restoring neutral spine and hip in sitting. (A) It is imperative that patients are taught to sit with their weight evenly distributed between the anterior, posterior left and right aspects of their pelvic girdle, i.e. centered. Most patients with low back pain and pelvic girdle pain tend to sit in a posterior pelvic tilt with a flexed lumbosacral junction. It is very difficult to achieve a neutral lumbar spine posture when the pelvis is seated in a posterior tilt and the buttock muscles are gripped. (B) Once the pelvic girdle position is correct [anterior superior iliac spines (ASISs) and pubic symphysis in the same coronal plane], and the femur is centrally seated in the acetabulum, the thoracolumbar posture can be addressed. (C) Cues to think of lengthening the spine (regionally and specifically) and letting the sternum 'sink' are often helpful to relax the global bracing strategies commonly used. For more information on specific verbal and tactile cues used for restoring the optimal pelvic base and neutral spine position, see Lee (2003) and Lee & Lee (2004b, 2004c).

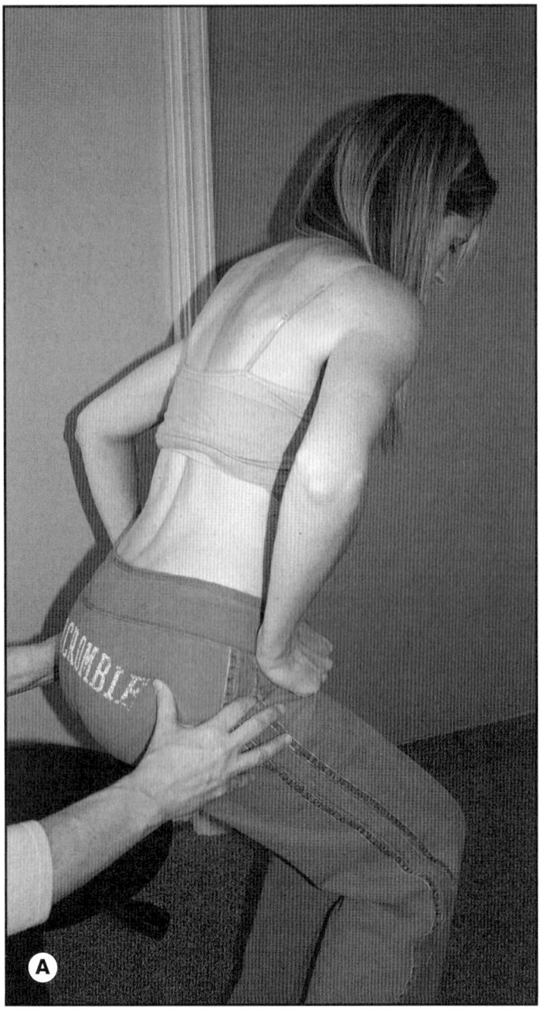

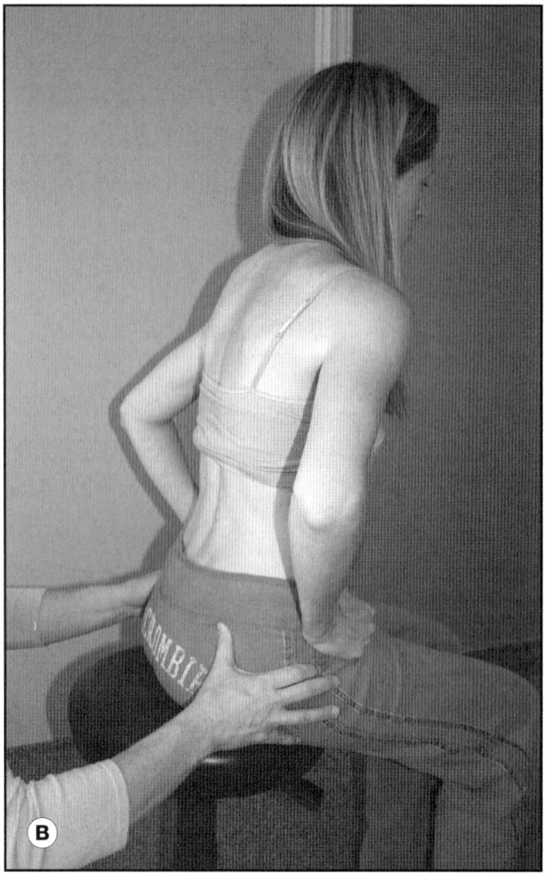

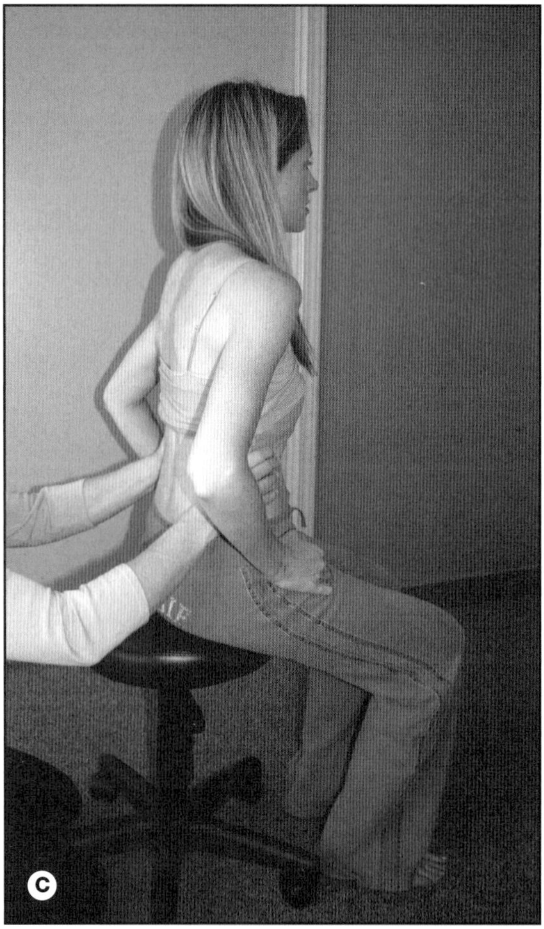

Fig. 39.29 Functional integration: squats, sit to stand training. Retraining integrated movement patterning during functional tasks is a significant part of this stage of rehabilitation. Living differently in your body requires not only learning how to be different statically (posture) but how to move differently (dynamic motion control). Exercises for moving from sitting to standing, squatting, lifting, etc. can be broken down into movement components and retrained with awareness. Cues for local system activation as well as thoracopelvic and pelvis/leg alignment are critical and patient specific. The therapist monitors the patient's areas of 'weakness' (joints that tend to fail under load) and provides verbal and tactile correction cues. When the loads are distributed throughout the body, movements appear effortless and the patient has a sense of control and strength. Making a habit of these new movement patterns requires commitment and practice. A good line to remember is 'If you always do what you've always done, you'll always get what you've always got! It takes time, awareness and commitment to make long-lasting changes in your body.'

References

Butler D, Moseley GL 2003 Explain pain. NOI Group, Adelaide, Australia

Buyruk HM, Snijders CJ, Vleeming A et al 1995a The measurements of SIJ stiffness with colour doppler imaging: a study on healthy subjects. European Journal of Radiology 21:117–121

Buyruk HM, Stam HJ, Snijders CJ et al 1995b The use of colour doppler imaging for the assessment of sacroiliac joint stiffness: a study on embalmed human pelvises. European Journal of Radiology 21:112–116

Damen L, Buyruk HM, Guler-Uysal F et al 2001 Pelvic pain during pregnancy is associated with asymmetric laxity of the sacroiliac joints. Acta Obstetrica Gynecologica Scandinavica 80:1019

Damen L, Stijnen T, Roebroeck ME et al 2002 Reliability of sacroiliac joint laxity measurement with Doppler imaging of vibrations. Ultrasound in Medicine and Biology 28:407

Ferreira PH, Ferreira ML, Hodges PW 2004 Changes in recruitment of the abdominal muscles in people with low back pain, ultrasound measurement of muscle activity. Spine 29:2560–2566

FitzGerald MP, Kotarinos A 2003a Rehabilitation of the short pelvic floor. I: background and patient evaluation. International Urogynecology Journal 14:261–268

FitzGerald MP, Kotarinos A 2003b Rehabilitation of the short pelvic floor. II: Treatment of the patient with the short pelvic floor. International Urogynecology Journal 14:269–275

Grimstone SK, Hodges PW 2003 Impaired postural compensation for respiration in people with recurrent low back pain. Experimental Brain Research 151: 218–224

Gunn CC 1996 The Gunn approach to the treatment of chronic pain. Intramuscular stimulation for myofascial pain of radicolopathic origin. Churchill Livingstone, New York

Hides JA, Richardson CA, Jull GA, Davies S 1995 Ultrasound imaging in rehabilitation. Australian Journal of Physiotherapy 41(3):187

Hodges PW 2003 Neuromechanical control of the spine. PhD thesis, Stockholm

Hodges PW, Richardson CA 1996 Inefficient muscular stabilization of the lumbar spine associated with low back pain. A motor control evaluation of transversus abdominis. Spine 21(22):2640–2650

Hodges PW, Richardson CA 1997 Contraction of the abdominal muscles associated with movement of the lower limb. Physical Therapy 77:132–144

Hungerford B, Gilleard W, Hodges PW 2003 Evidence of altered lumbopelvic muscle recruitment in the presence of sacroiliac joint pain. Spine 28(14):1593

Hungerford B, Gilleard W, Lee D 2004 Alteration of pelvic bone motion determined in subjects with posterior pelvic pain using skin markers. Clinical Biomechanics (19):456

Lee DG 2003 The thorax – an integrated approach. Diane G Lee Physiotherapist Corporation, Surrey, Canada. Online. Available: http://www.dianelee.ca

Lee DG 2004 The pelvic girdle, 3rd edn. Elsevier, Edinburgh

Lee DG, Lee LJ 2004a Diagnosing the lumbopelvic–hip dysfunction. In: Lee DG (ed) The pelvic girdle, 3rd edn. Elsevier Science, Edinburgh

Lee LJ, Lee DG 2004b Treating the lumbopelvic–hip dysfunction. In: Lee DG (ed) The pelvic girdle, 3rd edn. Elsevier Science, Edinburgh

Lee DG, Lee LJ 2004c An integrated approach to the assessment and treatment of the lumbopelvic–hip region. DVD. Online. Available: http://www.dianelee.ca

Mens JMA, Vleeming A, Snijders CJ et al 1999 The active straight leg raising test and mobility of the pelvic joints. European Spine 8:468–473

Mens JMA, Vleeming A, Snijders CJ et al 2001 Reliability and validity of the active straight leg raise test in posterior pelvic pain since pregnancy. Spine 26(10):1167–1171

Mens JMA, Vleeming A, Snijders CJ et al 2002 Validity of the active straight leg raise test for measuring disease severity in patients with posterior pelvic pain after pregnancy. Spine 27(2):196

Moseley GL 2003a A pain neuromatrix approach to patients with chronic pain. Manual Therapy 8(3):130–140

Moseley GL 2003b Unraveling the barriers to reconceptualization of the problem in chronic pain: the actual and perceived ability of patients and health professionals to understand the neurophysiology. Journal of Pain 4(4):184

O'Sullivan PB 2004 'Clinical instability' of the lumbar spine: its pathological basis, diagnosis and conservative management. In: Boyling JD, Jull GA (eds) Grieve's modern manual therapy: the vertebral column, 3rd edn. Elsevier, Edinburgh

O'Sullivan PB, Twomey L, Allison G 1997 Evaluation of specific stabilising exercise in the treatment of chronic low back pain with radiological diagnosis of spondylolysis and spondylolisthesis. Spine 15(24): 2959–2967

O'Sullivan PB, Beales D, Beetham JA et al 2002 Altered motor control strategies in subjects with SIJ pain during the active straight leg raise test. Spine 27(1):E1

Ostrzenski A, Osborne NG 1998 Ultrasonography as a screening tool for paravaginal defects in women with stress incontinence: A pilot study. International Urogynecology Journal 9:105–199

Richardson CA, Jull GA 1995 Muscle control – pain control. What exercises would you prescribe? Manual Therapy 1:2–10

Richardson CA, Jull GA, Hodges PW, Hides JA 1999 Therapeutic exercise for spinal segmental stabilization in low back pain – scientific basis and clinical approach. Churchill Livingstone, Edinburgh

Sapsford RR, Hodges PW, Richardson CA et al 2001 Co-activation of the abdominal and pelvic floor muscles during voluntary exercises. Neurourology and Urodynamics 20:31–42

Shirado O, Ito T, Kaneda K, Strax TE 1995 Flexion-relaxation phenomenon in the back muscles. A comparative study between healthy subjects and patients with chronic low back pain. American Journal of Physical Medicine and Rehabilitation 74(2):139–144

Spadoni G, Stratford PW, Solomen PE, Wishart LR 2004 The evaluation of change in pain intensity: a comparison of the P4 and single-item numeric pain rating scales. Journal of Orthopedic and Sports Physical Therapy 34(4):187–193

Stratford P, Gill C, Westaway M, Binkley J 1995 Assessing disability and change on individual patients: A report of a patient-specific measure. Physiotherapy Canada 47:258–263

Stuge B, Lærum E, Kirkesola G, Vøllestad N 2004 The efficacy of a treatment program focusing on specific stabilizing exercises for pelvic girdle pain after pregnancy. Spine 29(4):351

Sturesson B, Udén A, Vleeming A 2000 A radiosterometric analysis of movements of the sacroiliac joints during the standing hip flexion test. Spine 25(3):364–368

Van Wingerden JP, Vleeming A, Ronchetti I 2004 Physical compensation strategies in patients with chronic pelvic girdle pain. In: Proceedings from Fifth Interdisciplinary World Congress on Low Back and Pelvic Pain. Melbourne, Australia, p106

Vleeming A, de Vries HJ, Mens JM, van Wingerden JP 2002 Possible role of the long dorsal sacroiliac ligament in women with peripartum pelvic pain. Acta Obstetrica Gynecologica Scandinavica 81(5):430

Westaway MD, Stratford PW, Binkley JM 1998 The patient-specific functional scale: validation of its use in persons with neck dysfunction. Journal of Orthopedic and Sports Physical Therapy 27(5):331–338

Whittaker JL 2004a Real-time ultrasound analysis of local system function. In: Lee DG (ed) The pelvic girdle, 3rd edn. Elsevier Science, Edinburgh

Whittaker JL 2004b Abdominal ultrasound imaging of pelvic floor muscle function in individuals with low back pain. Journal of Manual and Manipulative Therapy 12(1):44

Whittaker JL 2004c Lumbo-pelvic segmental stabilization using technology to improve clinical skills. Course notes.

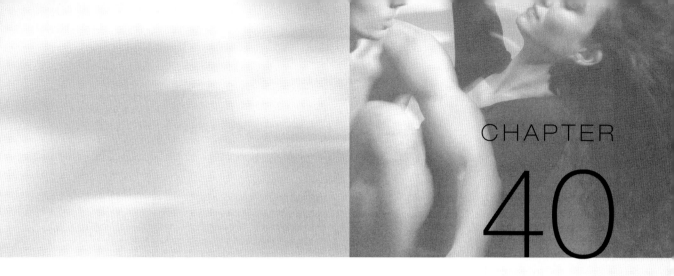

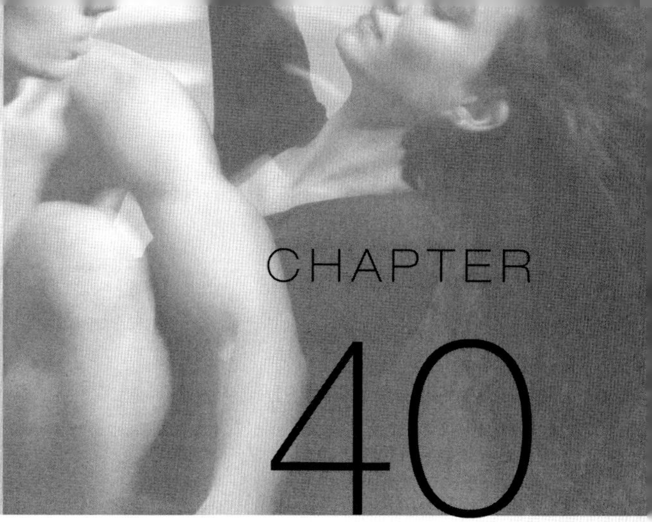

CHAPTER 40

An integrated therapeutic approach to the treatment of pelvic girdle pain

Diane Lee and Andry Vleeming

Introduction

The pelvic girdle is no longer considered the mystery it once was, due – in part – to the recent research on the role the pelvis plays in low back and pelvic girdle pain. Through interdisciplinary congresses and the research they have fostered, a consensus is arising as to the causes and treatment of pelvic girdle pain and dysfunction. Recently, guidelines for the diagnosis and treatment of pelvic girdle pain were presented by a European working group (Vleeming et al 2004). After an extensive review of the literature, this group recognized that although there is an increasing consensus of opinion, there is still the need for further research in all areas pertaining to pelvic girdle pain (epidemiology, biomechanics, diagnostics, and treatment).

This chapter presents the principles of an integrated multimodal approach for the management of pelvic girdle pain and dysfunction; it is drawn from anatomical and biomechanical studies of the pelvis, as well as from clinical experience of treating patients with lumbopelvic pain. The integrated model is evidence based where it can be and relies on sound clinical reasoning where the evidence is still lacking. This approach is a functional one that aims to address and clarify why the pelvic girdle is painful and no longer able to sustain and transfer loads in contrast to one which seeks to identify pain-generating structures. A model such as this requires an understanding of the function of the pelvic girdle.

Several studies have sought to understand the function of the pelvic girdle. The anatomical and biomechanical research (Barker et al 2004, Snijders et al 1993a, 1993b, Vleeming et al 1990a, 1990b, 1995, 1996) led to theories regarding form and force closure of joints and how stability could be achieved for effective load transfer. The timing of specific muscle activation (Barbic et al 2003, Hodges & Gandevia 2000a, 2000b, Hodges & Richardson 1996, 1997, Moseley et al 2002) and the pattern of muscular co-contraction (or lack thereof) in patients with low back pain (Hodges & Richardson 1996), posterior pelvic girdle pain (Hungerford et al 2003, O'Sullivan et al 2002) and groin pain (Cowan et al 2004) have further enhanced the force closure theory and suggested a crucial role for motor control. In addition, studies of muscle capacity in the low back pain population (McGill 2002) suggest that strength and endurance of trunk muscles is also important, especially for high load tasks. Based on this knowledge, functional tests of load transfer through the pelvic girdle were developed (Hungerford et al 2004, Mens et al 1999, 2001, 2002) and treatment protocols proposed (Lee & Vleeming 1998, Lee 2004, O'Sullivan et al 1997, Richardson & Jull 1995, Richardson et al 1999, Stuge et al 2004). Both clinically and scientifically, the impact of chronic pain and emotional states (stress, fear, anxiety) on motor control became evident and clinical outcomes are now known to be significantly influenced by the patient's thoughts and beliefs (Butler & Moseley 2003, Hodges & Moseley 2003, Holstege et al 1996, Moseley 2002, 2003a, 2003b, Moseley & Hodges 2005, Vlaeyen & Linton 2000, Watson et al 1997).

This integrated approach to the treatment of pelvic girdle pain has four components (Fig. 40.1): three that are physical (form closure, force closure, motor control) and one that is psychological (emotions). The proposal is that joint mechanics can be influenced by multiple factors including articular, neuromuscular and emotional and that the management of pain and dysfunction requires attention to all. The principles of the application of this model to the pelvic girdle will be outlined in this chapter. It draws from the substantial research cited above and previously presented in this text.

Function of the pelvic girdle

A primary function of the pelvis is to transfer the loads generated by body weight and gravity during standing, walking, sitting and other functional tasks. How well this load is managed dictates how efficient function will be. The word 'stability' is often used to describe effective load transfer and requires optimal function of three systems: the passive, active and control (Panjabi 1992). Collectively these systems produce approximation

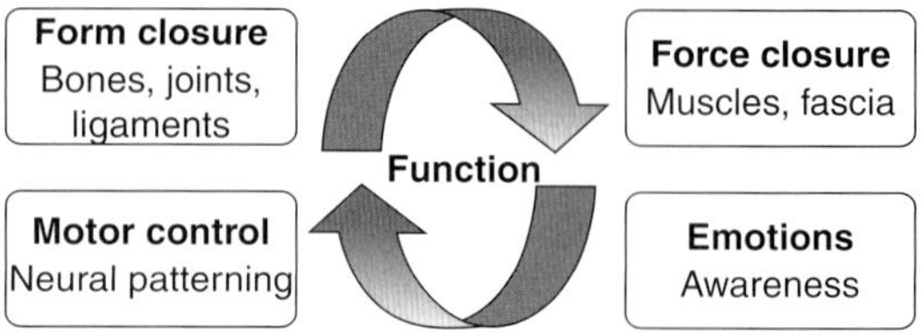

Fig. 40.1 The integrated model of function has four components: form closure (structure), force closure (forces produced by myofascial action), motor control (specific timing of muscle action/inaction during loading) and emotions.

of the joint surfaces (Snijders & Vleeming 1992a, 1992b). The amount of approximation required is variable and difficult to quantify because it depends on an individual's structure (form closure) and the forces they need to control (force closure). The following definition of joint stability comes from the European guidelines on the diagnosis and treatment of pelvic girdle pain (Vleeming et al 2004):

> *The effective accommodation of the joints to each specific load demands through an adequately tailored joint compression, as a function of gravity, coordinated muscle and ligament forces, to produce effective joint reaction forces under changing conditions. Optimal stability is achieved when the balance between performance (the level of stability) and effort is optimized to economize the use of energy. Nonoptimal joint stability implicates altered laxity/stiffness values leading to increased joint translations resulting in a new joint position and/or exaggerated/reduced joint compression, with a disturbed performance/effort ratio.*

Based on this definition, the analysis of pelvic girdle function will require tests for excessive/reduced joint compression as well as tests for motion control of the joints (sacroiliac and pubic symphysis) during functional tasks (one leg standing, active straight leg raise). Motion control of the joints requires the timely activation of various muscle groups such that the coactivation pattern occurs at minimal cost (minimal compression or tension loading and the least amount of effort) to the musculoskeletal system. Analysis of neuromuscular function will require tests for both motor control (timing of muscle activation) and muscular capacity (strength and endurance) because both are required for intersegmental or intrapelvic control, regional control (between thorax and pelvis, pelvis and legs) as well as the maintenance of whole-body equilibrium during functional tasks. Treatment protocols should include techniques to reduce joint compression where necessary, exercises to increase joint compression where and when necessary and education to foster understanding of both the mechanical and emotional components of the patient's experience.

Form closure: mobility and stability of the sacroiliac joint

The term 'form closure' was coined by Vleeming & Snijders (Snijders et al 1993a, 1993b, Vleeming et al 1990a, 1990b) to describe how a joint's structure, orientation, and shape contribute to its mobility and stability. All joints have a variable amount of form closure and the individual's anatomy will dictate how much additional force (force closure) is needed to ensure stability when loads are increased. The form of the sacroiliac joint (SIJ) evolves through life (Bowen & Cassidy 1981) and its shape adapts to the task of transferring high loads. The articular surfaces are relatively flat and this helps to transfer compression forces and bending moments. However, a relatively flat joint is theoretically more vulnerable to shear or translation forces. The SIJ is anatomically protected from shear in three ways:

1. The sacrum is wedge-shaped in both the anteroposterior and vertical planes and the orientation of the S1, S2, and S3 segments is variable (Solonen 1957).
2. The articular cartilage lining the ilium is irregular thus increasing the friction co-efficient of the joint when it is compressed (Bowen & Cassidy 1981, Sashin 1930, Vleeming et al 1990a, 1990b).
3. The SIJ has complementary intra-articular ridges and grooves (Vleeming et al 1990a).

For many decades, it was thought that the SIJ was immobile due to its anatomy. It is now known that mobility of the SIJ is not only possible (Egund et al 1978, Hungerford et al 2004, Lavignolle et al 1983, Sturesson et al 1989, 2000), but essential for shock absorption during weight-bearing activities and is maintained throughout life (Vleeming et al 1992). The quantity of motion is small (both for angular and translatoric motion) and variable between individuals (Jacob & Kissling 1995, Sturesson et al 1989, 2000).

To date, no manual diagnostic tests have shown reliability for determining *how much* an individual's SIJ is moving in either symptomatic or asymptomatic subjects (Carmichael 1987, Dreyfuss et al 1994, 1996, Herzog et al 1989, Laslett & Williams 1994, Potter & Rothstein 1985). There is considerable debate in the literature regarding the methods used, the subjects tested, the standardization of the technique, the skill of the tester and the statistical analysis used to determine the results in these studies.

The one leg standing, or Stork, test is commonly used to analyze the amplitude of motion of the SIJ. During this test posterior rotation of the non-weight-bearing innominate is compared bilaterally and often a diagnosis of hypermobility or hypomobility is assigned. This test has failed to show reliability and sensitivity for analyzing amplitude of motion. Both Jacob & Kissling (1995) and Sturesson et al (2000) investigated motion of the SIJ during this test. Healthy, pain-free subjects were tested in the Jacob & Kissling study whereas subjects with posterior pelvic girdle pain and a diagnosis of instability were tested in the study of Sturesson et al. Both studies found similar amplitudes of motion in their healthy and dysfunctional subjects. This suggests that this *active* mobility test cannot conclusively determine the *passive* mobility of the SIJ joint and that this test should not be used exclusively for analyzing amplitude of motion. Thus, we can confidently say that yes, the SIJ moves. However, how significant is the amplitude of SIJ motion in determining impaired function of the pelvic girdle? The research suggests that amplitude of motion is not an indicator of function or dysfunction in the pelvic girdle.

Buyruk et al (1995a) established that the Doppler imaging system could be used to measure the transference of vibration across the SIJ. The amplitude of transference reflects the stiffness of the SIJ. This research has been repeated and the results confirmed by Damen et al (2002a). Both Buyruk et al (1995b, 1997, 1999) and Damen et al (2001, 2002b) used this method to measure stiffness of the SIJ in subjects with and without pelvic girdle pain and noted a high degree of individual variance. *Within the same subject*, the asymptomatic individual demonstrated similar values for both SIJs, whereas the symptomatic individual demonstrated different stiffness values for the left and right SIJ. In other words, asymmetry of stiffness between sides correlated with the symptomatic individual. In keeping with this research, the emphasis of manual motion testing should focus less on *how much* (amplitude) the SIJ is moving and more on the symmetry, or asymmetry of the motion palpated. Form closure analysis for articular mobility/stability requires a comparison of the symmetry of stiffness of the right and left SIJ and should be done passively since the muscular system is known (Richardson et al 2002, van Wingerden et al 2004) to increase compression across the SIJ and thus would impact the findings. A clinical reasoning approach, which considers all of the findings from the examination, is required to determine if the amplitude of motion is less, or more, than optimal for that individual. To date, the passive tests for mobility for the SIJ or the pubic symphysis (Lee 1992, 2004) have not been properly tested for reliability, sensitivity and specificity for specific pelvic impairments.

Force closure/motor control: compression and stability of the pelvis

For every joint, there is a position called the close packed, or self-locked position in which there is maximum congruence of the articular surfaces and maximum tension of the major ligaments. This is the most stable position for the joint; however, it is also the most compressive and therefore primarily suitable for high loading tasks. For the SIJ, this position is nutation of the sacrum or posterior rotation of the innominate and occurs bilaterally whenever the lumbopelvic spine is loaded in sitting or standing (Hungerford 2004, Sturesson et al 2000). Counternutation of the sacrum (anterior rotation of the innominate) is thought to be a less stable position for the SIJ. The long dorsal sacroiliac ligament becomes taut when the sacrum is counternutated, however the other major ligaments (sacrotuberous, sacrospinous, and interosseus) are less tensed (Vleeming et al 1996).

Function would be significantly compromised if joints could only be stable in the close-packed position. Stability for load transfer is required throughout the entire range of motion and is provided by the active system when the joint is not in the close-packed position. Although the motion of the SIJ is small, control is still required if stability and effective load transfer are to be insured. Optimal force closure of the pelvic girdle requires just the right amount of force being applied at just the right time and this in turn requires a certain capacity (strength/endurance) of the muscular system as well as a finely tuned motor control system: one that is able to predict the timing of the load and to prepare the system appropriately. The amount of articular compression needed depends on the individual's form closure and the magnitude of the load. Therefore, there are multiple optimal strategies possible, some for low loading tasks and others for high loading tasks. The compression, or force closure, is produced by an integrated action and reaction between the muscle systems, their fascial and ligamentous connections, and gravity. The timing, pattern and amplitude of the muscular contraction depend on an appropriate efferent response of both the central and peripheral nervous systems, which in turn rely on appropriate afferent input from the joints, ligaments, fascia and muscles. It is indeed a complex system, often difficult to study, yet when one returns to the definition of joint stability (the ability to transfer loads with the least amount of effort which controls motion of the joints) it is not difficult to assess or treat.

An increasing body of evidence suggests that certain muscles function to prepare the system for loading whereas others are well-suited for generating movement. Bergmark (1989) classified these muscles into two systems, local and global, and the classification was based on certain anatomical features. The local muscles were thought to be deeper, more segmental and not necessarily aligned to produce articular motion but rather suited to apply compression across joints. The global muscles were thought to be more superficial with fewer segmental connections and to span regions of the body (i.e. thorax to pelvis). As the research advances, it is now known that this classification is too simple in that some muscles function both as local stabilizers and global movers during different functional tasks. Perhaps a more physiological or functional classification is required. A system of muscles is needed to prepare the musculoskeletal system against the buckling (compression) and shear (translation) that occur during loading. In addition, a system is required for generating torque and movement. A healthy, integrated neuro-myofascial system would ensure that loads are effectively transferred through the joints while mobility is maintained, continence is preserved and respiration supported. Nonoptimal strategies result in loss of motion control (excessive shearing or translation) and giving way, and/or excessive bracing (rigidity) of the hips, low back and/or rib cage. These strategies often create excessive increases in intra-abdominal pressure (Thompson et al 2005), which can compromise urinary and/or fecal continence. In addition, nonoptimal respiratory patterns, rate and rhythm can develop.

With respect to the low back and pelvis, there has been considerable research regarding the function of some of the deeper stabilizing muscles such as transversus abdominis (TrA), multifidus, the diaphragm, and the pelvic floor. It is well recognized that, in health, these muscles behave in a feedforward manner when loads are predictable and that their activation is absent, delayed, or inappropriately timed in the presence of low back and pelvic girdle pain. Often, patients with failed load transfer present with inappropriate force closure in that certain muscles become overactive while others remain inactive, delayed, or asymmetric in their recruitment (Hungerford et al 2003). This change in motor control (altering timing) means that the system is not prepared for the loads which reach it and repetitive strains of the passive soft tissue can result.

Hodges & Richardson (1996, 1997) have shown that, in health, TrA is recruited prior to the initiation of any movement of the upper or lower extremity. Saunders et al (2004) found that TrA was tonically active through all phases of the gait cycle and only turned off when speeds of running were greater than 3 m/s and only during the non-weight-bearing phases of the gait cycle. Although it does not cross the SIJ directly, TrA can impact stiffness of the pelvis through its direct anterior attachments to the ilium as well as its attachment to the middle layer and the deep lamina of the posterior layer of the thoracodorsal fascia (Barker & Briggs 1999, Barker et al 2004). Richardson et al (2002) propose that contraction of the TrA produces a force that acts on the ilia perpendicular to the sagittal plane (i.e. approximates the ilia anteriorly). They also propose that the 'mechanical action of a pelvic belt in front of the abdominal wall at the level of the TrA corresponds with the action of this muscle.' Theoretically, compression of the anterior aspect of the pelvic girdle [compressing the anterior superior iliac spines (ASISs) towards one another] could simulate the force produced by contraction of this muscle.

In a study of patients with chronic low back pain, a timing delay was found in which TrA failed to anticipate the initiation of arm and/or leg motion (Hodges & Richardson 1997). This delayed activation of TrA could also mean that the thoracodorsal fascia is not sufficiently pre-tensed and the pelvis therefore not optimally compressed in preparation for external loading. Therefore, it is potentially vulnerable to the loss of intrinsic stability during functional tasks. Cowan et al (2004) have also shown that TrA activation is delayed in patients with longstanding groin pain.

Moseley et al (2002) have shown that the deep fibers of the multifidus muscle are recruited prior to the initiation of any movement of the upper extremity. In contrast, the superficial fibers of the multifidus muscle were shown to be direction dependent. However, in walking and running, Saunders et al (2004) found the deep fibers of multifidus to be phasically active and more direction dependent. This research suggests that stabilization of the spine/pelvis is more about timing of muscle activation as opposed to tonic versus phasic contraction of specific muscles or their anatomy.

Hides et al (1994) and Danneels et al (2000) have studied the response of multifidus in low back and pelvic girdle pain patients and note that multifidus becomes inhibited and reduced in size in these individuals. The normal 'pump-up' effect of multifidus on the thoracodorsal fascia, and therefore its ability to compress the pelvis, is lost when the size or function of this muscle is impaired.

Using the Doppler imaging system, Richardson et al (2002) note that when the subject was asked to 'hollow' their lower abdomen (produce a co-contraction of TrA and multifidus) the stiffness of the SIJ increased. These authors state that: 'Under gravitational load, it is the transversely oriented muscles that must act to compress the sacrum between the ilia and maintain stability of the SIJ.' Although multifidus is not oriented transversely both it and several other muscles (erector spinae, gluteus maximus, latissimus dorsi, internal oblique) can generate tension in the thoracodorsal fascia and thus impart compression to the posterior pelvis (Barker et al 2004). Van Wingerden et al (2004) also used the Doppler imaging system to analyze the effect of contraction of the biceps femoris, erector spinae, gluteus maximus, and latissiumus dorsi on compression of the SIJ. None of these muscles directly crosses the SIJ yet each was found to effect compression (increase stiffness) of the SIJ. Theoretically, compression of the posterior aspect of the pelvic girdle could simulate the forces produced by contraction of these muscles.

The muscles of the pelvic floor play a critical role in both stabilization of the pelvic girdle as well as in the maintenance of urinary and fecal continence (Ashton-Miller et al 2001, Barbic et al 2003, Bø & Stein 1994, Constantinou & Govan 1982, Deindl et al 1993, 1994, Sapsford et al 2001). Constantinou & Govan (1982) measured the intraurethral and intrabladder pressures in healthy continent women during the Valsalva maneuver and coughing and found that during a cough the pressure in the urethra increased approximately 250 ms before any pressure increase was detected in the bladder. This did not occur during a Valsalva (bearing down or straining). This suggests that an anticipatory reflex (feedforward activity) exists and that the pelvic floor functions as a stabilizer for the urethra.

Barbic et al (2003) measured pressure in both the bladder and urethra as well as the electromyographic (EMG) activity in the levator ani (intramuscular) during both a cough and Valsalva in two subject groups, continent and incontinent women. They note that in the healthy group, an anticipatory contraction of the levator ani occurred prior to any measurable pressure increase in either the bladder or the urethra. In the incontinent group, a timing delay and/or absence of contraction of the levator ani was found. Again, this suggests that motor control (sequencing and timing of muscular activation) plays a critical role in the ability to effectively force close the urethra during loading tasks. There is also evidence that in health, the pubococcygeus should co-contract with transversus abdominis (Sapsford et al 2001). This research suggests that certain muscles function as a unit and that co-contraction is an important component of optimal function.

It is now recognized that although individual muscles are important for regional stabilization as well as for mobility, it is critical to understand how they connect and function together. A muscle contraction produces a force that spreads beyond the origin and insertion of the active muscle. This force is transmitted to other muscles, tendons, fasciae, ligaments, capsules and bones that lie both in series and in parallel to the active muscle. In this manner, forces are produced quite distant from the origin of the initial muscle contraction. These integrated muscle systems produce slings of forces that assist in the transfer of load. A muscle can participate in more than one sling and the slings might overlap and interconnect depending on the task being demanded. The hypothesis is that the slings have no beginning or end but rather connect to assist in the transference of forces. It is possible that the slings are all part of one interconnected myofascial system and that the particular sling that is identified during any motion is merely due to the activation of selective parts of the whole sling.

The identification and treatment of a specific muscle dysfunction within any sling (inappropriate timing, insufficient strength, lack of endurance) is important when restoring stability while ensuring adequate mobility between the pelvic girdle, thorax and hips for the task at hand.

Emotions, pain, and motor control

Emotional states play a significant role in human function, including the function of the musculoskeletal system. Many patients with chronic lumbopelvic pain present with traumatized life experiences in addition to their functional complaints. Some of these patients adopt motor patterns indicative of defensive posturing (fight or flight reactions). Negative emotional states, such as fear, anxiety, and insecurity, can express themselves in maladaptive postures and lead to further strain on the musculoskeletal system. Stress is a normal response intended to energize our system for quick 'fight or flight' reactions. When this response is sustained, high levels of adrenaline (epinephrine) and cortisol remain in the system (Holstege et al 1996), in part due to circulating stress-related neuropeptides (Sapolsky et al 1997a, 1997b), which are released in anticipation of defensive or offensive behavior.

Emotional states are necessarily expressed through muscle action and when sustained, influence basic muscle tone and patterning (Holstege et al 1996). If the muscles of the lumbopelvic region become hypertonic, this could increase force closure and therefore stiffening of the SIJs. Excessive compression of the joints can perpetuate pain and cause peripheral and/or central sensitization of the nervous system (Butler 2000, Butler & Moseley 2003, Moseley & Hodges 2005). This can subsequently result in altered sensory interpretation as well as motor output and therefore create substantial barriers to rehabilitation. The increased sensitivity of the peripheral system reduces the kinematic margin for error, such that even slight motor control abnormalities (inappropriately timed muscle contractions) can drive the nociceptor pathways (Moseley & Hodges 2005). Clinically, these patients present with frequent flare-ups of their pain and are easily exacerbated with minor exercise progressions. Moseley & Hodges (2005) propose (in their threat response model) that cortically mediated modulators increase and maintain pain (perceived threat). These modulators include patients' beliefs pertaining to pain in general, as well as their past experience, stress, hypervigilance, and fear of reinjury or lack of recovery (Fig. 40.2). Clinically, these patients avoid activities, initially to avoid flare-ups of pain; however, the avoidance can persist due to their fear of reinjury or an underlying belief that they are unable to perform because of their condition (fear avoidance) (Vlayen & Linton 2000).

It is important to understand patients' emotional state and their belief systems because the resultant detrimental motor patterns can often only be changed by affecting the emotional state.

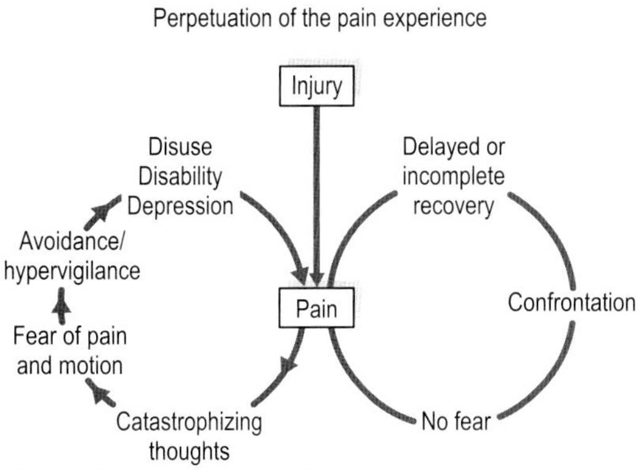

Fig. 40.2 Fear avoidance behavior can develop as a consequence of nonresolved pain. Patients require a program that addresses the emotional component of their experience and tools to take back control.

Sometimes it can be as simple as restoring hope through education (Butler & Moseley 2003), proper awareness of the underlying mechanical problem, and a clear understandable diagnosis. Other times, professional cognitive behavioral therapy is required to retrain more positive thought patterns.

The clinical diagnosis

Impaired pelvic function can be defined as an inability to optimally transfer forces through the pelvis. To reach this diagnosis, specific functional tests that analyze the ability of the pelvis to transfer load are required. To understand the precise cause for the impairment, specific tests that examine form closure, force closure, motor control, and the emotional state are required. Many of the tests often used clinically still require scrutiny for reliability, sensitivity and specificity for specific impairments of lumbopelvic function.

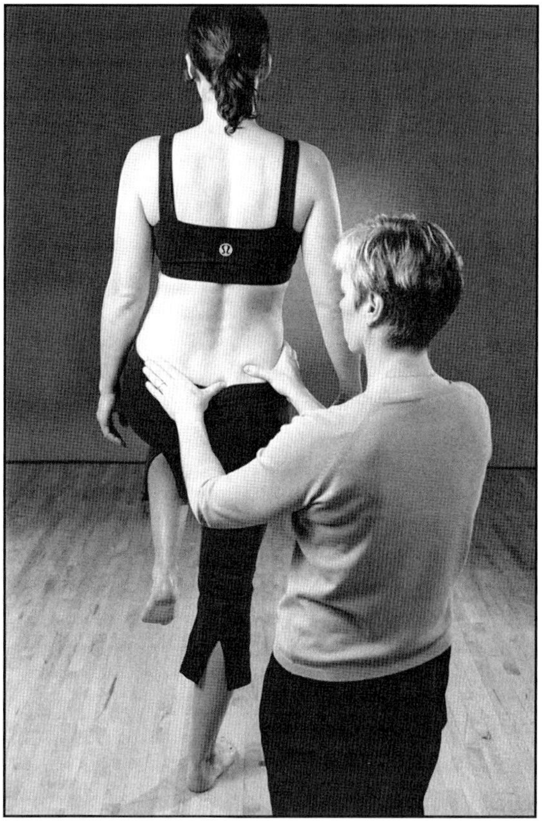

Fig. 40.3 The one leg standing or Stork test. The individual transfers weight through one leg and flexes the contralateral hip joint to approximately 90°. The innominates on both the non-weight-bearing and weight-bearing sides should posteriorly rotate relative to the sacrum (Hungerford et al 2004). Thus the sacroiliac joint remains in a self-locked position and loads are transferred through the pelvic girdle efficiently. (Reproduced with permission from Diane G. Lee Physiotherapist Corp ©.)

Functional tests of load transfer through the pelvis

One leg standing or Stork test

This test examines the ability of the patient to transfer load through the pelvis in standing. The patient is asked to stand on one leg and flex the contralateral hip (Fig. 40.3). During this task, the sacrum should nutate relative to the innominate on both the weight-bearing and non-weight-bearing sides (Hungerford et al 2004, Sturesson et al 2000). The load should be transferred to one leg smoothly and the pelvis should remain in its original coronal and transverse plane.

Hungerford et al (2004) investigated the pattern of innominate motion in both healthy (asymptomatic and functionally normal) and dysfunctional (symptomatic with signs of failed load transfer) groups during one leg standing. They found that in the healthy subjects, the innominate rotated posteriorly relative to the sacrum on both the weight-bearing and non-weight-bearing sides. In the dysfunctional group, they found that the innominate tended to *rotate anteriorly* relative to the sacrum on the weight-bearing side. This research suggests that the pattern of innominate motion may be a more relevant finding from this test and one which evaluates effective, or failed, load transfer.

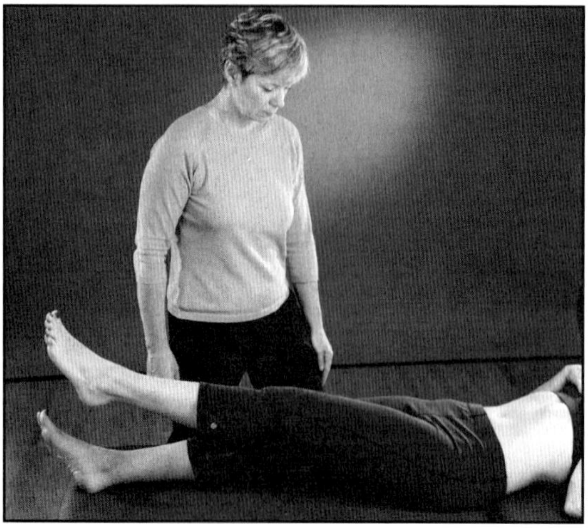

Fig. 40.4 Active straight leg raise test in a subject with excessive activation of the erector spinae causing the thorax to extend relative to the lumbar spine and pelvis. This subject has also lost the ability to control rotation of the pelvic girdle during this low load task (pelvis is left rotated). (Reproduced with permission from Diane G. Lee Physiotherapist Corp ©.)

The active straight leg raise test

The active straight leg raise test (ASLR) examines the ability of the patient to transfer load through the pelvis in supine lying and has been validated for reliability, sensitivity, and specificity for pelvic girdle pain (Mens et al 1999, 2001, 2002). It can also be used to identify nonoptimal stabilization strategies for load transfer through the pelvis in the supine position. The supine patient is asked to lift the extended leg 20 cm and to note any effort difference between the left and right leg (does one leg seem heavier or harder to lift). This is not a test for pain and the patient should only score the effort. The strategy used to stabilize the lumbopelvic region during this task is observed (Fig. 40.4). The leg should flex at the hip joint and the pelvis should not rotate, sidebend, flex, or extend relative to the lumbar spine. The rib cage should not draw in excessively (overactivation of the external oblique muscles), nor should the lower ribs flare out excessively (overactivation of the internal oblique muscles), nor should the abdomen bulge (breath holding – Valsalva). The pelvis is then compressed passively and the ASLR is repeated; any change in effort is noted. The location of the compression can be varied (anterior, posterior, oblique) to determine where more compression (force closure) is needed for optimal load transfer (Fig. 40.5) (Lee 2004).

Further specific tests are necessary to determine why the pelvic girdle is unable to sustain and transfer loads in patients with pelvic girdle pain. The tests include those for form closure (passive articular mobility and stability) and force closure/motor control analysis; essential for developing prescriptive management protocols that are specific to the patient's impairment.

Tests for form closure: neutral and elastic zone analysis

According to the European guidelines on the diagnosis and treatment of pelvic girdle pain:

> *Nonoptimal joint stability implicates altered laxity/stiffness values leading to increased joint translations resulting in a new joint position and/or exaggerated/reduced joint compression, with a disturbed performance/effort ratio. (Vleeming et al 2004)*

Therefore tests are required to determine if an individual has 'increased SIJ translations' and further tests are needed to determine if the laxity is due to impairment of the passive or active/control systems. With respect to the SIJ, the amplitude and resistance to motion should be symmetric in both the anteroposterior and craniocaudal planes (Buyruk et al 1995b, Damen et al 2001).

The neutral zone (Fig. 40.6) for anteroposterior and/or craniocaudal translation of the innominate relative to the sacrum is analyzed by comparing the sense of ease with which the innominate glides in a parallel manner relative to the sacrum until the point of first resistance (R1: Fig. 40.6) (Lee 1992, 2004). The elastic zone for anteroposterior and/or craniocaudal translation is analyzed from the point of first resistance (R1) to the end of the available motion (R2) and the quality of the resistance as well as the provocation of any pain or muscle spasm are noted. A judgment regarding the *amplitude of motion* (hypomobile, hypermobile, normal) should not be made because it has been shown that the SIJ range of motion is highly variable (Buyruk et al 1995b). Instead, the symmetry of resistance in each plane and in each zone (neutral and elastic) should be analyzed. The SIJ is then passively taken into the close-packed position (the sacrum is nutated while the innominate is simultaneously posteriorly rotated) and the translations are repeated. When the form closure mechanism is intact and the passive elements are healthy, no translation of the joint

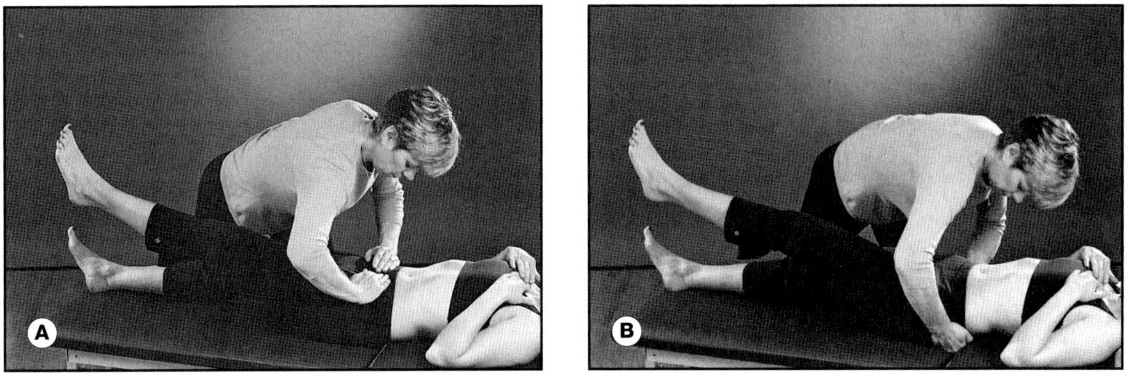

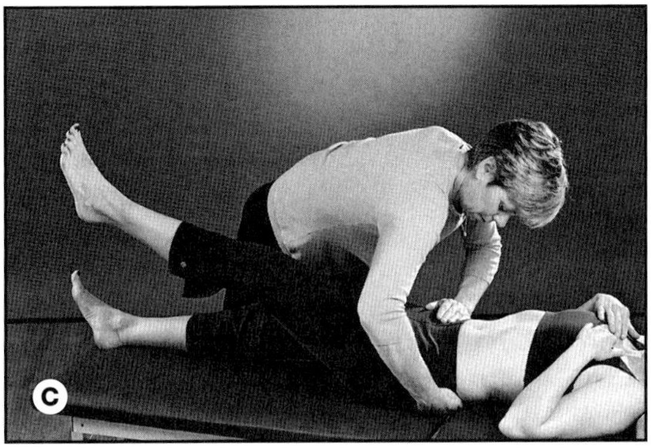

Fig. 40.5 Compression can be applied to the pelvic girdle bilaterally anteriorly, posteriorly, or obliquely to determine exactly where more compression facilitates optimal load transfer. The examiner observes the effort required to initiate a leg lift with and without the various compressions and correlates the findings to the patient's subjective response (score of the effort). (Reproduced with permission from Diane G. Lee Physiotherapist Corp ©.)

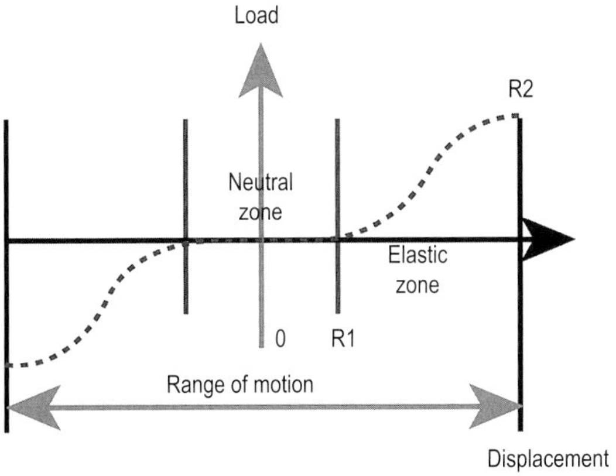

Fig. 40.6 The zones of articular motion: the neutral zone (0–R1) and the elastic zone (R1–R2) (Panjabi 1992). The neutral zone is a small region of the joint's range (in the center) where minimal resistance is given by the passive elements. The elastic zone is the region towards the end of the range of motion where a nonlinear increase to resistance occurs as the joint capsule and ligaments become progressively taut.

should occur in the close-packed, stable position. If there is increased laxity when the SIJ is in a neutral position, and stability (no translation) in the close-packed position, this suggests that the force closure or motor control system is impaired and that there is insufficient (or at least asymmetric) compression of the SIJ in neutral. Further tests are required to determine the specific deficit in the motor control system.

Tests for force closure and motor control

Richardson et al (2002) confirmed that a co-contraction of the TrA and multifidus can increase the stiffness of the SIJ. Sapsford et al (2001) noted that in healthy subjects the pelvic floor muscles co-contracted with TrA. Therefore, the ability of an individual to co-contract the TrA and the multifidus can be assessed by providing a verbal cue that results in a contraction of the pelvic floor. Real-time ultrasound imaging (Bø et al 2003, O'Sullivan et al 2003, Whittaker 2004) or internal pelvic floor examination should be used to confirm that the pelvic floor is contracting because a poor response to a verbal cue has been noted (Bump et al 1991, Thompson & O'Sullivan 2003).

To assess the ability of the left and right TrA to co-contract in response to a pelvic floor cue, the abdomen is palpated just medial to the ASISs bilaterally and the patient is instructed to gently squeeze the muscles around the urethra or to lift the vagina/testicles. When a bilateral contraction of TrA is achieved in isolation from the internal oblique, a deep tensioning will be felt symmetrically and the lower abdomen will flatten (hollow) (Richardson et al 1999).

The deep fibers of multifidus are palpated bilaterally close to the spinous processes or the median sacral crest. In a healthy system, a cue to contract the pelvic floor should result in a co-contraction of the deep fibers of multifidus. When a bilateral contraction of deep multifidus is achieved the muscle can be felt to swell symmetrically beneath the fingers (Richardson et al 1999). There should be no evidence of substitution from the multisegmental fibers of the multifidus, which will produce extension of the lumbar spine and a phasic bulge of the substituting muscle.

When the force closure mechanism is effective, co-contraction of these deep muscles should compress the joints of the lumbar spine (Hodges et al 2003b) and the SIJs (Richardson et al 2002) thereby increasing stiffness. To test the ability of the active force closure mechanism to sufficiently control motion in the neutral zone of the lumbar or pelvic joints, the patient is first instructed to co-contract the deep muscles. The form closure tests for neutral zone analysis (joint glides) are repeated while the patient maintains a gentle co-contraction. The joint stiffness should increase and no translation should occur even though the joint is in a neutral position. This means that an adequate amount of compression has occurred and that the force closure mechanism is effective for the amount of load being applied.

The previous tests for form closure analysis and the impact of optimal force closure still require scientific scrutiny for validity, sensitivity and specificity for impaired function of the lumbopelvic complex.

The management of pelvic impairment

Effective management of a patient with pelvic girdle pain first requires an understanding of the patient's specific impairment. Clinically, the patient might present with areas that are under too much compression and others that are under too little; in short, inappropriate force closure. The restoration of optimal function requires skills for releasing the joints as well as the ability to prescribe an exercise program for both motor control and muscle capacity according to the patient's needs/desires.

Excessive articular compression can be due to factors that are either intrinsic or extrinsic to the joint; both impact the neutral zone of motion. Panjabi (1992) notes that joints have nonlinear load–displacement curves, which results in a high degree of laxity in the neutral zone and a stiffening effect toward the end of the range of motion. He found that the size of the neutral zone can increase with injury, articular degeneration, and/or weakness of the stabilizing musculature and that this is a more sensitive indicator than angular range of motion for detecting instability. He used a ball and bowl illustration to represent this change in the neutral zone. Lee & Vleeming (1998) suggest that the neutral zone is not only affected quantitatively (bigger or smaller), but also qualitatively (more or less resistance) when compression is increased or decreased across the joint (Fig. 40.7). Consequently, motion of the SIJ can either be restricted (too much compression) or poorly controlled (too little compression) by both articular and myofascial factors. It is important to understand the cause of excessive/insufficient compression so that treatment protocols can be specific to the patient's impairment.

The next section describes some common clinical presentations for dysfunction of the SIJ and an integrated therapeutic approach for clinical management.

Excessive compression of the SIJ

Excessive compression of the SIJ can be the result of inflammatory pathology such as ankylosing spondylitis or due to fibrosis of the capsule secondary to trauma (Fig. 40.7C). These are intrinsic articular causes of excessive compression of the SIJ. The joint can also be compressed by overactivation of certain lumbopelvic muscles; extrinsic causes (Fig. 40.7D). When an individual habitually uses the piriformis, ischiococcygeus, and/or the erector spinae as a strategy for stabilization, the constant activation of these muscles can excessively compress the SIJ. In both instances (articular or myofascial), the stiffness of the SIJ is increased and the following is found on clinical examination. In the one leg

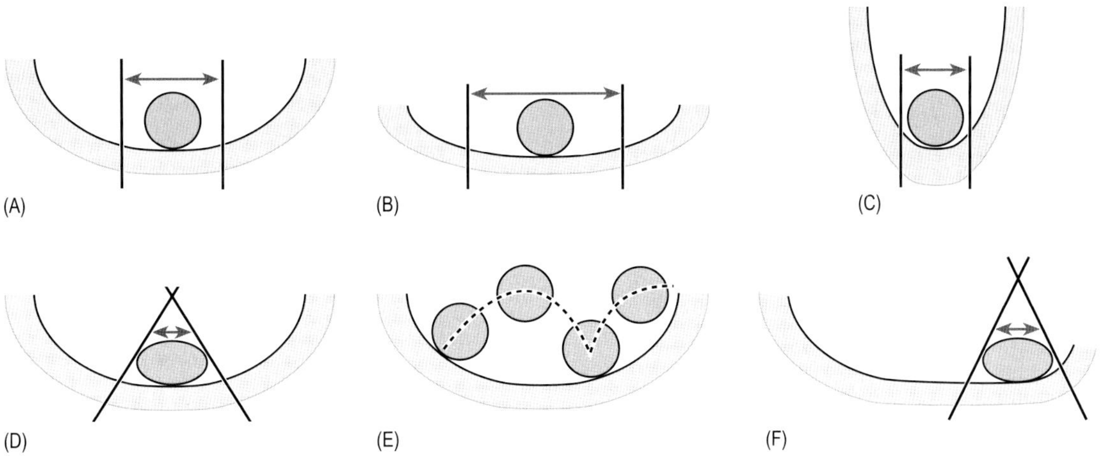

Fig. 40.7 The ball and bowl concept was introduced by Panjabi (1992) to represent differences in neutral zone motion. The distance the ball can roll represents the amplitude of the neutral zone of motion under varying conditions. The neutral zone can be affected by altering compression across the joint. (A) A graphic illustration of the neutral zone of motion in a hypothetically normal joint. (B) A joint that is insufficiently compressed due to the loss of either ligamentous (form closure) or myofascial (force closure) function will have a relative increase in the neutral zone of motion. (C) A joint that is excessively compressed due to fibrosis (or ankylosis) will have a relative decrease in the neutral zone of motion. (D) A joint that is excessively compressed due to sustained overactivation of certain muscles will also have a relative decrease in the neutral zone of motion. (E). When there is an intermittent motor control deficit, the neutral zone might be within normal limits because this is a dynamic intermittent impairment. (F) A joint that is 'fixated' is often excessively compressed with the joint held at one end of its available range of motion and no neutral zone exists – this is a complete joint block.

standing or Stork test the patient has no difficulty transferring load through the pelvic girdle if the SIJ is stiff; however, load transfer is often negatively affected when the problem is poor motor control (excessive compression due to myofascial causes). In both instances (stiff joint versus myofascial compression), the ASLR test reveals poor pelvic position control and more effort is usually required to lift the leg on the compressed/stiff side. Adding more compression to the pelvis rarely facilitates elevation of the leg since the pelvis is already overly compressed. When the problem is unilateral, the stiff joint has a decreased neutral zone of motion and a greater resistance to translation evident during the mobility/stability tests.

A fused SIJ cannot be mobilized with manual therapy techniques however; the fibrosed joint is easily mobilized in one or two treatments when specific, localized, passive techniques are used (DonTigny 1990, Hartman 1997, Lee 2004). Manual therapy is an essential part of the treatment for this individual. The SIJ that is excessively compressed due to imbalances in the muscle system requires a more comprehensive treatment protocol. Although manual therapy techniques can assist in relieving the compression, the impaired pattern is likely to recur unless the motor control strategy for stabilization is addressed. This individual would require a multimodal therapeutic approach including mobilization as well as exercises and education for long-term results.

Excessive compression of the SIJ with an underlying instability

When a force is applied to the SIJ sufficient to attenuate the articular ligaments (fall on the buttocks or a lift/twist injury), the muscles will respond to prevent dislocation and further trauma to the joint. The resulting spasm may fix the joint in an abnormal resting position (Fig. 40.7F) and marked asymmetry of the pelvic girdle (innominate and/or sacrum) can be present. This is an unstable joint under excessive compression. It commonly occurs unilaterally and presents with the following findings. The patient has marked difficulty standing on one leg and in the acute phase of the injury is often reluctant to do so. The ASLR test reveals poor pelvic position control and the patient frequently cannot lift the leg at all. There is no improvement in function (still cannot lift the leg) when compression is applied to the pelvis; in fact this often makes the

ASLR test worse. When the problem is unilateral, the SIJ is excessively compressed and no palpable motion can be found.

Treatment of this individual which focuses on exercise without first addressing the 'posture,' 'position,' or alignment' of the pelvis, tends to be ineffective and commonly increases symptoms. Conversely, if treatment only includes manual therapy (mobilization, manipulation, or muscle energy) for correction of 'posture,' 'position,' or 'alignment,' relief tends to be temporary and dependence on the healthcare practitioner providing the manual correction is common. This impairment requires a multimodal therapeutic approach to management which includes manual therapy to decompress and align the pelvic girdle followed by exercises and education for restoring optimal motor control, strength and endurance for functional tasks.

Insufficient compression of the sacroiliac joint

This pelvic impairment arises when there is either inadequate or inappropriate motor control such that there is insufficient compression of the SIJ during movement and loading (Fig. 40.7B,E). The patient often complains of sensations of giving way or a lack of trust when loading through the involved extremity. The following findings are noted on clinical examination: during one leg standing, or Stork test, the patient has difficulty transferring load through the dysfunctional side and the innominate anteriorly rotates as they attempt to do so (Hungerford et al 2004). The ASLR test reveals poor pelvic position control and is often associated with a dysfunctional motor control strategy for lumbopelvic stabilization. Function improves (decreased effort to lift the leg) when passive compression is applied (Mens et al 1999, 2001, 2002) to the anterior and/or posterior aspect of the pelvis (Lee 2004). The location of compression [bilaterally anterior, bilaterally posterior, oblique (unilateral anterior and unilateral posterior)], which results in decreased effort to lift the leg, assists the clinician in prescribing exercises for restoring motor control. The response of the deep muscles (TrA, deep multifudus) to a pelvic floor cue, combined with real-time ultrasound assessment, confirm the pattern of the motor control deficit. A variety of patterns will be found clinically (Lee 2004, O'Sullivan et al 2002, Richardson et al 1999).

Treatment for this pelvic impairment requires the restoration of both motor control and muscle capacity (strength/endurance) with specific exercises that initially train an optimal recruitment strategy for compression of the pelvic girdle, followed by exercises which challenge loads in functional tasks. The temporary application of a sacroiliac belt can be used to augment force closure during this stage of rehabilitation (Damen et al 2002c, 2002d, Vleeming et al 1992b).

Recent research has increased our understanding of muscle and joint function and consequently changed the way exercises for back pain and dysfunction are prescribed (Bergmark 1989, Bullock-Saxton et al 1993, Comerford & Mottram 2001, Danneels et al 2000, Hides et al 1994, 1996, Hodges 1997, 2003, Hodges & Richardson 1996, 1997, Hodges et al 2003, McGill 2002, Moseley 2002, Moseley et al 2002, O'Sullivan at al 1997, Richardson & Jull 1995, Richardson et al 1999, 2004, Stuge et al 2004). New concepts of how joints are stabilized and how load is transferred through the body highlight the importance of proprioception, automatic muscle activity, and motor control for regaining optimal movement after injury. It is clear from this body of evidence that successful rehabilitation of back and pelvic girdle pain and dysfunction requires exercises that differ from those used for conditioning and training the healthy, nonpainful population (Fig. 40.8, Lee & Lee 2004a, 2004b).

When planning injury rehabilitation, exercises should be prescribed as part of an integrated treatment plan, not as a standalone treatment. If exercise is prescribed without first restoring joint mobility (form closure), the patient's pain and dysfunction often get worse. This might lead to the conclusion that certain exercises are 'bad' or 'unsuccessful' for treating back pain, when it may merely be a problem of *inappropriately timed* exercise intervention.

Similarly, the *type* of exercise prescribed is of utmost importance. For lumbopelvic pain, the evidence cited above supports initially correcting deficits in motor control prior to focusing on strength and power of individual muscles. One randomized, controlled trial on a subgroup of pelvic girdle pain patients (insufficient compression after pregnancy) has shown efficacy with this approach to exercise intervention (Stuge et al 2004). In this trial considerable attention was paid to *how* the exercises were performed and each patient's program was specific to their needs. Patients who go mindlessly through a routine of exercises often have limited success in retraining motor patterns and can get worse with exercise if poor patterns and control are reinforced as this may result in irritation of joint structures and symptom exacerbation. The

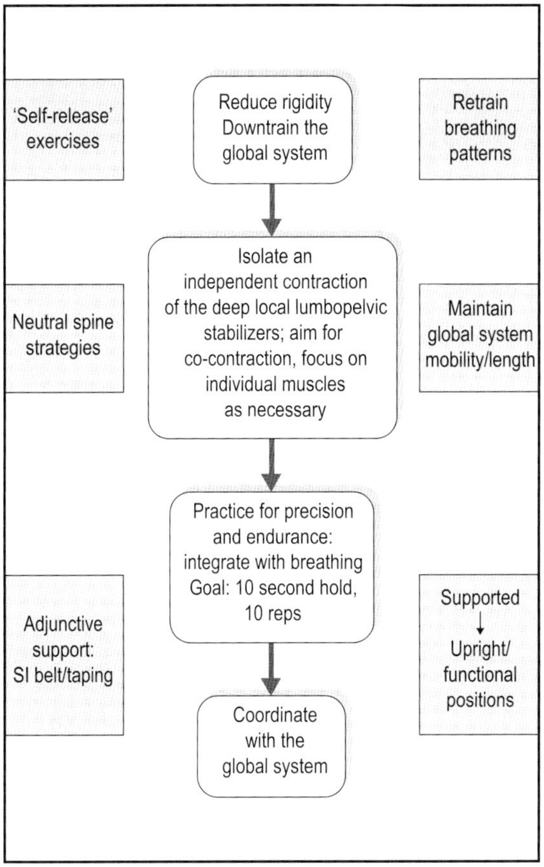

Fig. 40.8 Program for stabilization of the lumbar spine and pelvis. (From Lee & Lee 2004a, 2004b.)

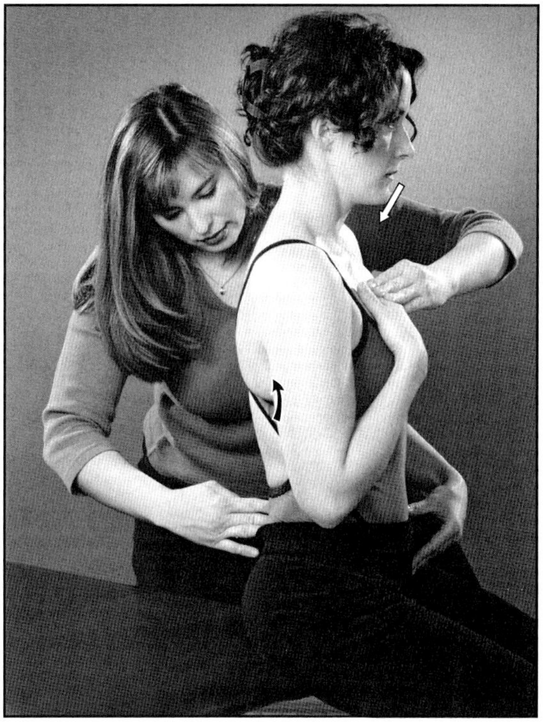

Fig. 40.9 Neutral spine in sitting. The therapist is correcting the following maladaptive posture: a flattened thoracic kyphosis, a decreased lumbar lordosis at L5–S1 and L4–L5 and a posterior pelvic tilt. The therapist's left hand helps the patient create a release of the sternum (think about sinking or softening) to facilitate an increase in the thoracic kyphosis in the upper thoracic spine and to bring the rib cage vertical over the pelvis. The therapist's right hand produces a gentle cranial and anterior pressure through the lumbar spinous processes to facilitate nutation of the sacrum and the restoration of a lumbar lordosis at L5–S1 and L4–L5 (only to neutral). In addition, this pelvic posture results in anterior tilting of the pelvis under the rib cage. Optimally the center of gravity falls midway between the pubic symphysis and the coccyx (Lee & Lee 2004a, 2004b). (Reproduced with permission from Diane G. Lee Physiotherapist Corp ©.)

problem is often not *which* exercise was prescribed, but *how* the exercise was performed.

The goal is to retrain strategies of muscular patterning such that load transfer is optimized through all joints of the kinetic chain. Optimal load transfer occurs when there is precise modulation of force, coordination, and timing of specific muscle contractions, ensuring control of the neutral zone for each joint (segmental control), the orientation of the spine (spinal curvatures, thorax on pelvic girdle, pelvis in relation to the lower extremity), and the control of postural equilibrium with respect to the environment (Hodges 2003). The result is stability with mobility, where there is stability without rigidity of posture, without episodes of collapse, and with fluidity of movement. Optimal coordination of the myofascial system will produce optimal stabilization strategies. These patients will have the ability to:

- find and maintain control of neutral spinal alignment both in the lumbopelvic region and in relationship to the thorax and hip (Fig. 40.9)
- consciously recruit and maintain a tonic, isolated contraction of the deep stabilizers of the lumbopelvis to ensure segmental control (control of the neutral zone) (Fig. 40.10) and then to maintain this contraction during loading (Fig. 40.11)
- move in and out of neutral spine (flex, extend, laterally bend, rotate) without segmental or regional collapse (Fig. 40.12)

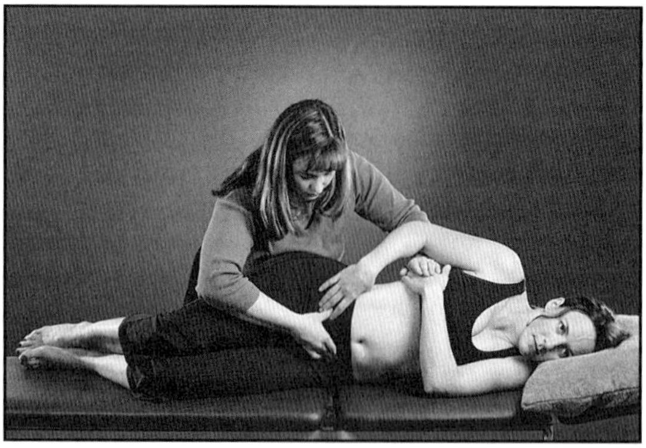

Fig. 40.10 Facilitation of transversus abdominis (TrA): sidelying position. The patient lies in a neutral spinal posture and is given a cue to activate the TrA (abdominal drawing in or activating the pelvic floor, etc.). The response to these verbal cues is palpated by both the therapist and the patient. The rib cage is monitored to prevent breath holding during the exercise session (Lee & Lee 2004a, 2004b). (Reproduced with permission from Diane G. Lee Physiotherapist Corp ©.)

- maintain all the above in coordination with the thorax and the extremities in functional, work-specific and sport-specific postures and movements (Fig. 40.13).

Treating the emotional component

The patient's emotional state can maintain a detrimental motor pattern and prevent a successful outcome. Anxiety regarding their current physical status and the future can be relieved with an explanation of the possible causal factors (Butler & Moseley 2003, Moseley 2002, 2003a, 2003b, Moseley & Hodges 2005). Restoring hope by providing a patient-specific treatment plan is often motivational and helps to build trust. When positive changes in function occur, the treatment plan is reinforced and this builds commitment. In the end, it is critical to teach people to accept responsibility for their health through education and motivation.

Summary

It has long been recognized that physical factors impact joint motion. The integrated therapeutic model presented here suggests that joint mechanics are influenced by multiple factors, some intrinsic to the joint itself while others are produced by

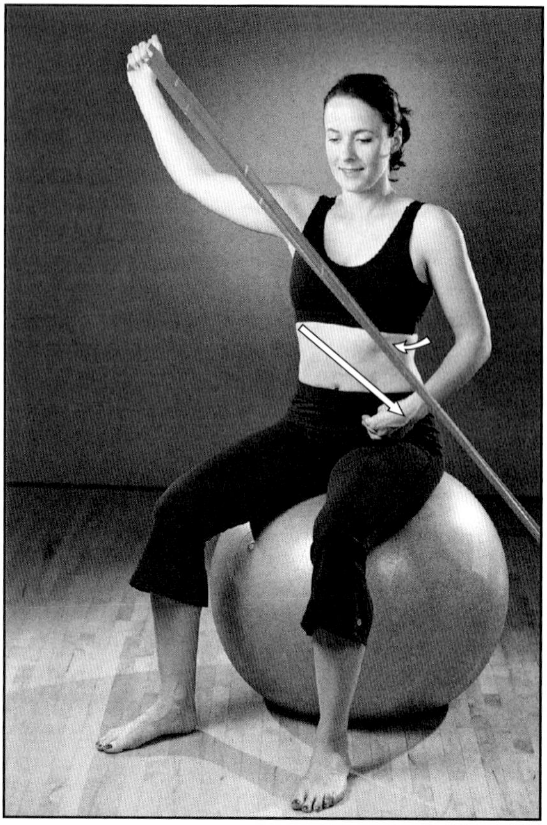

Fig. 40.11 Maintaining neutral spine with loading: unilateral flexion diagonal (combined extension and rotation control). The patient monitors contraction of the left transversus abdominis (TrA) throughout the exercise. The right hand starts just lateral to the left hip and then pulls against the resistive exercise band diagonally into flexion and abduction to the end position as shown. Note that there is a loss of the neutral position of the thorax over the pelvis into thoracolumbar extension and right rotation (short arrow). This should be corrected with a cue to connect the right rib cage to the left hand (diagonal arrow) (Lee & Lee 2004a, 2004b). (Reproduced with permission from Diane G. Lee Physiotherapist Corp ©.)

muscle action which in turn is influenced by the emotional state. More studies are required which identify subgroups of patients with pelvic girdle pain according to specific impairments recognizing that all patients with pelvic girdle pain do not have the same impairments. We need to develop more diagnostic tests relevant to motion and load transfer for both the SIJ and the pubic symphysis and then to test them for reliability, sensitivity and specificity for pelvic girdle pain. Only then will we have the ability to develop more sound studies (randomized and controlled) to test the efficacy of treatment

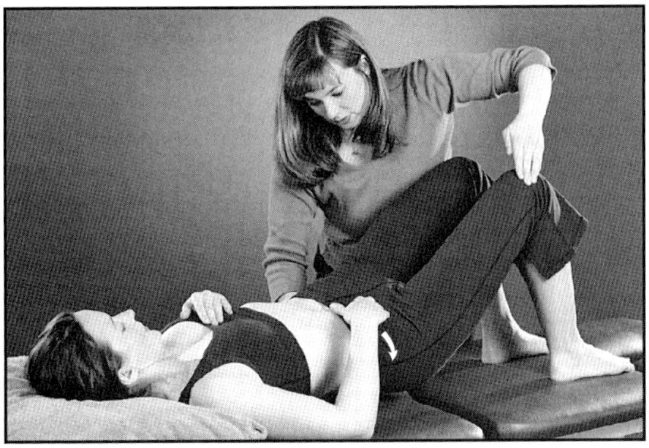

Fig. 40.12 Moving out of neutral spine: thoracopelvic control. Bridge and rotate. From neutral spine in a bridge position, the patient is rotating the pelvis to the right (arrow) while maintaining the thoracic position. The therapist cues control of the right femur in neutral alignment and palpates the lumbar multifidus. The pelvis returns to neutral by 'pulling the left ASIS back' (Lee & Lee 2004a, 2004b). (Reproduced with permission from Diane G. Lee Physiotherapist Corp ©.)

programs that are specific to each subgroup of impairment which leads to pelvic girdle pain. Until then, the best evidence-based treatment will be to use a multimodal approach which considers the biomechanical, neuromuscular and emotional needs of the patient with pelvic girdle pain.

This chapter has briefly outlined the principles for management of the articular (form closure) and muscular (force closure and motor control) factors which impact function of the SIJ and consequently the ability of the pelvic girdle to transfer load. The effective management of pelvic girdle pain and dysfunction requires attention to all four components – form closure, force closure, motor control, and emotions – with the ultimate goal being to guide patients towards a healthier way to live in their bodies.

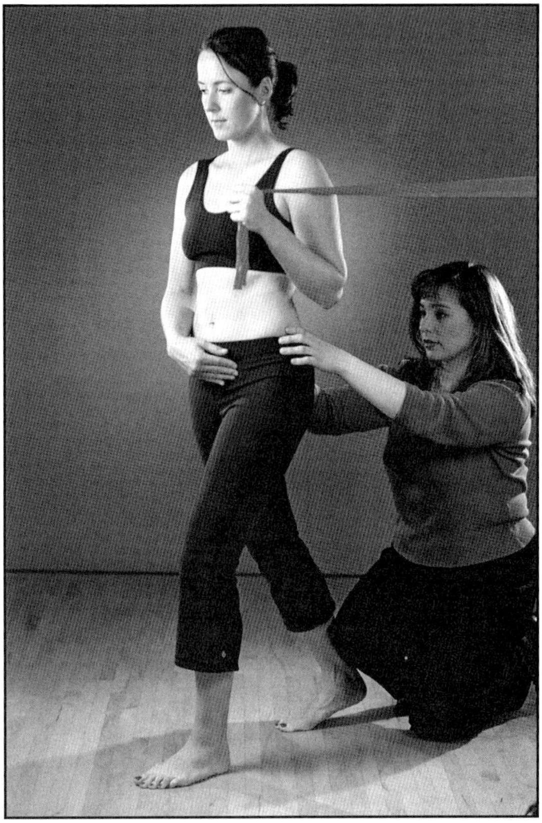

Fig. 40.13 A functional integration exercise: forward lunge against a resistive exercise band. As the lunge is performed the patient is cued to maintain the neutral spinal position and not allow rotation towards the band. This trains isometric control through the anterior oblique slings (against rotation and extension). In this example the therapist is palpating the left innominate and sacrum to ensure control of the left sacroiliac joint during the movement (Lee & Lee 2004a, 2004b). (Reproduced with permission from Diane G. Lee Physiotherapist Corp ©.)

References

Ashton-Miller JA, Howard D, DeLancey JOL 2001 The functional anatomy of the female pelvic floor and stress continence control system. Scandinavian Journal of Urology and Nephrology (suppl 207):1–7

Barbic M, Kralj B, Cor A 2003 Compliance of the bladder neck supporting structures: importance of activity pattern of levator ani muscle and content of elastic fibers of endopelvic fascia. Neurourology and Urodynamics 22:269

Barker PJ, Briggs CA 1999 Attachments of the posterior layer of the lumbar fascia. Spine 24(17):1757–1764

Barker PJ, Briggs CA, Bogeski G 2004 Tensile transmission across the lumbar fascia in unembalmed cadavers. Spine 29(2):129

Bergmark A 1989 Stability of the lumbar spine. A study in mechanical engineering. Acta Orthopedica Scandinavia 230 (60):20–24

Bø K, Stein R 1994 Needle EMG registration of striated urethral wall and pelvic floor muscle activity patterns during cough, valsalva, abdominal, hip adductor, and gluteal muscles contractions in nulliparous healthy females. Neurourology and Urodynamics 13:35–41

Bø K, Sherburn M, Allen T 2003 Transabdominal ultrasound measurement of pelvic floor muscle activity when activated directly or via a transversus abdominis muscle contraction. Neurourology and Urodynamics 22:582–588

Bowen V, Cassidy JD 1981 Macroscopic and microscopic anatomy of the sacroiliac joint from embryonic life until the eighth decade. Spine 6:620–628

Bullock-Saxton JE, Janda V, Bullock MI 1993 Reflex activation of gluteal muscles in walking: an approach to restoration of muscle function for patients with low back pain. Spine 18(6):704

Bump RC, Hurt GW, Fantl JA, Wyman JF 1991 Assessment of Kegal pelvic muscle exercise performance after brief verbal instruction. American Journal of Obstetrics and Gynecology 165:322

Butler D 2000 The sensitive nervous system. NOI Group, Adelaide, Australia

Butler D, Moseley GL 2003 Explain pain. NOI Group, Adelaide, Australia

Buyruk HM, Stam HJ, Snijders CJ et al 1995a The use of colour Doppler imaging for the assessment of sacroiliac joint stiffness: a study on embalmed human pelvises. European Journal of Radiology 21:112–116

Buyruk HM, Snijders CJ, Vleeming A et al 1995b The measurements of sacroiliac joint stiffness with colour Doppler imaging: a study on healthy subjects. European Journal of Radiology 21:117–121

Buyruk HM, Stam HJ, Snijders CJ et al 1997 Measurement of sacroiliac joint stiffness with color doppler imaging and the importance of asymmetric stiffness in sacroiliac pathology. In: Vleeming A et al (eds) Movement, stability and low back pain. Churchill Livingstone, Edinburgh

Buyruk HM, Stam HJ, Snijders CJ et al 1999 Measurement of sacroiliac joint stiffness in peripartum pelvic pain patients with Doppler imaging of vibrations (DIV). European Journal Obstetrics Gynecological Reproduction Biology 83(2):159–163

Carmichael JP 1987 Inter and intra examiner reliability of palpation for sacroiliac joint dysfunction. Journal Manipulative Physical Therapy 10(4):164–171

Comerford MJ, Mottram SL 2001 Movement and stability dysfunction – contemporary developments. Manual Therapy 6(1):15

Constantinou CE, Govan DE 1982 Spatial distribution and timing of transmitted and reflexly generated urethral pressures in healthy women. Journal of Urology 127:964–969

Cowan SM, Schache AG, Bennell KL et al 2004 Delayed onset of transversus abdominus in long-standing groin pain. Medicine and Science in Sports and Exercise December:2040–2045

Damen L, Buyruk HM, Guler-Uysal F et al 2001 Pelvic pain during pregnancy is associated with asymmetric laxity of the sacroiliac joints. Acta Obstetrica Gynecologica Scandinavica 80:1019

Damen L, Stijnen T, Roebroeck ME et al 2002a Reliability of sacroiliac joint laxity measurement with Doppler imaging of vibrations. Ultrasound in Medicine and Biology 28:407

Damen L, Buyruk HM, Guler-Uysal F et al 2002b Prognostic value of asymmetric laxity of the sacroiliac joints in pregnancy-related pelvic pain. Spine 27(24):2820

Damen L, Spoor CW, Snijders CJ, Stam HJ 2002c Does a pelvic belt influence sacroiliac joint laxity? Clinical Biomechanics 17(7):495

Damen L, Mens JMA, Snijders CJ, Stam JH 2002d The mechanical effects of a pelvic belt in patients with pregnancy-related pelvic pain. PhD thesis, Erasmus University, Rotterdam, the Netherlands

Danneels LA, Vanderstraeten GG, Cambier DC et al 2000 CT imaging of trunk muscles in chronic low back pain patients and healthy control subjects. European Spine 9(4):266–272

Deindl FM, Vodusek DB, Hesse U, Schussler B 1993 Activity patterns of pubococcygeal muscles in nulliparous continent women. British Journal of Urology 72:46

Deindl FM, Vodusek DB, Hesse U, Schussler B 1994 Pelvic floor activity patterns: comparison of nulliparous continent and parous urinary stress incontinent women. A kinesiological EMG study. British Journal of Urology 73:413

DonTigny RL 1990 Anterior dysfunction of the sacroiliac joint as a major factor in the etiology of idiopathic low back pain syndrome. Physical Therapy 70:250

Dreyfuss P, Dreyer S, Griffin J et al 1994 Positive sacroiliac screening tests in asymptomatic adults. Spine 19: 1138–1143

Dreyfuss P, Michaelsen M, Pauza D et al 1996 The value of history and physical examination in diagnosing sacroiliac joint pain. Spine 21:2594–2602

Egund N, Olsson TH, Schmid H 1978 Movements in the sacro-iliac joints demonstrated with roentgen stereophotogrammetry. Acta Radiologica 19:833–846

Hartman L 1997 Handbook of osteopathic technique, 3rd edn. Chapman & Hall, London

Herzog W, Read L, Conway PJW et al 1989 Reliability of motion palpation procedures to detect sacroiliac joint fixations. Journal Manipulative Physical Therapy 12(2):86–92

Hides JA, Stokes MJ, Saide M et al 1994 Evidence of lumbar multifidus muscles wasting ipsilateral to symptoms in patients with acute/subacute low back pain. Spine 19(2):165–177

Hides JA, Richardson CA, Jull GA 1996 Multifidus recovery is not automatic following resolution of acute first episode low back pain. Spine 21(23):2763–2769

Hodges PW 1997 Feedforward contraction of transversus abdominis is not influenced by the direction of arm movement. Experimental Brain Research 114:362–370

Hodges PW 2003 Core stability exercise in chronic low back pain. Orthopaedic Clinics of North America 34:245

Hodges PW, Gandevia SC 2000a Changes in intra-abdominal pressure during postural and respiratory activation of the human diaphragm. Journal Applied Physiology 89:967–976

Hodges PW, Gandevia SC 2000b Activation of the human diaphragm during a repetitive postural task. Journal of Physiology 522(1):165

Hodges PW, Moseley GL 2003 Pain and motor control of the lumbopelvic region: effect and possible mechanisms. Journal of Electromyography and Kinesiology 13:361

Hodges PW, Richardson CA 1996 Inefficient muscular

stabilization of the lumbar spine associated with low back pain. A motor control evaluation of transversus abdominis. Spine 21(22):2640–2650

Hodges PW, Richardson CA 1997 Contraction of the abdominal muscles associated with movement of the lower limb. Physical Therapy 77:132–144

Hodges PW, Kaigle Holm A, Holm S et al 2003 Intervertebral stiffness of the spine is increased by evoked contraction of transversus abdominis and the diaphragm: in vivo porcine studies. Spine 28(23):2594

Holstege G, Bandler R, Saper CB 1996 The emotional motor system. Elsevier Science, Edinburgh

Hungerford B, Gilleard W, Hodges PW 2003 Evidence of altered lumbopelvic muscle recruitment in the presence of sacroiliac joint pain. Spine 28(14):1593

Hungerford B, Gilleard W, Lee D 2004 Alteration of pelvic bone motion determined in subjects with posterior pelvic pain using skin markers. Clinical Biomechanics (19):456

Jacob HAC, Kissling RO 1995 The mobility of the sacroiliac joints in healthy volunteers between 20 and 50 years of age. Clinical Biomechanics 10(7):352–361

Laslett M, Williams W 1994 The reliability of selected pain provocation tests for sacroiliac joint pathology. Spine 19(11):1243–1249

Lavignolle B, Vital JM, Senegas J et al 1983 An approach to the functional anatomy of the sacroiliac joints in vivo. Anatomica Clinica 5:169–176

Lee DG 1992 Intra-articular versus extra-articular dysfunction of the sacroiliac joint – a method of differentiation. IFOMT Proceedings, Fifth International Conference. Vail, CO, p69

Lee DG 2004 The pelvic girdle, 3rd edn. Elsevier Science, Edinburgh

Lee DG, Lee LJ 2004a An integrated approach to the assessment and treatment of the lumbopelvic–hip region. DVD. Online. Available: http://www.dianelee.ca

Lee LJ, Lee DG 2004b Treating the lumbopelvic–hip dysfunction. In: Lee DG (ed) The pelvic girdle. Elsevier Science, Edinburgh

Lee DG, Vleeming A 1998 Impaired load transfer through the pelvic girdle – a new model of altered neutral zone function. In: Proceedings from the 3rd Interdisciplinary World Congress on Low Back and Pelvic Pain. Vienna, Austria

McGill S 2002 Low back disorders – evidence-based prevention and rehabilitation. Human Kinetics Publishers, Champaign, IL

Mens JMA, Vleeming A, Snijders CJ et al 1999 The active straight leg raising test and mobility of the pelvic joints. European Spine 8:468–473

Mens JMA, Vleeming A, Snijders CJ et al 2001 Reliability and validity of the active straight leg raise test in posterior pelvic pain since pregnancy. Spine 26(10): 1167–1171

Mens JMA, Vleeming A, Snijders CJ et al 2002 Validity of the active straight leg raise test for measuring disease severity in patients with posterior pelvic pain after pregnancy. Spine 27(2):196

Moseley GL 2002 Combined physiotherapy and education is efficacious for chronic low back pain. Australian Journal of Physiotherapy 48:297

Moseley GL 2003a A pain neuromatrix approach to patients with chronic pain. Manual Therapy 8(3):130–140

Moseley GL 2003b Unraveling the barriers to reconceptualization of the problem in chronic pain: the actual and perceived ability of patients and health professionals to understand the neurophysiology. Journal of Pain 4(4):184

Moseley GL, Hodges PW 2005 Chronic pain and motor control. In: Moseley GL (ed) Modern manual therapy. Elsevier Science, Edinburgh

Moseley GL, Hodges PW, Gandevia SC 2002 Deep and superficial fibers of the lumbar multifidus muscle are differentially active during voluntary arm movements. Spine 27(2):E29–E36

O'Sullivan PB, Twomey L, Allison G 1997 Evaluation of specific stabilising exercise in the treatment of chronic low back pain with radiological diagnosis of spondylolysis and spondylolisthesis. Spine 15(24):2959–2967

O'Sullivan PB, Beales D, Beetham JA et al 2002 Altered motor control strategies in subjects with sacroiliac joint pain during the active straight leg raise test. Spine 27(1):E1

O'Sullivan PB, Bryniolfsson G, Cawthorne A et al 2003 Investigation of a clinical test and transabdominal ultrasound during pelvic floor muscle contraction in subjects with and without lumbosacral pain. In: Fourteenth International WCPT Congress Proceedings. Barcelona, Spain. CD-ROM abstracts

Panjabi MM 1992 The stabilizing system of the spine. Part I: function, dysfunction, adaptation, and enhancement. Journal of Spinal Disorders 5(4):383–389

Potter NA, Rothstein J 1985 Intertester reliability for selected clinical tests of the sacroiliac joint. Physical Therapy 65(11):1671

Richardson CA, Jull GA 1995 Muscle control – pain control. What exercises would you prescribe? Manual Therapy 1:2–10

Richardson CA, Jull GA, Hodges PW, Hides JA 1999 Therapeutic exercise for spinal segmental stabilization in low back pain – scientific basis and clinical approach. Churchill Livingstone, Edinburgh

Richardson CA, Snijders CJ, Hides JA et al 2002 The relationship between the transversely oriented abdominal muscles, sacroiliac joint mechanics and low back pain. Spine 27(4):399–405

Richardson CA, Hodges PW, Hides JA 2004 Therapeutic exercise for lumbopelvic stabilization. Churchill Livingstone, Edinburgh

Sapolsky RM, Alberts RC, Altmann J 1997a Hypercortisolism associated with social subordinance isolation among wild baboons. Archives General Psychiatry 54(12):1137–1143

Sapolsky RM, Spencer EM 1997b Insulin growth factor 1 is suppressed in socially subordinate male baboons. American Journal Physiology 273 (4 Pt 2):1346–1351

Sapsford RR, Hodges PW, Richardson CA et al 2001

Co-activation of the abdominal and pelvic floor muscles during voluntary exercises. Neurourology and Urodynamics 20:31–42
Sashin D 1930 A critical analysis of the anatomy and the pathologic changes of the sacro-iliac joints. Journal of Bone and Joint Surgery 12:891–910
Saunders SW, Rath D, Hodges PW 2004 Postural and respiratory activation of the trunk muscles changes with mode and speed of locomotion. Gait and Posture 20:280
Snijders CJ, Vleeming A, Stoeckart R 1993a Transfer of lumbosacral load to iliac bones and legs. 1: Biomechanics of self-bracing of the sacroiliac joints and its significance for treatment and exercise. Clinical Biomechanics 8: 285–294
Snijders CJ, Vleeming A, Stoeckart R 1993b Transfer of lumbosacral load to iliac bones and legs. 2: Loading of the sacroiliac joints when lifting in a stooped posture. Clinical Biomechanics 8:295–301
Solonen KA 1957 The sacro-iliac joint in the light of anatomical roentgenological and clinical studies. Acta Orthopaedica Scandinavica Supplement 27:1–127
Stuge B, Lærum E, Kirkesola G, Vøllestad N 2004 The efficacy of a treatment program focusing on specific stabilizing exercises for pelvic girdle pain after pregnancy. Spine 29(4):351
Sturesson B, Selvik G, Uden A 1989 Movements of the sacroiliac joints a roentgen stereophotogrammetric analysis. Spine 14 (2):162–165
Sturesson B, Udén A, Vleeming A 2000 A radiosterometric analysis of movements of the sacroiliac joints during the standing hip flexion test. Spine 25(3):364–368
Thompson J, O'Sullivan PB 2003 Levator plate movement during voluntary pelvic floor muscle contraction in subjects with incontinence and prolapse: a cross-sectional study and review. International Urogynecology Journal 14:84
Thompson J, O'Sullivan PB, Briffa K, Neumann P 2005 Motor control strategies for activation of the pelvic floor. In: Proceedings of the Fifth Interdisciplinary World Congress on Low Back and Pelvic Pain. Melbourne, Australia, p116
Van Wingerden JP, Vleeming A, Buyruk HM, Raissadat K 2004 Stabilization of the sacroiliac joint in vivo: verification of muscular contribution to force closure of the pelvis. European Spine Journal 13(3):199
Vlaeyen JWS, Linton SJ 2000 Fear–avoidance and its consequences in chronic musculoskeletal pain: a state of the art. Pain 85:317–332
Vleeming A, Stoeckart R, Volkers ACW, Snijders CJ 1990a Relation between form and function in the sacroiliac joint. 1: clinical anatomical aspects. Spine 15(2):130–132
Vleeming A, Volkers ACW, Snijders CJ, Stoeckart R 1990b Relation between form and function in the sacroiliac joint. 2: biomechanical aspects. Spine 15(2):133–136
Vleeming A, van Wingerden JP, Dijkstra PF et al 1992a Mobility in the SI-joints in old people: a kinematic and radiologic study. Clinical Biomechanics 7:170–176
Vleeming A, Buyruk H, Stoechart R et al 1992b An integrated therapy for peripartum pelvic instability: a study of the biomechanical effects of pelvic belts. American Journal of Obstetrics and Gynecology 166(4):1243
Vleeming A, Pool-Goudzwaard AL, Stoeckart R et al 1995 The posterior layer of the thoracolumbar fascia: its function in load transfer from spine to legs. Spine 20:753–758
Vleeming A, Pool-Goudzwaard AL, Hammudoghlu D et al 1996 The function of the long dorsal sacroiliac ligament: its implication for understanding low back pain. Spine 21(5):556–562
Vleeming A, Albert HB, Östgaard HC et al 2004 European guidelines on the diagnosis and treatment of pelvic girdle pain. In: Proceedings of the Fifth Interdisciplinary World Congress on Low Back and Pelvic Pain. Melbourne, Australia, p6
Watson PJ, Booker CK, Main CJ, Chen AC 1997 Surface electromyography in the identification of chronic low back pain patients: the development of the flexion relaxation ratio. Clinical Biomechanics 12(3):165–171
Whittaker JL 2004 Abdominal ultrasound imaging of pelvic floor muscle function in individuals with low back pain. Journal of Manual and Manipulative Therapy 12(1):44

Coventry University Library

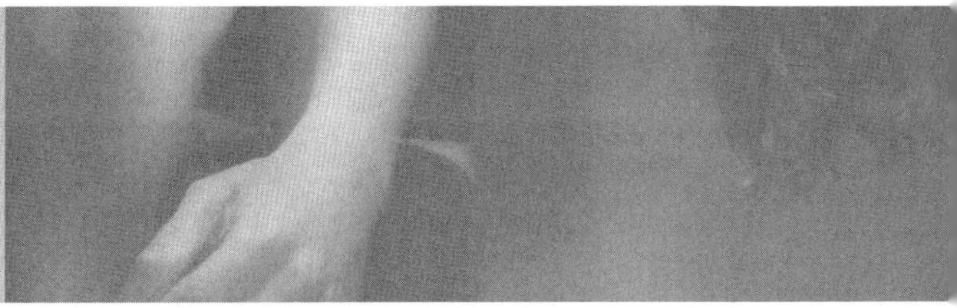

Index

Note: Page numbers in **bold** type refer to figures and tables; the abbreviation SIJ = sacroiliac joint.

A

B

C

F

G

H

I

J

K

M

Q

R

S

T

U

V

W

X

Y

Z